SECOND EDITION

ADVANCED MEDICAL NUTRITION THERAPY

Kelly Kane, MS, RD, LDN
Director of Nutrition and Dietetic Internship
Tufts Medical Center and Tufts University Friedman
School of Nutrition Science and Policy
Boston, Massachusetts

Kathy Prelack, PhD, RD
Associate Professor of Nutrition
Simmons University
Boston, Massachusetts

JONES & BARTLETT
LEARNING

World Headquarters
Jones & Bartlett Learning
25 Mall Road
Burlington, MA 01803
978-443-5000
info@jblearning.com
www.jblearning.com

Jones & Bartlett Learning books and products are available through most bookstores and online booksellers. To contact Jones & Bartlett Learning directly, call 800-832-0034, fax 978-443-8000, or visit our website, www.jblearning.com.

30850-1

Production Credits
Vice President, Innovative Learning and Assessment Solutions: Ada Woo
Senior Director, Content Production and Delivery: Christine Emerton
Director, Product: Melissa Kleeman-Moy
Product Manager: Sophie Fleck Teague
Manager, Content Development: Carol Brewer Guerrero
Senior Outsourcing Specialist: Elisabeth Williams
Content Manager: Jessica Covert
Content Coordinator: Rachelle Soden
Content Management: MPS Limited
Manager, Intellectual Properties and Content Production: Kristen Rogers
Content Production Manager: Roberta Sherman
Senior Intellectual Property Specialist (eBook): Colleen Lamy
Senior Product Marketing Manager: Susanne Walker
Director, Product Fulfillment: Aaron McKinzie
Purchasing Manager: Wendy Kilborn
Composition: S4Carlisle Publishing Services
Project Management: S4Carlisle Publishing Services
Cover Design: MPS Limited
Text Design: MPS Limited
Media Developer: Faith Brosnan
Intellectual Property Specialist: Lisa Passmore
Cover Image (Title Page, Section Opener, Chapter Opener): © Mooauan/Shutterstock
Printing and Binding: Sheridan Kentucky

Library of Congress Cataloging-in-Publication Data
Names: Kane, Kelly, 1969- author | Prelack, Kathy author
Title: Advanced medical nutrition therapy / Kelly Kane, Kathy Prelack.
Description: Second edition. | Burlington, MA : Jones & Bartlett Learning, [2027] | Includes bibliographical references and index.
Identifiers: LCCN 2025033220 | ISBN 9781284304213 paperback
Subjects: LCSH: Diet therapy | BISAC: HEALTH & FITNESS / Diet & Nutrition / Nutrition
Classification: LCC RM216 .K295 2027
LC record available at https://lccn.loc.gov/2025033220

6048

Printed in the United States of America
30 29 28 27 26 10 9 8 7 6 5 4 3 2 1

To my husband Dana and my two sons, Patrick and Jake, the reason behind all I do, who drive, challenge, and motivate me to set big goals and support me to reach them; to the staff of the Frances Stern Nutrition Center who are skillful and caring clinicians whose dedication to our patients and our students inspires me; and to my dietetic interns whose passion for the field of nutrition has shaped this textbook.

—Kelly

To my students who inspire me to work hard every day; to my colleagues and mentors who give me guidance and support; and to my family who give me strength, love, and purpose.

—Kathy

Brief Contents

Contents

Online-Only Chapters

Foreword

It is a delight to introduce readers to this second edition of *Advanced Medical Nutrition Therapy*. It is a major, timely contribution to the field of clinical nutrition and dietetics. It is the best introduction to the ins and outs of medical nutrition therapy that I am aware of. Both authors are superb clinical nutritionists associated with excellent teaching hospitals who update themselves on the fast-moving developments in the field.

Health professionals agree that, whenever possible, primary prevention of nutrition-related problems is preferable. Nutrition is important from the cradle to the grave, and so the text's extensive and holistic attention to health promotion and diet-related disease prevention over the entire life cycle is welcome.

However, primary prevention alone is not enough to stave off or control all of the adverse effects of diet-related diseases, and treatment, amelioration, and avoidance of further complications is also needed. The extensive coverage of medical nutrition therapy in the context of other preventive and treatment measures is a particular strength of *Advanced Medical Nutrition Therapy, Second Edition*. The chapters on nutritional assessment come alive with the inclusion of complex clinical case studies that help to clarify complex issues such as use of parenteral and enteral nutritional therapies. *Advanced Medical Nutrition Therapy* covers all of the common diet-related conditions such as under- and overweight; diabetes; cardiovascular disease; gastrointestinal problems; kidney, liver, and pulmonary disease; as well as the cancers, and more complex comorbidities.

Today's healthcare realities are well reflected in the chapters in this edition. There is increased emphasis in this edition on the use of evidence-based interventions, and on employing them using the nutrition care process for medical nutrition therapy. The growing recognition that health care is a collaborative enterprise that involves registered dietitians in multidisciplinary teams is reflected in the text's descriptions on how dietitians function in their roles as team members. Another bonus in this edition of *Advanced Medical Nutrition Therapy* is that more extensive coverage is paid to issues that are vitally important but also neglected in most textbooks, such as oral nutrition, food allergies, extremely premature infants, developmental disabilities, and the nutritional care of the aging and frail. All in all, this edition is an excellent update chock full of the latest information, and well worth reading.

Congratulations to the authors for producing this new edition, and to you the reader, for your wise choice of this authoritative textbook.

Johanna Dwyer, DSc, RD

Professor of Medicine and Community Health
School of Medicine and Friedman School of
Nutrition Science and Policy
Tufts University and Tufts Medical Center

Preface

Advanced Medical Nutrition Therapy is designed as the primary text for an upper-level undergraduate or graduate-level Medical Nutrition Therapy or Clinical Nutrition course for nutrition majors. The text is designed to be a current, evidence-based, and practical nutrition resource for nutrition students, dietetic interns, nutrition professionals, and non-nutrition clinicians. Other trainees, such as medical students or students enrolled in graduate programs in biomedical science, may also have an interest in such a text. This text will present information that meets the needs of those at the graduate nutrition level, as well as those who have advanced academic backgrounds, but limited clinical experience, or clinicians of other disciplines (nurses, physicians, physician assistants, etc.).

Conceptual Approach

Advanced Medical Nutrition Therapy utilizes a practice-oriented, case-based approach that incorporates problem-based learning and engages the reader in various clinically based scenarios that guide the narrative text. This approach is designed to encourage the reader to digest the didactic scientific information while applying it to a patient-based clinical situation. The cases in the text provide the framework around which the didactic information is presented. By understanding the importance of the subject matter through application, the reader will progress beyond the rote memorization approach that can be typical of science courses and integrate the science with the clinical scenario to gain a more complete understanding.

The text is practice-oriented with a strong clinical focus highlighting the treatment of the medical condition while incorporating the latest guidelines and research, with an emphasis on current topics. Commonly used formulas and equations are included to emphasize clinical application.

Organization

The first section of the text introduces the core concepts of nutrition, highlighting nutrition and biochemical assessment, enteral and parenteral nutrition support, and determination of energy requirements. These chapters provide the framework of the text. The next section gives an overview of the pathophysiology in various disease states including diabetes mellitus, cardiovascular disease, kidney disease, gastrointestinal and liver disease, and pulmonary disease. Students then apply the foundational aspects of medical nutrition therapy learned in the previous section to nutritional management of these various disease states. Clinical conditions such as critical illness and neurotraumatic injury resulting from stroke and traumatic brain injury are also included in this section. The last section examines application of medical nutrition therapy in pediatric patients. In this section, students explore nutritional needs and management of the preterm infant and of the general pediatric population, as well as in patients with cystic fibrosis, pediatric obesity, eating disorders, and developmental disabilities, thus providing a comprehensive summary of medical nutrition therapy in this nutritionally unique population. Additional supplemental online only chapters related to nutrition in wound healing, oral health, pregnancy and lactation, and geriatrics are also available to provide a comprehensive overview of medical nutrition therapy in various conditions as well as across the lifespan.

Features

Each chapter is designed to provide the reader the comprehension and skills to render effective nutrition care plans based on the fundamentals of diet and disease and existing research evidence. Each chapter introduces *Core Concepts*, which are important principles or themes that will be identified and highlighted to encourage functional learning. *Learning Objectives* are included at the beginning of each chapter to better assess student learning. A *Case Study* or clinical scenario introduces each topic and stimulates critical thinking by developing questions that are subsequently expanded upon in the text. Reliance on evidence-based practice via a *Clinical Controversy* is fostered through the introduction of research concepts in journal review. Discussion of clinical scenarios that do not have one clear, correct answer is covered in the *Clinical Roundtable*. *Practice Points* of useful clinical information are presented throughout each chapter to identify how it works "in the real world." *Key Terms* also help to familiarize the reader with new concepts in an organized fashion.

Benefits

The text is designed for students and practitioners who are fairly new to the clinical environment, as well as those who are new to addressing nutrition in the clinical environment and who have more recently studied and learned the basics of metabolism (anatomy; physiology; and carbohydrate, protein, and fat metabolism, for example). It incorporates a clinical case presentation, with discussion throughout each chapter calling upon details of the case in order to reinforce the didactic science information, thus challenging the student to think outside of the classroom. This approach will allow the student to apply this information and reinforce learning. In this edition, students who are training to become dietitians can implement various aspects of the nutrition care process. Students have the opportunity to develop formal problem statements, determine appropriate interventions, and establish methods for monitoring and evaluation of their nutrition care plan.

The text more broadly covers nutrition in the life cycle by integrating aspects of both adult and pediatric nutrition. This strong pediatric focus is reflected in chapters on general pediatrics, neonatology, pediatric obesity, developmental disabilities, and eating disorders. This *Second Edition* includes a newly added chapter on food allergies and intolerances providing current, evidence-based approaches to dietary management of common food allergies. The text also incorporates more specialized chapters on topics such as oral health, wound healing, and cystic fibrosis. This *Second Edition* includes a chapter dedicated to neurologic disease including Alzheimer's disease and other neurodegenerative diseases such as Parkinson's disease and amyotrophic lateral sclerosis. Use of the ketogenic diet and guidelines for the management of dysphagia using the International Dysphagia Diet Standardization Initiative framework are also provided in this edition. Chapters on maldigestion and malabsorption, historically covered through content related to "upper gastrointestinal" and "lower gastrointestinal" disorders, provide nutritional management of complex conditions such as short bowel syndrome. Also included are emerging topics in irritable bowel syndrome and non-celiac gluten sensitivity.

The text offers the versatility for use as both a classroom text as well as a clinical practice resource to integrate lectures with application and journal review. The text ties the clinical information directly with instruction in one text. Reliance on evidence-based practice is fostered through introduction of research concepts and exercises in journal review.

Supplement Package

Instructors using *Advanced Medical Nutrition Therapy* will have access to a full suite of supplemental resources, including the following:

- Test Bank in LMS-compatible formats, providing examination questions for each chapter as well as a Midterm and Final Exam
- Slides in PowerPoint format, including bulleted notes that can be easily customized
- Answer Key for In-Text Study Questions

Kelly Kane
Kathy Prelack

Features of This Text

Advanced Medical Nutrition Therapy incorporates a number of engaging pedagogical features in order to emphasize how the content can be applied in practice.

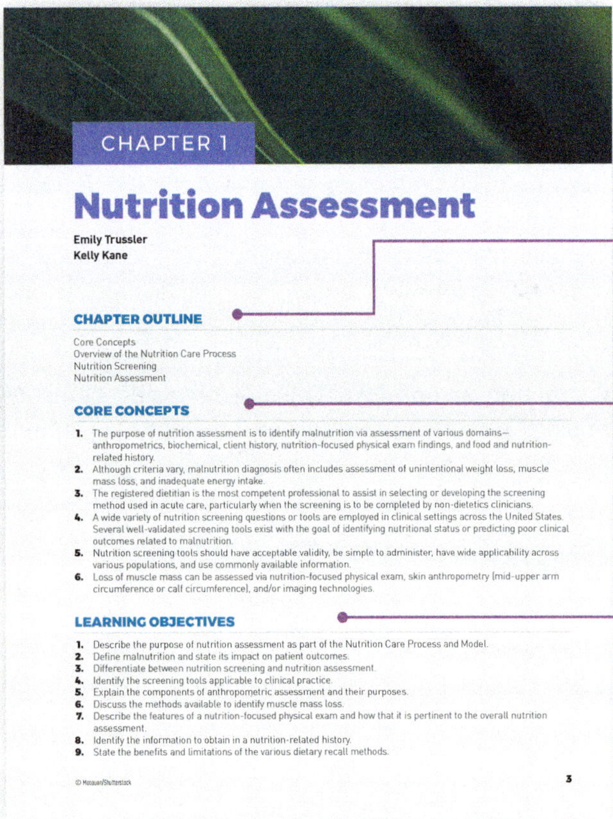

CHAPTER 1

Nutrition Assessment

Emily Trussler
Kelly Kane

CHAPTER OUTLINE

Core Concepts
Overview of the Nutrition Care Process
Nutrition Screening
Nutrition Assessment

CORE CONCEPTS

1. The purpose of nutrition assessment is to identify malnutrition via assessment of various domains—anthropometrics, biochemical, client history, nutrition-focused physical exam findings, and food and nutrition-related history.
2. Although criteria vary, malnutrition diagnosis often includes assessment of unintentional weight loss, muscle mass loss, and inadequate energy intake.
3. The registered dietitian is the most competent professional to assist in selecting or developing the screening method used in acute care, particularly when the screening is to be completed by non-dietetics clinicians.
4. A wide variety of nutrition screening questions or tools are employed in clinical settings across the United States. Several well-validated screening tools exist with the goal of identifying nutritional status or predicting poor clinical outcomes related to malnutrition.
5. Nutrition screening tools should have acceptable validity, be simple to administer, have wide applicability across various populations, and use commonly available information.
6. Loss of muscle mass can be assessed via nutrition-focused physical exam, skin anthropometry (mid-upper arm circumference or calf circumference), and/or imaging technologies.

LEARNING OBJECTIVES

1. Describe the purpose of nutrition assessment as part of the Nutrition Care Process and Model.
2. Define malnutrition and state its impact on patient outcomes.
3. Differentiate between nutrition screening and nutrition assessment.
4. Identify the screening tools applicable to clinical practice.
5. Explain the components of anthropometric assessment and their purposes.
6. Discuss the methods available to identify muscle mass loss.
7. Describe the features of a nutrition-focused physical exam and how that it is pertinent to the overall nutrition assessment.
8. Identify the information to obtain in a nutrition-related history.
9. State the benefits and limitations of the various dietary recall methods.

© Mooauan/Shutterstock

3

Each chapter opens with a **Chapter Outline** previewing the topics to be covered.

Core Concepts establish important principles that will be explored in the chapter; they later reappear within the chapter text once the relevant content has been broached.

Learning Objectives establish what the reader can expect to learn from the chapter.

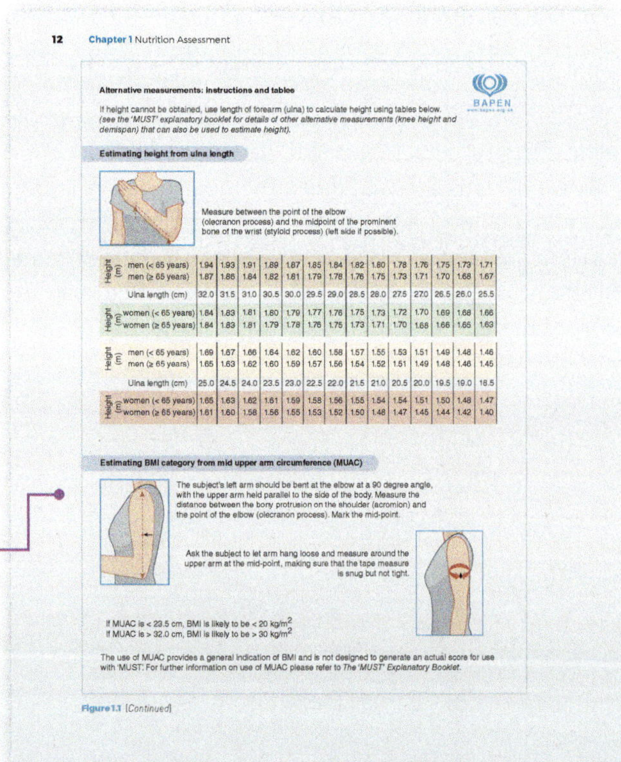

12 Chapter 1 Nutrition Assessment

Alternative measurements: instructions and tables

If height cannot be obtained, use length of forearm (ulna) to calculate height using tables below. *(see the 'MUST' explanatory booklet for details of other alternative measurements (knee height and demispan) that can also be used to estimate height).*

Estimating height from ulna length

Measure between the point of the elbow (olecranon process) and the midpoint of the prominent bone of the wrist (styloid process) (left side if possible).

Height (m)	men (< 65 years)	1.94	1.93	1.91	1.89	1.87	1.85	1.84	1.82	1.80	1.78	1.76	1.75	1.73	1.71
	men (≥ 65 years)	1.87	1.86	1.84	1.82	1.81	1.79	1.78	1.76	1.75	1.73	1.71	1.70	1.68	1.67
	Ulna length (cm)	32.0	31.5	31.0	30.5	30.0	29.5	29.0	28.5	28.0	27.5	27.0	26.5	26.0	25.5
Height (m)	women (< 65 years)	1.84	1.83	1.81	1.80	1.79	1.77	1.76	1.75	1.73	1.72	1.70	1.69	1.68	1.66
	women (≥ 65 years)	1.84	1.83	1.81	1.79	1.78	1.76	1.75	1.73	1.71	1.70	1.68	1.66	1.65	1.63
Height (m)	men (< 65 years)	1.69	1.67	1.66	1.64	1.62	1.60	1.58	1.57	1.55	1.53	1.51	1.49	1.48	1.46
	men (≥ 65 years)	1.65	1.63	1.62	1.60	1.59	1.57	1.56	1.54	1.52	1.51	1.49	1.48	1.46	1.45
	Ulna length (cm)	25.0	24.5	24.0	23.5	23.0	22.5	22.0	21.5	21.0	20.5	20.0	19.5	19.0	18.5
Height (m)	women (< 65 years)	1.65	1.63	1.62	1.61	1.59	1.58	1.56	1.55	1.54	1.54	1.51	1.50	1.48	1.47
	women (≥ 65 years)	1.61	1.60	1.58	1.56	1.55	1.53	1.52	1.50	1.48	1.47	1.45	1.44	1.42	1.40

Estimating BMI category from mid upper arm circumference (MUAC)

The subject's left arm should be bent at the elbow at a 90 degree angle, with the upper arm held parallel to the side of the body. Measure the distance between the bony protrusion on the shoulder (acromion) and the point of the elbow (olecranon process). Mark the mid-point.

Ask the subject to let arm hang loose and measure around the upper arm at the mid-point, making sure that the tape measure is snug but not tight.

If MUAC is < 23.5 cm, BMI is likely to be < 20 kg/m^2
If MUAC is > 32.0 cm, BMI is likely to be > 30 kg/m^2

The use of MUAC provides a general indication of BMI and is not designed to generate an actual score for use with 'MUST'. For further information on use of MUAC please refer to *The 'MUST' Explanatory Booklet*.

Figure 1.1 (Continued)

A comprehensive and instructional **art package** includes color photographs and illustrations throughout this text to add a visual dimension to the content being presented.

CASE STUDY REVISITED

On HD 6, Adam undergoes an urgent laparotomy for a severe gastric ulcer with perforation. On postoperative (postop) day 1/HD 7, you visit Adam for reassessment. He is currently in the ICU on mechanical ventilation with increased drainage from a nasogastric tube.

Anthropometric Data:

Weight: 77 kg on HD 7

Last weight: 73 kg on HD 3

Biochemical Data (postop day 1/HD 7):

Sodium 143 (136–145 mEq/L)
Potassium 3.5 (3.5–5.0 mEq/L)
Chloride 88 (96–106 mEq/L)
Carbon dioxide 41 (22–31 mEq/L)
Blood urea nitrogen 24 (8–20 mg/dL)

Creatinine 0.2 (0.7–1.3 mg/dL)
Glucose 139 (70–139 mg/dL)
Calcium 7.7 (8.5–10.5 mg/dL)
Phosphorus 3.0 (2.5–4.5 mg/dL)
Magnesium 1.4 (1.5–2.7 mg/dL)

Arterial Blood Gas:

pH 7.48 (7.35–.45)
PCO_2 48 (35–45 mm Hg)

PO_2 90 (80–100 mm Hg)
HCO_3 29 (22–26 mEq/L)

Dietary Data:

Diet Prescription: NPO

Questions

1. Describe Adam's acid-base status.
2. What specific acid-base disorder does he have?
3. What interventions would you recommend to manage this acid-base imbalance?

Each chapter begins with a **Case Study**, illustrating how topics discussed in the text might appear in practice. These case studies are revisited throughout the chapter, building in concert with the foundational material. Questions are incorporated to encourage active engagement with the scenarios.

The **Nutrition Care Process** is integrated throughout the case study and chapter content, including nutrition diagnosis and development of problem, etiology, and signs and symptoms phrases, evidenced based interventions appropriate for each clinical scenario, and guidelines for monitoring and evaluating the efficacy of nutrition interventions.

⚠ Clinical Controversy

The Relationship between Vitamin B12 Levels and Mortality Risk

While the biological importance of vitamin B12 is well established, recent evidence from epidemiological studies has sparked debate around the potential risks of excessive vitamin B12 levels. In a cohort study of over 5500 adults in the Netherlands, higher levels of plasma vitamin B12 were associated with an increased risk of all-cause mortality (25% increased risk for every 1 standard deviation rise in plasma vitamin B12), after adjusting for age, sex, kidney function, and other clinical and laboratory variables.[1] Additionally, in a systematic review and meta-analysis of 22 cohort studies (including over 92,000 individuals), Liu et al. found that each 100 pmol/L rise in serum vitamin B12 was associated with a 4% increased risk of all-cause mortality.[2] The mechanisms underlying this relationship are not fully understood. One proposed explanation is liver and/or kidney dysfunction, which can contribute to both elevated vitamin B12 levels and increased mortality risk. Nonetheless, findings on the topic have been mixed. For example, Wolffenbuttel et al.[3] found low serum B12 concentrations to be associated with a moderate increase in all-cause mortality, using data from the National Health and Nutrition Examination Survey. Overall, further research is needed to clarify the relationship between vitamin B12 levels and mortality, including the direction and magnitude of this association as well as its clinical significance.

Questions

1. What are some possible confounding factors that might explain the link between high vitamin B12 levels and mortality risk?
2. What are some other limitations to consider when interpreting the results of observational studies such as cohort studies?

References

1. Flores-Guerrero JL, Minovic I, Groothof D, et al. Association of plasma concentration of vitamin B12 with all-cause mortality in the general population in the Netherlands. *JAMA Netw Open*. 2020;3(1):e1919274.
2. Liu K, Yang Z, Lu X, et al. The origin of vitamin B12 levels and risk of all-cause, cardiovascular and cancer specific mortality: a systematic review and dose-response meta-analysis. *Arch Gerontol Geriatr*. 2024;117:105230.
3. Wolffenbuttel BHR, Heiner-Fokkema MR, Green R, Gans ROB. Relationship between serum B12 concentrations and mortality: experience in NHANES. *BMC Med*. 2020;18(1):307.

Clinical Controversy boxes emphasize engagement with evidence-based content by highlighting areas where there may be disagreements in the literature.

Clinical Roundtable boxes highlight clinical scenarios that invite a multitude of possible approaches.

Clinical Roundtable

Topic: C-Reactive Protein as a Biomarker of Cardiovascular Disease Risk

C-reactive protein (CRP) levels rise not only during acute inflammation, but also during chronic inflammation. In recent decades, CRP—specifically, high sensitivity CRP (hs-CRP)—has emerged as a potential predictor of cardiovascular disease (CVD) risk, since chronic, low-grade inflammation is known to contribute to the initiation, progression, and complications of CVD.[1] There is emerging evidence demonstrating an association between elevated hs-CRP and CVD risk, although the exact role of CRP in the pathogenesis of CVD is not fully understood. It is not clear whether CRP is a nonspecific marker of inflammation or a direct participant in CVD development. Unlike other markers of inflammation, CRP levels are stable over extended periods and can be measured using inexpensive, convenient, and high-sensitivity assays. Some experts recommend the inclusion of hs-CRP as part of routine CVD screening, while others recommend prioritizing traditional risk factors.[2,3] Further research is needed to clarify the role of CRP in CVD pathogenesis and the clinical utility of hs-CRP as an indicator of CVD risk.

Roundtable Discussion

1. What are some potential benefits of including CRP in routine CVD risk screenings, compared to traditional risk factors alone?
2. What are some limitations associated with using CRP as a biomarker for CVD risk?
3. What additional research is needed to validate the use of CRP in predicting cardiovascular events? For example, what types of studies should be conducted, and what research questions should they address?

References

1. Amezcua-Castillo E, González-Pacheco H, Sáenz-San Martín A, et al. C-reactive protein: The quintessential marker of systemic inflammation in coronary artery disease-advancing toward precision medicine. *Biomedicines*. 2023;11(9):2444.
2. Genest J, McPherson R, Frohlich J, et al. 2009 Canadian Cardiovascular Society/Canadian guidelines for the diagnosis and treatment of dyslipidemia and prevention of cardiovascular disease in the adult - 2009 recommendations. *Can J Cardiol*. 2009;25(10):567-579.
3. Lin JS, Evans CV, Johnson E, Redmond N, Coppola EL, Smith N. Nontraditional risk factors in cardiovascular disease risk assessment: Updated evidence report and systematic review for the US Preventive Services Task Force. *JAMA*. 2018;320(3):281-297.

PRACTICE POINT

Anthropometric measurements are only one piece of the nutrition assessment puzzle. Although changes in these measures are reliable predictors of nutritional outcome, they should always be considered in the context of the overall status of the patient.

Brief **Practice Points** provide additional details relevant to clinical dietetics practice.

Key Terms appear in bold-face type throughout the text and are collected at the end of each chapter.

Key Terms

static assays, functional assays, hemodilution, hemoconcentration, electrolytes, basic metabolic panel (BMP), comprehensive metabolic panel (CMP), lipid panel, renal function panel, hepatic function panel, complete blood count, differential count, osmolality, osmolarity, osmotic pressure, isotonic, hypertonic, hypotonic, third spacing, hypervolemia, hypovolemia, hyponatremia, osmotic demyelination syndrome (ODS), pseudohyponatremia, hypernatremia, hypokalemia, hyperkalemia, hemolysis, hypocalcemia, hypercalcemia, hypophosphatemia, hyperphosphatemia, hypomagnesemia, hypermagnesemia, refeeding syndrome, hypochloremia, hyperchloremia, acidemia, alkalemia, acidosis, alkalosis, arterial blood gases (ABGs), venous blood gases (VBGs), respiratory acidosis, respiratory alkalosis, metabolic acidosis, metabolic alkalosis, hypoglycemia, hyperglycemia, visceral protein, acute-phase proteins, positive acute-phase proteins, negative acute-phase proteins, marasmus, kwashiorkor, somatic protein, nitrogen balance, creatinine height index (CHI), anemia, microcytic anemia, macrocytic anemia, normocytic anemia, iron deficiency anemia, anemia of chronic disease, micronutrients, trace elements, order-writing privileges

Learning and Teaching Resources

Claire AI™ for Students

Included within the Navigate eBook, Claire AI is an AI-powered study tool that provides students with around-the-clock academic support and personalized guidance. Available at the point of learning, students can access instant, AI-driven assistance through a chat experience leveraging Jones & Bartlett Learning's trusted content to enhance their educational experience.

With Claire AI, learners will have the ability to clarify key content, generate flashcards, create memorable mnemonics, and quiz themselves with unique questions, all within their eBook.

Student Resources

Each new purchase of the print textbook comes with a Navigate eBook that includes:

- Four eBook-only chapters (not included in the printed text)
- Chapter Review Slides
- Medical Nutrition Therapy Interactive Simulations
- Flashcards

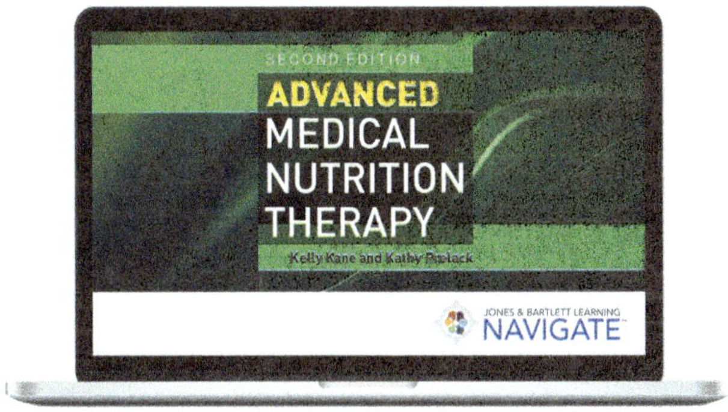

Instructor Resources

Qualified instructors can receive the full suite of Instructor Resources, including the following:

- Slides in PowerPoint format
- Test Bank in LMS-compatible formats
- Answer Key for In-Text Study Questions

We Value Your Feedback

Do you love this text? Spot an error you'd like to report? Follow this QR code to give us your observations and suggestions for improvement.

About the Authors

Kelly Kane, MS, RD, LDN, is the Director of Nutrition and Business Operations and Dietetic Internship Director at Tufts Medical Center and Assistant Professor in the Gerald J. and Dorothy R. Friedman School of Nutrition Science and Policy at Tufts University. She has been a Registered Dietitian for 30 years, over which time she has worked in the clinical setting providing medical nutrition therapy for acutely ill adults and children as well as educating patients on ways to improve their health with nutrition. She has taught nutrition to health professionals including dietetic interns, physician assistants, and medical students for over 25 years. She serves as Editor of the quarterly peer-reviewed journal, *Topics in Clinical Nutrition*. Kelly was awarded the 2022 Outstanding Faculty Member of the Year by the Tufts University Friedman School of Nutrition Science and Policy, 2022 Outstanding Dietitian of the Year by the Massachusetts Academy of Nutrition and Dietetics, as well as 2020 Outstanding Dietetics Educator of the northeast region by Nutrition and Dietetics Educators and Preceptors of the Academy of Nutrition and Dietetics.

Kathy Prelack, PhD, RD, is an Associate Professor at Simmons University and Adjunct Associate Professor at Tufts University with a primary academic focus on clinical nutrition, medical nutrition therapy, and interprofessional learning. Her research interests include energy and protein metabolism following burn injury and methods of body composition analysis in a clinical setting. Kathy is a registered Dietitian and is currently the Director of Clinical Nutrition at Shriners Children's Boston, a pediatric burn and surgical specialty hospital, where she has worked for over 30 years. She enjoys mentoring students, interns, and emerging investigators interested in pediatric critical care and clinical research. Kathy is actively involved in international outreach promoting the importance of early nutrition in children with burn injuries. She is a member of the Academy of Nutrition and Dietetics, and the American Society of Parenteral and Enteral Nutrition.

Contributors

Deena Altschwager, MS, RD, LDN, CNSC
Clinical Service Liaison, Nutrition Services
Coram Home Infusion
St. Louis, Missouri

Lisa Baxter, BSN, RN, CWOCN
Clinical Manager, Inpatient Support Services
Tufts Medical Center
Boston, Massachusetts

Katherine J. Best, BS
Dietetic Intern
Tufts University
Boston, Massachusetts

Xuemeng Chen, MS, RD, LDN, CDCES
Clinical Dietitian
Boston Medical Center, Brighton
Brighton, Massachusetts

Yijie (Claire) Cheng, MS, RD, CNSC
Medical Consultant
RB & Manon Business Co., Ltd
Shanghai, China

Alexa Cosgrove, MS, RDN, CSN
Registered Dietitian
Valley Health System Pediatric Endocrinology
Paramus, New Jersey

Maggie Dylewski Begis, PhD, RD
Clinical Professor
University of New Hampshire,
Durham, New Hampshire

Haley Follet, PA-C, MS, RD
Physician Assistant
Heart Center, Cook Children's Medical Center
Fort Worth, Texas

Katie Fort, MS, RD, CNSC
Advanced Level Practice Dietitian
US Department of Veteran's Affairs
Seattle, Washington

Nusheen Garrison, MS, RD, CSO, CNSC
Clinical Dietitian
Stanford Health Care
Palo Alto, California

Haewook Han, PhD, RD, LDN, FNKF
Kidney Nutrition Specialist
Atrius Health
Tufts University, Friedman School of Nutrition
Boston, Massachusetts

Sara Hendrix, MS, RD, LD
Certified Advanced Cystic Fibrosis Dietitian
Medical University of South Carolina
Charleston, South Carolina

Sora M. Johnson, MS
Dietetic Intern
NewYork-Presbyterian
New York, New York

Jillian Kaye, MS, RDN
Director of Nutrition and Interprofessional Education
Clinical Assistant Professor, Department of Pediatric Dentistry
New York University College of Dentistry
New York, New York

Judith Kirk, MS, RDN, CDN, FNKF
Nephrology Dietitian
Rochester Regional Health
Rochester, New York

Yu-Fang (Evonne) Lao, MS, RD
Clinical Dietitian
Cedars Sinai Medical Center
Los Angeles, California

John Leung, MD
CEO and Attending Physician, Boston Specialists
Adjunct Associate Professor, Tufts University Friedman School of Nutrition
Boston, Massachusetts

Jiawen Li, BS
Dietetic Intern
Tufts University
Boston, Massachusetts

Lily Lichtenstein-Swain, MS, RD
Clinical Dietitian
Tufts Medical Center
Boston, Massachusetts

Caroline MacDonald, MS, RDN, LDN
Clinical Dietitian, Weight Center
Massachusetts General Hospital
Boston, Massachusetts

Shibani Mallik, BS
Clinical Assistant
Boston Specialists, LLC
Boston, Massachusetts

Antoinette Maraglino, MS, RD, CSP, CDN
Clinical Nutrition Manager
Connecticut Children's Medical Center
Hartford, Connecticut

Lydia McGrath, MS, RD, LDN
Clinical Dietitian
Brigham & Women's Hospital
Boston, Massachusetts

Laura Padula, MS, RD, LDN
Senior Clinical Dietitian
Children's Hospital of Philadelphia
Philadelphia, Pennsylvania

Lauren Parsly Read-Button, MPH, RD, LDN
Transplant Dietitian
Tufts Medical Center
Boston, Massachusetts

Yvette Penner, MS, RD, LDN, CNSC
Clinical Nutrition Specialist II
Boston Children's Hospital
Boston, Massachusetts

Grace Phelan, MS, RD, LDN, CNSC
Nutrition Support Coordinator
Tufts Medical Center
Boston, Massachusetts

Natalie Pirolli, MS, RDN, LDN
Registered Dietitian Nutritionist
Naturally Natalie RDN, LLC
Providence, Rhode Island

Jessica Seltz Porto, MS, RD, LDN, CNSC
Transplant Dietitian, Clinical Inpatient Dietitian
Tufts Medical Center
Boston, Massachusetts

Jillian Reece, RDN, LDN
Clinical Bariatric Dietitian II/ Clinical Administration Manager
Tufts Medicine
Boston, Massachusetts

Anne-Marie Sandoval, BSN, RN, IBCLC
Lactation Consultant
Boston Children's Hospital
Boston, Massachusetts

Jennifer Shiel, MS, RD, LDN
Clinical Dietitian
Shriners Children's
Boston, Massachusetts

Nadine Tassabehji, PhD, RDN, LDN
Assistant Professor
Tufts School of Dental Medicine
Boston, Massachusetts

Emily Trussler, MS, RD, LDN CSR, CNSC
Senior Inpatient Clinical Dietitian
Brigham & Women's Hospital
Boston, Massachusetts

Molly Uebele Harrigan, PA-C, MS, RD
Physician Assistant
First Medical Associates
Germantown, Maryland

Kathleen Horrigan Walker, MDA, RDN, LDN, CSG
Assistant Professor of Practice
Simmons University
Boston, Massachusetts

Rachel Wilkinson-Bartlett, MS, RD, LDN, CSO
Registered Dietitian
Certified Specialist in Oncology Nutrition
Department of Veteran's Affairs
Portland, Maine

Jingwen Wu, BS
Dietetic Intern
Tufts University
Boston, Massachusetts

Yujia (Sandra) Zhang, MS, RDN
Pediatric Nutritionist
Tufts Medical Center
Boston, Massachusetts

Reviewers

Lauren Amaya, PhD, RD, LD, CDCES
Associate Professor/Diabetes Extension Specialist
Oklahoma State University
Stillwater, Oklahoma

Heather Frazier, PhD, RDN, LD
Associate Professor
University of the Incarnate Word
San Antonio, Texas

Neilann Horner, PhD, MPH, RDN
Associate Clinical Professor, Undergraduate Nutrition Program Director
Oregon State University
Corvallis, Oregon

Judith Lukaszuk, PhD, LDN, RDN
Professor Emeritus Nutrition
Northern Illinois University
DeKalb, Illinois

Sandra Mayol-Kreiser, PhD, RDN, CNSC
Clinical Professor
Arizona State University
Tempe, Arizona

Nadine Mikati, PhD, RDN, LDN
Associate Professor, MS-RDN Program Director
Nova Southeastern University
Davie, Florida

Stephanie N. Petrosky, DCN, MHA, RDN, LDN, FAND
Associate Professor and Chair, Department of Nutrition
Nova Southeastern University
Davie, Florida

Tania Rivera, PhD, RD, LD/N, FAND
Associate Clinical Professor
Florida International University
Miami, Florida

SECTION 1

Core Concepts

CHAPTER 1

Nutrition Assessment

Emily Trussler
Kelly Kane

CHAPTER OUTLINE

CORE CONCEPTS

1. The purpose of nutrition assessment is to identify malnutrition via assessment of various domains—anthropometrics, biochemical, client history, nutrition-focused physical exam findings, and food and nutrition-related history.
2. Although criteria vary, malnutrition diagnosis often includes assessment of unintentional weight loss, muscle mass loss, and inadequate energy intake.
3. The registered dietitian is the most competent professional to assist in selecting or developing the screening method used in acute care, particularly when the screening is to be completed by non-dietetics clinicians.
4. A wide variety of nutrition screening questions or tools are employed in clinical settings across the United States. Several well-validated screening tools exist with the goal of identifying nutritional status or predicting poor clinical outcomes related to malnutrition.
5. Nutrition screening tools should have acceptable validity, be simple to administer, have wide applicability across various populations, and use commonly available information.
6. Loss of muscle mass can be assessed via nutrition-focused physical exam, skin anthropometry (mid-upper arm circumference or calf circumference), and/or imaging technologies.

LEARNING OBJECTIVES

1. Describe the purpose of nutrition assessment as part of the Nutrition Care Process and Model.
2. Define malnutrition and state its impact on patient outcomes.
3. Differentiate between nutrition screening and nutrition assessment.
4. Identify the screening tools applicable to clinical practice.
5. Explain the components of anthropometric assessment and their purposes.
6. Discuss the methods available to identify muscle mass loss.
7. Describe the features of a nutrition-focused physical exam and how that it is pertinent to the overall nutrition assessment.
8. Identify the information to obtain in a nutrition-related history.
9. State the benefits and limitations of the various dietary recall methods.

Nutritional status affects virtually every individual's response to illness.[1] Those in a malnourished state benefit most if malnutrition is quickly identified. The importance of thorough and appropriate nutrition assessment is critical in both the prevention and treatment of illness. The process of assessment will provide the foundation from which any necessary nutrition-related intervention is built. The purpose of this chapter is to identify the specific components of recognizing and evaluating at-risk adult patients as the integral backbone of dietetics practice.

Overview of the Nutrition Care Process

To facilitate the provision of the highest quality of care, the Academy of Nutrition and Dietetics (AND) adopted the **Nutrition Care Process and Model (NCPM)** as a systematic framework to recognize, diagnose, and intervene upon nutrition-related problems for which a nutrition intervention is the primary treatment.[2,3] The NCPM was designed to provide a methodical structure for critically assessing patients across the wide spectrum of health and disease. The process consists of four steps to be completed in sequence—assessment, diagnosis, intervention, and monitoring and evaluation—each of which is linked to corresponding standardized terminology, called the **Nutrition Care Process Terminology (NCPT)**, for consistent documentation.[4–6] In all cases, assessment is preceded by screening, a separate but supportive task that triggers the entry of a patient into the NCPM.[2,7]

Nutrition assessment serves as the essential first step that provides a comprehensive evaluation of an individual's nutrition-related history. It is a systematic approach to collecting, recording, and interpreting all relevant data for the purpose of accurately diagnosing a nutrition-related problem. As part of the NCPM, nutrition assessment is organized into several domains, including anthropometric measurements; biochemical data, medical tests, and procedures; client history; nutrition-focused physical exam findings; food/nutrition-related history; and nutrition assessment, monitoring, and evaluation tools. This information may be obtained from a number of sources, including, but not limited to, the patient, family members, caregivers, medical care team, or medical record, depending upon the specific situation. The process of assessment

CASE STUDY INTRODUCTION

Marie is a 73-year-old Black female who recently emigrated from Haiti. She presents to the Emergency Department with weakness and reduced oral intake for the previous 3 months. Given her recent emigration, her medical record is limited.

Anthropometric Data:

Height: 160 cm
Weight: 65 kg
BMI: 25.4 kg/m^2

Biochemical Data:

Sodium 149 (136–145 mEq/L)
Potassium 3.4 (3.5–5.0 mEq/L)
Blood urea nitrogen 28 (8–20 mg/dL)
Creatinine 0.5 (0.7–1.3 mg/dL)
Glucose 105 (70–139 mg/dL)
Albumin 2.9 (3.5–5.5 g/dL)
Total cholesterol 150 (Desirable <200 mg/dL)

Clinical Data:

Past Medical History: Hypertension, osteoporosis
Medications: Alendronate, lisinopril
Vital Signs: Blood pressure 100/70 mm Hg, Temperature 99°F, Heart rate 85 beats/min

Questions

1. To determine whether Marie is at risk for malnutrition or warrants immediate nutrition assessment, what additional information would you like to consider?
2. What validated screening tool(s) would be appropriate to use to determine Marie's nutrition risk?

is not stagnant; instead, it should be viewed as an ongoing and continual analysis of an individual's nutritional status.[2,3]

The Purpose of Nutrition Assessment

The purpose of nutrition assessment is straightforward: to identify the presence of any nutrition-related problems, particularly malnutrition. However, over the past several decades, the topic of assessment has been surrounded by ongoing discussion, research, reworking, and redefining. Although researchers, clinicians, and public policymakers have invested significant energy into a unified approach for the identification and evaluation of malnutrition, no universally accepted approach has been determined. This may be attributed to the wide variation in existing definitions of the malnourished state.[8–11]

Defining Malnutrition

The relationship between malnutrition and nutrition assessment is critical. Any elements that influence the development of malnutrition and the manifestations that result should both comprise the steps of nutrition assessment and provide reliable identifiers for nutrition screening. Solidifying a transparent definition of the malnourished state is vital to understanding what and why specific signs and symptoms are assessed.

Consider the general concept of nutritional adequacy, the state of equilibrium in which an individual's dietary intake matches their requirements. In theory, malnutrition will occur when intake falls below (or exceeds) what is required. In practice, this process is significantly more complex. It is marked by a resulting succession of metabolic abnormalities, physiological changes, reduced organ and tissue function, and loss of critical body mass. For these reasons, malnutrition can be identified as any alteration in physiology, composition, or function attributable to a diet or to a disease that affects nutritional outcomes. Malnutrition for the purposes of nutrition assessment in the clinical setting refers to disease-related malnutrition that differs dramatically from that associated with natural disaster, conflict, or deprivation in the public health arena.[12–14]

Varying degrees of acute or chronic inflammation as part of the disease state are key factors in the pathogenesis of malnutrition. In clinical practice, malnutrition should be considered within one of three subcategories defined by a joint International Guidelines Committee of the American Society for Enteral and Parenteral Nutrition (ASPEN) and the European Society for Clinical Nutrition and Metabolism (ESPEN)[15]:

1. Chronic starvation without inflammation (e.g., anorexia nervosa)
2. Chronic disease–associated malnutrition, when inflammation is chronic and of mild-to-moderate degree (e.g., organ failure, pancreatic cancer)
3. Acute disease- or injury-associated malnutrition, when inflammation is acute and of severe degree (e.g., sepsis, burns, trauma, or closed head injury)

Per the AND/ASPEN Indicators to Diagnose Malnutrition (AAIM), malnutrition may be considered in the following contexts[9]:

1. Acute illness or injury (less than 3 months duration)
2. Chronic illness (3 months or longer duration)
3. Social or environmental circumstances (e.g., individuals without inflammation in a state of starvation or semi-starvation)

With these considerations in mind, one definition serves as a solid framework for the purposes of identifying and assessing clinical malnutrition: "Malnutrition is a subacute or chronic state of nutrition, in which a combination of varying degrees of overnutrition or undernutrition and inflammatory activity has led to a change in body composition and diminished function."[16]

Identifying Malnutrition

Identification of **malnutrition** and the entire purpose of the nutrition assessment process require a general understanding of its risk factors and manifestations. It is estimated that malnutrition affects between 20% and 50% of hospitalized patients and is thought to be underdiagnosed in many instances.[17] Among older adults, approximately 25% are malnourished or are at risk for malnutrition, and this has been identified as a key contributor to mortality in this population.[18] Specific disease states also exhibit a strong association with malnutrition. Among patients with cancer, 30–85% meet criteria for malnutrition.[19] Similarly, 20–85% of patients with inflammatory bowel disease (such as Crohn's disease or ulcerative colitis) are estimated to develop malnutrition.[20] Malnutrition prevalence is also notable in acute illnesses. Following the COVID-19 pandemic, it was found that in many countries, a high rate of malnutrition correlated with a high mortality rate from the infection.[21] Additionally, malnutrition was prevalent among patients hospitalized with the virus and was associated with prolonged and complicated hospital stays and increased mortality risk.[22] For these reasons, nutrition assessment is fundamental to the holistic evaluation of the acutely ill adult.

Parameters used for the identification of malnutrition within the screening and assessment processes should encompass both nutrition intake and severity of disease. Since no single clinical parameter is indicative of the malnourished state, data must be collected from a variety of domains.[8,9] Certain data are useful in the identification and documentation of malnutrition (**Table 1.1**).

The AAIM criteria propose specific diagnostic criteria that can be identified within the aforementioned contexts (**Table 1.2A - 1.2D**)[9]:

- Insufficient energy intake, established by determining the percentage of needs consumed (**Table 1.2A**)
- Unintended weight loss over a specific period of time (**Table 1.2B**)
- Indications of muscle mass and/or subcutaneous fat loss identified upon physical exam or fluid accumulation (generalized or localized) that may mask any recent weight loss (**Table 1.2C**)
- Diminished functional status as measured by handgrip strength (**Table 1.2D**)

A positive finding of any two characteristics in any one context (acute illness, chronic illness, or social/environmental circumstances) indicates malnutrition. Purposeful examination for these features should be present in every nutrition assessment.[9]

The Global Leadership in Malnutrition Criteria

It is important to note that the concept of malnutrition resulting from metabolic changes related to disease and injury is a subject not only of domestic research but also of global research. In 2016, a multinational Global Leadership Initiative on Malnutrition (GLIM) task force set out to further define malnutrition in clinical terms to allow for consistent identification

Table 1.1 Data Useful in the Identification of Malnutrition

Domain	Specific Data
Anthropometric	Standard measures of height, weight, and body composition, with particular focus on unintended weight loss
Biochemical	Biochemical assessment involves use of laboratory tests of patients' blood, urine, feces, and tissue samples to help determine nutritional status and organ function
Client History	Nutrition-focused past medical history, demographic data, clinical diagnosis, social history
Nutrition-Focused Physical Exam Findings	Nutrition-focused physical exam that may reveal the presence of several diagnostic characteristics of micronutrient deficiencies and malnutrition; declines in function measured via muscle strength and/or physical performance
Food/Nutrition-Related History	Information regarding food and nutrient intake will indicate the presence of any inadequacies or imbalances

Table 1.2A AAIM Interpretation of %Energy Indicator as a Key Indicator of Malnutrition

	Malnutrition in the Context of											
	Acute Illness or Injury				**Chronic Illness**				**Social/Environmental Circumstances**			
	Moderate Malnutrition		**Severe Malnutrition**		**Moderate Malnutrition**		**Severe Malnutrition**		**Moderate Malnutrition**		**Severe Malnutrition**	
Interpretation of Energy Intake	%	Time	%	Time	%	Time	%	Time	%	Time	%	Time
	Less than 75%	More than 7 days	50% or less	5 or more days	Less than 75%	1 or more months	75% or less	1 or more months	Less than 75%	3 or more months	50% or less	1 or more months

Data from White JV, Guenter P, Jensen G, et al. Consensus statement of the Academy of Nutrition and Dietetics/American Society for Parenteral and Enteral Nutrition: Characteristics recommended for the identification and documentation of adult malnutrition (undernutrition). *JPEN J Parenter Enteral Nutr.* 2012;36(3):275-283.
AAIM = Academy of Nutrition and Dietetics and American Society of Parenteral and Enteral Nutrition Indicators to Diagnose Malnutrition

Table 1.2B AAIM Interpretation of %Weight Loss as a Key Indicator of Malnutrition

	Malnutrition in the Context of							
	Acute Illness or Injury				Chronic Illness AND Social/Environmental Circumstances			
	Moderate Malnutrition		Severe Malnutrition		Moderate Malnutrition		Severe Malnutrition	
Interpretation of Weight Loss	%	Time	%	Time	%	Time	%	Time
	1–2	1 week	>2	1 week	5	1 month	>5	1 month
	5	1 month	>5	1 month	7.5	3 months	>7.5	3 months
	7.5	3 months	>7.5	3 months	10	6 months	>10	6 months
	–		–		20	1 year	>20	1 year

Data from White JV, Guenter P, Jensen G, et al. Consensus statement of the Academy of Nutrition and Dietetics/American Society for Parenteral and Enteral Nutrition: Characteristics recommended for the identification and documentation of adult malnutrition (undernutrition). *JPEN J Parenter Enteral Nutr.* 2012;36(3):275-283.
AAIM = Academy of Nutrition and Dietetics and American Society of Parenteral and Enteral Nutrition Indicators to Diagnose Malnutrition

Table 1.2C AAIM Interpretation of Physical Findings as a Key Indicator of Malnutrition

	Malnutrition in the Context of			
	Acute Illness or Injury		Chronic Illness AND Social/Environmental Circumstances	
Physical Findings	Moderate Malnutrition	Severe Malnutrition	Moderate Malnutrition	Severe Malnutrition
Body Fat	Mild Loss	Moderate Loss	Mild Loss	Severe Loss
Muscle Mass	Mild Loss	Moderate Loss	Mild Loss	Severe Loss
Fluid Accumulation	Mild	Moderate/Severe	Mild	Severe

Data from White JV, Guenter P, Jensen G, et al. Consensus statement of the Academy of Nutrition and Dietetics/American Society for Parenteral and Enteral Nutrition: Characteristics recommended for the identification and documentation of adult malnutrition (undernutrition). *JPEN J Parenter Enteral Nutr.* 2012;36(3):275-283.
AAIM = Academy of Nutrition and Dietetics and American Society of Parenteral and Enteral Nutrition Indicators to Diagnose Malnutrition

Table 1.2D AAIM Interpretation of Functional Status as a Key Indicator of Malnutrition

	Malnutrition in the Context of	
	Acute Illness or Injury and Chronic Illness and Social/Environmental Circumstances	
	Moderate Malnutrition	Severe Malnutrition
Reduced Grip Strength	—	Measurably Reduced

Data from White JV, Guenter P, Jensen G, et al. Consensus statement of the Academy of Nutrition and Dietetics/American Society for Parenteral and Enteral Nutrition: Characteristics recommended for the identification and documentation of adult malnutrition (undernutrition). *JPEN J Parenter Enteral Nutr.* 2012;36(3):275-283.
AAIM = Academy of Nutrition and Dietetics and American Society of Parenteral and Enteral Nutrition Indicators to Diagnose Malnutrition

and treatment worldwide. The resulting consensus report, endorsed by ESPEN, lists a number of diagnostic criteria known as the GLIM criteria[11]:

- Presence of non-volitional (unintentional) weight loss
- Low body mass index (BMI)
- Loss of muscle mass
- Reduction in intake
- Disease-related inflammation

Specific diagnostic thresholds will be discussed later in this chapter. The above elements are subtly different from the AAIM criteria[9] but are common across a number of screening and diagnostic tools.[8] The GLIM criteria, however, is the first consensus statement seeking to standardize criteria in clinical nutrition across countries.[11]

Consequences of Malnutrition

The importance of an appropriate assessment for the identification of malnutrition can be attributed to prevention of its far-reaching and damaging clinical impacts. It has long been understood that patients with poor nutritional status have inferior outcomes compared to their well-nourished counterparts.[13] In the acute care and critical care settings, malnutrition is a major contributor to increased morbidity and mortality, increased lengths of stay and rates of readmission, decreased function and quality of life, and higher healthcare costs.[23,24] Hospitalized patients who are malnourished have 34% higher costs compared to patients who are not malnourished.[25] Additionally, it has been estimated that the cost associated with treating patients with malnutrition in the United States is approximately $157 billion annually.[26] The presence of malnutrition alters the function and recovery of virtually every organ system, which can manifest as the development of pressure injuries, increased rates of infection, impaired wound healing, surgical complications, and increased ventilatory requirements, among others.[17] Patients who are malnourished are up to 5 times more likely to experience in-hospital death than those who are not malnourished.[23]

CORE CONCEPT 1

The purpose of nutrition assessment is to identify malnutrition via assessment of various domains—anthropometrics, biochemical, client history, nutrition-focused physical exam findings, and food and nutrition-related history.

CORE CONCEPT 2

Although criteria vary, malnutrition diagnosis often includes assessment of unintentional weight loss, muscle mass loss, and inadequate energy intake.

Performing the Nutrition Assessment: The Registered Dietitian (RD)

The Registered Dietitian (RD) or Registered Dietitian Nutritionist (RDN) credential is earned by a nutrition expert who has been trained in all domains of nutrition (clinical, community, and food service) and who has passed a national exam. This is in contrast to "nutritionist," a title that can be applied without qualification or credentialing. RDs must maintain their credential through ongoing education, and some states additionally require licensure to practice.[27] RDs can also acquire additional credentials in specialty areas including gerontology, sports nutrition, weight management, pediatrics, pediatric critical care, renal, and oncology through the Commission for Dietetic Registration (CDR).[28] The National Board of Nutrition Support Certification (NBNSC), established through ASPEN, offers specialty certification in nutrition support.[29]

The RD scope and standard of practice is set by the CDR and is updated regularly to adapt to the fast-developing field of nutrition science.[27] RDs must practice in an ethical, legal, and competent manner, and exhibit ongoing introspection, development, and quality improvement through continuing education and activities. Staying up to date with research, practice guidelines, and data management systems allows for care to stay current and evidence-based and ensures RDs are prepared to be active participants in broader conversations around the state of science and health policy. RDs should also be cognizant of health equity and disparities, social determinants of health (SDOH), sustainability, and the state of health at the global and the community level. RDs must work collaboratively in whichever setting they practice, and be able to actively and effectively screen, assess, evaluate, tailor interventions, and monitor their patients or clients.[28]

Due to the extensive training required, RDs are the only practitioners permitted to provide medical nutrition therapy (MNT) by the Centers for Medicare and Medicaid Services (CMS).[30] As noted, a thorough nutrition assessment is central to planning and implementing nutrition interventions within the Nutrition Care Process.[2,3]

The Role of the Clinician

"Clinician" can refer to a number of members of the multidisciplinary clinical healthcare team with whom the RD collaborates, as well as clinical dietitians themselves. A medical doctor (MD), Doctor of Osteopathic Medicine (DO), advanced practice providers (APPs, such as nurse practitioners [NPs] and physician assistants [PAs]), and the registered nurse (RN) are common clinician members of the interprofessional team. Clinicians often provide direct patient care and work collaboratively. Throughout the text, the term "clinician" is used to describe any of the above providers, including the RD.

Nutrition Screening

The Role of Nutrition Screening in the NCPM

Prior to the introduction of the NCPM, nutrition screening was recommended by AND as an integral component of care.[31] The process to identify those individuals at nutritional risk who would benefit from further assessment and intervention has evolved into a critical antecedent step of the NCPM. AND currently defines **nutrition screening** as "the process of identifying patients, clients, or groups who may have a nutrition diagnosis and benefit from nutrition assessment intervention by a registered dietitian (RD)."[7] The initial screen may not always be completed by a dietetics practitioner and is not actually considered to be part of the NCPM.[2,7]

AND supports nutrition screening as the preliminary step that triggers entrance into the NCPM. Given the impracticality of conducting a full assessment of all patients, RDs rely upon an appropriate screen to identify individuals who are either already malnourished or at risk of becoming malnourished. The goal in this case is not necessarily to *diagnose* malnutrition, but instead to identify the known characteristics associated with the malnourished state or other nutritional issues that would warrant a more thorough evaluation and potential intervention.[7,32]

Screening in Acute Care

The Joint Commission (JC) is the independent entity responsible for the accreditation and certification of healthcare organizations in the United States. In 1995, the JC mandated that the nutrition screen be performed when warranted by the patient's needs and conditions based upon organizational criteria.[33] When applicable to a patient's condition, the screen must be completed within 24 hours of an inpatient admission.[8,34] The JC does not require that a specific tool or criteria be used; the guidelines instead specify that each organization must have "defined criteria that identify when nutritional plans are developed."[33] In other words, there are no clear standards that dictate the screening tool itself, only that each organization screens within the designated time frame. As such, the methods used between sites vary considerably.[7,35]

The majority of acute care hospitals have incorporated screening into the admission process in order to help prioritize hospital resources, although the screening methods used to meet JC's mandate will vary from center to center. Several common denominators prevail among the multitude of tools utilized: validity and reliability, ease of use and convenience, speed (typically requiring less than 5 minutes), avoidance of complicated calculations or laboratory data, minimal expense, and noninvasiveness. To meet each of these characteristics, initial screening in most hospitals is based, at least in part, on height and weight collected upon admission.[7,31,34,36]

Any screening tool a hospital employs will be unable to account for the extreme variability observed in patients within an acute care setting. Other aspects of the disease state must be considered, in addition to nutritional measurements, to determine if and when intervention is warranted or is likely to be beneficial. Screening is not meant to replace the training and clinical judgment of the RD, but instead to assist in initiating the NCPM.[8] Although the use of a validated screening tool is the preferred method of screening, additional screening criteria, such as length of stay, specific disease states or treatments types, or prolonged period of NPO (nil per os) status, may be considered to detect patients at risk for malnutrition who may be missed by some screening tools.

Several existing screening tools are available for use in the clinical setting. These tools, which will be described in detail in the following sections, serve as exceptional resources for implementing a new, or revamping an existing, screening method. When selecting the tool or criteria to be used in acute care, there are two important considerations:

1. The screening of patients in the clinical setting differs greatly from that of the community setting. The primary purpose in this context is to identify those patients who will require further assessment of the need for nutrition support. Given that many of the developed tools were intended for use in the community setting, it is important

to ensure that the tool selected has been validated within the specific inpatient population for whom it will be used.[7]

2. Given the complexity of the malnourished state, there is no single parameter that is both sensitive and specific for malnutrition. Screening patients in acute care must be ongoing and should consider the routes for development of malnutrition (deficient intake, excessive losses, increased metabolic demand, etc.) to identify those who increase in risk over time or as they undergo treatment.[7,34]

Overall, the screening tool selected should identify all individuals at risk. To ensure this validity, a screening tool will have a high sensitivity (meaning that patients identified as at risk of malnutrition are actually malnourished) *and* a high specificity (patients not identified as at risk are, in fact, not malnourished). Furthermore, a screening tool should be reliable in that it consistently reproduces the same or similar results. The use of an inappropriate tool—or one that has not been validated or has been validated in a different population than the one for which it is currently being used—will negatively influence patient care and risk misdiagnosis of malnutrition.[7,34]

CORE CONCEPT 3

The registered dietitian is the most competent professional to assist in selecting or developing the screening method used in acute care, particularly when the screening is to be completed by non-dietetics clinicians.

Nutrition Screening Tools

Nutrition screening allows all patients at risk to receive the appropriate individualized nutrition care they require. When appropriate screening leads to appropriate intervention, outcomes are dramatically improved, including reduced readmissions, shorter lengths of hospital stay, and lower mortality rates.[36] Given this insight, a number of screening tools have been developed and validated for use in the acute care setting. Most validated tools will address four basic areas of nutrition risk: recent weight loss, recent dietary intake, current BMI, and current disease state. Depending on the tool, various other measurements of nutritional status may be included to further assist in the prediction of malnutrition risk.[37]

Although some screening tools have been endorsed by international nutrition societies, there is no universal or empirical agreement on a single best tool. The most well-known and widely used examples include the Malnutrition Universal Screening Tool (MUST), Nutritional Risk Screening (NRS-2002), the Short Nutritional Assessment Questionnaire (SNAQ), and the Malnutrition Screening Tool (MST). The Nutrition Risk in the Critically Ill (NUTRIC) score is another example but is only used in the critical care setting. Please note that while some of these tools were developed by professional groups outside of the United States, they are used widely across clinical practice.[38]

Malnutrition Universal Screening Tool (MUST)

To identify both undernutrition and overnutrition in adults of different ages and diagnoses, the Malnutrition Advisory Group, a standing committee of the British Association for Parenteral and Enteral Nutrition (BAPEN), convened to develop the **Malnutrition Universal Screening Tool (MUST)**. The MUST tool considers current weight status as BMI, unintentional changes in weight, and the presence of an acute disease that influences, or is likely to influence, dietary intake. Each of these three components can individually influence clinical outcomes, serving as a powerful predictor of nutrition risk when combined. To assess these variables, the MUST framework utilizes a simple five-step process to arrive at an overall score for malnutrition: either low, medium, or high risk (**Figure 1.1**). The tool then refers clinicians to management, which can be modified according to the specific healthcare setting and patient population.[32,34,36,38]

MUST has been deemed valid and reliable across a wide spectrum of adult patients, even among those requiring special interpretation for fluid disturbances, amputations, or inability to be measured for height and weight. In these situations, the MUST framework supplies instructions for alternative measurements that ensure reliability nearly identical to that of the original tool. Although originally developed for use in the community setting and supported by ESPEN as the preferred screening tool in this context, MUST has been considered suitable for use across the continuum of health care. When extended to the acute care setting, this framework demonstrates concurrent validity with other tools and strong predictive validity in terms of lengths of hospital stay, discharge destination, and mortality. MUST can be utilized by all members of the interdisciplinary team without concern for interrater variation (i.e., can be used by various professionals with similar results).[36,39–44] AND rates the MUST with high overall validity, moderate reliability and agreement, fair generalizability, with fair evidence quality.[45]

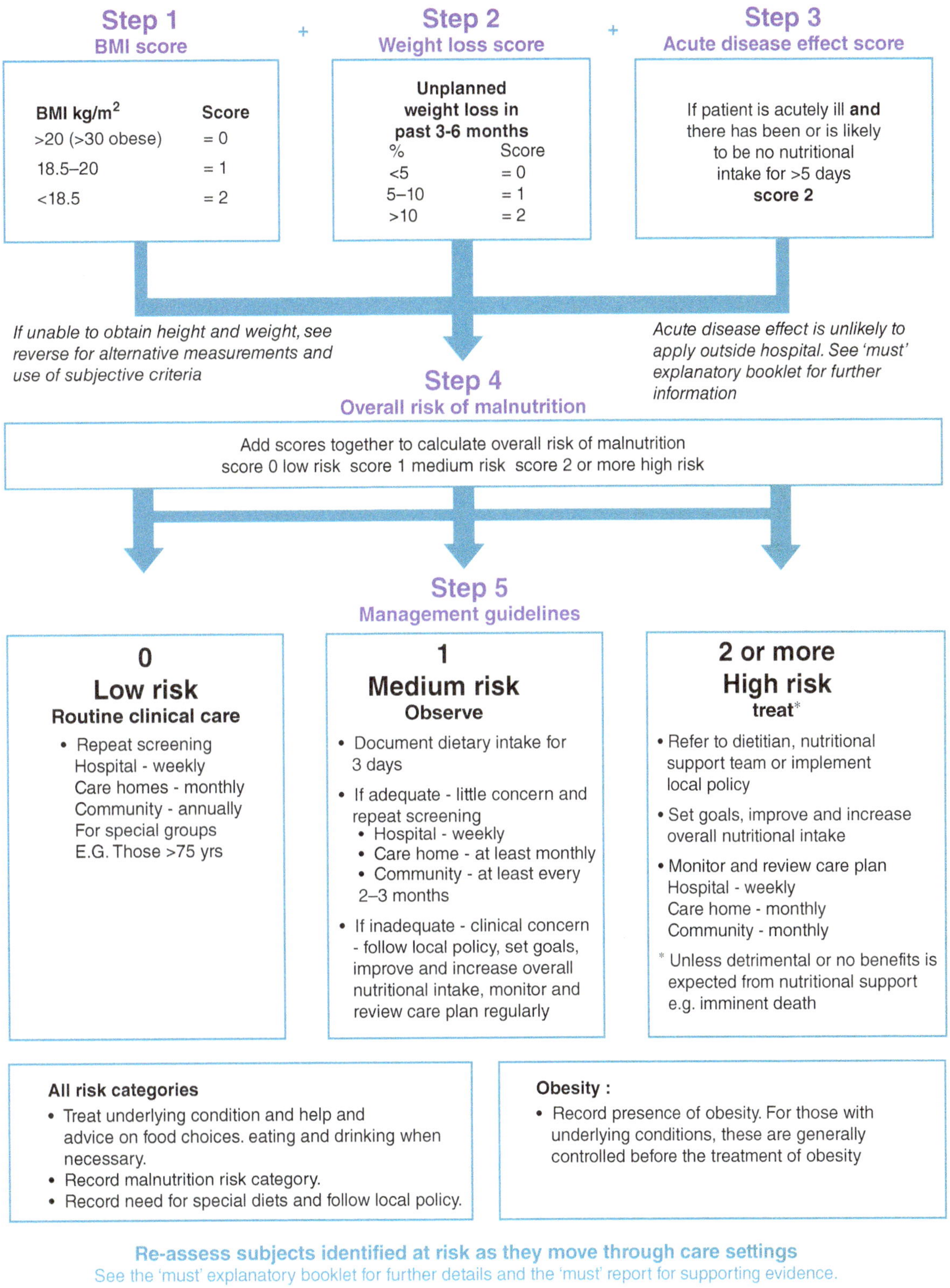

Figure 1.1 The Malnutrition Universal Screening Tool (MUST)

Reproduced from Elia M. The "MUST" report: *nutritional screening of adults: a multidisciplinary responsibility. Development and use of the Malnutrition Universal Screening Tool (MUST) for adults*. BAPEN; 2003. ISBN: 1-899467-70-X.'MUST' is reproduced here with the kind permission of BAPEN (British Association for Parenteral and Enteral Nutrition). For further information on 'MUST' see www.bapen.org.uk Copyright BAPEN 2012 (licence number LIC2206)

Alternative measurements: instructions and tables

If height cannot be obtained, use length of forearm (ulna) to calculate height using tables below.
(see the 'MUST' explanatory booklet for details of other alternative measurements (knee height and demispan) that can also be used to estimate height).

BAPEN
www.bapen.org.uk

Estimating height from ulna length

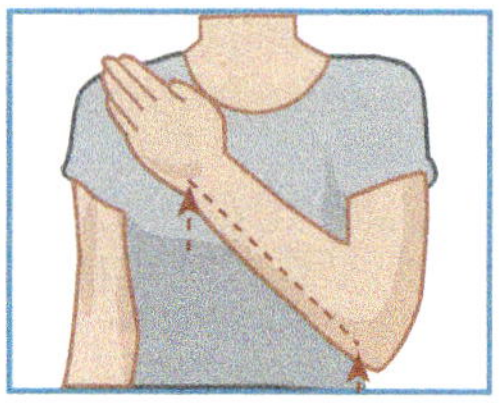

Measure between the point of the elbow (olecranon process) and the midpoint of the prominent bone of the wrist (styloid process) (left side if possible).

Height (m) men (< 65 years)	1.94	1.93	1.91	1.89	1.87	1.85	1.84	1.82	1.80	1.78	1.76	1.75	1.73	1.71
Height (m) men (≥ 65 years)	1.87	1.86	1.84	1.82	1.81	1.79	1.78	1.76	1.75	1.73	1.71	1.70	1.68	1.67
Ulna length (cm)	32.0	31.5	31.0	30.5	30.0	29.5	29.0	28.5	28.0	27.5	27.0	26.5	26.0	25.5
Height (m) women (< 65 years)	1.84	1.83	1.81	1.80	1.79	1.77	1.76	1.75	1.73	1.72	1.70	1.69	1.68	1.66
Height (m) women (≥ 65 years)	1.84	1.83	1.81	1.79	1.78	1.76	1.75	1.73	1.71	1.70	1.68	1.66	1.65	1.63

Height (m) men (< 65 years)	1.69	1.67	1.66	1.64	1.62	1.60	1.58	1.57	1.55	1.53	1.51	1.49	1.48	1.46
Height (m) men (≥ 65 years)	1.65	1.63	1.62	1.60	1.59	1.57	1.56	1.54	1.52	1.51	1.49	1.48	1.46	1.45
Ulna length (cm)	25.0	24.5	24.0	23.5	23.0	22.5	22.0	21.5	21.0	20.5	20.0	19.5	19.0	18.5
Height (m) women (< 65 years)	1.65	1.63	1.62	1.61	1.59	1.58	1.56	1.55	1.54	1.54	1.51	1.50	1.48	1.47
Height (m) women (≥ 65 years)	1.61	1.60	1.58	1.56	1.55	1.53	1.52	1.50	1.48	1.47	1.45	1.44	1.42	1.40

Estimating BMI category from mid upper arm circumference (MUAC)

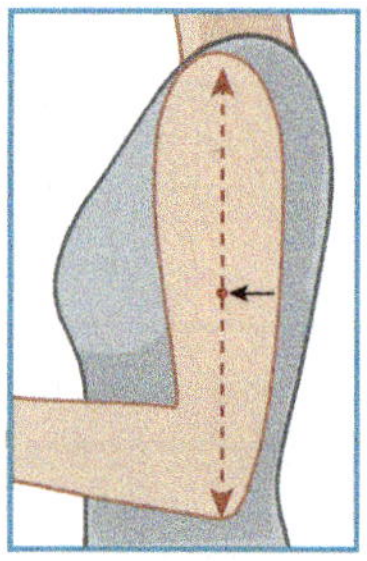

The subject's left arm should be bent at the elbow at a 90 degree angle, with the upper arm held parallel to the side of the body. Measure the distance between the bony protrusion on the shoulder (acromion) and the point of the elbow (olecranon process). Mark the mid-point.

Ask the subject to let arm hang loose and measure around the upper arm at the mid-point, making sure that the tape measure is snug but not tight.

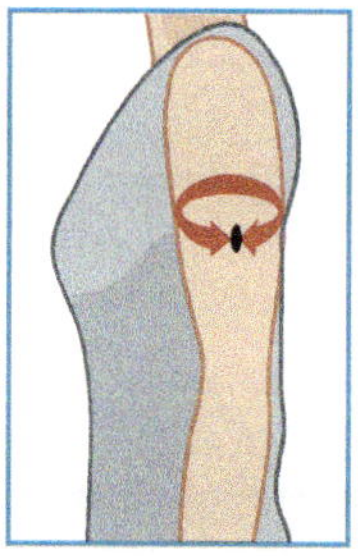

If MUAC is < 23.5 cm, BMI is likely to be < 20 kg/m^2
If MUAC is > 32.0 cm, BMI is likely to be > 30 kg/m^2

The use of MUAC provides a general indication of BMI and is not designed to generate an actual score for use with 'MUST'. For further information on use of MUAC please refer to *The 'MUST' Explanatory Booklet*.

Figure 1.1 *(Continued)*

Nutritional Risk Screening (NRS-2002)

When the Nutritional Risk Screening (NRS-2002) tool was developed by a working group of ESPEN, the goal was to establish a screening system based on the nutrition criteria or characteristics used in the current clinical trials.[46] The developers relied on the assumption that nutritional status and indication for nutrition support (based on undernutrition and/or increased nutritional requirements) relate directly to severity of disease. The tool measures disease impact in addition to the markers of current or potential malnutrition. It has been validated to identify not only patients who are malnourished at the time of screening, but also those at risk for malnutrition secondary to the disease state or associated treatment, thus emphasizing the need for preventing further deterioration of nutritional status as the clinical course progresses.[47]

The purpose of the NRS-2002 system is to detect either existing or anticipated malnutrition in the hospital setting. The initial screening tool consists of four simple, but strategic, questions that consider weight loss, BMI, and dietary intake history in the setting of illness. If there is a positive response to any of the questions in the initial screen, a second, more detailed screen is conducted. This second screen calculates two scores: one for current nutritional status and another for severity of disease and associated increase in metabolic demand. These scores are then combined and adjusted for age (with age older than 70 years as a risk factor) to result in a final evaluation of nutrition risk. Ultimately, this score is linked to an example intervention, although the content of the nutrition care plan is determined by the RD.[34,36,47,48]

Several studies have validated the NRS-2002 across a range of hospitalized patients, from surgical to cardiovascular to gastrointestinal, and can be applied in the acute care setting without concern for impracticality or inaccuracy.[47–55] ESPEN recommends NRS-2002 be used for all hospitalized patients[48] while ASPEN recommends its use for all patients who are critically ill.[49] AND rates the NRS-2002 with moderate validity and agreement with limited generalizability and fair strength of evidence.[45]

Short Nutritional Assessment Questionnaire (SNAQ)

The publication of the first ESPEN Screening Guidelines prompted international reevaluation of hospital-wide screening processes. Upon assessment of the tools available for use, many nations found that their current frameworks failed to meet the criteria recommended by the guidelines. In response, a committee of dietitians in the Netherlands developed the **Short Nutritional Assessment Questionnaire (SNAQ)**, a "quick and easy" screening tool intended for use during admission to an acute care facility. The development of SNAQ was based on an evaluation of mixed hospitalized medical and surgical adult patients. Following a statistical analysis of 26 questions related to nutritional status and disease state, the three questions identified with the highest predictive validity were included in the tool (refer to **Figure 1.2** for the complete tool)[47,56]:

1. Did you lose weight unintentionally? (scored according to the amount of weight loss)
2. Did you experience a decreased appetite over the last month?
3. Did you use supplemental drinks or tube feeding over the last month?

Based on response, the tool then classifies patients as well nourished, moderately malnourished, or severely malnourished. Using the validated tool, malnourished patients are recognized on admission and receive necessary intervention at an early stage. This early identification and intervention have been associated with a reduced length of hospital stay. The SNAQ screening tool has been validated in both outpatient and inpatient populations, with a simplicity that allows easy inclusion into the admission process.[35,36,56–59] This tool has shown a positive correlation with quality of life, functional status, and fat-free body composition during hospitalization.[56] AND rates SNAQ as moderate in overall validity and reliability with fair generalizability and fair quality of evidence.[45]

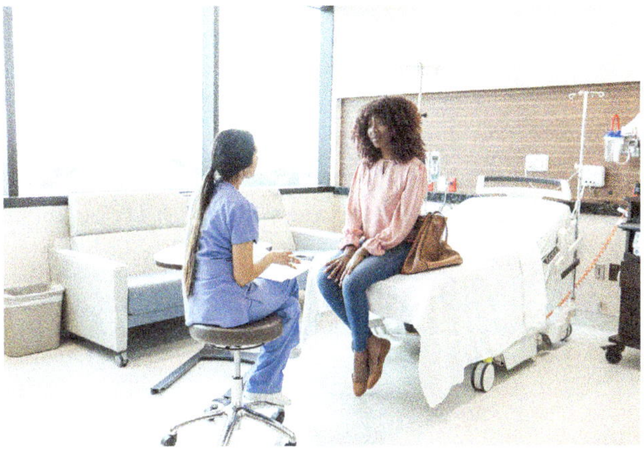

Malnutrition Screening Tool (MST)

Similar in concept to SNAQ, the **Malnutrition Screening Tool (MST)** is a three-question tool that was developed and validated for use based on general

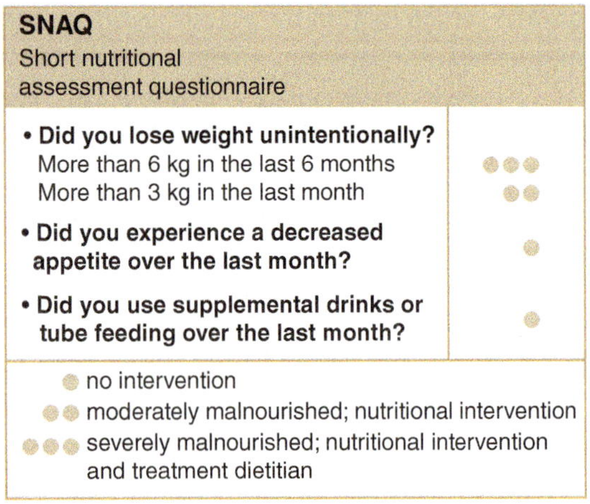

Figure 1.2 The Short Nutritional Assessment Questionnaire

Reproduced from Dutch Malnutrition Steering Group. SNAQ tools in English. Fight Malnutrition website. Updated 2017. Accessed February 10, 2017. https://www.fightmalnutrition.eu

medical and surgical hospitalized patients. It was created based on the need for a framework that used routinely available data, was noninvasive, convenient for non-dietetics staff, and could be employed across a heterogeneous adult population. In a process similar to that used for the development of SNAQ, 21 screening questions were selected based on the literature and clinical experience. Those with the highest sensitivity and specificity in predicting nutrition status were included in the final tool.[47]

Two questions—"Have you lost weight recently without trying?" and "Have you been eating poorly because of a decreased appetite?"—were deemed the best predictors of nutrition risk. In addition, a third question was incorporated to assess the degree of weight loss, if present. A score is allocated based on patient or caregiver response, which will categorize the patient as "not at risk" or "at risk." The scoring system can then be used to prioritize patient care, with those receiving the highest scores requiring the earliest intervention. Specifically, those who are screened with a score greater than or equal to 2 should be assessed by an RD.[34,60–62]

The MST is an attractive choice when selecting a screening tool due to its simplicity and ability to be completed without additional calculations. Despite its minimal nature, the tool is lauded as a strong predictor of nutritional status.[34,36,47,60,62,63] AND rates the MST as having moderate validity, good generalizability, moderate agreement, moderate reliability, strong quality of evidence, and recommends that the MST be used to screen all adults in all care settings regardless of age and medical history.[45]

CORE CONCEPT 4

A wide variety of nutrition screening questions or tools are employed in clinical settings across the United States. Several well-validated screening tools exist with the goal of identifying nutritional status or predicting poor clinical outcomes related to malnutrition.

NUTRIC Score

While the other screening tools explored in this chapter are designed for use regardless of disease state, the NUTRIC score is not a traditional screening tool since it was specifically designed for screening patients in the intensive care unit (ICU) setting to identify those who would benefit most from nutrition support. This screening tool incorporates more specific markers of inflammation including the interleukin-6 (IL-6) level, the Acute Physiology and Chronic Health Evaluation (APACHE) II score (describing illness severity), the Sequential Organ Failure Assessment (SOFA) score (for organ failure), as well as age, number of comorbidities, and days from hospital to ICU admission.[64] Scores of 6–10 out of 10 indicate high nutritional risk that may require nutrition support intervention.[49] A high NUTRIC score was positively correlated with 28-day mortality,[65] which has been consistently validated in other studies.[66] This tool requires more than 20 data points, making it difficult to administer. A newer version of the APACHE score (APACHE IV) is currently available that is not validated for the NUTRIC score. ASPEN recommends the NUTRIC score to screen patients who are critically ill.[49]

Assessment Tools Confused for Screening Tools

Two additional tools—the Subjective Global Assessment (SGA) and the Mini-Nutritional Assessment (MNA)—are often grouped with the list of screening tools previously discussed. These tools, however, can function as a means of nutrition assessment. In other words, the SGA and MNA should most readily be used to assess, not to screen, because they combine data on nutritional status with clinical observations, disease status, and/or biochemical values.[7,37]

Final Comparison of Screening Tools for Acute Care

As previously mentioned, there is no universal agreement in terms of nutrition screening tools. Comprehensive tools, like NRS-2002 and MUST, will require slightly more time and skill from the screening clinician because of the need for measurements, calculations, and evaluation of disease severity. Conversely, the "quick and easy" tools, such as SNAQ and MST, have adequate availability of screening components. The questions used in these tools are not only simple to complete but can identify malnutrition risk with similar accuracy as the comprehensive tools without the need for additional calculations or secondary screens.[45] The bottom line is that each of the screening tools may be employed based on individual hospital or clinical preferences. Because each is well validated and considered reliable, the RD must be careful to recommend the most appropriate tool for the specific setting, patient population, and/or screening goals (**Table 1.3**).[15,45,47]

Table 1.3 Comparison of Malnutrition Risk Screening Tools

Screening Tool	NRS-2002	MUST	SNAQ©	MST
Complexity	Comprehensive	Comprehensive	Abbreviated	Abbreviated
Intent	Developed for use in acute care settings.	Developed for use in the community setting.	Developed for use during admission to acute care facility.	Developed based on general medical and surgical inpatients.
Brief Description	Two-part tool that relates nutritional status to existing disease state.	Five-step framework that scores nutritional status in the setting of acute illness.	Three question tool that assesses simple and common indicators of malnutrition.	Two question tool that requires no measurements or additional calculations.
Parameters	▪ Unintentional weight loss ▪ BMI ▪ History of dietary intake ▪ Disease acuity ▪ Age	▪ Unintentional weight loss ▪ BMI ▪ Presence of an acute illness that may affect dietary intake	▪ Unintentional weight loss ▪ Decreases in appetite ▪ Need for supplemental or enteral nutrition	▪ Unintentional weight loss ▪ Decreases in appetite

NRS-20002, Nutritional Risk Screening 2002; MUST, Malnutrition Universal Screening Tool; SNAQ, Short Nutritional Assessment Questionnaire; MST, Malnutrition Screening Tool
Data from Jensen GL, Compher C, Sullivan DH, Mullin GE. Recognizing malnutrition in adults: Definitions, characteristics, screening, assessment, and team approach. *JPEN J Parenter Enteral Nutr.* 2013;37(6):802–807.

CASE STUDY REVISITED

After completing a nutrition screen, Marie is identified as being at high nutrition risk. You initiate a nutrition assessment for Marie, who is now on bedrest. You successfully obtain a weight history, but when you seek to confirm Marie's height, she states that she used to be 160 cm tall, but she is now shorter than that and is uncertain of her actual height.

Anthropometric Data:

Height: 160 cm
Weight: 65 kg
BMI: 25.4 kg/m^2

Weight history

66.5 kg 1 month ago
70 kg 3 months ago
77 kg 6 months ago (usual body weight)

Questions

1. Calculate Marie's percent usual body weight and percent weight loss.
2. Given the discrepancy in Marie's reported height, how do you proceed with your anthropometric evaluation?

CORE CONCEPT 5

Nutrition screening tools should have acceptable validity, be simple to administer, have wide applicability across various populations, and use commonly available information.

Modernizing Nutrition Screening: Social Determinants of Health (SDOH)

In 2023, CMS introduced a new high-priority quality measurement (#487) focused on screening for health-related social needs, also known as "social determinants of health (SDOH)."[67] SDOH have long been discussed as drivers of both over- and undernutrition and commonly include factors such as food security, infrastructure or built environment, transportation, education, historic systematic inequalities, socioeconomic status, and access to healthcare resources and healthful food.[68,69] These factors are now considered integral to effective public health interventions, and as such, are being included in national healthcare goals like Healthy People 2030[68] that marks objectives for advancement of population health. While challenging to compare research due to differences in exact definition and components included, SDOH have broadly been shown to impact prevalence and progression of several disease states including diabetes,[69] cardiovascular disease,[70] chronic kidney disease,[71] and steatotic liver disease.[72] Indeed, SDOH have been found to be responsible for up to 80% of health-related outcomes.[67] Quality measurement #487 for SDOH screening specifically requires institutions to assess adult patients for housing stability, food security, transportation, utilities, and safety to facilitate care with the goal of achieving optimal outcomes and cost reductions. It is anticipated that acute care facilities choosing to implement this quality metric for merit-based payment from CMS may observe increases in RD consultation to address malnutrition resulting from these factors. RDs should also consider SDOH when counseling patients on MNT to ensure patients have adequate resources to implement interventions, such as being able to access foods appropriate to their medically tailored diet and afford oral nutrition supplements or formulas after a hospital stay. RDs will benefit from fostering familiarity with local food pantries, "food pharmacies," supplemental food assistance programs such as SNAP and WIC, and nutrition support charities such as the Oley Foundation.[73,74] **Table 1.4** lists selected food security–related resources, programs, and organizations.

Table 1.4 Selected Food Security–Related Programs

Community Programs	Congressional Hunger Center, Feeding America, Food Recovery
Food Security Programs	USDA Food Atlas, Feeding America
Federal Programs	Child Nutrition, Child and Adult Care Food program, Farm to School, Fresh Fruit and Vegetable program, National School lunch, School Breakfast program, Special Milk program, Special Supplemental Nutrition Program for Women, Infants, and Children (WIC) program, Summer Foodservice program, Supplemental Nutrition Assistance (SNAP), USDA food distribution programs

Nutrition Assessment

Following the identification of nutrition risk via screening, a thorough assessment of a patient's nutritional status is the critical next step in identifying malnutrition. Since there is neither a single parameter nor gold standard that can determine nutritional status or the degree of malnutrition in an individual, a comprehensive nutrition assessment is needed. The remainder of this chapter will discuss the components of nutrition assessment as they are subdivided by the NCPM terminology with anthropometrics, biochemical, client history, nutrition-focused physical exam findings, and food and nutrition-related history. AND defines nutritional assessment as the process "to obtain, verify, and interpret data needed to identify nutrition-related problems, their causes, and significance."[7] It establishes the foundation for all other steps of the NCPM by providing the information necessary for determining a nutrition diagnosis and its etiology. The true purpose of the nutrition assessment is to collect all relevant information to identify nutrition-related problems and their causes.[7,36,75]

Anthropometric Measurements

One of the most obvious and indispensable components of nutrition assessment is the use of **anthropometry**, the assessment of measures and proportions of the human body.[76] Regardless of the setting, anthropometric assessment will involve obtaining and interpreting physical measurements as part of a comprehensive evaluation of nutritional status. These measures are essential to either determining the need for or monitoring the progress of an intervention. In this context, all anthropometric measures obtained should be compared to both of the following:

1. Population-specific standards that help reflect the current condition of the patient, e.g., BMI
2. The patient's previous measures to identify the loss or gain of body components, e.g., percent of usual body weight (UBW)

PRACTICE POINT

Trending anthropometric data points provides the most useful information. For example, a patient who may fall into the "normal" category by BMI may actually have experienced clinically significant weight loss in comparison to their usual body weight.

Height, weight, skinfold measures, and circumferences provide the most readily used data points, although there are additional assessment methods available for use. It is up to the clinician to determine which measures are most appropriate to the individual circumstance.[12,77,78]

PRACTICE POINT

Anthropometric measurements are only one piece of the nutrition assessment puzzle. Although changes in these measures are reliable predictors of nutritional outcome, they should always be considered in the context of the overall status of the patient.

Assessing Height

Measures of **height** (stature) are not particularly useful for assessing nutritional status without context. Body height remains an essential measure because it provides a necessary variable for calculating other useful parameters (including ideal body weight and BMI). Several important decisions, both nutrition related (i.e., the estimation of energy needs) and non-nutrition related (i.e., medication dosing), depend on the collection of an accurate measure of height.[78–81]

Ideally, height is measured with the patient in the standing position using either a wall-mounted or free-standing calibrated **stadiometer**, a piece of equipment designed to measure height constructed of a ruler and sliding horizontal headpiece adjusted to rest on the top of the head (**Figure 1.3**). Upright measures are not always feasible in the critical care setting due to the limitations of bed confinement or difficulties in maintaining the erect position. Obtaining an accurate measurement of the hospitalized patient who remains in the supine position attached to several intravenous lines, for example, must instead rely upon an alternate technique.[78–81]

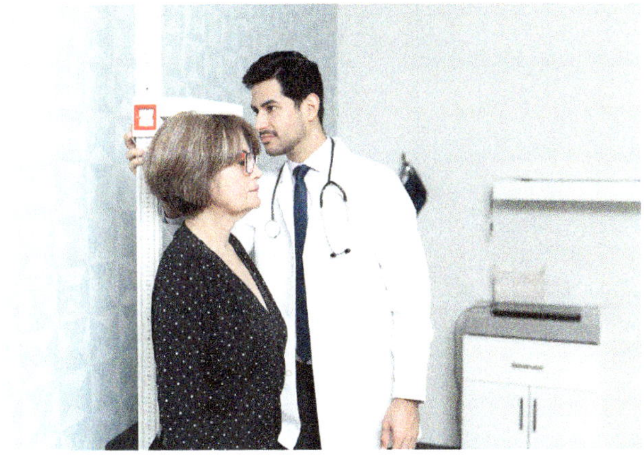

Figure 1.3 Measuring Height with a Stadiometer

PRACTICE POINT

For those able, height is measured in the upright position. To be most accurate, the individual should stand with bare feet flat on the floor and heels together; arms should hang loosely to the side with legs and back straight. The head should be in the Frankfort plane (i.e., outer corners of the eyes and tops of the ears parallel to the floor); height is measured after a deep in-breath, ensuring that the head remains in the correct position. Three points of contact—heels, scapula, and buttocks—should be touching the wall (**Figure 1.4**).

Alternate Measures to Assess Height. For all patients, an accurate measure of height must be obtained. Given the impracticability of the upright measure because of several conditions, such as immobility due to contractures, kyphosis, amputations, or quadriplegia, alternatives for estimating this value are often employed in clinical settings. These surrogate measures use the length of other body segments to predict or estimate standing height.[79,80,82–84]

Adult height records in the acute care setting are often based on verbal information provided by the patient instead of an actual measurement. Although this may appear to be an inaccurate substitute for assessing height, several studies have illustrated that the reliability of **self-reported height (SRH)** is comparable to, or often surpasses, other alternative measures. Given the ease and practicality of obtaining an SRH, it is much more likely to observe this surrogate measure than any other in the clinical setting. Despite the significant room for error, clinicians can feel comfortable using SRH as long as it is taken with the caveat that most individuals tend to overestimate height.[78,79,85,86]

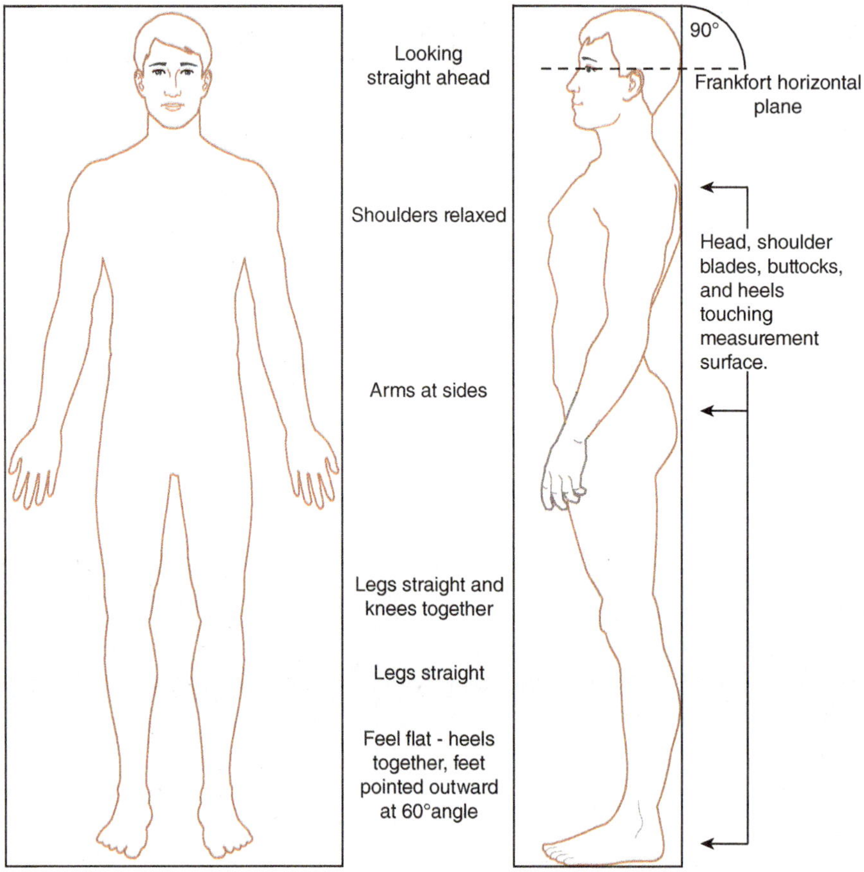

Figure 1.4 Upright Position for Accurate Measure of Adult Body Height

Reproduced from Centers for Disease Control and Prevention. *National Health and Nutrition Examination Survey (NHANES): anthropometry procedures manual.* 2007.

When neither standing height nor SRH is available (or to confirm an unlikely SRH), height can be estimated using one of the three most common surrogate measures—knee height, arm span, or arm length. These methods rely on the measurement of one or more long bones that do not lose length with aging in the same manner as the spine. Thereafter, a predictive equation specific to the body segment measured can be used to arrive at an estimate of stature. Each of these methods has demonstrated a reproducible and reliable correlation to standing height.[83,87]

Knee Height Measurement. Of the many available alternate measures of stature, measurement of **knee height** using a caliper device is perhaps the most acceptable and widely used in the clinical setting.[80] Due to its high correlation with upright height, this technique is often selected to assess the patient with critical illness given the ability to complete the measure while the patient is recumbent. The measurement itself is easily taken from the sole of the foot to the anterior surface of the thigh while the lower limb is flexed (**Figure 1.5**).[79]

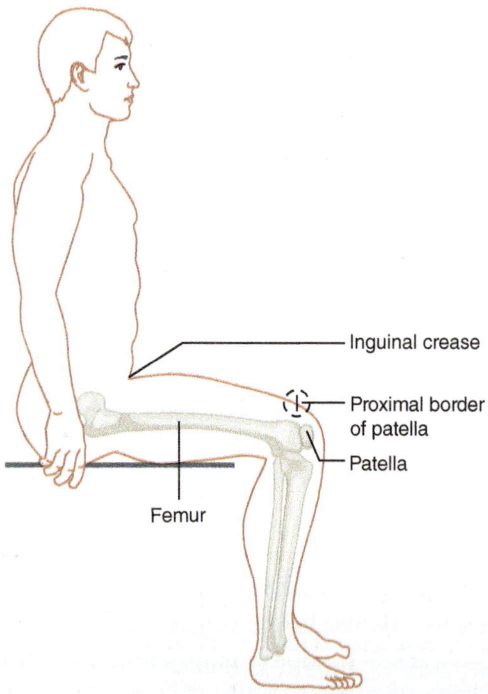

Figure 1.5 Positioning for the Measurement of Knee Height

Reproduced from Centers for Disease Control and Prevention. *National Health and Nutrition Examination Survey (NHANES): anthropometry procedures manual.* 2007.

The most accurate predictive equation for estimating standing height from knee height is that originally developed for use in nonambulatory older patients by Chumlea et al., otherwise known as the "Chumlea

Table 1.5 Equations for Predicting Stature from Knee Height*

White Male	Predicted height (cm) = [knee height (cm) × 1.88] + 71.85
Black Male	Predicted height (cm) = [knee height (cm) × 1.79] + 73.42
White Female	Predicted height (cm) = [knee height (cm) × 1.87] − [0.06 × age (y)] + 70.25
Black Female	Predicted height (cm) = [knee height (cm) × 1.86] − [0.06 × age (y)] + 68.10

*For use in those aged 18–60 years

Data from Chumlea WC, Guo SS, Steinbaugh ML. Prediction of stature from knee height for black and white adults and children with application to mobility-impaired or handicapped persons. *J Am Diet Assoc.* 1994;94(12):1385–1388.

PRACTICE POINT

Measurement of knee height requires positioning of the patient's lower limb at a 90-degree angle (i.e., the ankle and thigh must be flexed to this degree). Using the caliper device, measure the distance from the sole of the foot (under the heel) to the anterior surface of the thigh—above the level of the condyles of the femur and proximal to the patella.

method."[88] Despite its original intention, this method has been cross-validated for use in patients in the acute care setting and for those of other ethnic and age groups (such as older Korean adults and/or patients with immobility).[80,81,87,89] The original predictive equations are outlined in **Table 1.5**. Since its development, variations of the Chumlea equations have been published that allow for its use in a number of populations. Before applying this method, be sure to use the most appropriate equation specific to the individual patient.[89,90]

Total and Half Arm Span Measurements. For those adults who cannot safely stand and are unable to position the lower limb in the angle necessary for measurement of knee height, measurement of arm span can be used as a surrogate marker of standing height at maturity. Depending on the capacity of the patient, one of two measures can be taken:

1. With the patient's arm horizontal and in line with the shoulders, the length between the middle of the sternal notch and tip of the middle finger for each side is measured and then combined; this is called the **total arm span (TAS)**.
2. With one of the patient's arms extended horizontally, measure the extension from the tip of the middle finger to the sternal notch, maintaining the superior limb at a 90-degree angle to the body; this is called the **half arm span** (**HAS**; or arm length).

These measures, which are appropriate for use in adolescents, adults, and the older population, can be accurately obtained whether the patient is standing, sitting, or recumbent.[81,84]

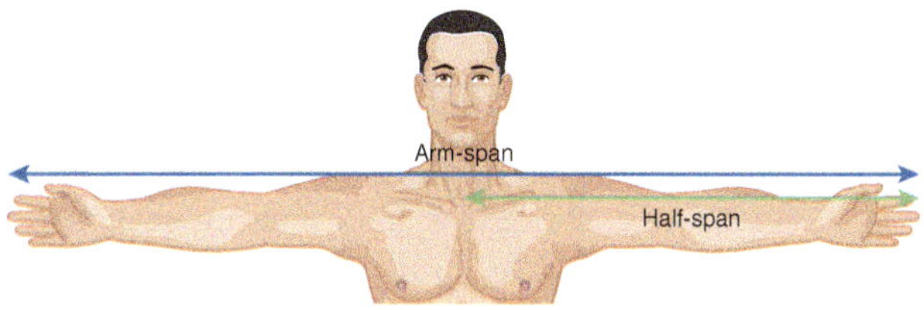

Figure 1.6 Measurement of Armspan

PRACTICE POINT

To achieve the most accurate TAS measurement, both of the patient's arms must be spread in a straight line; the fingertips of each hand must be equidistant from and parallel to the floor. For measuring HAS, only one arm must remain extended horizontally in a 90-degree angle.

Similar to the knee height estimate, the accuracy of an arm length or span measurement is dependent on the use of a predictive equation.[84,85] When TAS is measured, the following predictive equation can be used to estimate standing height[81]:

Females: Standing height (cm)
= [1.35 × total arm span (cm)] + 60.1*
Males: Standing height (cm)
= [1.40 × total arm span (cm)] + 57.8*

HAS (arm length) is recommended by the World Health Organization (WHO) for estimating the height of nonambulatory patients (**Figure 1.6**). The value obtained from this measure can either be multiplied by 2 to provide an estimate of TAS (and then plugged into the TAS predictive equation mentioned above) *or* can be used to estimate stature using the WHO equation[79]:

WHO Equation: Standing height (cm)
= 0.43 + [0.73 × (2 × HAS (cm))]*

*Of note, both the TAS and HAS equations may overestimate height when used in older adults. This occurs because arm measurements tend to give an estimate of maximal height rather than current height, which may change as the aging process progresses.

Overall, practicality is a critical factor in determining the alternate measure of standing height to be used. While some patients may have difficulty raising one or both arms, which would suggest knee height as the most appropriate method, others may be unable to bend the lower limb in the necessary angle and would be better assessed using an arm measurement. Since one surrogate measure is not superior to the other, clinicians are advised to consider all estimates of height and select the most appropriate for the individual circumstance.[78]

PRACTICE POINT

In all cases, when standing height cannot be obtained, the clinician must use the SRH, a surrogate measure, or both. Supine length measurement, which uses a flexible measuring tape to determine the length between the vertex of the head and the heel, has been proven inaccurate and unreliable (and as such should be used as a last resort). Instead, utilize TAS, HAS, or knee height, depending on the individual circumstance.

Assessing Weight

The assessment of **actual body weight** (actual BW) or body cell mass measurement, which represents the unadjusted sum of all body compartments without distinction between fat and fat-free mass, is fundamental to determining nutritional status. From a nutritional standpoint, an individual weight value provides limited information. Ideally, the value will be contextualized using an additional parameter. This may include the identification of individual trends, as in percentage changes from a usual body weight, or relation to other standards, such as ideal body weight. Given that actual BW is representative of muscle, fat, and fluid combined, the true value of the measure is found in its comparison to other criteria in the setting of the whole medical picture. Several conditions, such as those that induce fluid retention, will complicate the assessment of an actual BW.[77,78] The various adjustments to or calculations that involve actual BW measures will be discussed throughout this section.

Weight should be measured upon admission to any acute and chronic care facility and monitored throughout the length of stay. Serial measures are necessary for tracking trends in weight that may relate to nutritional and/or overall clinical status. The most accurate measure of current actual BW is that obtained from actually weighing the patient (**Figure 1.7**) instead of relying upon self-reported values, which tend to be underestimated. For those in the inpatient setting, this often requires the use of bed scales for those unable to transfer to the standing scale.[9,86]

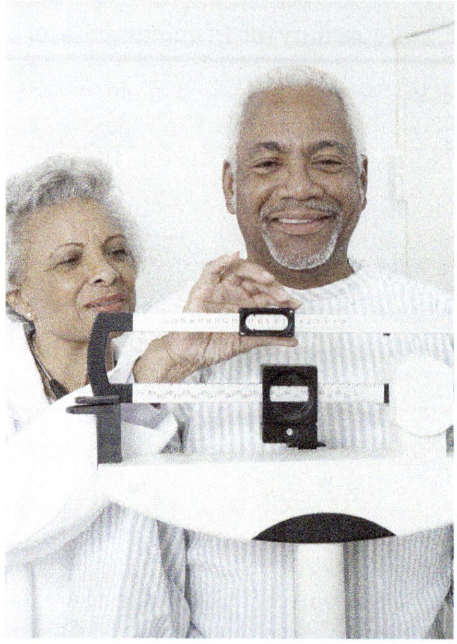

Figure 1.7 Measurement of Weight

PRACTICE POINT

Height and weight should never be visually estimated; an inaccurate weight may compromise application of effective medical nutrition therapy when used to assess energy and protein needs. Instead, employment of one of the surrogate measures to provide the best approximation is recommended.

PRACTICE POINT

Patients who can stand should be weighed on a standing digital or balanced mechanism scale without overgarments or shoes. To obtain an accurate actual BW measure, the patient should first remove all outer garments and empty pockets of loose change and/or keys. The patient will then step onto the digital or balanced mechanism scale with feet together in the center and arms hanging loosely at each side.

PRACTICE POINT

For hospitalized patients, an appropriately calibrated bed scale may be utilized instead of a standing scale. Standardized procedures (i.e., all bedding removed except for the bottom sheet and one pillow, along with any catheter bags, etc.) are often difficult to maintain for patients in acute care.

Usual Body Weight (UBW). In order to identify weight trends, it is necessary to understand a patient's typical weight range to compare to the current actual BW. This value, which can be obtained during the patient interview or estimated using serial measures documented in the medical record, is referred to as **usual body weight (UBW)**. In most cases, the UBW value is a self-reported measure of what the individual has weighed for the majority of their adult life. This is a critical comparison used to determine whether any change in weight has occurred. The deviation is quantified as percent UBW and/or percent weight change.

PRACTICE POINT

The majority of patients can respond appropriately to the question, "What have you weighed for most of your adult life?" It may also be helpful to discuss with family members or refer to documentation from primary care or past hospital admissions. If weight change is evident, always note the time frame in which the deviation from UBW occurred and if the change was intentional versus unintentional.

Percent Usual Body Weight (%UBW) and Percent Weight Change (%Weight Change). Obtaining repeated body weight measurements over time and/or comparing an actual BW measure to UBW are recommended for the identification of weight changes. In the clinical setting, these comparisons are made with specific attention to any losses that occurred unintentionally. Although any unintentional weight loss is concerning, it must be quantified as either **percent usual body weight (%UBW)** or **percent weight change (%weight change)** to be used as a nutrition assessment parameter; %UBW and %weight change can be calculated using the following equations:

$$\%\text{UBW} = (\text{actual body weight/usual body weight}) \times 100\%$$

For example, a male with a UBW of 91 kg is weighed as 85 kg upon admission to the hospital:

$$\%\text{UBW} = (85 \text{ kg}/91 \text{ kg}) \times 100\% = 93.4\% \text{ UBW}$$

$$\%\text{weight change} = (\text{amount of weight lost or gained/usual body weight}) \times 100\%$$

For this same patient, who has lost 6 kg:

$$\%\text{ weight change} = (6 \text{ kg}/91 \text{ kg}) \times 100\% = 6.6\% \text{ weight loss}$$

These values as measures of unintentional weight loss are the best-validated indicators for both the recognition of weight change and malnutrition. The clinical significance of these values can be determined by the degree and duration of weight loss. The time frame in which the loss occurred is necessary for interpretation of the data. For example, a 5% unintentional weight loss over 1 year may not be considered significant, but a 5% weight loss over the course of 1 month certainly would be. One of the key indicators of the AAIM criteria for malnutrition identification is interpretation of %weight loss in the context of the patient's clinical status and a specified length of time (Table 1.2B).[9]

As with any nutrition-related parameter, the interpretation of weight loss must also be considered in the context of the overall clinical picture. Weight changes often reflect more than just nutritional status. Loss may be an indication of the severity of underlying disease or inflammatory condition or may be a natural and intended effect of ongoing treatment, such as fluid removal via diuresis or dialysis. Gains could represent the intended outcome of a nutrition support intervention or could reflect a positive fluid status or an inaccurate weight measurement. Thinking about weight changes beyond simple increases and decreases is important beyond the assessment period when later determining the appropriate intervention.

Ideal Body Weight (IBW). In the clinical setting and beyond, comparisons of weight-to-height measures are the most commonly used anthropometric parameters. **Ideal body weight (IBW)** is a metric derived from historical data that examined the weight-for-height that correlated with the lowest risk of mortality. While the term "ideal" may be uncomfortable in modern clinical settings, it is important to remember that this term refers to reducing disease risk rather than to appearance or social pressures. For example, IBW can be useful when assessing the energy needs of a patient with obesity requiring nutrition support, as it allows for adequate nourishment of lean body mass and prevents overfeeding, which is associated with negative outcomes.[49] This is the same reason why IBW is used for medication dosing by clinicians in cases of severe obesity. It is important to recognize how the different anthropometric parameters can be applied within the nutrition care process.[91]

There are a number of ways to determine IBW, including height–weight tables such as the Metropolitan Life Ideal Weights Tables (1943 and 1983, based

Table 1.6 Summation of Ideal Body Weight Equations for Males and Females

Source	Equation
Rao and Balakrishna[196]	IBW (kg) = height (cm) − 100
Hamwi[197,*]	IBW (females) = 100 lb + 5 lb/inch over 5 feet IBW (males) = 106 lb + 6 lb/inch over 5 feet
Devine[198]	IBW (females) = 45.5 kg + 2.3 kg/inch over 5 feet IBW (males) = 50 kg + 2.3 kg/inch over 5 feet
Robinson et al.[199]	IBW (females) = 49 kg + 1.7 kg/inch over 5 feet IBW (males) = 52 kg + 1.9 kg/inch over 5 feet
Miller et al.[200,†]	IBW (females) = 53 kg + 1.33 kg/inch over 5 feet IBW (males) = 55.7 kg + 1.39 kg/inch over 5 feet
Hammond[201,*]	IBW (females) = 45 kg for 150 cm + 0.9 kg/cm IBW (males) = 48 kg for 150 cm + 1.1 kg/cm
Peterson et al.[202]	IBW (kg) = 2.2 × BMI + 3.5 × BMI (Height (m) − 1.5 m)

* *For Hamwi and Hammond methods, the calculated weight may be subtracted by 10% to account for a small frame or increased by 10% for a large frame.*

† *The Miller et al. formula is calculated for a medium frame.*

Data from Shah B, Sucher K, Hollenbeck CB. Comparison of ideal body weight equations and published height-weight tables with body mass index tables for healthy adults in the United States. *Nutr Clin Pract. 2006;21*(3):312-319.; Peterson CM, Thomas DM, Blackburn GL, Heymsfield SB. Universal equation for estimating ideal body weight and body weight at any BMI. *Am J Clin Nutr. 2016;103*(5):1197-1203.

on data obtained from policy holders between the ages of 25 and 59 years and later from NHANES), and predictive equations such as the Hamwi method and others (**Table 1.6**). There is controversy as to which provides the most appropriate or accurate calculation, although an equation is often selected for ease of use.[12,77] The Hamwi method is often described as the most appropriate measure for use in the clinical setting.[77,92–94]

IBW can also be determined using an equation based on the BMI that is associated with the lowest morbidity (22 kg/m^2, the middle value within the normal range). Estimates made using BMI (i.e., 22 kg/m^2 × height in m^2) are comparable to what is determined from other predictive equations and are desirable in the clinical setting due to the simplicity of the calculation.[77]

Percent of Ideal Body Weight. Similar to the use of %UBW as an indicator of weight status, **percent ideal body weight (%IBW)** can be used to compare current actual BW to the IBW value specific to the patient's height as a further metric to assess weight status.

$$\%\text{IBW} = (\text{actual body weight/ideal body weight}) \times 100\%$$

For example, a male who measures as 183 cm (72 in) tall would have an IBW of 81 kg (178 lb) based on the Hamwi method. If this patient actually weighs 97 kg (213 lb), %IBW is calculated as:

$$\begin{aligned}\%\text{IBW} &= (97\text{ kg}/81\text{ kg}) \times 100\% \\ &= 120\%\text{ IBW}\end{aligned}$$

Because IBW was standardized using healthy adult populations, %IBW should never be used as the sole basis for determination of nutritional status. Percent IBW is used much less frequently in the clinical setting when compared to the use of %UBW.

Adjusted Body Weight (Adjusted BW). In addition to assessing body weight as a measure of nutritional status, weight is an important component in the determination of energy expenditure. Body weight at the extremes (i.e., underweight or obese) complicates this calculation by resulting in a possible underestimation or overestimation of needs. Although this practice is significantly less common, utilizing **adjusted body weight** (adjusted BW) was previously a common method of preventing under- or overfeeding. Adjusted BW can be calculated for those with an actual BW greater than 115% of the calculated IBW.[95–97]

$$\text{Adjusted BW} = [(\text{actual body weight} - \text{ideal body weight}) \times 0.25] + \text{IBW}^{97}$$

For example, consider a female 170 cm (67 in) tall with an IBW of 61 kg (135 lb; per Hamwi method) and an actual BW of 95.5 kg (210 lb):

$$\text{Adjusted BW} = [(95.5\text{ kg} - 61\text{ kg}) \times 0.25] + 61\text{ kg} = 70\text{ kg}$$

Use of adjusted BW was first recommended to account for the percentage of excess weight that is most metabolically active (i.e., lean mass) instead of feeding based on actual BW. The underlying rationale is that subcutaneous fat is significantly less metabolically active than lean tissue and thus using actual BW to calculate needs will result in overprediction. It is important to note that adjusted BW, although sometimes used in practice, is *not* an evidence-based assessment. Recent studies have illustrated that utilizing adjusted BW actually results in a vast underestimation of energy needs. ASPEN and AND both urge against the use of adjusted BW despite its previous longstanding use in the clinical setting, recommending instead the use of actual BW and IBW based on the severity of obesity. It is also important for clinicians to adjust caloric provision based on clinical outcomes, as needed.[49,96,98]

Body Weight Modifications for Special Circumstance. As previously mentioned, body weight must always be considered in the setting of the overall clinical picture. There are two notable (and common) conditions that require special assessment of body weight measures: amputations and chronic fluid retention.

For those with extremity amputation(s), special weight adjustments are necessary in order to account for the body compartment that has been lost. An adjusted BW is calculated based on an estimate of the proportion of total body weight that the lost body segment represents.[99–101]

For many hospitalized patients, including those with liver disease, kidney failure, or malignancy, fluid overload precludes the use of actual BW. Increases in weight will often reflect overhydration, edema, ascites, or dialysate in the abdomen, instead of providing an accurate picture of actual body compartments. An estimate of **dry weight** is used to represent an individual's actual BW without the excess fluid. For those with chronic and fluctuating retention, dry weight may be estimated based on the UBW of the patient prior to onset of fluid retention *or* based on other clinical parameters, like the achievement of normotensive blood pressure.[12,102]

Calculating Body Mass Index (BMI)

The Quetelet's Index, better known as **body mass index (BMI)**, is the most common anthropometric comparison of body weight to body height independent of frame size. Defined by the equation weight (kg)/(height [m])^2, BMI offers a simple measure of body composition that can be interpreted (with caution) as an indirect measure of fat mass. The BMI classifications for interpretation of the adult patient population are outlined in **Table 1.7**, although all clinicians should be aware of the many caveats associated with this measure. Although sex, body type, and ethnicity influence BMI results, these factors are neither taken into account nor reflected in the measure. For example, BMI will often overestimate body fat for the muscular athlete and underestimate fat stores in the aging adult. As with any method of nutrition assessment, interpretation of the measure should be made in the context of the individual situation, and BMI should not be used as a sole metric of weight status.[103]

Table 1.7 Body Mass Index (BMI) Categories

BMI (kg/m^2)	Classification
<18.5	Underweight
18.5–24.9	Normal
25.0–29.9	Overweight
30.0–34.9	Class 1 Obesity
35.0–39.9	Class 2 Obesity
>40.0	Class 3 or Severe Obesity

Data from National Heart, Lung, and Blood Institute. *Classification of overweight and obesity by BMI, waist circumference, and associated disease risks.* National Heart, Lung, and Blood Institute. Accessed January 22, 2025. https://www.nhlbi.nih.gov/health/educational/lose_wt/BMI/bmi_dis.htm

Despite the known limitations of BMI, it remains widely used due to both its efficiency and its relatively high correlation with estimates of body fat mass.[78] Although malnutrition can occur in individuals of any BMI, measures at either extreme represent an increased likelihood of poor nutritional status and are associated with increased risk of mortality. This phenomenon is represented by a J-shaped relationship between mortality and BMI. Relative to normal weight, BMI values categorized as overweight or obese are associated with increased risk of cardiovascular disease and some cancers, while measures representing the underweight classification are associated with increased postsurgical complications, infection rates, and length of hospital stay.[9,78,103,104]

PRACTICE POINT

Use caution when applying BMI to patients with amputations.

PRACTICE POINT

Interpretation of BMI should involve consideration of age, sex, body type, and common confounders of body weight in the clinical setting, such as edema or ascites. BMI should be considered in the context of other metrics, nutrition-focused physical exam findings, and information from the client history.

Body Composition Measures

Classic anthropometric measurements, such as height, weight, and BMI, are extremely useful in the clinical setting but are unable to accurately represent body composition. As understanding of body composition and its impact on health risk and clinical outcome increases, so does the importance of obtaining its accurate measure. Clinicians turn to skinfold anthropometry and circumference measures for the most feasible representation of an individual's fat and muscle stores.[78] See Chapter 3, *Energy Expenditure and Body Composition in Health and Disease*, for more information on determining body composition.

Skinfold Anthropometry. **Skinfold anthropometry**, often referred to as "skinfold thickness," involves the measure of one or more anatomical sites using a skinfold caliper device to estimate body fat stores. The measures of skinfold thickness are representative of subcutaneous fat stores in the triceps, biceps, subscapular, and suprailiac regions (**Figure 1.8**). This measure is the most widely used method of indirectly estimating body fat percentage and, when used in an additional calculation, can provide an approximation of muscle mass.[78,105] Note that ethnic differences in adiposity based on skinfolds have been reported. In the United States, White males have been noted to have greater subcutaneous fat compared to Black males.[106] Such differences should be considered when interpreting results.

PRACTICE POINT

A "skinfold" measure represents the subcutaneous fat layer. Clinicians should take caution to avoid including the underlying muscle in this measure. Anatomic sites often used in this context are the biceps, triceps, subscapular, and suprailiac regions.

The procedure itself requires noncomplex portable equipment and can be applied to most clinical and public health settings. A variety of calipers—ranging from precision-engineered to plastic and disposable—are available for use. Validity of skinfold thickness depends less on the caliper used and more on the measurement technique and repetition over time. As with any anthropometric measure, differences in equipment can account for differences in measures. When used for serial measurements of the same individual, the same caliper tool should be used for each measure to best represent any changes (or lack thereof) in body composition.[78,107]

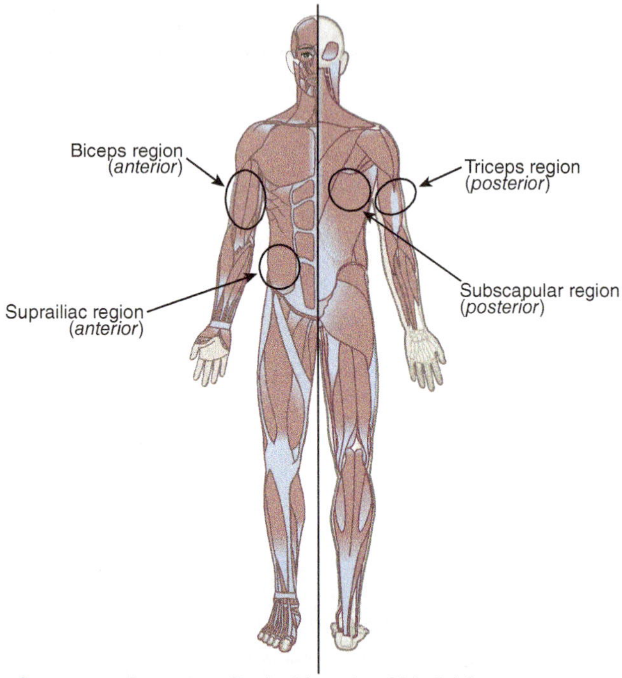

Figure 1.8 Common Body Sites for Skinfold Anthropometry

There are a variety of formulas to calculate body fat percentage using skinfold measurements. Consideration of age, sex, ethnicity, and physical condition (sedentary individual or athlete) is important in determining the appropriate formula.[108] There are also variations in the number and location of sites to assess with formulas that assess fewer (3–4) or more (7+) sites, in which the locations can vary by sex.[108–110] A reduced number of sites measured allows for a quicker evaluation but may reduce accuracy in determining body fat percentage due to variation in body fat distribution. Validation between 3 site measures and 7 site measures has shown variable accuracy in certain populations.[111–113]

PRACTICE POINT

Follow the procedures that accompany the skinfold caliper for the most accurate instructions on use. In general, at the given site, a lengthwise skinfold should be grasped and slightly lifted between the index and thumb of the hand (without including underlying muscle). The caliper is applied approximately 1 cm below the finger grasping the skinfold. All measurements should be repeated three times and averaged for the final value.

PRACTICE POINT

Accuracy of the skinfold measure decreases with increasing obesity. This technique is more useful in lean individuals (i.e., those with smaller fat stores) because skinfold caliper devices are unable to assess intra-abdominal adipose tissue.

Triceps Skinfold. For clinicians in the inpatient and outpatient settings, **triceps skinfold (TSF)** is the most common skinfold measure used for nutritional assessment. As with any other anatomic location mentioned above, TSF measures the amount of subcutaneous body fat, which represents ~50% of total body fat stores. TSF is the site found to be most reflective of actual body fatness when performed with strict adherence to measurement protocols by a trained professional. This site is not only the most convenient and accessible, but can be accurately measured in the supine position for patients unable to sit or stand (**Figure 1.9**).[78,107,114,115]

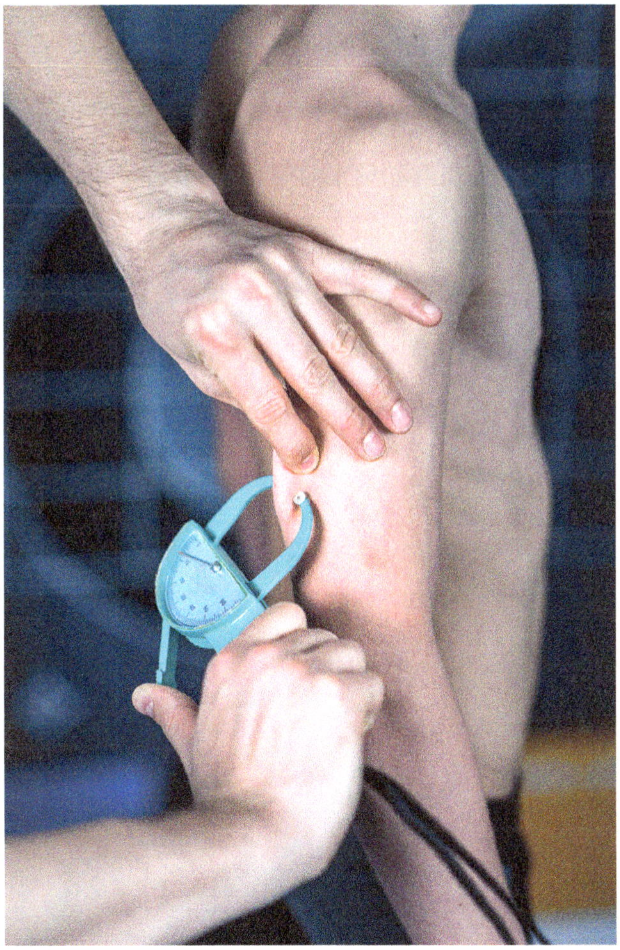

Figure 1.9 Measurement of Triceps Skinfold

PRACTICE POINT

Triceps skin fold measurements are taken using skinfold calipers on the nondominant arm of the individual, midway between the olecranon process and the acromion process (i.e., midway between the shoulder and the elbow). This measure may be difficult to implement in the critically ill if, for example, impeded by wound dressings or edema.

TSF measurements are interpreted in one of two ways: the measure can be compared against population standards due to abundant reference table availability that can vary by age, country, and ethnicity, or (preferably) by using serial measurements to assess change in the individual. Serial measures allow for estimates of body fat store changes and are more useful for assessment purposes than population comparisons. Depletion of this compartment can reflect chronic inadequate intake or nutrient depletion, which would be a critical consideration in determining future interventions. As with any other measure of assessment, TSF will be impacted by fluid retention; if edema is present, TSF measures cannot be considered reliable.[78,107]

Circumference Measurements. Depending on the anatomic location where the value is obtained, circumference measurements are used to measure skeletal muscle and/or fat mass. For example, mid-upper arm circumference can be used as an index of skeletal muscle mass (particularly when compared to other measures, like the TSF), whereas waist circumference provides a measure of central adiposity that is a significant marker of metabolic and cardiovascular risk.[107,116]

Mid-Upper Arm Circumference (MUAC). **Mid-upper arm circumference (MUAC)** is a measure of total arm circumference and provides a measure of both muscle and fat area (**Figure 1.10**). Measures of limb circumference, such as the MUAC, are used as indicators of nutrition status; in other words, MUAC is most often used to estimate malnutrition risk. MUAC is one of the indicators of pediatric malnutrition per the AAIM criteria.[117] The measure is simple, noninvasive, and feasible (even in patients who are acutely ill) because it can be completed in the supine position (if necessary) using only a tape measure. MUAC becomes particularly useful when height and weight measurements are inappropriate or impossible to obtain on a consistent basis.[1,118–120]

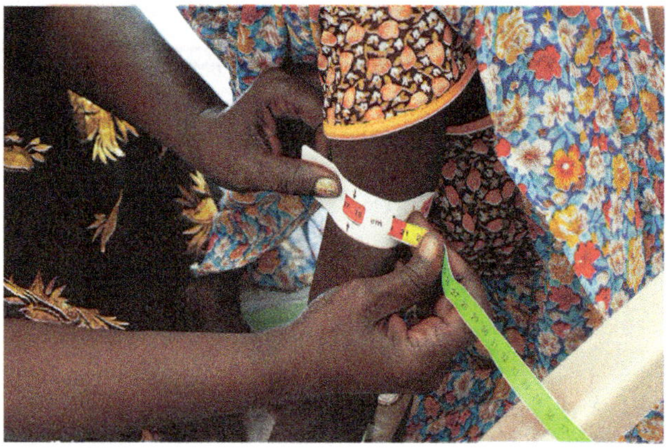

Figure 1.10 Measurement of Mid-Upper Arm Circumference

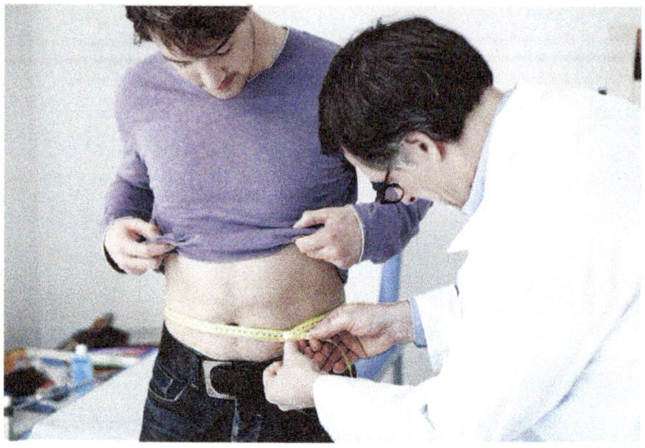

Figure 1.11 Measurement of Waist Circumference

PRACTICE POINT

To measure MUAC, a nonstretch tape measure is used at the midpoint between the acromion and olecranon processes.

For those who are critically ill and unable to assume the supine position for other anthropometric measures, MUAC provides an alternative index of nutritional status that is accurate and comparable to BMI.[107,121–123] MUAC can be used to calculate an estimate of an individual's BMI through a predictive equation; in general, MUAC measures of <25 cm for males and <24 cm for females will correlate with a BMI <20 kg/m^2, providing a substitute measure of potential adult undernutrition. Similarly, if a serial measure of MUAC changes by >10%, it can be assumed that the BMI has also changed by >10%. This solidifies the applicability of MUAC in identifying chronic energy deficiency and as a predictor of mortality.[120,124–126]

Predicting BMI with MUAC:

$$\text{Males: BMI (kg/m}^2) = 1.01 \times \text{MUAC (cm)} - 4.7$$

$$\text{Females: BMI (kg/m}^2) = 1.10 \times \text{MUAC (cm)} - 6.7$$

MUAC can be used in combination with a TSF measure to calculate **mid-arm muscle circumference (MAMC)**, a surrogate measure of lean body mass. MAMC cannot be measured directly by anthropometry but is instead obtained from the predictive equation:

$$\text{MAMC (cm)} = \text{MUAC (cm)} - [\text{TSF (mm)} \times 0.3142]$$

The value obtained provides an indication of muscle mass. Note that the equation provided will include the bone as well as the muscle; this should be considered in the assessment. MAMC equations that correct for bone are available, although these are not routinely used due to inherent issues with adjusting for bone size. Similar to other measures of body composition, interpretation of MAMC requires either comparison to reference standards specific to age, sex, and ethnicity or in the context of changes in serial measures. In general, lower MAMC values (MAMC <90% the reference value for the specific individual)[127] are associated with adverse outcomes including increased risk of mortality.[12,78,107]

Waist Circumference (WC). In contrast to limb circumference measures like the MUAC, **waist circumference (WC)** is utilized as an assessment of excess abdominal fat. This measure provides an indication of central adiposity, which can be interpreted in terms of obesity-related health risk, that is easily obtainable in the general population.[78,116] WC is more strongly associated with visceral adipose tissue and thus cardiometabolic risk than any other anthropometric measure.[128–131]

Several different anatomical sites can be used for measuring waist circumference. Four measurement sites are common, including the WHO's recommendation[132] for measuring the midpoint between the iliac crest and costal margin of the lowest rib (WC-mid) and the National Institutes of Health's (NIH) recommendation[133] for measuring in the horizontal plane of the superior border of the iliac crest (WC-IC). Other cited locations include the level of the umbilicus and the minimal waist, regardless of where on the abdomen it occurs. Studies indicate that a WC measured mid-abdominally (WC-mid) is the most accurate measure available for defining central obesity (**Figure 1.11**).[134] Because the various sites will yield drastic differences in interpretation of the measure,

Clinical Controversy

Is BMI a reliable indicator of cardiometabolic risk across various racial and ethnic groups?
Obesity as measured by BMI is associated with increased cardiometabolic risk, such as increased risk of cardiovascular disease and type 2 diabetes mellitus. BMI is an imperfect tool; it is limited in its ability to differentiate body composition or body fat distribution. The applicability of BMI as a disease risk indicator across different racial and ethnic groups has been more closely examined. In a study of a cardiometabolic risk phenotype described as "metabolic abnormality but normal weight" (MAN), Gujral et al. conducted a cross-sectional analysis of two community-based normal-weight cohorts to evaluate the prevalence of MAN in five racial/ethnic groups. BMI classification cutoffs can be noted in Table 1.7. BMI for South Asian and Chinese American participants was classified according to the WHO Asian cutoff points: normal weight BMI 18.5–22.9 kg/m^2; overweight BMI 23.0–24.7 kg/m^2; obese BMI ≥27.5 kg/m^2. The authors found that people with Indian and other South Asian ancestry had more than double the prevalence of MAN, followed by Hispanic Americans, Chinese Americans, and African Americans, who had greater prevalence of MAN compared to White people. It was estimated that the BMI values at which the expected equivalent numbers of metabolic abnormalities would equal those among White people at an overweight BMI of 25 kg/m^2, after adjusting for age, sex, and race–BMI interactions, were as follows:

1. >22.9 kg/m^2 for African Americans
2. 21.5 kg/m^2 for Hispanic Americans
3. 20.9 kg/m^2 for Chinese Americans
4. 19.6 kg/m^2 for South Asian Americans

These findings suggest that standard BMI categories may not be a useful screen for cardiometabolic risk in the non-White population.

Questions

1. How might BMI confound cardiometabolic screening in racial/ethnic minority groups?
2. What metabolic differences could be hypothesized to account for some of these risk variations?
3. How might these findings influence a clinician's ability to utilize BMI classification of overweight and obesity to identify cardiometabolic risk in a racially and ethnically diverse population?

References

1. Gujral UP, Vittinghoff E, Mongraw-Chafflin M, et al. Cardiometabolic abnormalities among normal-weight persons from five racial/ethnic groups in the United States: a cross-sectional analysis of two cohort studies. *Ann Intern Med.* 2017;166:628–636.
2. WHO Expert Consultation. Appropriate body-mass index for Asian populations and its implications for policy and intervention strategies. *Lancet.* 2004;363:157–163.

the clinician must be sure to document the location utilized to obtain accurate serial changes in the long term.[78,116,128,135]

PRACTICE POINT

Waist circumference is measured using a nonstretch tape placed directly on the skin, midway between the iliac crest and costal margin of the lowest rib at end expiration.

Abdominal obesity is associated with significantly greater health risks than fat deposited below the abdomen. For those with an android ("apple") body shape, a WC >102 cm (40 in) for males and >88 cm (34 in) for females has been illustrated to be an independent risk factor for type 2 diabetes mellitus, hypertension, and cardiovascular disease, even for individuals who are of normal weight by BMI standards. This risk has not been demonstrated for those with a gynoid ("pear") shape, indicating fat deposits below the waist (**Figure 1.12**).[78,132,133,136,137] The International Atherosclerosis Society (IAS) and the International Chair on Cardiometabolic Risk (ICCR) have proposed in their consensus statement that measuring

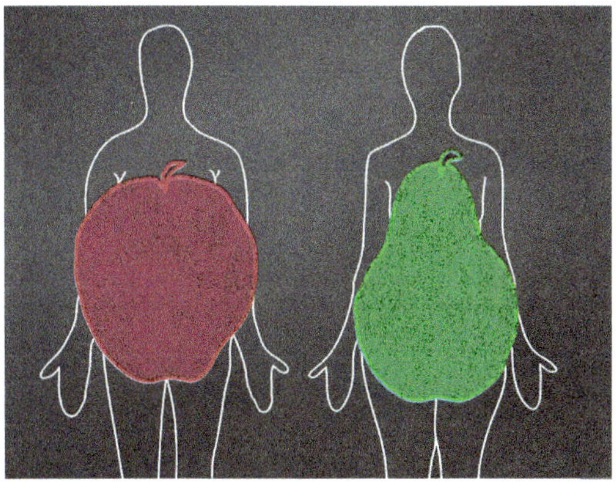

Figure 1.12 Android ("apple") versus Gynoid ("pear") Body Shapes

WC is an important "vital sign" in clinical practice and encourage its regular usage in the management of cardiometabolic risk.[138] The measurement of WC has evolved into a key diagnostic criterion for metabolic syndrome; according to the U.S. National Cholesterol Education Program and the International Diabetes Federation, the aforementioned sex-specific thresholds (>102 cm for males and >88 cm for females) are practical indicators of elevated risk.[133,135] However, additional thresholds exist stratified by BMI category as well as ethnicity.[138]

Hip Circumference. Similar to waist circumference, hip circumference will also provide an indication of adiposity, although its value in predicting disease risk and/or mortality is of significantly less importance. Although some studies indicate a significant and inverse relationship between hip circumference and cardiometabolic disease risk, this protective effect is not present in all ethnicities. Instead of using a direct measure of hip circumference as a marker of nutritional status, this value is typically interpreted as part of a **waist-hip ratio (WHR)**. WHR, the waist circumference value divided by the hip circumference value, provides an additional measure of body fat distribution as an index of both subcutaneous and intra-abdominal adipose tissue. WHR has been found to be a better tool than BMI for predicting chronic health problems. A higher WHR has been linked more strongly and consistently with increased mortality from any cause than BMI. In general, a WHR value ≥0.90 in males and ≥0.85 in females is associated with increased risk of cardiometabolic complications, although ethnic-specific cutoffs exist. While these cutoffs are not well researched, they may provide a general guideline for assessing different patient populations (examples of those acceptable for use are outlined in **Table 1.8**).[78,129,132,139–141]

Table 1.8 Suggested Waist-Hip Ratio Ethnic Cutoffs for Central Obesity

Ethnicity	Male	Female
Asian	>0.90	>0.80
African American	>0.90	>0.85
European	>0.90	>0.85
Hispanic	>0.90	>0.85
Middle Eastern	>0.90	>0.85

Data from Lear SA, James PT, Ko GT, Kumanyika S. Appropriateness of waist circumference and waist-to-hip ratio cutoffs for different ethnic groups. *Eur J Clin Nutr.* 2010;64:42–61.

PRACTICE POINT

When measuring hip circumference, the measuring tape should be positioned at the widest part over the buttocks and below the iliac crest. The subject should be asked not to contract their gluteal muscles before the measurement is taken.

Calf Circumference. Calf circumference (CC) is a practical and inexpensive marker that provides information about muscle mass. Low CC is a marker of low skeletal mass and may be confounded, as with other circumferences, by edema or obesity. Obesity confounding has been addressed through the development of a BMI adjustment factor developed by the NHANES general U.S. cohort.[142] CC is correlated with muscle strength, physical performance,[143] readmission rate,[144] and mortality risk.[145,146] If upper extremity edema precludes MUAC evaluation, CC may be considered as an alternate site to assess. Similarly, if lower extremity edema exists, MUAC may be checked instead of CC. CC <33 cm for males and <32 cm for females is considered a threshold for reduced muscle mass.[147]

PRACTICE POINT

When measuring calf circumference, a nonstretch measuring tape should be positioned at the widest part over the calf laying the tape on the skin without tightening. The measurement can be taken in the standing, seated, or supine position.

Imaging Technologies. Imaging techniques represent the most precise and reliable assessments of muscle mass when determining body composition. The most common methodologies—computerized tomography, magnetic resonance imaging, bioelectrical impedance analysis, dual-energy x-ray absorptiometry, and ultrasound—will be discussed briefly in this section. These technologies have gained greater interest since the introduction of the GLIM criteria to diagnose malnutrition that includes reduced muscle mass as a phenotypic criterion.[11]

Computed Tomography (CT). A **computed tomography (CT)** scan utilizes x-ray technology to provide quantitative data on muscle composition and distribution (**Figure 1.13**). CT scans are valuable due to the ability to measure fat and muscle content within a single abdominal cross-sectional slice; thereafter, the images obtained can be used to distinguish between fat mass, fat-free mass, and skeletal muscle, and even further between visceral and subcutaneous fat.

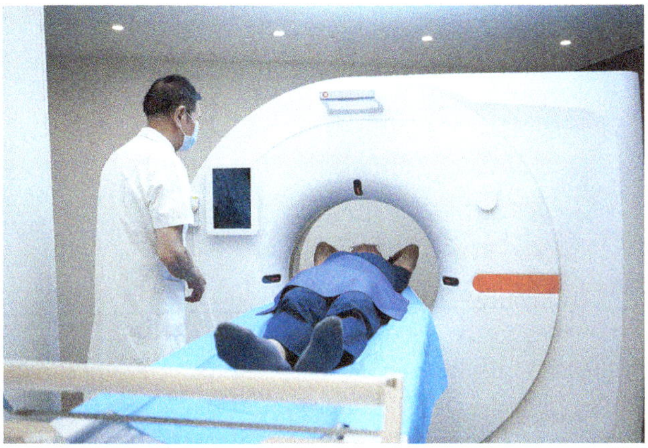

Figure 1.13 Computed Tomography Machine

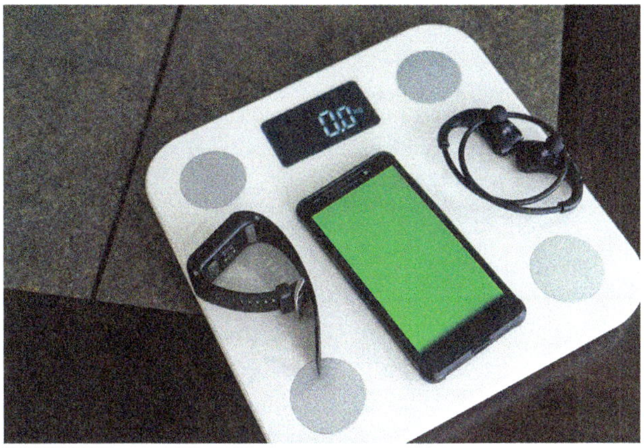

Figure 1.14 Bioelectrical Impedance Machine

The CT scan will provide an accurate quantification of whole-body composition. Although this technique may be routinely used for diagnosis and evaluation of several medical conditions, its application for nutrition assessment in the clinical setting is limited. CT scans are *not* recommended for the sole purpose of determining body composition due to expense and radiation exposure; however, CT scans are used frequently in certain conditions such as cancer and critical illness. Automated analysis software applications exist that may facilitate muscle assessment of available CT images.[147–149]

Magnetic Resonance Imaging (MRI). Body composition analysis can also be accomplished using **magnetic resonance imaging (MRI)**, utilizing what is referred to as a "free-ionizing radiation technique." Following either a whole-body or regional scan, an MRI will illustrate adipose tissue and lean mass (including skeletal muscle) distribution. Although widely used in research, the utility of MRI for assessing body composition in the clinical setting is limited due to long scan duration and extreme expense.[150]

Bioelectrical Impedance Analysis (BIA). Of the available technologies, **bioelectrical impedance analysis (BIA)** is perhaps the most widely used for body composition estimation. By measuring the resistance of a high-frequency, low-amplitude electrical current passed through the body, BIA allows for the distinction between fat-free mass (through determination of total body water) and fat mass. The scientific basis for this two-compartment model is based on conductivity of an electrical current, which is greater in compartments rich in fluid and electrolytes such as the fat-free mass. Conversely, bone and fat have poor conductivity and greater resistance to the electrical signal. Through conductivity and resistance, fat and fat-free mass can be differentiated. These values can be converted into body fat percentages using a variety of available regression equations. Within the realm of body composition analysis, this method can also be used to assess hydration status. BIA can only be applied to those without significant fluid or electrolyte abnormalities; in addition, a valid BIA equation appropriate to age, sex, and race must be available for the specific patient. When compared to other methods, BIA is attractive due to its relative simplicity, low cost, and portability (**Figure 1.14**). Previous research also suggests that changes in body composition as measured by BIA correlate directly with levels of energy and protein intake.[151] BIA cannot be recommended for use in the acutely ill patient population, for subjects at either BMI extreme, or for those with an abnormal hydration status (including kidney disturbances).[12,151–157]

Dual Energy X-ray Absorptiometry (DXA). Developed originally for the measurement of bone density and bone mass, **dual energy x-ray absorptiometry (DXA)** has quickly become a reference method for body composition assessment. Due to technological advancements, DXA can now be used to quantify soft-tissue composition, thus introducing the possibility for measuring total and regional body composition. The DXA scan divides the body into three compartments: bone, lean body mass, and fat mass. This method relies on the attenuation characteristics of tissues exposed to low levels of radiation at two peak energies, which are then converted into body assessment percentages using a number of available equations. Although DXA is not widely used in clinical practice for the assessment of body composition, DXA remains the method of choice for measuring bone mineral density, which, if available, may be an important consideration in a complete nutrition assessment. It is important to note that skeletal muscle

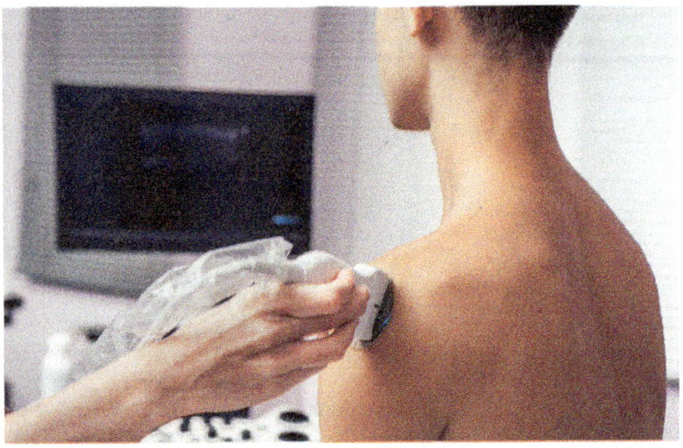

Figure 1.15 Ultrasound

is not measured directly but estimated from soft tissue. Other considerations include that the equipment is not mobile, may have height and weight restrictions, requires operation by a licensed technician, and may be associated with a high cost.[12,142,143,147,150,157,158]

Ultrasonography (US). Ultrasonography or **ultrasound (US)** (**Figure 1.15**) is a noninvasive, portable, widely available imaging technique that can estimate adipose tissue and muscle thickness. Advantages of US include lower cost, lack of radiation exposure, ability to assess various sites, and ability to provide repeated measurements on a patient. Limitations include the need for trained personnel, interoperator reproducibility, and lack of standardized techniques.[147,158,159]

Since access to these technologies may not be globally available, nutrition-focused physical examination and the use of MUAC and/or CC measurements are possible alternatives as a means to identify low muscle mass.[11]

PRACTICE POINT

Imaging techniques are gaining traction in the clinical setting for muscle mass assessment.

CORE CONCEPT 6

Loss of muscle mass can be assessed via nutrition-focused physical exam, skin anthropometry (mid-upper arm circumference or calf circumference), and/or imaging technologies.

Biochemical Data, Medical Tests, and Procedures

A number of critical biochemical values are important to consider as part of a complete nutrition assessment. Note that a variety of other tests and procedures, including gastric emptying time, may also fall into this category of assessment. Please refer to Chapter 2 *Biochemical Assessment* for information on biochemical assessment and its application to nutritional status.

Client History

A patient's nutritional status must be considered in the context of the overall clinical status. For that reason, a thorough nutrition assessment should always include an evaluation of client history, which includes personal as well as familial past medical history (PMH).

Nutrition-Focused Past Medical History

The relevance of the clinical picture to nutrition assessment cannot be overstated. Knowledge of an individual's medical and/or surgical history and current disease state(s) are particularly helpful in identifying a nutritional concern. Begin with an overview of the clinical diagnosis and its accompanying symptoms, particularly those that may affect intake. Note that any ongoing complaints or relevant PMH may represent a significant metabolic stressor or provide etiology behind poor appetite, decreased oral intake, or weight loss, all of which can indicate risk of malnutrition.[9] As a general guideline, a nutrition-focused PMH may include the following factors[6]:

- Personal demographic data: age, gender, sex, race, ethnicity, education level, literacy, physical ability differences
- Personal PMH: surgical history, previous acute or chronic illnesses, current or past treatments, prior need for enteral or parenteral nutrition support
- Family PMH: note the presence of any familial or genetic disorder that may impact nutritional status (cardiovascular disease, diabetes mellitus, cancer, etc.)
- Social history: socioeconomic status, occupation, social and medical support, relevant cultural and religious beliefs, daily stress level, living situation, food and housing insecurity, transportation, and any barriers to access food
- Chief complaint: a subjective statement of the problem, including onset and duration
- History of present illness (HPI): note all nutritionally relevant data, including recent diet and/or weight changes, UBW, appetite changes, gastrointestinal symptoms (nausea, vomiting, diarrhea, and/or constipation), abdominal pain, etc.

CASE STUDY REVISITED

As you continue your interview, you learn that Marie used to work as a schoolteacher prior to seeking asylum in the United States. She lives in an apartment with her son, but he works long hours, and she is often alone. She was widowed 6 months ago. Her neighborhood has one corner store that sells canned and packaged food and beverages, but the grocery store is a long walk from Marie's apartment, and she does not have a car. She reports worrying about affording food before the next paycheck.

Questions

1. How might Marie's social history impact her nutritional status?
2. What other questions might you pose to Marie to better assess barriers to her food security?

In general, note any chronic disease state, episode of acute or critical illness, and/or surgical procedure that may affect the nutritional status of the patient. Any number of conditions may increase the likelihood that the individual is malnourished. This may take the form of significantly increased metabolic demand, decreased appetite, compromised ability to ingest food by mouth (PO), and/or impaired nutrient absorption.[9,16]

PRACTICE POINT

A number of conditions, injuries, and/or complications cause significant metabolic demands.

Nutrition-Focused Physical Exam Findings

A **nutrition-focused physical exam (NFPE)** is an instrumental and informative component of nutrition assessment. The NFPE is a system-based examination of each region of the body that aids in the evaluation of nutrition status by identifying markers of malnutrition and/or nutrient deficiencies. The goal is to identify whether the fat, muscle, fluid, and/or micronutrient status of a patient has diminished due to inflammation, chronic disease, and/or poor nutrient intake. Because physical signs tend to be nonspecific, any findings should be considered in the context of other clinical parameters (including biomarkers) and the patient interview. Although the NFPE is only one component of a comprehensive nutrition assessment, it can provide the necessary supportive data to identify and/or diagnose malnutrition.[75,160–163]

Four out of the six necessary components of the AAIM criteria[9] include an evaluation of muscle and fat stores as part of the NFPE. In addition, the NFPE is included as part of the Standards of Practice for dietitians working in both adult and pediatric populations. If the NFPE is not performed, the nutrition assessment is incomplete.[162,163] In an AND/ASPEN multisite cohort study, RDs succeeded in completing all or most of an NFPE for a high proportion (>80%) of hospitalized adult and pediatric patients.[164]

Techniques of the NFPE

The NFPE is performed following the review of the PMH and any pertinent laboratory data using one or more of four techniques: inspection, palpation, percussion, and auscultation. The bulk of the examination employs the technique of **inspection**, which involves the visual observation of color, shape, texture, and size. **Palpation** is used to evaluate and assess texture, size, temperature, tenderness, and mobility; here, the tips and pads of the fingers should be used to assess pulsations and areas of sensitivity, whereas the back of the hand is used to assess temperature. **Percussion** describes the tapping of fingers against body surfaces for sounds that reflect solids, fluids, or gas (e.g., tympany can denote ascites). This technique provides minimal nutrition information but is important for abdominal assessment. **Auscultation** involves the assessment of sounds that reflect movement of fluid or air through organs and viscera using a stethoscope.[75,165]

PRACTICE POINT

The examination techniques most commonly used for identifying malnutrition as part of the NFPE include observation and palpation.

Using these techniques, the physical examination should begin with observation (i.e., inspection) of the general appearance of the patient, including

CASE STUDY REVISITED

As you continue your interview, you complete a nutrition-focused physical examination on Marie. Your findings are as follows:

Marie is alert but appears tired. Her hair is thin, dry, and easily plucked. Her face is notable for dark circles under both eyes, narrow facial appearance, and temporal muscle depression. Her eyes appear normal. Marie's oral exam is notable for dry oral mucosa and angular stomatitis. She has good dentition with no missing teeth and a normal tongue. She has evident clavicular muscle wasting. Her biceps reveal severe muscle wasting and triceps demonstrate moderate subcutaneous fat loss with loose and slightly hanging arm skin. Rib fat loss is evident. Marie's skin is dry with poor skin turgor. No wounds are evident. Abdominal exam is unremarkable. No lower extremity or pedal edema is evident. Nails are thin with slow capillary refill. Interosseous muscle is mildly wasted.

Questions

1. How would you assess Marie's nutrition-focused physical exam findings?
2. Can you corroborate your findings with Marie's anthropometric data?
3. Based on the nutrition-focused physical exam findings, what specific nutrients are of concern for Marie?

body type, mobility, skin color, and hair condition. Before initiating any hands-on assessment, the clinician should explain what the assessment will entail and request permission from the patient or healthcare proxy (if applicable) before proceeding. As previously mentioned, the clinician will check to identify any signs of poor nutritional status, including any physical manifestation of deficiency or malnutrition. Any notable observations are then compared to the nutrition-related concerns that were identified when reviewing the patient's PMH.[160,161]

PRACTICE POINT

In order to complete a thorough NFPE, it is recommended that the clinician follow a systematic approach. For example, the cephalocaudal order of examination is a guide to head-to-toe physical examination and includes these nutritionally relevant areas:

- Head, eyes, ears, nose, throat (HEENT)
- Hair
- Neck
- Upper extremities (including hands and fingernails)
- Chest and back
- Breast and axillae
- Abdomen
- Lower extremities

Note: Skin is checked throughout the assessment.

Components of the NFPE

A system-based evaluation of the body should include the following regions: general inspection, skin, hand and nails, head and hair, eyes and nose, oral cavity, neck and upper body, and musculoskeletal and lower extremities. Although the sections to follow will offer helpful hints on inspecting each region, refer to **Table 1.9** for general guidelines on the NFPE components and to **Table 1.10** for the specific deficiency that can be associated with physical findings.[165]

Skin. Findings of the skin examination are considered to be accurate reflections of nutrient deficiencies because rapidly proliferating tissues, such as skin, are thought to change simultaneously with developing nutritional abnormalities. Although several factors may affect the appearance of the skin, alterations in nutrition are often the culprit behind changes in fluid distribution (**Figure 1.16**), pigmentation, poor wound healing, development of dermatitis, and changes in turgor. These manifestations may be noted on the trunk or extremities, or on less obvious locations (as in the lips, mucous membranes, fingernails, and/or palms of hands and feet).[75,165]

PRACTICE POINT

When observing the skin, inspect the entire skin surface for changes in color, texture, temperature, moisture, lesions, mobility, and turgor.

Hands and Nails. A healthy nail plate should be firmly adhered to the nail bed, feel smooth to the touch, and appear uniformly thick and symmetric. The nail itself should be flat or slightly convex and translucent with a pink hue that is derived from the capillary system located underneath the nail plate.

Table 1.9 Components of the Nutrition-Focused Physical Exam

General Inspection	Observe overall appearance. Evaluate level of consciousness, demeanor, facial expression, body positioning, alterations in motor skills, body habitus, contractures, and/or amputations. Observe for wasting, cachexia, or obesity.
Skin	Observe for redness, pallor, cyanosis, jaundice or yellowing, bruising, and/or dark areas. Monitor for dry/moist skin, sweating, and temperature. Assess texture, thickness or hyperkeratosis, wounds or lesions, and turgor.
Hand and Nails	Inspect the hand and nails for color, texture, shape, and/or presence of lesions. Assess for transverse ridge, koilonychia. Observe and palpate the interosseous muscle for fullness and distribution.
Head and Hair	Inspect the scalp and hair for quantity, distribution, texture, and color. Evaluate for thinning, dryness, depigmentation, and corkscrew appearance. Assess temporalis muscle.
Eyes and Nose/Face	Interview to assess changes in dryness of eyes or night vision. Observe the color of the sclera and conjunctiva. Evaluate corners of eyes for fissures or redness. Assess fullness and color around the orbital region.
Oral Cavity	Evaluate lips for pallor, dryness, or redness. Inspect corners of the mouth for dryness or redness. Observe tongue for inflammation and atrophic lingual papilla. Assess mucous membranes for moisture or dryness. Observe gums for swelling or bleeding. Evaluate teeth for caries, loose/missing teeth, discoloration, or eroded dentition.
Neck and Upper Body	Inspect the neck for distention or masses. Assess for muscle and subcutaneous fat loss in these regions: clavicles, shoulders, scapula, fat overlying the ribs, and triceps. Note sagging skin. Evaluate for edema.
Musculoskeletal and Lower Extremity	Observe overall muscle appearance. Note size and shape of quadriceps and calf muscles. Rate fluid accumulation around ankles. Assess for atrophy.

Data from Pogatshnik C, Hamilton C. Nutrition-focused physical examination: Skin, nails, hair, eyes, and oral cavity. Support Line. 2011;33(2):7-13; and Esper DH. Utilization of nutrition-focused physical assessment in identifying micronutrient deficiencies. *Nutr Clin Pract. 2015;30*(2):194–202.

Table 1.10 Physical Assessment Nutrient Chart

Region	Abnormal Findings	Possible Deficiency or *Excess (in italics)*
Skin	Pallor (paleness) Cyanosis (bluish discoloration)	Iron Folate or vitamin B12 Biotin Copper
	Yellowing of skin	*Carotene or bilirubin (excess related)*
	Dermatitis Follicular hyperkeratosis (rough, cone-shaped, elevated papules around hair follicles)	B-complex vitamins Vitamin A Vitamin C Zinc
	Poor wound healing	Vitamin A Vitamin C Zinc
	Xerosis (abnormal dryness)	Vitamin A Essential fatty acid
	Perifolliculosis (pigmented plaques (thorax, abdomen, thighs, legs))	Vitamin C

(continues)

Table 1.10 Physical Assessment Nutrient Chart *(continued)*

Region	Abnormal Findings	Possible Deficiency or *Excess (in italics)*
	Pellagrous dermatitis (dermatitis with hyperpigmentation of areas exposed to sunlight)	Niacin Tryptophan
	Flaky paint dermatitis (hyperpigmented patches, usually on backs of thighs/buttocks, that peel to reveal hypopigmented skin)	Protein
	Edema **(Figure 1.16)** Poor turgor or tenting	*Fluid (hydration) in excess* Fluid (hydration)
	Acanthosis nigricans (dark patches of skin)	*Insulin excess due to insulin resistance*
Hand and Nails	Clubbing **(Figure 1.17)** Koilonychia: thin, spoon-shaped, concave nails **(Figure 1.18)**	Iron
	Excessive dryness Dark color of nails Curved nail ends	Vitamin B12
	Lackluster or dull nails Pallor or white coloring Ridging, transverse on 2+ extremities	Protein
	Mottled, pale, poor blanching	Vitamin A Vitamin C
	Splinter hemorrhages on distal ends of nails	Vitamin C
Head and Hair	Dull, lackluster color or depigmentation	Protein Copper
	Easily plucked Thinness Sparseness Alopecia	Protein Biotin Copper Essential fatty acids
	Scaly and/or flaky scalp	Essential fatty acids
	Corkscrew, coiled hairs	Vitamin C Copper
Eyes and Nose/ Face	Vision changes, particularly at night Excessive dryness Bitot spots: shiny gray spots on conjunctiva Keratomalacia (hazy, dry, softened cornea)	Vitamin A
	Itching Burning Corneal inflammation	Riboflavin Niacin
	Pallor conjunctiva	Iron Folate Vitamin B12
	Yellowish icterus **(Figure 1.19)**	*Bilirubin in excess*
	Diffuse pigmentation	Protein Energy

Region	Abnormal Findings	Possible Deficiency or *Excess (in italics)*
	Nasolabial seborrhea (scaling around nostrils)	Riboflavin Niacin Vitamin B6
	Temporal wasting (bilateral)	Protein Energy
Oral Cavity	Angular stomatitis (swollen corners of the mouth) **(Figure 1.20)**	Riboflavin Niacin Vitamin B6 Iron
	Glossitis (beefy red tongue, magenta color) Atrophied papillae	Riboflavin Niacin Folate Vitamin B12 Iron (severe)
	Pallor and generalized inflamed mucosa	Iron Vitamin B12 Folate B-complex
	Bleeding gums and poor dentition	Vitamin C
	Dysgeusia: distorted taste Hypogeusia: diminished taste	Zinc
	Cheilosis/Cheilitis (dry, swollen, or ulcerated lips) **(Figure 1.20)**	Riboflavin Vitamin B6 Niacin Iron (severe)
	Stomatitis: general inflammation of oral mucosa	B-complex Iron Vitamin C
	Edematous tongue	Niacin
	Atrophic filiform papillae (tongue is smooth or slick)	Niacin Folate Riboflavin Iron Vitamin B12
	Mottled teeth (whitish opaque-to-severe brown discoloration)	*Fluoride excess*
	Caries: tooth decay	Fluoride Vitamin C
Neck and Upper Body	Enlarged thyroid	Iodine
	Enlarged parotid	Protein Bulimia
	Muscle and fat wasting with prominent bony chest region **(Figure 1.22)**	Calorie and protein depletion

(*continues*)

Table 1.10 Physical Assessment Nutrient Chart *(continued)*

Region	Abnormal Findings	Possible Deficiency or *Excess (in italics)*
Musculoskeletal and Lower Extremity	Poor muscle control (ataxia) Numbness or tingling	Thiamine Vitamin B12 Copper
	Rickets, bowed legs	Vitamin D Calcium Phosphate
	Pitting edema	Protein Thiamine Vitamin C Fluid excess
	Swollen, painful joints	Vitamin C

Data from Pogatshnik C, Hamilton C. Nutrition-focused physical examination: Skin, nails, hair, eyes, and oral cavity. *Support Line. 2011;33*(2):7–13.

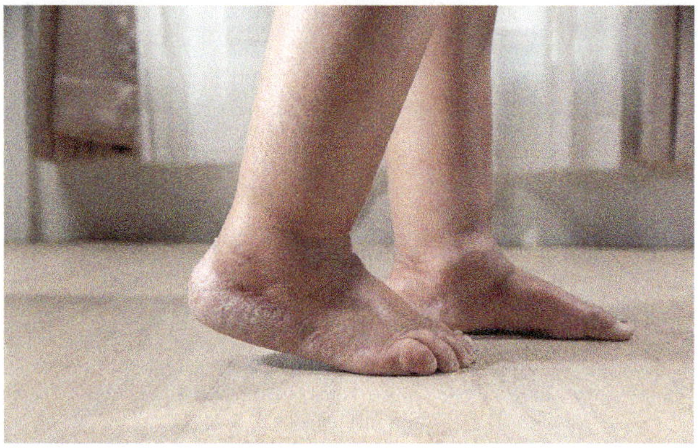

Figure 1.16 Lower Extremity Edema

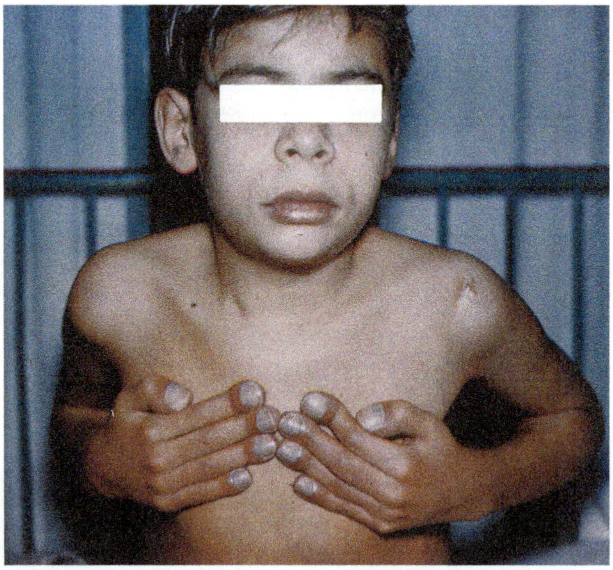

Figure 1.17 Child with Cyanosis and Clubbing of Fingernails

Crowley, An Introduction to Human Disease p 276 Fig 13-9

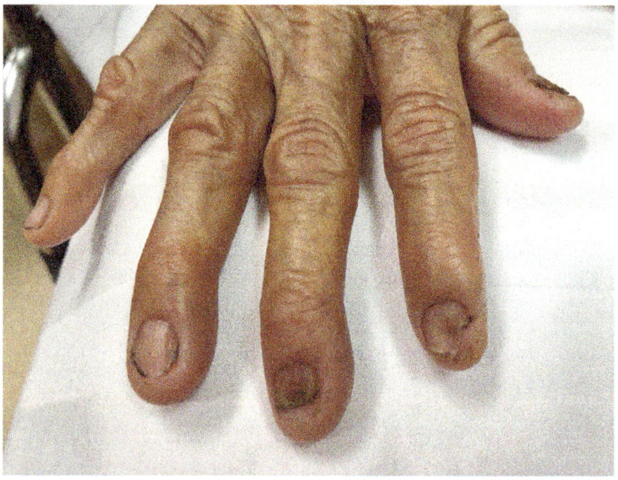

Figure 1.18 Koilonychia (spooned-shaped nails)

When palpating the nail by gently squeezing between the thumb and forefinger, the nail should blanch white and return to its pink color almost immediately (indicating normal capillary refill time indicating adequate hydration and blood flow to tissue). Any abnormalities in color or structure (**Figures 1.17** and **1.18**) may represent nutritional deficiency and/or dehydration and should be considered in the context of the overall clinical picture.[75]

PRACTICE POINT

Inspect the nails for color, length, configuration, symmetry, and cleanliness; nail hygiene often reflects a patient's self-care and emotional state.

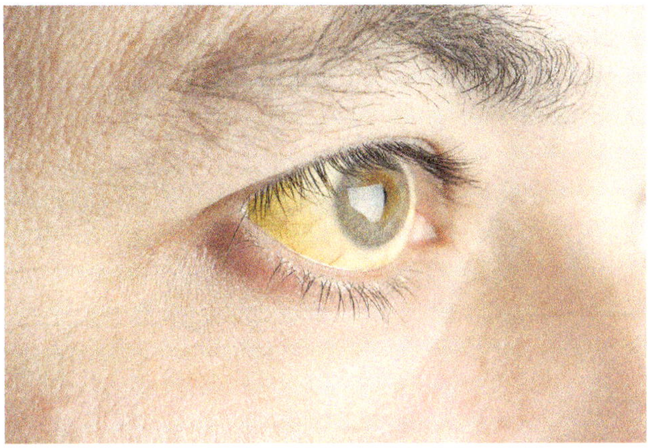

Figure 1.19 Scleral Icterus

© Oktay Ortakcioglu/Getty Images

Head and Hair. Inspection and palpation of the head, scalp, and hair should be performed to assess shape, quantity, distribution, and texture. Healthy scalp hair is shiny, smooth, resilient, and not easily plucked. Any abnormalities may indicate nutrient deficiency.[75]

PRACTICE POINT

Inspect the hair for color, pigmentation, distribution pattern, shine, texture, and quantity.

Eyes and Nose/Face. In general, the structure of the face should appear symmetric. Facial shape, particularly the temporal region, can also indicate deficiency in the form of protein-energy malnutrition. Be sure to note any temporal wasting upon inspection.[75]

The most common variations in eye health secondary to nutritional etiology include vitamin A deficiency, which manifests as night blindness or may be observed as Bitot spots in the eye conjunctiva (shiny gray spots). During the patient interview, note changes in scleral color (**Figure 1.19**) night vision, dryness, and/or inability to produce tears.[75]

Oral Cavity. The oral cavity is a critical region for identifying malnutrition. Due to the rapid turnover (3–5 days) of cells in the oral mucosa, deficiencies often manifest in the lips (**Figure 1.20**), tongue, gingiva, or mucosa. Any inflammation or infection in the oral cavity (**Figure 1.21**) that interferes with eating should be noted. NFPE of the oral cavity should also include assessment of the teeth. Prior to the oral examination, note any patient report of taste changes, pain or bleeding gums, and/or burning sensations. Refer

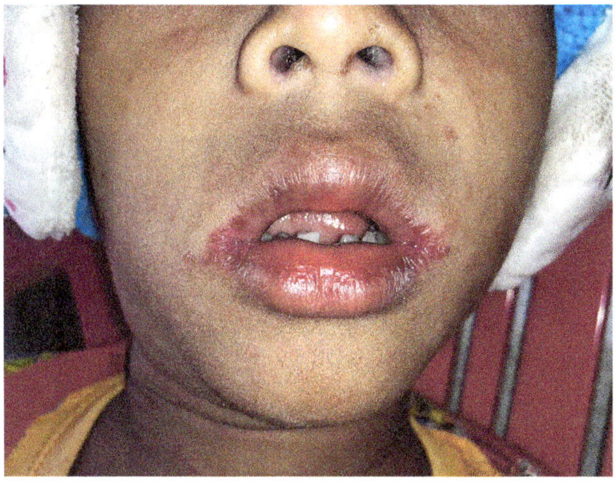

Figure 1.20 Cheilitis

© Zay Nyi Nyi/Shutterstock

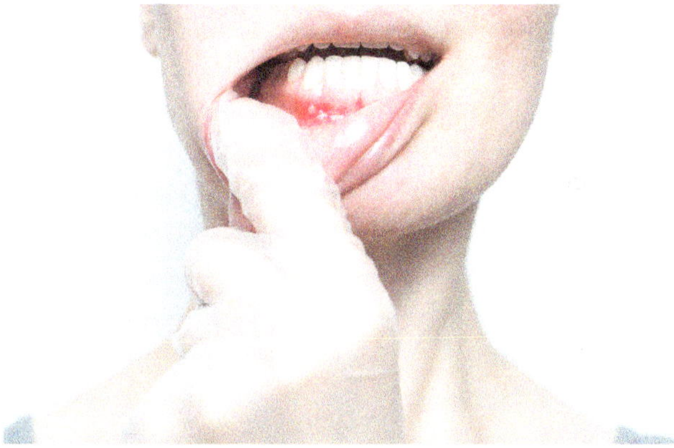

Figure 1.21 Aphthae on Gum

© Tatsiana Niamera/500px/Getty Images

to **Table 1.11** for specific locations of the oral cavity to inspect and the associated deficiencies.[75,161]

PRACTICE POINT

A small penlight, tongue depressor, and disposable gloves are recommended for the oral examination. Start by examining the lips, then assess the inside of the mouth, including the tongue, gums, and teeth.

Neck and Upper Body, Musculoskeletal, and Lower Extremities. The most important physical finding to identify on the trunk and extremities is muscle and/or fat wasting as an indicator of malnutrition. Incorporating the characteristics of malnutrition into the NFPE requires the evaluation of physical changes, including overt weight loss, shifts in body composition, loss of subcutaneous fat, and muscle wasting. Note that fluid retention in the form of edema or ascites may mask weight loss for many acutely ill patients. In addition, note that the AAIM

Table 1.11 Deficiencies Associated with Physical Findings of the Oral Cavity

Location	Signs/Symptoms	Possible Deficiency
Lips	Cheilosis (dry, swollen, ulcerated)	Vitamin B6
	Angular cheilosis (fissures in the corners of the mouth) **(Figure 1.20)**	Folate Riboflavin Niacin Vitamin B12 Iron
Mouth	Xerostomia (dry mouth)	Zinc
	Aphthous stomatitis (canker sores) **(Figure 1.21)**	Vitamin B12 Folate
	Candidiasis (thrush)	Vitamin C Iron
	Pale tissues	Iron
	Stomatopyrosis (painful, inflamed mouth)	Iron
	Dysesthesia (burning mouth syndrome)	Vitamin B12 Folate Magnesium
Teeth and Gums	Bleeding gums	Vitamin C
	Tooth loss	Vitamin C
	Dental caries	Fluoride Vitamin C
Tongue	Glossitis (inflamed) Magenta (red colored) Edematous Atrophic filiform Papillae (flattened protrusions on tongue, giving it a smooth, slick appearance)	Riboflavin Niacin Folate Vitamin B6 Vitamin B12 Iron

Data from Radler DR, Lister T. Nutrient deficiencies associated with nutrition-focused physical findings of the oral cavity. *Nutr Clin Pract. 2013;28*(6):710–721.

criteria[9] refer to several specific body areas that require assessment of fat, muscle, and/or fluid status. Per these guidelines, loss of subcutaneous fat is best identified in the orbital region, triceps, and/or overlying the ribs; muscle mass depletion manifests as wasting of the temples (temporalis muscle), clavicles (pectoralis and deltoids; **Figure 1.22**), shoulders (deltoids), interosseous muscles, scapula (latissimus dorsi, trapezius, deltoids), thigh (quadriceps), and calf (gastrocnemius); and generalized or localized fluid accumulation can be seen in the extremities, vulvar/scrotal region, or abdomen (as in ascites).[90,155]

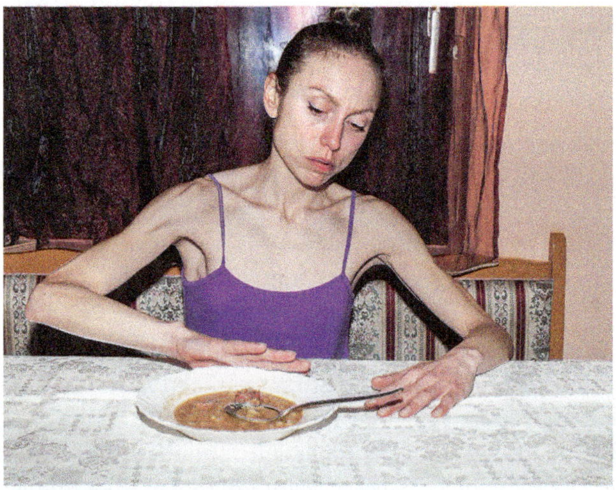

Figure 1.22 Clavicular Muscle Wasting

Telehealth and NFPE

The COVID-19 pandemic has led to an increase in telehealth visits where RDs may be tasked with performing nutrition assessments, including NFPEs, remotely. It is important to note that even with a virtual appointment with teleconferencing, significant information can be collected visually to support the NFPE component of the nutrition assessment. Examples include observation of dry skin, pallor, underweight or overweight status, patient's sitting or standing position, clothing fit, assistive devices (canes, walkers), etc. It may be helpful to ask to examine certain features (hair, nails, eyes, tongue) closer to the camera. The patient can also perform some of the NFPE tasks, such as a skin turgor check, on themselves.[166]

Malnutrition and NFPE Findings

Certain nutrition organizations have released standards for interpreting NFPE findings and correlating them to malnutrition, including AAIM[9] and the GLIM,[11] which is endorsed by ESPEN. It is important to note that each of these standards requires more than NFPE findings alone to diagnose malnutrition.

AAIM

In these guidelines, muscle and fat wasting are assessed separately and classified as mild, moderate, or severe. Different severity is required in the context of acute illness, chronic illness, and social/environmental circumstances to differentiate degrees of malnutrition.[9]

GLIM

The GLIM criteria utilize muscle wasting, but not fat wasting, for determining malnutrition severity. A mild-to-moderate loss of muscle classifies as stage 1/moderate malnutrition, and a severe loss as stage 2/severe malnutrition.[11]

Functional Assessment

Advanced malnutrition, often related to a decline in clinical status, is associated with loss of muscle mass and function that leads to measurable declines in strength and/or physical performance. The relationship is reciprocal: malnutrition can impair functioning and impaired functioning can lead to poor nutritional status through various avenues (e.g., inability to prepare meals). A functional assessment can be used to evaluate the degree of baseline impairment and should be repeated regularly thereafter for comparison of improvements with intervention or later declines in status. This assessment may include any abnormalities in body composition that interfere with normal function—including muscle strength and function. The functional assessment becomes particularly important when assessing the older patient population. Both physical performance and the ability to perform **activities of daily living** (ADLs; routine activities that most individuals complete daily including eating, bathing, dressing, toileting, and walking) have important nutritional implications for older adults.[16,167]

Muscle Function and Strength: Handgrip Strength. Declines in muscle strength will accompany loss of muscle mass that can result from advanced malnutrition. The most practical measure for the clinical assessment of muscle strength is that of **handgrip strength (HGS)** using a simple **handgrip dynamometer** (Figure 1.23). Other physical performance batteries include measures such as a timed gait (5-meter walk), chair stands, and stair steps, although these measures are generally outside the dietetics scope of practice.[16,167,168]

Muscle function reacts quickly to nutritional deprivation; changes in muscle function may manifest prior to visual depletions. Because the function most easily measured is muscle force, HGS, which is the simplest to measure and has been correlated with overall muscle strength,[169,170] can be used as a surrogate for voluntary muscle strength. A decline in HGS has been directly related to declines in nutrition status, especially in older adults,[47,171] and can be relied upon as a sensitive measurement of short-term response to nutritional therapy.[172] It has also been deemed a relevant predictor of prognosis, hospital length of stay, and readmission rates, and has been found to be a more useful functional measure than a 5-meter timed walk in the acute care setting. In general, HGS provides information on nutritional status, muscle mass, physical function, and overall health

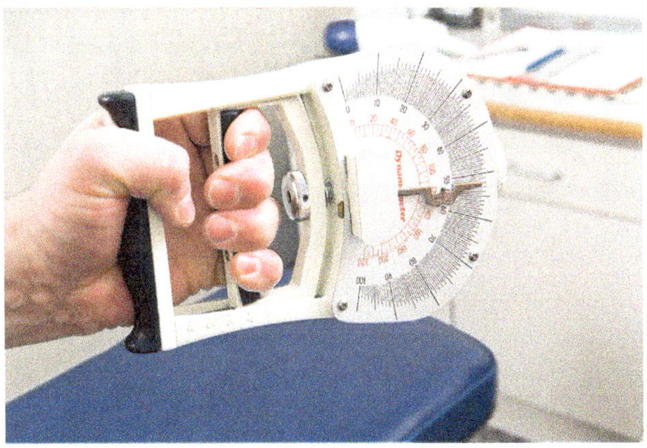

Figure 1.23 Handgrip Dynamometer

status. Moreover, handgrip dynamometry is rapid, cost-effective, and user-friendly with high test, retest, and interrater reliability.[16,167–169,173–178]

PRACTICE POINT

Although handgrip strength is a reliable marker of declining nutrition status, for some patients, declines in handgrip strength may be attributable to frailty with old age instead of overt malnutrition.

Procedure. In regard to technique, there is some evidence that posture, choice between dominant/nondominant hand, and different dynamometer models produce varying results. These factors can be avoided by following standardized procedures. The patient should perform the test while sitting comfortably with shoulder adducted and forearm neutrally rotated, elbow flexed to 90 degrees, and wrist in a neutral position. Ideally, the patient will be seated on a chair or at the side of the bed with feet on the floor. The grip on the dynamometer should be adjusted for hand size so that the dynamometer rests on the middle of the four fingers. The grip should be held for about 3–5 seconds with the patient being instructed to perform a maximal isometric contraction and exhaling during grip exertion. The test should be repeated, alternating hands (e.g., left hand then right hand then left hand) with about 15 seconds between each hand with a total of three tests per hand. An average value of the three tests should be recorded and compared to reference ranges specific to the dynamometer model that have been stratified by age and sex.[171,174,177,179]

Food/Nutrition-Related History

Dietary assessment is the portion of nutrition assessment that is used to identify inadequate, excessive, or imbalanced nutrient intakes. The most frequently used method for obtaining dietary history in both acute and outpatient care is the 24-hour dietary recall, although each of the most common techniques will be discussed later in this section. If dietary history cannot be obtained from direct patient interview, then medical records, family members, or caregivers can provide insight. It is not unusual for patients in the clinical setting to have compromised dietary intake for extended periods of time prior to assessment (particularly for those with acute medical events superimposed on chronic health conditions). The diet history can help to identify reasons behind changes in dietary intake, including disease-related symptoms.[16]

The food and nutrition-related history is also useful for providing average macronutrient and micronutrient intakes, as well as a depiction of general diet variety and eating patterns. When malnutrition is of concern, the current dietary recall should be compared to a normal dietary recall to provide the current percentage of normal intake. The dietary history will identify the contribution of poor dietary intake to the malnourished state. In general, a thorough food and nutrition history should address several areas.[6]

Food and Nutrient Intake

Assess for diet composition, adequacy of food and nutrient intake, meal and snack patterns, food preferences, environmental cues to eating, and current diets and/or food modifications; note that underreporting or overreporting are both common occurrences. Also note any influences on appetite, which should be assessed as within normal limits or for any relevant changes. Assess whether a patient requires nutrition support in the form of oral nutrition supplements, enteral nutrition, or parenteral support. If so, note the home regimen. In the acute care setting, dietary assessment must continue when nutrition support is initiated to monitor adequacy of nutrient provision. If a patient is receiving nutrition support in addition to oral feeding, it is important to track the adequacy of oral feeds to adjust the nutrition support provided.[16]

Food and Nutrient Administration

Identify current diet order, previous diet modifications, history of nutrition counseling, previous dieting attempts, history of fasting, and means of nutrition support administration (type of feeding tube, central line) and regimen. Note food allergies or intolerances, foods that are avoided, reason for the avoidance (description of associated symptoms), length of time of avoidance, and foods used to replace the avoided item.

Medication and Complementary/Alternative Medicine Use

Identify current medication regimen evaluating for medications with strong nutrition interactions (such as medications that may promote anorexia or interfere with the absorption, metabolism, or excretion of nutrients), including steroids, immunosuppressants, chemotherapy agents, antibiotics, and diuretics. Consider if medication use is a source of symptoms that affect intake (e.g., taste changes, gastrointestinal symptoms, swallowing ability, requirements for assistance or feeding). Assess for any herbal or dietary supplement use.

CASE STUDY REVISITED

As you continue to interview Marie, you ask about her dietary history. Marie reports struggling to cook at home due to fatigue. She also reports difficulty affording food for herself and her son. She typically eats a small breakfast but skips lunch. She eats dinner when she feels able to cook, which is about 5 out of 7 days/week.

24-hour Diet Recall:

Breakfast 8 am: 8 oz coffee black with ½ cup instant oatmeal with 2 oz added skim milk
Dinner 5 pm: ½ low-salt tuna sandwich with mayonnaise, 6 oz water
No lunch

Questions

1. How is Marie's intake influencing her nutritional status?
2. What other assessments can be conducted to assess Marie's functional status?
3. Does Marie classify as malnourished per the AAIM criteria?
4. Write two Problem/Etiology/Signs and Symptoms (PES) statements for Marie identifying Marie's active issues.
5. Identify the interventions you would like to initiate for Marie to address the problems identified in your PES statements.

Knowledge, Beliefs, and Attitudes

Assess general nutrition knowledge and beliefs about nutrition, including readiness for change. Consider any cultural or religious influence on eating habits. Identify attitudes toward food, eating patterns, body image, and perception of healthy weight.

Behaviors

Assess behaviors about nutrition recommendations, including self-monitoring principles; disordered eating or eating disordered behaviors (bingeing, purging, food restriction or avoidance); and general eating behavior (meal duration, food refusal or aversions, and fatigue associated with eating).

Access to Food and Related Supplies

Food availability and economics will have a significant impact on dietary habits for many patients. Assess food planning, purchasing, and preparation abilities; limitations; nutrition program utilization; and/or food insecurity. Tailor counseling to income and availability, but always be sensitive to the individual situation. Consider the number of people in the household, food storage and cooking facilities, and type of housing—each of these factors will certainly impact dietary habits.

Physical Activity and Function

Physical activity and exercise habits should be assessed. Other pertinent information includes functional status, activity patterns, amount of sedentary time, screen time, and sleep habits. If applicable, also note anything that would impact voluntary physical activity (such as perceived safety and walkability of neighborhood). Identify ability to shop, cook, self-feed, or administer nutrition support. Assess for breastfeeding initiation or difficulties.

Nutrition-Related Client-Centered Measures

Assess nutrition-related quality of life, concerns, experience, or outcomes.

PRACTICE POINT

When considering the acutely ill inpatient population, assessing dietary intake prior to hospital admission and duration of poor oral intake will be particularly pertinent to the assessment. It is not unusual for patients in acute care to have compromised dietary intakes for extended periods prior to admission.

Dietary Recall Methods/Methods of Obtaining Intake Data

The accurate assessment of dietary intake is an integral component of nutrition assessment. Self-reporting of intake via 24-hour dietary recalls, food records diary, and/or food frequency questionnaires are the most common methods for assessment. Because diet is inherently complicated to measure, any self-reported data are prone to errors attributed to memory, estimation of portion size, underreporting or overreporting, and distortion to socially desirable responses. These methods may be limited for use in the acutely ill or older patients who may be unable to self-report dietary intake. An additional observational method, the calorie count, is useful in the clinical setting but is often cumbersome, reliant on an accurate record, and cannot be applied to the outpatient setting. Despite these difficulties, assessment of nutrient intake is crucial to identifying individuals at risk for malnutrition and to estimating the contribution on decreased oral intake to the malnourished state.[180–184]

24-Hour Dietary Recall. The **24-hour dietary recall** is a retrospective tool that requires the client to recite all food intake during the previous 24 hours. To improve patient recall, a multiple-pass method is often employed; this involves multiple passes through the day ([1] collecting a quick list of foods; [2] assessing time, meal, and place; [3] reviewing a foods forgotten list; [4] revising food details; [5] final review) to provide additional memory cues. This method was developed to minimize underreporting of data by

Clinical Roundtable

Topic: Nutrition Assessment in the Intensive Care Unit

Background: Patients treated in the intensive care units are some of the highest acuity patients in the hospital. Many of the typical assessment criteria (weight status, dietary intake, biochemical markers, etc.) are difficult to reliably obtain or are confounded by factors like metabolic stress. Anthropometric measurements, which are fundamental to any nutrition assessment, may not be easily acquired from patients who are critically ill, intubated, and/or sedated, who may be both unable to be moved for measurement and unable to provide self-reported data. Other factors related to clinical status, like fluid shifts or edema, will further confound this assessment.

To help clinicians better assess those who are critically ill, Heyland et al. developed and validated a novel risk assessment tool based directly on the ICU patient population. This tool, the NUTrition Risk in the Critically ill (NUTRIC score), is based on variables that are easy to obtain in the critical care setting. Patients receive a score of 1–10 based on an algorithm that considers six variables: age, Acute Physiology and Chronic Health Evaluation scores (APACHE II), Sequential Organ Failure Assessment scores (SOFA), number of comorbidities, days from hospital to ICU admission, and serum interleukin-6 (IL-6). The following table outlines the NUTRIC score variables as they apply to the final evaluation:

To be most clinically applicable, the NUTRIC score provides interpretation guidelines based on whether or not the IL-6 marker is available (the other markers are routinely obtainable from the medical record of an ICU patient):

Variable	Range	Points
Age (years)	<50	0
	50–74	1
	≥75	2
APACHE II	<15	0
	15–19	1
	20–28	2
	≥28	3
SOFA	<6	0
	6–9	1
	≥10	2
Number of Comorbidities	0–1	0
	≥2	1
Days from Hospital to ICU Admission	<1	0
	≥1	1
IL-6	0–399	0
	≥400	1

Data from Heyland DK, Dhaliwal R, Jiang X, Day AG. Identifying critically ill patients who benefit the most from nutrition therapy: the development and initial validation of a novel risk assessment tool. *Crit Care.* 2011;15(6):R268.

If IL-6 is available:

High score (6–10 points): associated with worse clinical outcomes (i.e., mortality); these patients are most likely to benefit from aggressive medical nutrition therapy

Low score (0–5 points): low malnutrition risk

If IL-6 is *not* available:

High score (5–9 points): associated with worse clinical outcomes (i.e., mortality); these patients are most likely to benefit from aggressive medical nutrition therapy

Low score (0–4 points): low malnutrition risk

In general, the higher the sum of the scores from each component, the greater the likelihood of nutritional risk and anticipated benefit of nutrition intervention.

Roundtable Discussion

Given the difficulties with nutritional assessment in the critical care setting, how might the NUTRIC score be a valuable tool for clinicians in this setting?

Due to its validation, should the NUTRIC score supersede standard nutrition screening in this setting? Why or why not?

What are the advantages and disadvantages of using a nutrition risk assessment tool, such as the NUTRIC score, in the critical care setting?

How can you reconcile that ASPEN recommends the NUTRIC score be used to screen all patients in the ICU setting while AND recommends the Malnutrition Screening Tool (MST) be used to screen for all patients in all settings? Which tool would you use in the ICU setting?

References

1. Heyland DK, Dhaliwal R, Jiang X, Day AG. Identifying critically ill patients who benefit the most from nutrition therapy: the development and initial validation of a novel risk assessment tool. *Crit Care.* 2011;15(6):R268.
2. Bloomfield R, Steel E, MacLennan G, Noble DW. Accuracy of weight and height estimation in an intensive care unit: implications for clinical practice and research. *Crit Care Med.* 2006;34(8):2153–2157.
3. Rosa M, Heyland DK, Fernandes D, Rabito EL, Oliveira ML, Marcadenti A. Translation and adaptation of the NUTRIC score to identify critically ill patients who benefit the most from nutrition therapy. *Clin Nutr ESPEN.* 2016;14:31–36.
4. Kalaiselvan MS, Renuka MK, Arunkumar AS. Use of nutrition risk in critically ill (NUTRIC) score to assess nutritional risk in mechanically ventilated patients: a prospective observational study. *Indian J Crit Care Med.* 2017;21(5):253–256.
5. Rahman A, Hasan RM, Agarwala R, Martin C, Day AG, Heyland DK. Identifying critically-ill patients who will benefit most from nutritional therapy: further validation of the "modified NUTRIC" nutritional risk assessment tool. *Clin Nutr.* 2016;35(1):158–162.
6. Skipper A, Coltman A, Tomesko J, Charney P, Porcari J, Piemonte TA, Handu D, Cheng FW. Position of the Academy of Nutrition and Dietetics: malnutrition (undernutrition) screening tools for all adults. *J Acad Nutr Diet.* 2020;120(4):709–713. doi:10.1016/j.jand.2019.09.011
7. McClave SA, Taylor BE, Martindale RG, et al. Guidelines for the Provision and Assessment of Nutrition Support Therapy in the Adult Critically Ill Patient: Society of Critical Care Medicine (SCCM) and American Society for Parenteral and Enteral Nutrition (A.S.P.E.N.). *JPEN J Parenter Enteral Nutr.* 2016;40(2):159–211. doi:10.1177/0148607115621863. [Erratum in: *JPEN.* 2016;40(8):1200. doi:10.1177/0148607116670155.]

providing respondents with numerous opportunities to recall dietary intake. Visual aids may be used to assist subjects in estimating more accurate portion sizes.[180,182,185–187]

The 24-hour dietary recall is practical, quick, inexpensive, independent of literacy ability, and has a low respondent burden. With this type of recall, the patient or client is more likely to be honest about their dietary behavior. The known limitations include reliance on respondent memory, tendency to underestimate portion sizes, and high interrater variability. The 24-hour recall has several limitations to its use in the inpatient clinical setting; be sure to clarify whether the recall depicts a typical day and, if not, determine what makes it atypical. As with any 24-hour recall, engage in a discussion on how that intake compares to usual intake. Bear in mind that this method of recall portrays a snapshot in time; it will be beneficial to combine the information obtained from the recall with information on typical intake to better understand eating habits and any changes in usual patterns. The reliability of dietary assessment increases when 24-hour dietary recalls are repeated on several occasions.[16,180,181,188]

Food Records Diary. The **food records diary** is applicable to the outpatient setting. As a prospective tool, this method requires the client to record food intake for a specific time period (usually several days to 1 week). The diary provides greater precision than the 24-hour dietary recall and is not reliant on client memory. It can be considered more reflective of an "actual intake" because it will typically encompass several days, including weekdays and weekend days. The most notable limitation is that participants tend to modify eating behavior based on what they feel is an "acceptable" dietary intake for the duration of the food record. This method has a much higher client burden when compared to the 24-hour dietary recall and is dependent on literacy and numeracy with knowledge of portion sizes.[181]

Food Frequency Questionnaire (FFQ). The **food frequency questionnaire (FFQ)** is utilized most often in the outpatient setting or for national survey data collection, although modified versions may be useful for assessing intake patterns of the hospitalized patient. The FFQ is a retrospective tool that requires the client to complete a survey about food intake over a specific period of time in an attempt to depict "usual" intake. This method has several benefits, including low client burden, ease of administration, low cost, ease of standardization, and ability to examine specific nutrients. The data provided are qualitative. The tool also requires that the client be literate and numerate and is significantly memory-dependent. The tool may be cognitively difficult because it relies on a foods list and is not meal-based.[181,189,190]

Observation of Food Intake: "Calorie Counts." Observation of food intake in the form of "calorie counts" can only be employed in controlled settings (like an inpatient hospital unit). This method will not represent usual intake, but instead a picture of current intake that is often useful when diagnosing malnutrition or assessing the need for nutrition support in the clinical setting. Observation methods have a low client burden (i.e., the client is generally unaware of the dietary assessment) and are not memory or literacy dependent. In addition to increasing staff burden, this tool is intrusive and may be difficult to implement and interpret. This tool should not serve as the first choice for a dietary assessment method and should be saved for instances when other dietary recall methods are not feasible.[181,184]

Technological Advancements for Tracking Dietary Intake and Other Metrics

Technological advancements have begun to change the way dietary assessment is implemented in the outpatient setting. Innovative dietary assessment technologies using smartphones and web-based platforms have grown in popularity and now tend to replace traditional pen-and-paper versions of dietary assessment. The application of technology in this setting has recently been demonstrated to reduce issues associated with accuracy, client burden, and time of data collection. It should be noted, however, that food databases within different applications can have variable accuracy of nutritional information for the same foods. Being aware of the current technologies and their function may help facilitate better data collection when compared to the traditional methods.[182,183,186,191]

Telehealth and Technology

Technology can be especially useful for RDs counseling remotely via telehealth. There are various direct-to-consumer technologies that can be used to monitor certain metrics, such as weight and diet composition for self-monitoring. Additional reportable metrics include activity level, sleep pattern, blood pressure, and blood glucose levels. This information can be shared with the RD or, in some cases, reported directly to the clinician. Although there is great potential for technology to enhance nutrition assessment via telehealth, cost may be a barrier to some clients.[166] Note that providing nutrition counseling in the home setting provides a unique opportunity for the client to visually share, if they desire, their home food environment, including food choices and contents of their food pantry.

Nutrition Assessment Tools

There are assessment tools available to RDs to assist in completing nutrition assessments, although these are not as thorough as the full assessment detailed above. Most common are the Subjective Global Assessment (SGA)[192] and the Mini Nutrition Assessment (MNA).[193] These can provide a clear structure to RDs completing assessments and create a score-based system for determining malnutrition. These tools are more commonly used in the research setting, where numerical scores are often preferred for statistical analysis and comparison to other study results.

Subjective Global Assessment

The SGA includes seven points of evaluation. While termed a "screening tool," it is in fact a diagnostic tool for malnutrition rather than nutrition risk. It encompasses many of the domains outlined above:

- Weight and weight change
- Route, amount, and changes in dietary intake
- Gastrointestinal symptoms (nausea, vomiting, diarrhea)
- Extent of and changes in functional capacity

- Nutrition-related conditions/PMH
- Nutrition-focused physical findings (muscle wasting, fat stores, and edema)

Each domain is scored on a scale from 1 to 7 according to a predetermined scale, yielding a composite number that correlates with well-nourished/very mild risk (6–7), mild-to-moderate risk (3–5), and severe malnutrition (1–2). Scores may change over an admission or intervention, and tracking these changes allows for ongoing monitoring. The SGA has been validated in many different disease states and clinical conditions to predict patient outcomes, including survival, length of stay, and malnutrition.[192,193]

Mini Nutrition Assessment

The MNA was initially developed for older adults in a variety of settings. The original full MNA is 18 points and includes specific questions regarding dietary intake; however, in 2001, a "Short Form" (MNA-SF) was validated for use alone and as a "prescreen" to the full MNA. The MNA-SF contains six central elements:

- Decreased food intake (due to low appetite, issues chewing or swallowing, or gastrointestinal symptoms)
- Weight change
- BMI or calf circumference
- Mobility
- Recent psychological or physiological stress
- Presence of dementia or other psychological disorders

The full-form MNA includes calf and mid-upper arm circumference but does not include other nutrition-focused physical findings as are noted above.[194,195]

Next Step: Nutrition Diagnosis: Writing Problem/Etiology/Signs and Symptoms (PES) Statements

Once a nutrition assessment has been completed, the next step is to identify a nutrition diagnosis per the NCPM.[6] Using standardized terminology, a nutrition diagnostic statement requires identification of a nutrition problem (P), its etiology (E), and accompanying signs and symptoms (S) or PES statement. Throughout the text, you will be asked to write a PES statement within the context of each case study. The nutrition diagnosis, which is distinct from a medical diagnosis, seeks to identify a nutrition issue (P), its contributing factor(s) (E), and defining characteristics (S). When writing a PES statement, one starts with choosing a nutrition diagnosis from the eNCPT reference manual[6] that best captures the nutrition issue or challenge to be addressed. The second step is to identify the etiology or the most specific cause of the nutrition problem and ideally one which can be addressed. The third or final step is to identify the signs and symptoms of the issue, which is something the clinician observes or the patient or family reports. The PES statement is written via the format of "Problem" *related to* "Etiology" *as evidenced by* "Signs and Symptoms." An example of a PES statement for malnutrition would be, "Severe chronic disease-related malnutrition related to poor oral intake as evidenced by 8% weight loss over 1 month and food records revealing patient consuming 60% of estimated energy needs for 2 months."[6]

Chapter Summary

Nutrition assessment is an integral part of patient care because it involves obtaining and interpreting information needed to identify and then treat nutrition-related issues, such as malnutrition. It is a multifactorial process that utilizes various data sources including anthropometric, biochemical, client history, nutrition-focused physical exam findings, and food/nutrition-related history data to compare specific criteria. Although there is a broad range of evaluation parameters, assessment of nutritional status requires interpretation of data compared to standards made within the context, interpreted, and adjusted for the individual clinical situation. Nutrition assessment is supported by, but does not include, nutrition screening, which seeks to identify individuals who would benefit most from a complete assessment.

Key Terms

nutrition care process and model (NCPM), nutrition care process terminology (NCPT), malnutrition, nutrition screening, malnutrition universal screening tool (MUST), short nutritional assessment questionnaire (SNAQ), malnutrition screening tool (MST), anthropometry, height, stadiometer, self-reported height (SRH), knee height, total arm span (TAS), half arm span (HAS), actual body weight, usual body weight (UBW), percent usual body weight (%UBW), percent weight change (%weight change), ideal body weight (IBW), percent ideal body weight (%IBW), adjusted body weight, dry weight, body mass index (BMI), skinfold anthropometry, triceps skinfold (TSF), mid-upper arm circumference (MUAC), mid-arm muscle circumference (MAMC), waist circumference, waist-hip ratio (WHR), calf circumference (CC), computed tomography (CT), magnetic resonance imaging (MRI), bioelectrical impedance analysis (BIA), dual energy x-ray absorptiometry (DXA), ultrasound (US), nutrition-focused physical exam (NFPE), inspection, palpation, percussion, auscultation, activities of daily living, handgrip strength, handgrip dynamometer, 24-hour dietary recall, food records diary, food frequency questionnaire (FFQ)

Acknowledgments

The authors acknowledge V. Paige Murphy for contributions to the previous version of this chapter.

References

1. Ravasco P, Camilo ME, Gouveia-Oliveira A, Adam S, Brum G. A critical approach to nutritional assessment in critically ill patients. *Clin Nutr*. 2002;21(1):73–77.
2. Lacey K, Pritchett E. Nutrition care process and model: ADA adopts road map to quality care and outcomes management. *J Am Diet Assoc*. 2003;103(8):1061–1072.
3. Swan WI, Pertel DG, Hotson B, et al. Nutrition care process (NCP) update part 2: developing and using the NCP terminology to demonstrate efficacy of nutrition care and related outcomes. *J Acad Nutr Diet*. 2019;119(5):840–855. doi:10.1016/j.jand.2018.10.025
4. Nutrition Care Process and Terminology Committee. Editorial guidance for the Nutrition Care Process Terminology (NCPT). Accessed December 20, 2024. https://www.cdrnet.org/vault/2459/web//NCPTEditorialGuide-2023.pdf
5. Nutrition Care Process and Model Web Resources. Accessed December 20, 2024. https://www.cdrnet.org/nutrition-care-process-and-terminology.
6. Academy of Nutrition and Dietetics. Nutrition Terminology Reference Manual (eNCPT). Accessed December 20, 2024. https://www.ncpro.org.
7. Field LB, Hand RK. Differentiating malnutrition screening and assessment: a nutrition care process perspective. *J Acad Nutr Diet*. 2015;115(5):824–828.
8. Mueller C, Compher C, Ellen DM. American Society for Parenteral and Enteral Nutrition (A.S.P.E.N.) Board of Directors. A.S.P.E.N. Clinical guidelines: nutrition screening, assessment, and intervention in adults. *JPEN J Parenter Enteral Nutr.* 2011;35(1):16–24.
9. White JV, Guenter P, Jensen G, Malone A, Schofield M. Consensus statement of the Academy of Nutrition and Dietetics/American Society for Parenteral and Enteral Nutrition: Characteristics recommended for the identification and documentation of adult malnutrition (undernutrition). J Acad Nutr Diet. 2012;112(5):730-738. doi:10.1016/j.jand.2012.03.012
10. Cederholm T, Bosaeus I, Barazzoni R, et al. Diagnostic criteria for malnutrition—an ESPEN consensus statement. *Clin Nutr.* 2015;34(3):335–340.
11. Cederholm T, Jensen GL, Correia MITD, et al. GLIM criteria for the diagnosis of malnutrition—A consensus report from the global clinical nutrition community. *Clin Nutr.* 2019;38(1):1–9. doi:10.1016/j.clnu.2018.08.002
12. Jeejeebhoy KN. Nutrition assessment. *J Nutr*. 2000;16(7/8): 585–590.
13. Guenter P, Jenson GL. Patel V, et al. Addressing disease-related malnutrition in hospitalized patients: a call for a national goal. *Jt Comm J Qual Pat Saf.* 2015;41(10):469–473.
14. Guenter P, Abdelhadi R, Anthony P, et al. Malnutrition diagnoses and associated outcomes in hospitalized patients: United States, 2018. *Nutr Clin Pract.* 2021;36(5):957–969. doi:10.1002/ncp.10771
15. Jensen GL, Mirtallo J, Compher C, et al. Adult starvation and disease-related malnutrition: a proposal for etiology-based diagnosis in the clinical practice setting from the International Consensus Guideline Committee. *JPEN.* 2010;34(2):156–159.
16. Soeters PB, Schols AM. Advances in understanding and assessing malnutrition. Curr Opin Clin Nutr Metab Care. 2009;12(5):487-494.
17. Barker LA, Gout BS, Crowe TC. Hospital malnutrition: prevalence, identification, and impact on patients and the healthcare system. *Int J Environ Res Public Health.* 2011;8:514–527.
18. Mostafa N, Sayed AA, Rashad O, Baqal OJ. Malnutrition-related mortality trends in older adults in the United States from 1999 to 2020. *BMC Med.* 2023;21(1). doi:10.1186/s12916-023-03143-8
19. National Cancer Institute. Nutrition in Cancer Care (PDQ®)–Health Professional Version - National Cancer Institute. www.cancer.gov. Updated September 20, 2024. Accessed December 16, 2024. https://www.cancer.gov/about-cancer/treatment/side-effects/appetite-loss/nutrition-hp-pdq#_12_toc.
20. Balestrieri P, Ribolsi M, Guarino MPL, Emerenziani S, Altomare A, Cicala M. Nutritional aspects in inflammatory bowel diseases. *Nutrients.* 2020;12(2):372. doi:10.3390/nu12020372
21. Matteo Tosato, Calvani R, Ciciarello F, et al. Malnutrition in COVID-19 survivors: prevalence and risk factors. *Aging Clin Exp Res.* 2023;35(10):2257–2265. doi:10.1007/s40520-023-02526-4
22. Guðnadóttir SD, Gunnarsdóttir I, Hernandez UB, Ingadóttir ÁR. High risk of malnutrition among hospitalised coronavirus disease 2019 (COVID-19) patients is associated with mortality and other clinical outcomes. *Clin Nutr ESPEN.* 2024;61:1–7. doi:10.1016/j.clnesp.2024.02.023
23. Barrett ML, Bailey MK, Owens PL, Brown MH. Non-maternal and Non-neonatal Inpatient Stays in the United States Involving Malnutrition, 2016. August 30, 2018. U.S. Agency for Healthcare Research and Quality. https://hcup-us.ahrq.gov/reports/ataglance/HCUPMalnutritionHospReport_083018.pdf

24. Hejazi N, Mazloom Z, Zand F, Rezaiazadeh A, Amini A. Nutrition assessment in critically ill patients. *Iran J Med Sci.* 2016;41(3):171–179.
25. Curtis LJ, Bernier P, Jeejeebhoy K, et al. Costs of hospital malnutrition. *Clin Nutr.* 2017;36(5):1391–1396.
26. Dobak S, Peterson S, Corrigan, M, Lefton J. Current practices and perceived barrier to diagnosing, documenting, and coding for malnutrition. *J Acad Nutr Diet.* 2018; 118(6):978–983.
27. Academy of Nutrition and Dietetics. About RDNs and NDTRs. Published 2024. Accessed December 20, 2024. https://www.eatright.org/about-rdns-and-ndtrs
28. Commission on Dietetic Registration, Scope and Standards of Practice Task Force. Revised 2024 Scope and Standards of Practice for the Registered Dietitian Nutritionist Commission on Dietetic Registration Scope and Standards of Practice Task Force. 2024. Accessed December 20, 2024. https://www.cdrnet.org/vault/2459/web//Scope%20Standards%20of%20Practice%202024%20RDN_FINAL.pdf
29. National Board of Nutrition Support Certification. Accessed December 26, 2024. https://www.nutritioncare.org/nbnsc/
30. Welcome to Medicare. Medical Nutrition Therapy Services. Accessed December 26, 2024. https://www.medicare.gov/coverage/medical-nutrition-therapy-services#:~:text=Only%20a%20registered%20dietitian%20(or,of%20your%20overall%20dialysis%20care
31. Skipper A, Ferguson M, Thompson K, Castellanos VH, Porcari J. Nutrition screening tools: an analysis of the evidence. *JPEN.* 2012;36(3):292–298.
32. Poulia KA, Klek S, Doundoulakis I, et al. The two most popular malnutrition screening tools in light of the new ESPEN consensus definition of the diagnostic criteria for malnutrition. *Clin Nutr.* 2017;36(4):1130–1135.
33. The Joint Commission. Standards FAQs. Updated November 17, 2022. Accessed December 26, 2024. https://www.jointcommission.org/standards/standard-faqs/critical-access-hospital/provision-of-care-treatment-and-services-pc/000001652/
34. Phillips W, Zechariah S. Minimizing false-positive nutrition referrals generated from the malnutrition screening tool. *J Acad Nutr Diet.* 2017;117(5):665–669.
35. Patel V, Romano M, Corkins MR, et al. Nutrition screening and assessment in hospitalized patients: a survey of current practice in the United States. *Nutr Clin Pract.* 2014;29(4):483–490.
36. Jensen GL, Compher C, Sullivan DH, Mullin GE. Recognizing malnutrition in adults: definitions, characteristics, screening, assessment, and team approach. *JPEN J Parenter Enteral Nutr.* 2013;37(6):802–807.
37. Reber E, Gomes F, Vasiloglou MF, Schuetz P, Stanga Z. Nutritional risk screening and assessment. *J Clin Med.* 2019;8(7):1065. doi:10.3390/jcm8071065.
38. House M, Gwaltney C. Malnutrition screening and diagnosis tools: implications for practice. *Nutr Clin Pract.* 2022;37(1):12–22. doi:10.1002/ncp.10801.
39. Malnutrition Advisory Group. The 'MUST' report. Nutritional screening of adults: a multidisciplinary responsibility. Development and use of the malnutrition universal screening tool (MUST) for adults. *BAPEN*; 2003. https://www.health.gov.il/download/ng/N500-19.pdf
40. Stratton RJ, Hackston A, Longmore D, et al. Malnutrition in hospital outpatients and inpatients: Prevalence, concurrent validity, and ease of use of the 'malnutrition universal screening tool' ('MUST') for adults. *Br J Nutr.* 2004;92:799–808.
41. Stratton RJ, King CL, Stroud MA, Jackson AA, Elia M. 'Malnutrition universal screening tool' predicts mortality and length of hospital stay in acutely ill elderly. *Br J Nutr.* 2006;95:325–330.
42. Cooper PL, Raja R, Golder J, et al. Implementation of nutrition risk screening using the malnutrition universal screening tool across a large metropolitan health service. *J Hum Nutr Diet.* 2016;29(6):697–703.
43. Rahman A, Wu T, Bricknell R, Muqtadir Z, Armstrong D. Malnutrition matters in Canadian hospitalized patients: malnutrition risk in hospitalized patients in a tertiary care center using the malnutrition universal screening tool. *Nutr Clin Pract.* 2015;30(5):709–713.
44. Boléo-Tomé C, Monteiro-Grillo I, Camilo M, Ravasco P. Validation of the malnutrition universal screening tool (MUST) in cancer. *Br J Nutr.* 2012;108(2):343–348.
45. Skipper A, Coltman A, Tomesko J, et al. Position of the Academy of Nutrition and Dietetics: Malnutrition (Undernutrition) Screening Tools for All Adults. *J Acad Nutr Diet.* 2020;120(4):709–713. doi:10.1016/j.jand.2019.09.011.
46. Kondrup J, Rasmussen HH, Hamberg O, Stanga Z, an ad hoc ESPEN Working Group. Nutritional risk screening (NRS 2002): a new method based on an analysis of controlled clinical trials. *Clin Nutr.* 2003;22(3):321–336.
47. Anthony PS. Nutrition screening tools for hospitalized patients. *Nutr Clin Pract.* 2008;23(4):373–382.
48. Kondrup J, Allison SP, Elia M, Vellas B, Plauth M. ESPEN guidelines for nutrition screening 2002. *Clin Nutr.* 2003;22(4):415–421.
49. McClave SA, Taylor BE, Martindale RG, et al. Guidelines for the Provision and Assessment of Nutrition Support Therapy in the Adult Critically Ill Patient: Society of Critical Care Medicine (SCCM) and American Society for Parenteral and Enteral Nutrition (A.S.P.E.N.). *JPEN J Parenter Enteral Nutr.* 2016;40(2):159-211. doi:10.1177/0148607115621863. [Erratum in: *JPEN* J Parenter Enteral Nutr. 2016;40(8):1200. doi:10.1177/0148607116670155]
50. Rasmussen HH, Holst M, Kondrup J. Measuring nutritional risk in hospitals. *Clin Epidemiol.* 2010;21(2):209–216.
51. Gur AS, Atahan K, Aladag I, et al. The efficacy of nutrition risk screening-2002 (NRS-2002) to decide on the nutritional support in general surgery patients. *Bratisl Lek Listy.* 2009;110(5):290–292.
52. Mercadal-Orfila G, Lluch-Taltavull J, Campillo-Artero C, Torrent-Quetglas M. Association between nutritional risk based on the NRS-2002 test and hospital morbidity and mortality. *Nutr Hosp.* 2012;27(4):1248–1254.
53. Boban M, Laviano A, Persic V, Rotim A, Jovanovic Z, Vcev A. Characteristics of NRS-2002 nutritional risk screening in patients hospitalized for secondary cardiovascular prevention and rehabilitation. *J Am Coll Nutr.* 2014;33(6):466–473.
54. Orell-Kotikangas H, Österlund P, Saarilahti K, Ravasco P, Schwab U, Mäkitie AA. NRS-2002 for pre-treatment nutritional risk screening and nutritional status assessment in head and neck cancer patients. *Support Care Cancer.* 2015;23(6):1496–1502.
55. Guo W, Ou G, Li X, Huang J, Liu J, Wei H. Screening of the nutritional risk of patients with gastric carcinoma before operation by NRS 2002 and its relationship with postoperative results. *J Gastroenterol Hepatol.* 2010;25(4):800–803.
56. Kruizenga HM, Seidell JC, de Vet HC, Wierdsma NJ, van Bokhorst-de van der Schueren MA. Development and validation of a hospital screening tool for malnutrition: the short nutritional screening questionnaire (SNAQ©). *Clin Nutr.* 2005;24(1):75–82.

57. Kruizenga HM, de Jonge P, Seidell JC, et al. Are malnourished patients complex patients? Health status and care complexity of malnourished patients detected by the short nutritional assessment questionnaire (SNAQ). *Eur J Intern Med.* 2006;17(3):189–194.
58. Neelemaat F, Kruizenga HM, de Vet HC, Seidell JC, Butterman M, van Bokhorst-de van der Schueren MA. Screening malnutrition in hospital outpatients. Can the SNAQ malnutrition screening tool also be applied to this population? *Clin Nutr.* 2008;27(3):439–446.
59. van Venrooij LM, de Vos R, Borgmeijer-Hoelen AM, Kruizenga HM, Jonkers-Schuitema CF, de Mol BA. Quick-and-easy nutritional screening tools to detect disease-related undernutrition in hospital in- and outpatient settings: a systematic review of sensitivity and specificity. *e-SPEN Eur E J Clin Nutr Metab.* 2007;2:21–37.
60. Ferguson M, Capra S, Bauer J, Banks M. Development of a valid and reliable malnutrition screening tool for adult acute hospital patients. *Nutrition.* 1999;15(6):458–464.
61. Malnutrition screening tool (MST). Accessed December 26, 2024. https://static.abbottnutrition.com/cms-prod/abbottnutrition-2016.com/img/Malnutrition%20Screening%20Tool_FINAL_tcm1226-57900.pdf.
62. Ferguson ML, Bauer J, Gallagher B, Capra S, Christie DR, Mason BR. Validation of a malnutrition screening tool for patients receiving radiotherapy. *Australas Radiol.* 1999;43(3):325–327.
63. Isenring E, Cross G, Daniels L, Kellett E, Koczwara B. Validity of the malnutrition screening tool as an effective predictor of nutritional risk in oncology outpatients receiving chemotherapy. *Support Care Cancer.* 2006;14(11):1152–1156.
64. Critical Care Connections. NUTRIC Score—Critical Care Nutrition. Published December 16, 2015. Accessed December 20, 2024. https://www.criticalcarenutrition.com/resources/nutric-score.
65. Heyland DK, Dhaliwal R, Jiang X, Day AG. Identifying critically ill patients who benefit the most from nutrition therapy: the development and initial validation of a novel risk assessment tool. *Crit Care.* 2011;15(6):R268. doi:10.1186/cc10546.
66. Jeong DH, Hong SB, Lim CM, et al. Comparison of Accuracy of NUTRIC and Modified NUTRIC Scores in Predicting 28-Day Mortality in Patients with Sepsis: a Single Center Retrospective Study. *Nutrients.* 2018;10(7):911. doi:10.3390/nu10070911.
67. Centers for Medicare & Medicaid Services. Quality ID #487: Screening for Social Drivers of Health; November 2022:1–6. https://qpp.cms.gov/docs/QPP_quality_measure_specifications/CQM-Measures/2023_Measure_487_MIPSCQM.pdf.
68. Office of Disease Prevention and Health Promotion. Healthy People 2030. Health.gov. Published 2024. Accessed December 20, 2024 https://odphp.health.gov/healthypeople/priority-areas/social-determinants-health.
69. Ogunwole SM, Golden SH. Social determinants of health and structural inequities—root causes of diabetes disparities. *Diabetes Care.* 2020;44(1):11–13. doi:10.2337/dci20-0060
70. Howell CR, Zhang L, Yi N, Mehta T, Cherrington AL, Garvey WT. Associations between cardiometabolic disease severity, social determinants of health (SDoH) and poor COVID-19 outcomes. *Obesity.* 2022;30(7). doi:10.1002/oby.2344.
71. Ozieh MN, Garacci E, Walker RJ, Palatnik A, Egede LE. The cumulative impact of social determinants of health factors on mortality in adults with diabetes and chronic kidney disease. *BMC Nephrology.* 2021;22(1). doi:10.1186/s12882-021-02277-2.
72. Chen V, Song M, Suresh D, Wadhwani SI, Perumalswami PV. Effects of social determinants of health on mortality and incident liver-related events and cardiovascular disease in steatotic liver disease. *Aliment Pharmacol Ther.* 2023;58(5):537–545. doi:10.1111/apt.17631
73. Oley Foundation. Accessed December 26, 2024. https://oley.org/
74. Holben DH, Marshall MB. Position of the Academy of Nutrition and Dietetics: Food Insecurity in the United States. *J Acad Nutr Diet.* 2017;117(12):1991–2002. doi:10.1016/j.jand.2017.09.027.
75. Pogatshnik C, Hamilton C. Nutrition-focused physical examination: skin, nails, hair, eyes, and oral cavity. *Support Line.* 2011;33(2):7–13.
76. Gorstein J, Akré J. The use of anthropometry to assess nutritional status. *World Health Stat Q.* 1988;41(2):48–58.
77. Shah B, Sucher K, Hollenbeck CB. Comparison of ideal body weight equations and published height-weight tables with body mass index tables for healthy adults in the United States. *Nutr Clin Pract.* 2006;21(3):312–319.
78. Madden AM, Smith S. Body composition and morphological assessment of nutritional status in adults: a review of anthropometric variables. *J Hum Nutr Diet.* 2016;29(1):7–25.
79. Beghetto MG, Fink J, Luft VC, de Mello ED. Estimates of body height in adult inpatients. *Clin Nutr.* 2006;25(3):438–443.
80. Cereda E, Bertoli S, Battezzati A. Height prediction formula for middle-aged (30-55 y) Caucasians. *Nutrition.* 2010;26(11-12):1075–1081.
81. Venkataraman R, Ranganathan L, Nirmal V, et al. Height measurement in the critically ill patient: a tall order in the critical care unit. *Indian J Crit Care Med.* 2015;19(11):665–668.
82. Centers for Disease Control and Prevention (CDC). National Health and Nutrition Examination survey (NHANES): Anthropometry procedures manual. Updated January 2007. Accessed December 26, 2024. https://stacks.cdc.gov/view/cdc/50334
83. Hickson M, Frost G. A comparison of three methods for estimating height in the acutely ill elderly population. *J Hum Nutr Diet.* 2003;16(1):13–20.
84. Brown JK, Whittemore KT, Knapp TR. Is arm span an accurate measure of height in young and middle-age adults? *Clin Nurs Res.* 2000;9(1):84–94.
85. Brown JK, Feng J, Knapp TR. Is self-reported height or arm span a more accurate alternative measure of height? *Clin Nurs Res.* 2002;11(4):417–432.
86. Gorber SC, Tremblay M, Moher D, Gorber B. A comparison of direct vs. self-report measures for assessing height, weight, and body mass index: a systematic review. *Obes Rev.* 2007;8(4):307–326.
87. Berger MM, Cayeux M, Schaller M, Soguel L, Piazza G, Chioléro RL. Stature estimation using the knee height determination in critically ill patients. *e-SPEN Eur E J Clin Nutr Metab.* 2008;3(2):e84–e88.
88. Chumlea WC, Guo SS, Steinbaugh ML. Prediction of stature from knee height for black and white adults and children with application to mobility-impaired or handicapped persons. *J Am Diet Assoc.* 1994;94(12):1385–1388.
89. Hwang IC, Kim KK, Kang HC, Kang DR. Validity of stature-predicted equations using knee height for elderly and mobility impaired persons in Koreans. *Epidemiol Health.* 2009;31:e20009004.

90. Chumlea WC, Guo SS, Wholihan K, Cockram D, Kuczmarski RJ, Johnson CL. Stature prediction equations for elderly non-Hispanic white, non-Hispanic Black, and Mexican-American persons developed from NHANES III. *J Am Diet Assoc.* 1998;98(2):137–142.
91. Müller MJ. Ideal body weight or BMI: so, what's it to be? *Am J Clin Nutr.* 2016;103(5):1193–1194.
92. Peterson CM, Thomas DM, Blackburn GL, Heymsfield SB. Universal equation for estimating ideal body weight and body weight at any BMI. *Am J Clin Nutr.* 2016;103(5):1197–1203.
93. Hamwi GJ. Changing dietary concepts. In: Donowski TS, ed. *Diabetes Mellitus: Diagnosis and Treatment.* American Diabetes Association; 1964:73–78.
94. Pai MP, Paloucek FP. The origin of the "ideal" body weight equations. *Ann Pharmacother.* 2000;34(9):1066–1069.
95. Ireton-Jones C. Adjusted body weight, con: why adjust body weight in energy-expenditure calculations? *Nutr Clin Pract.* 2005;20(4):474–479.
96. Kohn JB. Adjusted or ideal body weight for nutrition assessment? *J Acad Nutr Diet.* 2015;115(4):680.
97. Barak N, Wall-Alonso E, Sitrin MD. Evaluation of stress factors and body weight adjustments currently used to estimate energy expenditure in hospitalized patients. *JPEN J Parenter Enteral Nutr.* 2002;26(4):231–238.
98. Krenitsky J. Adjusted body weight, pro: Evidence to support the use of adjusted body weight in calculating calorie requirements. *Nutr Clin Pract.* 2005;20(4):468–473.
99. Andrews AM, Pruziner AL. Guidelines for using adjusted versus unadjusted body weights when conducting clinical evaluations and making clinical recommendations. *J Acad Nutr Diet.* 2017;117(7):1011–1015.
100. Osterkamp LK. Perspective on assessment of human body proportions of relevance to amputees. *J Am Diet Assoc.* 1995;95(2):215–218.
101. Mozumdar A, Roy SK. Method for estimating body weight in persons with lower-limb amputation and its implication for their nutritional assessment. *Am J Clin Nutr.* 2004;80(4):868–875.
102. Gunal A. How to determine 'dry weight'? *Kidney Int Suppl.* 2013;3(4):377–379.
103. Frankenfield DC, Rowe WA, Cooney RN, Smith JS, Becker D. Limits of body mass index to detect obesity and predict body composition. *Nutrition.* 2001;17(1):26–30.
104. Flegal KM, Kit BK, Orpana H, Graubard BI. Association of all-cause mortality with overweight and obesity using standard body mass index categories. *JAMA.* 2013;309(1):71–82.
105. Zin T, Yusuff ASM, Myint T, Naing DKS, Htay K, Wynn AA. Body fat percentage, BMI and skinfold thickness among medical students in Sabah, Malaysia. *South East Asia J Public Health.* 2014;4(1):35–40.
106. Addo OY, Himes JH. Reference curves for triceps and subscapular skinfold thicknesses in US children and adolescents. *Am J Clin Nutr.* 2010: 91(3): 635–642.
107. Jensen TG, Dudrick SJ, Johnston DA. A comparison of triceps skinfold and upper arm circumference measurements taken in standard and supine positions. *JPEN J Parenter Enteral Nutr.* 1981;5(6):519–521.
108. Heyward V. ASEP Methods Recommendation: body composition assessment. *JEPOnline.* 2001;4(4):1–12.
109. Jackson AS, Pollock ML. Generalized equations for predicting body density in men. *Br J Nutr.* 1978;40:497–504.
110. Jackson AS, Pollock ML, Ward A. Generalized equations for predicting body density of women. *Med Sci Sports Exerc.* 1980;12:175–182.
111. Margoti T. Comparison of results between the equations of body composition of Jackson & Pollock of three and seven skinfolds. *Fit Perf J.* 2009;8(3):191–198.
112. Baranauskas MN, Johnson KE, Juvancic-Heltzel JA, et al. Seven-site versus three-site method of body composition using BodyMetrix ultrasound compared to dual-energy X-ray absorptiometry. *Clin Physiol Funct Imag.* 2017; 37(3):317–321. doi:10.1111/cpf.12307
113. Elsey AM, Lowe AK, Cornell AN, Whitehead PN, Conners RT. Comparison of the three-site and seven-site measurements in female collegiate athletes using BodyMetrix™. *Int J Exerc Sci.* 2021;14(4):230–238
114. Burden ST, Stoppard E, Shaffer J, Makin A, Todd C. Can we use mid upper arm anthropometry to detect malnutrition in medical inpatients? A validation study. *J Hum Nutr Diet.* 2005;18(4):287–294.
115. Zuchinali P, Souza GC, Alves FD, et al. Triceps skinfold as a prognostic predictor in outpatient heart failure. *Arq Bras Cardiol.* 2013;101(5):434–441.
116. University of Colorado Denver. Waist circumference measurements in clinical research. Accessed December 20, 2024. https://cctsi.cuanschutz.edu/docs/librariesprovider28/ctrc/nutrition/waist_circumference_web.pdf?sfvrsn=ceb765b9_2. 93
117. Becker PJ, Nieman Carney L, Corkins MR, et al. Consensus statement of the Academy of Nutrition and Dietetics/American Society for Parenteral and Enteral Nutrition: indicators recommended for the identification and documentation of pediatric malnutrition (undernutrition). *J Acad Nutr Diet.* 2014;114(12):1988–2000.
118. Jeyakumar A, Ghugre P, Gadhave S. Mid-upper-arm circumference (MUAC) as a simple measure to assess the nutritional status of adolescent girls as compared with BMI. *ICAN.* 2013;5(1):22–25.
119. Cattermole GN, Graham CA, Rainer TH. Mid-arm circumference can be used to estimate weight of adult and adolescent patients. *Emerg Med J.* 2017;34(4):231–236.
120. Sultana T, Karim N, Ahmed T, Hossain I. Assessment of under nutrition of Bangladeshi adults using anthropometry: can body mass index be replaced by mid-upper-arm-circumference? *PLoS One.* 2015;10(4):1–8.
121. Powell NJ, Collier B. Nutrition and the open abdomen. *Nutr Clin Pract.* 2012;27(4):499–506.
122. Mei Z, Grummer-Strawn LM, de Onis M, Yip R. The development of a MUAC-for-height reference, including a comparison to other nutritional status screening indicators. *Bull World Health Organ.* 1997;75(4):333–341.
123. Powell-Tuck J, Hennessy EM. A comparison of mid upper arm circumference, body mass index and weight loss as indices of undernutrition in acutely hospitalized patients. *Clin Nutr.* 2003;22(3):307–312.
124. Tang AM, Chung M, Dong KR, et al. Determining a global mid-upper arm circumference cutoff to assess underweight in adults (men and non-pregnant women). *Public Health Nutr.* 2020;23(17): 3104–3113.
125. Hymers R. The use of mid upper arm circumference in the nutritional assessment of the critically ill patient. Scottish Intensive Care Society. Updated 2009. Accessed December 26, 2024. http://www.scottishintensivecare.org.uk/uploads/2014-05-28-23-52-56-TheuseofMidUpperArmCircum-59986.pdf.
126. Weng CH, Tien CP, Li CI, et al. Mid-upper arm circumference, calf circumference and mortality in Chinese long-term

care facility residents: a prospective cohort study. *BMJ Open*. 2018; 8(5):e020485.
127. Tartari RF, Ulbrich-Kulczynski JM, Filho AF. Measurement of mid-arm muscle circumference and prognosis in stage IV non-small cell lung cancer patients. *Oncol Lett*. 2013;5(3):1063–1067.
128. Wang J, Thornton JC, Bari S, et al. Comparisons of waist circumferences measured at 4 sites. *Am J Clin Nutr*. 2003; 77(2):379–384.
129. de Koning L, Merchant AT, Pogue J, Anand SS. Waist circumference and waist-to-hip ratio as predictors of cardiovascular events: meta-regression analysis of prospective studies. *Eur Heart J*. 2007;28(7):850–856.
130. Janssen I, Katzmarzyk PT, Ross R. Waist circumference and not body mass index explains obesity-related health risk. *Am J Clin Nutr*. 2004;79(3):379–384.
131. Vazquez G, Duval S, Jacobs Jr. DR, Silventoinen K. Comparison of body mass index, waist circumference, and waist /hip ratio in predicting incident diabetes: a meta-analysis. *Epidemiol Rev*. 2007;29:115–128.
132. World Health Organization Expert Consultation. Waist circumference and waist-hip ratio: report of a WHO Expert Consultation. December 2008. Accessed December 20, 2024. https://iris.who.int/bitstream/handle/10665/44583/9789241501491_eng.pdf?sequence=1
133. NHLBI Obesity Education Initiative. The practical guide to the identification, evaluation and treatment of overweight and obesity in adults (NIH, 2000). Accessed December 20, 2024. https://www.govinfo.gov/content/pkg/GOVPUB-HE20-PURL-LPS16589/pdf/GOVPUB-HE20-PURL-LPS16589.pdf
134. Ma W, Yang C, Shih S, et al. Measurement of waist circumference: Midabdominal or iliac crest? *Diabetes Care*. 2013;36(6):1660–1666.
135. Mason C, Katzmarzyk PT. Variability in waist circumference measurements according to anatomic measurement site. *Obesity (Silver Spring)*. 2009;17(9):1789–1795.
136. Cerhan JR, Moore SC, Jacobs EJ, et al. A pooled analysis of waist circumference and mortality in 650,000 adults. *Mayo Clin Proc*. 2014;89(3):335–345.
137. Britton KA, Massaro JM, Murabito JM, Kreger BE, Hoffmann U, Fox CS. Body fat distribution, incident cardiovascular disease, cancer, and all-cause mortality. *J Am Coll Cardiol*. 2013;62(10):921–925.
138. Ross R, Neeland IJ, Yamashita S, et al. Waist circumference as a vital sign in clinical practice: a Consensus Statement from the IAS and ICCR Working Group on Visceral Obesity. *Nat Rev Endocrinol*. 2020;16:177–189. doi:10.1038/s41574-019-0310-7
139. Price GM, Uauy R, Breeze E, Bulpitt CJ, Fletcher AE. Weight, shape, and mortality risk in older persons: Elevated waist-hip ratio, not high body mass index, is associated with a greater risk of death. *Am J Clin Nutr*. 2006;84(2):449–460.
140. Lear SA, James PT, Ko GT, Kumanyika S. Appropriateness of waist circumference and waist-to-hip ratio cutoffs for different ethnic groups. *Eur J Clin Nutr*. 2010;64:42–61.
141. Khan I, Chong M, Le A, et al. Surrogate adiposity markers and mortality. *JAMA Netw Open*. 2023;6(9):e2334836. doi:10.1001/jamanetworkopen.2023.34836
142. Gonzalez MC, Mehrnezhad A, Razaviarab N, Barbosa-Silva TG, Heymsfield SB. Calf circumference: cutoff values from the NHANES 1999-2006. *Am J Clin Nutr*. 2021;113(6):1679–1687.
143. Mamphwe P, Kruger HS, Moss SJ, et al. The association between anthropometric measures and physical performance in black adults of the North West Province, South Africa. *Am J Hum Biol*. 2020;32:e23324. doi:10.1002/ajhb.23324
144. Real GG, Frühauf IR, Sedrez JHK, Dall'Aqua EJF, Gonzalez MC. Calf circumference: a marker of muscle mass as a predictor of hospital readmission. *JPEN J Parenter Enteral Nutr*. 2018;42(8):1272–1279. doi:10.1002/jpen.1170.
145. Camargo Pereira C, Pagotto V, de Oliveira C, Silveira EA. Low muscle mass and mortality risk later in life: a 10-year follow-up study. *PLoS One*. 2022;17(7):e0271579.
146. Li X, Lang X, Peng S, et al. Calf circumference and all-cause mortality: a systematic review and meta-analysis based on trend estimation approaches. *J Nutr Health Aging*. 2022:26(9):826–838.
147. Compher C, Cederholm T, Correia MITD, et al. Guidance for assessment of the muscle mass phenotypic criterion for the Global Leadership Initiative on Malnutrition diagnosis of malnutrition. *JPEN*. 2022;46(6):1232–1242. doi:10.1002/jpen.2366
148. Silver HJ, Welch EB, Avison MJ, Niswender KD. Imaging body composition in obesity and weight loss: challenges and opportunities. *Diabetes Metab Syndr Obes*. 2010;3:337–347.
149. Andreoli A, Scalzo G, Masala S, Tarantino U, Guglielmi G. Body composition assessment by dual-energy X-ray absorptiometry (DXA). *Radiol Med*. 2009;114:286–300.
150. Ross R, Goodpaster B, Kelley D, Boada F. Magnetic resonance imaging in human body composition research from quantitative to qualitative tissue measurement. *Ann N Y Acad Sci*. 2000;904:12–17.
151. Lee Y, Kwon O, Shin CS, Lee SM. Use of bioelectrical impedance analysis for the assessment of nutritional status in critically ill patients. *Clin Nutr Res*. 2015;4(1):32–40.
152. Kyle UG, Boseaus I, De Lorenzo AD, et al. Bioelectrical impedance analysis - part I: review of principles and methods. *Clin Nutr*. 2004;23(5):1225–1243.
153. Kyle UG, Boseaus I, De Lorenzo AD, et al. Bioelectrical impedance analysis - part II: utilization in clinical practice. *Clin Nutr*. 2004;23(5):1430–1453.
154. Walter-Kroker A, Kroker A, Mattiucci-Guehlke M, Glaab T. A practical guide to bioeletrical impedance analysis using the example of chronic obstructive pulmonary disease. *Nutr J*. 2011;10(35):1–8.
155. Savalle M, Gillaizeau F, Maruani G, et al. Assessment of body cell mass at bedside in critically ill patients. *Am J Physiol Endocrinol Metab*. 2012;303:E389–E396.
156. Chahar PS. Comparison of skinfold thickness measurement and bioelectrical impedance method for assessment of body fat. *World Appl Sci J*. 2013;28(8):1065–1069.
157. Andreoli A, Garaci F, Cafarelli FP, Guglielmi G. Body composition in clinical practice. *Eur J Radiol*. 2016;85(8): 1461–1468.
158. Prado CM, Ford KL, Gonzalez MC, et al. Nascent to novel methods to evaluate malnutrition and frailty in the surgical patient. *JPEN*. 2023;47 Suppl 1(Suppl 1):S54–S68. doi:10.1002/jpen.2420.
159. Fischer A, Hertwig A, Hahn R, et al. Validation of bedside ultrasound to predict lumbar muscle area in the computed tomography in 200 non-critically ill patients: the USVALID prospective study. *Clin Nutr*. 2022;41(4):829–837.
160. Litchford M. Putting the nutrition focused physical assessment into practice in long-term care settings. *Ann Longterm Care*. 2013;21(11):38–41.

161. Radler DR, Lister T. Nutrient deficiencies associated with nutrition-focused physical findings of the oral cavity. *Nutr Clin Pract*. 2013;28(6):710–721.
162. Mordarski BA, Hand RK, Wolff J, Steiber AL. Increased knowledge, self-reported comfort, and malnutrition diagnosis and reimbursement as a result of the nutrition-focused physical exam hands-on training workshop. *J Acad Nutr Diet*. 2017;117(11):1822–1828. doi:10.1016/j.jand.2017.06.362
163. Fischer M, JeVenn A, Hipskind P. Evaluation of muscle and fat loss as diagnostic criteria for malnutrition. *Nutr Clin Pract*. 2015;30(2):239–248.
164. Jimenez EY, Lamers-Johnson E, Long JM, Mordarski BA, Ma X, Steiber A. Completion of a nutrition-focused physical exam with hospitalized adults and pediatric patients: secondary analysis of a prospective cohort study. *Nutr Clin Pract*. 2024;39(4):888–902. doi:10.1002/ncp.11137
165. Esper DH. Utilization of nutrition-focused physical assessment in identifying micronutrient deficiencies. *Nutr Clin Pract*. 2015;30(2):194–202.
166. Mauldin K, Gieng J, Saarony D, Hu C. Performing nutrition assessment remotely via telehealth. *Nutr Clin Pract*. 2021;36(4):751–768. doi:10.1002/ncp.10682
167. Russell MK. Functional assessment of nutrition status. *Nutr Clin Pract*. 2015;30(2):211–218.
168. Norman K, Stobäus N, Gonzalez MC, Schulzke J, Pirlich M. Hand grip strength: outcome predictor and marker of nutritional status. *Clin Nutr*. 2011;30(2):135–142.
169. Bohannon RW. Muscle strength: clinical and prognostic value of hand-grip dynamometry. *Curr Opin Clin Nutr Metab Care*. 2015;18(5):465–470.
170. Wang AY, Sea MM, Ho ZS, Lui S, Li PK, Woo J. Evaluation of handgrip strength as a nutritional marker and prognostic indicator in peritoneal dialysis patients. *Am J Clin Nutr*. 2005;81(1):79–86.
171. Hillman TE, Nunes QM, Hornby ST, et al. A practical posture for hand grip dynamometry in the clinical setting. *Clin Nutr*. 2005;24(2):224–228.
172. Matos LC, Tavares MM, Amaral TF. Handgrip strength as a hospital admission nutritional risk screening method. *Eur J Clin Nutr*. 2007;61(9):1128–1135.
173. Jakobsen LH, Rask IK, Kondrup J. Validation of handgrip strength and endurance as a measure of physical function and quality of life in healthy subjects and patients. *Nutrition*. 2010;25(5):542–550.
174. Mendes J, Azevedo A, Amaral TF. Handgrip strength at admission and time to discharge in medical and surgical inpatients. *JPEN J Parenter Enteral Nutr*. 2014;38(4):481–488.
175. Flood A, Chung A, Parker H, Kearns V, O'Sullivan TA. The use of hand grip strength as a predictor of nutrition status in hospital patients. *Clin Nutr*. 2014;33(1):106–114.
176. Garcia MF, Meireles MS, Führ LM, Donini AB, Wazlawik E. Relationship between hand grip strength and nutritional assessment methods used of hospitalized patients. *Rev Nutr*. 2013;26(1):49–57.
177. Norman K, Stobäus N, Smoliner C, et al. Determinants of hand grip strength, knee extension strength and functional status in cancer patients. *Clin Nutr*. 2010;29(5):586–591.
178. McNicholl T, Dubin JA, Curtis L, et al. Handgrip strength, but not 5-meter walk, adds value to a clinical nutrition assessment. *Nutr Clin Pract*. 2019;34(3):428–435.
179. Luna-Heredia E, Martín-Peña G, Ruiz-Galiana J. Handgrip dynamometry in healthy adults. *Clin Nutr*. 2005;24:250–258.
180. Jonnalagadda SS, Mitchell DC, Smiciklas-Wright H, et al. Accuracy of energy intake data estimated by a multiple-pass, 24-hour dietary recall technique. *J Am Diet Assoc*. 2000;100(3):303–308.
181. Kubena KS. Accuracy in dietary assessment: on the road to good science. *J Am Diet Assoc*. 2000;100(7):775–776.
182. Timon CM, van den Barg R, Blain RJ, et al. A review of the design and validation of web- and computer-based 24-h dietary recall tools. *Nutr Res Rev*. 2016;29(2):260–280.
183. Kirkpatrick SI, Collins CE. Assessment of nutrient intakes: introduction to the special issue. *Nutrients*. 2016;8(4):184–187.
184. Subar AF, Freedman LS, Tooze JA, et al. Addressing current criticism regarding the value of self-report dietary data. *J Nutr*. 2015;145(12):2639–2645.
185. Moshfegh AJ, Rhodes DG, Baer DJ, et al. The US Department of Agriculture automated multiple-pass method reduces bias in the collection of energy intakes. *Am J Clin Nutr*. 2008;88(2):324–332.
186. Blanton CA, Moshfegh AJ, Baer DJ, Kretsch MJ. The USDA automated multiple-pass method accurately estimates group total energy and nutrient intake. *J Nutr*. 2006;136(10):2594–2599.
187. Conway JM, Ingwersen LA, Moshfegh AJ. Accuracy of dietary recall using the USDA five-step multiple-pass method in men: an observational validation study. *J Am Diet Assoc*. 2004;104(4):595–603.
188. Chambers EI, McGuire B, Godwin S, McDowell M, Vecchio F. Quantifying portion sizes for selected snack foods and beverages in 24-hour dietary recalls. *Nutr Res*. 2000;20(3):315–326.
189. Subar AF. Developing dietary assessment tools. *J Am Diet Assoc*. 2004;104(5):769–770.
190. National Cancer Institute. Usual dietary intakes: The NCI method. Epidemiology and Genomics Research Program. Updated August 19, 2024. Accessed December 26, 2024. https://epi.grants.cancer.gov/diet/usualintakes/method.html
191. Sharp DB, Allman-Farinelli M. Feasibility and validity of mobile phones to assess dietary intake. *Nutrition*. 2014;30(11–12):1257–1266.
192. Lim SL, Lin XH, Daniels L. Seven-point subjective global assessment is more time sensitive than conventional subjective global assessment in detecting nutrition changes. *JPEN*. 2016;40(7):966–972. doi:10.1177/0148607115579938
193. Duerksen DR, Laporte M, Jeejeebhoy K. Evaluation of nutrition status using the subjective global assessment: malnutrition, cachexia, and sarcopenia. *Nutr Clin Pract*. 2021;36(5):942–956. doi:10.1002/ncp.10613
194. Nestle Nutrition Institute. Development and Validation of the MNA. Accessed December 26, 2024. https://www.mna-elderly.com/development-and-validation
195. Vellas B, Guigoz Y, Garry PJ, et al. The Mini Nutritional Assessment (MNA) and its use in grading the nutritional state of elderly patients. *Nutrition*. 1999;15(2):116–122. doi:10.1016/s0899-9007(98)00171-3.
196. Rao KV, Balakrishna N. Feasibility of Broka's index for the nutritional status of adults. *Indian J Med Res*. 1995;102:173–178.
197. Hamwi GJ. Therapy: changing dietary concepts. In: Danowski TS, ed. *Diabetes Mellitus: Diagnosis and Treatment*. American Diabetes Association; 1964:73–78.

198. Devine BJ. Gentamicin therapy. *Drug Intell Clin Pharm.* 1974;8:650–655. Reference for Robinson (1983):
199. Robinson JD, Lupkiewicz SM, Palenik L, Lopez LM, Ariet M. Determination of ideal body weight for drug dosage calculations. *Am J Hosp Pharm.* 1983;40:1016–1019.
200. Miller DR, Carlson JD, Lyod BJ, Day BJ. Determining ideal body weight [and mass]. *Am J Hosp Pharm.* 1983;40:1622.
201. Hammond KA. Dietary and clinical assessment. In: Mahan LK, Stump SE, eds. Krause's Food, Nutrition Therapy. 10th ed. Saunders; 2000:353–379.
202. Peterson CM, Thomas DM, Blackburn GL, Heymsfield SB. Universal equation for estimating ideal body weight and body weight at any BMI. *Am J Clin Nutr.* 2016;103(5):1197–1203.

CHAPTER 2

Biochemical Assessment

Lydia McGrath
Kelly Kane

CHAPTER OUTLINE

Core Concepts
Introduction
Specimen and Assay Types
Routine Medical Laboratory Tests
Fluid and Electrolytes
Acid-Base Physiology
Glucose and Glycosylated Hemoglobin
Protein Assessment
Lipid Profile
Hematology
Vitamins and Trace Elements
Clinical Applications: Order-Writing Privileges
Chapter Summary

CORE CONCEPTS

1. Biochemical assessment is an essential component of the nutrition care process and must be interpreted alongside other assessment data (e.g., physical findings, patient history, anthropometrics) for accuracy.
2. Nutrient concentrations in plasma do not necessarily reflect total body nutrient stores, and may be influenced by factors such as disease, inflammation, and recent dietary intake.
3. Refeeding syndrome can result in nutritional abnormalities due to carbohydrate intake triggering a sudden release of insulin and subsequent intracellular shift of potassium, phosphorus, and magnesium, as well as fluid retention.
4. Fluid, electrolyte, and acid-base imbalances can lead to serious complications, ranging from metabolic and gastrointestinal problems to cardiovascular, respiratory, and neurological concerns, each requiring careful evaluation, monitoring, and treatment.
5. Visceral proteins can be altered by acute and chronic metabolic stress, making them more accurate indicators of inflammation than indicators of nutritional status.
6. Lipid profile results can be used to assess risk of cardiovascular and metabolic disorders as well as overall nutritional status.
7. Deficiencies of iron, vitamin B12, and folate can all compromise red blood cell functioning and contribute to anemia.

LEARNING OBJECTIVES

1. Describe the role of biochemical assessment in the nutrition care process.
2. Identify the causes and treatments of serum electrolyte and fluid imbalances.
3. Explain the metabolic changes that occur during refeeding syndrome.
4. Identify the causes and treatments of metabolic and respiratory acid-base imbalances.
5. Specify two biomarkers used to assess each of the following: endocrine, kidney, liver, and cardiovascular functioning.
6. Name two protein biomarkers used to assess nutritional status and the advantages and disadvantages of each.
7. Define the components of a lipid profile and describe how nutrition can influence blood lipid levels.
8. Identify the components of a hematological test and the role of each in the diagnosis of anemias.
9. Explain the physiologic roles of vitamins and minerals and the signs and consequences of micronutrient deficiencies and toxicities.

Introduction

Biochemical assessment is an essential component of nutrition assessment, the first step in implementing the Nutrition Care Process (NCP) in clinical practice. Laboratory tests of blood, urine, feces, and tissue samples are important indicators of nutritional status and organ function. Evaluation of laboratory values is critical in patients with acute and chronic diseases. Patients with acute illness or injury may experience dramatic changes in laboratory results, while patients with chronic illness may develop laboratory abnormalities more gradually. Comparing laboratory results to reference values and interpreting discrepancies in the context of patients' clinical symptoms and medical history helps clinicians develop appropriate interventions. Laboratory values are essential for monitoring the effectiveness of medical treatments and nutrition interventions and determining when adjustments to the care plan are needed. Biochemical assessment is a carefully controlled process that provides objective, quantitative indicators of nutritional status. However, no single parameter provides a complete picture of nutritional status. Biochemical data should always be interpreted in conjunction with other forms of assessment data such as physical findings, patient history, and anthropometrics. This chapter will review biochemical data such as electrolytes, glucose measures, proteins, enzymes, lipids, hematological tests, and micronutrients, and their significance in identifying fluid and electrolyte imbalances, organ dysfunction, and nutritional abnormalities in clinical practice.

CORE CONCEPT 1

Biochemical assessment is an essential component of the Nutrition Care Process and must be interpreted alongside other assessment data (e.g., physical findings, patient history, anthropometrics) for accuracy.

Specimen and Assay Types

Specimens

There are many types of specimens used for nutrient and nutrient-related analyses. The most common specimens used in nutrition assessment include the following (**Figure 2.1**):

- **Whole blood**: Contains red blood cells (RBCs), white blood cells (WBCs), and platelets suspended in plasma; collected with an anticoagulant when the entire content of the blood is evaluated and none of the elements are removed
- **Serum**: Fluid remaining in blood after blood has been clotted and centrifuged to remove coagulation proteins and blood cells

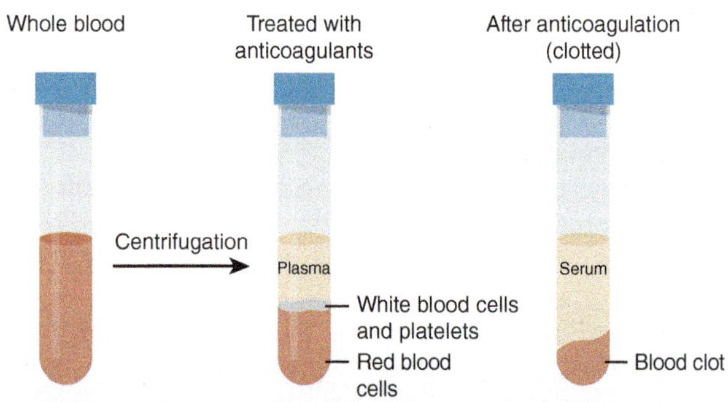

Figure 2.1 Examples of Blood Specimens Collected for Biochemical Assessment

Data from Bartnik K, Janik M, Koba M, Rygiel T, Musolf P, Śmietana M. Biosensing solutions for protein measurement in blood-derived media: a review. *Measurement*. 2025;253:117756. doi:10.1016/j.measurement.2025.117756

CASE STUDY INTRODUCTION

Adam is a 68-year-old male admitted to the hospital with a 1-month history of nausea, vomiting, and diarrhea resulting in weight loss and fatigue. He presents tachycardic with abdominal pain, fever, and chills. Adam is a retired engineer and lives at home with his partner.

Anthropometric Data:

Height: 165 cm
Weight: 75 kg
BMI: 27.5 kg/m^2

Weight History:
Usual body weight: 82 kg (1 year ago)

Biochemical Data:

Sodium 129 (136–145 mEq/L)
Potassium 3.2 (3.5–5.0 mEq/L)
Chloride 90 (96–106 mEq/L)
Carbon dioxide 43 (22–31 mEq/L)
Blood urea nitrogen 30 (8–20 mg/dL)
Creatinine 0.5 (0.7–1.3 mg/dL)
Glucose 166 (70–139 mg/dL)
Magnesium 1.3 (1.5–2.7 mg/dL)
Calcium 8.0 (8.5–10.5 mg/dL)
Phosphorus 2.7 (2.5–4.5 mg/dL)
Albumin 2.6 (3.5–5.5 g/dL)

Total cholesterol 233 (Desirable <200 mg/dL)
LDL-cholesterol 41 (Desirable <100 mg/dL)
HDL-cholesterol 52 (Desirable ≥40 mg/dL)
Triglycerides 40 (Desirable <150 mg/dL)
Hemoglobin 11.1 (14–18 g/dL)
Hematocrit 36.4 (40–50%)
White blood cells 6×10^9 ($5–10 \times 10^9$/L)
Mean corpuscular volume 89 (80–100 fL)
Mean corpuscular hemoglobin concentration 32 (32–36 g/dL)
Serum osmolality 250 (275–295 mOsm/kg)
Red cell distribution width 50 (39–46 fL)

Clinical Data:

Past Medical History: Hypertension, dyslipidemia, hypertriglyceridemia, gastroesophageal reflux disease
Medications: aspirin, atorvastatin, captopril, loperamide, omeprazole
Vital Signs: Blood pressure 110/50 mm Hg, Temperature 99.5°F, Heart rate 115 beats/min, tachycardic
Nutrition-focused Physical Exam: Patient noted to be pale with dry skin and poor skin turgor. Temporal muscles mildly wasted. Upper arm fat loss and lower extremity muscle wasting evident. Abdomen appears slightly distended. Oral exam notable for a dry tongue and good dentition. No wounds observed and no edema noted. No shortness of breath evident.
Dietary Data:
Dietary History: Normal appetite. Adam reveals that he has avoided high-fat foods for the past year and limits his sodium intake. He reports that he has had minimal intake for 3–4 days prior to admission.
Usual Diet Recall:
Breakfast: 8 oz orange juice, hard-boiled egg, 1/2 bagel with 2 oz cream cheese
Lunch: Sandwich with 3–4 oz turkey or ham and mustard on white bread, canned soup, 1 oz potato chips, 1% milk, apple
Dinner: 4 oz baked chicken, 2/3 cup rice, 1/2 cup cooked green beans
Diet Prescription: NPO (nil per os)

Questions

1. What are Adam's nutritional risk factors?
2. Describe the possible pathophysiologic etiology associated with Adam's electrolyte abnormalities.
3. Write two Problem/Etiology/Signs and Symptoms (PES) statements for Adam identifying Adam's active issues.
4. Identify the interventions you would like to initiate for Adam to address the problems identified in your PES statements.
5. What biochemical indices should be included in your monitoring and evaluation plan? Why?

- **Plasma**: Component of blood composed of water, blood proteins, organic electrolytes, and clotting factors
- **Blood cells**: Measurement of cellular components, separated from anticoagulated whole blood

In addition to blood, other specimens can also be used for analysis:

- **Urine**: Contains a concentrate of excreted metabolites from a random sample or timed collection

- **Feces**: Used to evaluate the composition of gut flora and extent of nutrient absorption; obtained from random sample or timed collection
- **Hair and nails**: Identifies exposure to toxic metals (e.g., cadmium, lead) and may be an indicator of levels of trace elements (e.g., zinc, copper, chromium, and manganese)
- **Saliva**: Noninvasive medium with a high turnover, used to evaluate functional adrenal stress and hormone levels
- **Breath tests**: Performed on the air generated from exhalation; less common and less invasive tool to assess nutrient metabolism; can help identify intolerance to sugars such as lactose, fructose, and sucrose

Assays

Two types of laboratory assays are available to measure nutrient levels in specimens: static and functional assays. **Static assays** are used to measure the actual level of a nutrient in the specimen. This type of assay is specific to the nutrient of interest, although the concentration of the nutrient within the specimen does not always reflect its amount stored in body pools and tissues. Serum levels of nutrients may be influenced by the status of their protein carriers, which may be altered by inflammation. Additionally, the concentration of a nutrient in serum, plasma, or another fluid or tissue may be influenced by recent dietary intake. To address this limitation, overnight (8–12 hours) fasting is often recommended when collecting static assays.[1] Examples of static assays include serum iron, serum ascorbic acid, serum alpha tocopherol, plasma 25-hydroxy vitamin D, total red blood cell folate, and urinary riboflavin excretion.[2]

Functional assays evaluate the biochemical or physiological functions influenced by a nutrient, rather than the concentration of the nutrient itself. These tests can help provide a comprehensive view of nutritional status by evaluating the body's functional capacity, rather than just nutrient levels. Functional assays are not always specific for one nutrient of interest, as many physiological processes and enzymatic activities depend on multiple nutrients. Examples of functional assays include the following:

- Serum methylmalonic acid (MMA): used to detect vitamin B12 deficiency, since MMA levels increase when vitamin B12 is not present in sufficient amounts
- Erythrocyte transketolase (ETK) activity test: measures the ability of the ETK enzyme to catalyze a thiamine-dependent reaction, with a significant rise in ETK activity after the addition of exogenous thiamine indicating thiamine insufficiency
- Prothrombin time (PT): measures the time it takes for blood to clot; can help assess vitamin K status, as vitamin K deficiency impairs coagulation, causing prolonged PT

CORE CONCEPT 2

Nutrient concentrations in plasma do not necessarily reflect total body nutrient stores, and may be influenced by disease, inflammation, and recent dietary intake.

Decreased red blood cell concentrations and increased plasma levels (**hemodilution**) and increased red blood cell concentrations and decreased plasma levels (**hemoconcentration**) can result from a gain or loss of plasma volume, respectively. As with abnormalities in fluid volume, an imbalance of plasma volume can contribute to an imbalance in **electrolytes**, or substances that dissolve into ions in solution. This can in turn interfere with accurate interpretation of biochemical assessment tests. For instance, during pregnancy, an increase in total cell and plasma volume can cause hemodilution and create an artificial anemia known as "physiologic anemia of pregnancy."[3] Additionally, in cases of extreme edema, hemodilution may decrease serum sodium levels, providing a false indication of hyponatremia that warrants different treatment than true hyponatremia.

PRACTICE POINT

Biochemical assessment in patients with hemodilution or hemoconcentration requires careful interpretation and management, due to the confounding effects of plasma volume.

Routine Medical Laboratory Tests

Blood Chemistry Tests

Most laboratory tests can be ordered as a panel, a grouping of tests, or as individual tests. The **basic metabolic panel (BMP)** and **comprehensive metabolic panel (CMP)** are the most commonly ordered laboratory panels. The BMP, also referred to as the "CHEM-7," measures glucose, sodium, potassium, carbon dioxide, chloride, blood urea nitrogen (BUN),

Table 2.1 Components of Common Laboratory Panels

BMP	CMP	Lipid Panel	RFP	HFP
Glucose Na^+ K^+ CO_2 Cl^- BUN Creatinine	Glucose Na^+ K^+ CO_2 Cl^- BUN Creatinine Albumin Total protein ALP ALT AST Bilirubin	Total cholesterol LDL-cholesterol HDL-cholesterol TG	Albumin BUN BUN:Creatinine Calcium CO_2 Cl^- Creatinine Glucose PO_4^{2-} Na^+ K^+	ALT Albumin ALP AST Bilirubin Total protein

ALP, alkaline phosphate; ALT, alanine aminotransferase; AST, aspartate aminotransferase; BMP, basic metabolic panel; BUN, blood urea nitrogen; Cl^-, chloride; CMP, comprehensive metabolic panel; CO_2, carbon dioxide; K^+, potassium; LDL, low-density lipoprotein; HDL, high-density lipoprotein; TG, triglycerides; RFP, renal function panel; HFP, hepatic function panel; Na^+, sodium

and creatinine. The CMP includes all components of the BMP plus albumin, total protein, alkaline phosphatase, alanine transaminase, aspartate transaminase, and bilirubin.

A **lipid panel** typically measures total cholesterol, low-density lipoprotein (LDL)-cholesterol, high-density lipoprotein (HDL)-cholesterol, and triglycerides. Lipid panels are frequently used to screen for dyslipidemia, a condition characterized by any abnormality of the blood lipids, as well as cardiovascular disease risk.

Various organ- or disease-oriented panels may also be ordered. A **renal function panel**, which assesses kidney function, typically includes albumin, BUN, BUN:creatinine ratio, calcium, carbon dioxide, chloride, creatinine, glucose, phosphorus, potassium, and sodium.[4] A **hepatic function panel**, which assesses liver function, typically includes alanine aminotransferase, albumin, alkaline phosphatase, aspartate aminotransferase, direct bilirubin, total bilirubin, and total serum protein.[4] Components of common laboratory panels are summarized in **Table 2.1**.

Complete Blood Count

A **complete blood count** (CBC) provides information on the general composition of all formed elements in the peripheral blood (white blood cells, platelets, and red blood cells). **Table 2.2** outlines the components of a CBC. A **differential count** is a CBC that measures the number of each type of white blood cell. A CBC can be helpful in evaluating a wide range of conditions, including infection, bleeding, and certain types of cancer.

Table 2.2 Components of a Complete Blood Count

Hemoglobin (Hgb)
Hematocrit (Hct)
Red Blood Cell (RBC) Count
Mean Corpuscular Volume (MCV)
Mean Corpuscular Hemoglobin (MCH)
MCH Concentration (MCHC)
Red Cell Distribution Width (RCDW)
Platelet Count
Mean Platelet Volume (MPV)

Data from El Brihi J, Pathak S. *Normal and abnormal complete blood count with differential*. In: StatPearls [Internet]. Treasure Island, FL: StatPearls Publishing; 2025. Updated June 8, 2024. Available from: https://www.ncbi.nlm.nih.gov/books/NBK604207

Stool Tests

Stool tests may be performed to assess the presence of blood, pathogens, and gut flora, especially among adults older than 50 years and individuals with unexplained anemia. Stool culture testing may also be ordered for patients with prolonged diarrhea, suspected food-borne illness, chronic gastrointestinal (GI) symptoms, or unexplained weight loss.

Urinalysis

A urinalysis measures urine color, appearance, specific gravity, pH, and chemical parameters such as protein, glucose, ketones, blood, and bilirubin. A urine specific gravity test compares the density of urine to the density of water, providing information on the kidneys' capacity to dilute or concentrate urine.

Fluid and Electrolytes

Bodily fluids can vary widely in the concentration and distribution of dissolved substances. To maintain an environment necessary for normal cell functioning, numerous regulatory mechanisms work simultaneously to achieve electrolyte and fluid balance, which can be disrupted by acute and chronic illnesses. Evaluation and treatment of fluid and electrolyte imbalance is critical in practice, as these imbalances can have significant consequences on numerous organ systems.

Fluid Distribution

Water constitutes approximately 50–60% of body weight, with a higher percentage among infants and children and a lower percentage among women and individuals with obesity. Those with more body fat have proportionally less water because adipose tissue contains less water than lean body mass. Therefore, total body water (TBW) is a function of weight, age, sex, and lean body mass. TBW is divided into two main compartments: intracellular fluid (ICF) and extracellular fluid (ECF) (**Figure 2.2**). ICF is contained within cells and accounts for about two-thirds of TBW, and ECF is outside cells and accounts for one-third of TBW. ECF is further divided into three compartments: interstitial fluid, blood plasma, and transcellular fluid. Interstitial fluid, which makes up about 75% of ECF (25% of TBW), is the fluid that lies between blood vessels. Plasma, which accounts for 20% of ECF (7% of TBW), is fluid within blood vessels. The remaining 5% of ECF (1% of TBW) is transcellular fluid, which is fluid contained in body cavities, such as within joints and in the space surrounding the brain and spinal cord.[5]

ECF is the most clinically important fluid compartment because it contains interstitial fluid (surrounding cells) and intravascular fluid (within blood). The distribution of water between each fluid compartment is determined primarily by **osmotic pressure**, which is the pressure needed to maintain equilibrium with no net movement of solvent. Each compartment has one major active solute that determines its osmotic pressure and holds water within the compartment. Sodium is the dominant extracellular osmole, potassium is the dominant intracellular osmole, and plasma proteins are the primary substances in intravascular space. Under normal conditions, the sodium-potassium-adenosine triphosphate (Na^+–K^+-ATPase) pump maintains the solute compositions of ECF and ICF. **Table 2.3** provides the ionic composition of intracellular and extracellular fluid.

Osmotic pressure is expressed using **osmolality**, which represents the number of osmotically active particles per kilogram of solvent (mOsm/kg). Osmolality may be confused with **osmolarity**, which is a measure of the number of dissolved particles per liter of solution (mOsm/L). Direct measurements (using an osmometer) measure osmolality, while calculated measurements are estimates of osmolarity. For practical purposes, however, these measurements may be considered interchangeable. The term "osmolality" will be used throughout this discussion for consistency. Normal serum osmolality ranges from 275 to 295 mOsm/kg.[6] Serum osmolality (in mOsm/kg) can be calculated using the following equation[7]:

$$S_{osm} = (2 \times \text{Sodium, in mEq/L}) + (\text{Glucose, in mg/dL}/18) + (\text{BUN, in mg/dL}/2.8)$$

Sample Calculation: Sodium 135 mEq/L, Glucose 105 mg/dL, BUN 33 mg/dL

$$S_{osm} = (2 \times 135) + (105/18) + (33/2.8)$$
$$S_{osm} = 288 \text{ mOsm/kg}$$

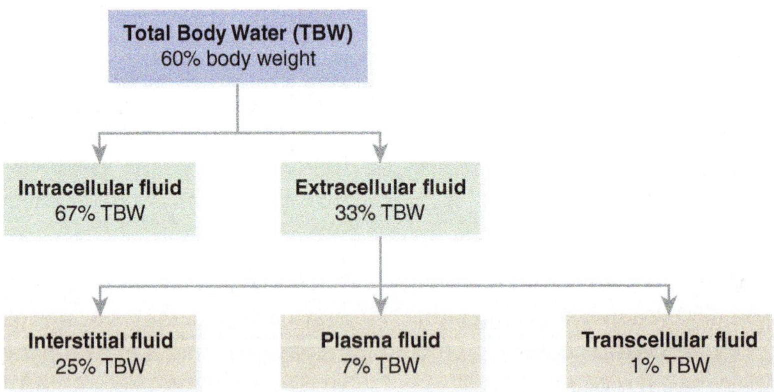

Figure 2.2 Intracellular and Extracellular Fluid

Data from Aronson PS, Boron WF, Boulpaep EL. Transport of solutes and water. In: Boron WF, Boulpaep EL, eds. *Medical Physiology*. 3rd ed. Elsevier; 2017.

Table 2.3 Ionic Composition of Intracellular and Extracellular Fluid

Electrolytes	Extracellular* Fluid Concentration (mEq/L)	Intracellular† Fluid Concentration (mEq/L)
Cations		
Sodium (Na^+)	140	13
Potassium (K^+)	5	140
Calcium (Ca^{2+})	5	Minimal
Magnesium (Mg^{2+})	2	7
Total	**151**	**160**
Anions		
Chloride (Cl^-)	104	3
Bicarbonate (HCO_3^-)	24	10
Sulfate (SO_4^{2-})	1	—
Phosphate (PO_4^{2-})	2	107
Proteins	15	40
Organic anions	5	—
Total	**151**	**160**

* Values are for plasma. Interstitial fluid concentration varies slightly (about 4%).

† Values are for cell water in muscle.

Data from Shils ME, Shike M, Ross AC, et al, eds. *Modern Nutrition in Health and Disease*.10th ed. Lippincott Williams & Wilkins; 2005:149-193.

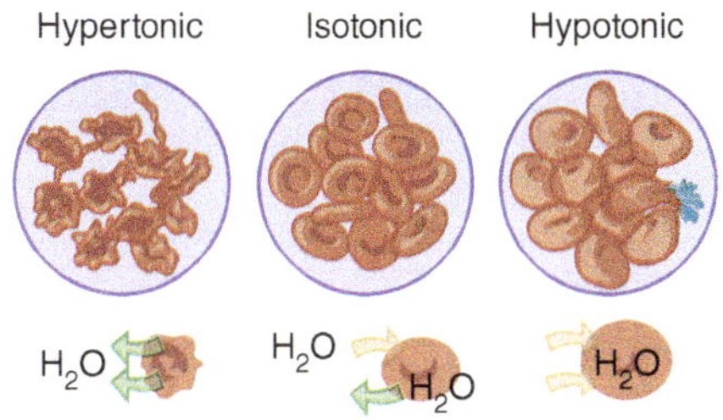

Figure 2.3 Fluid Distribution Based on Tonicity: Red Blood Cells in Hypertonic, Isotonic, and Hypotonic Solution

For example, a patient with a sodium level of 135 mEq, glucose of 105 mg/dL, and BUN of 33 mg/dL would have a serum osmolality level of 288 mOsm/kg, which is considered normal.

Osmolalities of ECF and ICF are assumed to be equal (**isotonic**) under normal conditions. When cells are exposed to solutions with an osmolality greater than that of blood (**hypertonic**), fluids move out of cells in an attempt to establish equilibrium, resulting in cellular dehydration. In contrast, when cells are exposed to solutions with an osmolality less than that of blood (**hypotonic**), fluid moves into cells, causing swelling. **Figure 2.3** illustrates the red blood cell responses to solutions of varying tonicities.

Osmolality is affected by solutes such as glucose, amino acids, and electrolytes (e.g., sodium, chloride, potassium, bicarbonate). Lipids, which are complex and water-insoluble, do not influence osmolality. Thus, in cases where osmolality needs to be limited (e.g., for patients receiving peripheral parenteral nutrition support), lipids may be used to increase total energy supply without raising osmolality.

To better understand the mechanisms of water distribution in ECF and ICF, consider the composition of commonly used intravenous (IV) fluids administered in practice (**Table 2.4**). When 1000 mL of 5% dextrose (hypotonic, solute-free water) is infused, the dextrose is metabolized and the free water distributes evenly across all compartments. Approximately two-thirds (667 mL) of the solution goes to the ICF, where water enters the cell, and one-third (333 mL) goes to the ECF. Alternatively, if 1000 mL of 0.9% sodium chloride (normal saline) is administered, the water is distributed completely to the ECF because sodium is found mainly in the ECF. Approximately 25% (250 mL) goes to intravascular space and 75% (750 mL) goes to interstitial space. In contrast, administration of 3% sodium chloride (hypertonic saline) causes water to move out of cells and into ECF until osmotic equilibrium is reached. The addition of sodium chloride to ECF and the loss of water to ICF would eventually lead to increased osmolalities of both compartments, with the change in volume proportional to the degree of increase in ECF osmolality.

While osmotic pressure determines the distribution of fluid between ECF and ICF, plasma oncotic and hydrostatic pressures influence the movement of fluid between the plasma and interstitial fluid. Under normal conditions, these compartments are maintained in a steady state and the pressures are generally balanced, despite large fluid exchanges between compartments.

When disruption in oncotic and/or hydrostatic pressure favors fluid movement from intravascular to interstitial fluid, **third spacing** occurs. Third spacing is the accumulation of fluid in the interstices (edema) or in the potential fluid spaces (effusion) between body cavities. An example of edema is displayed in **Figure 2.4**. Third spacing is common in critical

Table 2.4 Composition of Commonly Used Intravenous Fluids

Solution	Dextrose (g/L)	Sodium (mEq/L)	Tonicity	Free Water (mL/L)	Uses
D5W (5% Dextrose)	50	0	Hypotonic	1000	Provides free water
0.45% NaCl (1/2 Normal Saline)	0	77	Hypotonic	500	Provides free water and sodium
0.9% NaCl (Normal Saline)	0	154	Isotonic	0	Replaces ECF volume
Lactated Ringer's	0	130	Isotonic	0	Replaces ECF volume; provides electrolyte content similar to plasma
3% NaCl (Hypertonic Saline)	0	513	Hypertonic	Negative (loss of free water)	Treats severe, symptomatic hyponatremia

ECF: extracellular fluid
Data from Bruno JJ. *ASPEN Fluids, Electrolytes, and Acid-Base Disorders Handbook*. 2nd ed. American Society for Parenteral and Enteral Nutrition; 2020.

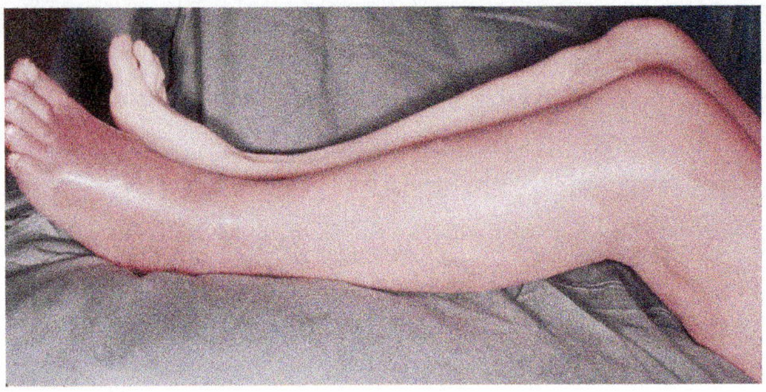

Figure 2.4 Localized Edema

illness, as increased capillary permeability may cause albumin to leak into interstitial space, leading to a decline in plasma oncotic pressure. Although fluid will be reabsorbed into extracellular compartments over a period of days, the acute drop in blood volume is associated with severe volume depletion. Thus, fluid intake and output should be monitored carefully in these circumstances.

Fluid and Electrolyte Disorders

Fluid and electrolyte disorders can be classified by disturbances of volume, concentration, or composition, which often occur concurrently in clinical practice. Volume overload (**hypervolemia**) and volume depletion (**hypovolemia**) occur when there is a gain or loss in fluid, respectively, which alters extracellular fluid volume. Disorders of fluid balance can occur simultaneously with imbalances of electrolytes such as sodium, potassium, magnesium, calcium, phosphorus, chloride, bicarbonate, and hydrogen ions. For example, a change in sodium concentration leading to a change in plasma osmolality contributes to a gain or loss of water (overhydration or dehydration, respectively). Excessive losses from the GI tract and abnormalities in kidney function are often the primary contributors to electrolyte imbalances.[8] Understanding the composition of specific body fluids can be helpful in managing fluid and electrolyte disorders, as many causes of water loss may also lead to significant electrolyte losses.

Management of Electrolyte Disorders

Safe and effective treatment of electrolyte disorders requires careful assessment of the etiology of the electrolyte imbalance. If laboratory results are inconsistent with the patient's clinical condition, the accuracy of the specimen sample must be reassessed prior to initiating treatment. This is critical to prevent improper treatment of electrolyte values that could arise from errors in sample collection or handling. Only after laboratory results are validated should clinicians develop a treatment plan.

Generally, when electrolyte levels are above the normal range, removal of exogenous sources or facilitation of electrolyte elimination is recommended. The severity of the electrolyte disorder and presence or absence of symptoms will determine the most appropriate treatment approach. Treatment may include removal of electrolyte supplementation from IV fluids or parenteral/enteral nutrition, discontinuation of medications that may contribute to electrolyte imbalances, and/or inducing renal or GI elimination of the electrolyte(s).

When electrolyte levels are below the normal range, oral or IV electrolyte replacement may be indicated. Intravenous electrolyte replacement is considered optimal for patients with critically low electrolyte levels who are NPO ("nil per os," meaning nothing by mouth) or who have impaired GI functioning or difficulty swallowing. Patients with impaired kidney function should receive conservative electrolyte replacement, unless actively receiving renal replacement therapy. Patients with volume overload should receive volume-restricted electrolyte replacement or oral therapy when possible. Identifying peripheral or central venous access is also important because peripheral administration may limit the volume and rate of administration. Tissue damage may result from exceeding these limits in patients with peripheral access.

Because patients often have more than one electrolyte abnormality, all electrolyte values should be reviewed. The presence of concurrent electrolyte abnormalities requires clinicians to consider optimizing and minimizing replacement. For example, optimizing treatment should be considered if a patient has both hypomagnesemia and hypokalemia. This is because potassium repletion can rarely occur if magnesium is deficient, so magnesium should be corrected before potassium to optimize replacement.[9] Minimizing replacement applies when patients have conditions such as hypokalemia and hypophosphatemia, where potassium phosphate can be used to correct both imbalances simultaneously. Clinicians should also consider product availability and shortages to determine whether conservation or alternate therapy may be required.

Sodium

Sodium (Na^+) is the principal cation in the ECF, with a normal serum concentration of 136–145 mEq/L.[10] Adequate sodium intake for adults is approximately 65 mEq or 1500 mg/day.[11] Sodium is the major osmotic determinant regulating volume and water distribution in the body. Sodium also assists in acid-base balance; activation of enzyme reactions; nerve impulse conduction; and contraction of myocardial, skeletal, and smooth muscles. Sodium levels in the body are regulated primarily by the kidneys, which adjust urinary sodium excretion under the influence of hormones such as aldosterone, to maintain fluid balance and blood pressure.

Hyponatremia

Hyponatremia, or low serum sodium, is the most common electrolyte disorder seen in medical care facilities, affecting 20–35% of hospitalized patients.[12]

Signs and Symptoms. Evaluation of symptoms, rate of onset, and etiology can help clinicians determine the most effective treatment. Most patients with chronic hyponatremia have serum sodium levels ranging from 125 to 135 mEq/L and are asymptomatic or have mild symptoms such as nausea, malaise, vomiting, and disorientation. Headaches, lethargy, agitation, confusion, and altered mental status are common in patients with lower sodium levels in the range of 115–125 mEq/L. Severe symptoms such as seizures, coma, respiratory distress, and death may present when serum sodium falls below 115 mEq/L, due to an inability to maintain blood pressure and support nerves and muscles, which are critical for respiratory and cardiac functioning.

By determining the rate of onset of hyponatremia and assessing medical history and patient symptom information, clinicians can more effectively correct the disorder at a rate similar to that at which it developed. Acute hyponatremia (developing in <48 hours) is more likely to result in cerebral edema, herniation of the brain, and cardiopulmonary arrest. These

CASE STUDY REVISITED

Adam requires treatment for his hyponatremia (Na^+ 129 mEq/L; normal: 136–145 mEq/L). The medical team asks for possible means of correcting his sodium through nutritional modifications of his diet.

Questions

1. What are the possible causes of Adam's hyponatremia?
2. What labs might help you determine its cause?
3. How would you recommend his hyponatremia be treated? Explain your rationale.

rapid adaptations to decreased intracellular osmolality increase the risk of **osmotic demyelination syndrome (ODS)**, which can also develop in patients with chronic hyponatremia when sodium correction is too rapid.[13] To prevent ODS, sodium correction rate should not exceed 10–12 mEq/L/day, or 8 mEq/L for patients at heightened risk of ODS (e.g., those with malnutrition, alcohol use disorder, or advanced liver disease).[13]

Etiology and Treatment. After initial identification of hyponatremia, clinicians should assess serum osmolality to determine the etiology and appropriate treatment. Calculated serum osmolality should be compared to measured serum osmolality. Hyponatremia can occur with high plasma osmolality (hypertonicity), normal osmolality (isotonicity), and low plasma osmolality (hypotonicity).

Hypertonic hyponatremia (serum osmolality >295 mOsm/kg) can be caused by the presence of other osmotically active substances in the ECF, in addition to sodium. This is most often caused by severe hyperglycemia with dehydration or retention of hypertonic infusions of mannitol.[13] The following equation can be used to estimate the correction of serum sodium in hyperglycemia[14]:

$$\text{Corrected Sodium} = \text{Serum Sodium (mEq/L)} + 0.016\,[\text{Serum Glucose (mg/dL)} - 100]$$

Sample Calculation: Sodium 125 mEq/L, Glucose 350 mg/dL

$$\text{Corrected Sodium} = 125 + 0.016\,[350 - 100]$$

$$\text{Corrected Sodium} = 129 \text{ mEq/L}$$

For example, for a patient with a serum sodium of 125 mEq/L and serum glucose of 350 mg/dL, the corrected serum sodium would be 129 mEq/L. The correction factor of 0.016 is based on the assumption that for every 100 mg/dL increase in blood glucose above 100 mg/dL, serum sodium drops by about 1.6 mEq/L.[15]

Isotonic hyponatremia (serum osmolality 275–295 mOsm/kg), also called **pseudohyponatremia**, involves an increased concentration of plasma solutes other than sodium salts (e.g., proteins and lipids). When the concentration of lipids or proteins increases, the water content in a collected specimen declines, resulting in a low measured sodium concentration. This condition is often caused by hyperlipidemia, hyperproteinemia, infusion of hypertonic solutions, or mannitol. Pseudohyponatremia does not reflect true hyponatremia because the concentration of sodium in plasma is normal. Thus, treatment for this condition does not involve administration of exogenous sodium, but rather correction of the underlying cause. With laboratory analysis advancing, pseudohyponatremia is less frequently observed in practice.[16] For practical purposes, hyponatremia in the presence of normal serum osmolality is usually attributed to pseudohyponatremia.

Hypotonic hyponatremia (serum osmolality <275 mOsm/kg) is the most common form of hyponatremia. Once this determination is made, a more detailed assessment of volume status is needed. Hypovolemic (low ECF volume), hypervolemic (high ECF volume), and euvolemic (normal ECF volume) hyponatremia each require distinct treatments.

Hypovolemic hypotonic hyponatremia (low volume, low osmolality) is characterized by a deficit of both sodium and fluid, with a relative excess of sodium loss. Common signs of hypovolemia include decreased blood pressure, tachycardia, dry tongue, flattened neck veins, sunken eyeballs, increased body temperature, and acute weight loss. The causes of fluid losses are divided into two categories: renal and extrarenal. Renal losses, identified by a urine sodium >20 mmol/L, include fluid loss from diuretic excess, osmosis diuresis, mineralocorticoid deficiency, salt-wasting nephritis, pseudohypoaldosteronism, bicarbonaturia, renal tubular acidosis, and ketonuria. Extrarenal losses, identified by a urine sodium <20 mmol/L, are often caused by vomiting, diarrhea, fistula output, excess sweating, burns, open wounds, and fluid drains.

Treatment for hypovolemic hypotonic hyponatremia typically involves volume repletion with isotonic saline, although hypertonic saline may be indicated in cases of acute or severe and symptomatic hyponatremia. The following equation can be used to approximate the sodium deficit[17]:

$$\text{Sodium Deficit (mEq)} = [\text{Desired Sodium (mEq/L)} - \text{Actual Sodium (mEq/L)}] \times \text{TBW}$$

where TBW = Weight (kg) × % body water, and % body water is 0.6 in adult males and 0.5 in adult females

Sample Calculation:
Desired Sodium 135 mEq/L, Actual Sodium 129 mEq/L, Weight 70 kg

$$\text{Sodium Deficit (mEq)} = (135 - 129) \times 70 \times 0.6$$

$$\text{Sodium Deficit} = 252 \text{ mEq}$$

For example, a 70-kg male patient with hyponatremia (sodium 129 mEq/L) would require a gradual administration of 252 mEq of sodium (sodium deficit) to obtain the desired serum sodium of 135 mEq/L.

The constant in this equation is 0.6 to reflect the fact that approximately 60% of body weight is water. Due to variations in body water with age and sex, some formulas will adjust this constant for females, children, and older adults. This formula can be used to determine the amount of sodium needed to reach appropriate serum sodium levels. With 154 mEq/L of sodium, isotonic or normal saline increases sodium gradually at approximately 1 mEq/L for each liter administered. Clinicians should be cautious not to replenish sodium too quickly because this can lead to fluid shifts in the brain and cause central nervous system disturbances.

For patients receiving nutrition support, clinicians should consider changes to fluids or sodium content of formulas. Sodium can be increased using a formula with a higher sodium content, administering sodium chloride tablets, or replacing water flushes with saline solution. For patients receiving parenteral nutrition (PN), changing the formula can increase both fluid and sodium levels. If diuretics are the cause of hypovolemia, clinicians should consider possible medication changes as part of treatment.

Potassium supplementation should be considered when estimating sodium deficit, because potassium can increase plasma sodium and osmolality in hyponatremic patients. The following equation can be used to calculate this effect[17]:

$$\Delta \text{ Plasma Sodium} = [\text{Infusate Sodium} + \text{Infusate Potassium} - \text{Plasma Sodium}]/(\text{TBW} + 1)$$

where TBW = Weight (kg) × % body water, and % body water is 0.6 in adult males and 0.5 in adult females

Sample Calculation:
Infusate Sodium 154 mEq,
Infusate Potassium 30 mEq,
Plasma Sodium 129 mEq/L,
Body Weight 70 kg

$$\Delta \text{ Plasma Sodium} = (154 + 30 - 129)/(70 \times 0.6 + 1)$$

$$\Delta \text{ Plasma Sodium} = 55/43$$

$$\Delta \text{ Plasma Sodium} = 1.3$$

For a 70-kg patient with hyponatremia (sodium 129 mEq/L), infusing 1 L of normal saline (containing 154 mEq sodium) and 30 mEq potassium will raise the plasma sodium by 1.3 units, to approximately 130 mEq/L.

Euvolemic hypotonic hyponatremia (normal volume, low osmolality) often occurs in patients with syndrome of inappropriate antidiuretic hormone (SIADH), a condition characterized by uncontrolled release of antidiuretic hormone (ADH). These patients have stable sodium intake and output but retain large amounts of water due to excess ADH. Common causes of SIADH include central nervous system disturbances, head trauma, lung malignancies, and pneumonia. Fluid restriction of 10–15 mL/kg/day and administration of exogenous salt is the primary treatment for SIADH.[18] Pharmacological therapy with vasopressin receptor antagonists may be required for SIADH refractory to conventional therapy. Other causes of euvolemic hypotonic hyponatremia include psychogenic polydipsia (ingestion of large amounts of water), hypothyroidism, hypopituitarism, medications, and reset osmostat, a condition that occurs when the kidneys adequately concentrate and dilute urine but the threshold for ADH secretion is reset downward.[13,18] In these patients, euvolemia is identified based on the absence of signs of hypovolemia (e.g., tachycardia, decreased skin turgor, dry mucous membranes) or hypervolemia (e.g., edema, ascites).[13] Treatment for euvolemic hypotonic hyponatremia involves restricting fluids to <1–1.5 L/day and correcting the underlying disorder.[15]

Hypervolemic hypotonic hyponatremia (high volume, low osmolality) is observed in patients with kidney failure, heart failure, and other conditions associated with fluid retention and edema. A urine sodium >20 mmol/L suggests hyponatremia due to kidney failure, and a urine sodium <20 mmol/L suggests extrarenal causes such as heart failure, hepatic cirrhosis, and nephritic syndrome. Sodium and fluid restriction and diuretic therapy are the mainstays of treatment for hypervolemic hypotonic hyponatremia. Patients may also be prescribed a vasopressin receptor antagonist (e.g., tolvaptan), a type of medication that causes a selective diuresis of water, without impacting sodium or potassium excretion. **Figure 2.5** and **Figure 2.6** provide an algorithm to define hyponatremia. Treatment approaches for hyponatremia are outlined in **Table 2.5**.

Hypernatremia

Hypernatremia, or increased serum sodium, occurs in approximately 1–4% of hospitalized patients,[19] with values >160 mEq/L associated with increased mortality.[20]

Signs and Symptoms. Clinical manifestations of hypernatremia are similar to those of hyponatremia and include neurologic problems ranging from headaches and dizziness to more severe symptoms of

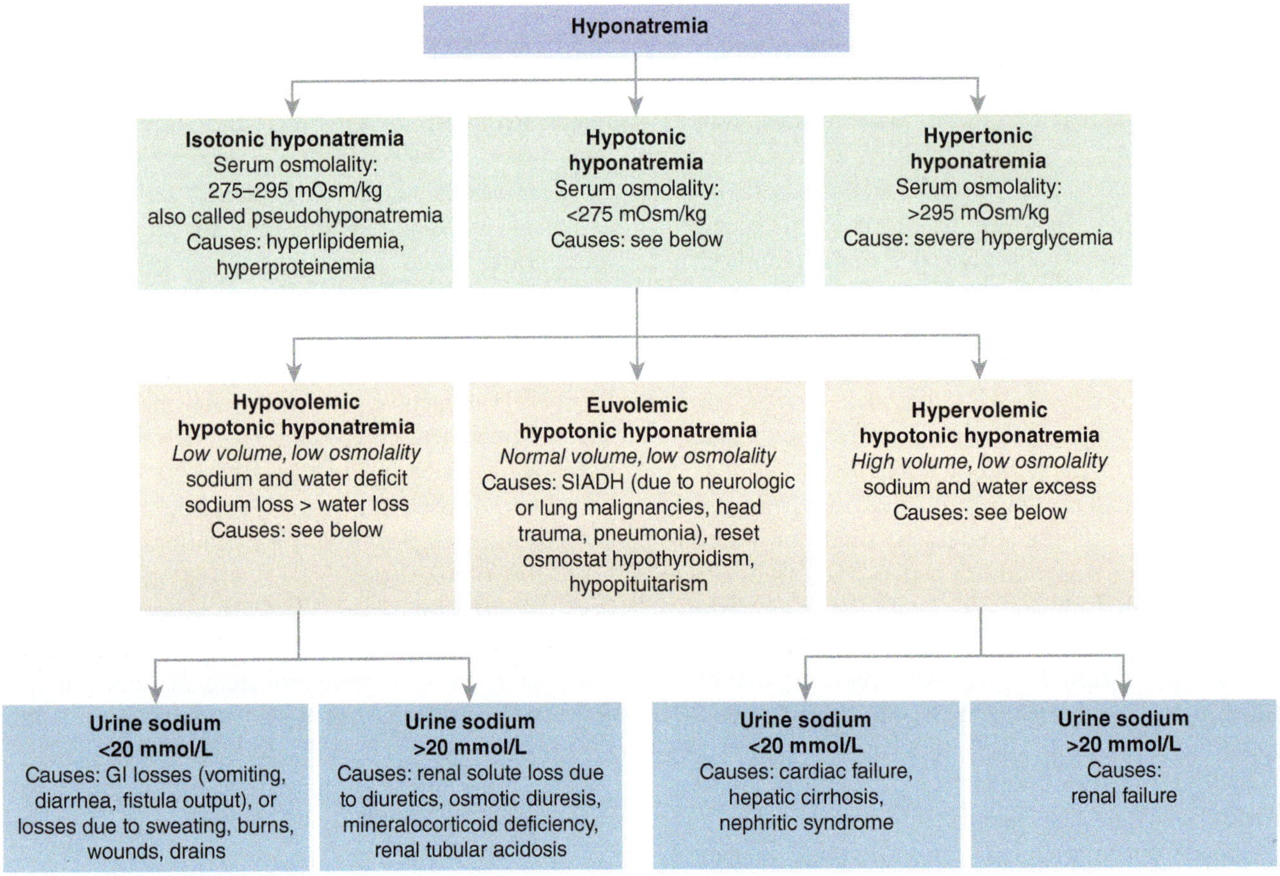

Figure 2.5 Algorithm to Define Hyponatremia

Table 2.5 Treatment for Hyponatremia

Condition	Treatment
Isotonic hyponatremia	Correct the underlying cause (e.g., insulin for hyperglycemia, statin therapy for hyperlipidemia); avoid attempting to correct serum sodium
Hypotonic hyponatremia	Assess volume status ■ If hypovolemic: repletion with isotonic saline, or with hypertonic saline for urgent correction ■ If euvolemic: fluid restriction ■ If hypervolemic: sodium and fluid restriction; diuretic therapy Correct the underlying cause
Hypertonic hyponatremia	Correct the underlying cause (e.g., insulin for hyperglycemia)

Data from Bruno JJ. *ASPEN Fluids, Electrolytes, and Acid-Base Disorders Handbook*. 2nd ed. American Society for Parenteral and Enteral Nutrition; 2020.

seizures, coma, or death. Like hyponatremia, assessment of volume status is the first step in diagnosing hypernatremia.

Etiology and Treatment. *Hypovolemic hypernatremia* occurs when patients have higher sodium levels relative to fluid volumes. Hypovolemic hypernatremia may be due to renal losses (characterized by urine sodium >20 mmol/L) or extrarenal losses (characterized by urine sodium <20 mmol/L). Causes of renal losses include diuretic use, solute diuresis, and acute tubular necrosis. Causes of extrarenal losses include diarrhea and excessive sweating. Treatment for hypovolemic hypernatremia typically begins with administration of isotonic IV fluids (e.g., normal saline or Lactated Ringer's solution) to expand the extracellular fluid volume and stabilize blood pressure. Once blood pressure stabilizes, hypotonic fluids may be provided (orally, enterally, or parenterally) to correct the remaining water deficit.[15]

Euvolemic hypernatremia occurs when patients lose large amounts of dilute, electrolyte-free water.

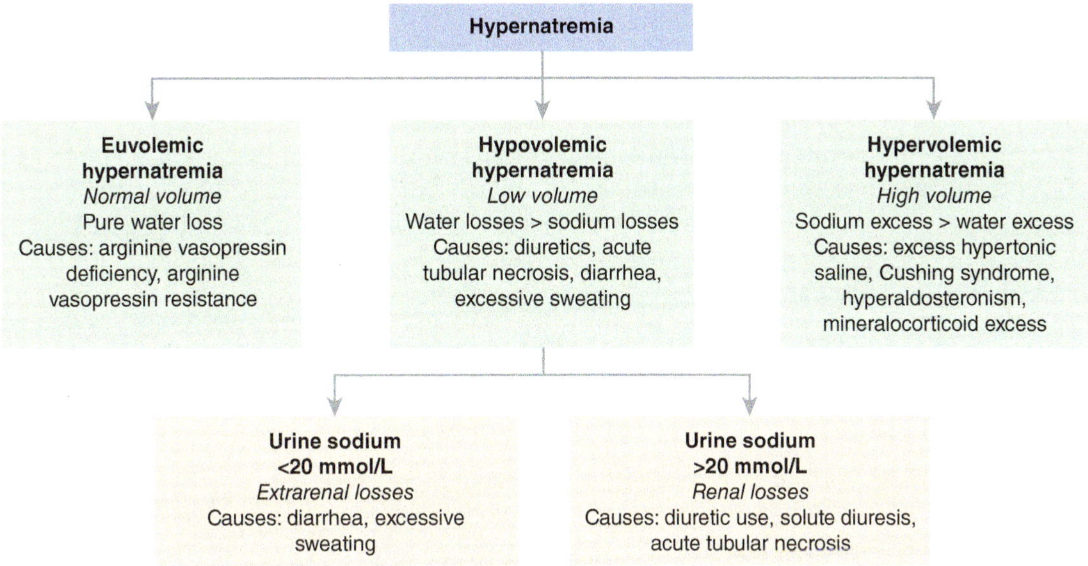

Figure 2.6 Algorithm to Define Hypernatremia

Data from Douglas I. Hyponatremia: why it matters, how it presents, how we can manage it. *Cleve Clin J Med*. 2006;73(suppl 3):S4-S12. doi:10.3949/ccjm.73.suppl_3.s4

This is commonly caused by arginine vasopressin (AVP) disorder, formerly known as "diabetes insipidus."[21] AVP disorder includes AVP deficiency (AVP-D, formerly called "central diabetes insipidus"), which involves impaired ADH secretion in the brain, and AVP resistance (AVP-R, formerly called "nephrogenic diabetes insipidus"), which involves an inability of the kidneys to respond to ADH. The etiology of AVP-D is often idiopathic, inherited, or related to acute trauma to the brain. Possible etiologies of AVP-R include genetic mutations, lithium toxicity, hypercalcemia, and hypokalemia.[22] While treatment differs depending on the etiology, all cases of euvolemic hypernatremia require replacement of water via oral, enteral, or parenteral routes.

Hypervolemic hypernatremia occurs when there is an excess of sodium that is greater than the excess of water. It is most often due to iatrogenic causes such as excess hypertonic fluid administration. For instance, hypernatremia is commonly observed in critically ill patients who receive large amounts of fluid to correct hypovolemia or hypotension. Other potential causes include Cushing syndrome, hyperaldosteronism, and mineralocorticoid excess.[23] Treatment involves correcting the underlying disorder, minimizing fluids, eliminating sodium, and, in some cases, administering diuretics. To evaluate and treat hypernatremia, free water deficit may be calculated as follows:[24]

$$\text{Free Water Deficit (L)} = \text{TBW} \times [\text{Serum Sodium (mEq/L)}/140 - 1]$$

where TBW = Weight (kg) × % body water, and % body water is 0.6 in adult males and 0.5 in adult females

Sample Calculation: Weight 70 kg, Sodium 153 mEq/L

$$\text{Free Water Deficit (L)} = 70 \times 0.6 \times (153/140 - 1)$$

$$\text{Free Water Deficit (L)} = 42 \times 0.09$$

$$\text{Free Water Deficit (L)} = 3.8\ \text{L}$$

For example, a male 70-kg patient with hypernatremia (sodium 153 mEq/L) has a fluid deficit of 3.8 L, meaning a gradual infusion of 3.8 L would be required to lower the serum sodium to normal.

As with hyponatremia, sodium correction should not exceed 10–12 mEq/L/day, or an average of 0.5 mEq/L/hour, due to the risk of cerebral edema and neurological impairment associated with overcorrection.[25] Regular monitoring of serum sodium is necessary to guide appropriate repletion, with the frequency of monitoring proportional to the severity of the hypernatremia.

PRACTICE POINT

Sodium is considered a critical electrolyte because high and low serum levels can lead to serious, potentially irreversible complications. Careful monitoring of sodium is crucial, especially in the acute care setting.

Potassium

Potassium (K^+) is the major intracellular cation, with 98% of total body potassium located within cells.

Normal serum potassium ranges from 3.5 to 5.0 mEq/L, and the recommended adequate intake is 66-87 mEq (2600–3400 mg)/day.[11] Potassium homeostasis is regulated by the Na^+-K^+-ATPase pump, which imports two K^+ ions in exchange for three Na^+ ions, for every molecule of ATP consumed. Factors that influence potassium balance include extracellular pH, exercise, and hormones such as insulin, epinephrine, and aldosterone. Potassium plays an important role in cellular metabolism, transportation of glucose into the cell, and protein and glycogen synthesis, among other processes. The ratio of intracellular to extracellular potassium concentration is essential for maintaining the resting membrane potential and thus supporting neurotransmission and muscle contraction function. Minor shifts in plasma potassium concentration can have significant consequences, so maintaining potassium balance is vital.

Hypokalemia

Hypokalemia, or low serum potassium, is one of the most common electrolyte disorders in clinical practice.[25] It occurs in up to 20% of hospitalized patients, although most cases are mild.[26]

Signs and Symptoms. Patients with mild hypokalemia (serum potassium 3–3.5 mEq/L) are typically asymptomatic but may present with nonspecific symptoms such as generalized weakness, lethargy, muscle cramping, anorexia, and constipation. Symptoms of severe hypokalemia (serum potassium <3 mEq/L) can include muscle necrosis, ascending paralysis, arrhythmias, and possible death.

Etiology. Hypokalemia may be caused by three general mechanisms: increased losses, intracellular shifts, and inadequate intake. Increased losses are the most common cause and include urinary losses and GI losses. Urinary losses are often due to loop diuretics and thiazide diuretics, which act proximal to the potassium secretory site at the kidneys. Although uncommon, chronic licorice ingestion may also cause abnormal urinary potassium loss.[27] This is because licorice contains a compound called "glycyrrhizic acid," which inhibits an enzyme that catalyzes the inactivation of cortisol. Excess glycyrrhizic acid can thus lead to a buildup of cortisol, which has mineralocorticoid activity similar to aldosterone, promoting sodium reabsorption and potassium secretion. Hypokalemia may also be caused by GI losses (e.g., vomiting, diarrhea, and nasogastric suction) and the associated compensatory changes in acid-base balance. For example, the loss of gastric acid from vomiting can lead to metabolic alkalosis, which triggers increased bicarbonate excretion and subsequent renal potassium wasting.[28] Hypokalemia may also result from transcellular shifts of potassium from the ECF to ICF, which may be caused by increased release of insulin or catecholamines (epinephrine), metabolic alkalosis, or refeeding syndrome. Inadequate potassium intake may contribute to hypokalemia, although it is rarely a sole cause.

Treatment. The goals of hypokalemia treatment include preventing or treating life-threatening complications, restoring serum potassium concentrations, correcting the underlying cause, and preventing hyperkalemia. Oral correction of hypokalemia is often preferred due to its safety and relatively low risk of causing rebound hyperkalemia. Oral supplements of potassium chloride are available as a capsule, tablet, or liquid. Potassium preparations include potassium chloride, potassium phosphate, and potassium acetate. Potassium chloride is generally the preferred preparation, as patients with hypokalemia are often chloride-depleted as well (e.g., due to vomiting or diuresis). Potassium acetate is used for patients with metabolic acidosis, and potassium phosphate (the least common preparation) may be considered in cases of coexisting hypokalemia and hypophosphatemia.[29] Oral supplementation of 60–80 mmol/day, provided in divided doses over days to weeks, is generally sufficient to correct mild or moderate hypokalemia.[30]

Only patients with severe hypokalemia or GI disturbances require IV potassium supplementation, with dosing based on kidney function and deficiency severity. For patients requiring IV replacement, potassium chloride given in 40 mmol doses every 3–4 hours is generally preferred.[30] Serum potassium levels are expected to rise by about 0.25 mEq/L with every 20 mEq of IV potassium administered.[30] In most cases, infusion rates should not exceed 20 mEq/hour, although higher rates have been used in emergent cases.[31] Saline should be used as the diluent instead of dextrose, as dextrose can promote an intracellular shift of potassium due to increased insulin release. Continuous cardiac monitoring is recommended if infusion rates exceed 10 mEq/hour, to detect potential signs of hyperkalemia.[31] A central venous catheter is the preferred administration route to minimize phlebitis and burning. **Table 2.6** outlines guidelines for hypokalemia treatment through IV replacement.

Patients with hypokalemia should also be evaluated for hypomagnesemia, since hypomagnesemia may impede potassium repletion and potentially

Table 2.6 Empirical Treatment of Hypokalemia

Serum Potassium Concentration (mEq/L)	Intravenous Potassium Dose (mEq)
3–3.4	20–40
2.5–2.9	40–80
<2.5	80–120

Data from Kraft MD, Btaiche IF, Sacks GS, Kudsk KA. Treatment of electrolyte disorders in adult patients in the intensive care unit. *Am J Health Syst Pharm*. 2005;62(16):1663-1682.

exacerbate hypokalemia-induced cardiac arrhythmias.[31] In patients with severe hypokalemia, repletion of both potassium and magnesium may be required even in the absence of hypomagnesemia, to support maintenance of intracellular potassium levels.[32]

Hyperkalemia

Hyperkalemia, or increased serum potassium, is rare in the general population due to the body's efficient regulatory mechanisms. Individuals are often asymptomatic until serum potassium levels exceed 6.5 mEq/L.[33]

Signs and Symptoms. The clinical manifestations of hyperkalemia are cardiac and neurological in nature, resulting from the inactivation of electrical transmissions across the cell membrane. Signs and symptoms may include muscle twitching, cramping, weakness, ascending paralysis, electrocardiogram changes, and arrhythmias. Other electrolyte imbalances (e.g., hypocalcemia, hyponatremia) and acid-base imbalances can exacerbate the adverse effects of hyperkalemia.

Etiology. Hyperkalemia may be caused by inadequate potassium excretion, increased potassium movement out of cells, and/or increased potassium intake. Inadequate renal excretion is common in patients with acute or chronic kidney disease, due to factors such as reduced glomerular filtration, reduced tubular potassium secretion, and reduced secretion of or responsiveness to aldosterone.[34] Decreased potassium excretion may be due to potassium-sparing diuretics, which are commonly used for heart failure and high blood pressure treatment. Other examples of medication-related hyperkalemia are outlined in **Table 2.7**.

Increased movement of potassium out of cells can be caused by metabolic acidosis, in which potassium moves to the ECF to maintain electroneutrality. In general, serum potassium is expected to increase by 0.6 mEq/L for every 0.1-unit reduction in pH.[35] Extracellular shifts can also result from insulin deficiency, hyperosmolality, tissue catabolism, and strenuous exercise. Another possible cause is pseudohyperkalemia, a condition in which potassium is released from cells following a blood draw. This is commonly due to trauma during venipuncture or hemolysis of blood samples. **Hemolysis**, a term that describes the pathological process of breakdown of red blood cells, can be caused by a variety of technical errors during blood collection, storage, processing, and transport. If a laboratory sample is identified as being hemolyzed (e.g., through visual inspection where the sample may appear tinged with pink or red), it may be rejected and recollected, or reported with a comment on its clinical interpretation.[36] Falsely high potassium levels may also be observed in hematological disorders such as leukocytosis or thrombocytosis.[37] If there is no apparent cause for hyperkalemia, a repeat potassium level should be obtained to confirm a hyperkalemia diagnosis.

Excessive potassium intake rarely causes hyperkalemia in patients with normal kidney function, but it can be an important cause in those with impaired kidney function. Potassium-containing salt substitutes are a notable source of dietary potassium that may be easily overlooked when assessing potassium intake. For patients with kidney disease, consideration of all possible dietary sources of potassium (including natural food sources and potassium-enriched products) is critical for preventing and treating hyperkalemia.

Treatment. Treatment goals differ based on the degree of hyperkalemia and the severity of symptoms. As with other electrolyte disorders, treating the underlying cause is crucial. Intravenous calcium gluconate is recommended as a first-line therapy for hyperkalemic emergencies, as it helps stabilize the cardiac response to hyperkalemia.[15] If excess exogenous potassium or other medications may have contributed to hyperkalemia, these should be discontinued or decreased if feasible. Insulin, dextrose, sodium bicarbonate, and beta-2 adrenergic agents such as albuterol may be administered, as these medications drive potassium intracellularly. To increase potassium excretion, diuretics and GI cation exchangers such as patiromer may be used.[33] Dietary restrictions of potassium may be considered for patients with kidney disease, depending on the patient's individual needs and clinician judgment.[38]

Serum potassium should be closely monitored during treatment, as patients are susceptible to redeveloping hyperkalemia until the underlying etiology is addressed and excess potassium is eliminated. Additionally, blood glucose should be monitored in patients receiving insulin, with dextrose provision adjusted accordingly to prevent or treat hypoglycemia.

Table 2.7 Potential Causes of Drug-Induced Hyperkalemia

Mechanism	Examples
Impaired renal potassium excretion	■ ACE-inhibitors ■ Angiotensin-II receptor blockers ■ Aripiprazole ■ Canagliflozin ■ Cyclosporine ■ Everolimus ■ Potassium-sparing diuretics (spironolactone, epleronone, triamterene, amiloride) ■ Heparin ■ Nonsteroidal anti-inflammatory agents ■ Pentamidine ■ Tacrolimus ■ Trimethoprim
Increased potassium input	■ Packed red blood cells ■ Penicillin G potassium ■ Potassium supplements ■ Salt substitutes
Movement of potassium out of cells	■ Beta-blockers ■ Digoxin intoxication ■ Succinylcholine

Data from Perazella MA. Drug-induced hyperkalemia: Old culprits and new offenders. *Am J Med.* 2000;109(4):307–314.

Phosphorus and Calcium

Phosphorus (P^{3-}) and calcium (Ca^{2+}) are closely interrelated in the body. Homeostasis of these minerals depends on many factors, including clinical conditions and medications. Phosphorus and calcium are regulated primarily through serum phosphorus levels, serum calcium levels, and the actions of three hormones: parathyroid hormone (PTH), calcitriol (the active form of vitamin D), and calcitonin. PTH is released by the parathyroid gland in response to low serum calcium levels. PTH acts directly on two major sites: the bones, where it increases calcium resorption, and the kidneys, where it stimulates calcitriol formation (i.e., vitamin D activation) and increases renal calcium resorption and urinary phosphorus excretion.[39] Calcitriol upregulates intestinal absorption of phosphorus and calcium, thereby increasing serum calcium concentration. Through a negative feedback mechanism, the increase in serum calcium suppresses PTH release, thus lowering vitamin D activation. The increase in serum calcium also stimulates thyroid cells to release **calcitonin**, which inhibits bone resorption and lowers serum calcium levels. Magnesium can also affect calcium homeostasis, as hypermagnesemia may inhibit PTH secretion and hypomagnesemia can stimulate PTH secretion.[40] **Figure 2.7** illustrates the processes involved in phosphorus and calcium homeostasis, and **Table 2.8** summarizes the actions of PTH, active vitamin D, and calcitonin.

Calcium

Calcium (Ca^{2+}) is the most abundant divalent cation in the body and plays a key role in bone structure, blood

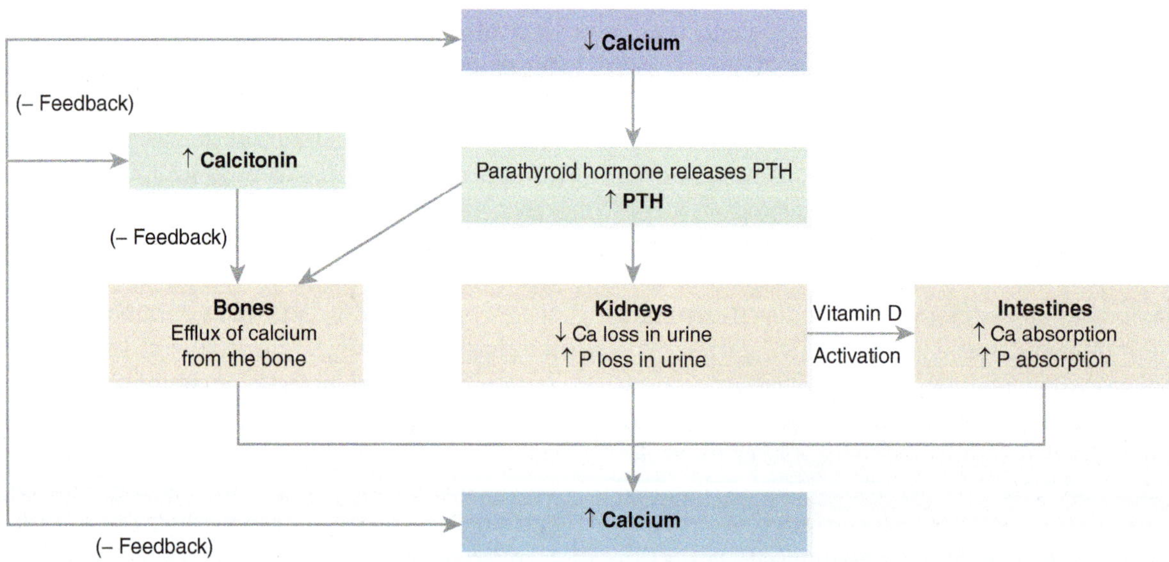

Figure 2.7 Mechanisms Involved in Phosphorus and Calcium Homeostasis

Data from Kraft MD. Phosphorus and calcium: a review for the adult nutrition support clinician. *Nutr Clin Pract.* 2015;30(1):21–33.

Table 2.8 Effects of Parathyroid Hormone (PTH), Calcitriol, and Calcitonin on Calcium Balance

	PTH	Calcitriol	Calcitonin
Serum calcium	↑	↑	↓
Bone calcium	↓	**	↑
Renal calcium reabsorption	↑	↑	↓
Intestinal calcium reabsorption	*	↑	No effect

*Indirect effect via calcitriol production
**Indirect effect via PTH release
Data from Gropper SG, Smith JL, Carr TP. *Advanced Nutrition and Human Metabolism*, 7th ed. Cengage Learning; 2018.

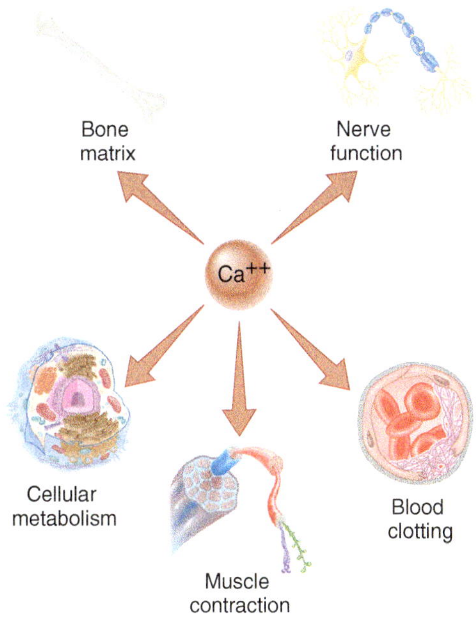

Figure 2.8 Essential Functions of Calcium

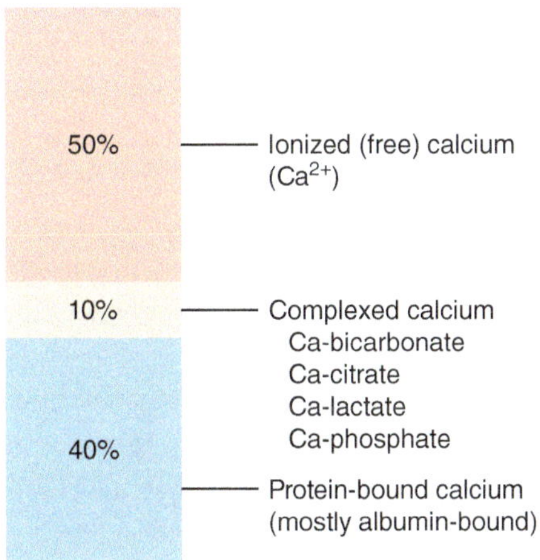

Figure 2.9 Distribution of Extracellular Calcium

Data from Koeppen B. Potassium, calcium, and phosphate homeostasis. In: *Berne & Levy Physiology*. 8th ed. Elsevier; 2024:chap 36.

coagulation, platelet adhesion, endocrine and exocrine functioning, neuromuscular activity, and cardiac and smooth muscle functioning. **Figure 2.8** illustrates the major functions of calcium. Calcium is closely regulated by PTH, calcitonin, and calcitriol. Ninety-nine percent of the body's calcium resides in bones and teeth, and the remaining 1% in body fluids. In serum, 40% of calcium is bound to proteins (mostly albumin), 10% is complexed (typically with citrate and phosphate), and 50% is ionized (**Figure 2.9**).[39] The normal range for total serum calcium is 8.5–10.5 mg/dL (2.12–2.62 mmol/L), and *ionized calcium* has a normal range of 4.65–5.25 mg/dL (1.16–1.31 mmol/L).[41] Since much of serum calcium is bound to albumin, calcium levels decline when albumin levels are low. On average, serum calcium is expected to drop by 0.8 mg/dL for every 1 g/dL drop in serum albumin.[39] The following equation can be used to correct serum calcium due to hypoalbuminemia[42]:

$$\text{Corrected Serum Calcium (mg/dL)} = 0.8 \times [4.0 - \text{Albumin (g/dL)}] + \text{Serum Calcium}$$

Sample Calculation: Albumin: 3.0 g/dL, Calcium 8.0 mg/dL

$$\text{Corrected Serum Calcium (mg/dL)} = 0.8 \times (4.0 - 3.0) + 8.0$$

$$\text{Corrected Serum Calcium} = 0.8 \times 1 + 8.0$$

$$\text{Corrected Serum Calcium} = 8.8 \text{ mg/dL}$$

For example, a patient with a serum albumin level of 3.0 g/dL and a measured serum calcium level of 8.0 mg/dL has a corrected serum calcium of 8.8 mg/dL.

The value of 4.0 in the equation reflects the typical desired serum albumin level in g/dL. The value of 0.8 in this equation reflects the 0.8 mg/dL decline in serum calcium per 1 g/dL decline in serum albumin. Hypoalbuminemia causes total serum calcium to drop but has less of an impact on ionized calcium. Ionized calcium is thus considered a better indicator of the functional status of calcium metabolism than serum calcium. This is particularly true for critically ill patients, as ionized calcium is weakly correlated with total calcium in this population, due to factors such as hypoalbuminemia and acid-base disturbances. Therefore, ionized calcium is often the preferred measure of calcium status in the critical care setting.[43,44]

The recommended adequate intake for calcium is approximately 1000–1200 mg/day for healthy adults, depending on age and sex.[45] Most enteral nutrition (EN) formulas contain approximately 700–1200 mg/L (~17–30 mmol) of calcium, and most adult patients with normal kidney function require a dose of 10–15 mEq/day for maintenance with PN admixtures. Calcium doses can be adjusted by approximately 20–50%, depending on the daily calcium dose, serum calcium levels, responses to dose changes, and underlying medical conditions. Calcium absorption from foods is generally around 30%, although this varies by type of food. For instance, food compounds such as phytate, oxalate, and fiber can lower calcium bioavailability.

Calcium is available in various supplemental forms, with calcium carbonate and calcium citrate being the most common. Calcium citrate is often recommended over calcium carbonate, as it appears to have better absorption and is associated with fewer GI side effects. Calcium citrate is also less dependent on stomach acid and is thus useful for patients taking histamine-2 receptor blockers or proton pump inhibitors.[45] Calcium carbonate should be taken with food for maximal absorption, while calcium citrate may be taken on an empty stomach. The percentage of calcium absorbed tends to decline with increasing supplement doses, so individual doses of 500 mg or less are recommended for optimal absorption.[45]

Hypocalcemia. **Hypocalcemia**, or low serum calcium, has been estimated to occur in approximately 18–28% of hospitalized patients and up to 85% of those in the intensive care unit.[46–48]

Etiology. Hypocalcemia is rarely due to low dietary calcium intake, due to the body's efficient regulatory mechanisms. Common causes of hypocalcemia include hypoparathyroidism, vitamin D deficiency, chronic kidney disease (CKD), and hypomagnesemia. Other possible causes include hyperphosphatemia, sepsis, and pancreatitis. Drugs such as loop diuretics, corticosteroids, chemotherapeutic agents, and contrast dye may also contribute to hypocalcemia. Other examples of drug-related hypocalcemia are summarized in **Table 2.9**.

Signs and Symptoms. The clinical manifestations of hypocalcemia range from asymptomatic in mild-to-moderate cases to life-threatening in severe cases. Mild-to-moderate hypocalcemia may cause neuromuscular, cardiovascular, and central nervous system symptoms such as muscle cramps, paresthesias (tingling, numbness of extremities), and mental status changes. Patients with chronic hypocalcemia may experience dermatologic manifestations including dermatitis, eczema, brittle or grooved nails, and hair loss. Severe hypocalcemia (serum calcium <7 mg/dL) may manifest as tetany (intermittent muscle spasms), seizures, and arrhythmias.[41]

Treatment. Treatment of hypocalcemia varies depending on the severity and underlying cause. For patients with symptomatic hypocalcemia, treatment with IV calcium is indicated until symptoms resolve.

Table 2.9 Drugs Commonly Associated with Hypocalcemia

Mechanism	Examples
Decreased intestinal calcium absorption	■ Corticosteroids ■ Histamine-2 receptor blockers ■ Proton pump inhibitors
Calcium chelators	■ Citrate (used to inhibit coagulation in banked blood) ■ Excess fluoride ■ Foscarnet ■ Sodium ethylenediaminetetraacetic acid
Drug-related vitamin D deficiency	■ Carbamazepine ■ Isoniazid ■ Phenobarbital ■ Phenytoin
Decreased bone resorption	■ Amphotericin B ■ Bisphosphates ■ Calcitonin ■ Chemotherapeutic agents (cisplatin, cyclophosphamide) ■ Ethanol
Increased urinary calcium excretion	■ Corticosteroids ■ Loop diuretics

Data from Ravioli S, Lafranchi A, Exadaktylos AK, Haidinger M, Lindner G. Characteristics and outcome of severe hypercalcemia on admission to the emergency department: a retrospective cohort study. Swiss Med Wkly. 2023;153:40069. doi:10.57187/smw.2023.40069; Stewart AF. Clinical practice. Hypercalcemia associated with cancer. N Engl J Med. 2005;352(4):373-379. doi:10.1056/NEJMcp042806; Sadiq NM, Naganathan S, Badireddy M. Hypercalcemia. In: *StatPearls* [Internet]. StatPearls Publishing; 2024.

Intravenous calcium may be provided as calcium gluconate or calcium citrate. Calcium gluconate is generally the preferred form because it is less likely to cause injury if extravasation (leakage of fluid out of a blood vessel) occurs.[41] Calcium chloride provides three times more elemental calcium than an equivalent dose of calcium gluconate. To prevent dosing errors, orders should specify the type of calcium salt and the dose in grams, milligrams, or milliequivalents. Clinicians must also be sure not to infuse calcium in the same IV line as solutions containing phosphate, due to the risk of calcium-phosphorus precipitation. Fixed IV doses are determined by symptoms and ionized calcium levels, rather than weight-based calculations. Calcium repletion typically involves 1–2 g calcium gluconate (equivalent to 90–180 mg elemental calcium) administered over 10–20 minutes, followed by additional boluses as needed until symptoms subside.[41]

Oral calcium supplements may be considered in patients with mild-to-moderate hypocalcemia who are receiving EN or can tolerate oral medication. Vitamin D and PTH status may need to be evaluated prior to oral administration. For patients receiving PN, daily calcium maintenance doses in PN formulations or daily oral supplements may be adjusted based on the patient's laboratory values and clinical condition.

As previously discussed, hypoalbuminemia can produce a falsely low serum calcium. If a patient has asymptomatic hypocalcemia due to hypoalbuminemia with normal ionized calcium levels, then no treatment is needed to correct hypocalcemia. Although there is debate over the need to correct asymptomatic hypocalcemia, most clinicians treat hypocalcemia to avoid the potential negative consequences of severe hypocalcemia, particularly in critically ill patients.

Other disease-specific treatments may be indicated depending on the underlying etiology. For patients with hypomagnesemia, for example, magnesium levels should be corrected before correcting hypocalcemia.[41] When hypocalcemia is due to hyperphosphatemia, phosphate binders may be recommended to lower serum phosphorus levels.

Hypercalcemia. **Hypercalcemia**, or increased serum calcium, is observed in approximately 3–5% of hospitalized patients and up to 30% of those with cancer.[46,49,50]

Etiology. Hypercalcemia occurs when the amount of calcium entering circulation exceeds the amount excreted via urine or deposited in bone. Primary hyperparathyroidism and malignancy are the most common causes of hypercalcemia, accounting for 90% of cases.[51] Primary hyperparathyroidism, which is commonly due to a parathyroid adenoma, causes increased bone resorption and increased intestinal calcium absorption. Malignancy can cause hypercalcemia in various ways, including increased PTH secretion, osteoclastic activation, and calcitriol overproduction. Other possible causes of hypercalcemia include vitamin A or D toxicity, chronic ingestion of milk and/or calcium carbonate-containing antacids in patients with renal insufficiency (milk-alkali syndrome), and adrenal insufficiency. Immobilization, tuberculosis, Paget's disease, rhabdomyolysis, and medications such as thiazide diuretics, estrogens, and tamoxifen may also cause hypercalcemia.

Signs and Symptoms. Early signs and symptoms of hypercalcemia are nonspecific and include fatigue, nausea, vomiting, constipation, anorexia, and confusion. Chronic hypercalcemia may lead to calcium-phosphate precipitation, metastatic calcification, and kidney failure. Severe hypercalcemia may cause cardiac manifestations such as bradycardia (slow heart rate) or arrhythmias with electrocardiograph changes. Immediate treatment is required for severe hypercalcemia because acute kidney injury, ventricular arrhythmias, coma, and death are potential consequences. Prolonged hypercalcemia can lead to tissue calcification, which may be irreversible.

Treatment. As with other electrolyte disorders, treatment of hypercalcemia depends on severity and etiology. Patients with asymptomatic, mild hypercalcemia (total serum calcium $<$12 mg/dL) typically do not require immediate therapy. However, they should avoid factors that could worsen hypercalcemia, such as thiazide diuretics, calcium supplementation, high dietary calcium intake, and prolonged bed rest. Patients receiving PN may benefit from temporary reduction or removal of calcium from the PN prescription. Patients with symptomatic, severe hypercalcemia (total serum calcium $>$14 mg/dL) should be treated immediately with IV fluids to correct hypovolemia. Saline hydration may also be combined with loop diuretics such as furosemide (which increase urinary calcium excretion), although this approach should be used with caution due to risks of worsened electrolyte derangements and volume depletion.[52] Calcitonin, which inhibits bone resorption and increases renal calcium excretion, may be used to treat severe, symptomatic hypercalcemia. Calcitonin is used as an early treatment, as its onset of action is within 2 hours of being administered and its effectiveness appears to decline with repeated administration.[52] Bisphosphonates, which inhibit bone resorption, are commonly used to treat malignancy-related hypercalcemia. Serum calcium levels should be monitored every 4–24 hours during active treatment of severe, symptomatic hypercalcemia, and every 24–48 hours after levels return to normal and symptoms subside.[15]

Phosphorus

Phosphorus (P^{3-}) is the primary intracellular anion in the body. Approximately 85% of total body phosphorus is found in the skeleton, 14% in soft tissue, and only 1% in ECF.[53] Phosphorus exists mainly as phosphate (PO_4) in serum. Phosphate is also the primary form ingested from dietary and supplemental sources.

Phosphorus has many important functions in the body, including supporting skeletal health and maintaining cell membrane composition. Phosphorus also provides energy bonds in the form of adenosine triphosphate (ATP), which supplies energy needed for many cellular processes and functions. Phosphorus is a key component of 2,3-diphosphoglycerate (2,3-DPG), which is essential for oxygen release from hemoglobin and delivery to tissues. Maintaining normal total body phosphorus is crucial for neurologic function, muscle contractility, electrolyte transport, and hematologic status.

Serum phosphorus concentration is determined by the amount of intestinal absorption, renal excretion, hormonally regulated bone resorption and deposition, and distribution within intracellular and extracellular compartments. Intracellular phosphorus shifts may be caused by insulin administration, catecholamines, and alkalosis, and extracellular shifts may occur from cellular destruction and acidosis. Normal serum phosphorus concentration ranges from 2.5 to 4.5 mg/dL.[53] However, serum phosphorus levels may not correlate well with total body phosphorus, as serum phosphorus is only a small percentage of total body phosphorus. Thus, when interpreting phosphorus laboratory values, clinicians must consider factors that affect total body phosphorus homeostasis, including kidney function, malnutrition, and certain medications.

Hypophosphatemia. **Hypophosphatemia**, or low serum phosphorus, is estimated to occur in up to 3.1% of hospitalized patients and at least 15% of critically ill patients.[54,55]

Etiology. Hypophosphatemia generally occurs by three possible mechanisms: decreased intestinal phosphate absorption, increased urinary phosphate excretion, and increased movement of extracellular phosphate into cells. Decreased intestinal absorption may be due to medications (particularly those containing magnesium or aluminum), phosphate binders, vitamin D deficiency, chronic diarrhea, vomiting, and malabsorptive disorders. Causes of increased urinary phosphate losses include vitamin D deficiency, hyperparathyroidism, and renal tubular defects. Acute intracellular shifts of phosphate may be caused by respiratory and metabolic alkalosis, due to an intracellular shift of hydrogen ions, resulting in an increased production of phosphorylated metabolites within cells.[56] Increased insulin secretion (e.g., during carbohydrate refeeding in malnourished patients) may also induce hypophosphatemia via intracellular phosphate shifts. Hypophosphatemia is frequently observed in patients receiving nutrition support due to factors such as inadequate phosphate supplementation, increased metabolic demands, refeeding syndrome, and altered phosphate metabolism due to medications or medical conditions.[57] Hypophosphatemia is also common in patients with alcohol use disorder, likely due to a combination of factors such as inadequate phosphorus and vitamin D intake, correction of metabolic acidosis (leading to an intracellular shift of phosphate), kidney dysfunction (causing increased phosphate excretion), and refeeding syndrome.[56]

Signs and Symptoms. Patients with mild hypophosphatemia (serum phosphorus 1.8–2.5 mg/dL) are typically asymptomatic but may experience generalized muscle weakness and fatigue. Severe hypophosphatemia (serum phosphorus <0.9 mg/dL) can be life-threatening and is associated with a wide range of neurological, cardiac, and respiratory abnormalities.[58] Signs and symptoms of severe hypophosphatemia may include altered mental status, seizures, numbness, muscle pain, heart failure, cardiac arrhythmias, and difficulty weaning from mechanical ventilation. Low phosphate levels can also cause calcium and phosphorus to mobilize from bone, contributing to osteomalacia in adults and rickets in children.[58]

Treatment. Treatment of hypophosphatemia depends on the underlying cause and severity of deficiency. Mild and moderate hypophosphatemia can usually be treated with increased dietary phosphate intake or oral phosphate supplementation. Oral phosphate is rapidly absorbed and excreted within several hours, so it should be administered in divided doses (e.g., three or four times per day).[58] Intravenous phosphorus repletion is indicated in patients with severe hypophosphatemia, as well as in those unable to tolerate oral therapy. Estimating IV phosphate doses is largely empirical because serum phosphorus levels may not correlate well with total body phosphorus stores. To minimize potential adverse effects such as calcium-phosphate precipitation and thrombophlebitis, IV phosphate should be infused over 4–6 hours at a maximum rate of 7 mmol/hour, with careful monitoring of serum phosphate concentrations.[15] For patients at risk for refeeding syndrome (discussed later in this chapter), hypophosphatemia should be corrected prior to initiating any form of nutrition support.

Hyperphosphatemia

Etiology. **Hyperphosphatemia**, or elevated serum phosphorus, may result from decreased phosphate excretion, increased phosphate load, increased renal phosphate absorption, and extracellular phosphate shifts. Kidney disease commonly causes hyperphosphatemia via decreased phosphate excretion, particularly when glomerular filtration rate falls below 30 mL/min/1.73 m^2.[59] Acute increases in phosphate load may occur from exogenous sources (e.g., excessive administration of phosphate supplementation or intake of phosphate-containing laxatives) or endogenous sources (e.g., in the setting of tumor lysis syndrome or muscle injury).[56] Increased renal phosphate reabsorption may occur in patients with hypoparathyroidism, acromegaly, and vitamin D toxicity. Lactic acidosis and diabetic ketoacidosis may also contribute to hypophosphatemia, by triggering the movement of phosphate out of cells.

Signs and Symptoms. The clinical manifestations of hyperphosphatemia are generally few and nonspecific. They include muscle weakness, anorexia, nausea, vomiting, and tachycardia. Hyperphosphatemia may induce hypocalcemia via calcium-phosphate precipitation, thereby contributing to hypocalcemia-related symptoms such as tetany, muscle cramping, paresthesias, and seizures. Calcium-phosphorus crystals can cause further organ damage, particularly in the lungs, myocardium, and blood vessels, and may deposit in soft tissue. Evaluation of both serum calcium and phosphorus is essential to guide treatment plans and prevent such complications.

Treatment. The approach to therapy should be tailored to the underlying cause and acuity of hyperphosphatemia. In cases of acute severe hyperphosphatemia, saline infusion may be provided to increase phosphate excretion. Hemodialysis may be initiated for patients with severe hyperphosphatemia with symptomatic hypocalcemia, particularly if kidney function is impaired. Additionally, medications that may be responsible for hyperphosphatemia should be discontinued, and phosphate intake should be adjusted or restricted (e.g., by reducing doses in PN prescription, initiating a renal EN formula, or providing counseling on a low-phosphorus diet). For patients with CKD and persistent hyperphosphatemia despite dietary phosphate restriction, phosphate binder medications may be recommended. Phosphate binders, when taken with meals and snacks, can help lower serum phosphate levels by binding dietary phosphate in the GI tract and reducing its absorption. Common phosphate binders include calcium-, aluminum-, and magnesium-containing antacids. Aluminum-based phosphate binders, while effective, are not recommended for long-term use given their potential to cause aluminum toxicity.[60]

Magnesium

Magnesium (Mg^{2+}) is a highly abundant mineral in the ICF. Approximately 50–60% of total body magnesium is in bone, and the remaining 40–50% in soft tissues. Only 1% of total body magnesium is found in ECF. In serum, about 55% of magnesium is ionized (i.e., free), 30% is protein-bound (mostly to albumin), and 15% is complexed with anions such as phosphate or citrate.[61]

Magnesium is a required cofactor in more than 300 cellular reactions, including those relating to glucose metabolism, fatty acid synthesis, and DNA and protein metabolism. Magnesium is a cofactor of the Na^+-K^+-ATPase system, which is necessary for nerve impulse conduction, muscle contraction, and normal heart rhythm. Magnesium also influences the movement of calcium and potassium across cell membranes, meaning alterations in magnesium levels can have downstream effects on the regulation of other key electrolytes.

Magnesium homeostasis is maintained by the intestine, kidneys, and bones. Approximately 30–40% of dietary magnesium is absorbed, which occurs primarily in the jejunum and ileum.[62] Intestinal absorption is dependent on magnesium status, as the amount of dietary magnesium absorbed increases when intake is low. About one-third of magnesium in bone is exchangeable, serving as a reservoir to help maintain normal extracellular magnesium levels.[61] Kidney function is vital for magnesium homeostasis, as about 70% of serum magnesium is filtered by the kidneys, and about 95% of this filtered magnesium is reabsorbed.[63]

Normal serum magnesium ranges from 1.5 to 2.7 mg/dL.[64] However, since serum contains only about 1% of total body magnesium, it may not accurately reflect total magnesium stores. In addition, hypoalbuminemia may produce a falsely low serum magnesium since much of magnesium in serum is bound to albumin.

Hypomagnesemia

Hypomagnesemia, or low serum magnesium, is estimated to occur in approximately 20% of hospitalized patients and up to 65% of critically ill patients.[65,66]

Etiology. Mechanisms of hypomagnesemia include decreased intake, GI malabsorption, increased renal or GI losses, and cellular redistribution. Hypomagnesemia secondary to decreased intake may be observed in patients with malnutrition, alcohol use disorder, eating disorders, and those receiving magnesium-free IV fluids or PN.[64,67] Chronic diarrhea, inflammatory bowel disease, short bowel syndrome, steatorrhea, and intestinal bypass surgeries can cause hypomagnesemia through reduced absorption and GI losses.[68] Renal losses may occur in patients with renal tubular disorders, poorly controlled diabetes, hyperaldosteronism, and inherited conditions such as Bartter syndrome and Gitelman syndrome. Medications such as loop diuretics, cyclosporine, tacrolimus, laxatives, cisplatin, amphotericin B, aminoglycosides, and omeprazole may also induce hypomagnesemia through increased renal losses.[67] In addition, hypomagnesemia may occur when magnesium is redistributed from extracellular to intracellular compartments, which can be caused by pancreatitis, refeeding syndrome, diabetic ketoacidosis, hyperthyroidism, and alcohol withdrawal.[64]

Signs and Symptoms. Neuromuscular hyperexcitability is often the first clinical manifestation of hypomagnesemia. Tetany, muscular weakness, and seizures may also occur.[64] Cardiac complications, including electrocardiogram changes, arrhythmias, and increased sensitivity to cardiac glycosides, are also common.[64] General symptoms may include depression, anorexia, nausea, vomiting, and ileus. Many of the signs and symptoms of hypomagnesemia are difficult to differentiate from those of hypokalemia and hypocalcemia, both of which are refractory to treatment in the presence of hypomagnesemia. Reports indicate that approximately 40% of patients with hypokalemia and 20% of patients with hypocalcemia also present with hypomagnesemia.[69]

Treatment. Since serum magnesium may not correlate with total body magnesium, treatment goals for hypomagnesemia are largely empirical. Treatment should focus on addressing the underlying cause and correcting coexisting electrolyte imbalances following magnesium repletion. Oral salts are recommended for mild-to-moderate depletion, although they should be used with caution because they may cause diarrhea. For symptomatic, severe hypomagnesemia, IV magnesium (typically in the form of magnesium sulfate) should be provided. Intravenous repletion may also be used for patients who are unable to tolerate oral supplementation. For patients with impaired kidney function, recommended empirical doses should

CASE STUDY REVISITED

On hospital day (HD) 3, you visit Adam and learn that he has been NPO since admission due to his medical GI evaluation. Because Adam is feeling better and his GI symptoms have resolved, the medical team has just advanced Adam to a regular diet. Adam reports an excellent appetite and is looking forward to eating.

Anthropometric Data:

Weight: 73 kg

Last weight: 75 kg at admission

Biochemical Data (HD 3):

Sodium 134 (136–145 mEq/L)
Potassium 3.3 (3.5–5.0 mEq/L)
Blood urea nitrogen 22 (8–20 mg/dL)
Creatinine 0.2 (0.7–1.3 mg/dL)
Glucose 95 (70–139 mg/dL)
Phosphorus 2.9 (2.5–4.5 mg/dL)
Magnesium 1.4 (1.5–2.7 mg/dL)

Clinical Data:

Medications: atorvastatin, captopril, pantoprazole

Dietary Data:

Diet Prescription: Regular

Questions

1. Is Adam at risk for refeeding syndrome? Explain.
2. What factors mediate the refeeding process?
3. Assess Adam's PES statement(s) from his initial RD encounter. Identify if each statement remains an active issue or if the PES statement has been resolved. If the PES statement remains an active issue, is it being addressed and/or has improvement in the issue been noted? If the issue has been resolved, write a new PES statement.
4. Identify the interventions you would like to initiate for Adam to address the problems identified in your PES statements.
5. What biochemical indices should be included in your monitoring and evaluation plan? Why?

be reduced by about 50% to minimize the risk of hypermagnesemia.[64]

Hypermagnesemia

Hypermagnesemia, or high serum magnesium, is uncommon, primarily occurring in patients with impaired kidney function.

Etiology. In addition to renal insufficiency, hypermagnesemia may be caused by excessive administration of magnesium infusions, laxatives, and magnesium enemas. Less common causes include lithium toxicity (which can decrease urinary magnesium excretion), primary hyperparathyroidism (which causes increased tubular reabsorption of magnesium), and tumor lysis syndrome (which can cause extracellular magnesium shifts).[70]

Signs and Symptoms. Dehydration, nausea, vomiting, diaphoresis (excessive sweating), flushing, drowsiness, depressed mental status, hypotension, and bradycardia are common symptoms of mild-to-moderate hypermagnesemia. Neuromuscular functions can also be impaired, leading to decreased reflexes, muscle weakness, and paralysis. In severe cases, hypermagnesemia may cause respiratory depression, coma, and cardiac arrest.[67]

Treatment. If kidney function is normal, removal of all exogenous magnesium sources is typically sufficient to treat hypermagnesemia. Patients with severe, symptomatic hypermagnesemia may be treated with IV calcium gluconate (typically 1–2 g infused over 5–10 minutes) to alleviate neuromuscular and cardiovascular symptoms.[15] For patients with kidney failure, hemodialysis may be recommended. Clinicians may also consider administering diuretics to increase magnesium excretion.

Refeeding Syndrome

Refeeding syndrome is a condition that can occur in malnourished patients during the initiation of concentrated calorie delivery. While there is no universally accepted definition of refeeding syndrome, the condition is generally characterized by metabolic complications that result from derangements in phosphorus, potassium, magnesium, and glucose control in the setting of aggressive nutritional rehabilitation. In a 2020 American Society for Parenteral and Enteral Nutrition (ASPEN) consensus recommendation, two main criteria for refeeding syndrome diagnosis were proposed: (1) a decrease in phosphorus, potassium, and/or magnesium levels by at least 10% and/or the presence of organ dysfunction resulting from a reduction in any of these and/or a result of thiamine deficiency; and (2) the occurrence of these impairments within 5 days of nutrition reintroduction.[71]

Reintroduction of carbohydrates (oral, enteral, or parenteral) after a prolonged period of inadequate nutrition triggers a sudden release of insulin and subsequent shift from using ketones as the primary energy source to glucose. During this shift from catabolism to anabolism, phosphorus, potassium, and magnesium shift intracellularly, leading to low serum levels of these electrolytes. The carbohydrate delivery also enables massive phosphorylation of ADP to ATP, leading to a rapid depletion of stored phosphorus, as well as thiamine. The sudden introduction of carbohydrate may also cause renal excretion of sodium and water to decline, thereby increasing the risk of fluid overload. **Figure 2.10** outlines the metabolic changes associated with refeeding syndrome. According to case reports, refeeding syndrome can continue for up to 5 days after feeding initiation.[72]

Populations at increased risk for refeeding syndrome include patients with anorexia nervosa, alcohol use disorder, malabsorptive syndromes, malignancy, and critical illness.[71] According to consensus recommendations, refeeding syndrome risk among adults may be classified as moderate or severe, based on the degree of weight loss, decreased intake, electrolyte abnormalities, fat/muscle loss, and high-risk comorbidities. Criteria for identifying adult patients at risk for refeeding syndrome are outlined in **Table 2.10**.

Refeeding syndrome can have a wide range of potentially life-threatening consequences. Hypophosphatemia can lead to neurological symptoms such as seizures, delirium, and encephalopathy; cardiorespiratory symptoms such as arrhythmias or respiratory failure; and hematologic symptoms such as tissue hypoxia (due to decreased production of 2,3-diphosphoglycerate, resulting in increased hemoglobin oxygen affinity).[73] Hypokalemia may cause neurological abnormalities (e.g., paralysis), cardiac arrhythmias, and GI disturbances.[74] Hypomagnesemia may cause neurological symptoms such as muscle twitching, tetany, and altered mental status, as well as cardiac and GI dysfunction.[73] Thiamine deficiency may cause encephalopathy, oculomotor abnormalities, and lactic acidosis.[71] Additionally, sodium retention can contribute to pulmonary edema and cardiac decompensation.

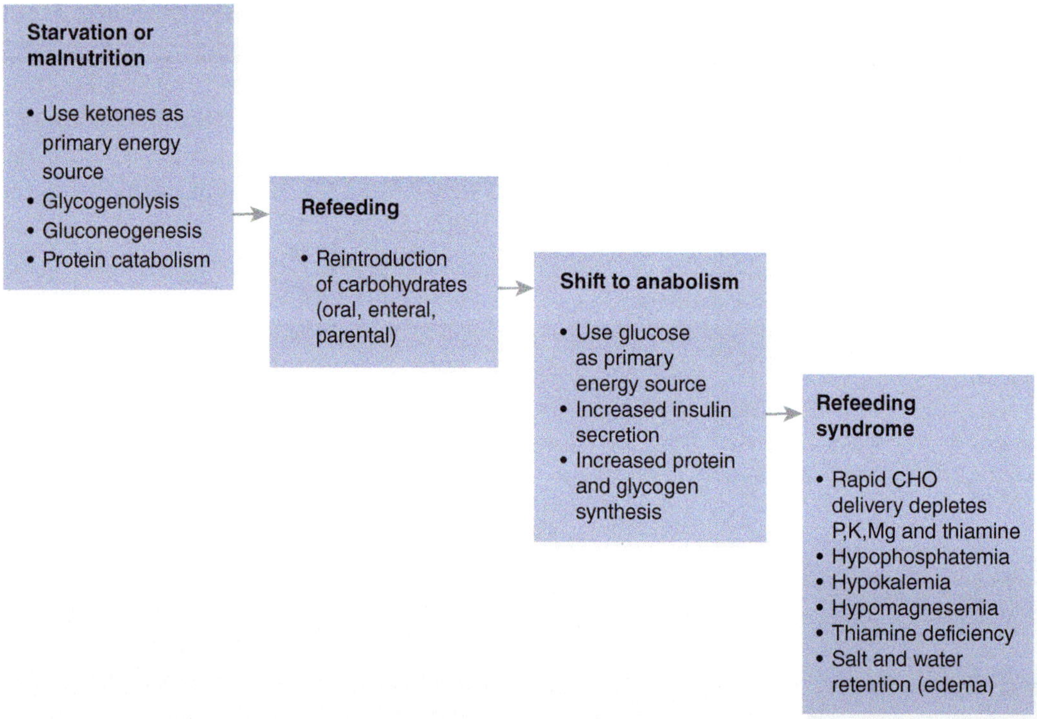

Figure 2.10 Metabolic Changes During Refeeding Syndrome

Table 2.10 Criteria for Identifying Adult Patients at Risk for Refeeding Syndrome

BMI (kg/m^2)	■ <18.5
Weight Loss	■ 5–10% in 1 month–6 months
Food Intake	■ < 50–75% estimated energy needs for > 5–7 days
Electrolyte (Potassium, Phosphorus, Magnesium) Levels Prior to Feeding	Low levels before initiating nutrition/requiring supplementation after feeding
Subcutaneous Fat Loss	Moderate-Severe
Muscle Loss	Mild-Severe

Data from da Silva JSV, Seres DS, Sabino K, et al. ASPEN consensus recommendations for refeeding syndrome. *Nutr Clin Pract*. 2020;35(2):178-195. doi:10.1002/ncp.10474

Many strategies have been suggested to prevent the adverse effects of refeeding syndrome. In patients at risk for refeeding syndrome, feeding should be initiated gradually alongside close monitoring of electrolyte and fluid status. ASPEN guidelines recommend initiating feeding at 10–20 kcal/kg in the first 24 hours, then increasing by 33% of the energy goal every 1–2 days.[71] Additionally, thiamine is commonly supplemented before and during the first few days of refeeding to prevent thiamine deficiency and its associated complications. The typical dose for thiamine supplementation is 100 mg daily for 5–7 days.[71] If refeeding syndrome is detected, clinicians should slow nutrition repletion and aggressively correct electrolyte abnormalities, while carefully monitoring cardiorespiratory function. Clinicians should use clinical judgment to develop an individualized plan for feeding advancement, considering patient-specific factors such as illness acuity, baseline electrolyte levels, and severity of malnutrition.

CORE CONCEPT 3

Refeeding syndrome can result in nutritional abnormalities due to carbohydrate intake triggering a sudden release of insulin and subsequent intracellular shift of potassium, phosphorus, and magnesium, as well as fluid retention.

PRACTICE POINT

Screening patients for malnutrition (i.e., evaluating anthropometrics, functional indicators, diet history) prior to initiating feeds is critical to minimize the adverse effects of refeeding syndrome. Initiating feeding at 10–20 kcal/kg and advancing gradually every 1–2 days to the goal is recommended.

Chloride

Chloride (Cl^-) is the most abundant anion in the ECF, with approximately 88% of total body chloride found in extracellular compartments.[75] Normal serum chloride ranges from approximately 96–106 mEq/L, and serum levels are closely regulated by the kidneys. Chloride exists mainly as sodium chloride (NaCl) and hydrochloric acid (HCl) in the body. Chloride works alongside sodium to maintain cell membrane integrity via regulation of fluid balance and serum osmolality. Chloride also plays a critical role in acid-base balance, as chloride ions migrate into extracellular space in response to a loss of bicarbonate.[76] Thus, alterations in serum chloride can cause acid-base imbalances. High serum chloride can result in metabolic acidosis, and low serum chloride can result in metabolic alkalosis. Chloride also has important GI functions, as HCl is necessary for protein digestion, nutrient absorption (e.g., vitamin B12, folate, ascorbic acid, non-heme iron), and preventing the growth of harmful bacteria in the small intestine.[77]

Hypochloremia

Etiology. **Hypochloremia**, or low serum chloride, may be caused by GI losses (e.g., vomiting, diarrhea, nasogastric suction), excessive sweating, and renal losses (e.g., due to thiazide or loop diuretics).[78] Hypochloremia may also occur in the setting of congestive heart failure, due to hemodilution and/or depletion due to loop diuretics.[79]

Signs and Symptoms. Patients with hypochloremia are often asymptomatic, with symptoms only present at extremely low levels. Symptoms may include muscle cramps, tremors, tetany, slowed breathing, and hypotension resulting from fluid loss. In severe cases, hypochloremia may cause seizures, life-threatening respiratory depression, cardiac arrhythmias, and coma.[80]

Treatment. Treatment of hypochloremia must be directed toward the underlying etiology. For instance, this may involve treating the cause of vomiting, reducing gastric suctioning, and reducing loop or thiazide diuretic administration. Assessment of hydration status, severity of hypochloremia, and presence of concurrent electrolyte disorders (e.g., hypokalemia, hyponatremia) and metabolic alkalosis is critical. Hypochloremia is typically corrected with isotonic saline, with doses determined by patients' serum chloride levels. The chloride deficit can be calculated using the following equation[81]:

$$\text{Chloride Deficit (mEq)} = 0.2 \times \text{Weight (kg)} \times [103 - \text{Chloride level (mEq/L)}]$$

Sample Calculation: Weight 70 kg, Chloride 92 mEq/L

$$\text{Chloride Deficit in mEq} = 0.2 \times 70 \times (103 - 92)$$

$$\text{Chloride Deficit} = 154 \text{ mEq}$$

For example, a 70-kg patient with hypochloremia (chloride 92 mEq/L) has a chloride deficit of 154 mEq. The value of 103 in the equation represents the typical desired chloride level (in mEq/L). An infusion of approximately 1 L normal saline (which contains 154 mEq NaCl) would be needed to raise the patient's serum chloride to normal.

Hyperchloremia

Etiology. **Hyperchloremia**, or increased serum chloride, may be caused by severe diarrhea, renal tubular acidosis, kidney failure, pancreatic fistulas, chronic laxative use, and excessive fluid resuscitation with normal saline.[76,77] Medications such as corticosteroids, acetazolamide, and triamterene may also contribute to hyperchloremia.[77]

Signs and Symptoms. The clinical manifestations of hyperchloremia are typically nonspecific and overlap with those of metabolic acidosis or other electrolyte disorders. Common symptoms include weakness, lethargy, confusion, nausea, and vomiting. In severe cases, patients may experience unconsciousness and Kussmaul respirations, which are deep and labored breaths, often associated with diabetic ketoacidosis.[80,82]

Treatment. Treatment for hyperchloremia varies based on etiology. Treatment may involve removing contributing medications (e.g., chloride-containing IV fluids), supplementing with bicarbonate to restore acid-base balance, and addressing other underlying causes (e.g., diarrhea, renal tubular acidosis) as indicated. If chronic acidosis is present with hyperchloremia due to diarrhea, long-term therapy with sodium and potassium citrate solutions may be recommended.

Bicarbonate

Bicarbonate is a compound in the blood that works closely with chloride to maintain acid-base balance. Bicarbonate commonly refers to HCO_3^- or carbon dioxide (CO_2), with normal serum levels ranging from 22 to 31 mEq/L.[83] High serum bicarbonate causes metabolic alkalosis, while low serum bicarbonate causes metabolic acidosis. Metabolic acidosis is typically treated with sodium bicarbonate ($NaHCO_3$) via IV administration. For patients receiving PN, however, treatment with sodium bicarbonate is discouraged due to compatibility and stability concerns.[84] In these cases, metabolic acidosis is typically treated using acetate, which is metabolized to bicarbonate by the liver. To estimate the amount of bicarbonate needed to correct metabolic acidosis, the bicarbonate deficit can be calculated as follows[85]:

$$\text{Bicarbonate Deficit (mEq)} = 0.5 \times \text{Weight (kg)} \times [24\text{-Measured } HCO_3 \text{ (mEq/L)}]$$

Sample Calculation: Weight 70 kg, Serum HCO_3^- 17 mEq/L

$$\text{Bicarbonate Deficit} = 0.5 \times 70 \times (24 - 17)$$

$$\text{Bicarbonate Deficit} = 245 \text{ mEq}$$

For example, a 70-kg patient with a serum bicarbonate of 17 mEq/L has a bicarbonate deficit of 245 mEq, indicating that approximately 245 mEq of bicarbonate would be needed to normalize the patient's bicarbonate levels. The value of 0.50 in this equation represents the bicarbonate volume of distribution, which is generally 50% of body weight. The value of 24 in the equation represents the typical desired bicarbonate level (in mEq/L).

Acid-Base Physiology

An acid is any substance that releases hydrogen ions (H^+) in solution, whereas a base is a substance that accepts or combines with H^+. The free hydrogen ion concentration, represented by the pH, determines the acidity of body fluids. The pH is inversely related to hydrogen ion concentration, meaning a drop in hydrogen ion concentration raises the pH and an increase in hydrogen ion concentration lowers the pH. In arterial blood, the pH is normally maintained within a narrow range of 7.35–7.45. A blood pH below 7.35 is called **acidemia**, while a blood pH above 7.45 is called **alkalemia**. **Acidosis** occurs when there is an increased concentration of hydrogen ions, and **alkalosis** occurs when there is a decreased hydrogen ion concentration. These terms are important to understand when evaluating acid-base status, as multiple types of acid-base disorders can exist simultaneously. **Figure 2.11** illustrates the pH scale and hydrogen ion concentration range.

As with fluid and electrolyte balance, acid-base balance is critical for many physiologic functions and biochemical reactions. Serum chloride and bicarbonate levels are the most common electrolytes associated with acid-base imbalance. In a healthy individual, acid-base balance is maintained by the lungs, kidneys, and several buffering systems. Metabolic and respiratory disorders can disrupt this homeostasis, resulting in alkalosis and/or acidosis. Acid-base disorders can have many adverse effects, which can be life-threatening

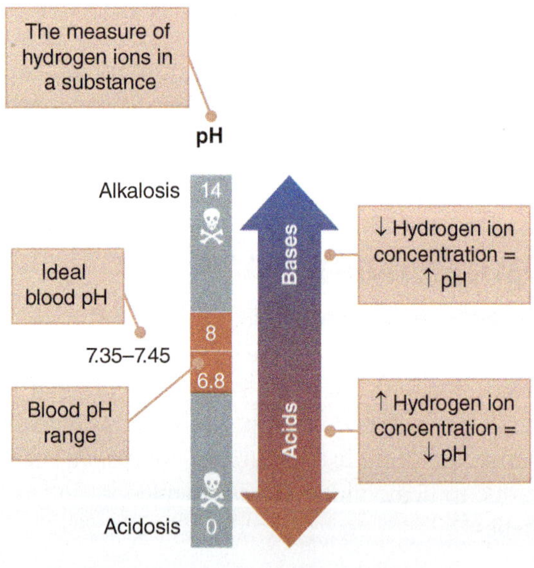

Figure 2.11 pH Scale in Relation to Hydrogen Ion Concentration

CASE STUDY REVISITED

On HD 6, Adam undergoes an urgent laparotomy for a severe gastric ulcer with perforation. On postoperative (postop) day 1/HD 7, you visit Adam for reassessment. He is currently in the ICU on mechanical ventilation with increased drainage from a nasogastric tube.

Anthropometric Data:

Weight: 77 kg on HD 7

Last weight: 73 kg on HD 3

Biochemical Data (postop day 1/HD 7):

Sodium 143 (136–145 mEq/L)
Potassium 3.5 (3.5–5.0 mEq/L)
Chloride 88 (96–106 mEq/L)
Carbon dioxide 41 (22–31 mEq/L)
Blood urea nitrogen 24 (8–20 mg/dL)

Creatinine 0.2 (0.7–1.3 mg/dL)
Glucose 139 (70–139 mg/dL)
Calcium 7.7 (8.5–10.5 mg/dL)
Phosphorus 3.0 (2.5–4.5 mg/dL)
Magnesium 1.4 (1.5–2.7 mg/dL)

Arterial Blood Gas:

pH 7.48 (7.35–.45)
PCO_2 48 (35–45 mm Hg)

PO_2 90 (80–100 mm Hg)
HCO_3 29 (22–26 mEq/L)

Dietary Data:

Diet Prescription: NPO

Questions

1. Describe Adam's acid-base status.
2. What specific acid-base disorder does he have?
3. What interventions would you recommend to manage this acid-base imbalance?

in severe cases. Clinicians must understand the physiological processes underlying acid-base disorders to accurately diagnose and correct these conditions.

Most hydrogen ions originate as a byproduct or end product of cellular metabolism, although a small amount of acidic substance may enter the body via ingested food. Each day, oxidation of carbohydrates and fats produces approximately 15,000 mmol of CO_2, which forms carbonic acid when combined with water.[86] Without tight regulation, progressive accumulation of acids can be detrimental. Acid-base regulation occurs through three primary mechanisms: (1) chemical buffering systems, (2) carbon dioxide release by the lungs, and (3) hydrogen ion excretion and bicarbonate resorption by the kidneys. Each mechanism is described in further detail hereunder.

Chemical Buffers: Buffering systems prevent large changes in hydrogen ion concentration and are the first line of defense, occurring immediately to resist changes in pH. In general, the buffering systems consist of weak acid and base pairs that take up or release hydrogen ions to minimize changes in free concentration. The carbonic acid/bicarbonate (H_2CO_3/HCO_3^-) system is the most abundant buffer system in the body. Others include the plasma protein, hemoglobin, phosphate, and ammonia buffering systems.

Lungs: The primary role of the respiratory system in maintaining acid-base balance is to control the amount of carbon dioxide in blood. The lungs do this by adjusting both the rate and depth of respirations, which can occur within minutes of acid-base disturbances.[87] As a result, any condition that impairs respiratory system functioning can contribute to acid-base imbalances.

Kidneys: The renal system is the final, slowest mechanism involved in acid-base homeostasis. The kidneys regulate pH by reabsorbing bicarbonate (to make the pH more alkaline) and excreting acids (to make the pH more acidic). Figure 2.12 illustrates the primary mechanisms involved in acid-base regulation.

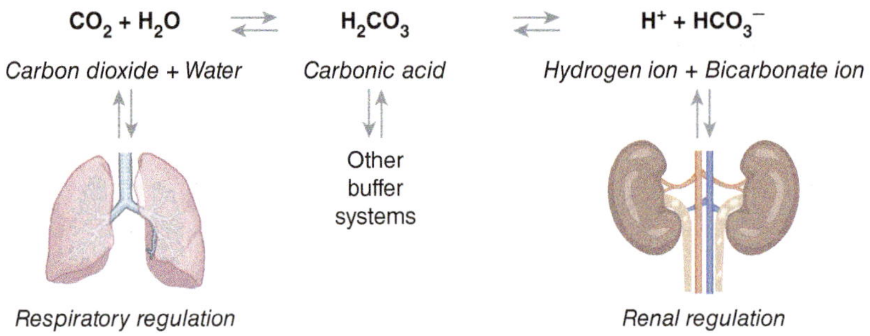

Figure 2.12 Respiratory and Renal Acid-Base Regulation

Data from Tucker AM, Johnson TN. Acid-base disorders: a primer for clinicians. *Nutr Clin Pract. 2022;37*(5):980-989. doi:10.1002/ncp.10881

Table 2.11 Normal Blood Gas Values

Laboratory Test	Arterial	Venous
pH	7.35–7.45	7.33–7.43
PCO_2 (mm Hg)	35–45	41–51
PO_2 (mm Hg)	80–100	35–40
HCO_3^- (mEq/L)	22–26	24–28
SO_2 (%)	>93	70–75
Base excess	−2 to +2	−2.4 to +2.3

PCO_2, partial pressure of carbon dioxide; PO_2, partial pressure of oxygen; HCO_3^-, bicarbonate; SO_2, oxygen saturation

Data from Tucker AM, Johnson TN. Acid-base disorders: a primer for clinicians. *Nutr Clin Pract. 2022;37*(5):980-989. doi:10.1002/ncp.10881

Arterial Blood Gases

Blood gas values are used to assess a patient's oxygenation and acid-base status. **Arterial blood gases (ABGs)** reflect the lung's ability to oxygenate blood, while **venous blood gases (VBGs)** reflect tissue oxygenation. Common blood gas measurements include pH, partial pressure of carbon dioxide (PCO_2), partial pressure of oxygen (PO_2), calculated bicarbonate, oxygen saturation (SO_2), and base excess. As indicated in **Table 2.11**, the normal ranges of these measurements differ for ABGs and VBGs.

PCO_2 reflects the lung's ability to excrete carbon dioxide. Changes in PCO_2 are associated with respiratory processes that can cause acid-base disorders. Because CO_2 is the acid component of the carbonic acid/bicarbonate buffer system, an increase in PCO_2 reflects an acidosis and a decrease in PCO_2 reflects an alkalosis. PO_2 describes the amount of oxygen dissolved in the blood and is directly related to SO_2, which represents the percentage of hemoglobin bound to oxygen molecules. In other words, when PO_2 is high, SO_2 is also high, and vice versa.

Changes in bicarbonate are associated with metabolic processes that can lead to acid-base disorders. Bicarbonate may be measured directly from plasma or calculated using pH and CO_2 partial pressure measurements. Since bicarbonate is the base component of the carbonic acid/bicarbonate buffer system, an increase in serum or calculated bicarbonate reflects an alkalosis, and a decrease reflects an acidosis. Another value that can be calculated is base excess, which estimates the metabolic component of an acid-base disorder. An increase in base excess occurs in metabolic alkalosis, while base deficit occurs in metabolic acidosis.

Acid-Base Disorders

Stepwise Approach to Evaluating Acid-Base Disorders

Acid-base disorders must be assessed using a careful, systematic approach to ensure accurate diagnosis. The following steps can be useful when evaluating acid-base disorders:

1. Use the pH value to determine if the patient is acidemic (pH <7.4) or alkalemic (pH >7.4). A pH of 7.4 should not be excluded from assessment because compensation or a mixed acid-base disorder could contribute to a normal pH range.
2. Assess PCO_2 to determine respiratory status. Elevated PCO_2 indicates respiratory acidosis, while low PCO_2 indicates respiratory alkalosis (refer to **Table 2.12** for a summary of the characteristics of primary acid-base imbalances).
3. Assess HCO_3^- to determine metabolic status. Elevated HCO_3^- indicates metabolic alkalosis, while low HCO_3^- indicates metabolic acidosis.
4. Calculate the anion gap to help determine the etiology of metabolic acidosis. The anion gap represents the difference between the concentration

(in mEq/L) of serum cations (Na^+) and anions (Cl^- and HCO_3^-):

$$\text{Anion gap} = Na^+ - (Cl^- + HCO_3^-)$$

Note: The HCO_3^- used in this calculation is the serum HCO_3^-, not the HCO_3^- from the blood gas measurement.

5. Determine whether the acid-base disorder is acute or chronic. Acute disorders typically develop over minutes to hours, while chronic disorders develop over several days or longer.[88]
6. Assess the degree of compensation. For example, if the imbalance is primarily metabolic, consider whether respiratory compensation has occurred (refer to Table 2.12 for expected compensatory responses). If adequate compensation is not evident, it is likely that more than one acid-base disorder is present.

Table 2.12 Characteristics of Primary Acid-Base Imbalances

Disorder	pH	Primary Disturbance	Compensatory Response
Metabolic Acidosis	Low	↓ HCO_3^-	↓ PCO_2
Metabolic Alkalosis	High	↑ HCO_3^-	↑ PCO_2
Respiratory Acidosis	Low	↑ PCO_2	↑ HCO_3^-
Respiratory Alkalosis	High	↓ PCO_2	↓ HCO_3^-

Data from Raymond & Morrow. *Krause and Mahan's Food & the Nutrition Care Process*. 15th edition. Elsevier; 2021.

Metabolic Disorders. **Metabolic acidosis** is characterized by a low pH, low HCO_3^- concentration, and compensatory hyperventilation that leads to a decreased PCO_2. **Figure 2.13** illustrates the bicarbonate and carbonic acid imbalance that occurs in metabolic acidosis, and the compensatory response. Metabolic acidosis can result from either the inability of kidneys to excrete the dietary hydrogen ion load, or an increase in hydrogen ion generation due to an addition of hydrogen ions or a loss of bicarbonate. Calculating the anion gap (using the calculation presented above) can assist in the diagnosis of metabolic acidosis, allowing clinicians to differentiate between normal anion gap acidosis and high anion gap acidosis. Normal anion gap values commonly range from 4 to 12 mEq/L, although reference ranges vary depending on the specific analyzer used.[89]

Normal anion-gap acidosis, also known as "hyperchloremic metabolic acidosis," occurs when there is a milliequivalent-for-milliequivalent replacement of extracellular bicarbonate by chloride. As a result, there is a normal anion gap because the sum remains constant for the major measured anions. This disorder is commonly caused by GI loss of bicarbonate (e.g., chronic diarrhea) or a failure of kidneys to excrete acid (e.g., renal tubular acidosis).[89]

High anion-gap metabolic acidosis occurs when there is an accumulation of "unmeasured anions," or anions other than chloride and bicarbonate. Common causes of high anion-gap metabolic acidosis include lactic acidosis, ketoacidosis (e.g., from uncontrolled diabetes mellitus), kidney failure, salicylate (aspirin) poisoning, and chronic acetaminophen use.[89] **Table 2.13** summarizes possible causes of normal and high anion gap metabolic acidosis.

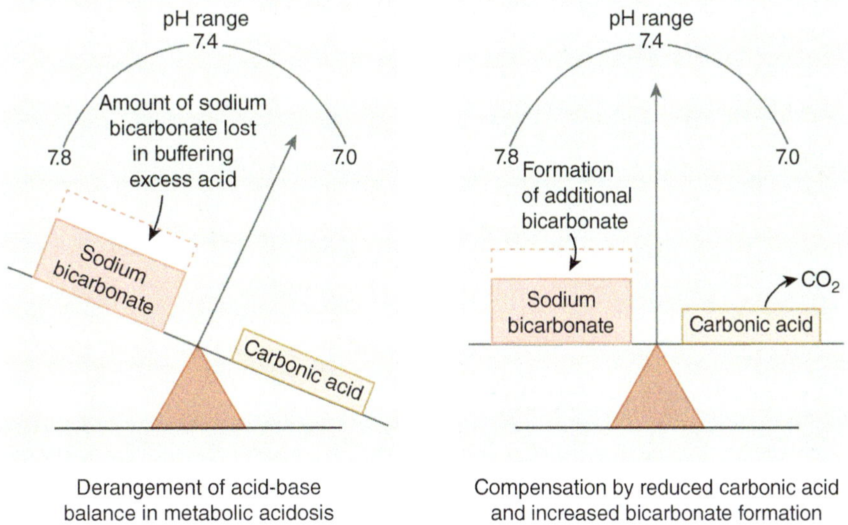

Figure 2.13 Metabolic Acidosis: Bicarbonate and Carbonic Acid Imbalance

Table 2.13 Common Causes of Metabolic Acidosis

Normal Anion Gap	Increased Anion Gap
■ Gastrointestinal loss of HCO_3^- • Diarrhea • Pancreatic fistula • Urinary diversion procedures ■ Ingestions • Ammonium chloride • Parenteral nutrition (chloride salts) ■ Renal loss of HCO_3^- • Carbonic anhydrase inhibitors • Hyperparathyroidism • Renal tubular acidosis	■ Failure to excrete acids • Kidney failure ■ Increased production of endogenous acid • Inborn errors of metabolism • Ketoacidosis • Lactic acidosis ■ Ingestion of exogenous acid • Salicylates, methanol, ethanol

Data from Canada T, Lord LM. Fluid, electrolytes, and acid-base disorders. In: Chan LN, ed. *ASPEN Adult Nutrition Support Core Curriculum*. 4th ed. Silver Spring, MD: The American Society for Parenteral and Enteral Nutrition; 2025:159-192.

Table 2.14 Causes of Saline-Responsive and Saline-Resistant Metabolic Alkalosis

Saline-Responsive (Urine Chloride <20 mEq/L)	Saline-Resistant (Urine Chloride >20 mEq/L)
■ Diuretic therapy ■ Excessive bicarbonate administration ■ Gastrointestinal loss ■ Nasogastric suction ■ Rapid correction of hypocapnia ■ Renal losses ■ Vomiting	■ Cushing syndrome ■ Excess mineralocorticoids ■ Excessive licorice ingestion (e.g., from chewing tobacco) ■ Hyperaldosteronism ■ Profound potassium depletion

Data from Canada T, Lord LM. Fluid, electrolytes, and acid-base disorders. In: Chan LN, ed. ASPEN *Adult Nutrition Support Core Curriculum*. 4th ed. Silver Spring, MD: The American Society for Parenteral and Enteral Nutrition; 2025:159-192.

Treatment of both normal and high anion-gap metabolic acidosis requires correcting the underlying cause. For instance, this may involve fluid repletion for patients with hypovolemia and insulin therapy for patients with diabetic ketoacidosis. Sodium bicarbonate infusion may be used to treat severe acidemia (pH <7.1), although the current evidence suggests limited benefit from this approach.[90]

Metabolic alkalosis is characterized by a high pH, high HCO_3^-, and compensatory hypoventilation that results in an increased PCO_2. Common causes of this disorder include loss of gastric acid from vomiting or nasogastric suction and loss of intravascular volume and chloride from diuretic use. In hospital settings, metabolic alkalosis is frequently caused by excessive bicarbonate administration (e.g., in the treatment of metabolic acidosis) and an excess of acetate (a precursor to bicarbonate) in PN.[91] Hypokalemia can also contribute to the development of metabolic alkalosis, by causing a transcellular shift of hydrogen ions. Normally, the kidneys are able to correct metabolic alkalosis by excreting excess bicarbonate in urine. Thus, maintenance of metabolic alkalosis indicates some degree of impairment in renal bicarbonate excretion. Urine chloride concentration can be used to classify metabolic alkalosis into two major types: saline-responsive and saline-resistant.

Saline-responsive metabolic alkalosis (urine chloride <20 mEq/L) is a metabolic alkalosis associated with decreased extracellular volume and low urine chloride. To treat this disorder, administration of normal saline is recommended to reverse the increase in bicarbonate reabsorption that maintains alkalosis. While sufficient repletion of sodium chloride can typically normalize bicarbonate concentration, metabolic alkalosis will not be reversed if associated with hypokalemia. Potassium chloride is required to correct this underlying disorder.

Saline-unresponsive metabolic alkalosis (urine chloride >20 mEq/L) is characterized by normal to increased extracellular volume and high urine chloride, and is commonly caused by mineralocorticoid excess. Treatment of this disorder involves addressing the underlying cause (i.e., reversing or blocking mineralocorticoid excess, if possible) and correcting electrolyte abnormalities such as hypokalemia. **Table 2.14** outlines common causes of saline-responsive and saline-resistant metabolic alkalosis.

Mixed acid-base disorders occur when patients have more than one acid-base disturbance occurring simultaneously. Diagnosing a mixed acid-base disorder involves identifying the primary acid disorder, then evaluating whether the degree of compensation is appropriate. When a set of blood gases does not fall within the range of expected responses for a simple acid-base disturbance, then clinicians should suspect that a mixed disorder exists. Mixed acid-base disorders can include combinations of metabolic disorders (e.g., vomiting-induced metabolic alkalosis and hypovolemia-induced lactic acidosis), mixed metabolic and respiratory disorders (e.g., metabolic acidosis and respiratory alkalosis in the setting of salicylate intoxication), and more complex combinations.[92]

Respiratory Disorders. **Respiratory acidosis** is characterized by a low pH, high PCO_2, and variable increase in plasma HCO_3^- concentration. This disorder is most often due to conditions or situations that cause a decrease in CO_2 exhalation, such as pulmonary diseases, neuromuscular disorders, and drugs that cause respiratory depression. Although less common, respiratory acidosis may also be caused by increased CO_2 production, such as in cases of chronic overfeeding.[87] Treatment of respiratory acidosis should focus on addressing the underlying cause (e.g., removing offending medication, providing bronchodilators to patients with asthma or COPD, etc.). In patients with severely impaired CO_2 excretion and/or life-threatening hypoxemia, adequate oxygenation should be provided. In cases of overfeeding, reduction of total caloric provision may be indicated. Sodium bicarbonate infusion may be provided when acidosis is severe (pH <7.2) and not responsive to other treatments.[15]

Respiratory alkalosis is characterized by a high pH, low PCO_2, and variable decrease in plasma HCO_3^- concentration. This occurs when the rate of CO_2 removal via ventilation exceeds the rate of CO_2 production, leading to hyperventilation. Common causes of respiratory alkalosis include pulmonary disease, hypoxemia, and increased respiratory stimulation. **Table 2.15** outlines additional causes of respiratory acid-base imbalances. Treatment of respiratory alkalosis depends on the underlying cause, and may involve discontinuation of offending medication, provision of analgesic agents (e.g., for patients with pain or inadequate sedation), and supportive counseling (e.g., for patients with hyperventilation due to anxiety). Refer to Chapter 14, *Nutrition in Pulmonary Disease*, for more information on nutritional therapy for respiratory disorders.

Table 2.15 Causes of Respiratory Acid-Base Disorders

Respiratory Acidosis	Respiratory Alkalosis
▪ Acute respiratory distress syndrome (ARDS) ▪ Aspiration ▪ Asthma ▪ Bronchitis ▪ Chronic obstructive pulmonary disease (COPD) ▪ Head injury ▪ Hypoventilation ▪ Malignancy ▪ Medications (e.g., opioids, anesthetics, sedatives, neuromuscular blockers) ▪ Neuromuscular diseases (e.g., amyotrophic lateral sclerosis, Guillain-Barré syndrome, multiple sclerosis) ▪ Overfeeding ▪ Pulmonary edema ▪ Sleep apnea ▪ Spinal cord injury ▪ Stroke	▪ Altitudes (high) ▪ Anemia (severe) ▪ Anxiety ▪ Asthma ▪ Brain tumor ▪ Cirrhosis ▪ Fever ▪ Head trauma ▪ Hyperventilation ▪ Hypoxemia ▪ Medications (e.g., catecholamines, nicotine, salicylate, xanthine derivatives) ▪ Meningitis ▪ Pain ▪ Pregnancy ▪ Pulmonary edema or embolus ▪ Pneumonia ▪ Vascular accident

Data from Bruno JJ. *ASPEN Fluids, Electrolytes, and Acid-Base Disorders Handbook*. 2nd ed. American Society for Parenteral and Enteral Nutrition; 2020.

CORE CONCEPT 4

Fluid, electrolyte, and acid-base imbalances can lead to serious complications, ranging from metabolic and gastrointestinal problems to cardiovascular, respiratory, and neurological concerns, each requiring careful evaluation, monitoring, and treatment.

Glucose and Glycosylated Hemoglobin

Glucose values are important in screening and diagnosing endocrine disorders and in monitoring patients with acute stress and critical illness. Evaluating trends in glucose measures is essential to determine glucose tolerance and prevent adverse, potentially fatal consequences associated with glycemic abnormalities.

Blood glucose, the measure of glucose in plasma (also known as "plasma glucose" [PG]), is a short-term indicator of glycemic response and glucose tolerance. Normal *fasting plasma glucose* (FPG) values range from 70 to 100 mg/dL (3.9–5.6 mmol/L), and normal *2-hour postprandial plasma glucose* (2-h PG) values are less than 140 mg/dL (7.8 mmol/L). FPG >100 mg/dL or 2-h PG >140 mg/dL suggest impaired glucose metabolism.[93] Diagnostic criteria for diabetes mellitus (DM) include FPG ≥126 mg/dL (7.0 mmol/L), 2-h PG ≥200 mg/dL (11.1 mmol/L), or classic symptoms of hyperglycemia or hyperglycemic crises with random plasma glucose ≥200 mg/dL.[88] Blood glucose measurements provide valuable information in every step of the nutrition care process, from assessing nutritional risk, to establishing a nutrition-related diagnosis, to monitoring and evaluating the effectiveness of nutrition interventions.

Urine glucose, while not a diagnostic criterion, may also be abnormal in patients with DM. Normal urine glucose tests should be negative, while patients with DM may have positive tests. Glucosuria (the presence of glucose in the urine) can develop when the filtered load of glucose exceeds the kidneys' reabsorption capacity, which may occur at blood glucose levels over 180 mg/dL.[94] Treatment of glucosuria includes managing DM and improving hydration status, due to the loss of water that follows when glucose is present in urine.

Urine ketones may be evaluated when glucose levels are elevated during periods of illness or stress. For patients with DM, urine ketones should be tested if blood glucose is consistently above 240 mg/dL.[95] In healthy patients without diabetes, urine ketones should be negative. Uncontrolled DM is the most common cause of ketonuria (the presence of ketones in the urine).[96] Other potential causes include fever, anorexia, GI disturbances, persistent vomiting, cachexia, fasting, and starvation. Ketonuria can be a possible indication of diabetic ketoacidosis, a condition characterized by dehydration and electrolyte imbalances due to osmotic diuresis. Without immediate treatment, diabetic ketoacidosis can be fatal. Treatment includes correction of severe hyperglycemia with IV fluids, insulin, and electrolytes. Doses of supplemental insulin are required until metabolic stability returns.[97]

Glycosylated hemoglobin (HbA1c) reflects the amount of glucose in the bloodstream that is bound to hemoglobin. HbA1c provides a measure of the average blood glucose levels over 3 months (the average lifespan of red blood cells). A 1% change in HbA1c correlates with an approximate 35 mg/dL change in plasma glucose.[98] **Table 2.16** demonstrates the correlations between HbA1c and average blood glucose levels. Unlike blood glucose levels, an HbA1c test does not reflect recent changes, making it a useful measure to differentiate between short-term hyperglycemia (e.g., due to physiologic stress) and long-term hyperglycemia in patients with DM. HbA1c may be tested in a fasting or fed state, and it should be measured in a certified laboratory using a standardized assay (i.e., not by a finger stick test). In adults with normal glycemic control, HbA1c values range from 4.3% to 5.6%.[99] HbA1c values of 5.7–6.4% fall in the prediabetic range, and values ≥6.5% can be used to diagnose DM.[88] Diagnosis of DM is confirmed when there are two abnormal screening test results (i.e., HbA1c ≥6.5%, FBG ≥126 mg/dL, or 2-h PG ≥200 mg/dL) measured either together or at two different times.[88]

Table 2.16 Hemoglobin A1c and Estimated Equivalent Average Blood Glucose

Hemoglobin A1c	Mean Blood Glucose
6%	126 mg/dL
7%	154 mg/dL
8%	183 mg/dL
9%	212 mg/dL
10%	240 mg/dL
11%	269 mg/dL
12%	298 mg/dL

Data from Nathan DM, Kuenen J, Borg R, Zheng H, Schoenfeld D, Heine RJ; A1c-Derived Average Glucose Study Group. Translating the A1C assay into estimated average glucose values. *Diabetes Care.* 2008;31:1473–1478.

Conditions that increase or decrease red blood cell turnover may alter the results of the HbA1c test. For example, conditions that reduce red blood cell production, such as iron, vitamin B12, or folate deficiency anemias, can lead to falsely elevated HbA1c levels.[100] Conversely, conditions that increase red blood cell turnover, such as pregnancy, blood transfusions, and use of erythropoiesis-stimulating agents or iron-replacement therapies, can lead to falsely low HbA1c.[101,102] Thus, HbA1c should be used as a secondary measure (after blood glucose) of glycemic status during pregnancy.[102] In addition to being diagnostic criteria, HbA1c and trends in blood glucose levels are considered preferred indicators of glycemic control in patients with DM.[103] Clinicians can interpret trends in these levels and use this information to make recommendations for improved nutrition and DM management.

Hypoglycemia, or low blood glucose, may be due to fasting, glycogen storage disease, liver disease, renal insufficiency, excessive alcohol intake, abrupt PN cessation, cancer, and prolonged exercise, among other possible causes. Hypoglycemia is defined as a plasma glucose level below 70 mg/dL, although signs and symptoms may not appear until plasma glucose falls below 54 mg/dL.[103] The clinical manifestations of hypoglycemia include irritability, confusion, tremors, sweating, and fatigue. In severe cases, hypoglycemia may lead to loss of consciousness, seizure, coma, and potential death if not immediately corrected. Treatment for hypoglycemia involves the provision of a fast-acting carbohydrate source (e.g., fruit juice), followed by ongoing blood glucose monitoring and further carbohydrate intake as needed. Patients who are unable or unwilling to consume carbohydrates by mouth may be prescribed glucagon, which may be administered intramuscularly or intranasally.

Hyperglycemia, or high blood glucose, can result from conditions such as uncontrolled diabetes, pancreatic insufficiency, obesity, acute stress, and cirrhosis. Hyperglycemia is generally defined as an FPG above 125 mg/dL or 2-h PG above 180 mg/dL.[104] Severe hyperglycemia may be observed with diabetic ketoacidosis and hyperglycemic hyperosmolar state, which are serious, potentially life-threatening complications of DM. Symptoms of severe hyperglycemia may include increased urine output, glucosuria, hypernatremia, and headaches. Treatment of severe hyperglycemia requires replacement of fluids and electrolytes and insulin administration. Refer to Chapter 8, *Nutrition in Diabetes Mellitus*, for further discussion of blood glucose, HbA1c, and diabetes management.

Protein Assessment

Adequate protein in the body is essential for cellular growth and metabolism. Despite the large amount of protein in muscle and viscera, the body strives to avoid using protein as an energy source by drawing primarily from fat and glycogen stores. In the setting of acute or chronic metabolic stress, protein may be drawn from muscle to meet energy needs. Protein status can be assessed using a combination of anthropometric, dietary, physical, and biochemical measures. Biochemical assessment of protein focuses on evaluation from two compartments: somatic (muscle) and visceral (non-muscle) protein. **Somatic protein**, or protein within skeletal muscle, makes up most of the total body protein pool. **Visceral protein** represents a small portion of total body protein and includes non-muscular protein in organs, structural components, serum proteins, and blood cells.

Total serum protein measures the total amount of protein in the blood and includes two major categories of plasma protein: albumin and globulins. Globulins are produced by the liver and immune cells and include hundreds of serum proteins such as immunoglobulins, carrier proteins, and enzymes. Normal total serum protein levels range from 5.5 to 9 g/dL.[105] Abnormalities may be caused by changes in total plasma volume or the concentration of one or more plasma proteins. Low total serum protein, or hypoproteinemia, can result from decreased protein production or increased protein losses. Common causes of hypoproteinemia include liver disorders, kidney disorders, and GI malabsorption disorders such as celiac disease or inflammatory bowel disease. Low total protein levels may also be seen in patients with severe malnutrition. High total protein levels, or hyperproteinemia, can result from chronic inflammation or infection, such as viral hepatitis or human immunodeficiency virus (HIV), as well as bone marrow disorders such as multiple myeloma. Medications, inflammation, infection,

CASE STUDY REVISITED

It is now postop day 6/HD 12 and Adam remains in the ICU. He is currently receiving enteral nutrition support since postop day 3, which provides him with 1700 calories and 100 g protein.

Anthropometric Data:

Weight: 76 kg
Last Weight: 77 kg postop day 1/HD 7

Admit weight 75 kg

Biochemical Data:

Albumin 2.1 (3.5–5.5 g/dL)
Prealbumin 14 (16–30 mg/dL)

Urine urea nitrogen (UUN) 10 g/24 hours

Questions

1. How do you interpret Adam's current albumin and prealbumin levels? What information does this provide for your assessment of Adam's nutritional status?
2. Calculate Adam's nitrogen balance. Is he in positive or negative nitrogen balance?
3. What biochemical indices should be included in your monitoring and evaluation plan to further assess nutritional adequacy?

prolonged bed rest, chronic illness, and pregnancy can also impact total serum protein levels. If patients have abnormal total serum protein levels, clinicians must further assess serum globulin and albumin levels to evaluate the etiology and determine the appropriate nutrition therapy.

Visceral Proteins

Visceral protein indirectly measures protein stores by assessing the proteins made by the viscera, or the internal organs of the body (primarily the liver). When acute illness or trauma causes inflammation and metabolic stress, hormones and cell-mediated responses trigger muscle breakdown. **Acute-phase proteins** respond to inflammation by either increasing (positive acute-phase proteins) or decreasing (negative acute-phase proteins) in concentration. As a result, protein status can be difficult to assess in acutely ill patients because these acute-phase proteins do not accurately reflect changes in protein status. Inflammation, which can be identified by serum visceral proteins, can contribute to numerous nutrition-related issues, including loss of lean body mass due to muscle catabolism, reduced intake due to inflammation-associated anorexia, and altered levels of **micronutrients** such as iron, copper, and zinc.[106,107] Clinicians must consider the specificity, sensitivity, and reliability of each visceral protein measurement when assessing and treating patients with acute illnesses.

Positive acute-phase proteins such as C-reactive protein, ferritin, and ceruloplasmin increase during inflammation. *C-reactive protein (CRP)* is a nonspecific inflammatory biomarker, with a normal level defined as ≤ 0.8 mg/dL.[105] CRP increases as levels of transport proteins (e.g., prealbumin and albumin) decrease. While the exact function of CRP is unclear, it increases rapidly in response to inflammation, trauma, or infection. Generally, a higher CRP indicates increased nutritional risk.

Negative acute-phase proteins include serum albumin, prealbumin, retinol binding protein, and transferrin. These transport proteins are synthesized in the liver and decrease during acute-inflammatory stress, injury, or illness.

Albumin accounts for approximately 50–60% of total serum proteins.[108] Normal serum albumin levels range from 3.5 to 5.5 g/dL.[105] Albumin has many important functions in the body, such as serving as a carrier of circulating molecules and regulating vascular fluid and electrolyte balance. Major blood constituents, hormones, enzymes, medications, minerals, ions, fatty acids, and metabolites are all transported via albumin. Maintenance of colloidal osmotic pressure also requires albumin, with albumin accounting for about 80% of colloidal osmotic pressure of the plasma.[109] Serum albumin is widely used in hospital settings, as low serum albumin levels have been shown to be predictors of morbidity and mortality.[110–112] However, while albumin can help characterize inflammation (and thus, overall nutritional risk), it is not an indicator of malnutrition per se. Albumin has a relatively long half-life of 18–21 days, meaning it can take several weeks for albumin levels to reflect changes in nutritional status. Thus, the use of serum albumin as a marker of nutritional status is not recommended in acute illness.[113]

Several non-dietary factors can alter serum albumin levels. Hypoalbuminemia (low serum albumin) may be caused by changes in fluid distribution, increased albumin losses, and (although rare) decreased albumin synthesis. For instance, hypoalbuminemia may be caused by renal losses (e.g., nephrotic syndrome or CKD), GI losses (e.g., protein-losing enteropathy, malabsorptive disorders), and extravascular losses (e.g., burns, sepsis).[114] Hypoalbuminemia is also common in patients with cirrhosis, which may be related to decreased albumin production.[114] Additionally, hydration status affects serum albumin levels because water in the plasma shifts between the interstitial compartment if patients are overhydrated (leading to decreased albumin) or dehydrated (leading to increased albumin).

Albumin may also be abnormal in patients with **kwashiorkor**, a type of protein-energy malnutrition characterized by protein deficiency with or without caloric deficit. In this condition, inadequate protein intake is associated with deranged protein metabolism. Specifically, insulin will stimulate muscle protein anabolism and decrease catabolism, leading to reduced release of amino acids from muscle. Inadequate amino acids lead to insufficient hepatic albumin synthesis, resulting in low albumin levels. Given the importance of albumin for fluid balance, patients with kwashiorkor commonly experience edema due to hypoalbuminemia. As a result, these patients may have low serum albumin levels, while their weight may be normal or elevated due to fluid retention (**Figure 2.14**). In contrast, in patients with **marasmus**, which is a type of protein-energy malnutrition characterized by severe caloric depletion, the body uses fat and somatic protein (i.e., muscle) as fuel, but conserves visceral protein (which is presumably more critical for survival).[115] Thus, despite severe fat and muscle loss, albumin levels may remain normal in patients with marasmus.

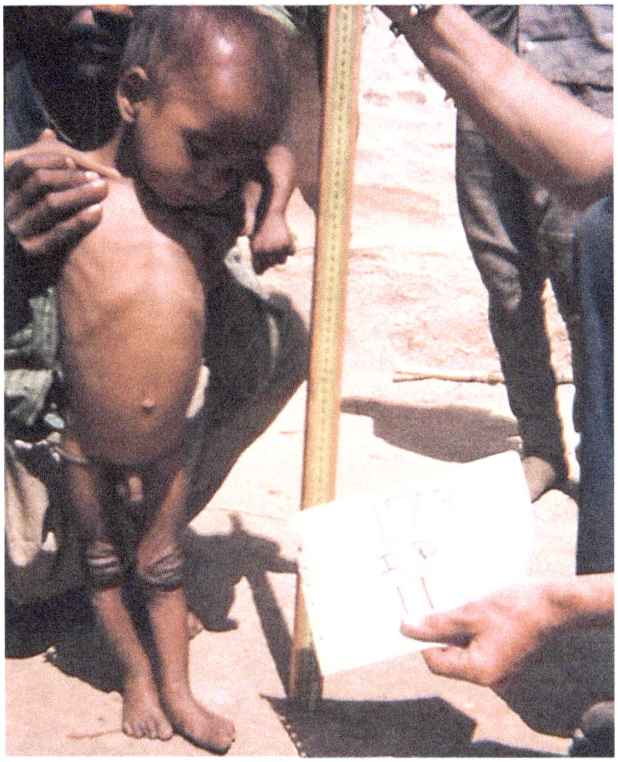

Figure 2.14 Extremity Edema and a Bloated Abdomen are Common in Kwashiorkor

Courtesy of CDC/Dr. Lyle Conrad.

Table 2.17 Factors Affecting Serum Albumin and Prealbumin Levels

Serum Protein	Factors that Increase	Factors that Decrease
Albumin	■ Anabolic hormones ■ Corticosteroids ■ Dehydration ■ Exogenous albumin	■ Burns ■ Chronic kidney disease ■ Cirrhosis ■ Malabsorptive disorders ■ Nephrotic syndrome ■ Overhydration ■ Protein-losing enteropathy ■ Sepsis
Prealbumin	■ Corticosteroids ■ Nonsteroidal anti-inflammatory agents ■ Oral contraceptives ■ Severe kidney failure	■ Burns ■ Hyperthyroidism ■ Infection ■ Liver dysfunction ■ Trauma

Data from Delliere S, Cynober L. Is transthyretin a good marker of nutritional status? *Clin Nutr.* 2017;36(2):364–370. doi:10.1016/j.clnu.2016.06.004

Increased albumin levels (hyperalbuminemia) can result from dehydration and exogenous albumin administration. Anabolic hormones and corticosteroids can also raise albumin levels higher than normal. Clinicians must interpret changes in albumin level with caution, recognizing that low albumin is likely an indicator of stress or inflammation., if present, and not overall protein status.

Prealbumin (PAB) is a hepatic protein transported in the serum bound to retinol-binding protein and vitamin A. PAB received its name after it was found to migrate ahead of albumin on electrophoresis. Normal PAB levels range from 16 to 30 mg/dL.[105] PAB is also known as transthyretin due to its role in transporting thyroid hormones (triiodothyronine and thyroxine) and retinol binding protein. It is synthesized in the liver and is renally excreted, although it is not influenced by hydration status. With a relatively short half-life of 2–3 days, PAB is considered a more sensitive indicator of nutritional status than albumin.[113,116] However, since PAB levels are influenced by inflammation, the reliability of PAB as a marker of nutritional status is limited during acute inflammatory states. Thus, it has been proposed that PAB should not be used for nutritional assessment when CRP (an inflammatory biomarker) exceeds 15 mg/L.[117]

Low PAB levels may be caused by illness, infection, trauma, burns, metabolic stress, liver dysfunction, and hyperthyroidism. Serum PAB may also decrease in the presence of zinc deficiency, as zinc is necessary for the synthesis and secretion of PAB in the liver.[118] Serum PAB may increase due to severe kidney failure, corticosteroids, nonsteroidal anti-inflammatory agents, and oral contraceptives.[117] **Table 2.17** summarizes factors that can increase or decrease serum albumin and PAB levels. Clinicians must consider the etiology of abnormal PAB or albumin levels to assess and monitor the condition appropriately.

Retinol-binding protein (RBP) is an acute-phase protein produced in the liver whose main function is to transport vitamin A in the blood. Normal RBP levels range from 3 to 6 mg/dL.[116] With a short half-life of approximately 12 hours, RBP is considered a relatively sensitive indicator of protein status. RBP is a small protein that does not pass through the renal glomerulus because it circulates bound to PAB. Once RBP releases retinol in peripheral tissue, the PAB-RBP complex dissociates. RBP is then filtered by the glomerulus and catabolized by the renal tubule.

As with other negative acute-phase proteins, RBP decreases in the presence of inflammatory stress. Serum RBP levels are reduced in acute catabolic states, post-surgery, hyperthyroidism, and liver diseases such as hepatitis and cirrhosis.[119] Low RBP levels may also be seen with vitamin A deficiency (since most of vitamin A circulating in blood is bound to RBP) as well as zinc deficiency, as low levels of zinc may inhibit mobilization of RBP in the liver.[119] RBP therefore cannot reliably assess protein status until such deficiencies are addressed. Also, since RBP is catabolized in the kidneys, high levels are common when kidney function is impaired. Thus, RBP does not accurately reflect protein-energy status in patients with renal insufficiency.

Transferrin is a globulin protein that transports iron in blood to bone marrow for hemoglobin production. Transferrin also helps prevent the growth of harmful bacteria by binding free iron and removing it from bacteria that require iron for survival. Normal serum transferrin levels range from 200 to 400 mg/dL.[105] Serum transferrin can be measured directly or derived from total iron binding capacity (TIBC), which is an estimate of the blood's capacity to bind iron with transferrin. Refer to the "Hematology" section of this chapter for more information on TIBC.

Serum transferrin levels are highly dependent on the size of the iron storage pool. Transferrin levels increase when iron stores are depleted (e.g., in iron deficiency anemia), to accommodate the need for increased levels of iron transport. In contrast, transferrin levels fall in response to a decreased need for iron transport (e.g., due to decreased iron absorption), which may occur with infection, iron overload, malignancies, and liver dysfunction. Although transferrin has a shorter half-life (~10 days) than albumin, it does not respond fast enough to changes in intake to be a useful indicator of protein status in acutely ill patients. Transferrin is thus not a specific indicator for malnutrition, nor a valid measure for iron deficiency anemia.

CORE CONCEPT 5

Visceral proteins can be altered by acute and chronic metabolic stress, making them more accurate indicators of inflammation than indicators of nutritional status.

PRACTICE POINT

During acute stress, exogenous protein alone will not attenuate the loss of endogenous protein.

Somatic Proteins

Like visceral proteins, assessment of somatic (skeletal muscle) proteins can provide clinicians with a more in-depth understanding of protein status and requirements, while recognizing how certain conditions may influence interpretation of these values.

Nitrogen balance occurs when nitrogen input (Nin) or intake (oral, enteral, or parenteral) is equal to nitrogen output (Nout) or excretion (urinary, fecal, or wound drainage). Since nitrogen is a key component of proteins, it can be a useful measure when evaluating protein status. Urine urea nitrogen (UUN) is the primary biochemical measure used to calculate Nout. UUN is the end-product of protein breakdown in the body and thus signifies protein catabolism. One gram of nitrogen loss is thought to equal about 30 g of lean tissue loss.[120] Thus, during severe illness, up to about 0.5 kg of lean mass could be lost per day as a result of excess protein catabolism.[120]

To calculate nitrogen balance (Nbal) a 24-hour urine collection is needed for analysis of UUN. Because urea nitrogen only represents approximately 85% of total urine nitrogen (TUN), with ammonia being the other significant contributor of nitrogen in the urine, a correction factor of 0.85 is applied. In addition, a factor of 2 g of nitrogen is added to Nout to represent non-urinary nitrogen losses that occur in sweat, stool, and wound exudate. To calculate Nin, a 24-hour dietary intake of protein is collected. Since protein contains approximately 16% nitrogen by weight, 1 g of nitrogen is equivalent to 6.25 g of protein. Thus, total protein intake is converted to grams of nitrogen using a factor of 6.25. The following equation is used to calculate Nbal[121]:

$$\text{Nbal} = \text{Nin} - \text{Nout}$$

$$\text{Nbal} = \text{Dietary protein intake(g)}/6.25\text{ g Nitrogen} - [(\text{UUN}/0.85) + 2]$$

Sample Calculation: Protein intake = 94 g; UUN = 13 g/24 hours;
Non-urinary nitrogen losses = 2 g/24 hours

$$\text{Nbal} = 94/6.25 - [(13/0.85) + 2]$$

$$\text{Nbal} = 15 - 17$$

$$\text{Nbal} = -2\text{ g nitrogen}$$

For example, a patient with a protein intake of 94 g and a UUN of 13 g/24 hours would have a Nbal of negative 2 g, meaning they are in negative nitrogen balance. Protein intake would have to be increased by 2 g nitrogen (or ~12 g protein) to reach nitrogen balance. Since the nitrogen balance goal for anabolism is positive 2–4 g nitrogen, an additional 12–25 g of protein would be added to their protein intake goal.

Nitrogen balance can be used for critically ill patients receiving nutrition support. If patients have a negative nitrogen balance, recommendations typically include increasing protein and caloric intake. However, nitrogen balance carries numerous limitations, particularly in acute care settings. For instance, a valid 24-hour urine collection can be inconvenient and tedious to collect unless a patient has a urinary catheter. Urine collection also fails to account for nitrogen losses from wounds, burns, diarrhea, and vomiting. Equally confounding is the use of a factor of 0.85 to determine TUN from UUN, as this is flawed in patients with variable excretion of ammonia (e.g., during trauma, kidney disease, and liver failure). True protein status can be better described by protein turnover or flux, which requires labeled protein (stable isotope) to measure protein synthesis and breakdown. This is typically done as part of a research protocol rather than as part of routine protein assessment. If nitrogen balance is used to estimate protein status in critically ill patients or those with conditions that alter urinary nitrogen excretion, clinicians must recognize the limitations of UUN as a measure of nitrogen output. TUN should be measured when possible, although this is often not practical in a clinical setting.

Creatinine is a nitrogen-containing compound that is produced endogenously and obtained from dietary sources. The endogenous formation of creatine begins in the kidneys, where the amino acids arginine and glycine react to form guanidinoacetate. The second step occurs in the liver, where guanidinoacetate is methylated using S-adenosyl methionine.[122] Once synthesized, creatinine enters the blood and travels to tissues. About 95% of creatinine resides in muscle, and the remaining 5% in organs such as the heart, brain, and testes.[123] In muscle, about two-thirds of creatinine exists as creatinine phosphate (the phosphorylated form of creatinine), and the remainder as free creatinine.[123] Creatine phosphate serves as an energy transport system, providing high-energy phosphates from ATP production to support muscle contraction. Creatine phosphate is degraded to form free creatinine, which is then cleared from muscle and excreted by the kidneys, and this occurs at a fairly constant rate. As a result, daily urine output of creatinine has been found to correlate with total muscle mass.[124]

Although urinary creatinine can help with assessing somatic protein status in some patients, it is confounded by many variables. First, dietary creatinine cannot be distinguished from endogenously produced creatinine in the body. Thus, creatinine clearance may be a poor reflection of somatic muscle status in patients with a high dietary creatinine intake (e.g., from red meat, fish, or creatine supplements). Additionally, urinary creatinine is influenced by other factors such as sex, with higher clearance rates among males than females, as well as drugs such as trimethoprim-sulfamethoxazole (Bactrim), which can increase circulating creatinine levels.[125]

Creatinine height index (CHI) compares a patient's urinary creatinine to the amount expected in patients of the same sex and height. A calculated CHI >90% is considered normal; 80–90% suggests mild skeletal muscle depletion; 60–80% suggests moderate skeletal muscle depletion; and <60% suggests severe skeletal muscle depletion.[126] CHI is calculated using the following equation[127]:

$$\text{CHI} = \text{Actual 24-hour urine creatinine (mg)}/\text{Expected 24-hour urine creatinine (mg)}$$

where expected creatinine excretion is:

Female: 18 mg/kg
Male: 23 mg/kg

Sample Calculation: 66 kg female;
24-hour creatinine excretion: 890 mg

$$\text{Expected 24-hour urine creatinine (mg)} = 18 \text{ mg/kg} \times 66 \text{ kg} = 1188 \text{ mg}$$

$$\text{CHI} = 890 \text{ mg}/1188 \text{ mg}$$

$$\text{CHI} = 75\%$$

For example, a female weighing 66 kg with a 24-creatinine excretion of 890 mg/24 hours has CHI of 75%, suggesting mild muscle depletion.

CHI also has some limitations that clinicians must consider. As with UUN excretion, a test of urine creatinine excretion can be difficult to obtain. Furthermore, standards in the calculations for urinary creatinine do not account for variations in age, disease, physical training, body frame size, or weight status. In addition, factors such as incomplete urine collection, impaired kidney function, high meat or milk intake, and glucocorticoid use can impact creatinine excretion independently of changes in muscle mass.[120] Clinicians must account for these potential confounding factors when using urine creatinine values to evaluate protein status.

While urinary creatinine has been used to assess somatic proteins status, *serum creatinine* is more commonly used (alongside blood urea nitrogen) to assess kidney function. Normal serum creatinine levels range 0.5–1.1 mg/dL in females and 0.7–1.3 mg/dL in males.[105] Since serum creatinine is maintained within a relatively narrow range by the kidneys, elevated levels are most commonly due to impaired kidney function, which leads to poor creatinine clearance. In contrast, low serum creatinine levels may result from decreased muscle mass, such as from advanced age or chronic disease (e.g., cancer, liver disease). Clinicians must evaluate serum creatinine with other measures to determine the etiology of and treatment for abnormal values.

Blood urea nitrogen (BUN) is a serum byproduct of protein metabolism, commonly used to help assess kidney function. Normal BUN levels are 8–20 mg/dL.[105] BUN reflects the amount of circulating urea, which is a nitrogen-containing compound formed in the liver through protein metabolism. Specifically, through a series of biochemical reactions called the "urea cycle," ammonia, which is produced through protein catabolism and generated by intestinal bacteria, is converted to urea. This urea then enters the bloodstream and travels to the kidneys, where it is filtered and excreted through the urine. In healthy individuals, there is usually a small amount of urea nitrogen in the blood, although many factors can alter BUN levels.

High BUN levels may result from conditions that reduce urea excretion (e.g., renal insufficiency) or increase urea production (e.g., excessive protein intake, GI bleeding, hypercatabolic states). BUN should be interpreted in conjunction with creatinine to assess kidney function. In kidney and liver disease, BUN levels may rise and then return to normal. Clinicians should be careful in interpreting this drop, as it does not suggest improved renal excretory function, but rather may reflect the inability of the liver to form urea. In these patients, BUN may remain normal or only slightly elevated, while blood ammonia levels may rise as liver function declines. Hydration status is also important to consider when interpreting BUN levels, as dehydration may cause BUN to be temporarily elevated. Increased BUN levels are also common in patients with acute myocardial infarction, since decreased cardiac function may impair renal blood flow, thus reducing urea nitrogen excretion and leading to an accumulation of BUN.

Low BUN is less common and is not typically a cause for concern. Low BUN levels may occur in patients with protein-energy malnutrition, severe liver damage, malabsorption, and overhydration.[128] However, low BUN levels are rarely used to diagnose or monitor these conditions.

A BUN:creatinine ratio can provide further insight into the etiology of abnormal BUN levels. Normal BUN:creatinine ratios typically range from approximately 10:1 to 20:1.[129] An elevated BUN:creatinine ratio is common in hypovolemic states due to increased urea reabsorption. A high BUN:creatinine ratio may also be observed with GI bleeding, catabolic states, and steroid medications.[129] Conversely, a low BUN:creatinine ratio may be caused by low protein intake, advanced liver disease, rhabdomyolysis, and sickle cell anemia.[130] Patients with renal insufficiency may have a normal BUN:creatinine ratio, due to both BUN and creatinine levels being elevated. Thus, both BUN and BUN:creatinine values must be interpreted cautiously. Clinicians must consider the etiology of abnormal BUN levels alongside other protein assessment measures when determining the appropriate treatment.

Enzymes

Biochemical assessment of serum enzymes can aid in the evaluation of a wide range of conditions affecting various organ systems. Aspartate aminotransferase, alanine aminotransferase, alkaline phosphatase, and lactate dehydrogenase are among the most common enzymes found within the blood that may be abnormal in conditions such as liver, kidney, cardiac, and bone disorders. Clinicians must evaluate these serum enzymes in conjunction with the serum proteins discussed above when assessing and treating patients.

Aspartate aminotransferase (AST), also known as "aspartate transaminase," is an enzyme found primarily in the heart, liver, skeletal muscle cells, and to a lesser extent in the kidneys and pancreas. Normal serum AST values range from 10 to 40 U/L.[105] Elevated AST levels may be seen in hepatocellular disease and coronary occlusive heart disease. An increase in AST is directly correlated to the number of cells affected by the disease or injury. During a myocardial infarction, AST levels begin to rise within 6–8 hours of symptom onset, peak at 24–36 hours, and return to normal in 3–7 days unless another cardiac injury occurs.[131] Therefore, AST levels are often evaluated to estimate the time of myocardial infarction. Acute liver damage also increases AST levels, peaking at up to 25 times the normal value.[132] In chronic liver disease, high AST levels persist. Other conditions that may increase AST levels include celiac disease, thyroid disorders, strenuous exercise, and Wilson disease.[132]

Low serum AST is common in patients with vitamin B6 deficiency, since AST requires vitamin B6 as a cofactor. Other possible causes of low AST levels include diabetic ketoacidosis, chronic liver disease, and hemodialysis.[128] Treatment of abnormal AST values will vary based on the underlying cause. Monitoring

AST levels in combination with other serum enzyme tests is important in determining etiology and guiding the appropriate treatment.

Alanine aminotransferase (ALT), also known as "alanine transaminase," is an enzyme found mostly in the liver and to a lesser extent in the kidneys, heart, and skeletal muscle. Since its concentration is highest in the liver, ALT is considered a more specific indicator of liver injury than AST. Normal serum ALT ranges from 29 to 33 IU/L in males and 19 to 25 IU/L in females.[133] High ALT levels are most associated with disorders that involve the liver such as cholestasis, hepatitis, hepatic ischemia, cirrhosis, liver cancer, and obstructive jaundice. Very high ALT levels (>1000 U/L) may be caused by acute viral hepatitis, acute ischemic liver injury, or severe drug-induced liver injury.[134] Mild-to-moderate elevations in ALT (<15 times the upper limit of normal) may be caused by chronic hepatitis, metabolic dysfunction-associated fatty liver disease (formerly called "non-alcoholic fatty liver disease"[135]), myocardial infarction, thyroid disorders, strenuous exercise, and genetic disorders such as Wilson disease and hemochromatosis.[133] Elevated ALT levels may also be caused by a wide range of medications, including antibiotics, antiepileptics, nonsteroidal anti-inflammatory drugs, statins, anti-tuberculosis drugs, anti-retroviral treatment for HIV, and certain chemotherapeutic agents.[133]

The AST to ALT ratio is frequently used to help characterize the etiology of abnormal liver enzyme values. In most types of liver diseases, the elevation of ALT is higher than that of AST, meaning the AST:ALT ratio is less than 1. When liver damage is alcohol-induced, however, the rise in AST is typically greater than the rise in ALT. Thus, an AST:ALT ratio greater than 2 is suggestive of alcohol-related liver injury.[133] Although AST and ALT are often referred to as "liver function tests," they are better measures of hepatocellular damage rather than function. Certain proteins, such as albumin and clotting factors, which can reflect the liver's synthetic function, may be better indicators of actual liver function.

While low AST levels are not typically a concern, low ALT has been correlated with poor nutritional status.[136] One possible reason for this is malnutrition-related vitamin B6 deficiency, since vitamin B6 is required as a cofactor for ALT metabolism.[137] Treatment of abnormal ALT values will depend on the etiology and severity of the abnormalities. Clinicians must search for other markers for a comprehensive assessment.

Alkaline phosphatase (ALP) is an enzyme found primarily in the liver and bones. Normal serum ALP ranges from 30 to 120 U/L,[105] and elevated levels are observed in a variety of liver and bone disorders. In patients with cholestasis, ALP levels are typically elevated to at least four times the upper limit of normal. Lesser degrees of elevation are noticed in other types of liver disease, such as viral hepatitis, and infiltrative diseases of the liver, such as sarcoidosis, fungal infection, and cancer metastasis.[133] Since ALP is also present in bone, high levels of ALP can result from conditions affecting bone cell activity, including osteomalacia, osteoblastic tumors, rickets, Paget's disease, and hyperparathyroidism. In cases of bone cancer or Paget's disease, ALP levels may increase initially but return to normal over time in response to treatment. ALP levels may also be temporarily elevated during periods of growth, including pregnancy, infancy, and adolescence. Additionally, patients with O and B blood types may experience elevated ALP levels following the consumption of a fatty meal, which is why serum ALP levels are recommended to be collected in the fasting state.[132]

In contrast, low ALP levels may be caused by conditions such as malnutrition, zinc deficiency, vitamin B12 deficiency, hypothyroidism, vitamin D intoxication, hypophosphatasia, and Wilson disease.[138] Additionally, low ALP levels may be caused by medications such as oral contraceptives and estrogen replacement therapy.[139] Treatment of abnormal ALP values varies based on etiology, and must address the underlying cause and associated clinical manifestations (e.g., vitamin or mineral deficiencies). Monitoring ALP can provide clinicians with important insight into progression and treatment of certain diseases.

Lactate dehydrogenase (LDH) is an enzyme present in almost all body tissues, with concentrations highest in the muscle, liver, and kidney. LDH is released into the bloodstream in response to cell damage or death, and is thus used as a biomarker of tissue injury. Normal serum LDH values range from 140 to 280 U/L.[140] Since it is widely distributed throughout the body, an abnormal LDH value is not specific for damage to any particular organ. However, there are five isoenzymes of LDH (LDH-1 through LDH-5) that help differentiate LDH among various organs. LDH-1 is expressed primarily in the heart, LDH-2 in the reticuloendothelial system, LDH-3 in the lungs, LDH-4 in the kidneys, and LDH-5 in skeletal muscle and the liver.[140]

The ratio of LDH-1 to LDH-2 is typically less than 1. An LDH-1: LDH-2 greater than 1 (a so-called "flipped" LDH ratio) is common in patients with myocardial infarction, although this is not the primary measure used for this diagnosis. The flipped LDH ratio may also be seen with hemolytic anemia, megaloblastic anemia, and renal cell carcinoma.[141] Elevations in LDH-3 and LDH-4 may be observed in patients with pulmonary disease or white blood cell malignancies, while an elevated LDH-5 in isolation most often suggests hepatocellular injury or disease.[140,141] Elevations in all LDH isoenzymes may suggest tissue damage to multiple organ sites, and may be observed in patients with shock, metastatic carcinoma, or multiorgan failure. Abnormally low LDH levels are extremely rare and not typically considered harmful.

Troponin is a complex consisting of three subunits (troponin C, troponin I, and troponin T) that plays a crucial role in skeletal and cardiac muscle cell function. A troponin test is most commonly performed to assess heart conditions because troponin is released into the blood when the heart muscle is damaged. In most healthy individuals, the amount of troponin in the blood is significantly low or undetectable. Elevated troponin is typically suggestive of cardiac damage, with very high levels often concerning for myocardial infarction. Specifically, myocardial injury (which is part of the diagnostic criteria for myocardial infarction) is defined as an elevated troponin value above the 99th percentile upper reference limit, with the condition considered acute if there is a rise and/or fall of the troponin value.[142] In patients experiencing myocardial infarction, troponin levels typically begin rising within 2–3 hours of symptom onset, peak around 12–48 hours, and decline to normal over the next 4–10 days.[142] Elevated troponin may also be caused by other cardiac conditions such as myocarditis, pericarditis, pulmonary embolism, stroke, heart failure, and cardiac arrhythmias, as well as noncardiac conditions such as kidney failure, extreme physical exertion, and critical illness. As with other serum enzymes, nutrition interventions for patients with abnormal troponin levels will vary according to the patient's underlying condition and clinical status.

Lipid Profile

Lipids serve many critical functions in the body. Triglycerides are a source of stored energy, and cholesterol is an important structural component of hormones, cell membranes, and bile acids. Abnormalities in lipid metabolism can be detected through a lipid profile, which typically consists of total cholesterol, LDL-cholesterol, HDL-cholesterol, and triglycerides. Both low and elevated lipid levels can have a wide range of negative effects throughout the body. The term *dyslipidemia* refers to a condition of abnormal blood lipid levels; this may include total cholesterol, LDL-cholesterol, HDL-cholesterol, and/or triglycerides. *Hyperlipidemia* is another common term, typically referring to an elevation of total cholesterol, LDL-cholesterol, and/or triglycerides. Medical nutrition therapy can play an important role in the prevention, treatment, and management of various lipid disorders, so it is important that dietitians are skilled at interpreting lipid abnormalities.

Lipoproteins are complex particles that transport lipids such as cholesterol and triglycerides throughout the body. Lipoproteins are comprised of a central hydrophobic core containing cholesterol and triglycerides, surrounded by a hydrophilic membrane containing charged molecules that interact with the aqueous external environment. The surface of lipoproteins contains phospholipids, free cholesterol, and apolipoproteins, which are proteins that provide structural support and help lipoproteins interact with cellular receptors and enzymes in the environment. There are four major classes of lipoproteins, varying in their size, density, and lipid/protein composition: chylomicrons, VLDL, LDL, and HDL. As the density of the particle increases, the size and the relative amount of lipid decrease. For example, large VLDLs contain a higher percentage of triglyceride and lower percentage of protein than small HDLs. **Table 2.18** provides an overview of the major lipoprotein classes. **Figure 2.15** illustrates the pathways involved in lipoprotein metabolism.

VLDL is a triglyceride-rich lipoprotein that transports endogenous lipids (mainly triglycerides) from the liver to other tissues for storage and utilization. VLDL levels are typically calculated based on triglyceride levels, since there is no direct way of measuring VLDL in blood. VLDL can be estimated by dividing triglyceride levels (in mg/dL) by five. However, this method is not valid when triglyceride levels exceed 400 mg/dL. VLDL is considered atherogenic, as high levels may promote the development of plaque in arterial walls.[143] VLDL levels must be assessed in conjunction with other lipid values to determine appropriate nutrition therapy. Low VLDL levels are generally not of concern and do not require dietary intervention.

LDL transports cholesterol to peripheral tissues and is eventually recycled back to the liver. If there is too much LDL-cholesterol in the blood, these particles can adhere to the walls of arteries, forming plaque. Plaque can narrow arteries, contribute to high blood pressure, and initiate the process of atherosclerosis (the buildup of fatty deposits in artery walls). For these reasons, LDL-cholesterol is commonly known as the "bad" cholesterol. Optimal LDL-cholesterol is

Table 2.18 Major Lipoprotein Classes

Lipoprotein	Origin	Major Lipid	Protein Content	Function
Chylomicron	Intestine	TG (90%)	1%	Transport dietary fat from the intestine to peripheral tissues
VLDL	Liver	TG (90%)	10%	Transport TG from liver to peripheral tissues
LDL	Derived from VLDL	Cholesterol (50%)	20%	Transport cholesterol to peripheral tissues
HDL	Liver and intestine	Phospholipid (25%) Cholesterol (20%)	50%	Transport cholesterol from peripheral tissues to liver

VLDL, very low-density lipoprotein; LDL, low-density lipoprotein; HDL, high-density lipoprotein; TG, triglyceride
Data from Damjanov I. *Pathophysiology*. Elsevier; 2009.

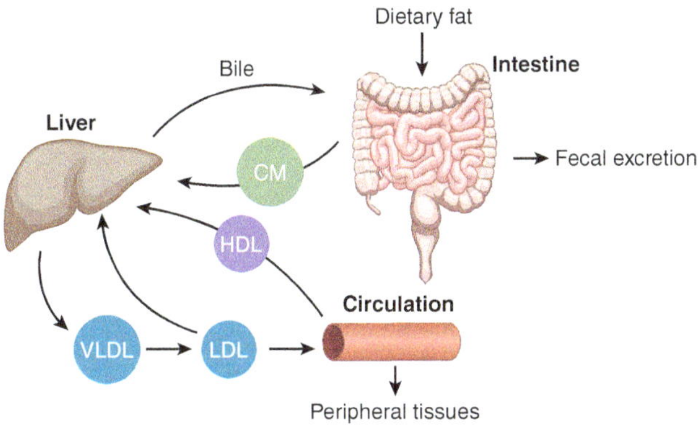

Figure 2.15 Overview of Lipoprotein Metabolism

CM: chylomicron. HDL: high-density lipoprotein. LDL: low-density lipoprotein. VLDL: very low-density lipoprotein.

defined as less than 100 mg/dL.[144] LDL-cholesterol can be measured directly or calculated using the following equation[145]:

$$\text{LDL-cholesterol (mg/dL)} = (\text{total cholesterol}) - (\text{HDL-cholesterol}) - (\text{triglycerides}/5)$$

Sample Calculation: Total cholesterol 170 mg/dL, HDL-cholesterol 55 mg/dL, triglycerides 100 mg/dL

$$\text{LDL-cholesterol} = (170) - (55) - (100/5) = 95 \text{ mg/dL}$$

For example, a patient with a total cholesterol level of 170 mg/dL, HDL-cholesterol level of 55 mg/dL, and triglyceride level of 100 mg/dL would have an LDL-cholesterol level of 95 mg/dL. As with VLDL estimations, this equation should only be used when triglyceride levels are less than 400 mg/dL.

Diet and lifestyle play a crucial role in treating high LDL-cholesterol. Nutrition interventions for elevated LDL-cholesterol levels include limiting saturated fat, avoiding trans-fat, and increasing unsaturated fat intake. For example, replacement of 5% of calories from saturated fat with unsaturated fat is associated with a 5–10% reduction in LDL-cholesterol.[146] Interventions may also include increasing soluble fiber and plant protein intake, increasing physical activity, and encouraging smoking cessation. Depending on the severity and response to lifestyle interventions, cholesterol-lowering drugs such as hydroxymethylglutaryl (HMG) CoA reductase inhibitors (statins), bile acid sequestrants, nicotinic acid, and fibric acids may be prescribed in conjunction with dietary therapy.

Low LDL-cholesterol (<50 mg/dL) is less common but can occur due to various genetic or acquired causes. Possible etiologies include inherited lipid disorders, malignancies, malabsorption, cirrhosis, and infection.[147–149] Additionally, acute myocardial infarction and stress from surgery or trauma can cause LDL-cholesterol to drop temporarily. Low LDL is not generally a concern and should be evaluated with other measures to determine the appropriate nutrition therapy.

HDL mobilizes cholesterol from tissues and transports it back to the liver for excretion, through a process called "reverse cholesterol transport." In contrast to VLDL- and LDL-cholesterol, HDL-cholesterol is considered anti-atherogenic (i.e., protective against atherosclerosis) because it helps remove excess cholesterol from the body and prevent the formation of arterial plaque. Thus, HDL-cholesterol is often referred to as the "good" cholesterol. Normal HDL levels are defined as ≥40 mg/dL in males and ≥50 mg/dL in females.[150] Low HDL-cholesterol is associated with increased cardiovascular disease risk, independent of LDL-cholesterol.[150] Possible causes of low HDL-cholesterol include insulin resistance, physical inactivity, overweight/obesity, diabetes mellitus, cigarette smoking, excessive carbohydrate intake, certain medications (e.g., beta blockers, anabolic steroids, and benzodiazepines), acute illness, and inherited lipid disorders.[150–152] Low HDL-cholesterol is not typically a direct target of treatment. Rather, interventions should focus on reducing overall cardiovascular risk, such as through physical activity, smoking cessation, and substitution of saturated fat with unsaturated fat.

Total cholesterol represents the total amount of circulating cholesterol, encompassing cholesterol in VLDL, LDL, and HDL. Total cholesterol less than 200 mg/dL is considered desirable, 200–239 mg/dL is considered borderline high, and 240 mg/dL or higher is considered high.[150] The ratio of *total/HDL-cholesterol* is considered a better predictor of cardiovascular disease risk than total cholesterol or LDL-cholesterol alone.[153] A total cholesterol/HDL-cholesterol ratio less than 5:1 is considered desirable, and less than 3.5:1 is considered optimal.[154] Treatment for elevated total/HDL ratio and elevated total cholesterol varies depending on the underlying etiology, and may include strategies aimed at reducing LDL-cholesterol and/or raising HDL-cholesterol.

PRACTICE POINT

Interpreting LDL- and HDL-cholesterol levels in the context of total cholesterol provides more clinical significance than any one lipid value alone. For example, a patient with elevated total cholesterol but normal HDL-cholesterol may be at lower cardiovascular risk than a patient with elevated total cholesterol but low HDL-cholesterol.

Triglycerides make up the largest percentage of fat in the body and are an important source of stored energy. Plasma triglycerides include exogenous triglycerides, which come from dietary fat and are carried in chylomicrons, and endogenous triglycerides, which are synthesized in the liver and carried in VLDL particles. A normal plasma triglyceride level is less than 150 mg/dL.[144] A level of 150–199 mg/dL is considered borderline high, 200–499 mg/dL is considered high, and ≥500 mg/dL is considered very high.[150] Hypertriglyceridemia is associated with an increased risk of cardiovascular disease and events such as myocardial infarction and stroke.[155,156] Hypertriglyceridemia may also lead to acute pancreatitis in severe cases. The risk for hypertriglyceridemia-induced pancreatitis increases progressively with serum triglyceride levels over 500 mg/dL and becomes particularly elevated when triglyceride levels exceed 1000–2000 mg/dL.[157,158]

Causes of hypertriglyceridemia include genetic factors (e.g., mutations in genes involved in lipoprotein metabolism) as well as acquired factors such as metabolic syndrome, diabetes, excessive alcohol consumption, obesity, and kidney disease. Drugs such as corticosteroids, oral estrogens, thiazide diuretics, beta blockers, and bile acid sequestrants may also increase hypertriglyceridemia risk.[159] In patients receiving PN, hypertriglyceridemia may occur due to dextrose overprovision, or when the infusion rate of lipids exceeds the capacity of plasma fat clearance. Treatment for hypertriglyceridemia depends on the causes of the elevation and its severity. Nutrition therapy should focus on a diet low in saturated fat, added sugar, refined grains, and alcohol. For patients receiving PN, treatment for hypertriglyceridemia may involve lowering the dextrose and/or lipid emulsion dose to prevent overfeeding.

CORE CONCEPT 6

Lipid profile results can be used to assess risk of cardiovascular and metabolic disorders as well as overall nutritional status.

Hematology

A hematological assessment is used to detect and treat a variety of blood disorders, many of which have important nutritional implications. **Anemia** is a condition characterized by a reduced oxygen-carrying capacity of blood, reflected by a low hemoglobin concentration or low hematocrit. Anemia is a major public health concern, affecting nearly a quarter of the worldwide population.[160] The causes of anemia are multifactorial and include excessive blood loss (e.g., due to acute or chronic bleeding), excessive red blood cell destruction (e.g., due to autoimmune conditions, infection, enzymatic abnormalities, and certain medications), and decreased red blood cell production (e.g., due to bone marrow failure, micronutrient deficiency, or erythropoietin deficiency). **Figure 2.16** provides an overview of the etiologies of anemia. Populations that are considered particularly vulnerable to anemia include young children, pregnant women, older adults, and patients with kidney

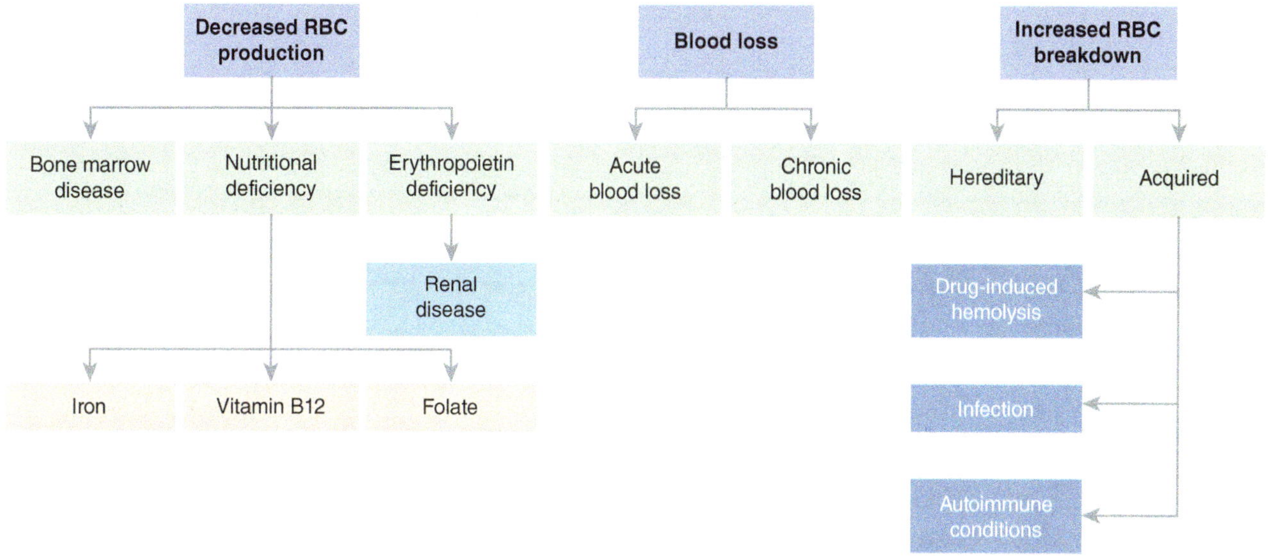

Figure 2.16 Etiologies of Anemia

Data from Damjanov I. *Pathophysiology*. Elsevier; 2009.

Table 2.19 Micronutrients Involved in Red Blood Cell Production

Micronutrient	Role in Red Blood Cell Production
Iron	Key component of hemoglobin
Folate	Required for DNA synthesis
Vitamin B12	Required for DNA synthesis
Copper	Promotes intestinal absorption of iron and distribution of iron to tissues
Zinc	Cofactor for enzymes involved in hemoglobin synthesis and red blood cell maturation

Data from Chan LN, Mike LA. The science and practice of micronutrient supplementations in nutritional anemia: an evidence-based review. *JPEN J Parenter Enteral Nutr*. 2014;38(6):656–672. doi:10.1177/0148607114533726

disease, uncontrolled chronic illness, cancer, extensive GI surgeries, and malnutrition.

Anemia is often nutritional in origin, meaning it is caused by a deficiency in one or more of the nutrients that are essential for red blood cell formation. Nutritional anemia most commonly involves deficiencies of iron, folate, or vitamin B12, although copper and zinc deficiency may also contribute. Iron is a key component of hemoglobin, the protein responsible for carrying oxygen in red blood cells. Vitamin B12 and folate are necessary for DNA synthesis in red blood cell production. Copper supports dietary iron absorption and iron distribution among tissues, and zinc is a cofactor for several enzymes involved in the synthesis of hemoglobin and the maturation of red blood cells.

Table 2.20 Clinical Manifestations of Anemia

Organ/System	Clinical Manifestation
General	Weakness, fatigue, cold intolerance
Cardiovascular	Tachycardia, palpitations, dyspnea
Pulmonary	Shortness of breath, rapid breathing
Cerebral	Dizziness, vertigo, headache, depression, anxiety
Renal	Proteinuria, edema
Gastrointestinal	Ulcers, malabsorption, glossitis
Dermatological	Pallor, cold skin

Data from Pirker R. Symptoms of anemia. In: Nowrousian MR, ed. Recombinant Human Erythropoietin (rhEPO) in Clinical Oncology. Springer; 2008:307-315.

Table 2.19 summarizes the roles of iron, folate, vitamin B12, copper, and zinc in red blood cell production.

A CBC provides information on the size, shape, and number of blood cells. Components of the CBC include hemoglobin, red blood cell count, hematocrit, mean corpuscular volume, mean corpuscular hemoglobin concentration, red cell distribution width, and white blood cell count, each described in further detail below. Biochemical assessment alongside evaluation of clinical signs and symptoms (**Table 2.20**) and medical status can help clinicians determine the etiology, severity, and appropriate treatment of anemia and other hematologic conditions.

Clinical Roundtable

Topic: C-Reactive Protein as a Biomarker of Cardiovascular Disease Risk

C-reactive protein (CRP) levels rise not only during acute inflammation, but also during chronic inflammation. In recent decades, CRP—specifically, high sensitivity CRP (hs-CRP)—has emerged as a potential predictor of cardiovascular disease (CVD) risk, since chronic, low-grade inflammation is known to contribute to the initiation, progression, and complications of CVD.[1] There is emerging evidence demonstrating an association between elevated hs-CRP and CVD risk, although the exact role of CRP in the pathogenesis of CVD is not fully understood. It is not clear whether CRP is a nonspecific marker of inflammation or a direct participant in CVD development. Unlike other markers of inflammation, CRP levels are stable over extended periods and can be measured using inexpensive, convenient, and high-sensitivity assays. Some experts recommend the inclusion of hs-CRP as part of routine CVD screening, while others recommend prioritizing traditional risk factors.[2,3] Further research is needed to clarify the role of CRP in CVD pathogenesis and the clinical utility of hs-CRP as an indicator of CVD risk.

Roundtable Discussion

1. What are some potential benefits of including CRP in routine CVD risk screenings, compared to traditional risk factors alone?
2. What are some limitations associated with using CRP as a biomarker for CVD risk?
3. What additional research is needed to validate the use of CRP in predicting cardiovascular events? For example, what types of studies should be conducted, and what research questions should they address?

References

1. Amezcua-Castillo E, González-Pacheco H, Sáenz-San Martín A, et al. C-reactive protein: The quintessential marker of systemic inflammation in coronary artery disease-advancing toward precision medicine. *Biomedicines*. 2023;11(9):2444.
2. Genest J, McPherson R, Frohlich J, et al. 2009 Canadian Cardiovascular Society/Canadian guidelines for the diagnosis and treatment of dyslipidemia and prevention of cardiovascular disease in the adult - 2009 recommendations. *Can J Cardiol*. 2009;25(10):567-579.
3. Lin JS, Evans CV, Johnson E, Redmond N, Coppola EL, Smith N. Nontraditional risk factors in cardiovascular disease risk assessment: Updated evidence report and systematic review for the US Preventive Services Task Force. *JAMA*. 2018;320(3):281-297.

CASE STUDY REVISITED

It is now HD 15 and Adam is recovering well. He has been moved out of the ICU to the medical ward and is preparing for discharge home. His appetite and oral intake are improving. Based on his labs and symptoms of fatigue, an iron supplement is ordered.

Biochemical Data (HD 15):

Hemoglobin 12.0 (14–18 g/dL)
Hematocrit 34 (40–50%)
Mean corpuscular volume 98 (80–100 fL)
Red cell distribution width (RDW-SD) 50 (39–46 fL)

Clinical Data:

Medications: atorvastatin, captopril, iron, pantoprazole

Dietary Data:

Diet Prescription: Regular

Questions

1. Describe the abnormalities in Adam's biochemical data.
2. What type of anemia or anemias might Adam have? What are his risk factors?
3. What biochemical indices would be required to make a more accurate assessment?

Hemoglobin (Hgb) concentration is a measure of the total amount of hemoglobin in blood. Hemoglobin is a protein in erythrocytes that delivers oxygen to cells and picks up CO_2 for expiration by the lungs. **Figure 2.17** depicts the structure of hemoglobin. Hgb concentration is considered the principle biochemical indicator of anemia. According to the World Health Organization, anemia is defined as Hgb levels <13.0 g/dL in men, <12.0 g/dL in non-pregnant women, and <11.0 g/dL in pregnant women.[161]

Hgb concentration is not a sensitive or specific test for differentiating between nutritional anemias, and it can be influenced by many non-nutritional factors. For example, Hgb levels may decrease due to cancer, chronic infection, bone marrow failure, renal insufficiency, blood loss, overhydration, and pregnancy. Hgb levels also commonly decline with age, due to factors such as chronic disease and age-related physiological changes. Additionally, low Hgb may be caused by intense physical activity, especially when involving repetitive, forceful striking of the hands or feet. For instance, endurance running may lead to blood cell lysis in the feet, resulting in intravascular hemolysis and subsequent decline in circulating Hgb concentration (a phenomenon known as "foot strike hemolysis" or "march anemia"). In contrast, elevated Hgb concentration may be due to dehydration, smoking, and certain medications such as sodium-glucose co-transporter 2 inhibitors.[162] Hgb may also become elevated at high altitudes, as a means of adapting to the reduced availability of oxygen.

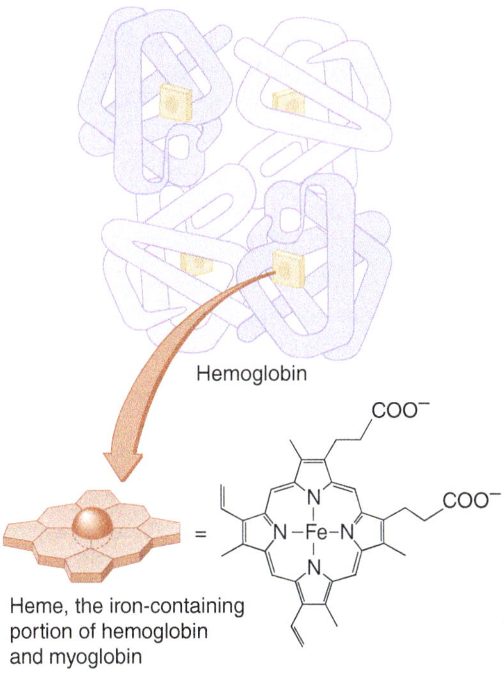

Figure 2.17 Structure of Hemoglobin

Hematocrit (Hct) is another parameter commonly used to evaluate anemia. Hct represents the percentage of red blood cells in relation to the total volume of blood. In healthy individuals, Hct (expressed as a percentage) is typically three times Hgb concentration (expressed in g/dL). Normal Hct values are approximately 42–50% in males and 37–47% in females.[105] Hct is affected by factors similar to those affecting Hgb concentration. For example, low Hct may occur due to chronic diseases, bone marrow disorders, genetic aberrations, blood loss, and pregnancy, and high Hct may occur due to smoking or high altitude. Additionally, since Hct and Hgb are both dependent on plasma volume, they may appear elevated in the setting of dehydration and low in the setting of overhydration. Similar to Hgb, Hct is not a sensitive or specific test for anemia. Hct should be evaluated alongside other laboratory values and a recent medical history to determine the appropriate nutrition therapy.

Red blood cell (RBC) count measures the number of RBCs per unit volume of blood, typically expressed as millions of cells per microliter. RBCs contain hemoglobin and are the most common type of cell found in blood. They are regenerated every 4 months on average, with production, development, and function dependent on a wide range of nutritional, genetic, and environmental factors. Normal RBC count ranges from 4.7 to 6.1 $\times$ 10^6/μL in males and 4.2 to 5.4 $\times$ 10^6/μL in females.[10] Like Hgb and Hct, a low RBC count may result from nutritional deficits or other factors such as hemorrhage, hemolysis, inherited conditions, kidney disease, and certain medications. As with Hgb, an RBC count is not sensitive to nutritional causes of anemia.

Mean corpuscular volume (MCV) measures the average volume of RBCs, expressed in femtoliters (fL). Normal serum MCV ranges from 80 to 100 fL.[163] MCV can be used to classify anemia into three categories: microcytic (MCV <80), normocytic (MCV 80–100), and macrocytic (MCV >100), each described in further detail below.

- **Microcytic anemia** is characterized by small RBC size, reflecting an abnormality in cellular Hgb synthesis. Common causes of microcytic anemia include iron deficiency, thalassemia (a genetic disorder that causes impaired Hgb synthesis), lead poisoning, and chronic diseases such as rheumatoid arthritis, congestive heart failure, and CKD.
- **Normocytic anemia** is a type of anemia characterized by normal-sized RBCs. Normocytic anemia is associated with many chronic and inflammatory conditions including kidney disease, infection, cancer, autoimmune disorders, and

endocrine dysfunction. These conditions cannot be treated effectively with iron supplementation.

- **Macrocytic anemia** is characterized by abnormally large RBCs, most commonly due to impairments in cell division. Macrocytic anemia can be further classified into two categories: megaloblastic and non-megaloblastic. *Megaloblastic anemia* is characterized by impaired DNA synthesis and is commonly caused by folate or vitamin B12 deficiency. Other possible causes of megaloblastic macrocytic anemia include congenital disorders of DNA synthesis and medications that interfere with DNA synthesis. *Non-megaloblastic anemia* is characterized by normal DNA synthesis, and may be caused by liver disease, alcohol use disorder, and congenital hematologic disorders. **Table 2.21** summarizes the common causes of anemia according to MCV classification.

Care should be taken when interpreting MCV, as it may be confounded by various nutritional and non-nutritional factors. For example, MCV may appear within normal range in the early stages of iron, folate, or vitamin B12 deficiency. MCV may also appear normal when iron deficiency is present in conjunction with folate and/or vitamin B12 deficiency, as the small cell volume associated with iron deficiency is masked by the large cell volume associated with folate and/or vitamin B12 deficiency. Additional laboratory values are necessary to distinguish between nutritional and non-nutritional causes of anemia and determine the appropriate treatment.

Table 2.21 Common Causes of Anemia Based on MCV Classification

Anemia Type	Causes
Microcytic (MCV <80)	Iron deficiency Thalassemia Chronic disease (e.g., kidney disease, rheumatoid arthritis, congestive heart failure) Lead poisoning
Normocytic (MCV 80–100)	Kidney disease Autoimmune conditions Infection Endocrine disorders
Macrocytic (MCV >100)	Megaloblastic ▪ Vit B12 deficiency ▪ Folate deficiency Non-megaloblastic ▪ Chronic liver disease ▪ Alcohol use disorder ▪ Congenital hematologic disorders

Data from Vieth JT, Lane DR. Anemia. *Emerg Med Clin North Am. 2014;32*(3):613–628. doi:10.1016/j.emc.2014.04.007

PRACTICE POINT

Evaluation of mean corpuscular volume (MCV) is important in determining a patient's type of anemia (microcytic, macrocytic, normocytic) and guiding the appropriate nutrition intervention.

Mean corpuscular hemoglobin concentration (MCHC) is the average concentration of Hgb within RBCs. It is calculated by dividing Hgb concentration (g/dL) by Hct (%). Normal MCHC is defined as 32–36 g/dL.[164] Since macrocytic cells generally have more hemoglobin and microcytic cells have less hemoglobin, the etiologies of MCHC abnormalities closely resemble those of MCV abnormalities. When MCHC is low, RBCs are said to be hypochromic (i.e., deficient in hemoglobin), which is often seen with iron deficiency or thalassemia. Elevated MCHC may reflect spherocytosis, an inherited blood disorder characterized by spherical-shaped RBCs that are more prone to hemolysis.

Red cell distribution width (RDW) measures the degree of *anisocytosis*, or variation in RBC size. It may be expressed as the RDW-coefficient of variation (RDW-CV) or RDW-standard deviation (RDW-SD). RDW-CV represents the width of the distribution curve of RBC volumes relative to the MCV and is calculated by dividing the standard deviation of the MCV by the MCV and multiplying this value by 100. RDW-SD, in contrast, is a direct measure of the actual width of the distribution curve. RDW-SD is not affected by MCV, and is therefore considered a more accurate indicator of RBC size variations than RDW-CV.[165] Normal adult RDW values are 11.6–14.6% for RDW-CV and 39–46 fL for RDW-SD.[166] A high RDW reflects a large variation in RBC sizes, while a low RDW reflects a more homogeneous population of RBCs. A high RDW is common in anemias caused by nutritional deficiencies (e.g., iron, folate, vitamin B12), but it is not specific for any abnormality.

Evaluation of RDW in conjunction with MCV can help clinicians determine the etiology of anemia. For example, in patients with microcytic anemia (low MCV), an elevated RDW may suggest iron deficiency, while a normal RDW may suggest thalassemia or anemia of chronic disease and inflammation. In patients with macrocytic anemia (high MCV), an elevated RDW is associated with vitamin B12 and/or folate deficiency, while a normal RDW is suggestive of non-megaloblastic anemia. RDW and MCV are useful in evaluating the etiology of blood disorders, but these measures should be interpreted alongside other biochemical data as well as clinical signs and symptoms to accurately identify and address the underlying cause.

Platelet count measures the number of circulating platelets (thrombocytes), which are small cell fragments that are essential for blood clotting. A normal platelet count is defined as 150,000–400,000 per microliter (150–400 × 10^9/L). A low platelet count (thrombocytopenia) may be due to bone marrow failure, inherited platelet disorders, acute or chronic infection, hemorrhage, and dilution from blood transfusions. An elevated platelet count (thrombocytosis) may occur with iron deficiency anemia or malignancy (e.g., leukemia, lymphoma, or solid tumors).

Reticulocyte count provides information on the rate of RBC production. Reticulocytes are immature RBCs that are released from bone marrow into the bloodstream, where they mature into RBCs within a few days. A normal reticulocyte count in adults is 0.5–2%.[10] The reticulocyte can help distinguish between anemias due to underproduction of RBCs and those related to shortened survival of RBCs in circulation. A decreased reticulocyte count may be noticed in nutritional anemia (e.g., iron, folate, or vitamin B12 deficiency anemias), as well as anemia due to bone marrow failure. An increased reticulocyte count is commonly associated with hemolytic anemia or blood loss. The reticulocyte count may be included in a CBC or obtained as a follow-up laboratory test.

White blood cell (WBC) count is another component of the CBC that can help to detect and evaluate hematological disorders. WBCs (leukocytes) are produced in bone marrow and play a critical role in immune system function. The WBC count measures the number of WBCs in the blood, with normal values ranging from 5000 to 10,000 WBCs per microliter (5–10 × 10^9/L).[10] An elevated WBC count, or *leukocytosis*, may be caused by infection, inflammation (e.g., due to inflammatory bowel disease or arthritis), leukemia, neoplasm, allergies, and stress (e.g., due to trauma, burns, surgery). A decreased WBC count, or *leukopenia*, may result from bone marrow disorders, lymphoma or other cancers spreading to bone marrow, autoimmune disease, protein-energy malnutrition, sepsis, and is associated with chemotherapy or radiation therapy. The WBC count may be accompanied by a *differential*, which measures the relative amounts of each leukocyte type: neutrophils, lymphocytes, monocytes, eosinophils, and basophils. The differential can help determine the etiology of a WBC abnormality, thus aiding in the diagnosis and treatment of various conditions such as infections, autoimmune disorders, and leukemia.

Interpretation of Anemia

Microcytic Anemia from Iron Deficiency

Iron is essential for a wide range of metabolic processes. In addition to its role in oxygen transport, iron is crucial for growth and development, particularly in the brain. It helps form myelin, a protective layer that coats the brain cells. Iron also serves as a cofactor for enzymes involved in immune function, energy metabolism, and regulation of gene expression, among other processes. There are two major dietary forms of iron: heme iron, which is found in foods of animal origin, and non-heme iron, which is found in both plant and animal foods, as well as iron-enriched or fortified foods. **Table 2.22** provides examples of common dietary sources of iron. Non-heme iron is generally less readily absorbable than heme iron.

Iron deficiency can result from inadequate dietary iron intake, decreased iron absorption, excessive losses, or a combination of these and other factors. Iron deficiency progresses through three stages: iron storage depletion, functional iron depletion, and iron deficiency anemia.[167] In the first stage, iron stores in the liver, spleen, and bone marrow become diminished. At this stage, there may be no obvious signs or symptoms of deficiency, and Hgb levels remain

Table 2.22 Dietary Sources of Iron

Food Source	Iron (mg)	% DV*
Heme Iron		
Clams (3 oz)	2.3	13
Beef, cooked (3 oz)	2.6	14
Sardines, canned (3 oz)	2.5	14
Tuna, canned (3 oz)	1.3	7
Poultry, cooked (3 oz)	1.1	6
Non-Heme Iron		
Fortified cereal (1 cup)	8.1	45
Spinach, cooked (1 cup)	6.4	36
Lentils (1/2 cup)	3.3	18
Chickpeas (1/2 cup)	2.4	13
Pumpkin seeds (1 oz)	2.3	13
Kidney beans (1/2 cup)	1.9	11
Tahini (1 tbsp)	1.3	7
Bread, whole wheat (1 slice)	0.8	4

*DV = Daily Value. The DV for iron is 18 mg for adults.

Data from U.S. Department of Agriculture, Agricultural Research Service. FoodData Central. 2019. https://fdc.nal.usda.gov

normal. In the second stage, functional iron (i.e., the iron that circulates in blood and is available for utilization) begins to decline, as the iron storage pool becomes exhausted. Symptoms may start to arise at this stage, and Hgb levels may drop slightly or remain within normal limits. If left untreated, iron deficiency commonly progresses to iron deficiency anemia.

Iron deficiency anemia is the most prevalent type of anemia worldwide. Infants, young children, adolescents, and women of child bearing age are among those at highest risk. Other risk factors include vegan or vegetarian dietary patterns, conditions associated with decreased iron absorption (e.g., celiac disease, bariatric surgery, atrophic gastritis), and conditions associated with increased iron losses (e.g., heavy menstrual bleeding, frequent blood draws, gastric ulcer disease, hemodialysis).[168] Common clinical manifestations of iron deficiency anemia include fatigue, hair loss, headache, exercise intolerance, koilonychia (spoon-shaped nails), pallor, and atrophic glossitis (smooth, glossy surface over the tongue). Iron deficiency anemia may also cause behavioral disturbances such as "pica," which is the craving to eat nonfood items such as dirt or ice. Iron deficiency anemia can have many functional consequences, including weakened immune function, reduced work capacity, pregnancy complications, and potentially irreversible effects on neurological and behavioral development.[169]

Low Hgb, low Hct, and low MCV are characteristic biochemical indicators of iron deficiency anemia. However, these measures are subject to certain limitations. For example, folate and vitamin B12 deficiency may mask iron deficiency by keeping MCV levels within a normal range. In addition, these tests are not sensitive to marginal deficiencies and thus cannot detect early stages of iron deficiency. Furthermore, Hgb and Hct are concentrations that depend on RBC mass and plasma volume, meaning they may decline with hemodilution (e.g., in patients who are volume overloaded) and increase with hemoconcentration (e.g., in patients who are volume depleted). If abnormal results are found on a CBC test, iron studies may be obtained to confirm the presence of iron deficiency anemia. Such iron studies include serum iron, ferritin, transferrin, and total iron binding capacity, each described in detail below.

Serum iron measures the amount of circulating iron, most of which is bound to the transport protein *transferrin*. Normal serum iron levels are 50–160 μg/dL (9–29 μmol/L).[170] Low serum iron may be due to iron deficiency as well as infection and inflammatory disorders. This is because serum iron depends on the efficiency of iron recycling by bone marrow and macrophages, which is reduced in these conditions. High serum iron may be related to iron overload, liver disease, massive blood transfusions, and lead toxicity. Oral contraceptives may also increase serum iron levels. Serum iron is considered a relatively poor index of iron status because it varies greatly day to day, even in healthy individuals. In addition, a natural diurnal variation in serum iron occurs, with highest values in the morning and lowest values late in the day.[170] Serum iron may also transiently increase after recent intake of iron-rich foods or oral iron supplements, which is why it is most reliable when obtained in a fasting state.[10] Serum iron by itself cannot be used to diagnose iron deficiency, and should be interpreted alongside other iron studies for a comprehensive evaluation of iron status.

Serum transferrin measures the total amount of transferrin in blood. Normal serum transferrin levels are 200–400 mg/dL.[105] Increased transferrin levels are associated with iron deficiency anemia, as transferrin synthesis is upregulated in response to diminished iron stores. Since transferrin is a negative acute-phase protein, it may be low in patients with acute inflammation. Low levels may also be observed in patients with liver disease, malignancy, infection, protein-energy malnutrition, and iron overload.[10] Thus, when these conditions are present, other iron biomarkers are necessary to accurately assess iron stores and determine the underlying cause of anemia.

Total iron binding capacity (TIBC) is a measure of all proteins available for binding circulating iron. Since transferrin is the predominant iron-binding protein, TIBC is an indirect measure of transferrin. Thus, TIBC typically increases in iron deficiency and decreases in iron overloaded states. Like serum transferrin, TIBC may remain normal or decrease in response to acute or chronic inflammation. Normal TIBC values range from 250 to 460 μg/dL.[10] TIBC is calculated by summing the serum iron and unsaturated iron binding capacity (a measure of how much transferrin is not bound to iron), or by multiplying the serum transferrin concentration by 1.389.[171]

Transferrin saturation represents the percentage of transferrin and other iron-binding proteins saturated with iron. Generally, about one-third of transferrin in the blood is saturated with iron. Transferrin saturation is calculated as a ratio of serum iron to TIBC[172]:

$$\text{Transferrin saturation (\%)} = \text{Serum iron } (\mu g/dL)/\text{TIBC } (\mu g/dL) \times 100$$

Sample Calculation: Serum iron: 48 μg/dL;
TIBC: 352 μg/dL
Transferrin saturation = 48/352 × 100
Transferrin saturation = 14%

For example, a patient with a serum iron of 48 and TIBC of 352 has a total iron binding capacity of 14%, suggesting iron deficiency.

Normal transferrin saturation generally ranges from 20% to 50%.[10] Low transferrin saturation is common in iron deficiency anemia, due to decreased serum iron and elevated TIBC. A low transferrin saturation (typically, <15%) is considered characteristic of iron deficiency, although not diagnostic by itself.[171] In contrast, high transferrin saturation may be seen with hemolytic or megaloblastic anemias, as well as iron overload and sudden increases in iron intake.[10]

Serum ferritin measures the amount of circulating ferritin, a storage protein that holds iron within hepatocytes and other storage cells for later use. Serum ferritin is considered a strong indicator of iron stores, with levels rising as iron stores increase, and declining as iron stores become diminished. Every 1 ng/mL of serum ferritin corresponds to approximately 8 mg of stored iron.[10] Normal ferritin levels are 12–300 ng/mL in males and 10–150 ng/mL in females.[10] A low serum ferritin combined with a low transferrin saturation generally supports the diagnosis of iron deficiency.[171] Unlike serum iron, serum ferritin levels do not display diurnal variation. As a positive acute-phase protein, ferritin levels rise during inflammation. Thus, serum ferritin may appear falsely normal in patients with liver disease, heart failure, malignancy, infection, and other disorders or conditions associated with inflammation. In these cases, other iron biomarkers must be used to evaluate the presence of iron deficiency.

Anemia of chronic disease (ACD), also known as "anemia of inflammation," is the second leading cause of anemia after iron deficiency anemia.[173] ACD is most often associated with infection, inflammatory conditions, and malignancy, although it may also be related to other acute and chronic disorders such as diabetes and heart failure. The pathological mechanisms of ACD are multifactorial and include decreased RBC survival, diminished RBC production, and impaired iron utilization. For instance, the presence of high levels of proinflammatory cytokines may trigger upregulation of *hepcidin*, a key iron-regulatory hormone. Elevated hepcidin interferes with the release of stored iron and inhibits intestinal iron absorption, thus reducing the availability of iron for Hgb synthesis. In addition, proinflammatory cytokines may diminish the production of erythropoietin, a hormone that stimulates RBC production in bone marrow. **Figure 2.18** illustrates the pathological mechanisms underlying ACD.

Being able to distinguish iron deficiency anemia from ACD is critical, as the treatment for these conditions differs. ACD is often normocytic and normochromic, reflected by normal MCV and normal MCHC, respectively. Iron deficiency anemia, in contrast, is typically microcytic (low MCV) and hypochromic (low MCHC). Additionally, while low ferritin is a characteristic feature of iron deficiency, serum ferritin is often normal or increased in ACD, since ferritin is a positive acute-phase protein that is elevated during inflammation. Similarly, transferrin (a negative acute-phase protein) is often low in ACD but elevated in iron deficiency anemia. In some cases, ACD and iron deficiency anemia may occur simultaneously. When this happens, iron deficiency is typically secondary to blood losses, such as in patients with inflammatory

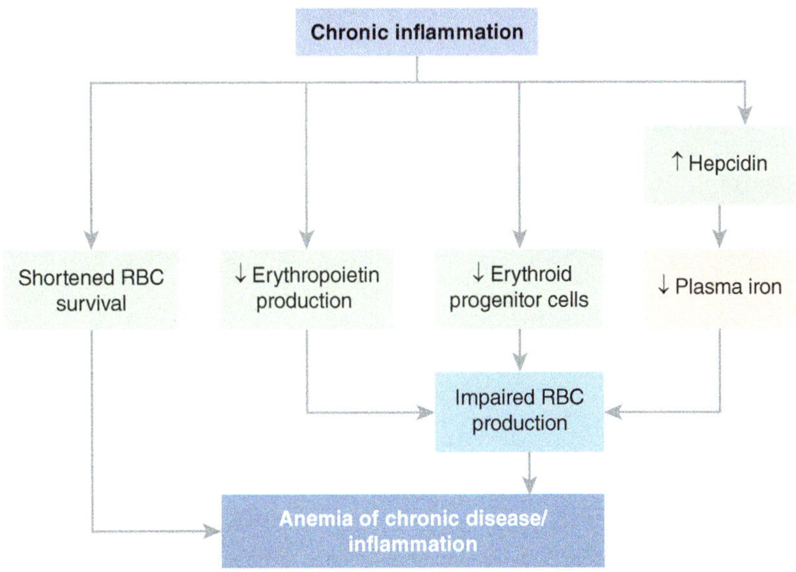

Figure 2.18 Pathogenesis of Anemia of Chronic Disease

Data from Macciò A, Madeddu C. Management of anemia of inflammation in the elderly. *Anemia*. 2012;2012:563251.

bowel disease who have chronic bleeding with inflammation. **Table 2.23** outlines common laboratory measures in iron deficiency anemia and ACD. Clinicians must carefully evaluate clinical history and laboratory findings to accurately diagnose and differentiate between ACD and iron deficiency anemia.

Treatment of iron deficiency anemia involves addressing the underlying cause, restoring Hgb concentrations, and replenishing iron stores. Iron supplementation can be administered orally or intravenously. Oral iron should ideally be taken on an empty stomach, when gastric acid levels are high. Consuming vitamin C (ascorbic acid) or vitamin C-containing foods may also increase the acidity of the GI tract. The low gastric pH facilitates iron absorption by promoting the conversion of insoluble ferric (Fe^{3+}) to absorbable ferrous (Fe^{2+}) iron. Numerous oral iron preparations are available, with the most commonly used being ferrous sulfate, ferrous gluconate, and ferrous fumarate. In general, the effectiveness of these preparations in treating iron deficiency is comparable.[171]

Oral iron is commonly given in three divided doses daily, with each dose containing about 50–60 mg of elemental iron.[171] Gastrointestinal side effects such as nausea, constipation, diarrhea, and metallic taste are common in patients taking oral iron supplements, which can impair adherence to treatment. Strategies to improve the tolerability of iron supplements include taking iron with food or milk (although this may reduce absorption), using a formulation with a lower amount of elemental iron, and switching from a tablet to a liquid formulation. A rise in Hgb levels is often noticed within 2 weeks of oral iron supplementation. However, repletion of iron stores (measured by serum ferritin) takes longer to occur. Thus, iron supplementation should continue for at least 3 months to replenish tissue iron stores.[174]

Parenteral iron administration may be indicated for patients who are intolerant to oral iron, or with conditions where oral iron is likely to be ineffective (e.g., malabsorptive disorders or excessive iron losses). Parenteral iron supplementation carries the potential to cause adverse safety events, including potentially life-threatening anaphylaxis. However, such allergic reactions have been primarily associated with older products such as high molecular weight iron dextran, which has been removed from the market due to safety concerns.[175] Of note, low molecular weight iron dextran is the only IV iron that is compatible and can be added to PN. More recent data suggest that IV iron is generally well tolerated, and the risk of serious allergic reactions with this treatment method is exceedingly low.[176]

Table 2.23 Laboratory Measures in Iron Deficiency Anemia and Anemia of Chronic Disease

Laboratory Measure	IDA	ACD
Hemoglobin	Reduced	Reduced
Mean corpuscular volume	Reduced	Reduced to normal
Serum iron	Reduced	Reduced
Serum ferritin	Reduced	Normal to increased
Serum transferrin	Increased	Reduced to normal
Transferrin saturation	Reduced	Reduced
Cytokine levels	Normal	Increased

IDA, Iron deficiency anemia; ACD, anemia of chronic disease

Data from Clark SF. Iron deficiency anemia. *Nutr Clin Pract.* 2008;23(2):128–141.

Macrocytic Anemias from B Vitamin Deficiencies

Macrocytic anemia can be caused by either folate deficiency or vitamin B12 deficiency, since both folate and vitamin B12 are involved in DNA synthesis and cell division. In the folate cycle, dietary folate (folic acid) is required to produce tetrahydrofolate, the active form of folate. Tetrahydrofolate is involved in the synthesis of purines and pyrimidines, which are essential for DNA synthesis. The folate cycle is catalyzed by methionine synthase, an enzyme that requires vitamin B12 as a coenzyme (**Figure 2.19**). Thus, a deficiency of

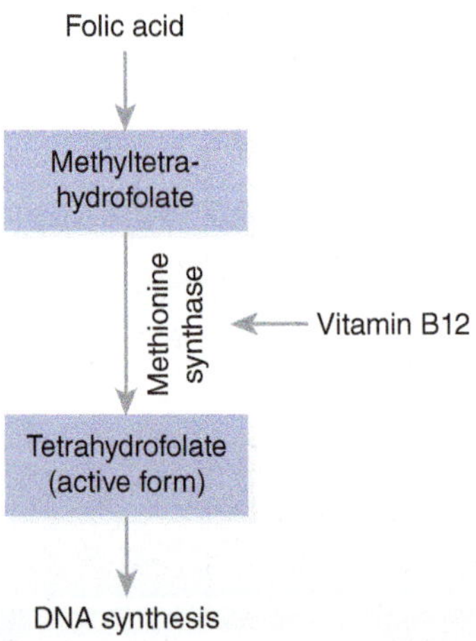

Figure 2.19 Role of Folic Acid and Vitamin B12 in DNA Synthesis

Data from Antony A. Megaloblastic anemias. In: Hoffman R, Benz EJ, Silberstein LE, et al, eds. Hematology: Basic Principles and Practice. 8th ed. Elsevier; 2023:524–554. Chapter 40.

either folate or vitamin B12 can impair DNA synthesis and in turn disrupt the formation and maturation of RBCs. As a result, RBCs may become abnormally large and few in number, reducing their capacity to adequately deliver oxygen to tissues.

Clinicians must assess patients further for vitamin B12 and folate deficiencies if abnormal CBC results (high MCV, low Hgb) indicate that macrocytic anemia may be present. The clinical symptoms of vitamin B12 and folate deficiency are similar, so biochemical assessment of vitamin B12 and folate status is necessary to distinguish between these deficiencies. Vitamin B12 and folate status can be evaluated using various static and functional indicators, common examples of which are reviewed below.

Vitamin B12 (cobalamin) is a water-soluble vitamin that functions as a cofactor for enzymes involved in the synthesis of DNA, lipids, and myelin. Absorption of vitamin B12 requires an acidic environment as well as the presence of intrinsic factor, a protein that is secreted by the parietal cells of the stomach. When vitamin B12 combines with intrinsic factor, the resulting complex binds to receptors on the ileum, where vitamin B12 absorption occurs. Vitamin B12 absorption may decrease with age since gastric acid production declines. In addition to inadequate dietary intake, vitamin B12 deficiency may be caused by conditions or medications that interfere with vitamin B12 absorption. For instance, deficiency may be seen in patients with pernicious anemia (an autoimmune condition that causes a lack of intrinsic factor) and patients who have undergone bariatric or intestinal surgeries that interfere with intrinsic factor production. Medications such as antacids, proton pump inhibitors, metformin, and nitrous oxide may also contribute to vitamin B12 deficiency.

Serum cobalamin is the most commonly used measure of vitamin B12 status. A serum cobalamin above 300 pg/mL is considered normal, 200–300 pg/mL is considered borderline low, and <200 pg/mL is consistent with deficiency.[177] Serum cobalamin is subject to both false negatives and false positives. For instance, falsely low values may be seen with pregnancy, multiple myeloma, and HIV infection, and spuriously high values may occur with liver disease, kidney disease, and malignant blood disorders.[177–180] Generally, low serum cobalamin levels indicate macrocytosis and are associated with high MCV, high RDW, and low Hgb.

Serum levels of *homocysteine* and *methylmalonic acid (MMA)* may also be used to evaluate vitamin B12 status. These are examples of functional assays, as they

⚠ Clinical Controversy

The Relationship between Vitamin B12 Levels and Mortality Risk

While the biological importance of vitamin B12 is well established, recent evidence from epidemiological studies has sparked debate around the potential risks of excessive vitamin B12 levels. In a cohort study of over 5500 adults in the Netherlands, higher levels of plasma vitamin B12 were associated with an increased risk of all-cause mortality (25% increased risk for every 1 standard deviation rise in plasma vitamin B12), after adjusting for age, sex, kidney function, and other clinical and laboratory variables.[1] Additionally, in a systematic review and meta-analysis of 22 cohort studies (including over 92,000 individuals), Liu et al. found that each 100 pmol/L rise in serum vitamin B12 was associated with a 4% increased risk of all-cause mortality.[2] The mechanisms underlying this relationship are not fully understood. One proposed explanation is liver and/or kidney dysfunction, which can contribute to both elevated vitamin B12 levels and increased mortality risk. Nonetheless, findings on the topic have been mixed. For example, Wolffenbuttel et al.[3] found low serum B12 concentrations to be associated with a moderate increase in all-cause mortality, using data from the National Health and Nutrition Examination Survey. Overall, further research is needed to clarify the relationship between vitamin B12 levels and mortality, including the direction and magnitude of this association as well as its clinical significance.

Questions

1. What are some possible confounding factors that might explain the link between high vitamin B12 levels and mortality risk?
2. What are some other limitations to consider when interpreting the results of observational studies such as cohort studies?

References

1. Flores-Guerrero JL, Minovic I, Groothof D, et al. Association of plasma concentration of vitamin B12 with all-cause mortality in the general population in the Netherlands. *JAMA Netw Open.* 2020;3(1):e1919274.
2. Liu K, Yang Z, Lu X, et al. The origin of vitamin B12 levels and risk of all-cause, cardiovascular and cancer specific mortality: a systematic review and dose-response meta-analysis. *Arch Gerontol Geriatr.* 2024;117:105230.
3. Wolffenbuttel BHR, Heiner-Fokkema MR, Green R, Gans ROB. Relationship between serum B12 concentrations and mortality: experience in NHANES. *BMC Med.* 2020;18(1):307.

describe the physiologic functioning of vitamin B12, rather than just its presence in blood. Vitamin B12 serves as a cofactor in the conversion of MMA to succinyl-CoA, a key step in the tricarboxylic acid (TCA) or Krebs cycle. Vitamin B12 is also a cofactor in the conversion of homocysteine to the essential amino acid methionine. When vitamin B12 is not present in sufficient quantities, these enzymatic reactions cannot occur, leading homocysteine and MMA to accumulate in the blood. Thus, high levels of serum MMA and homocysteine are common in vitamin B12 deficiency. Reference ranges for MMA and homocysteine vary by laboratory; examples of typical normal ranges are 70–270 nmol/L for MMA and 5–15 μmol/L for homocysteine. For patients with kidney disease, MMA is considered a more specific marker than homocysteine because homocysteine may be elevated due to decreased kidney function.[181] MMA is elevated in vitamin B12 deficiency but not in folate deficiency, making it a helpful indicator to differentiate these deficiencies. In contrast, homocysteine may be elevated in both vitamin B12 and folate deficiencies, since both vitamins are required in the conversion of homocysteine to methionine. **Figure 2.20** illustrates the role of folate and vitamin B12 in homocysteine and MMA metabolism.

For patients who are deficient due to inadequate vitamin B12 intake, oral vitamin B12 supplementation (most commonly available as cyanocobalamin) is adequate for repletion. Parenteral repletion may be indicated for patients with vitamin B12 deficiency that is related to lack of intrinsic factor. In these cases, 1000 μg of vitamin B12 delivered intramuscularly once a month is recommended.[182] More aggressive therapy may be necessary in cases of severe deficiency with neurologic symptoms. If the underlying cause of deficiency is irreversible (e.g., lack of intrinsic factor due to gastric bypass surgery or pernicious anemia), lifelong replacement is necessary. If the cause of deficiency is reversible (e.g., inadequate dietary intake), supplementation may be discontinued once the deficiency is corrected.

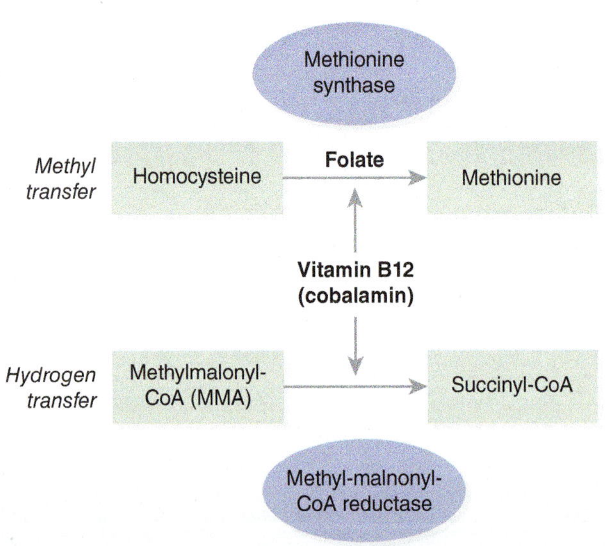

Figure 2.20 Role of Folate and Vitamin B12 in Homocysteine and Methylmalonyl-CoA Metabolism

Data from Means RT, Fairfield KM. Clinical manifestations and diagnosis of vitamin B12 and folate deficiency. *UpToDate*. Wolters Kluwer. Accessed January 9, 2026. https://www.uptodate.com

Folate (vitamin B9) is a water-soluble vitamin that plays an essential role in the synthesis of DNA and metabolism of amino acids. Mechanisms of folate deficiency include inadequate dietary intake, malabsorption (e.g., due to celiac disease, short bowel syndrome, gastric bypass, tropical sprue), and medications that interfere with folate metabolism (e.g., methotrexate, phenytoin, sulfasalazine, trimethoprim). *Serum folate* measures the concentration of folate in the blood. Generally, a serum folate level >4 ng/mL is considered normal, 2–4 ng/mL is borderline low, and <2 ng/mL is deficient.[183] However, serum folate is highly influenced by dietary folate intake, meaning it may appear falsely normal after recent intake, or falsely low after poor intake.

Red blood cell folate (RBC folate) measures the amount of folate in RBCs. Unlike serum folate, RBC folate is not influenced by transient changes in folate intake. RBC folate reflects folate status over the preceding 4 months (i.e., the lifespan of RBCs), and is considered a more accurate indicator of tissue folate stores than serum folate. Normal RBC folate ranges from 360 to 1400 nmol/L.[10]

Elevated homocysteine levels may also be suggestive of folate deficiency. However, homocysteine is not a specific marker of folate deficiency, since elevated levels may also be seen in vitamin B12 deficiency. **Table 2.24** summarizes the laboratory values associated with iron, vitamin B12, and folate deficiency anemias.

Vitamin B12 status must be assessed prior to treating folate deficiency, as large doses of folic acid may mask vitamin B12 deficiency until its neurological consequences become irreversible. This is because, when vitamin B12 deficiency is present, folate may partially compensate for the lack of vitamin B12 in erythropoiesis but cannot compensate for the essential role of vitamin B12 in the nervous system. Thus, treatment with folic acid may improve hematologic status, but cannot improve neurological deficits associated with vitamin B12 deficiency, which may, if untreated, progress and cause permanent neurological damage.[183]

Treatment of folate deficiency should focus on correcting anemia and replenishing folate stores.

Table 2.24 Summary of Laboratory Indicators of Nutritional Anemias

Micronutrient Deficiency	Laboratory Values	Considerations
Iron	↓ MCV ↓ Serum iron ↓ Transferrin saturation ↑ TIBC ↓ Ferritin	■ Ferritin increases with inflammation (not accurate indicator in patients with acute inflammation) ■ MCV may appear normal if concurrent deficiency in vitamin B12 and/or folate
Vitamin B12	↑ MCV ↓ Serum cobalamin ↑ MMA ↑ Homocysteine	■ Homocysteine may increase due to kidney dysfunction ■ High homocysteine may also reflect folate deficiency ■ MCV may appear normal if concurrent with iron deficiency
Folate	↑ MCV ↓ Serum folate ↓ RBC folate ↑ Homocysteine	■ Serum folate may be elevated after recent dietary intake ■ MCV may appear normal if concurrent with iron deficiency

MCV, mean corpuscular volume; TIBC, total iron binding capacity; MMA, methylmalonic acid; RBC, red blood cell
Data from Chan LN, Mike LA. The science and practice of micronutrient supplementation in nutritional anemias: an evidence-based review. *JPEN J Parenter Enteral Nutr*. 2014;38(6):656-672.

Folate deficiency is typically treated with oral folic acid supplementation provided in doses of 1–5 mg daily. The duration of therapy varies according to the underlying cause of deficiency. One to four months is generally sufficient when the cause of deficiency is reversible, and lifelong therapy may be needed when the cause is chronic. Intravenous folic acid may be indicated for patients who cannot tolerate oral supplementation or who require more urgent correction.

Ensuring adequate folate status during pregnancy is crucial to protect against neural tube defects, which are severe birth defects of the brain or spine. To help prevent neural tube defects, women of childbearing age are recommended to obtain 400 μg of folic acid per day, in addition to the folate consumed through dietary sources.[184] Folic acid is the synthetic form of folate that is used in supplements and fortified foods, and its bioavailability is higher than that of naturally occurring food folates. Dietary folate equivalents (DFEs) are a unit of measure that account for the differences in bioavailability between food folate and folic acid, with 1 DFE equivalent to 1 μg of food folate; 0.6 μg of folic acid taken with food; and 0.5 μg of folic acid taken on an empty stomach.

CORE CONCEPT 7

Deficiencies of iron, vitamin B12, and folate can all compromise red blood cell functioning and contribute to anemia.

Vitamins and Trace Elements

Fat-Soluble Vitamins

Fat-soluble vitamins (vitamins A, D, E, and K) are processed similarly to fat. In the duodenum, they are incorporated into micelles, taken up by enterocytes, and then repackaged into chylomicrons before traveling to extrahepatic tissues. Fat-soluble vitamins can be stored in tissues, so deficiency is unlikely under normal physiological circumstances, but may occur from diseases or conditions that impair fat absorption. **Table 2.25** provides an overview of the functions, food sources, and deficiency signs/syndromes associated with each fat-soluble vitamin.

Vitamin A

Vitamin A plays a crucial role in vision, immune function, and cellular growth and differentiation. Dietary vitamin A exists in two main forms: preformed vitamin A (retinoids), which includes retinol and retinyl esters and is found in animal sources (e.g., liver, kidney, egg yolk, butter), and provitamin A carotenoids, which are plant pigments that include beta-carotene, alpha-carotene, and beta-cryptoxanthin. Vitamin A deficiency may lead to xerophthalmia, a vision disorder that has the potential to cause permanent blindness. In the United States, vitamin A deficiency is relatively rare and is usually due to malabsorptive processes (e.g., inflammatory bowel disease, pancreatic insufficiency,

Table 2.25 Fat-Soluble Vitamins: Functions, Food Sources, and Associated Deficiencies

Vitamin	Biochemical or Physiological Function	Food Sources	Deficiency Signs/Syndromes
Vitamin A	Vision, cell growth/differentiation, bone development, immune function	Retinoids: liver, dairy products, fortified foods Provitamin A carotenoids: yellow and orange fruits, leafy green vegetables	Night blindness, xerophthalmia, Bitot's spots, hyperkeratosis (dry, scaly skin)
Vitamin D	Calcium and phosphorus homeostasis, bone mineral metabolism, cell growth/differentiation	Fatty fish, fortified foods, egg yolks	Osteomalacia, rickets
Vitamin E	Antioxidant defense, cell membrane integrity	Vegetable oils, nuts, seeds, whole grains	Hemolytic anemia
Vitamin K	Blood clotting, calcium metabolism	Leafy green vegetables	Hemorrhage

Data from Gropper SG, Smith JL, Carr TP. *Advanced Nutrition and Human Metabolism*, 7th ed. Cengage Learning; 2018.

post-bariatric surgery) rather than inadequate dietary intake.[185]

Vitamin A status may be assessed using serum retinol concentration, levels less than 20 μg/dL suggesting deficiency.[185] However, serum retinol concentration may be falsely low in the setting of acute inflammation. Clinical signs of vitamin A deficiency, such as night blindness and impaired dark vision adaptation, should be evaluated alongside biochemical markers to aid in accurate diagnosis.

Acute or chronic vitamin A toxicity may occur with excessive vitamin A supplementation. Since most vitamin A in the body is stored in the liver, circulating vitamin A concentrations do not consistently reflect vitamin A stores and are thus not a reliable indicator of toxicity. Instead, serum retinyl ester concentrations are often used as a marker of hypervitaminosis A.

Vitamin D

Vitamin D is essential for calcium-phosphorus balance, neuromuscular and immune function, and other cellular processes. There are two major forms of vitamin D: vitamin D2 (ergocalciferol), which is found in dietary supplements and vitamin D-fortified foods, and vitamin D3 (cholecalciferol), which is synthesized in the skin after exposure to sunlight and naturally occurs in certain animal-based foods. Both forms are converted in the body to calciferol, the active form of vitamin D.

Vitamin D status is assessed using 25-hydroxy vitamin D (25-OH vitamin D; also known as "calcifediol" or "calcidiol"), with levels ≥20 ng/mL (50 nmol/L) considered optimal.[45] Vitamin D insufficiency is defined as a 25-OH vitamin D level of 12 to <20 ng/mL (30–50 nmol/L), and deficiency is defined as a 25-OH vitamin D level <12 ng/mL (30 nmol/L).[45] Populations at risk of vitamin D deficiency include individuals with inadequate sunlight exposure, older adults, individuals with dark skin, and individuals with fat malabsorptive disorders or kidney disease.[186]

Vitamin E

Vitamin E is a fat-soluble antioxidant that protects cells from free radical damage. Vitamin E exists in eight forms, with alpha-tocopherol being the most biologically active form in humans. Vitamin E status is assessed using serum alpha-tocopherol, with levels less than 5 μg/mL indicative of deficiency.[187] Alpha-tocopherol is transferred through the bloodstream by lipoproteins such as VLDL and LDL, so serum alpha-tocopherol levels are closely associated with serum lipid levels.[188] Thus, vitamin E status may be assessed using a ratio of alpha-tocopherol (mg) to total lipids (g), with a ratio less than 0.8 suggestive of vitamin E deficiency.[187] Vitamin E deficiency is rare under normal physiological conditions but may be observed in patients with fat malabsorption or genetic lipid disorders. Clinical manifestations of vitamin E deficiency include ataxia, anemia, and poor reflex control.

Vitamin K

Vitamin K is an essential cofactor for proteins involved in blood clot formation, bone mineralization, and vascular health. Vitamin K refers to a group of compounds that include phylloquinone (vitamin K1), which is obtained from plant-based foods, and menaquinones (vitamin K2), which are obtained from animal foods and synthesized by intestinal bacteria.[189] There is currently no single biomarker established to evaluate vitamin K status. Prothrombin time (PT), which represents the time it takes for a clot to form in a blood sample, is a commonly used functional measure of vitamin K status. Normal PT is approximately 11–13 seconds,[105] and prolonged PT is common in vitamin K deficiency. Serum phylloquinone may also be used to assess vitamin K status, with concentrations <0.15 μg/L considered indicative of deficiency.[190]

Common causes of vitamin K deficiency include fat malabsorption (e.g., due to cystic fibrosis, celiac disease, inflammatory bowel disease, liver disease) and antibiotic or anticoagulant treatments. Vitamin K deficiency may contribute to uncontrolled bleeding, reduced bone mineralization, osteoporosis, and increased cardiovascular disease risk. Vitamin K deficiency bleeding (VKDB) is a potentially life-threatening condition that may occur in newborns due to inadequate vitamin K stores during infancy. To prevent VKDB, all newborns are recommended to receive a single intramuscular dose of vitamin K within 6 hours of birth.[191]

Water-Soluble Vitamins

Water-soluble vitamins (B-complex vitamins, vitamin C) are essential for energy production, nutrient metabolism, RBC formation, and gene expression. Water-soluble vitamins are absorbed primarily in the proximal small intestine and are stored in small quantities in body tissues. Generally, any excess of these vitamins is excreted in the urine, meaning the risk for toxicity is lower with water-soluble vitamins than with fat-soluble vitamins. **Table 2.26** outlines the absorption sites, functions, food sources, and deficiencies associated with each of the water-soluble vitamins.

Table 2.26 Water-Soluble Vitamins: Absorption Sites, Functions, Food Sources, and Associated Deficiencies

Vitamin	Absorption Site	Biochemical or Physiological Function	Food Sources	Deficiency Signs/Syndromes
Thiamine (B1)	Duodenum, jejunum	Carbohydrate metabolism, nervous system function	Pork, grains, legumes	Beriberi (nervous system and cardiac dysfunction)
Riboflavin (B2)	Duodenum, jejunum	Electron transfer reactions for nutrient metabolism and energy production	Meat, dairy, eggs	Cheilosis (cracked lips), glossitis, angular stomatitis (cracked corners of mouth), magenta tongue
Niacin (B3)	Small intestine	Electron transfer reactions for nutrient metabolism and energy production	Meat, fish, peanut butter	Pellagra (dermatitis, diarrhea, confusion), beefy red tongue
Pantothenic Acid (B5)	Jejunum	Acetylation of proteins/ sugars, gene expression	Animal foods, grains, legumes	Burning sensation in feet
Pyridoxine (B6)	Jejunum	Nutrient metabolism, energy production, gene expression	Meat, fish, grains	Dermatitis, glossitis, nervous system dysfunction
Biotin (B7)	Proximal small intestine	Nutrient metabolism, energy production, gene expression	Liver, soybeans, eggs	Dermatitis, nervous system dysfunction, alopecia
Folate (B9)	Duodenum, jejunum	Nutrient metabolism, energy production, hematopoiesis	Green vegetables, fortified grains	Megaloblastic anemia
Cobalamin (B12)	Ileum	Nutrient metabolism, energy production, hematopoiesis	Meat, fish, poultry, milk	Megaloblastic anemia
Vitamin C	Small intestine, jejunum	Antioxidant defense	Citrus fruits, potatoes, green and yellow vegetables	Scurvy, bleeding gums, petechiae, poor wound healing

Data from Gropper SG, Smith JL, Carr TP. *Advanced Nutrition and Human Metabolism*, 7th ed. Cengage Learning; 2018.

B Vitamins

B vitamins serve as cofactors for enzymes involved in neurological function, RBC production, macronutrient metabolism, and a wide range of other cellular and physiologic processes. Vitamin B12, folate (B9), and thiamine (B1) are among the most common B vitamin deficiencies. Thiamine deficiency may result in Beriberi and Wernicke-Korsakoff syndrome and may be seen in individuals with alcohol use disorder or malabsorptive conditions. Thiamine status may be assessed using erythrocyte transketolase (ETK) activity, which measures the ability of the ETK enzyme to catalyze a thiamine-dependent reaction. In this test, basal ETK activity is measured, then exogenous thiamine is added to the erythrocyte sample, and then ETK activity is measured again. When thiamine status is adequate, the change in ETK activity is expected to be minimal (since thiamine would already be present to facilitate ETK activity), whereas a significant rise in ETK activity would indicate thiamine insufficiency. This test is an indirect, functional measure of thiamine status because it assesses the availability of thiamine to carry out one of its essential functions. However, the ETK test is not readily available outside of research settings. Thus, direct measurement of blood thiamine concentration may also be used, although this method has limited sensitivity and specificity and may be falsely low in the setting of inflammation.[192]

Other B vitamins such as riboflavin (B2) and pyridoxine (B6) may also be assessed by measuring the activation of enzymes that require these vitamins as cofactors. For instance, erythrocyte glutathione reductase activity can be used to assess riboflavin status, and the activity of erythrocyte amino acid transferase enzymes can be used to assess vitamin B6 status. For vitamin B6, direct measurement of pyridoxal 5-phosphate, the biologically active form of vitamin B6, is often preferred.[189] Niacin (B3) status is generally assessed using urinary niacin metabolites such as N-methylnicotinamide.

Vitamin C

Vitamin C, or ascorbic acid, supports immune function, aids in iron homeostasis, protects against free radical damage, and participates in a variety of enzymatic processes. Plasma and leukocyte vitamin C levels are the most common biomarkers of vitamin C status. Normal plasma vitamin C is approximately 0.4–1.5 mg/dL,[105] although symptoms of deficiency usually do not appear until levels fall below 0.2 mg/dL.[193] Vitamin C deficiency results in scurvy, which manifests as bleeding gums, poor wound healing, diminished immune function, fatigue, and petechiae. Vitamin C levels decline rapidly during acute inflammation, so low levels are common in critically ill patients.[189] Thus, higher dosages of vitamin C might be needed to counteract disease-related deficiencies in these patients.

Trace Elements

Trace elements serve a variety of structural, regulatory, and catalytic roles in the body. **Table 2.27** outlines the key functions, food sources, and deficiencies associated with the trace elements. Deficiencies of trace elements may be due to inadequate intake, inadequate supplementation in PN, or a disease state that interferes with trace element absorption, utilization, or excretion. Abnormalities of selected trace elements are described below:

- **Copper**: Copper deficiency is seen with malabsorption (e.g., following bariatric surgery or intestinal resection), Menkes disease (a genetic disorder that impairs copper transport), and prolonged PN or EN without adequate copper. Copper deficiency may also be induced by zinc oversupplementation, as zinc and copper compete for absorption in the small intestine.[194] Serum copper and serum ceruloplasmin (the main copper-carrying protein in blood) are common biomarkers of copper status. Unlike most micronutrients, copper levels increase during acute inflammation.[189] Thus, in patients with inflammatory conditions, serum copper should be interpreted alongside a surrogate marker of inflammation such as CRP. Copper is regulated primarily through its excretion in the bile, so impaired biliary excretion or cholestasis can cause copper accumulation in the liver, which can lead to liver damage and dysfunction.[195] Significant hepatic copper overload has been observed in patients receiving long-term PN, highlighting the importance of monitoring plasma copper status in long-term PN patients and adjusting doses as needed.[196]
- **Selenium**: Selenium deficiency is uncommon but has been reported in geographic regions with low selenium levels in soil, as well as in patients receiving PN not supplemented with selenium.[197] Total plasma selenium is the most widely used biomarker of selenium status. Cardiomyopathy and skeletal muscle dysfunction are the primary clinical manifestations of selenium deficiency.
- **Iodine**: Iodine deficiency is characterized by goiter and hypothyroidism and is seen in areas with a

Table 2.27 Trace Elements: Functions, Food Sources, and Associated Deficiencies

Trace Element	Biochemical or Physiological Function	Food Sources	Deficiency Signs/Syndromes
Chromium	Insulin signaling, glucose metabolism	Meat, cereals, yeast	Insulin resistance
Copper	Iron utilization, collagen synthesis, antioxidant defense	Meat, fish, nuts, seeds, legumes	Anemia, impaired immune function
Iodine	Thyroid hormone synthesis	Iodized salt, salt-water seafood	Goiter (enlarged thyroid gland)
Iron	Oxygen transport, hormone synthesis	Meat, leafy green vegetables, enriched grains	Microcytic anemia
Manganese	Central nervous system function	Grains, legumes, nuts, seafood	Poor growth, central nervous system function (deficiency unlikely)
Molybdenum	Purine metabolism, breakdown of toxins	Legumes, meat, poultry, fish, grains	Neurological dysfunction
Selenium	Antioxidant defense	Meat, fish, grains, Brazil nuts	Cardiomyopathy, myalgia
Zinc	Cell growth/replication, DNA and RNA metabolism, nutrient metabolism	Meat, liver, poultry, grains, legumes	Abnormal taste, poor wound healing, subnormal growth, impaired reproductive system development

Data from Gropper SG, Smith JL, Carr TP. *Advanced Nutrition and Human Metabolism*, 7th ed. Cengage Learning; 2018.

low concentration of iodine in food products. Urinary iodine concentration is considered a strong indicator of iodine status, since more than 90% of ingested iodine is excreted in the urine.[189]

- **Zinc**: Zinc deficiency can cause impaired growth, alopecia, dysgeusia (impaired taste), immune dysfunction, impaired wound healing, and skin lesions, among other clinical consequences. Zinc deficiency is observed in malabsorptive conditions such as short bowel syndrome, bariatric surgery, cystic fibrosis, chronic pancreatitis, and inflammatory bowel disease, as well as in patients receiving long-term PN without zinc supplementation.[189] Plasma or serum zinc concentrations are commonly used to evaluate zinc status, with normal plasma zinc defined as 75–140 μg/dL.[105] Zinc concentrations may decline significantly with low albumin levels or systemic inflammation, so care must be taken when interpreting zinc status in patients with hypoalbuminemia or inflammatory disease states.

See **Table 2.28** for a summary of the biochemical indicators of nutritional status discussed throughout this chapter.

Clinical Applications: Order-Writing Privileges

Clinical privileges granted to registered dietitian nutritionists (RDNs) vary according to state professional licensure regulations and institutional policies. In 2014, the Centers for Medicare and Medicaid Services (CMS) announced a final rule that authorized nutrition-related ordering privileges for qualified RDNs in hospital settings.[198] Under this rule, RDNs are permitted to become privileged to order patient diets, order laboratory tests to monitor the effectiveness of dietary plans and orders, and modify diets based on the lab tests, if consistent with state law and healthcare regulations and specifically authorized by the facility's medical staff. The rule does not specifically include

Table 2.28 Summary of Biochemical Indicators and Nutritional Implications

Test	Reference Range*	Comments
I. Electrolytes and Hydration Status		
Sodium (Na^+)	136–145 mEq/L	■ Influenced by hydration/volume status; may be low or elevated in dehydration and overhydration, respectively
Potassium (K^+)	3.5–5 mEq/L	■ May appear falsely high if sample is hemolyzed
Calcium (Ca^{2+})	8.5–10.5 mg/dL	■ Ionized calcium may be measured when serum albumin is low (normal ionized calcium: 4.65–5.25 mg/dL)
Phosphorus (PO_4)	2.5–4.5 mg/dL	■ Does not necessarily reflect total body PO_4 content
Magnesium (Mg^{2+})	1.5–2.7 mg/dL	■ Does not necessarily reflect total body Mg^{2+} content
Chloride (Cl^-)	96–106 mEq/L	■ Low levels may cause metabolic alkalosis; high levels may cause metabolic acidosis
Bicarbonate (HCO_3^-)	22–31 mEq/L	■ Low levels may cause metabolic acidosis; high levels may cause metabolic alkalosis
Osmolality, serum	275–295 mOsm/kg	■ Affected by solutes such as glucose, amino acids, and electrolytes (e.g., sodium, chloride, potassium, bicarbonate)
II. Acid-Base Status		
pH	7.35–7.45	■ <7.35 indicates acidemia; >7.45 indicates alkalemia
PCO_2	Arterial: 35–45 mm Hg Venous: 41–51 mm Hg	■ Increased in respiratory acidosis and in response to metabolic alkalosis; decreased in respiratory alkalosis and in response to metabolic acidosis
HCO_3^-	Arterial: 22–26 mEq/L Venous: 24–28 mEq/L	■ Increased in metabolic alkalosis and in response to respiratory acidosis; decreased in metabolic acidosis and in response to respiratory alkalosis
PO_2	Arterial: 80–100 mm Hg Venous: 35–40 mm Hg	■ Represents the amount of oxygen dissolved in blood
O_2 saturation	Arterial: >93% Venous: 70–75%	■ Represents the percentage of hemoglobin bound to oxygen molecules
III. Glycemic Status		
Blood glucose, fasting	70–100 mg/dL	■ ≥126 mg/dL diagnostic for diabetes
2-h postprandial blood glucose	<140 mg/dL	■ ≥200 mg/dL diagnostic for diabetes
HbA1c	4.3–5.6%	■ 5.7–6.4% indicates prediabetes; ≥6.5% indicates diabetes
IV. Protein Status		
Total serum protein	5.5–9 g/dL	■ Measures two major types of proteins: albumin and globulin
CRP	≤0.8 mg/dL	■ Elevated in both acute and chronic inflammation
Albumin	3.5–5.5 g/dL	■ Can help characterize inflammation, but is not a direct indicator of malnutrition
Prealbumin	16–30 mg/dL	■ Considered a more sensitive indicator of nutritional status than albumin due to its relatively short half-life, but is still influenced by non-dietary factors such as acute inflammation ■ Low levels may be found in zinc deficiency

Test	Reference Range*	Comments
RBP	3–6 mg/dL	■ Low levels may be found with vitamin A and/or zinc deficiencies
Transferrin	200–400 mg/dL	■ Elevated when iron stores are low
		■ Decreased in inflammation (negative acute-phase protein)
Creatinine, serum	Females: 0.5–1.1 mg/dL	■ Influenced by renal function and muscle mass
	Males: 0.7–1.3 mg/dL	
BUN	8–20 mg/dL	■ Elevated with dehydration
V. Enzymes		
AST	10–40 U/L	■ Decreased in vitamin B6 deficiency
		■ An elevation of AST that is higher than that of ALT may indicate alcohol-induced liver damage
ALT	Females: 19–25 IU/L	■ Decreased in vitamin B6 deficiency
	Males: 29–33 IU/L	
ALP	30–120 U/L	■ Decreased in malnutrition
VI. Lipid Status		
LDL-cholesterol	<100 mg/dL	■ Calculated using the Friedewald formula, which is only valid when TG concentration is <400 mg/dL
		■ Correlated with atherosclerotic cardiovascular disease risk
HDL-cholesterol	Females: ≥50 mg/dL	■ Considered anti-atherogenic
	Males: ≥40 mg/dL	
Total cholesterol	<200 mg/dL	■ Correlated with atherosclerotic cardiovascular disease risk
Triglycerides	<150 mg/dL	■ Correlated with atherosclerotic cardiovascular disease risk
		■ Severe elevations associated with acute pancreatitis
VII. Hematological Status		
Hemoglobin	Females: 12–16 g/dL	■ Not sensitive to nutritional causes of anemia
	Males: 14–18 g/dL	
Hematocrit	Females: 35–43%	■ Not sensitive to nutritional causes of anemia
	Males: 40–50%	
RBC count	Females: 3.8–5.0 × 10^6/μL	■ Not sensitive to nutritional causes of anemia
	Males: 4.2–5.7 × 10^6/μL	
VII. Hematological Status		
MCV	80–100 fL	■ Used to classify anemia as microcytic (MCV <80), normocytic (MCV 80–100), and macrocytic (MCV >100)
		■ May appear normal when iron deficiency is present in conjunction with folate and/or vitamin B12 deficiency

(*continues*)

Table 2.28 Summary of Biochemical Indicators and Nutritional Implications (continued)

Test	Reference Range*	Comments
MCHC	32–36 g/dL	■ Low values indicate hypochromic RBCs, often seen in iron deficiency anemia
RDW	RDW-SD: 39–46 fL	■ RDW-SD considered a more accurate indicator of RBC size variations than RDW-CV
	RDW-CV: 11.6–14.6%	■ Elevated in nutritional anemias
Platelet count	$(150–400 \times 10^9/L)^9$	■ Elevated in iron deficiency anemia
Reticulocyte count	0.5–2%	■ Decreased in iron, folate, or vitamin B12 deficiency anemias
WBC count	5–10 × 109/L	■ Elevated in infection and inflammation
		■ Decreased in bone marrow disorders
Iron, serum	50–160 μg/dL	■ Considered a relatively poor indicator of iron status due to natural diurnal variation and influence of dietary iron intake
Transferrin	Refer to "Transferrin" under Protein Status	
TIBC	250–460 μg/dL	■ Elevated in iron deficiency anemia
Transferrin saturation	20–50%	■ Decreased in iron deficiency anemia
Ferritin	Females: 10–150 ng/mL	■ Considered a strong indicator of iron stores
	Males: 12–300 ng/mL	■ Elevated in inflammation (positive acute-phase protein)
Cobalamin, serum	>300 pg/mL	■ Low levels associated with macrocytic anemia
MMA	70–270 nmol/L	■ Elevated in vitamin B12 deficiency
Homocysteine	5–15 μmol/L	■ Elevated in vitamin B12 and folate deficiency
Folate, serum	>4 ng/mL	■ Low levels associated with macrocytic anemia
		■ Highly influenced by dietary folate intake
Folate, RBC	360–1400 nmol/L	■ Considered a more accurate indicator of folate stores than serum folate
VIII. Micronutrient Status		
A. Fat-Soluble Vitamins		
Vitamin A	Serum retinols: 20–60 μg/dL	■ <20 μg/dL suggests vitamin A deficiency
Vitamin D	25-OH vitamin D: ≥20 ng/mL	■ 12 to <20 ng/mL suggests vitamin D insufficiency; <12 ng/mL suggests deficiency
Vitamin E	Alpha tocopherols: 5.7–20 mg/L	■ May be interpreted alongside total lipids; a low alpha-tocopherol to lipid ratio (<0.8) suggests vitamin E deficiency
Vitamin K	1. PT: 11–13 seconds	■ Functional indicator of vitamin K status; often prolonged in vitamin K deficiency
	2. Phylloquinone: 0.15–1 μg/L	■ The major circulating form of vitamin K

Test	Reference Range*	Comments
B. Water-Soluble Vitamins		
Thiamine (B1)	1. ETK activity: <15%	■ Functional indicator of thiamine status; not commonly used outside of research settings
	2. Whole blood thiamine: 70–180 nmol/L	■ Limited sensitivity and specificity; may be falsely low during inflammation
Riboflavin (B2)	EGR activity test ratio: <1.2	■ Functional indicator of riboflavin status; >1.4 indicates deficiency
Niacin (B3)	Urinary NMN: 17–115 µmol/day	■ One of the major niacin urinary metabolites
Pyridoxine (B6)	1. Erythrocyte AST activation coefficient <1.6; erythrocyte ALT activation coefficient: <1.25 (measuring the change in AST/ALT activity with added PLP)	■ Functional indicator of vitamin B6 status, as vitamin B6 is a cofactor in AST and ALT metabolism ■ Confounded by diseases and medications that affect liver or cardiac function
	2. PLP: 5–50 µg/L	■ The biologically active form of vitamin B6
Folate	Refer to "Folate" under Hematological Status	
Cobalamin (B12)	Refer to "Cobalamin" under Hematological Status	
Vitamin C	0.4–1.5 mg/dL	■ Decreased in inflammation ■ Deficiency signs typically do not appear until <0.2 mg/dL
C. Trace Elements		
Copper	1. Serum copper: 10–25 µmol/L	■ Elevated in inflammation
	2. Ceruloplasmin: 180–400 mg/L	■ The main copper-carrying protein in blood; influenced by the same factors that affect serum copper (e.g., inflammation)
Selenium	Plasma selenium: 120–160 µg/L	■ Includes selenium found in selenoproteins and in the enzyme glutathione peroxidase
Iodine	1. Urinary iodine: 100–199 µg/L	■ Sensitive indicator of recent iodine intake
	2. Thyroglobulin: 2–10 ng/mL	■ Precursor to thyroid hormones thyroxine (T4) and triiodothyronine (T3), which require iodine for their synthesis
Zinc	75–140 µg/dL	■ Reduced in inflammation

CRP, C-reactive protein; BUN, blood urea nitrogen; AST, aspartate aminotransferase; ALT, alanine aminotransferase; ALP, alkaline phosphatase; LDH, lactate dehydrogenase; LDL, low-density lipoprotein; HDL, high-density lipoprotein; RBC, red blood cell; MCV, mean corpuscular volume; MCHC, mean corpuscular hemoglobin concentration; RDW, red cell distribution width; WBC, white blood cell; TIBC, total iron binding capacity; MMA, methylmalonic acid; 25 OH vitamin D, 25-hydroxy vitamin D; PT, prothrombin time; ETK, erythrocyte transketolase; EGR, erythrocyte glutathione reductase; NMN, N-methyl-nicotinamide; PLP, pyridoxal 5-phosphate

*Ranges vary by laboratory, patient populations, and the assays, equipment, and techniques used. The values presented in this table may differ from ranges reported from a local laboratory.

Data from Shrimanker I, Bhattarai S. Electrolytes. [Updated 2023 Jul 24]. In: StatPearls [Internet]. Treasure Island (FL): StatPearls Publishing; 2025 Jan–. Available from: https://www.ncbi.nlm.nih.gov/books/NBK541123/; El Brihi J, Pathak S. Normal and abnormal complete blood count with differential. [Updated 2024 Jun 8]. In: StatPearls [Internet]. Treasure Island (FL): StatPearls Publishing; 2025 Jan–. Available from: https://www.ncbi.nlm.nih.gov/books/NBK604207/; American Diabetes Association Professional Practice Committee. 2. Diagnosis and classification of diabetes: standards of care in diabetes-2024. *Diabetes Care*. 2024;47(Suppl 1):S20–S42. doi:10.2337/dc24-S002; Rice M, Ismail B, Pillow MT. Approach to metabolic acidosis in the emergency department. *Emerg Med Clin North Am*. 2014;32(2):403–420. doi:10.1016/j.emc.2014.01.002; ABIM Laboratory Test Reference Ranges. American Board of Internal Medicine (ABIM). Accessed March 30, 2024. https://www.abim.org/Media/bfijryql/laboratory-reference-ranges.pdf

privileges for ordering lab or other diagnostic services but does not state that these cannot be ordered by an RDN. Thus, the scope of an RDN's privileges can vary considerably by state and institution. It is essential for RDNs to understand the specific definitions of **order-writing privileges** within their healthcare institution to ensure regulatory compliance. RDNs in hospital settings interested in petitioning for ordering privileges must review state laws (e.g., licensure, certification, and title protection) and healthcare regulations to identify possible barriers that may need to be addressed.[199]

Chapter Summary

Biochemical assessment is a vital component of the nutrition care process, providing important information regarding an individual's nutritional status as it relates to pertinent underlying health conditions. Interpreting trends in electrolyte, fluid, and acid-base levels can provide critical information about the progression of health conditions and aid in determining appropriate nutrition therapy plans. Consideration of these values in the context of other assessment measures (e.g., anthropometrics, functional assessment, and diet history) is crucial to accurately evaluate a patient's condition and nutritional needs. A collective evaluation of endocrine biomarkers, liver function tests, lipid levels, and visceral proteins can help clinicians evaluate endocrine, liver, and cardiovascular function, as well as the presence of inflammatory stress, all of which can significantly impact a patient's nutritional status and needs. Numerous biochemical values are also used to assess hematological status, and understanding how to interpret these values and differentiate between types of anemia and treatment methods is critical. Prioritizing a patient's most severe and pertinent abnormal laboratory values in the context of nutritional status and needs is essential to provide the most effective nutrition therapy.

Key Terms

static assays, functional assays, hemodilution, hemoconcentration, electrolytes, basic metabolic panel (BMP), comprehensive metabolic panel (CMP), lipid panel, renal function panel, hepatic function panel, complete blood count, differential count, osmolality, osmolarity, osmotic pressure, isotonic, hypertonic, hypotonic, third spacing, hypervolemia, hypovolemia, hyponatremia, osmotic demyelination syndrome (ODS), pseudohyponatremia, hypernatremia, hypokalemia, hyperkalemia, hemolysis, hypocalcemia, hypercalcemia, hypophosphatemia, hyperphosphatemia, hypomagnesemia, hypermagnesemia, refeeding syndrome, hypochloremia, hyperchloremia, acidemia, alkalemia, acidosis, alkalosis, arterial blood gases (ABGs), venous blood gases (VBGs), respiratory acidosis, respiratory alkalosis, metabolic acidosis, metabolic alkalosis, hypoglycemia, hyperglycemia, visceral protein, acute-phase proteins, positive acute-phase proteins, negative acute-phase proteins, marasmus, kwashiorkor, somatic protein, nitrogen balance, creatinine height index (CHI), anemia, microcytic anemia, macrocytic anemia, normocytic anemia, iron deficiency anemia, anemia of chronic disease, micronutrients, trace elements, order-writing privileges

Acknowledgments

The authors acknowledge Katelyn Castro for contributions to the previous version of this chapter.

References

1. Stephenson T, Schiff W. *Human Nutrition Science for Healthy Living*. 1st ed. McGraw-Hill Education; 2016.
2. Pfeiffer CM, Schleicher RL, Caldwell KL. Biochemical Indices. In: Caballero B, ed. *Encyclopedia of Human Nutrition (Third Edition)*. Academic Press; 2013:156–174.
3. Gandhi MH, Gupta V. Physiology, maternal blood. *StatPearls*. StatPearls Publishing; 2023.
4. Laboratory panels – Coding and billing. Centers for Medicare & Medicaid Services. Accessed January 25, 2024. https://www.cms.gov/medicare-coverage-database/view/article.aspx?articleid=56486&ver=6&=
5. Aronson PS, Boron WF, Boulpaep EL. Transport of solutes and water. In: Boron WF, Boulpaep EL, eds. *Medical Physiology*. 3rd ed. Elsevier; 2017.

6. Najem O, Shah MM, De Jesus O. Serum osmolality. *StatPearls*. StatPearls Publishing; 2024.
7. Purssell RA, Pudek M, Brubacher J, Abu-Laban RB. Derivation and validation of a formula to calculate the contribution of ethanol to the osmolal gap. *Ann Emerg Med*. 2001;38(6):653–659. doi:10.1067/mem.2001.119455
8. Shrimanker I, Bhattarai S. Electrolytes. *StatPearls*. StatPearls Publishing; 2024.
9. Ahmed F, Mohammed A. Magnesium: The forgotten electrolyte–A review on hypomagnesemia. *Med Sci (Basel)*. 2019;7(4):56. doi:10.3390/medsci7040056
10. Pagana KD, Pagana TJ, Pagana TN. *Mosby's Diagnostic and Laboratory Test Reference*. 15th ed. Elsevier; 2021.
11. National Academies of Sciences, Engineering, and Medicine. *Dietary Reference Intakes for Sodium and Potassium*. National Academies Press (US); 2019.
12. Rondon H, Badireddy M. Hyponatremia. *StatPearls*. StatPearls Publishing; 2024.
13. Verbalis JG, Goldsmith SR, Greenberg A, et al. Diagnosis, evaluation, and treatment of hyponatremia: Expert panel recommendations. *Am J Med*. 2013;126(10 Suppl 1):S1–42. doi:10.1016/j.amjmed.2013.07.006
14. Hillier TA, Abbott RD, Barrett EJ. Hyponatremia: Evaluating the correction factor for hyperglycemia. *Am J Med*. 1999;106(4):399–403. doi:10.1016/s0002-9343(99)00055-8
15. Bruno JJ. *ASPEN Fluids, Electrolytes, and Acid-Base Disorders Handbook*. 2nd ed. American Society for Parenteral and Enteral Nutrition; 2020.
16. Theis SR, Khandhar PB. Pseudohyponatremia. *StatPearls*. StatPearls Publishing; 2024.
17. Adrogue HJ, Madias NE. Hyponatremia. *N Engl J Med*. 2000;342(21):1581–1589.doi:10.1056/NEJM200005253422107
18. Faber M. Clinical overview: Syndrome of inappropriate antidiuresis. ClinicalKey. Accessed https://www.clinicalkey.com/nursing/#!/content/derived_clinical_overview/76-s2.0-B9780323755764008863 (updated January 1, 2024). Accessed July 31, 2025.
19. Arzhan S, Roumelioti ME, Litvinovich I, Bologa CG, Myers OB, Unruh ML. Hypernatremia in hospitalized patients: a large population-based study. *Kidney360*. 2022;3(7):1144–1157. doi:10.34067/KID.0000702022
20. Aiyagari V, Deibert E, Diringer MN. Hypernatremia in the neurologic intensive care unit: How high is too high? *J Crit Care*. 2006;21(2):163–172. doi:10.1016/j.jcrc.2005.10.002
21. Arima H, Cheetham T, Christ-Crain M, et al. Changing the name of diabetes insipidus: a position statement of the Working Group for Renaming Diabetes Insipidus. *J Clin Endocrinol Metab*. 2022;108(1):1–3. doi:10.1210/clinem/dgac547
22. Hui C, Khan M, Khan Suheb MZ, Radbel JM. Arginine vasopressin disorder (diabetes insipidus). *StatPearls*. StatPearls Publishing; 2024.
23. Yun G, Baek SH, Kim S. Evaluation and management of hypernatremia in adults: clinical perspectives. *Korean J Intern Med*. 2023;38(3):290–302. doi:10.3904/kjim.2022.346
24. Sonani B, Naganathan S, Al-Dhahir MA. Hypernatremia. *StatPearls*. StatPearls Publishing; 2024.
25. Kumbar L, Sahota RJ. Clinical overview: hypernatremia. ClinicalKey. Accessed July 31, 2025. https://www.clinicalkey.com/nursing/#!/content/derived_clinical_overview/76-s2.0-B9780323755764004634
26. Kardalas E, Paschou SA, Anagnostis P, Muscogiuri G, Siasos G, Vryonidou A. Hypokalemia: a clinical update. *Endocr Connect*. 2018;7(4):R135–R146. doi:10.1530/EC-18-0109
27. Gallacher SD, Tsokolas G, Dimitropoulos I. Liquorice-induced apparent mineralocorticoid excess presenting in the emergency department. *Clin Med (Lond)*. 2017;17(1):43–45. doi:10.7861/clinmedicine.17-1-43
28. Oh MS, Briefel G, Pincus MR. Evaluation of renal function, water, electrolytes, and acid-base balance. In: McPherson RA, Pincus MR, eds. *Henry's Clinical Diagnosis and Management by Laboratory Methods*. Elsevier; 2022:182–207.e2.
29. Asmar A, Mohandas R, Wingo CS. A physiologic-based approach to the treatment of a patient with hypokalemia. *Am J Kidney Dis*. 2012;60(3):492–497. doi:10.1053/j.ajkd.2012.01.031
30. Castro D, Sharma S. Hypokalemia. *StatPearls*. StatPearls Publishing; 2024.
31. Viera AJ, Wouk N. Potassium disorders: hypokalemia and hyperkalemia. *Am Fam Physician*. 2015;92(6):487–495.
32. Clinical overview: hypokalemia. ClinicalKey. Accessed July 31, 2025. https://www.clinicalkey.com/nursing/#!/content/clinical_overview/67-s2.0-f493c228-fe54-486c-8bb1-a49f1fc99f48
33. Simon LV, Hashmi MF, Farrell MW. Hyperkalemia. *StatPearls*. StatPearls Publishing; 2024.
34. Hunter RW, Bailey MA. Hyperkalemia: pathophysiology, risk factors and consequences. *Nephrol Dial Transplant*. 2019;34(Suppl 3):iii2–iii11. doi:10.1093/ndt/gfz206
35. Adrogué HJ, Madias NE. Changes in plasma potassium concentration during acute acid-base disturbances. *Am J Med*. 1981;71(3):456–467. doi:10.1016/0002-9343(81)90182-0
36. Wan Azman WN, Omar J, Koon TS, Tuan Ismail TS. Hemolyzed specimens: major challenge for identifying and rejecting specimens in clinical laboratories. *Oman Med J*. 2019;34(2):94–98. doi:10.5001/omj.2019.19
37. Meng QH, Wagar EA. Pseudohyperkalemia: a new twist on an old phenomenon. *Crit Rev Clin Lab Sci*. 2015;52(2):45–55. doi:10.3109/10408363.2014.966898
38. Ikizler TA, Burrowes JD, Byham-Gray LD, et al. KDOQI Clinical Practice Guideline for Nutrition in CKD: 2020 update. *Am J Kidney Dis*. 2020;76(3, Supplement 1):S1–S107. doi:10.1053/j.ajkd.2020.05.006
39. Koeppen B. Potassium, calcium, and phosphate homeostasis. In: Hall, JM, Koeppen BM, Swiatecka-Urban A, Stanton BA, eds. *Berne & Levy Physiology*. 8th ed. Elsevier; 2024.
40. Shaker JL, Deftos L. Calcium and phosphate homeostasis. In: Feingold KR, Anawalt B, Blackman MR, et al, eds. *Endotext*. MDText.com, Inc.; 2000.
41. Goyal A, Anastasopoulou C, Ngu M, Singh S. Hypocalcemia. *StatPearls*. StatPearls Publishing; 2024.
42. Payne RB, Little AJ, Williams RB, Milner JR. Interpretation of serum calcium in patients with abnormal serum proteins. *Br Med J*. 1973;4(5893):643–646. doi:10.1136/bmj.4.5893.643
43. Sanaie S, Mahmoodpoor A, Hamishehkar H, et al. Association between disease severity and calcium concentration in critically ill patients admitted to intensive care unit. *Anesth Pain Med*. 2018;8(1):e57583. doi:10.5812/aapm.57583
44. Calvi LM, Bushinsky DA. When is it appropriate to order an ionized calcium? *J Am Soc Nephrol*. 2008;19(7):1257–1260. doi:10.1681/ASN.2007121327
45. IOM (Institute of Medicine). *Dietary Reference Intakes for Calcium and Vitamin D*. National Academies Press (US); 2011.
46. Catalano A, Chila D, Bellone F, et al. Incidence of hypocalcemia and hypercalcemia in hospitalized patients: is it changing? *J Clin Transl Endocrinol*. 2018;13:9–13. doi:10.1016/j.jcte.2018.05.004

47. Aishah AB, Foo YN. A retrospective study of serum calcium levels in a hospital population in Malaysia. *Med J Malaysia*. 1995;50(3):246–249.
48. Hastbacka J, Pettila V. Prevalence and predictive value of ionized hypocalcemia among critically ill patients. *Acta Anaesthesiol Scand*. 2003;47(10):1264–1269. doi:10.1046/j.1399-6576.2003.00236.x
49. Ravioli S, Lafranchi A, Exadaktylos AK, Haidinger M, Lindner G. Characteristics and outcome of severe hypercalcemia on admission to the emergency department: a retrospective cohort study. *Swiss Med Wkly*. 2023;153:40069. doi:10.57187/smw.2023.40069
50. Stewart AF. Clinical practice. Hypercalcemia associated with cancer. *N Engl J Med*. 2005;352(4):373–379. doi:10.1056/NEJMcp042806
51. Sadiq NM, Naganathan S, Badireddy M. Hypercalcemia. *StatPearls*. StatPearls Publishing; 2024.
52. Minisola S, Pepe J, Piemonte S, Cipriani C. The diagnosis and management of hypercalcaemia. *BMJ*. 2015;350:h2723. doi:10.1136/bmj.h2723
53. Qadeer HA, Bashir K. Physiology, phosphate. *StatPearls*. StatPearls Publishing; 2024.
54. Larsson L, Rebel K, Sorbo B. Severe hypophosphatemia–a hospital survey. *Acta Med Scand*. 1983;214(3):221–223. doi:10.1111/j.0954-6820.1983.tb08598.x
55. Berger MM, Appelberg O, Reintam-Blaser A, et al. Prevalence of hypophosphatemia in the ICU - Results of an international one-day point prevalence survey. *Clin Nutr*. 2021;40(5):3615–3621. doi:10.1016/j.clnu.2020.12.017
56. Koumakis E, Cormier C, Roux C, Briot K. The causes of hypo- and hyperphosphatemia in humans. *Calcif Tissue Int*. 2021;108(1):41–73. doi:10.1007/s00223-020-00664-9
57. López MTF, Amarelle CG, Mato JAM. Hypophosphatemia in adults with nutritional support, a literature review. *Med Res Arch*. 2019;7(2). doi:10.18103/mra.v7i2.1819
58. Florenzano P, Cipriani C, Roszko KL, et al. Approach to patients with hypophosphataemia. *Lancet Diabetes Endocrinol*. 2020;8(2):163–174. doi:10.1016/S2213-8587(19)30426-7
59. Barreto FC, Barreto DV, Massy ZA, Drueke TB. Strategies for phosphate control in patients with CKD. *Kidney Int Rep*. 2019;4(8):1043–1056. doi:10.1016/j.ekir.2019.06.002
60. Kidney Disease: Improving Global Outcomes CKDMBDUWG. KDIGO 2017 Clinical Practice Guideline Update for the Diagnosis, Evaluation, Prevention, and Treatment of Chronic Kidney Disease-Mineral and Bone Disorder (CKD-MBD). *Kidney Int Suppl (2011)*. 2017;7(1):1–59. doi:10.1016/j.kisu.2017.04.001
61. Klemm KM, Klein MJ, Zhang Y. Biochemical markers of bone metabolism. In: McPherson RA, Pincus MR, eds. *Henry's Clinical Diagnosis and Management by Laboratory Methods*. 24th ed. Elsevier; 2022:208–224.e2.
62. Noronha JL, Matuschak GM. Magnesium in critical illness: metabolism, assessment, and treatment. *Intensive Care Med*. 2002;28(6):667–679. doi:10.1007/s00134-002-1281-y
63. van de Wal-Visscher ER, Kooman JP, van der Sande FM. Magnesium in chronic kidney disease: should we care? *Blood Purif*. 2018;45(1-3):173–178. doi:10.1159/000485212
64. Gragossian A, Bashir K, Bhutta BS, Friede R. Hypomagnesemia. *StatPearls*. StatPearls Publishing; 2024.
65. Cheungpasitporn W, Thongprayoon C, Qian Q. Dysmagnesemia in hospitalized patients: prevalence and prognostic importance. *Mayo Clin Proc*. 2015;90(8):1001–1010. doi:10.1016/j.mayocp.2015.04.023
66. Ryzen E, Wagers PW, Singer FR, Rude RK. Magnesium deficiency in a medical ICU population. *Crit Care Med*. 1985;13(1):19–21. doi:10.1097/00003246-198501000-00006
67. Jahnen-Dechent W, Ketteler M. Magnesium basics. *Clin Kidney J*. 2012;5(Suppl 1):i3–i14. doi:10.1093/ndtplus/sfr163
68. Reddy ST, Yaseen M. Hypomagnesemia. In Ferri F, ed. *Ferri's Clinical Advisor 2024*. Elsevier; 2024:765.e4-765.e7.
69. Whang R, Oei TO, Aikawa JK, et al. Predictors of clinical hypomagnesemia. Hypokalemia, hypophosphatemia, hyponatremia, and hypocalcemia. *Arch Intern Med*. 1984;144(9):1794–1796.
70. Cascella M, Vaqar S. Hypermagnesemia. *StatPearls*. StatPearls Publishing; 2024.
71. da Silva JSV, Seres DS, Sabino K, et al. ASPEN consensus recommendations for refeeding syndrome. *Nutr Clin Pract*. 2020;35(2):178–195. doi:10.1002/ncp.10474
72. Skipper A. Refeeding syndrome or refeeding hypophosphatemia: a systematic review of cases. *Nutr Clin Pract*. 2012;27(1):34–40. doi:10.1177/0884533611427916
73. Persaud-Sharma D, Saha S, Trippensee AW. Refeeding syndrome. *StatPearls*. StatPearls Publishing; 2024.
74. Kraft MD, Btaiche IF, Sacks GS. Review of the refeeding syndrome. *Nutr Clin Pract*. 2005;20(6):625–633. doi:10.1177/0115426505020006625
75. Efsa Panel on Nutrition NF, Food A, Turck D, et al. Dietary reference values for chloride. *EFSA J*. 2019;17(9):e05779. doi:10.2903/j.efsa.2019.5779
76. Sharma S, Hashmi MF, Aggarwal S. Hyperchloremic acidosis. *StatPearls*. StatPearls Publishing; 2024.
77. Berend K, van Hulsteijn LH, Gans RO. Chloride: the queen of electrolytes? *Eur J Intern Med*. 2012;23(3):203–211. doi:10.1016/j.ejim.2011.11.013
78. Signorelli GC, Bianchetti MG, Jermini LMM, et al. Dietary chloride deficiency syndrome: pathophysiology, history, and systematic literature review. *Nutrients*. 2020;12(11). doi:10.3390/nu12113436
79. Kataoka H. Chloride in heart failure syndrome: its pathophysiologic role and therapeutic implication. *Cardiol Ther*. 2021;10(2):407–428. doi:10.1007/s40119-021-00238-2
80. Powers F. The role of chloride in acid-base balance. *J Intraven Nurs*. 1999;22(5):286–291.
81. Harken AH, Gabel RA, Fencl V, Moore FD. Hydrochloric acid in the correction of metabolic alkalosis. *Arch Surg*. 1975;110(7):819–821. doi:10.1001/archsurg.1975.01360130051010
82. Gallo de Moraes A, Surani S. Effects of diabetic ketoacidosis in the respiratory system. *World J Diabetes*. 2019;10(1):16–22. doi:10.4239/wjd.v10.i1.16
83. Kamel KS, Halperin ML. Principles of acid–base physiology. In: Kamel KS, Halperin ML, eds. *Fluid, Electrolyte and Acid-Base Physiology*. 5th ed. Elsevier; 2017:3–32.
84. Boullata JI, Mirtallo JM, Sacks GS, et al. Parenteral nutrition compatibility and stability: a comprehensive review. *JPEN*. 2022;46(2):273–299. doi:10.1002/jpen.2306
85. Velissaris D, Karamouzos V, Ktenopoulos N, Pierrakos C, Karanikolas M. The use of sodium bicarbonate in the treatment of acidosis in sepsis: a literature update on a long term debate. *Crit Care Res Pract*. 2015;2015:605830. doi:10.1155/2015/605830
86. Palmer BF, Clegg DJ. Respiratory acidosis and respiratory alkalosis: core curriculum 2023. *Am J Kidney Dis*. 2023;82(3):347–359. doi:10.1053/j.ajkd.2023.02.004
87. Tucker AM, Johnson TN. Acid-base disorders: a primer for clinicians. *Nutr Clin Pract*. 2022;37(5):980–989. doi:10.1002/ncp.10881

88. American Diabetes Association Professional Practice C. 2. Diagnosis and Classification of Diabetes: Standards of Care in Diabetes-2024. *Diabetes Care*. 2024;47(Suppl 1):S20–S42. doi:10.2337/dc24-S002
89. Rice M, Ismail B, Pillow MT. Approach to metabolic acidosis in the emergency department. *Emerg Med Clin North Am*. 2014;32(2):403–420. doi:10.1016/j.emc.2014.01.002
90. Jaber S, Paugam C, Futier E, et al. Sodium bicarbonate therapy for patients with severe metabolic acidaemia in the intensive care unit (BICAR-ICU): a multicentre, open-label, randomised controlled, phase 3 trial. *Lancet*. 2018;392(10141):31–40. doi:10.1016/S0140-6736(18)31080-8
91. Chan LN, ed. *ASPEN Adult Nutrition Support Core Curriculum*. 4th ed. The American Society for Parenteral and Enteral Nutrition; 2025.
92. Cao S, Cao S. Diabetic ketoalkalosis: a common yet easily overlooked alkalemic variant of diabetic ketoacidosis associated with mixed acid-base disorders. *J Emerg Med*. 2023;64(3):282–288. doi:10.1016/j.jemermed.2022.12.023
93. Mean fasting blood glucose. World Health Organization, Global Health Observatory Indicators. Accessed March 27, 2024. https://www.who.int/data/gho/indicator-metadata-registry/imr-details/2380#
94. Echeverry G, Hortin GL, Rai AJ. Introduction to urinalysis: historical perspectives and clinical application. *Methods Mol Biol*. 2010;641:1–12. doi:10.1007/978-1-60761-711-2_1
95. Diabetes & DKA (ketoacidosis). American Diabetes Association. Accessed March 28, 2024. https://diabetes.org/about-diabetes/complications/ketoacidosis-dka/dka-ketoacidosis-ketones
96. Comstock JP, Garber AJ. Ketonuria. In: Walker HK, Hall WD, Hurst JW, eds. *Clinical Methods: The History, Physical, and Laboratory Examinations*. 3rd ed. Butterworth-Heinemann Ltd; 1990.
97. Lizzo JM, Goyal A, Gupta V. Adult diabetic ketoacidosis. *StatPearls*. StatPearls Publishing; 2024.
98. Rohlfing CL, Wiedmeyer HM, Little RR, England JD, Tennill A, Goldstein DE. Defining the relationship between plasma glucose and HbA(1c): analysis of glucose profiles and HbA(1c) in the Diabetes Control and Complications Trial. *Diabetes Care*. 2002;25(2):275–278. doi:10.2337/diacare.25.2.275
99. Sherwani SI, Khan HA, Ekhzaimy A, Masood A, Sakharkar MK. Significance of HbA1c test in diagnosis and prognosis of diabetic patients. *Biomark Insights*. 2016;11:95–104. doi:10.4137/BMI.S38440
100. Radin MS. Pitfalls in hemoglobin A1c measurement: when results may be misleading. *J Gen Intern Med*. 2014;29(2):388–394. doi:10.1007/s11606-013-2595-x
101. Kidney Disease: Improving Global Outcomes Diabetes Work G. KDIGO 2020 Clinical Practice Guideline for Diabetes Management in Chronic Kidney Disease. *Kidney Int*. 2020;98(4S):S1–S115. doi:10.1016/j.kint.2020.06.019
102. American Diabetes Association Professional Practice C. 15. Management of Diabetes in Pregnancy: Standards of Care in Diabetes-2024. *Diabetes Care*. 2024;47(Suppl 1):S282–S294. doi:10.2337/dc24-S015
103. American Diabetes Association Professional Practice C. 6. Glycemic Goals and Hypoglycemia: Standards of Care in Diabetes-2024. *Diabetes Care*. 2024;47(Suppl 1):S111–S125. doi:10.2337/dc24-S006
104. Mouri M, Badireddy M. Hyperglycemia. *StatPearls*. StatPearls Publishing; 2024.
105. ABIM laboratory test reference ranges. American Board of Internal Medicine (ABIM). Accessed March 30, 2024. https://www.abim.org/Media/bfijryql/laboratory-reference-ranges.pdf
106. Gautron L, Laye S. Neurobiology of inflammation-associated anorexia. *Front Neurosci*. 2009;3:59. doi:10.3389/neuro.23.003.2009
107. McMillan DC, Maguire D, Talwar D. Relationship between nutritional status and the systemic inflammatory response: micronutrients. *Proc Nutr Soc*. 2019;78(1):56–67. doi:10.1017/S0029665118002501
108. Kubota K, Nakayama A, Takehana K, Kawakami A, Yamada N, Suzuki E. A simple stabilization method of reduced albumin in blood and plasma for the reduced/oxidized albumin ratio measurement. *Int J Biomed Sci*. 2009;5(3):293–301.
109. Darwish A, Lui F. Physiology, colloid osmotic pressure. *StatPearls*. StatPearls Publishing; 2024.
110. Vincent JL, Dubois MJ, Navickis RJ, Wilkes MM. Hypoalbuminemia in acute illness: is there a rationale for intervention? A meta-analysis of cohort studies and controlled trials. *Ann Surg*. 2003;237(3):319–334. doi:10.1097/01.SLA.0000055547.93484.87
111. Jellinge ME, Henriksen DP, Hallas P, Brabrand M. Hypoalbuminemia is a strong predictor of 30-day all-cause mortality in acutely admitted medical patients: a prospective, observational, cohort study. *PLoS One*. 2014;9(8):e105983. doi:10.1371/journal.pone.0105983
112. Akirov A, Masri-Iraqi H, Atamna A, Shimon I. Low albumin levels are associated with mortality risk in hospitalized patients. *Am J Med*. 2017;130(12):1465.e11-1465.e19. doi:10.1016/j.amjmed.2017.07.020
113. Evans DC, Corkins MR, Malone A, et al. The use of visceral proteins as nutrition markers: an ASPEN position paper. *Nutr Clin Pract*. 2021;36(1):22–28. doi:10.1002/ncp.10588
114. Gounden V, Vashisht R, Jialal I. Hypoalbuminemia. *StatPearls*. StatPearls Publishing; 2024.
115. Kumar V, Abbas AK, Aster JC, Deyrup AT, Das A. Environmental and nutritional diseases. In: Kumar V, Abbas AK, Aster JC, Deyrup AT, eds. *Robbins & Kumar Basic Pathology*. 11th ed. Elsevier; 2023:235–273.
116. Keller U. Nutritional laboratory markers in malnutrition. *J Clin Med*. 2019;8(6). doi:10.3390/jcm8060775
117. Delliere S, Cynober L. Is transthyretin a good marker of nutritional status? *Clin Nutr*. 2017;36(2):364–370. doi:10.1016/j.clnu.2016.06.004
118. Bates J, McClain CJ. The effect of severe zinc deficiency on serum levels of albumin, transferrin, and prealbumin in man. *Am J Clin Nutr*. 1981;34(9):1655–1660. doi:10.1093/ajcn/34.9.1655
119. Gibson RS. *Principles of Nutritional Assessment*. 2nd ed. Oxford University Press; 2005.
120. Mason J. Nutritional principles and assessment of the gastroenterology patient. In: Feldman M, Friedman LS, Brandt LJ, eds. *Sleisenger and Fordtran's Gastrointestinal and Liver Disease*. 11th ed. Elsevier; 2021:52–73.e3.
121. Wilmore DW. *Metabolic Management of the Critically Ill*. Plenum Publishing; 1977:193.
122. Gropper SAS, Smith JL, Carr TP. *Advanced Nutrition and Human Metabolism*. 7th ed. Cengage Learning; 2018.
123. Kreider RB, Stout JR. Creatine in health and disease. *Nutrients*. 2021;13(2):447. doi:10.3390/nu13020447

124. Baxmann AC, Ahmed MS, Marques NC, et al. Influence of muscle mass and physical activity on serum and urinary creatinine and serum cystatin C. *Clin J Am Soc Nephrol*. 2008;3(2):348–354. doi:10.2215/CJN.02870707
125. Shahbaz H, Gupta M. Creatinine clearance. *StatPearls*. StatPearls Publishing; 2024.
126. Datta D, Foley R, Wu R, Grady J, Scalise P. Can creatinine height index predict weaning and survival outcomes in patients on prolonged mechanical ventilation after critical illness? *J Intensive Care Med*. 2018;33(2):104–110. doi:10.1177/0885066616648133
127. Heimburger DC. 10 - Nutritional assessment. In: Heimburger DC, Ard JD, eds. *Handbook of Clinical Nutrition (Fourth Edition)*. Mosby; 2006:242–261.
128. Daniels R. *Delmar's Manual of Laboratory and Diagnostic Testing*. Delmar; 2003.
129. Brown RS, Goldfarb-Rumyantzev A, Raines NH. Acute kidney injury. In: Brown RS, ed. *Clinical Handbook of Nephrology*. Elsevier; 2024:73–91.
130. Hosten AO. BUN and creatinine. In: Walker HK, Hall WD, Hurst JW, eds. *Clinical Methods: The History, Physical, and Laboratory Examinations*. 3rd ed. Butterworth-Heinemann Ltd; 1990.
131. Ndrepepa G. Aspartate aminotransferase and cardiovascular disease—A narrative review. *JLPM*. 2020;6. doi:10.21037/jlpm-20-93
132. Pratt DS. Liver chemistry and function tests. In: Feldman M, Friedman LS, Brandt LJ, eds. *Sleisenger and Fordtran's Gastrointestinal and Liver Disease*. 11th ed. Elsevier; 2021:1154-1163.e2.
133. Kwo PY, Cohen SM, Lim JK. ACG Clinical Guideline: Evaluation of Abnormal Liver Chemistries. *Am J Gastroenterol*. 2017;112(1):18–35. doi:10.1038/ajg.2016.517
134. Moriles KE, Azer SA. Alanine amino transferase. *StatPearls*. StatPearls Publishing; 2024.
135. Eslam M, Newsome PN, Sarin SK, et al. A new definition for metabolic dysfunction-associated fatty liver disease: an international expert consensus statement. *J Hepatol*. 2020;73(1):202–209. doi:10.1016/j.jhep.2020.03.039
136. Saito Y, Okumura Y, Nagashima K, et al. Low alanine aminotransferase levels are independently associated with mortality risk in patients with atrial fibrillation. *Sci Rep*. 2022;12(1):12183. doi:10.1038/s41598-022-16435-5
137. Vespasiani-Gentilucci U, De Vincentis A, Ferrucci L, Bandinelli S, Antonelli Incalzi R, Picardi A. Low alanine aminotransferase levels in the elderly population: frailty, disability, sarcopenia, and reduced survival. *J Gerontol A Biol Sci Med Sci*. 2018;73(7):925–930. doi:10.1093/gerona/glx126
138. Riancho JA. Diagnostic approach to patients with low serum alkaline phosphatase. *Calcif Tissue Int*. 2023;112(3):289–296. doi:10.1007/s00223-022-01039-y
139. Naz F, Jyoti S, Rahul, Akhtar N, Siddique YH. Effect of oral contraceptive pills on the blood serum enzymes and DNA damage in lymphocytes among users. *Indian J Clin Biochem*. 2016;31(3):294–301. doi:10.1007/s12291-015-0533-x
140. Farhana A, Lappin SL. Biochemistry, lactate dehydrogenase. *StatPearls*. StatPearls Publishing; 2024.
141. Pincus MR, Carty RP. Clinical enzymology. In: McPherson RA, Pincus MR, eds. *Henry's Clinical Diagnosis and Management by Laboratory Methods*. Elsevier 2022:291–313.e3.
142. Stark M, Kerndt CC, Sharma S. Troponin. *StatPearls*. StatPearls Publishing; 2024.
143. Lee HC, Akhmedov A, Chen CH. Spotlight on very-low-density lipoprotein as a driver of cardiometabolic disorders: implications for disease progression and mechanistic insights. *Front Cardiovasc Med*. 2022;9:993633. doi:10.3389/fcvm.2022.993633
144. Grundy SM, Stone NJ, Bailey AL, et al. 2018 AHA/ACC/AACVPR/AAPA/ABC/ACPM/ADA/AGS/APhA/ASPC/NLA/PCNA Guideline on the Management of Blood Cholesterol: a Report of the American College of Cardiology/American Heart Association Task Force on Clinical Practice Guidelines. *Circulation*. 2019;139(25):e1082–e1143. doi:10.1161/CIR.0000000000000625
145. Friedewald WT, Levy RI, Fredrickson DS. Estimation of the concentration of low-density lipoprotein cholesterol in plasma, without use of the preparative ultracentrifuge. *Clin Chem*. 1972;18(6):499–502.
146. Kirkpatrick CF, Sikand G, Petersen KS, et al. Nutrition interventions for adults with dyslipidemia: a clinical perspective from the National Lipid Association. *J Clin Lipidol*. 2023;17(4):428–451. doi:10.1016/j.jacl.2023.05.099
147. Welty FK. Hypobetalipoproteinemia and abetalipoproteinemia. *Curr Opin Lipidol*. 2014;25(3):161–168. doi:10.1097/MOL.0000000000000072
148. Henriksson P, Eriksson M, Ericsson S, et al. Hypocholesterolaemia and increased elimination of low-density lipoproteins in metastatic cancer of the prostate. *Lancet*. 1989;2(8673):1178–1180. doi:10.1016/s0140-6736(89)91790-x
149. Soran H, Ho JH, Durrington PN. Acquired low cholesterol: diagnosis and relevance to safety of low LDL therapeutic targets. *Curr Opin Lipidol*. 2018;29(4):318–326. doi:10.1097/MOL.0000000000000526
150. National Cholesterol Education Program (NCEP) Expert Panel on Detection E, and Treatment of High Blood Cholesterol in Adults (Adult Treatment Panel III). Third Report of The National Cholesterol Education Program (NCEP) Expert Panel on Detection, Evaluation, And Treatment of High Blood Cholesterol in Adults (Adult Treatment Panel III). *Circulation*. 2002;17(106):3143–3421. doi:10.1161/circ.106.25.3143
151. van Leeuwen HJ, Heezius EC, Dallinga GM, van Strijp JA, Verhoef J, van Kessel KP. Lipoprotein metabolism in patients with severe sepsis. *Crit Care Med*. 2003;31(5):1359–1366. doi:10.1097/01.CCM.0000059724.08290.51
152. Cohen JC, Kiss RS, Pertsemlidis A, Marcel YL, McPherson R, Hobbs HH. Multiple rare alleles contribute to low plasma levels of HDL cholesterol. *Science*. 2004;305(5685):869–872. doi:10.1126/science.1099870
153. Millan J, Pinto X, Munoz A, et al. Lipoprotein ratios: physiological significance and clinical usefulness in cardiovascular prevention. *Vasc Health Risk Manag*. 2009;5:757–765.
154. Bailey A, Mohiuddin SS. Biochemistry, high density lipoprotein. *StatPearls*. StatPearls Publishing; 2024.
155. Nordestgaard BG, Benn M, Schnohr P, Tybjaerg-Hansen A. Nonfasting triglycerides and risk of myocardial infarction, ischemic heart disease, and death in men and women. *JAMA*. 2007;298(3):299–308. doi:10.1001/jama.298.3.299
156. Freiberg JJ, Tybjaerg-Hansen A, Jensen JS, Nordestgaard BG. Nonfasting triglycerides and risk of ischemic stroke in the general population. *JAMA*. 2008;300(18):2142–2152. doi:10.1001/jama.2008.621
157. Tung YC, Hsiao FC, Lin CP, et al. High triglyceride variability increases the risk of first attack of acute pancreatitis. *Am J Gastroenterol*. 2023;118(6):1080–1090. doi:10.14309/ajg.0000000000002198

158. Feingold KR. Pancreatitis secondary to hypertriglyceridemia. In: Feingold KR, Anawalt B, Blackman MR, et al, eds. *Endotext*. MDText.com, Inc.; 2000.
159. Hegele RA, Ginsberg HN, Chapman MJ, et al. The polygenic nature of hypertriglyceridaemia: implications for definition, diagnosis, and management. *Lancet Diabetes Endocrinol*. 2014;2(8):655–666. doi:10.1016/S2213-8587(13)70191-8
160. Collaborators GBDA. Prevalence, years lived with disability, and trends in anaemia burden by severity and cause, 1990-2021: findings from the Global Burden of Disease Study 2021. *Lancet Haematol*. 2023;10(9):e713–e734. doi:10.1016/S2352-3026(23)00160-6
161. Guideline on haemoglobin cutoffs to define anaemia in individuals and populations. World Health Organization. Accessed April 18, 2024. https://www.who.int/publications/i/item/9789240088542
162. Chin-Yee B, Matyashin M, Cheong I, et al. Secondary causes of elevated hemoglobin in patients undergoing molecular testing for suspected polycythemia vera in southwestern Ontario: a chart review. *CMAJ Open*. 2022;10(4):E988–E992. doi:10.9778/cmajo.20210322
163. Maner BS, Moosavi L. Mean corpuscular volume. *StatPearls*. StatPearls Publishing; 2024.
164. Sarma PR. Red cell indices. In: Walker HK, Hall WD, Hurst JW, eds. *Clinical Methods: The History, Physical, and Laboratory Examinations*. 3rd ed. Butterworth-Heinemann Ltd; 1990.
165. Hoffmann J, Urrechaga E. Role of RDW in mathematical formulas aiding the differential diagnosis of microcytic anemia. *Scand J Clin Lab Invest*. 2020;80(6):464–469. doi:10.1080/00365513.2020.1774800
166. Briggs C, Bain BJ. Basic haematological techniques. In: Bain BJ, Bates I, and Laffan MA, eds. *Dacie and Lewis Practical Haematology*. 12th ed. Elsevier; 2017:18–49.
167. Crichton R. Iron deficiency, iron overload and therapy. In: Crichton R, ed. *Iron Metabolism: From Molecular Mechanisms to Clinical Consequences*. John Wiley & Sons; 2016:376–417.
168. Evans S. Iron deficiency anemia. In: Kellerman RD, Heidelbaugh JJ, eds. *Conn's Current Therapy 2024*. Elsevier; 2024:470–472.
169. Georgieff MK, Krebs NF, Cusick SE. The benefits and risks of iron supplementation in pregnancy and childhood. *Annu Rev Nutr*. 2019;39:121–146. doi:10.1146/annurev-nutr-082018-124213
170. Elghetany MT, Banki K. Erythrocytic disorders. In: McPherson RA, Pincus MR, eds. *Henry's Clinical Diagnosis and Management by Laboratory Methods*. 24th ed. Elsevier 2022:588–635.e2.
171. Auerbach M, Adamson JW. How we diagnose and treat iron deficiency anemia. *Am J Hematol*. 2016;91(1):31–38. doi:10.1002/ajh.24201
172. Elsayed ME, Sharif MU, Stack AG. Chapter four - Transferrin saturation: a body iron biomarker. In: Makowski GS, ed. *Advances in Clinical Chemistry*. Elsevier; 2016:71–97.
173. Weiss G, Ganz T, Goodnough LT. Anemia of inflammation. *Blood*. 2019;133(1):40–50. doi:10.1182/blood-2018-06-856500
174. Warner MJ, Kamran MT. Iron deficiency anemia. *StatPearls*. StatPearls Publishing; 2024.
175. Auerbach M, Macdougall I. The available intravenous iron formulations: history, efficacy, and toxicology. *Hemodial Int*. 2017;21 Suppl 1:S83–S92. doi:10.1111/hdi.12560
176. Arastu AH, Elstrott BK, Martens KL, et al. Analysis of adverse events and intravenous iron infusion formulations in adults with and without prior infusion reactions. *JAMA Netw Open*. 2022;5(3):e224488. doi:10.1001/jamanetworkopen.2022.4488
177. Antony A. Megaloblastic anemias. In: Hoffman R, Benz EJ, Silberstein LE, et al., eds. *Hematology: Basic Principles and Practice*. 8th ed. Elsevier; 2023:524–554.
178. Obeid R, Murphy M, Sole-Navais P, Yajnik C. Cobalamin status from pregnancy to early childhood: lessons from global experience. *Adv Nutr*. 2017;8(6):971–979. doi:10.3945/an.117.015628
179. Kavitha K, Saharia GK, Singh AK, Mangaraj M. Association of serum vitamin B(12) with immuno-hematological parameters in treatment-naive HIV positive cases. *J Family Med Prim Care*. 2022;11(7):3784–3789. doi:10.4103/jfmpc.jfmpc_2490_21
180. Andrès E, Serraj K, Zhu J, Vermorken AJM. The pathophysiology of elevated vitamin B12 in clinical practice. *QJM*. 2013;106(6):505–515. doi:10.1093/qjmed/hct051
181. Chan LN, Mike LA. The science and practice of micronutrient supplementations in nutritional anemia: an evidence-based review. *JPEN*. 2014;38(6):656–672. doi:10.1177/0148607114533726
182. Ankar A, Kumar A. Vitamin B12 deficiency. *StatPearls*. StatPearls Publishing; 2024.
183. Khan KM, Jialal I. Folic acid deficiency. *StatPearls*. StatPearls Publishing; 2024.
184. Folic acid recommendations. Centers for Disease Control and Prevention. Accessed April 27, 2024. https://www.cdc.gov/ncbddd/folicacid/recommendations.html
185. Hodge C, Taylor C. Vitamin A deficiency. *StatPearls*. StatPearls Publishing; 2024.
186. Chang SW, Lee HC. Vitamin D and health - The missing vitamin in humans. *Pediatr Neonatol*. 2019;60(3):237–244. doi:10.1016/j.pedneo.2019.04.007
187. Kemnic TR, Coleman M. Vitamin E deficiency. *StatPearls*. StatPearls Publishing; 2024.
188. Albahrani AA, Greaves RF. Fat-soluble vitamins: clinical indications and current challenges for chromatographic measurement. *Clin Biochem Rev*. 2016;37(1):27–47.
189. Berger MM, Shenkin A, Schweinlin A, et al. ESPEN micronutrient guideline. *Clin Nutr*. 2022;41(6):1357–1424. doi:10.1016/j.clnu.2022.02.015
190. David John C, Renata G, Dominic Jon H. Laboratory assessment of vitamin K status. *J Clin Pathol*. 2020;73(2):70. doi:10.1136/jclinpath-2019-205997
191. Hand I, Noble L, Abrams SA. Vitamin K and the newborn infant. *Pediatrics*. 2022;149(3):e2021056036. doi:10.1542/peds.2021-056036
192. Lima LFPd, Leite HP, Taddei JAdAC. Low blood thiamine concentrations in children upon admission to the intensive care unit: risk factors and prognostic significance. *The American Journal of Clinical Nutrition*. 2011;93(1):57–61. doi:10.3945/ajcn.2009.29078
193. IOM (Institute of Medicine). *Dietary Reference Intakes for Vitamin C, Vitamin E, Selenium, and Carotenoids*. National Academies Press (US); 2000.
194. Wahab A, Mushtaq K, Borak SG, Bellam N. Zinc-induced copper deficiency, sideroblastic anemia, and neutropenia: a perplexing facet of zinc excess. *Clin Case Rep*. 2020;8(9):1666–1671. doi:10.1002/ccr3.2987

195. Vanek VW, Borum P, Buchman A, et al. A.S.P.E.N. position paper: recommendations for changes in commercially available parenteral multivitamin and multi-trace element products. *Nutr Clin Pract*. 2012;27(4):440–491. doi:10.1177/0884533612446706
196. Blaszyk H, Wild PJ, Oliveira A, Kelly DG, Burgart LJ. Hepatic copper in patients receiving long-term total parenteral nutrition. *J Clin Gastroenterol*. 2005;39(4):318–320. doi:10.1097/01.mcg.0000155135.35315.05
197. Shenkin A. Selenium in intravenous nutrition. *Gastroenterology*. 2009;137(5 Suppl):S61–69. doi:10.1053/j.gastro.2009.07.071
198. Medicare and Medicaid Programs; Regulatory Provisions to Promote Program Efficiency, Transparency, and Burden Reduction; Part II, FR 27106-27157 (2014). Accessed May 5, 2024. https://www.federalregister.gov/documents/2014/05/12/2014-10687/medicare-and-medicaid-programs-regulatory-provisions-to-promote-program-efficiency-transparency-and
199. Practice tips: Implementation steps – ordering privileges for the RDN. Commission on Dietetic Registration. Accessed May 5, 2024. https://www.cdrnet.org/vault/2459/web/Case%20Studies%20Practice%20Tips%20Credentialing%20Tips/6%20Practice%20Tips-Implementation%20Steps%20Ordering%20Privileges.pdf

CHAPTER 3

Energy Expenditure and Body Composition in Health and Disease

Kathy Prelack

CHAPTER OUTLINE

CORE CONCEPTS

1. Total energy expenditure is composed primarily of basal metabolic rate, energy cost of physical activity, and diet-induced thermogenesis.
2. Basal metabolic rate is primarily determined by body cell mass, the metabolically active component of the body.
3. During illness, resting energy expenditure can be increased due to disease burden and inflammation.
4. Energy and substrate metabolism is altered during periods of stress or starvation impacting body composition.
5. Expansion in extracellular water during illness confounds interpretation of weight, lean body cell mass, and erosion of body cell mass.

LEARNING OBJECTIVES

1. Outline the components of energy expenditure and body composition and their changes during health and metabolic stress.
2. Determine factors both metabolic and clinical that impact total energy expenditure and its components.
3. Distinguish the metabolic differences between stress and starvation and the impact on nutritional status.
4. Describe methods for determining estimates based on energy expenditure—including empirical equation, indirect calorimetry, and experimental models.
5. Identify the effects of the inflammatory response on body composition and its measurement.
6. Identify techniques that may be used to assess body composition in a clinical setting, their advantages, and their limitations.
7. Determine appropriate goals for nutrition support using information related to energy expenditure, protein turnover, and substrate utilization during metabolic stress.

Introduction

The goals of medical nutrition therapy are to support the metabolic demands of a specific disease state, uphold nutritional status, and improve clinical outcomes. Differences in cell energetics arise based on the physiology of any given condition, preexisting nutritional status, degree of inflammation, and nutritional intake. Understanding the impact of pathophysiologic conditions on energy metabolism is necessary for guiding nutrition support. Although indirect calorimetry is considered the gold standard for determining energy needs, predictive equations are most commonly used in a clinical setting. Numerous equations exist, making it important to know which equation to use for any given population or condition. Equally, applying the appropriate stress and/or activity factors can prevent both over- and underfeeding and their consequences. Energy needs should be reassessed and adjusted based on monitoring parameters such as weight, metabolic response, healing, and recovery. Unfortunately, methods of assessing efficacy of nutritional therapy are lacking. Measures of weight can be confounded and do not provide information about lean body and fat mass. Measures of body composition exist ranging from two to multiple compartment models. More complex models include imaging techniques that provide valuable information about muscle quality, fatty infiltration of muscle, and type of adipose tissue. Body composition tools in a hospital setting are limited. Measures of circumference and skinfold thickness are convenient, noninvasive, and inexpensive compared with more sophisticated methods. Although lacking in precision, these, along with bioelectrical impedance and air displacement plethysmography, can be useful in a variety of patient settings. Interpretation of results should always include consideration of hydration, technical error, and assumptions made by any given method.

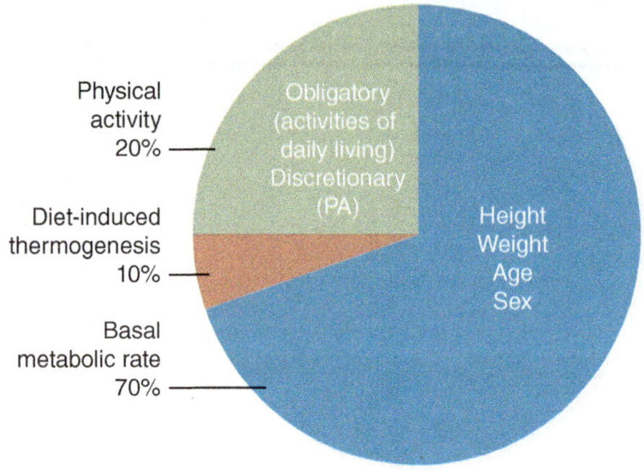

Figure 3.1 Components of Total Energy Expenditure. Total energy expenditure is comprised of basal metabolic rate, diet-induced thermogenesis, and physical activity.

Determinants of Total Energy Expenditure: Basal Metabolic Rate, Diet-Induced Thermogenesis, and Physical Activity

Total daily energy expenditure is comprised of three main components: basal metabolic rate, diet-induced thermogenesis, and activity energy expenditure (Figure 3.1). **Basal metabolic rate (BMR)** refers to energy expenditure associated with maintaining the metabolic activities of the body's cells and tissues.[1] These activities represent functions that are essential for life, such as cell function and replacement; hormone and protein synthesis; maintenance of body core temperature; and work associated with cardiac, respiratory, muscle, and brain function. BMR represents a postabsorptive state (for at least 12–14 hours) with the subjects measured awake, before rising, in a thermoneutral environment. Measures of BMR should be at least 8 hours after physical activity and in the absence of mental or psychological stress. Once BMR is obtained, it can be expressed in kilocalories (kcal) per 24 hours, then becoming basal energy expenditure (BEE). Achieving optimal conditions for true measure of BEE is difficult; therefore, **resting energy expenditure (REE)** is most commonly described and used in many energy expenditure equations. REE is approximately 10% greater than BMR, and typically represents 60%–70% of **total energy expenditure (TEE)**.[1]

The major determinants of REE are age, sex, weight, and height. These indicators essentially serve as proxies for differences in body composition, primarily with respect to **body cell mass (BCM)**. The BCM is that component within the **lean body mass (LBM)** compartment that encompasses all metabolically active organs and tissues. Among them, the brain and skeletal muscle have high metabolic rates per mass, each contributing to 25% of REE. Next, digestive, cardiac, respiratory, and urinary organ systems have high rates of metabolic activity, collectively contributing to the remaining proportion of REE. Adipose tissue is the least metabolically active by mass, contributing less than 5 kcal/kg of weight.[2]

CASE STUDY INTRODUCTION

Josephine is a 65-year-old female admitted to the hospital with major trauma after falling down the stairs. She has returned from major surgery for repair of her injuries, which include multiple rib and long bone fractures. She will be at complete bed rest for the next 7 days to allow for healing. She is ordered for a full liquid diet due to her fractured jaw. Her anthropometric data are as follows.

Anthropometric Data:

Admission height: 160 cm
Admission weight: 69 kg
Body mass index (BMI): 27 kg/m^2

Biochemical Data:

Sodium 138 (136–145 mEq/L)
Potassium 4.5 (3.5–5.0 mEq/L)
Chloride 100 (96–106 mEq/L)
Carbon dioxide 27 (22–31 mEq/L)
Blood urea nitrogen 12 (8–20 mg/dL)
Creatinine 1.1 (0.7–1.3 mg/dL)
Glucose 180 (70–139 mg/dL)
Calcium 9.2 (8.5–10.5 mg/dL)
Phosphorus 4.2 (2.5–4.5 mg/dL)
Magnesium 2.1 (1.3–2.1 mg/dL)
Albumin 3.5 (3.5–5.5 g/dL)

Clinical Data:

Past Medical History: HTN
Prior Medications: ACE inhibitor (angiotensin-converting enzyme)
Vital Signs: Blood pressure 177/52 mm Hg, Temperature 99.6°F
Nutrition-Focused Physical Exam: Appears well nourished. Limited exam due to patient experiencing pain. No evidence of muscle or fat wasting. Good handgrip strength. Nasogastric tube in place.

Dietary Data:

Diet History: Good appetite, follows low-sodium heart-healthy diet at home.

Usual Diet Recall:

Breakfast: 8 oz coffee (milk and sugar), two slices of toast with butter, one scrambled egg
Lunch: Sandwich (turkey or tuna on whole wheat), mustard, lettuce, tomato, diet soda
Afternoon: Tea with milk, two cookies
Dinner: 5–6 oz chicken or fish, one cup rice or pasta, broccoli, carrots or kale
Diet Prescription: Full liquid diet × 4 weeks

Questions

1. What are Josephine's nutritional risk factors?
2. Describe how Josephine's injury will impact her energy expenditure? What stress and activity factors do you use?
3. Write two Problem/Etiology/Signs and Symptoms (PES) statements for Josephine identifying Josephine's active issues.
4. Calculate Josephine's total energy requirement using the MSJ equation for REE. Apply the appropriate stress and activity factors.
5. Identify the interventions you would like to initiate for Josephine to address the problems identified in your PES statements.
6. What indices should be included in your monitoring and evaluation plan to be sure your intervention is working?

CORE CONCEPT 1

Total energy expenditure is composed primarily of basal metabolic rate, energy cost of physical activity, and diet-induced thermogenesis.

Energy expenditure and body composition are inextricably linked. Differences in REE across the lifespan or by sex are often explained by differences in LBM. **Table 3.1** defines energy expenditure terms and components of body composition. **Fat-free mass (FFM)**

Table 3.1 Definition of Terms Related to Total Energy Expenditure and Its Determinants

Term	Definition
Basal Metabolic Rate (BMR)	Energy expenditure associated with maintaining the metabolic activities of the body's cells and tissues. It is the amount of energy needed to maintain structure and function of cells that is essential for life. It includes maintenance of body core temperature, protein synthesis, and the energy cost of cardiac, respiratory, muscle, and brain function.
Basal Energy Expenditure (BEE)	Basal metabolic rate expressed as energy expenditure over a 24-hour period. It is measured after awakening from sleep, in a thermoneutral environment, 12–14 hours after fasting, 8 hours after physical activity. It represents energy expenditure at complete mental, physical, and digestive rest.
Resting Energy Expenditure (REE)	Energy derived from oxygen uptake when the body is awake, rested, at least 4–6 hours after eating or engaging in physical activity. It includes basal metabolic rate. REE is 10% greater than BEE and makes up approximately 60–70% of total energy expenditure.
Activity Energy Expenditure (AEE)	Energy expenditure with physical activity that includes energy cost of both obligatory physical activity such as those associated with daily living as well as exercise-related energy expenditure which depends on the degree and type of activity. Activity energy expenditure is highly variable in an ambulatory setting. It contributes less to energy expenditure in hospitalized patients.
Diet-Induced Thermogenesis (DIT)	Also known as the thermic effect of food, this represents the increase in metabolic rate associated with digestion, absorption, storage, and processing of nutrients. It represents approximately 10% of total energy expenditure.
Total Energy Expenditure (TEE)	This is a 24-hour energy expenditure that includes the sum of REE, TEF, and AEE.
Metabolic Stress	The increase above REE that is associated with the energy cost of injury, disease, or condition. It is often incorporated using stress factors based on the magnitude of the insult.
Body Cell Mass (BCM)	Includes all cellular components of the body involved in biochemical processes and energy metabolism. It includes the nonfat portion of tissues including organs, skeletal muscle, viscera, blood, and brain. It does not include bone.
Lean Body Mass (LBM)	That portion of the body that includes BCM as well as extracellular mass, which includes bone and extracellular fluid. LBM is 73% water. It includes intracellular water within the BCM and extracellular water that makes up plasma and interstitial fluid.
Fat Mass (FM)	That portion of the body that includes adipose tissue, circulating lipids, and components of cell membranes.
Fat-Free Mass (FFM)	That compartment that includes muscles, bones, organs, ligaments, tendons, and water. It is that component after all fat has been extracted from the body. It does not include the fat that is found in cell membranes.

refers to that portion of the body after all the fat has been extracted. It differs from LBM in that it does not include fat in cell membranes. In this chapter, we will use the terms according to how they have been reported in the original research. For clinical purposes, they can be considered interchangeable.

Age and Sex

Age-related differences can be appreciated throughout the life cycle and are largely related to changes in body size and BCM. A larger BMR per unit of body weight in neonates through infancy is attributable to a relatively larger brain, skin, and viscera than in older children and adults.[3] Although skeletal mass is less during the infancy stages, rapid growth and tissue deposition contribute to energy expenditures 150% of that of adults when adjusting for body size and FFM. Throughout childhood, total and basal energy expenditures steadily increase in proportion to gains in FFM, plateauing at age 20 where energy expenditure remains stable through most of adulthood. Birth sex does not impact total and resting energy expenditures in adults once adjusting for FFM. In other words, differences in REE between males and females are largely due to differences in FFM, where males tend to have a higher FFM than females after puberty. Accordingly, when adjusting for FFM, sex is not a factor in determining REE. After age 60, there is a decline in energy expenditure associated with a decline in FFM as well as a decrease in organ metabolism. After age 90, energy expenditure per unit of FFM is significantly lower than middle-aged adults.[4]

Race and Ethnicity

Few studies have been done related to energy expenditure across race and ethnicity. A number of studies have indicated that Black individuals tend to have a lower REE per FFM as compared to White individuals. Differences in REE seem to be related to the metabolic activity of regional body composition differences. Studies of energy expenditure in racial and ethnic groups beyond Black and White individuals are limited.[5]

CORE CONCEPT 2

Basal metabolic rate is primarily determined by body cell mass, the metabolically active component of the body.

Certain conditions may lead to increased REE unrelated to an individual's FFM or LBM. During pregnancy, REE increases in proportion to fetal weight gain (although this may reflect an actual increase in LBM contributed by the fetus). Milk production during lactation also increases REE independently of LBM. Thermoregulation contributes to energy expenditure. Usually, this contribution is minor because humans can adjust clothing and environment to maintain ambient temperature. However, in certain endocrine disorders such as hypo- and hyperthyroid and central nervous system disorders such as brain injury or neurological diseases, the impact of thermoregulation on REE is more prominent. In the case of burn injury, where extensive water losses result in evaporative cooling and a drop in body core temperature, energy associated with thermoregulation is a significant contributor to increased REE.[4]

Diet-Induced Thermogenesis

Diet-induced thermogenesis (DIT), also referred to as the **thermic effect of food (TEF)**, is the production of heat associated with the digestion and metabolism of food. This includes energy required for absorption, transport, cellular oxidation, and nutrient deposition. Although it is the smallest component of the three main contributing factors to TEE, DIT can be significant in the development of obesity. DIT is most often determined by measuring REE before and after a meal using indirect calorimetry. DIT can also be measured in a respiratory chamber, allowing for timing and duration of postprandial response. DIT increases TEE by 8%–10% of BMR over a 24-hour period in a healthy individual eating a normal mixed diet. Diet composition differentially affects DIT, with protein and alcohol resulting in the largest increase in DIT and carbohydrate and fat contributing the least to DIT. Other factors that can alter DIT include weight gain (increase) or weight loss (decrease), intermittent versus continuous feeding (with DIT significantly reduced with continuous feeds), and ambient temperature.[1]

Activity Energy Expenditure

Activity energy expenditure (AEE) is the energy expenditure associated with physical activity. In healthy individuals, this can be the second largest (after BMR), albeit most variable, component of TEE. AEE includes both obligatory physical activity and discretionary physical activity. Obligatory physical activity includes daily activities such as going to work or school, tending to children, household activities, and other demands an individual faces from their environment. Discretionary activities are not imposed on the individual but rather are chosen for recreational or physical fitness. This component of AEE can vary dramatically based on the type, frequency, and intensity of activity.[3]

Estimating Energy Requirements in Health and Disease

Energy Requirements Under Normal Conditions

Other than in research settings, TEE is typically estimated using standardized equations or formulas. Here, a value for REE can be obtained according to standard evidence-based references that incorporate weight, height, age, and sex. **Table 3.2** presents common equations for REE throughout the lifespan.[6–10] Using a factorial approach, the energy costs of various activities are summed to account for physical activity or AEE. In 2004, the Institute of Medicine developed physical activity levels (PALs) according to the general classification of sedentary, low active, active, and very active. Numbers assigned to each PAL could then be multiplied by REE to get TEE.[11] However, this factorial approach for determining TEE was flawed primarily due to the many assumptions about the energy cost associated

Table 3.2 Estimation of Daily Basal or Resting Energy Expenditure by Age and Gender in Healthy Individuals

Reference	Age (years)	Equation
Schofield[6]	0–3	M: 59.5 (W) – 30.4 F: 58.3 (W) – 31.1
	3–10	M: 22.7 (W) + 504.3 F: 20.3 (W) + 485.9
	10–18	M: 17.7 (W) + 658.2 F: 13.4 (W) + 692.6
	18–30	M: 15.1 (W) + 692.2 F: 14.8 (W) + 486.6
	30–60	M: 11.472 (W) + 873.1 F: 8.126 (W) + 845.6
	>60	M: 11.7 (W) + 587.7 F: 9.1 (W) + 658.5
Mifflin-St Jeor[7]	>18	M: 10(W) + 6.25 (H) – 5(A) + 5 W: 10(W) + 6.25 (H) – 5(A) – 161
Harris-Benedict[8]	>18	M: 66 + (13.7 W) + (5 H) – (6.8 A) F: 655 + (9.7 W) + (1.85H) – (4.7A)
Owen[9]	>18	M: 10.2 (W) + 879 F: 7.18 (W) + 795
WHO[10]	18–30 y	M: 15.057 (W) + 692.2 F: 14.818 (W) + 486.6

Note: M= Male; F= Female; W = weight in kg; H = height in cm; A = age in years

Data from Schofield WN. Predicting basal metabolic rate: new standards and review of previous work. *Hum Nutr Clin Nutr.* 1985;39C(1 suppl):5-42.; Mifflin MD, St Jeor ST, Hill LA, Scott BJ, Daugherty SA, Koh YO. A new predictive equation for resting energy expenditure in healthy individuals. *Am J Clin Nutr.* 1990;51(2):241-247.; Harris JA, Benedict FG. *A Biometric Study of Basal Metabolism in Man.* Washington, DC: Carnegie Institution of Washington; 1919.; Owen OE, Holup JL, D'Alessio DA, et al. *A reappraisal of the caloric requirements of men. Am J Clin Nutr.* 1987;46(6):875-885.; Alam DS, Hulshof PJM, Roordink D, et al. Validity and reproducibility of resting metabolic rate measurements in rural Bangladeshi women: comparison of measurements obtained by Medgem and by Deltatrac device. *Eur J Clin Nutr.* 2005;59(5):651-657. doi:10.1038/sj.ejcn.160212

with various activities, particularly across the lifespan. A growing database of measured TEE using the doubly water method (DLW) has led to more representative estimates of TEE and AEE, currently reported in the Dietary Reference Intakes (DRI) for energy.[12] Because TEE is made up of REE, DIT, and AEE, then:

$$\text{TEE} - (\text{REE} + \text{DIT}) = \text{AEE}$$

where REE is measured using indirect calorimetry and DIT is assumed to be 10% of TEE.

Table 3.3 shows the different physical activity levels (PALs) according to age group derived by the DLW method. Calculation of TEE in adults can be easily performed using an equation to predict REE multiplied by the PAL. For example, TEE for a female who is 52 years old, weighs 65 kg, and is relatively inactive can be calculated as follows. REE is derived using the Schofield equation for a female 30–60 years of age (F: 8.126 (W) + 845.6) and then a PAL of 1.25 (mid-range of inactive) is applied:

$$\text{TEE} = 1374\ (\text{REE}) \times 1.25\ (\text{PAL})$$
$$= 1718\ \text{kcal/day}$$

In addition, the DRI provides age and sex specific equations for determining TEE based on the DLW data (**Table 3.4**). Using the age and sex specific equation for the same female weighing 65 kg, with a height 150 cm who is inactive, we find:

$$\text{TEE} = 584.90 - (7.01 \times \text{age}) + (5.72 \times \text{height}) + (11.71 \times \text{weight}) \text{ or } 1840\ \text{kcal/day}$$

Note that a measure of height is needed.

In children, calculating energy requirements using this method does not incorporate energy cost associated with deposition of tissue and bone during growth. Therefore, the DRIs provide estimated energy requirements (EERs), which in children is the sum of TEE and energy deposition. An additional physical activity factor can be added for children 3 years and older (**Table 3.5**).[12]

Table 3.3 Physical Activity Level (Pal) by Age Group

Age Group	PAL Category	PAL Range Definition
3–8.99 years	Inactive	1.0 ≤ PAL <1.31
	Low active	1.31 ≤ PAL < 1.44
	Active	1.44 ≤ PAL < 1.59
	Very active	1.59 ≤ PAL < 2.50
9–13.99 years	Inactive	1.0 ≤ PAL <1.44
	Low active	1.44 ≤ PAL < 1.59
	Active	1.59 ≤ PAL < 1.77
	Very active	1.77 ≤ PAL < 2.50
14–18.99 years	Inactive	1.0 ≤ PAL <1.56
	Low active	1.56 ≤ PAL < 1.73
	Active	1.73 ≤ PAL < 1.92
	Very active	1.92 ≤ PAL < 2.50
>19 years	Inactive	1.0 ≤ PAL <1.53
	Low active	1.53 ≤ PAL < 1.68
	Active	1.68 ≤ PAL < 1.85
	Very active	1.85 ≤ PAL < 2.50

Data from National Academies of Sciences, Engineering, and Medicine. *Dietary Reference Intakes for Energy*. Washington, DC: The National Academies Press; 2023. doi:10.17226/26818

Table 3.4 Equations for Estimating Total Energy Expenditure

Males, 0–2 years	TEE = –716.45 – (1.00 × age) + (17.82 × height) + (15.06 × weight)
Females, 0–2 years	TEE = –69.15 + (80.0 × age) + (2.65 × height) + (54.15 × weight)
Males, 3–18 years	
Inactive	TEE = – 447.51 + (3.68 × age) + (13.01 × height) + (13.15 × weight)
Low active	TEE = 19.12 + (3.68 × age) + (8.62 × height) + (20.28 × weight)
Active	TEE = – 388.19 + (3.68 × age) + (12.66 × height) + (20.46 × weight)
Very active	TEE = – 671.75 + (3.68 × age) + (15.38 × height) + (23.25 × weight)
Females, 3–18 years	
Inactive	TEE = 55.59 – (22.25 × age) + (8.43 × height) + (17.07 × weight)
Low active	TEE = – 297.54 – (22.25 × age) + (12.77 × height) + (14.73 × weight)
Active	TEE = – 189.55 – (22.25 × age) + (11.74 × height) + (18.34 × weight)
Very active	TEE = – 709.59 – (22.25 × age) + (18.22 × height) + (14.25 × weight)
Males, > 19 years	
Inactive	TEE = 753.07 – (10.83 × age) + (6.50 × height) + (14.10 × weight)
Low active	TEE = 581.47 – (10.83 × age) + (8.30 × height) + (14.94 × weight)
Active	TEE = 1004.82 – (10.83 × age) + (6.52 × height) + (15.91 × weight)
Very active	TEE = – 517.88 – (10.83 × age) + (15.61 × height) + (19.11 × weight)
Females, > 19 years	
Inactive	TEE = 584.90 – (7.01 × age) + (5.72 × height) + (11.71 × weight)
Low active	TEE = 575.77 – (7.01 × age) + (6.60 × height) + (12.14 × weight)
Active	TEE = 710.25 – (7.01 × age) + (6.54 × height) + (12.34 × weight)
Very active	TEE = 511.83 – (7.01 × age) + (9.07 × height) + (12.56 × weight)

Note: W = weight in kg; H = height in cm; A = age in years

Modified from National Academies of Sciences, Engineering, and Medicine. *Dietary Reference Intakes for Energy*. Washington, DC: National Academies Press; 2023. doi:10.17226/26818

Table 3.5 Estimated Total Energy Requirements in Children

Age	EER = TEE + Energy Deposition
0–3 months	(89W – 100) + 175
4–6 months	(89W – 100) + 56
7–12 months	(89W – 100) + 22
13–35 months	(89W – 100) + 20
3–8 years	M: 88.5 – (61.9 × A) + PA × [(26.7 × W) + (903 × H)] + 20 F: 135.3 – (30.8 × A) + PA × [(10 × W) + (934 × H)] + 20
9–18 years	M: 88.5 – (61.9 × A) + PA × [(26.7 × W) + (903 × H)] + 25 F: 135.3 – (30.8 × A) + PA × [(10 × W) + (934 × H)] + 25

Note: M = Male; F = Female; W = weight in kg; H = height in m; A = age in years; PA = physical activity
Data from National Academies of Sciences, Engineering, and Medicine. *Dietary Reference Intakes for Energy*. Washington, DC: National Academies Press; 2023. doi:10.17226/26818

Factorial Approach in Determining Energy Requirements During Disease and Illness

Use of DRI for estimates of TEE is not recommended during acute illness or various conditions and disease states. Energy expenditure under these conditions does not parallel values obtained in healthy individuals. DRIs do not incorporate energy cost associated with disease- or condition-related pathophysiology. Furthermore, DRIs incorporate increased needs for tissue building such as during growth and pregnancy and variations in activity level. These do not consistently apply in hospitalized, acutely ill patients, who often have lost mobility. Estimates of REE poorly correlate with measured REE in hospitalized, acutely ill patients, a finding that has been consistent in the scientific literature. Prediction accuracy of most formulas rarely falls within 10% of measured REE.[13–16] This can be explained by the fact that in many disease states, particularly those associated with an inflammatory response, an additional component of TEE emerges representing increased energy requirement associated with metabolic stress. Actual measures of REE "capture" this additional component of stress, whereas when using the factorial approach, this component must be estimated and added on as a stress factor. **Figure 3.2** illustrates the factors contributing to each component of TEE in a metabolically stressed, hospitalized individual.

As it is apparent, while the stress component increases, AEE and DIT decrease. The decrease in AEE is primarily due to limited physical activity other than that associated with physical therapy and positioning.[17] Decline in DIT is most often attributed to a lower energy cost of nutrient storage and retrieval when administering nutrition continuously.[18] Although DIT is a component of TEE, due to its variability, it is often not incorporated into routine estimates of daily energy expenditure.

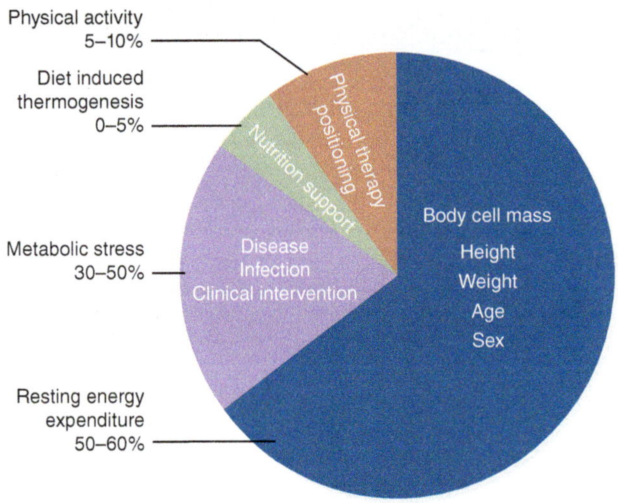

Figure 3.2 Components of Total Energy Expenditure During Metabolic Stress. While the stress component increases, AEE and DIT decrease. The decrease in AEE is primarily due to limited physical activity other than that associated with physical therapy and positioning. Decline in DIT is most often attributed to a lower energy cost of nutrient storage and retrieval when administering nutrition continuously.

Numerous predictive equations exist for energy assessment during critical illness (**Table 3.6**).[7,8,19–24] These equations vary based on the number of subjects used to develop them, as well as the subject's medical

Table 3.6 Predictive Equations Used During Critical Illness and Metabolic Stress

Source	Population	TEE Component Measured	Equation
Harris–Benedict[25]	N = 239 healthy subjects	BEE	M: 66 + (13.7W) + (5H) − (6.8A) F: 655 + (9.7W) + (1.85H) − (4.7A)
Revised Harris–Benedict[26]	N = 239 healthy subjects from original study plus additional 98 healthy subjects	BEE	M:88 + (13.4W) + (5H) − (5.7A) F:448 + (9.2W) + (3H) − (4.3A)
Mifflin–St Jeor[27]	N = 498 healthy subjects	REE	M: 10(W) + 6.25 (H)-5(A) + 5 W: 10(W) + 6.25 (H)-5(A) − 161
Penn State 2003b[20]	N = 74 mechanically ventilated trauma/medical/surgical patients	REE, metabolic stress	Mifflin Equation (0.96) + Tmax (167) + Ve (31) − 6212
Penn State 2010[20]	N = 50 mechanically ventilated trauma/medical/surgical patients	REE, metabolic stress	Mifflin Equation (0.71) + Ve (64)+ Tmax (85) − 3085
Swinamer[28]	N = 112 mechanically ventilated, critically ill trauma/medical/surgical patients	REE, metabolic stress	945 (BSA) − 6.4(A) + 108(T) + 24.2(RR) + 817 (Vt) − 4349
American College of Chest Physicians[29]	29 mechanically ventilated patients aged 16–79 years	TEE	25 W If BMI 16–25 use UBW If BMI >25 use IBW If BMI <16 use existing weight for 7–10 days, then use IBW

Note: M = Male; F = Female: W = weight in kg; H = height in cm; A = age in years; Tmax = maximum body temperature in the previous 24 hours (degrees Centigrade); T = temperature. Ve = minute ventilation recorded from ventilator in liters per minute; Vt = tidal volume (mL); BSA = body surface area

or clinical condition. The larger the study population, the greater likelihood of predictive accuracy of the equation. Similarly, it is useful to choose equations developed in the population type representative of the patient of interest. For example, equations such as the Penn State equation are best to use in patients who are critically ill and mechanically ventilated.

When relying on standardized equations, prediction of REE, which is highly variable, is required, as well as factors associated with metabolic stress of disease and AEE. Heterogeneity among hospitalized patients with respect to disease burden, clinical interventions, and degree of inflammation exists, often making predictions of energy needs using the factorial approach for the individual patient challenging. Differences in body composition can impact REE, resulting in the inclusion of BMI categories for estimating needs. In patients who are overweight or obese, certain predictive equations such as the Mifflin–St Jeor (MSJ) and Penn State equations are known to correlate with measured REE across BMI categories. However, the prediction error can be high, risking both over- and underfeeding.[14,15] Some of these equations regard clinical status by incorporating factors that would impact REE, such as temperature or ventilatory variables.[20,21,24] However, during critical illness, clinical status is inconstant from day to day and patient to patient, and general stress factors may not capture these differences. Commonly used stress factors and clinical conditions that can have changeable effects on energy expenditure are presented in **Tables 3.7** and **3.8**. Clinical interventions targeting infection control, pain management, and anxiety reduce energy expenditure, while sepsis, fever, and respiratory effort increase energy expenditure.

CASE STUDY REVISITED

After 2 weeks of intensive care, another weight is obtained. Despite meeting 100% of her calorie goal on the blenderized diet, Josephine has lost 3 kg. The team consults you for a reassessment of energy requirements using indirect calorimetry. Her activity level has increased to allow physical therapy 30 minutes/day.

Your findings are below.

Anthropometric Data:

Current weight: 65 kg
Last Weight: 68 kg (dry)

Admission weight: 69 kg

Estimated Goals Upon Initial Assessment:

Energy goal = 1204 kcal (REE predicted by MSJ; using 68 kg) × 1.5 (stress factor) = 1791 kcal
No activity factor—bedrest

Protein goal (based on 1.5 g/kg) = 102 g/day
Energy intake (5 days mean): 1780 kcal/100 g protein

Indirect Calorimetry Results:

Patient was measured while fasting, rested, lying in bed. Following achievement of a steady state, a 40-minute measurement was performed. Conditions for measurement are considered to be ideal; the results are presumed to be accurate.
Measured REE (MREE): 2400 kcal
Respiratory quotient (RQ): 0.79

Questions

1. What are the reasons for the difference between Josephine's measured versus predicted REE by MSJ?
2. Calculate Josephine's MREE/MSJREE. What is the percent increase in metabolic rate above predicted?
3. What stress factor if any will you use to adjust your indirect calorimetry measurement? Would you add an activity factor?
4. What is your new estimation for Josephine's total energy requirement?

PRACTICE POINT

Energy goals should be routinely reassessed to accommodate changes in the patient's clinical condition that may alter energy expenditure.

Measuring Energy Expenditure—Direct and Indirect Calorimetry

Use of calorimetry to determine energy expenditure is based on the construct that human metabolism involves the combustion of nutrients, a process that requires oxygen and produces carbon dioxide (which is eventually eliminated) and heat (which is used for cellular processes). Calorimetry relies on the first principle of thermodynamics, which states that energy cannot be created or destroyed, only transferred. Several methods can be employed for determining TEE via calorimetry. One method, **direct calorimetry**, involves direct measurement of heat produced or lost from this combustion reaction. Considered the gold standard, direct calorimetry assumes that metabolic rate is the sum of heat production and work or physical activity. In controlled circumstances, where the subject is not performing work of physical activity, the heat loss is considered to represent the subject's metabolic rate. Direct calorimetry requires the subject to be contained in a thermally controlled chamber for direct measure of heat produced. This is impractical in a clinical setting, making this tool more likely to exist in a research environment.[30]

Indirect calorimetry (IC) is the measure of respiratory gas exchange. In this process, volume of oxygen (VO_2) consumed and volume of carbon dioxide (VCO_2) produced are determined. These variables can be used to calculate both respiratory quotient

Table 3.7 Stress and Activity Factors for Use with Predictive Equations in Hospitalized Patients

Activity	Factor
Bed Rest	1–1.2 [hospitalized]
Ambulatory	1.3
Fever	12% increase in REE for every degree >37°C
Disease State or Condition	
Mild Surgery	1.1–1.3
Mild Stress	1.1–1.3
Moderate Stress	1.3–1.5
Infection	1.3
Long Bone Fracture	1.3
Major Surgery	1.5
Major Trauma	1.5–1.7
Sepsis	1.2–1.4
Burn Injury	1.5–2
Traumatic Brain Injury	1.3–1.5
Cardiac Failure	1.0–1.3

Additional increase for fever may not be needed and can be accounted for by the stress factors. Sepsis represents a condition that increases energy expenditure above current state. It should be included along with other stress factors. Not to exceed 40% increase to avoid overfeeding.

Table 3.8 Clinical Factors That Contribute to Stress Factor in Estimating Energy Expenditure

Decrease	Increase
Heated environment	Sepsis
Infection control	Fever
Pain control	Increased work of breathing
Sedation	Psychological stress/anxiety
Medications: Adrenergic blockade, muscle relaxants, opiates, barbiturates, antipyretics	Medications: Epinephrine

and energy expenditure using calorimetric equations. **Doubly labeled water (DLW)** is a form of IC. It assumes an exponential disappearance of hydrogen and oxygen isotopes from the body. Because oxygen atoms in exhaled carbon dioxide and body water are in isotopic equilibrium, the kinetics of water elimination and respiration are interdependent. Experimentally, a dose of water containing the combined stable isotopes deuterium oxide and oxygen 18 (hence, doubly labeled water or D_2O^{18}) is consumed. Following equilibrium, DLW is eliminated from the body in the urine and breath. The H_2O^{18} is eliminated as both CO_2 and H_2O, while the D_2O is eliminated only as H_2O. Thus, the difference between these elimination rates is a measure of CO_2 flux, which can be related to energy expenditure using standard calorimetric equations (**Figure 3.3**).[31]

DLW is well validated for reproducibility and its ability to determine longitudinal changes in energy expenditure, intake, and body composition.[32] It serves as the gold standard by which other methods of determining TEE are compared. DLW provides an estimation of TEE over a period of 1–3 weeks, ideal for the study of energy metabolism in free-living individuals. The DLW method does rely on certain assumptions, including a constant rate of CO_2 production and a constant total body water pool. These assumptions can be confounded in patients with respiratory failure or significant evaporative water losses, as might be the case in patients with large wounds or burn injury. Combined with its expense and turnover time for results, it is not ideal in a clinical setting.

The more common form of IC in a hospital setting is the use of a portable "metabolic cart." In this form of IC, measures of VO_2 and VCO_2 in mL/min are obtained through breath analysis. These values are used to calculate REE using the Weir equation[33]:

Abbreviated Weir Equation:

$$\text{REE (kcal/day)} = 1.44\,([3.9 \times VO_2] + [1.1 \times VCO_2])$$

IC can be performed at the bedside in both mechanically ventilated and spontaneously breathing patients. Patients breathing on their own can be measured using an attached canopy hood (**Figure 3.4**). Patients who are on a mechanical ventilator can be measured by attaching the metabolic cart to the expiratory port of a mechanical ventilator. Mechanically ventilated patients with a partial fraction of oxygen (FiO_2) greater than 60% should not be measured. Strategies for successful IC measurement are mentioned in **Table 3.9**. Breath-to-breath measures are captured and provided in minute-by-minute intervals. Ideally, measurements should be taken for a minimum of 30 minutes once a steady state has been achieved (as defined by less than a 10% minute-to-minute variability). Steady-state measures, while important, are

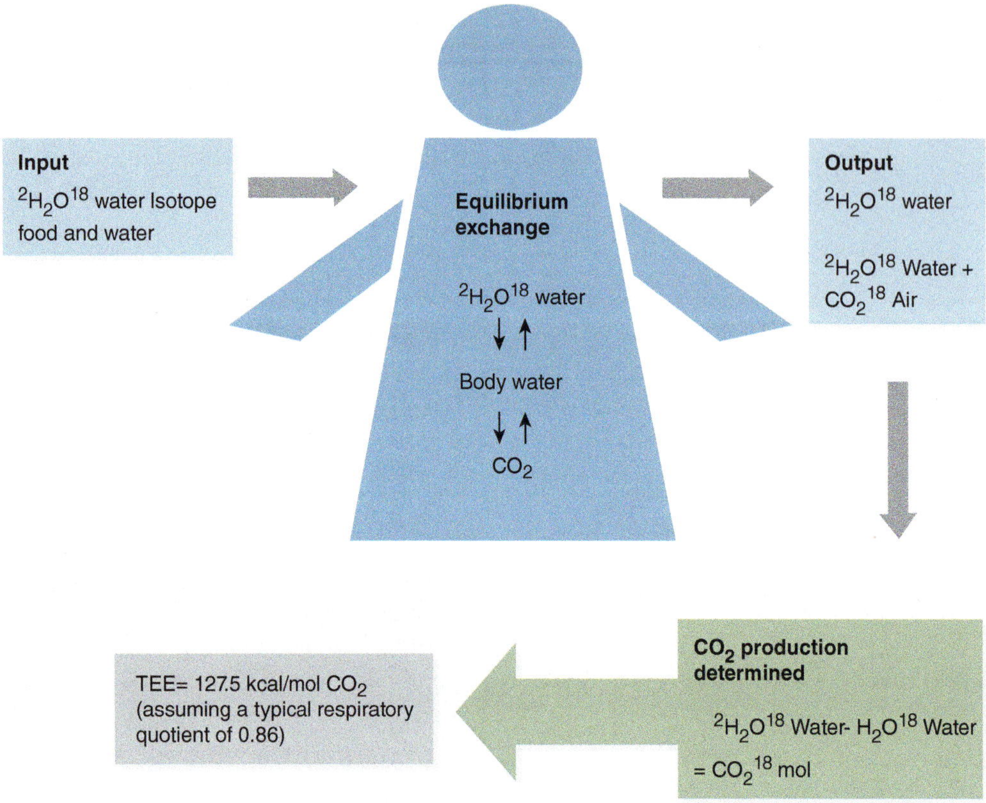

Figure 3.3 Doubly Labeled Water Method. The doubly labeled water method measures the elimination of CO_2 (in both air and water) and H_2O (water only) to determine, through subtraction, CO_2 production. CO_2 production is then used to calculate TEE.

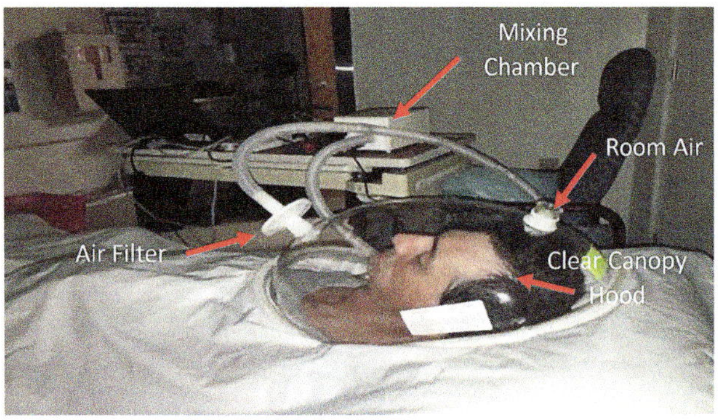

Figure 3.4 Indirect Calorimetry in Spontaneously Breathing Patient Using a Canopy Hood. Indirect calorimetry can be done at the bedside using a canopy hood. In this system, room air enters the hood. Expired air from the patient will travel through an air filter into a mixing chamber where the volume of oxygen and carbon dioxide is measured.

Reproduced from Alazzam AM, Alrubaye MW, Goldsmith JA, Gorgey AS. Trends in measuring BMR and RMR after spinal cord injury: a comprehensive review. Br J Nutr. 2023;130(10):1720-1731. doi:10.1017/S0007114523000831. Published by Cambridge University Press on behalf of The Nutrition Society. "Reproduced with permission of The Licensor through PLSclear"

difficult to obtain in a clinical environment, which is a common frustration among clinicians. Studies examining the validity of shorter measurements may offer ease and practicality in the future.[34]

Table 3.9 Conditions for Optimal Indirect Calorimetry Measurement

Indirect Calorimetry Device	Patient Status	Environment
Precise calibration	Stable respiratory status Positive end expiratory pressure >12 FiO_2 <60%	Thermoneutral
Adequate machine warm-up	Hemodynamically stable	Same ventilatory setting for past 2 hours
Steady state achieved	No airway leaks, chest tubes	At least 24 hours postoperative

Because measured REE (MREE) encompasses increases in REE due to inflammation and stress, it is greater than predicted REE, which requires an additional factor to account for these variables of stress that are not included in its estimate. The clear advantage of using MREE is the actual measurement of the stress associated with the disease as opposed to an estimated stress factor component that is prone to error. Usually, as a result, MREE in the metabolically stressed population represents up to 90% of TEE. **Figure 3.5** shows the elements captured by MREE. As components of metabolic stress, factors such as fever, pain, anxiety, and respiratory stress are measured. Additionally, if the patient is measured in a fed state (or during continuous feeding, which is customary), DIT is included in the measurement as well. By virtue of the fact that a larger component of TEE is measured versus estimated, IC provides greater accuracy than predictive equations.[35–37] However, while most of TEE is captured by IC, MREE represents a moment in time (as opposed to a 24-hour measurement). Changes that occur in the components of metabolic stress during the day (such as change in ventilator status, fever, or feeding regimen) will alter the REE throughout the day. Also, physical activity associated with bedside interventions, physical therapy, and activity level as prescribed will impact TEE. A small factor may be incorporated to account for additional "activities" as well as changes that take place when the patient is not at rest. A common factor for this is 1.2 times MREE, which has been shown to compare well with measures of TEE.[38,39]

PRACTICE POINT

A factor of 1.2 times MREE by indirect calorimetry may need to be used to accommodate for "physical activity."

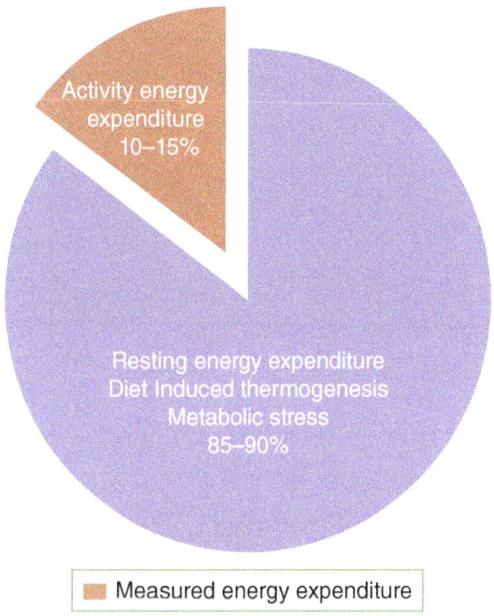

Figure 3.5 Components of Energy Expenditure Captured by Indirect Calorimetry. Measures of resting energy expenditure (MREE) incorporate the stress of disease and diet-induced thermogenesis. By capturing these elements, only physical activity must be estimated and included with MREE to determine total energy expenditure.

CORE CONCEPT 3

During the inflammatory response, resting energy expenditure incorporates the energy cost associated with the physiologic and metabolic stress of disease and clinical interventions.

⚠ Clinical Controversy

Topic: Indirect Calorimetry-Guided Therapy

Assessing energy requirements in hospitalized patients is a cornerstone of medical nutrition therapy. It is well known that predictive equations are imprecise with an associated error that may result in significant over-or underfeeding. Indirect calorimetry is considered to be a gold standard for determination of energy needs. However, the impact of nutrition therapy guided by IC versus predictive equations on clinical outcomes has not been extensively studied. Furthermore, current guidelines recommend or allow for lower energy intake during the first week of care. One systematic review showed that IC-guided therapy was not associated with reduced mortality or hospital length of stay. This approach improved the days of mechanical ventilation in one study. A subsequent systematic review demonstrated that lower rates of mortality were associated with energy intakes assessed using IC versus predictive equations. IC-guided therapy can prevent underfeeding in this population, possibly improving outcomes.

1. Based on the results of this systematic approach, how might you evaluate the need for indirect calorimetry in your population?
2. Are there specific populations that may benefit more?
3. How does the quality of the research on IC-guided nutrition therapy impact your decision?

References

1. Tatucu-Babet OA, Fetterplace K, Lambell K, Miller E, Deane AM, Ridley EJ. Is energy delivery guided by indirect calorimetry associated with improved clinical outcomes in critically ill patients? A systematic review and meta-analysis. *Nutr Metab Insights*. 2020;13. doi:10.1177/1178638820903295
2. Moonen HPFX, Beckers KJH, van Zanten ARH. Energy expenditure and indirect calorimetry in critical illness and convalescence: current evidence and practical considerations. *J Intensive Care*. 2021;9(1):8. doi:10.1186/s40560-021-00524-0.

Use of Indirect Calorimetry to Prevent Over- and Underfeeding

Not surprisingly, studies show that predictive equations in critically ill, metabolically stressed patients are inaccurate. Because they both under- and overestimate measured REE, they contribute to morbidity risk factors such as hyperglycemia, hepatic steatosis, and difficulty weaning from the ventilator in the case of overfeeding. In the case of underfeeding, malnutrition, prolonged intensive care stay, impaired immune function, and delayed healing can occur. Nutrition support regimens guided by energy prescription according to IC measures of REE show improved mortality and outcomes.[30] Current guidelines suggest measurement of energy expenditure whenever possible.[27] It is understood that not all patient care settings have the resources or expertise for routine measurement of energy expenditure. Patients who benefit the most from measured energy expenditure include those who are malnourished or obese, critically ill, and mechanically ventilated.

PRACTICE POINT

Patients who are malnourished, obese, or critically ill and mechanically ventilated should have their energy expenditure measured by indirect calorimetry when possible.

Interpretation of Respiratory Quotient

The **respiratory quotient (RQ)** is a measure of VCO_2/VO_2 and is useful for interpretation of both composition and adequacy of feeds. **Table 3.10** presents the physiologic range of RQs and their interpretation. RQ values for pure fat, protein, and carbohydrate oxidation are shown. When measuring a patient on a mixed diet, RQ values are usually in the range of 0.85–087; in fed patients, RQ values of less than 0.67 are considered nonphysiologic and suggest the need for a repeated measure. When fat oxidation is increased, RQ values are low. This may represent a hypocaloric state, or diet composition high in fat, both accelerating fat oxidation and ketogenesis. Lipogenesis occurs with excessive caloric or high carbohydrate intake and is associated with increased CO_2. When RQ values exceed 1.0, feedings may need to be decreased to avoid the consequences of hepatic fat deposition and/or excessive CO_2 production on respiratory function.[25]

Table 3.10 RQ Values and Interpretation for Substrate Utilization

RQ Value	Interpretation
<0.67	Nonphysiologic
0.7	Fat oxidation
0.8	Protein oxidation
0.8–0.87	Mixed diet
1.0	Carbohydrate oxidation
>1.0	Lipogenesis

While interpretation of RQ is useful to determine dietary intake and substrate utilization, several non-nutritional factors influence the VCO_2 and therefore RQ. Among these are hyper- or hypoventilation and acid–base balance, where RQ is altered in

Clinical Roundtable

Topic: Predictive Equations: Which Weight Should Be Used?

Background: Formulas for predicting energy requirements require inclusion of a patient's weight. Unfortunately, actual weight upon assessment may be unknown or skewed by edema or fluid overload. Many patients upon admission may have already experienced weight loss, which could be mild, moderate, or severe, designating some to a malnourished status in which weight gain is desired. In obese patients, using actual weight may lead to overestimation of energy requirements. The latter has prompted the use of adjusted body weight, which is the use of ideal body weight adjusted with a 25% increase to account for increased FFM associated with obesity. Unfortunately, research evidence does not support the use of adjusted body weight, nor is it definitive as to which weight to use for estimating energy needs.

Roundtable Discussion:

Consider the use of actual, usual, ideal, and adjusted body weight when using predictive equations in critically ill patients.

1. When might you use each?
2. What are the risks or possible negative outcomes associated with your choices?
3. How might the weight you use alter the stress factor, if any, that you select?

response to shifts in associated respiratory dynamics and CO_2 elimination. Nutritional factors such as high carbohydrate feedings; inefficient substrate utilization; use of alternative, nonoxidative pathways; and defects in fat metabolism can also result in misinterpretation of the energy adequacy of feedings. Therefore, interpretation of RQ should primarily be used to assess if IC measurements are within physiologic range, and to avoid the burden of nutrition support on respiratory function. It lacks the sensitivity and specificity to determine over- and underfeeding and should not be used to adjust feedings.[25]

The Effect of Inflammation on Energy Expenditure and Metabolism

Inflammation impacts energy expenditure in a manner that is well described. Whether chronic or acute, inflammation instigates a complex series of metabolic and physiologic changes. It occurs when there is significant insult or injury to the cell. The impact of this insult on energy expenditure varies in proportion to the magnitude of the injury. For example, inflammation that takes place following major trauma, disease, sepsis, or surgery results in extreme physiologic changes that are observed at every major organ level, including cardiac, respiratory, and gastrointestinal. These patients are considered to be **hypermetabolic** and will require a higher adjustment for stress. Inflammation in chronic disease may be less extreme, but over time, persistent levels result in the same ultimate outcome of wasting and malnutrition. Regardless of the initial cause, the ensuing response is universally the same, driven by an inflated **systemic immune response** with macrophage activation and the subsequent release of proinflammatory mediators. These mediators upregulate **acute-phase reactants** with concomitant downregulation of visceral proteins. Endocrine changes lead to an accelerated catabolic state with major changes in energy, protein, and substrate metabolism. In those with major inflammatory responses, such as in critical illness, nutrition support is required to alleviate severe lean body mass (LBM) wasting.[40–44]

Energy Cost Associated with Altered Metabolism

Table 3.11 shows the energy cost associated with increased reliance on biochemical pathways including lipolysis, gluconeogenesis, and muscle protein breakdown. The cost of inefficient substrate recycling contributes to a 21% increase in energy expenditure above that of healthy individuals.[26] Without consideration of other requirements such as wound healing and immunity, energy expenditure at baseline simply due to altered metabolism is greater than 50% above normal. The preponderance of **counterregulatory hormones** and cytokines that stimulate increased reliance on these ATP-consuming biochemical pathways such as glucagon, cortisol, and the **catecholamines** (epinephrine and norepinephrine) synergistically act to increase gluconeogenesis. Concurrently, they promote insulin and growth hormone resistance, ensuring available amino acids and glucose for tissue and wound repair. Additional breakdown of endogenous adipose stores, mediated primarily by epinephrine and norepinephrine, completes the picture of this autocatabolism that favors injury repair and survival.[44]

Table 3.11 Contribution of ATP Requiring Metabolic Pathways to Increased Energy Expenditure

Biochemical	Percent Increase from Healthy
Protein synthesis	22
Urea synthesis	3
Gluconeogenesis	11
Substrate cycling:	
Fat recycling	17
Glycolytic-gluconeogenic	4
Total increase in energy expenditure	57

Data from Yu YM, Tompkins RG, Ryan CM, Young VR. The metabolic basis of the increase in energy expenditure in severely burned patients. *JPEN J Parenter Enteral Nutr*. 1999;23(3):160-168.

CORE CONCEPT 4

Metabolic effects of the inflammatory response manifest as increased energy expenditure related to gluconeogenesis, protein synthesis and breakdown, and altered substrate utilization.

Hormonal and Metabolic Response to Stress Versus Starvation

Comparing stress to **starvation** essentially represents the difference between a state of adaptation, which occurs in starvation, and autocatabolism,

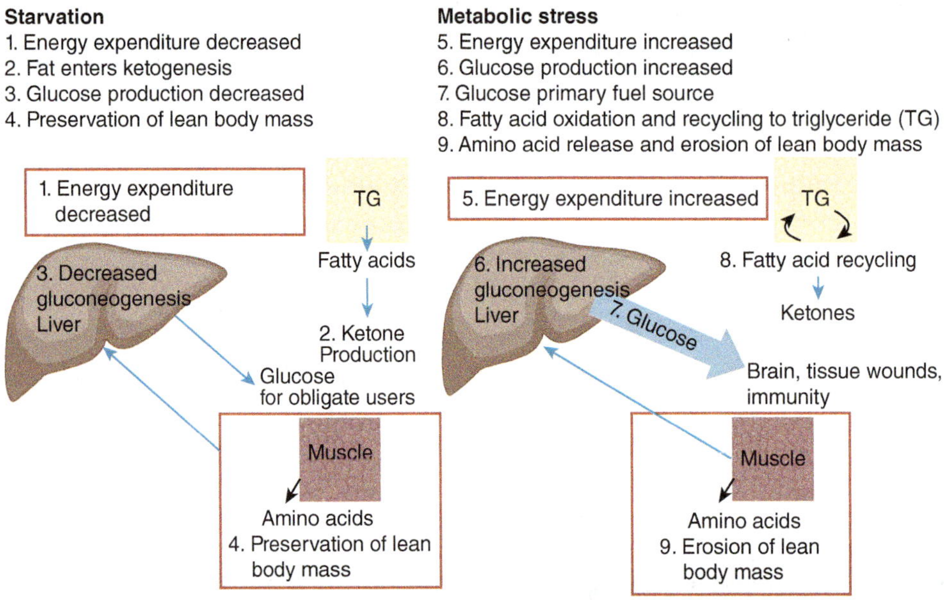

Figure 3.6 Metabolic Changes in Starvation Versus Stress. Decreased energy expenditure and minimized gluconeogenesis help to preserve muscle mass while ketones provide glucose for obligate users. This process is reversed in stress, where energy expenditure and oxidation of substrate result in loss of muscle mass.

which occurs in stress (**Figure 3.6**). In the later stages of starvation, after glycogen stores have been depleted, **gluconeogenesis** provides necessary glucose for the brain and obligate users such as red blood cells and renal medulla. Energy expenditure is decreased to minimize loss of body stores, primarily LBM. Lipolysis increases with accompanying **ketone production**. Beta-hydroxybutyrate is the ketone that becomes the primary fuel source for the brain. Muscle provides alanine as a source of glucose, but ultimately

CASE STUDY REVISITED

Four weeks later, Josephine had healed her injuries. She will soon be transferred to an inpatient rehabilitation unit to help her regain her strength. At her discharge planning meeting, it was noted that Josephine's follow-up CT scan showed that she has had a significant reduction in muscle mass since her admission. This is not consistent with body composition monitoring that was done during her inpatient stay. According to weekly weight and BIA measures, her LBM has not significantly changed. Furthermore, her discharge weight is increased. Provide your interpretation of these findings.

Anthropometric Data:

Weight History	BIA Readings
Admission Weight: 69 kg	
Week 1 Weight: 68 kg	LBM: 60.5 kg
Week 2 Weight: 65 kg	LBM: 60.5 kg
Week 4 Weight: 68 kg	LBM: 60.5 kg

Questions

1. What are the limitations of each of these body composition methods? Which is considered a gold standard method of body composition assessment?
2. How do you explain a stable LBM by BIA and increase in weight despite the CT findings?
3. What is the most important component of body composition to maintain?
4. What tools are available to determine body composition and its change in a hospital versus a research setting?

these biochemical pathways are kept to a minimum. Insulin levels are decreased due to the ultimate lack of substrate, and glucagon is increased to promote the gluconeogenesis and glycolysis that are needed.[41]

During **stress**, the body goes into a state of autocatabolism. Energy expenditure is increased, with glucose, amino acids, and fat all serving as primary fuel sources. Fat is broken down, but rather than contributing to large ketone production, it is oxidized to support the energy cost of gluconeogenesis. Much of the hydrolyzed fat enters a recycling process to ultimately be resynthesized in to triglycerides. Glucose production is increased. In the metabolically stressed state, insulin and glucagon are both increased. Insulin increases as the body tries to accommodate the increased hyperglycemia but is ineffective. Protein breakdown is substantial. In addition to alanine, other amino acids that are likely needed during times of stress, such as glutamine, branched chain amino acids, and arginine, are released, leading further to the erosion of LBM.[40–42]

Body Composition Assessment in Clinical Practice

Traditional Assessment of Nutritional Status

Although prevention of malnutrition is a priority in care planning for hospitalized patients, appropriate indicators for assessing nutritional status are lacking. Among those most used are anthropometrics, energy intake, and nitrogen balance. These indicators provide only crude estimates of nutritional status because they rely on many assumptions that are inaccurate due to the pathophysiology of most disease states. In a hospital setting, measures of weight and weight changes as proxies for the adequacy of nutritional intake are important. However, they are often confounded and complicated by derangements in fluid homeostasis. Similarly, the presence of wound dressings, therapeutic garments, and IV tubing can also influence weight measures. Overexpansion of fluid volume and erroneous weight gain may result even while tissue stores are being depleted.

Body mass index (BMI), which is an index of weight proportional to height, is sometimes used to classify weight status. BMI is used to define weight ranging from undernutrition to obesity (**Table 3.12**). However, BMI is not a measure of body composition and does not distinguish between fat and FFM, which can vary dramatically among individuals of the same height. In this context, BMI may falsely identify obesity among individuals with increased muscle mass. In aging individuals, both the size and composition of muscle mass change, which would not be appreciated with BMI alone. Such changes can only be seen with in-depth body composition analysis.[45]

Table 3.12 Mid-Upper Arm Circumference (MUAC) Cutoffs and BMI Category

BMI (kg/m^2)	MUAC (Male/Female)	Weight Classification
$<$18.5	25/23	Underweight
23	26/25	Normal Weight
25	28/27	Overweight
$>$30	30/28	Obese

Data from U.S. Centers for Disease Control and Prevention. *Adult BMI categories.* https://www.cdc.gov/cdc-info/index.html. Accessed August 2, 2025.

Protein nutritional status is also difficult to measure. Biochemical indicators of nutritional status do not exist. Common protein markers such as albumin and visceral proteins are also confounded during stress and disease. Hypoalbuminemia can be the result of hemodilution, leakage from wound exudate, and marked protein catabolism, which includes enhanced albumin degradation. This is concurrent with diminished albumin synthesis due to the acute-phase response, making albumin a poor marker of protein nutritional status in stressed patients. Other serum proteins, such as retinol binding protein, transthyretin (prealbumin), sex hormone–binding globulin, fibronectin, and somatomedin C, have shorter half-lives and thus are more sensitive indicators of protein nutritional status. However, their production is also affected by the acute-phase response. Moreover, gains in these clinical markers do not necessarily correspond with improved clinical outcomes.[46]

Nitrogen balance studies are often flawed by overestimates of nitrogen intake and underestimation of nitrogen output, which lead to falsely positive results. Nitrogen balance is also a poor predictor of protein metabolic state as measured by isotope kinetics.[28] Isotopic amino acid kinetic studies have been used to determine rates of protein synthesis and breakdown during illness or in response to a specific dietary intervention. They provide valuable information about the alterations in metabolism that accompany disease and the inflammatory response. Comparisons of the relative rates of protein synthesis and breakdown only imply the extent of protein catabolism or anabolism that may be associated with nutritional therapy, but do not quantify changes in lean tissue.[29] Changes in body composition throughout the course of hospital stay are not routinely assessed in metabolically stressed patients, despite the common understanding that losses in LBM are associated with adverse clinical outcomes in other diseased populations.[47] A lack of reliable tools for measuring body composition at the bedside is largely to blame. Given that most hospitalized patients, particularly those who are critically ill, are not easily transported to a lab for more sophisticated and accurate techniques, body composition and its change often go unmeasured. Advances in technology including the use of imaging techniques at the bedside are promising. The ability to accurately measure LBM change in response to nutritional therapy and other interventions could benefit patient outcomes.

Models of Body Composition

Understanding the body's composition and its alterations during disease is fundamental for proper nutritional assessment and for gauging the efficacy of diet therapy. Various models for the analysis of body composition exist based on elemental, anatomical, or hydrational compartmentalization of the body.[48] While use of these sophisticated multicompartment methods of body composition analysis is predominantly limited to a research environment, certain less-invasive techniques such as **anthropometry**, bioelectrical impedance, dual energy absorptiometry, and imaging techniques have been validated, enabling them to be applied in a clinical setting.[48–52] When interpreted appropriately, they give the clinician tools for measuring patient progress and outcome (**Table 3.13**).

Table 3.13 Body Composition Tools Available in a Clinical Setting

Tool	Body Compartment Measured	Equipment	Strengths	Limitations
Skinfold Thickness and Circumference	Combined measures provide estimates of fat and fat-free mass	Skinfold calipers Tape measure	Convenient Inexpensive Accurate interrater reliability with training	Measures impacted by edema, dehydration
Bioelectrical Impedance Analysis (BIA)	Two-compartment model: total body water	BIA instrument (various models and types exist)	Easy to use Inexpensive Regional analysis	Sensitive to hydration Does not differentiate between tissue type
Dual Energy X-ray Absorptiometry (DXA)	Three-compartment model: bone, fat mass, and lean body mass	DEXA machine	Gold standard for bone mineral density Accurate	Expensive Certified technician required Low-dose radiation involved
Air Displacement Plethysmography (ADP)	Two-compartment model: total body density, fat mass, and fat-free mass	BOD POD	Automated Minimal expertise required	Expensive
Computed Tomography (CT)	Multicompartment model: tissue analysis	CT Scanner	High precision and validity	Expensive Technician required Radiation exposure
Magnetic Resonance Imaging (MRI)	Multicompartment model: tissue analysis	MRI scanner	High precision and validity No radiation	Expensive Technician required
Ultrasonography (US)	Muscle quantity and quality	Ultrasound machine	Available in most clinical settings No radiation	Technically difficult More validation studies needed

Data from Holmes CJ, Racette SB. The utility of body composition assessment in nutrition and clinical practice: an overview of current methodology. *Nutrients*. 2021;13:2493. doi:10.3390/nu13082493

Anthropometry

The simplest model, and one that is most commonly utilized in a clinical setting, is the single compartment model represented by total body weight. Measures of total body weight do not provide information about LBM or FM. Moreover, in clinical settings, expansion of fluid volume commonly results in weight gain, even while tissue stores are being depleted. Despite this, measures of total body weight remain clinically useful, particularly when taken routinely so that trends can be followed. Measurements should be documented with additional information related to the presence of edema or other confounding factors for better interpretation.

Anthropometric tools such as **skinfold thickness (SFT)** and **mid-upper arm circumference (MUAC)** measures are resurfacing as useful tools in clinical practice. Historically, as a means of body composition analysis, they were criticized for their lack of precision and large interrater variability. However, with proper training, these measures have proven to be useful in nutritional assessment across multiple populations. MUAC measures correlate well with BMI and have been successfully applied as a screening tool for services, to evaluate change in nutritional status, and to diagnose malnutrition.[53–55] Measures involve finding the midpoint between the shoulder and elbow (**Figure 3.7**). A tape measure is then wrapped around the arm at that point, and the circumference is measured to the nearest 0.1 cm. MUAC cutoff values according to BMI classification are presented in Table 3.12. MUAC can identify losses in skeletal muscle mass and is accepted as a criteria for diagnosing malnutrition.[53] MUAC is sensitive to change in nutritional status with treatment in children, correlating well with changes in weight during recovery from malnutrition. The World Health Organization recommends use of MUAC as a means of diagnosing malnutrition in children, making this measure useful in both initial assessment as well as an indicator of response to nutritional intervention in this population.[54] Severe malnutrition as identified by MUAC measures is associated with a high risk of mortality, lending credibility to this measure as a prognostic indicator.[55] Note that circumference measures are affected by edema and are not sensitive to acute changes in body composition, which are common in metabolically stressed patients.

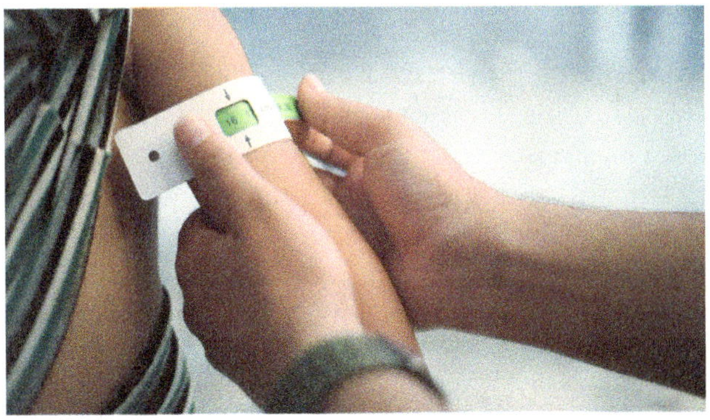

Figure 3.7 Mid-Upper Arm Circumference Measurement. Measurement of mid-arm muscle circumference using a measuring tape. Circumference measurements are made at the midpoint between the shoulder and elbow.

Analysis of total body fat using SFT relies on the assumption that the thickness of skin and underlying subcutaneous fat in various segments of the body is consistent with total body fat (**Figure 3.8**). Equations exist for SFT using three, four, and seven site-specific locations. SFT measures are summed to determine body density, which is then used in sex-specific equations to estimate % fat, FM, and FFM.[45] The use of many skinfold measures improves prediction of total body fat but still does not provide a measure of visceral fat, which does not necessarily vary in the same fashion. The advantages of SFT and circumference measures are simplicity, portability, and low cost. Combined measures of MUAC and SFT allow crude estimates of subcutaneous fat and muscle mass. The advantage of having reference normals and percentile curves for children increases their applicability.[56]

Two-Compartment Model

The two-compartment model divides the body into its fat mass and LBM as presented in **Figure 3.9**.[50] FFM is often used interchangeably with LBM. FFM differs in that it does not include the fat that is contained within cell membrane structures. In addition to the BCM, LBM includes bone, which does not contribute to energy expenditure. LBM also includes total body water. Measurement of the two-compartment model relies on the assumption that these compartments are constant and not influenced by hydration. This is important to recognize when applying these techniques during inflammation and illness, where derangements in fluid homeostasis confound interpretation of LBM and its change. A variety of techniques for measuring LBM using the two-compartment model exist and are applicable in the clinical setting, including bioelectrical impedance, dual x-ray absorptiometry, and imaging techniques.

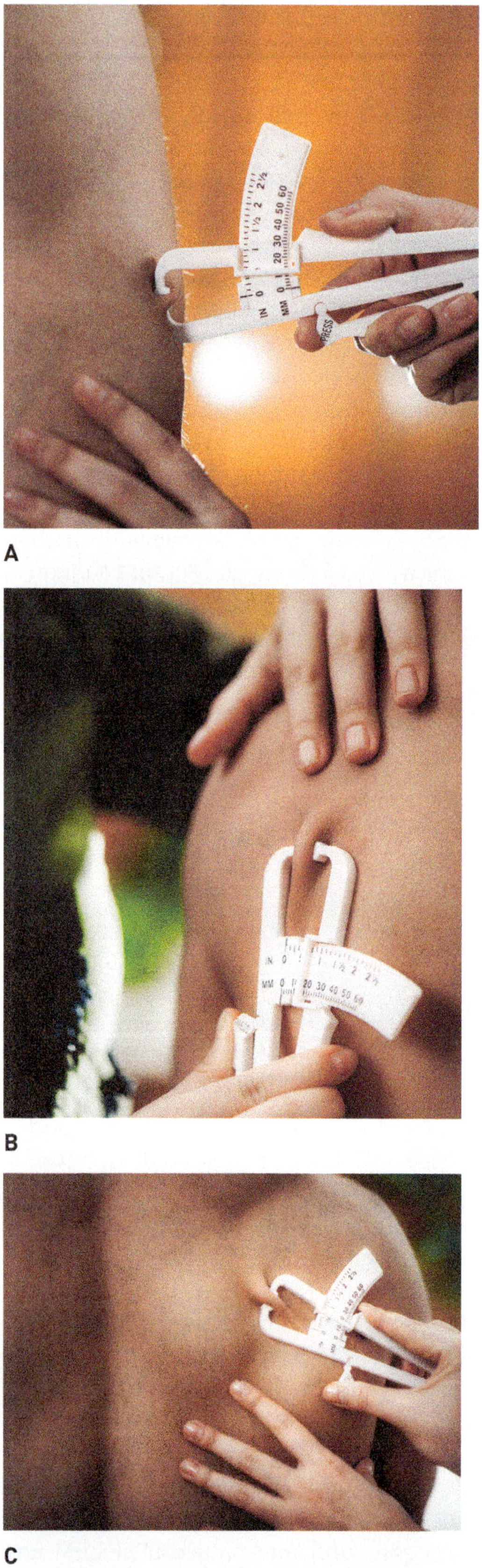

Figure 3.8 Skinfold Thickness. Measurement of subcutaneous fat in different segments of the body using skinfold calipers. **A.** Tricep **B.** Subscapular **C.** Pectoralis TB

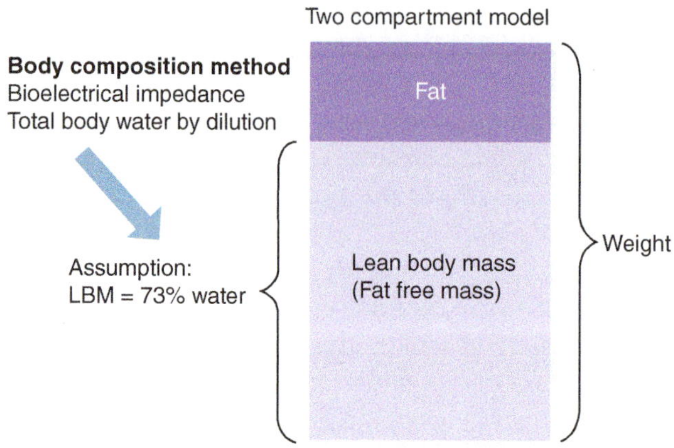

Figure 3.9 The Two-Compartment Model for Assessing Fat and Fat-free Mass. The two-compartment model divides the body into fat and lean body mass (LBM). This method relies on the assumption of normal hydration of LBM (73%). Measures of total body water (TBW) can be divided by 0.73 to determine LBM. For example, in a 70 kg male, whose TBW is 39 kg, LBM = 53 kg (39 kg LBM/0.73% water = 53 kg LBM).

Methods Relying on Measures of Total Body Water

Bioelectrical Impedance

Because water comprises up to two-thirds of total body weight, models of body composition based on total body water and its properties are common. **Bioelectrical impedance analysis (BIA)** has become an increasingly popular method that relies on TBW to estimate body composition. It combines safety and noninvasiveness with the ease of portability. With BIA, a weak electrical current is applied to the body and impedance or resistance to the flow of current is measured (**Figure 3.10**). The current will flow with less resistance through aqueous compartments since fluid and electrolytes will conduct the current. This provides a measure called "reactance." These BIA measures can be used to determine LBM and FM. Resistance to conduction of the electric current increases in proportion to body fatness because fat is a poor conductor. Therefore, individuals with a higher percent body fat will have increased resistance, whereas individuals with a lower percent of body fat will have less resistance and more reactance to the current.[45] BIA analysis resembles a series of conducting cylinders. If the length and diameter of a cylinder are known, summing measures of resistance and reaction can be used to determine impedance. From there, impedance is used to determine intracellular and extracellular water, TBW, FM, and FFM. There are a number of types of BIA instruments that vary in

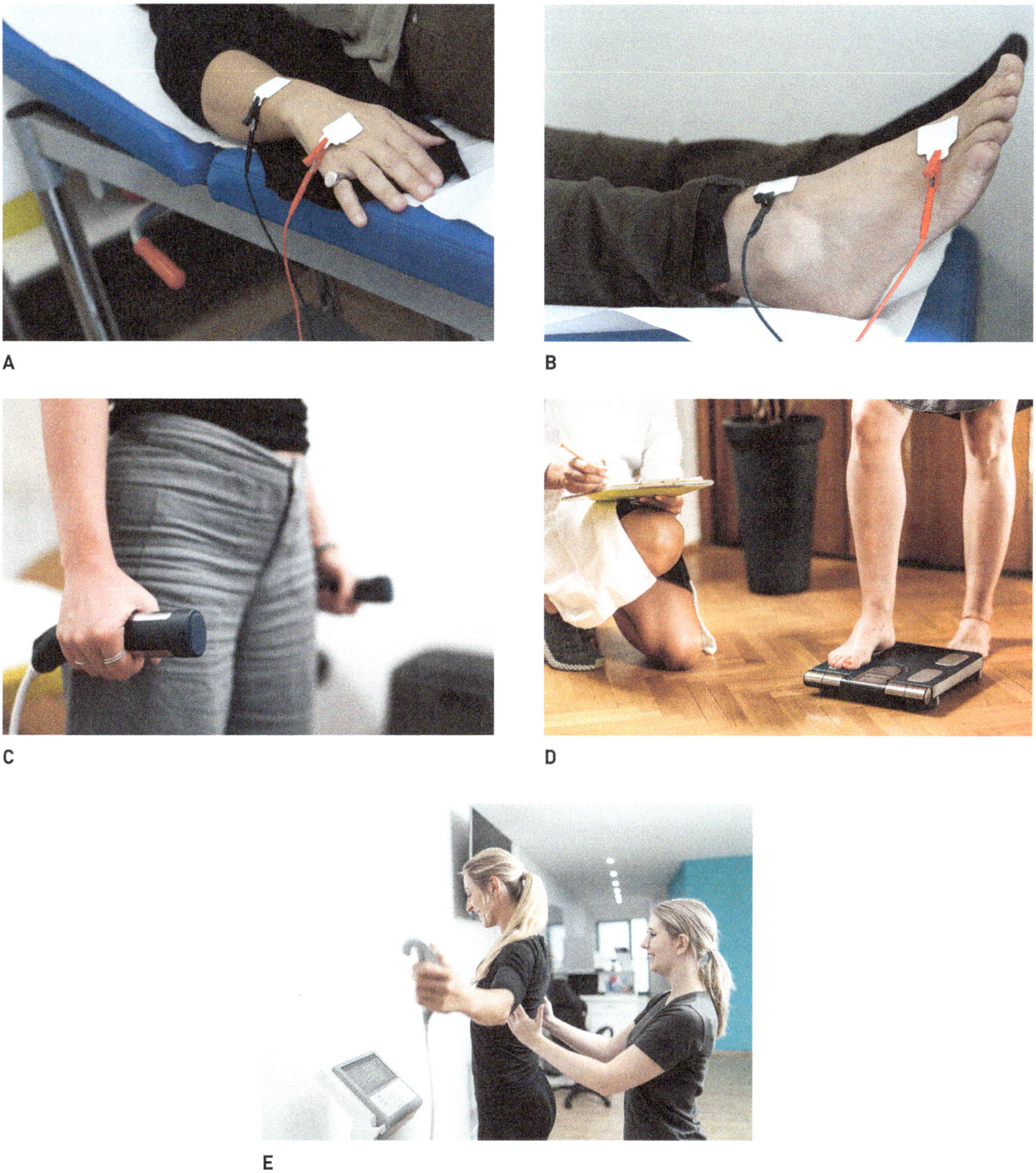

Figure 3.10 Bioelectrical Impedance Analysis. Several different models of bioelectrical impedance analyzers exist. **A, B.** Whole body BIA using the placement of electrodes on the hands and feet. **C.** Hand-to-hand bioelectrical impedance. **D.** Foot-to-foot bioelectrical impedance scale. **E.** Multiple frequency, segmental bioelectrical impedance.

A,B: © Noiel/Shutterstock; **C:** © oscarloperamartos/Shutterstock; **D:** © Microgen/Shutterstock; **E:** © r.classen/Shutterstock

their level of sophistication, reliability, and validity.[57] Some BIA instruments can measure the whole body as well as segmental FM and FFM in the limbs and trunk. There are both single and multiple frequency instruments. Multifrequency BIA (MFBIA) allows for greater penetration of different tissues with greater accuracy. MFBIA has been used to estimate skeletal muscle mass (SMM) with good agreement and correlation with other body composition techniques such as computed tomography (CT), magnetic resonance imaging (MRI), and dual energy x-ray absorptiometry (DXA) equations.[58–60] Because MFBIA can be used to distinguish bone mass, it is being investigated as a model for predicting sarcopenia. This underscores the need and potential future for MFBIA as a noninvasive, convenient tool in identifying conditions associated with aging and disease.[61] Technological differences, lack of standardization in methodology, differences in equations used, and heterogeneity of populations studied must still be factored when applying in a clinical setting.[57]

Isotope Dilution Techniques

The **isotope dilution technique** is the classic method for measuring TBW. The main assumption involved in using this method is that isotopes of oxygen or hydrogen (either as deuterium or tritium) are exchanged in the body in a manner similar to water. Following ingestion of a known amount of tracer and allowing for an equilibration period, samples of blood, urine, or saliva can be used to determine the amount of TBW. The equation is $C1V1 = C2V2$, where C1V1 reflects the concentration of tracer ingested, C2 reflects the concentration of tracer in sampling fluid, and V1 represents TBW. When applying deuterium, adjustments must be made for nonaqueous exchange of hydrogen. The precision of this method is 3%.[62]

Labeled oxygen is more precise than deuterium, with a coefficient of variation of less than 1%. However, both methods for determining LBM, like all methods based on the two-compartment model, are flawed by the presumption that the hydrational status of the fat-free body is constant at 73%. While this assumption is sufficiently precise to be acceptable in healthy populations, in diseased individuals, where derangements in fluid homeostasis are suspected, it is likely to be invalid.[63] An extension of the two-compartment model is to use combined measurements of TBW and ECW to compensate for fluid alterations that are observed in the critically ill. To specifically measure ECW, a marker that exists exclusively (or nearly so) in the extracellular fluid component is needed. Bromide (Br) exchanges rapidly with chloride within the body and has essentially the same distribution as chloride, making it well suited for measuring ECW. Following the administration of a known quantity of Br and allowing for an equilibration period, corrected bromide space (CBS) is determined from the serum Br concentration. CBS can then be used to determine ECW. This technique has been successfully applied to measure ECW in children who are hospitalized and acutely ill.[64] The results of such studies have been useful in detecting abnormal states of hydration. Once measurements of both ECW and TBW are obtained, they can be used to estimate intracellular water (ICW), which is an indicator of the BCM.[65–68]

Air Displacement Plethysmography

Air displacement plethysmography (ADP) relies on the basic principles of densitometry as does a more familiar method, underwater weighing. This method relies on the concept that the amount of weight that is lost when placed under water is equal to the weight of the volume that is displaced. ADP follows a similar principle; however, in this case, the volume of displaced air is measured to determine body volume. Like underwater weighing, ADP can be used to determine LBM and FM. With ADP, subjects are placed in a chamber of known pressure and volume. Any changes are attributed to the subject's total body volume, which is then used to derive total body density (**Figure 3.11**).[45] One of the advantages of ADP is that it can accommodate individuals of varying age and size, enabling the tracking of body composition throughout the lifespan. ADP devices are easy to use and do not include radiation. Manufactured devices such as BOD, POD, and PEA POD (CosMed, Inc; Concord, CA) are available in a number of clinical settings. Perhaps most appealing is that ADP can consider crying and movements of infants and young children without compromising precision and validity. This is one of the few methods that are available to measure body composition and growth in neonates through childhood.[69,70] Despite its reliability in healthy children and young adults, ADP may be inaccurate in certain pediatric patient populations, needing further

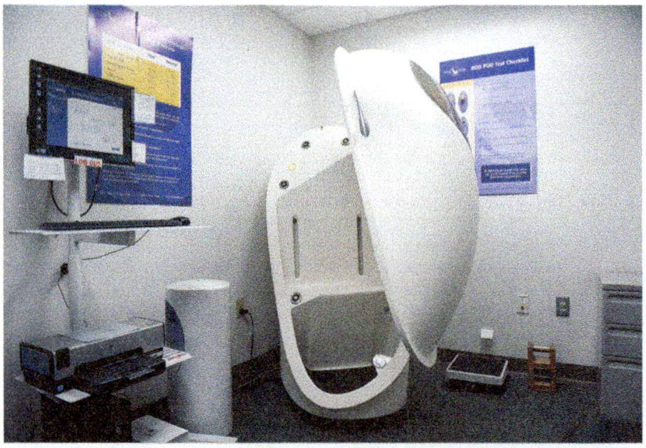

Figure 3.11 Air Displacement Plethysmography. ADP is conducted by placing the subject in a pressure-controlled chamber. The amount of air displaced in the chamber is used to calculate the subject's total body volume, where the volume of subject equals the volume of empty chamber minus the volume of chamber with subject.

Courtesy of U.S. Air Force photo by Airman 1st Class Joshua T. Crossman.

validation in certain disease states or conditions.[71] It should be noted that ADP, like underwater weighing, relies on the assumptions of the two-compartment model, meaning that it only measures LBM and FM. It does not provide information about the quality of the LBM, which can vary based on hydration, amount of skeletal muscle mass, or the contribution of bone. Similarly, ADP cannot distinguish the type of fat in adipose tissue. More sophisticated multicompartment models are needed for that.[50]

The Effect of Catabolic Disease on Body Composition Implications for the Two-Compartment Model

When moving toward more complex, multicompartment models, it becomes evident that in addition to BCM, LBM consists of extracellular solids that consist of the structural proteins of the body, including skeleton, fascia, cartilage, dermis, and ECW. The extracellular solid mass remains relatively unchanged during acute injury, although the ECW can vary.

Figure 3.12 shows that significant changes in LBM and FM result from the prolonged inflammatory state that occurs in catabolic disease; this state may continue for days, weeks, or years in certain chronic inflammatory conditions. Fat represents a significant fuel source to aid in recovery from illness, and its losses account for approximately one-half of the weight loss experienced during severe catabolic injury. The remaining half of weight loss occurs within the LBM compartment, primarily within the soft tissue component. In this component, there is a decrease in BCM accompanied by an expansion of ECW. While the etiology of this fluid expansion is not completely understood, it is thought that increased membrane permeability induced by shock of injury or sepsis allows the efflux of plasma proteins and cellular constituents, which is accompanied by the efflux of water into the interstitium. Increased levels of aldosterone and vasopressin occur following injury or starvation, suggesting that sodium and fluid retention are hormonally mediated as well. These alterations can mask the diminution of BCM that results from accelerated nitrogen losses. Not uncommonly, weight loss is marginal; however, the quality of LBM is diminished because its proportion of BCM to ECW is decreased.[63]

CORE CONCEPT 5

Expansion in extracellular water during illness confounds interpretation of weight, lean body cell mass, and erosion of body cell mass.

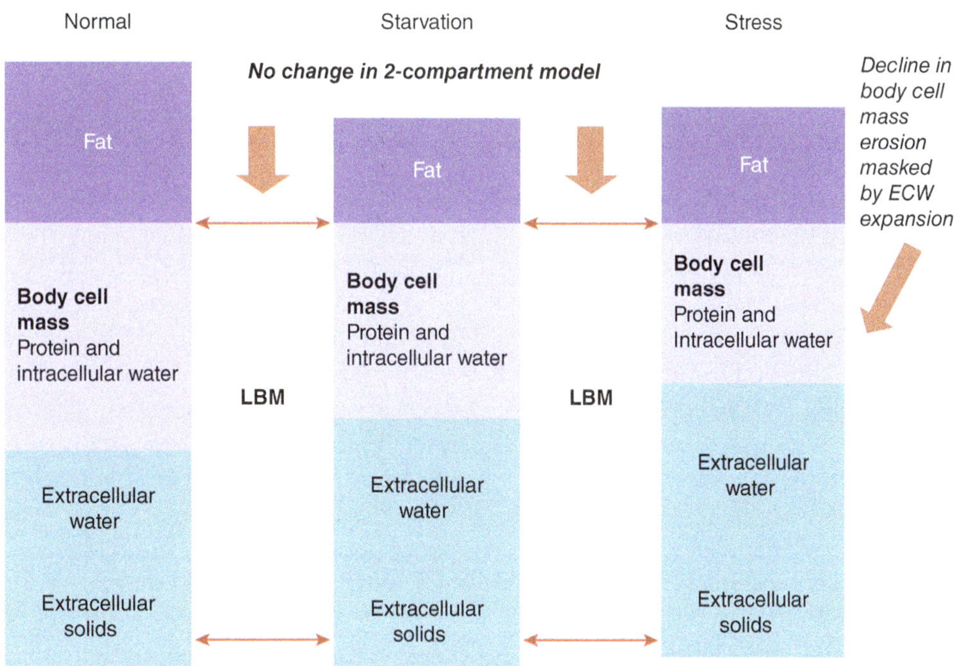

Figure 3.12 The Effect of Starvation and Stress on Body Composition: The Two-Compartment Model. Differences in metabolism between stress and starvation manifest in changes in body composition. While both demonstrate a decrease in fat mass from normal health, body cell mass (BCM) is diminished to a greater extent. When measuring lean body mass using the two-compartment model, the loss in BCM cannot be appreciated due to the expansion of extracellular water.

Because significant depletion of the BCM has a direct, negative impact on immune competence, functional capacity, and, ultimately, survival, losses of BCM increase risks of adverse outcomes in metabolically stressed patients. The actual extent of BCM wasting is directly related to the degree and duration of the catabolic stimuli that are present. Therefore, individuals suffering from major trauma or sepsis can be expected to have greater losses than those with minor trauma. Measuring changes in various tissues and body compartments during stress can identify those patients at extremely high risk for BCM wasting and may serve as a better compartment to assess response to nutritional therapy. Unfortunately, at this time, convenient noninvasive measures of BCM do not exist.

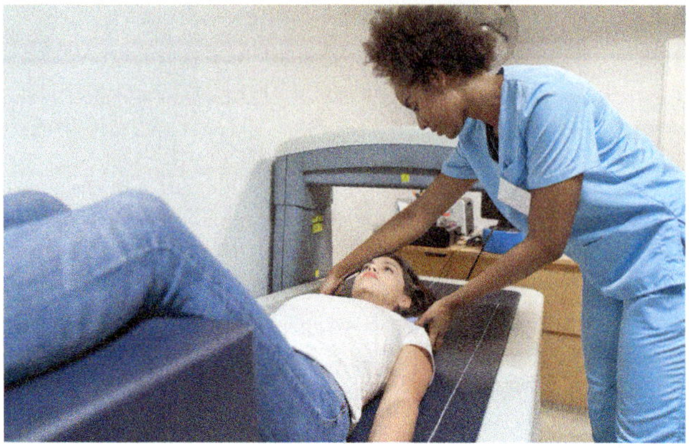

Figure 3.13 Measurement of Body Composition by Dual Energy X-ray Absorptiometry

Body Composition Analysis Using Imaging Techniques in Multicompartmental Models

Dual Energy X-ray Absorptiometry

Dual energy x-ray absorptiometry (DXA) has evolved as a well-accepted tool for measuring body composition. Traditionally used for measures of bone mineral density, the precision and accuracy of DXA has gained distinction for estimating soft tissue as well, such as LBM and FM. Hence, DXA utilizes a three-compartment model, where three components are measured: LBM, FM, and bone mineral density. This tool demonstrates good reliability for body composition measurement when compared with imaging studies of body fat by CT and magnetic resonance imaging (MRI), although its accuracy declines in individuals with obesity.[71,72]

The DXA method involves the use of x-ray beams at two photon energies to estimate body composition. As the energy from these beams passes through the bone or soft tissue, some of it is absorbed, while the rest passes through the body and is detected on the other side, providing information on the density of the bone or tissue. Although it is not portable, it is common in many clinical settings (**Figure 3.13**).[72] Other advantages include providing a rapid measure (3–10 minutes for lumbar spine and whole-body measures) with a minimal radiation dose. It also provides regional body composition analysis, although this is not based on direct measure, but rather on assumptions based on anatomical models. DXA measures can be confounded in that it assumes a constant hydration factor for soft tissue within the LBM, which can vary particularly with age; therefore, standardization of timing, fasting state, population differences, and factors such as exercise or edema should be considered.[72]

DXA is capable of measuring both regional and whole-body muscle mass. Its ability to quantify appendicular skeletal muscle mass (ASM), which is the sum of muscle in the four limbs, has led to its inclusion as a proper measurement tool to quantify muscle mass in the diagnosis of sarcopenia. Because muscle quantity is also a function of body size, the appendicular skeletal muscle index (ASMI) is derived by dividing ASM/height in m^2. This index, along with measures of muscle strength and function, is used in the operational definition of sarcopenia.[73,74] DXA can also provide information on both the type and distribution of adipose. Measures of visceral adipose tissue (VAT), a marker of chronic disease, are considered to be more accurate than BMI and WC and have been validated by MRI (considered to be the gold standard). DXA therefore allows assessment of bone mineral density as well as visceral and somatic fat mass. As a screening tool, there can be significant advantages, particularly in the aging population where the risk of osteoporosis and other chronic diseases is increased.[75]

Development of imaging techniques such as MRI, CT, and ultrasonography (US) has benefited body composition assessment as well as clinical medicine. These methods assess body composition at the tissue level. Their use can provide information on both the quantity and quality of skeletal muscle, the type of adipose tissue, and the contribution of visceral organs, bone, and brain. Apart from their superior images and reliability, these techniques offer cross-sectional views. This is especially useful in evaluating visceral adipose tissue and its distribution. Another advantage is that these techniques are available in most medical centers. They are not influenced by hydration status. Lack of radiation exposure with US and MRI allows it to be used longitudinally. MRI and CT are both considered to be gold standard techniques by which other measures are compared and validated.[73,76,77]

Computerized Tomography

In a hospital setting, CT is generally used for diagnosis or targeted interventions. It provides useful information about body composition such as fatty infiltration and muscle attenuation, which are predictors or manifestations of chronic conditions including sarcopenia, hepatomegaly, and fragility due to muscle loss.[78]

CT can provide cross-sectional "slices" of a particular region of interest. On this slice, CT can identify muscle mass and quality, as well as fatty infiltration that often accompanies a reduction in muscle mass. In this way, CT imaging has been instrumental for identifying sarcopenia, which is becoming significantly more prevalent, particularly in the aging population. Furthermore, because sequential measures of CT are common for staging tumors and monitoring of various disease conditions, assessment of sarcopenia and its progression can be followed as part of clinical care without the need for additional scans.[79–81]

Magnetic Resonance Imaging

While both CT and MRI can quantify muscle and adipose tissue with great sophistication and reliability, MRI does not involve radiation (**Figure 3.14**). This makes it the preferable choice, particularly for repeated measures. MRI measures of body composition are included in a number of long-term epidemiological studies and databases including the UK Biobank and the Dallas Heart Study.[81] MRI can quantify different body compartments with high accuracy and reproducibility.[82–84] Like CT, MRI can determine muscle volume and identify myosteatosis, which is fatty infiltration of muscle fibers (**Figure 3.15**). MRI's ability to differentiate soft tissue shows promise with respect to identifying different muscle fiber types. Technical difficulty and time-consuming data analysis limit MRI use to research settings.[81]

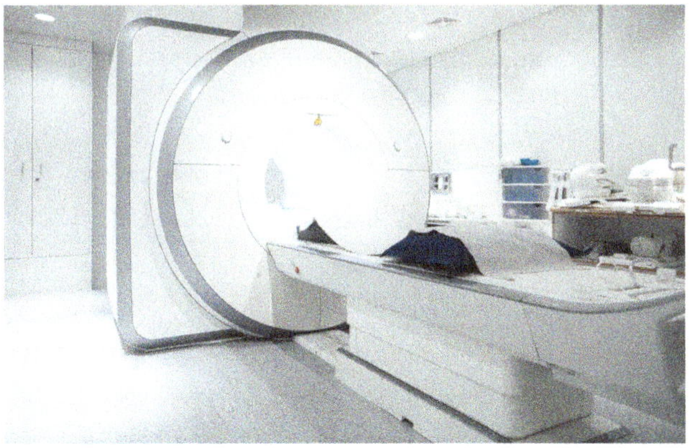

Figure 3.14 Body Composition Can Be Measured Using Imaging Techniques such as Magnetic Resonance Imaging

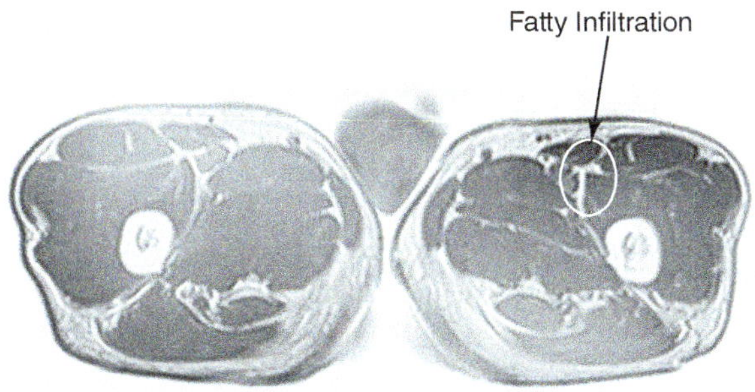

Figure 3.15 MRI cross sectional image of thigh muscle with fatty infiltration. Subcutaneous fat can be seen in the perimeter.

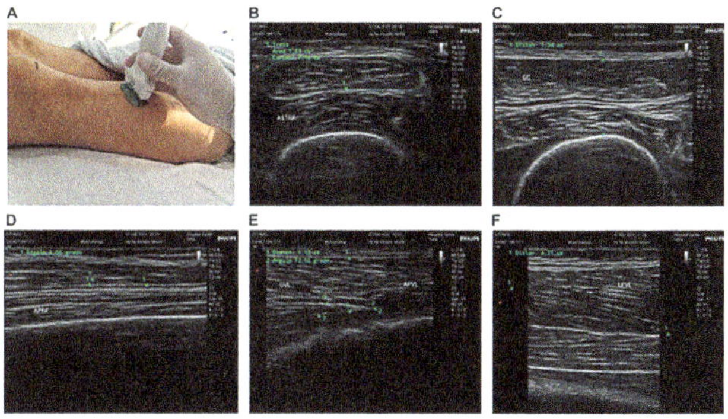

Figure 3.16 Assessment of quantitative and qualitative measurements of the quadriceps using ultrasound. A) Measurement of the midpoint and distal third of the quadriceps, skin marking for sequential measurements, and muscle evaluation in the transverse axis with a high-frequency linear transducer. B) Cross-sectional area of the rectus femoris. C) Thickness of the rectus femoris and vastus internus. D) Pennation angle of the rectus femoris. E) Thickness and pennation angle of the vastus lateralis. F Length of the fascicle of the vastus lateralis using a linear extrapolation technique

Ultrasonography

Ultrasonography (US) has recently emerged as a tool for body composition analysis in a clinical setting. It serves as a noninvasive tool that can be used conveniently at the bedside (**Figure 3.16**). Thickness and cross-sectional area of upper and lower body muscles are determined. One of the most commonly measured muscles is the quadricep femoris due to its sensitivity to change. US can also measure fat thickness, which can be used to derive percent body fat.[85] US has proven validity both in healthy and injured subjects, with good interrater reliability.[86–88] Because it does not require radiation, longitudinal measures of US can be used to quantify muscle mass and change in muscle mass in a hospital setting. In patients with critical illness, repeated US measures identified a daily muscle loss of 1–2% during the first week of critical illness. Whether US will be useful for measuring response to nutritional therapy and outcome remains to be determined.[89,90]

Chapter Summary

Determination of energy needs is central to medical nutrition therapy. TEE is essentially the sum of REE, DIT, and AEE. REE is approximately 70% of TEE and parallels lean body mass (more specifically BCM). During illness, the metabolic stress associated with disease or injury also contributes to TEE. Predictive equations allow for TEE to be estimated using validated equations for REE along with stress factors to account for the impact of disease on energy expenditure. Similarly, factors for physical activity are also incorporated. AEE is sometimes ignored when patients are at bedrest and/or sedated. Otherwise, consideration should be made for ambulation and physical activity, particularly during rehabilitative care or in ambulatory patients.

Much of the increase in REE with disease and illness is associated with inflammation. With severe trauma, the magnitude of inflammation, often termed "inflammatory response," is great. Stress factors should ultimately be gauged to match the degree of stress and its impact on metabolism. Whether acute or chronic, inflammation leads to the production and release of cytokines that stimulate the endocrine system to produce glucagon, glucocorticoids, and catecholamines, which, in turn, have widespread effects on glucose, amino acid, and fatty acid metabolism. These aberrations in metabolism are clinically manifested by increased energy expenditure, impaired nutrient utilization, and LBM losses. This differs from the metabolic response to semi-starvation. In this scenario, gluconeogenesis and hence protein breakdown are minimized. There is an increased reliance on lipolysis and ketones as an energy source. These, in turn, lower energy expenditure. Reliance on these metabolic pathways helps to preserve the erosion of lean body mass.

Monitoring response to nutritional therapy is limited to a few indicators including weight, estimated intake, healing, and function. Preservation of LBM is associated with improved clinical outcomes. Unfortunately measures of LBM are often confounded during illness. Certain tools have proven effective in a clinical setting. Skinfold thickness and mid-upper arm circumference measures are convenient, inexpensive, and reliable with effective measurement training. Both measures have reference standards for comparison that are helpful in diagnosis of malnutrition and response to therapy. BIA is also an option for assessment of TBW and subsequently fat and fat-free mass. Changes related to hydration can impact interpretation of LBM. Erosion of BCM while LBM is constant is possible depending on the models used. Imaging studies with CT and MRI have played a role in validating tools for body composition assessment. For example, DXA has been validated as an appropriate measure of sarcopenia. This is advantageous given that DXA scans are often done in the aging population for monitoring bone mineral density. In this way, muscle mass and quality can also be assessed, leading to interventions that can improve muscle size and strength.

Key Terms

Total energy expenditure (TEE), basal metabolic rate (BMR), thermic effect of food, activity energy expenditure (AEE), resting energy expenditure (REE), body cell mass (BCM), lean body mass (LBM), fat-free mass (FFM), indirect calorimetry (IC), Doubly labeled water (DLW), direct calorimetry, respiratory quotient (RQ), inflammation, systemic immune response, hypermetabolic, acute-phase reactants, gluconeogenesis, counterregulatory hormones, catecholamines, stress, starvation, ketone production, anthropometry, mid-upper arm circumference (MUAC), skinfold thickness (SFT), dual energy x-ray absorptiometry (DXA), bioelectrical impedance analysis (BIA), isotope dilution technique, air displacement plethysmography (ADP)

References

1. Westerterp, K. Control of energy expenditure in humans. *Eur J Clin Nutr*. 2017;71:340–344. doi:10.1038/ejcn.2016.237
2. Heymsfield SB, Thomas DM, Bosy-Westfal A, Muller MJ. The anatomy of resting energy expenditure: body composition mechanisms. *Eur J Clin Nutr.* 2019;73:166–171.
3. Human energy requirements. Report of the joint FAO/WHO/UNU Expert Consultation, October 17–24, 2001; Rome, Italy.
4. Pontzer H, Yamada Y, Sagayama H, et al. Daily energy expenditure through the human life course. *Science*. 2021;373(6556):808–812. doi:10.1126/science.abe5017
5. National Academies of Sciences, Engineering, and Medicine. Factors affecting energy expenditure and requirements. In: *Dietary Reference Intakes for Energy.* The National Academies Press; 2023.
6. Schofield WN. Predicting basal metabolic rate, new standards and review of previous work. *Hum Nutr Clin Nutr.* 1985;39c(1s):5–42.
7. Mifflin D, St Jeor ST, Hill LA, Scott BJ, Daugherty SA, Koh YO. A new predictive equation for resting energy expenditure in healthy individuals. *Am J Clin Nutr*. 1990;51:241–247.
8. Harris JA, Benedict FG. *A Biometric Study of Basal Metabolism in Man*. Carnegie Institution; 1919.
9. Owen OE, Holup JL, D'Alessio DA, et al. A reappraisal of the caloric requirements of men. *Am J Clin Nutr*. 1987;46:875–885.
10. Alam DS, Hulshof PJ, Roordink D, et al. Validity and reproducibility of resting metabolic rate measurements in rural Bangladeshi women: comparison of measurements obtained by Medgem and by Deltatrac device. *Eur J Clin Nutr.* 2005;59:651–657. doi:10.1038/sj.ejcn.1602122
11. Institute of Medicine. Dietary Reference Intakes for Energy, Carbohydrate, Fiber, Fat, Fatty Acids, Cholesterol, Protein, and Amino Acids. The National Academies Press; 2005.
12. National Academies of Sciences, Engineering, and Medicine. Development of prediction equations for estimated energy requirements. In: *Dietary Reference Intakes for Energy*. The National Academies Press; 2023.
13. Houmoller C, Hellerup SH, Nohr NK, et al. Measured vs estimated energy requirement in hospitalized patients. *Clin Nutr ESPEN*. 2024;59:312–319.
14. Murray G, Thomas S, Dunlea T, et al. Comparison of predictive equations and indirect calorimetry in critical care: does the accuracy differ by body mass index classification? *Nutr Clin Pract*. 2023;38:1124–1132.
15. Madden AM, Mulrooney HM, Shah S. Estimation of energy expenditure using prediction equations in overweight and obese adults: a systematic review. *J Hum Nutr Diet*. 2016;29:458–476. doi:10.1111/jhn.12355
16. De Waele E, Opsomer T, Honore PM, et al. Measured versus calculated resting energy expenditure in critically ill adult patients. Do mathematics match the gold standard? *Minerva Anestesiol*. 2015;81(3):272–282.
17. Hickmann CE, Roeseler J, Castanares-Zapatero D, Herrera EI, Mongodin A, Laterre PF. Energy expenditure in the critically ill performing early physical therapy. *Intensive Care Med*. 2014; 40(4):548–555.
18. Nacht CA, Schutz Y, Vernet O, Christin L, Jequier E. Continuous versus single bolus enteral nutrition: comparison of energy metabolism in humans. *Am J Physiol Endocrinol Metab*.1986; 251(5):E524–E529.
19. Roza AM, Shizgal HM. The Harris Benedict equation reevaluated: resting energy requirements and the body cell mass. *Am J Clin Nutr*. 1984;40(1):168–182.
20. Walker RN, Heuberger RA. Predictive equations for energy needs for the critically ill. *Respir Care*. 2009;54:509–521.
21. Frankenfield D. Validation of an equation for resting metabolic rate in older obese, critically ill patients. *JPEN*. 2011;35(2):264–269.
22. Swinamer DL, Grace MG, Hamilton SM, Jones RL, Roberts P, King G. Predictive equation for assessing energy expenditure in mechanically ventilated critically ill patients. *Crit Care Med*. 1990;18(6):657–661.
23. Cerra FB, Benitez BR, Blackburn GL, Irwin RS, Jeejeebhoy K, Katz DP. Applied nutrition in ICU patients: a consensus statement of the American College of Chest Physicians. *Chest*. 1997;111:769–778.
24. Ireton-Jones C. Improved equations for predicting energy expenditure in patients: the Ireton-Jones Equations. *Nutr Clin Pract*. 2002;17:29–31.
25. McClave SA, Lowen CC, Kleber MJ, et al. Clinical use of respiratory quotient obtained from indirect calorimetry. *JPEN*. 2003;27(1):21–26.
26. Yu YM, Tompkins RG, Ryan CM, Young VR. The metabolic basis of the increase of the increase in energy expenditure in severely burned patients. *JPEN*. 1999;23(3):160–168.
27. McClave SA, Taylor BE, Martindale RG, et al. Guidelines for the provision and assessment of nutrition support therapy in the adult critically ill patient: Society of Critical Care Medicine (SCCM) and American Society for Parenteral and Enteral Nutrition (A.S.P.E.N.). *JPEN*. 2016;40(2):159–211. doi:10.1177/0148607115621863
28. Prelack K, Dwyer J, Yu YM, Sheridan RL, Tompkins RG. Urinary urea nitrogen is imprecise as a predictor of protein balance in burned children. *J Am Diet Assoc*. 1997;97: 489–495.
29. Picou D, Taylor-Roberts T. The measurement of total protein synthesis and catabolism and nitrogen turnover in infants in different nutritional states and receiving different amounts of dietary protein. *Clin. Sci Land*. 1969;36:283–301.
30. Levine J. Measurement of energy expenditure. *Pub Health Nutr.* 2005;87(A):1123–1132.
31. Schoeller DA, Ravussin E, Schutz Y, et al. Energy expenditure by doubly labeled water: validation in humans and proposed calculation. *Am J Physiol*. 1986; 250:R823–R830.
32. Schoeller DA, Hnilicka J. Reliability of the doubly labeled water method for measurement of total daily energy expenditure in free-living subjects. *J Nutr.*1996;126:348S–354S.
33. Weir JB de V. New methods for calculating metabolic rate with special reference to protein metabolism. *J Physiol*. 1949;109(1-2):1–9.
34. Smallwood CD, Mehta NM. Accuracy of abbreviated indirect calorimetry protocols for energy expenditure measurement in critically ill children. *JPEN*. 2012;36(6):693–699.
35. Frankenfield D, Roth-Yousey L, Compher C. Comparison of predictive equations for resting metabolic rate in healthy nonobese and obese adults: a systematic review. *J Am Diet Assoc*. 2005;105(5):775–789.
36. Mehta NM. Energy expenditure: how much does it matter in infant and pediatric chronic disorders? *Pediatr Res*. 2015;77(1-2):168–172.

37. Kross EK, Sena M, Schmidt K. A comparison of predictive equations and measured energy expenditure in critically ill patients. *J Crit Care*. 2012;27(3):321.e5–321.e12.
38. Goran MI, Peters EJ, Herndon DN, Wolfe RR. Total energy expenditure in burned children using the doubly labeled water technique. *Am J Physiol*. 1990;259(4 Pt 1):E576–E585.
39. Prelack K, Yu YM, Dylewski M, Lydon M, Keaney TJ, Sheridan RL. Measures of total energy expenditure and its components using the doubly labeled water method in rehabilitating burn children. *JPEN*. 2017;41(3):470–480.
40. Williams FN, Jeschke MG, Chinkes DL, Suman OE, Branski LK, Herndon DN. Modulation of the hypermetabolic response to trauma: temperature, nutrition, and drugs. *J Am Coll Surg*. 2009;208(4):489–502.
41. Finnerty CC, Mabvuure NT, Ali A, Kozar RA, Herndon DN. The surgically induced stress response. *JPEN*. 2013;37(5 Suppl):21S–29S.
42. Simsek T, Simsek HU, Canturk NZ. Response to trauma and metabolic changes: posttraumatic metabolism. *Ulus Cerrahi Derg*. 2014;30(3):153–159.
43. Stahel PF, Flierl MA, Moore EE. "Metabolic staging" after major trauma: a guide for clinical decision making? *Scand J Trauma Resusc Emerg Med*. 2010;18:34.
44. Porter C, Tompkins RG, Finnerty CC, Sidossis LS, Suman OE, Herndon DN. The metabolic stress response to burn trauma: current understanding and therapies. *Lancet*. 2016;388:1417–1426.
45. Holmes CJ, Racette SB. The utility of body composition assessment in nutrition and clinical practice: an overview of current methodology. *Nutrients*. 2021;13:2493. doi:10.3390/nu13082493
46. Shields BA, Pidcoke HF, Chung KK, et al. Are visceral proteins valid markers for nutritional status in the burn intensive care unit? *J Burn Care Res*. 2015;36(3):375–380.
47. Kotler DP. Nutritional considerations in AIDS. *Bol Asoc Med P R*. 1991;83(2):81–83.
48. Heymsfield SB, Ebbeling CB, Zheng J, et al. Multi-component molecular-level body composition reference methods: Evolving concepts and future directions. *Obes Rev*. 2015; 16(4):282–294.
49. Adreoli A, Garaci F, Pio Cafarelli F, Guglielmi. G. Body composition in clinical practice. *Eur J Radiol*. 2016;85:1461–1468.
50. Borga M, West J, Bell JD, et al. Advanced body composition assessment: from body mass index to body composition profiling. *J Investig Med*. 2018;66(5):1–9. doi:10.1136/jim-2018-000722
51. Flegal KM, Shepherd JA, Looker AC, et al. Comparisons of percentage body fat, body mass index, waist circumference, and waist-stature ratio in adults. *Am J Clin Nutr*. 2009;89(2):500–508.
52. Price KL, Earthman CP. Update on body composition tools in clinical settings: computed tomography, ultrasound, and bioimpedance applications for assessment and monitoring. *Eur J Clin Nutr*. 2019; 73:187–193.
53. Barazzoni R, Jenssen GL. Correia MITD. Guidance for assessment of the muscle mass phenotypic criterion for the Global Leadership Initiative on Malnutrition (GLIM) diagnosis of malnutrition. *Clin Nutr*. 2022; 41:1425–1433.
54. Binns P, Dale N, Hoq M, Banda C, Myatt M. Relationship between mid upper arm circumference and weight changes in children aged 6-59 months. *Arch Public Health*. 2015;73:54-015-0103-y.
55. Wu T, Xu H, Zou Y, et al. Mid-arm muscle circumference or body weight-standardized hand grip strength in the GLIM superiorly predicts survival in Chinese colorectal cancer patients. *Nutrients*. 2022;4(23):5166. doi:10.3390/nu14235166
56. Nagy P, Kovacs E, Moreno L, et al. Percentile reference values for anthropometric body composition indices in European children from the IDEFICS study. *Int J Obes*. 2013;38 (Suppl 2): S15–S25. doi:10.1038/ijo.2014.131
57. Csiernik B, Edgar M, DeGraauw C, Howitt S, Hogg-Johnson S. The utility of bioelectrical impedance analysis in the diagnosis of sarcopenia: a systematic review. *J Can Chiropr Assoc*. 2022; 66(2):118–129.
58. Kim EY, Kim SR, Won DD, Choi MH, Lee K. Multifrequency bioelectrical impedance analysis compared with computed tomography for assessment of skeletal muscle mass in primary colorectal malignancy: a predictor of short-term outcome after surgery. *Nutr Clin Pract*. 2020;35(4);664–674.
59. Buch A, Ben-Yehuda A, Rouach V, et al. Validation of a multi-frequency bioelectrical impedance analysis device for the assessment of body composition in older adults with type 2 diabetes. *Nutr Diab*. 2022;12(45). doi:10.1038/s41387-022-00223-1
60. Tinsley GM, LaValle C, Rodriguez C, Siedler MR, Heymsfield SB. Skeletal muscle estimation using magnetic-resonance-imaging based equations for dual-energy X-ray absorptiometry and bioelectrical impedance analysis. *Eur J Clin Nutr*. 2023;77:1151–1159. doi:10.1038/s41430-023-01331-6
61. Konoshita N, Onishi H, Mizukami Y, et al. Can bone mass measured via bioelectrical impedance analysis be used to diagnose sarcopenia? *J Clin Biochem Nutr*. 2024;74(2): 154–161. doi:10.3164/jcbn.23-88
62. Schoeller DA, van Santen E, Peterson DW, Dietz W, Jaspan J, Klein PD. Total body water measurement in humans with 18O and 2H labeled water. *Am J Clin Nutr*. 1980;33(12):2686–2693.
63. Roubenoff R, Kehayias JJ. The meaning and measurement of lean body mass. *Nutr Rev*. 1991;49(6):163–175.
64. Prelack K, Sheridan R, Yu YM, et al. Sodium bromide by instrumental neutron activation analysis quantifies change in extracellular water space with wound closure in severely burned children. *Surgery*. 2003;133(4):396–403.
65. Prelack K, Dwyer J, Sheridan R, et al. Body water in children during recovery from severe burn injury using a combined tracer dilution method. *J Burn Care Rehabil*. 2005;26(1):67–74.
66. Monk DN, Plank LD, Franch-Arcas G, Finn PJ, Streat SJ, Hill GL. Sequential changes in the metabolic response in critically injured patients during the first 25 days after blunt trauma. *Ann Surg*. 1996;223(4):395–405.
67. Plank LD, Hill GL. Sequential metabolic changes following induction of systemic inflammatory response in patients with severe sepsis or major blunt trauma. *World J Surg*. 2000;24(6):630–638.
68. Finn PJ, Plank LD, Clark MA, Connolly AB, Hill GL. Progressive cellular dehydration and proteolysis in critically ill patients. *Lancet*. 1996;347(9002):654–656.
69. Fields DA, Gunatilake R, Kalaitzoglou E. Air displacement plethysmography. *Nutr Clin Pract*. 2015;30:219–226. doi:10.1177/0884533615572443.
70. Wiechers C, Kirchhof S, Maas C, Poets CF, Franz AR. Neonatal body composition by air displacement plethysmography in healthy term singletons: a systematic review. *BMC Pediatr*. 2019;19(1):489. doi:10.1186/s12887-019-1867-y
71. Bijlsma A, van Beijsterveldt IALP, Vermeulen MJ, et al. Challenges in body composition assessment using air-displacement

plethysmography by BOD POD in pediatric and young adult patients. *Clin Nutr*. 2023;42(9):1588–1594. doi:10.1016/j.clnu.2023.07.003

72. Cheung AS, de Rooy C, Hoermann R, et al. Correlation of visceral adipose tissue measured by Lunar Prodigy dual X-ray absorptiometry with MRI and CT in older men. *Int J Obesity*. 2016;40(8):1325–1328.
73. Bredella M, Ghomi RH, Thomas BJ, et al. Comparison of DXA and CT in the assessment of body composition of premenopausal women with obesity and anorexia nervosa. *Obesity*. 2010;18(11):2227–2233.
74. Toomey CM, McCormack WG, Jakeman P. The effect of hydration status on the measurement of lean tissue mass by dual-energy X-ray absorptiometry. *Eur J Appl Physiol*. 2017;117:567–574.
75. Cruz-Jentoft AJ, Bahat G, Bauer J, et al. Sarcopenia: revised European consensus on definition and diagnosis. *Age Ageing*. 2019;48(1):16–31. doi:10.1093/ageing/afy169 [Erratum in: *Age Ageing*. 2019;48(4):601. doi:10.1093/ageing/afz046]
76. Messina C, Albano D, Gitto S, et al. Body composition with dual energy X-ray absorptiometry: from basics to new tool. *Quant Imaging Med Surg*. 2020;10(8):1687–1698. doi:10.21037/qims.2020.03.02
77. Bea JW, Chen Z, Blew RM, et al. MRI based validation of abdominal adipose tissue measurements from DXA in postmenopausal women. *J Clin Densit*. 2022;25(2):189–197.
78. Ohliger MA. Body composition at CT and risk of future disease. *Radiology*. 2023;306(2):e222162. doi:10.1148/radiol.222162
79. Lacoste Jeanson A, Dupej J, Villa C, Brůžek J. Body composition estimation from selected slices: equations computed from a new semi-automatic thresholding method developed on whole-body CT scans. *PeerJ*. 2017;5:e3302.
80. Chianca V, Albano D, Messina C, et al. Sarcopenia: imaging assessment and clinical application. *Abdom Radiol (NY)*. 2022;47(9):3205–3216. doi:10.1007/s00261-021-03294-3
81. Borga M. MRI adipose tissue and muscle composition analysis-a review of automation techniques. *Br J Radiol*. 2018;91(1089):20180252. doi:10.1259/bjr.20180252
82. Huber FA, Del Grande F, Rizzo S, Guglielmi G, Guggenberger R. MRI in the assessment of adipose tissues and muscle composition: how to use it. *Quant Imaging Med Surg*. 2020;10(8):1636–1649. doi:10.21037/qims.2020.02.06
83. Nordez A, Jolivet E, Südhoff I, Bonneau D, de Guise JA, Skalli W. Comparison of methods to assess quadriceps muscle volume using magnetic resonance imaging. *J Magn Reson Imaging*. 2009;30:1116–1123. doi:10.1002/jmri.21867
84. Faron A, Sprinkart AM, Kuetting DLR, et al. Body composition analysis using CT and MRI: intra-individual intermodal comparison of muscle mass and myosteatosis. *Sci Rep*. 2020;10(1):11765. doi:10.1038/s41598-020-68797-3
85. Smith-Ryan AE, Blue MNM, Trexler ET, Hirsch KR. Utility of ultrasound for body fat assessment: validity and reliability compared to a multicompartment criterion. *Clin Physiol Funct Imaging*. 2018;38(2):220–226. doi:10.1111/cpf.12402
86. Fazzini B, Märkl T, Costas C, et al. The rate and assessment of muscle wasting during critical illness: a systematic review and meta-analysis. *Crit Care*. 2023;27(1):2. doi:10.1186/s13054-022-04253-0
87. Dresen E, Weißbrich C, Fimmers R, Putensen C, Stehle P. Medical high-protein nutrition therapy and loss of muscle mass in adult ICU patients: a randomized controlled trial. *Clin Nutr*. 2021;40(4):1562–1570. doi:10.1016/j.clnu.2021.02.021
88. Miclos-Balica M, Muntean P, Schick F, et al. Reliability of body composition assessment using A-mode ultrasound in a heterogeneous sample. *Eur J Clin Nutr*. 2021;75(3):438–445. doi:10.1038/s41430-020-00743-y
89. Hendrickson N, Davison J, Schiller L, Willey M. Reliability and validity of A-mode ultrasound to quantify body composition. *J Orthop Trauma*. 2019;33(9):472–477. doi:10.1097/BOT.0000000000001498
90. Chandler AJ, Cintineo HP, Sanders DJ, et al. Agreement between B-mode ultrasound and air displacement plethysmography in preprofessional ballet dancers. *Med Sci Sports Exerc*. 2021;53(3):653–657. doi:10.1249/MSS.0000000000002489

CHAPTER 4

Enteral Nutrition Therapy

Nusheen Garrison
Kathy Prelack

CHAPTER OUTLINE

CORE CONCEPTS

1. Enteral nutrition includes food, oral supplements, and formulas created specifically to prevent malnutrition and accommodate nutrient needs in various disease states.
2. A patient's specific disease state and anticipated length of feeding time determine the route of enteral nutrition.
3. Gastric feeding more closely mimics how the gastrointestinal tract functions physiologically, which offers a metabolic and lifestyle benefit.
4. Small bowel feedings are recommended for patients with gastric complications, gastroparesis, or increased aspiration risk.
5. The feeding–fasting environment associated with bolus feeding induces a favorable hormonal and nutrient response that promotes protein synthesis and anabolism.
6. Enteral nutrition formulas include carbohydrate, fat, protein, vitamins, minerals, and fiber, and are nutritionally complete.
7. Disease-specific formulas that deviate from standard formulations can be used in many disease states to aid patients in meeting their nutritional needs.
8. Patients must be monitored closely for complications related to enteral feeding or side effects to medical treatment. Feeding method and formula should be adjusted as needed.

LEARNING OBJECTIVES

1. Explain the evolution of today's enteral nutrition.
2. Identify a patient's enteral nutrition route based on the current disease state and anticipated length of feeding time.
3. Explore the various short-term and long-term tube placements.
4. Describe the types of tubes and devices available for tube feeding.
5. State the advantages and disadvantages of gastric versus small bowel feeding.
6. Identify three different formula delivery methods.
7. Describe the standard composition of enteral formulas.
8. Explain characteristics of specialty formulas and indications for their use.
9. Recognize complications associated with enteral nutrition and strategies to manage them.

Introduction

Enteral nutrition (EN) refers to the delivery of nutrients into the gastrointestinal (GI) tract either by mouth or through a feeding tube. EN includes food, oral supplements, and formulas created specifically to prevent malnutrition and accommodate nutrient needs in various disease states.[1,2] The development of EN has transformed nutritional care in a hospital setting, where the inability to receive adequate nutrition by normal means is common. Obstacles to oral intake have many causes, including GI disease, swallowing inabilities, or increased nutrient needs related to critical illness or wound healing.[3] The use of EN to target specific immune-related and physiologic processes and alter the course of disease is an exciting aspect of EN support that is supported by a robust research platform.

The Evolution of Enteral Nutrition

Enteral nutrition has a long history that dates back to the early 20th century. The first nasoduodenal tube was placed in 1910 and had a formula of raw egg, milk, and lactose.[4] In 1918, the first reported jejunal feeding took place using a formula of peptonized milk, dextrose, and whiskey.[4] It was not until the 1950s that the first commercial formulas were used.[4] It was at this time that flexible polyethylene tubes were developed as well. The 1970s brought increased food technology, including the formulation of more synthetic tube feeds (TFs). Low-residue and lactose-free TFs were developed, as well as TFs with a range of osmolalities.

In the 1980s, EN resurged and became more clinically formalized to support nutrition and digestion, aid wound healing, help the immune system, and support the critically ill.[5] Around this time, the first **percutaneous endoscopic gastrostomy (PEG) tube** was placed.[6,7] Tube placement capabilities became more advanced, and TF products proliferated. Formula began to be fortified with fiber, predigested to include di- and tripeptides, and enhanced to be more calorically dense. Product developers soon began to create more specialized formulas specific to certain diseases.

EN technology continued to advance in the 1990s. The potential pharmacologic role of micronutrients in modulating cellular and systemic physiology demonstrated a clear connection among disease, inflammation, and nutrient metabolism. The era of **immunonutrition**, marked by the predominance of specialty formulas enhanced with glutamine, arginine, and omega-3 fatty acids, had arrived. Research on the safety and efficacy of these formulas in altering the progression of disease, at times lagging industrial gains, continues to help guide the appropriate use of these immune-enhancing enteral products.

CORE CONCEPT 1

Enteral nutrition includes food, oral supplements, and formulas created specifically to prevent malnutrition and accommodate nutrient needs in various disease states.

Determining the Route of Enteral Nutrition

Determining the site and route of EN should consider an individual's anticipated length of feeding time; their medical condition or disease state, including anatomical barriers within the GI tract; and the surgical options for that individual (**Figure 4.1**).

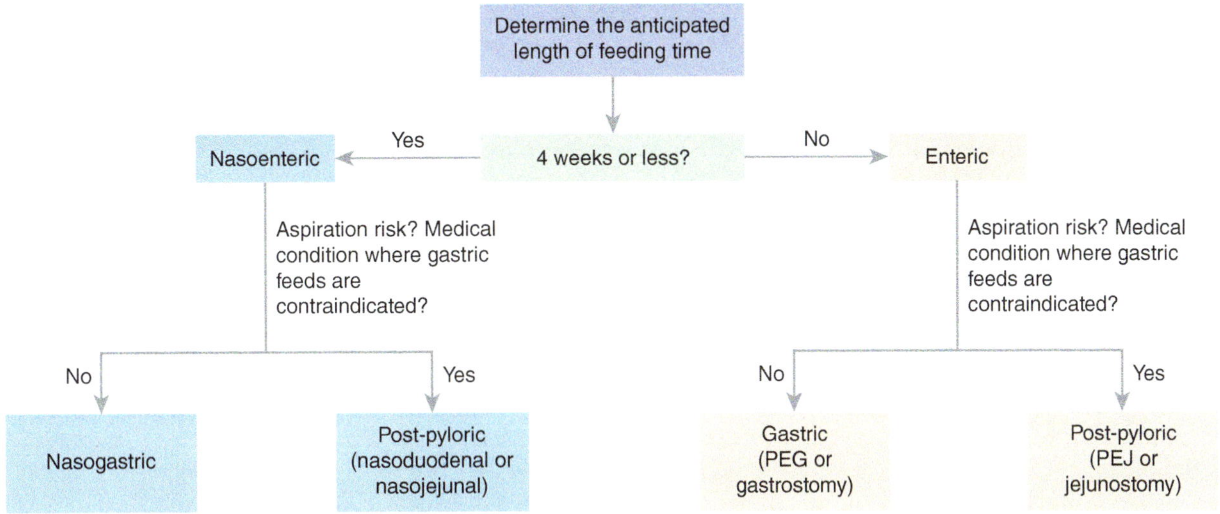

Figure 4.1 Algorithm for Selection of Feeding Tube Placement

Data from Gorman RC, Morris JB. Minimally invasive access to the gastrointestinal tract. In: Rombeau JL, Rolandelli RH, eds. *Clinical Nutrition: Enteral and Tube Feeding*. 3rd ed. Philadelphia, PA: WB Saunders; 1997.

The timing of enteral delivery is determined according to several considerations. First is the anticipated duration of enteral support. If a person is expected to require short-term tube feeding, generally 4 weeks or fewer, then a **nasoenteric** or **oroenteric** tube may be used.[1,8] Nasoenteric or oroenteric feeds require that a tube be placed in the nose or mouth and advanced into the stomach or past the pylorus. Nasoenteric tubes are used more often than oroenteric tubes for short-term feeding because they are better tolerated by the patient. If a person is in need of long-term nutrition care, or nutrition care lasting for longer than 4 weeks, then a more permanent gastrostomy or jejunostomy method is used.[2,8,9] A patient's specific needs or GI function determines the specific enteral route, as presented in **Figure 4.2**.

CORE CONCEPT 2

A patient's specific disease state and anticipated length of feeding time determine the route of enteral nutrition.

PRACTICE POINT

If a patient requires tube feeding for 4 weeks or fewer, utilize a nasoenteric tube. If a patient requires significantly more than 4 weeks of nutrition care, a gastric or postpyloric percutaneous tube placement can be considered.

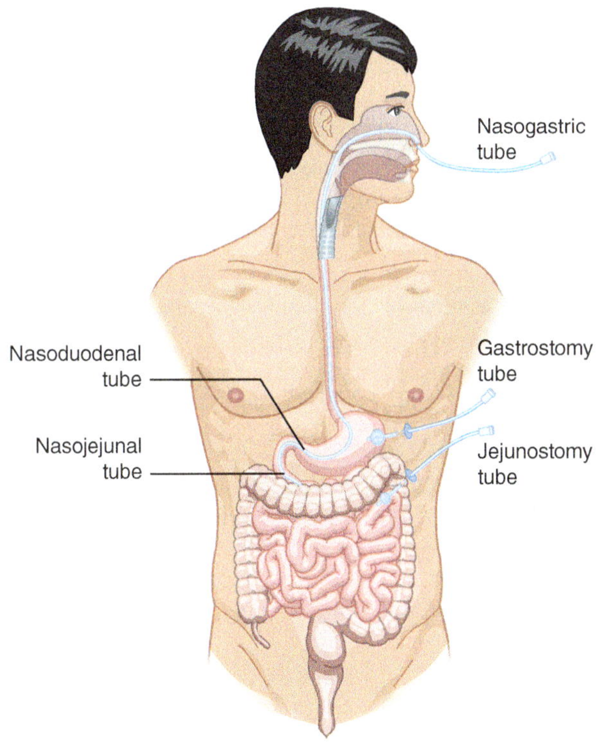

Figure 4.2 Basic Tube Placement Options

Short-Term Placement

As mentioned, for patients who need short-term feeding, a nasoenteric or oroenteric method is used.[1,8,10–12] Nasoenteric tubes can be placed at the bedside, endoscopically, or fluoroscopically. **Nasogastric tube** placement is appropriate for patients who have normal gastric function. A tube enters through the nose

CASE STUDY INTRODUCTION

Laura is a 58-year-old female admitted to the hospital following a motor vehicle accident. She is planned for cranial facial surgery to repair her broken jaw. A feeding tube will be placed as Laura will be NPO for 3 weeks while her jaw heals. Laura was well nourished prior to her injury. Laura lives with her husband. She has two adult children, and her oldest daughter is a nurse and lives nearby.

Anthropometric Data:

Height: 149 cm
Weight: 69 kg
Body mass index: 31 kg/m^2

Weight History
Usual weight: 69 kg

Biochemical Data:

Sodium 140 (133–145 mEq/L)
Potassium 4.7 (3.5–5.0 mEq/L)
Chloride 101 (96–106 mEq/L)
Carbon dioxide 23 (22–31 mEq/L)
Blood urea nitrogen 21 (8–20 mg/dL)
Creatinine 0.5 (0.7–1.3 mg/dL)
Glucose 101 (70–139 mg/dL)
Hemoglobin 11.1 (12.0–15.5 g/dL)
Hematocrit 30 (35–42%)

Calcium 8.7 (8.5–10.5 mg/dL)
Phosphorus 4.0 (2.5–4.5 mg/dL)
Magnesium 1.6 (1.5–2.7 mg/dL)
Total protein 6.0 (6.4–8.3 g/dL)
Albumin 3.2 (3.5–5.5 g/dL)

Clinical Data:

Past Medical History: Gastroesophageal reflux
Medications: None
Vital Signs: Blood pressure 155/77 mm Hg, Temperature 99.0°C, Heart rate 98 beats/min
Nutrition-Focused Physical Exam: Patient appears tired. Abdominal exam within normal limits. Skin, hair, nail and oral exam appear normal. Patient noted to have adequate fat and muscle stores. No edema noted.

Dietary Data:

Dietary History: Laura typically has a good appetite. "I tend to eat healthy. I typically eat 3 meals per day and an afternoon snack. I last had a meal yesterday evening."

24-Hour Diet Recall:

Breakfast: Coffee (cream and sugar), oatmeal with honey, or fruit with yogurt
Lunch: Turkey on whole grain bread with mustard, chocolate chip cookies, diet soda
Afternoon snack: fruit (apple or banana) with a handful of nuts
Dinner: Salmon, rice pilaf, garden salad, glass of wine
Diet Prescription: NPO (nothing by mouth). Nutrition consult is placed for suggestion for enteral tube feeding recommendation.

Questions

1. What are Laura's nutritional risk factors?
2. Specify the enteral feeding placement (NG, PEG, NJ, J-tube), formula type (intact, semi-elemental, elemental), and method of delivery (continuous, intermittent, bolus). Explain your rationale.
3. Write two Problem/Etiology/Signs and Symptoms (PES) statements for Laura identifying Laura's active issues.
4. Identify the interventions you would like to initiate for Laura to address the problems identified in your PES statements.
5. What indices should be included in your monitoring and evaluation plan to be sure your tube feed intervention is working?

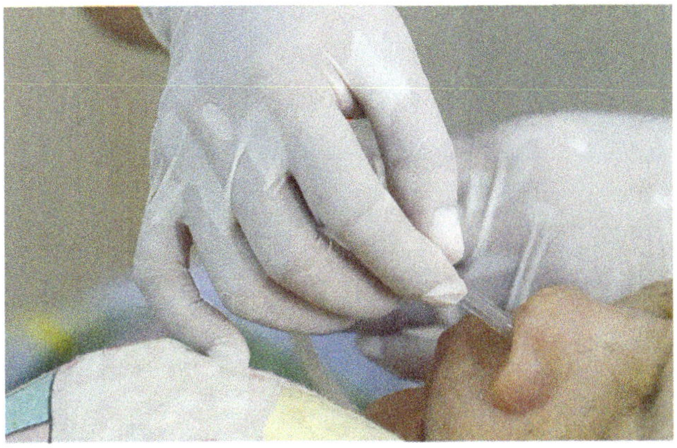

Figure 4.3 Insertion of Nasoenteric Feeding Tube

or mouth and is placed directly into the stomach. Postpyloric placement of nasoenteric tubes is used if a patient has gastric complications or aspiration risk but otherwise normal small intestine function. **Nasoduodenal tube** feeding requires the tube be placed from the nose, through the stomach, to the duodenum of the small intestine, and **nasojejunal tube** feedings require that the tube is placed from the nose and advanced to the jejunum of the small intestine. While nasogastric tubes can usually be placed at the bedside, nasojejunal tubes are better placed with endoscopic or fluoroscopic methods.[10,11]

Bedside Nasoenteral Technique

The bedside nasogastric tube placement begins by obtaining a small-bore tube, about 8–12 French (1 French [Fr] is equal to 0.33 mm in diameter). A large-bore tube can also be used and is thought to prevent clogging; however, if feeding is to resume for greater than 5–7 days, the small-bore tube can be more comfortable for the patient.[13] The length of the tube is determined by first measuring the distance from the patient's nose to the earlobe, and then from the earlobe to the xiphoid.[14] The patient lies on their right side and, as air is insufflated, the tube is bent and slowly enters through the patient's nose (**Figure 4.3**).

Prokinetics, which are medications that promote motility by increasing small intestine contractions (such as metoclopramide and erythromycin), are often used to facilitate this technique.[15,16] Auscultation, pH monitoring, and aspiration of gastric content have been used to assess whether the nasoenteric tube is placed correctly; however, these are not foolproof. For blind bedside feeding tube placements (although generally not recommended unless it is the only option), radiographic confirmation of tip location is necessary. This can be done via chest x-ray or kidney ureter bladder (KUB) x-ray, which visualizes the gastric body.[11,13,17,18] For postpyloric nasoenteric tube placement, electromagnetically guided feeding tubes have the advantage of being able to immediately confirm tube placement or identify tube misplacement so that the tube can be adjusted. Not only does this alleviate the need for an additional chest x-ray, it also allows for feedings to be initiated sooner.[19] If an electromagnetic imaging system is not available, a CT of the abdomen and pelvis area can visualize the small intestine and confirm placement. Camera-assisted feeding tubes allow for placement of the tube to be visualized in real time (**Figure 4.4**). This newly emerged technique provides direct visualization of bronchial structures and immediate removal of the feeding tube if incorrectly placed. Feeding tube misplacements can lead to serious complications such as pneumothorax, vocal cord injury, bronchial fistula, and death. These technologies help ensure safety by lowering the risk of complications.[20,21] One disadvantage of nasoenteric tubes is that they can be easily dislodged. One safeguard to prevent dislodgement of a nasoenteric tube is the use of a nasal bridle (**Figure 4.5**).

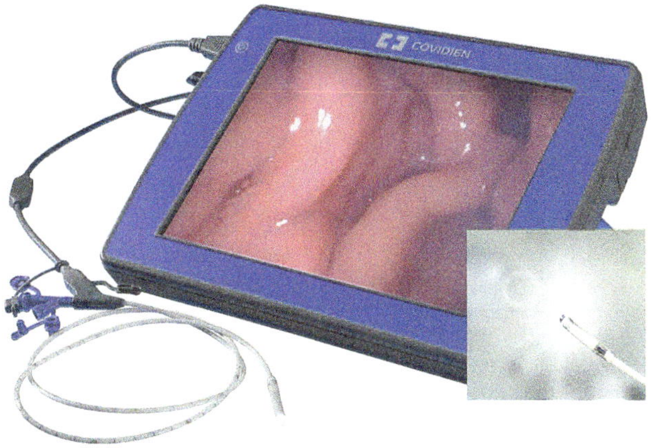

Figure 4.4 Integrated Realtime Imaging System (IRIS) Tube Placement from Anatomical Structures That Were Reliably Visible

Endoscopic Nasoenteral Technique

Nasoduodenal and nasojejunal tube placements are most easily done by endoscopic insertion. A drag and pull technique is often utilized, where a suture is placed at the end of the nasoenteric tube and pushed with the tube from the patient's nostril to the stomach. Meanwhile, an endoscope, with forceps, is advanced orally to the stomach. In the stomach, the endoscopic forceps take hold of the nasoenteric tube and suture, and the entire unit then enters the duodenum, or even the jejunum, if possible.

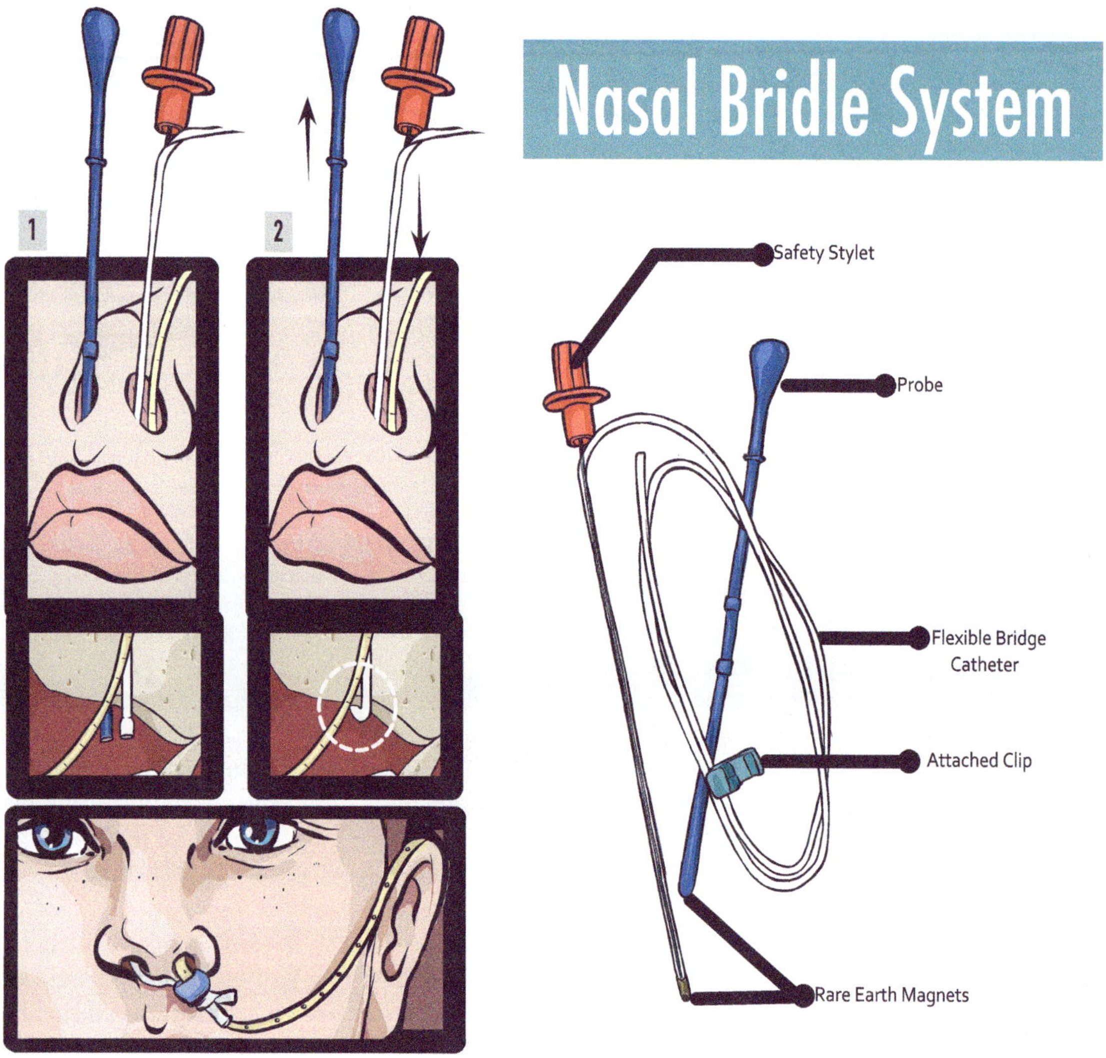

Figure 4.5 Nasal Bridle

In the small intestine, the forceps release the tube and the endoscope retracts. Many studies suggest that there is greater placement success if the tube is placed after the ligament of Treitz. With endoscopic aid, the nasoenteral tube is now properly placed in the small intestine.

Another endoscopic nasoenteral technique involves pushing an endoscope all the way to the small intestine with a guidewire to allow tube entry. The guidewire is pushed through the transnasal channel with the endoscope and then remains in the small intestine while the endoscope is removed. The feeding tube is advanced over the guidewire to ultimately be placed in the small intestine through the same passage.[11,13,17]

Fluoroscopic Nasoenteric Technique

Fluoroscopic nasoenteric tube placement involves using x-ray imaging as a guide when placing the feeding tube from the nose to the stomach or small intestine. While there is success with this technique, it is not used as often as the bedside or endoscopic techniques because of radiation exposure or if the patient requires bedside attention due to critical illness.[22,23]

PRACTICE POINT

Nasogastric tubes are commonly placed at the patient's bedside. Nasoduodenal and nasojejunal tubes are more easily placed using endoscopic, and less commonly, fluoroscopic methods.

Long-Term Placement

Percutaneous Endoscopic Gastrostomy Technique

Percutaneous endoscopic gastrostomy is the most common long-term tube placement method and can be performed at the bedside. In what is called

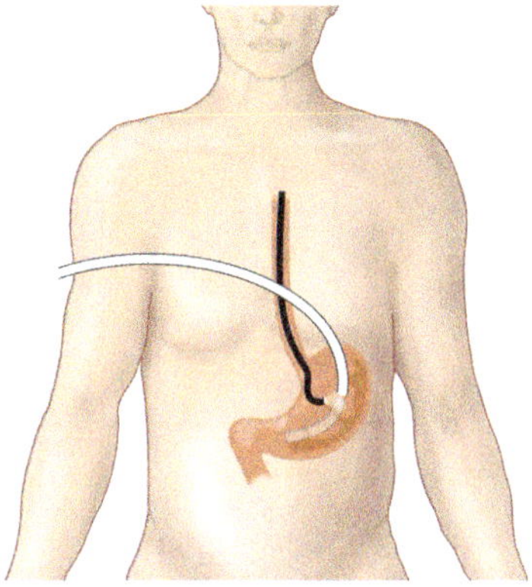

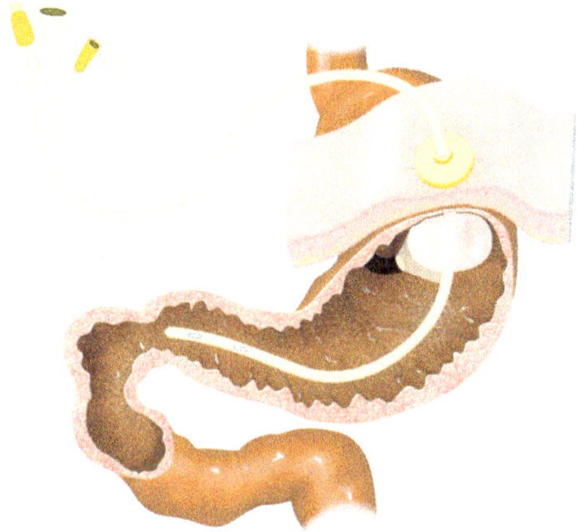

Figure 4.6 Percutaneous Endoscopic Gastrostomy Is the Most Common Long-Term Tube Placement Method and Can Be Performed at the Bedside

the "pull technique," an endoscope is placed into the abdomen (**Figure 4.6**). Air is insufflated into the abdomen through the endoscope. The abdomen is then transilluminated to find the optimal spot for the tube placement, and an indentation is placed on that spot. After a small incision is made, a needle is placed through the abdominal wall and into the stomach so that a guidewire can be placed through the needle. An endoscopic snare is attached to the needle. The endoscope, needle, and snare are pulled back through the mouth, and the feeding tube is attached to the guidewire or placed over the guidewire. The guidewire and tube are then pulled back through the esophagus and to the stomach. The tube is internally held in place by a bumper. An external bumper also ensures secure gastronomic placement.

Percutaneous Endoscopic Jejunostomy Technique

If the patient has gastric complications, a **percutaneous endoscopic jejunostomy (PEJ)** can be performed.

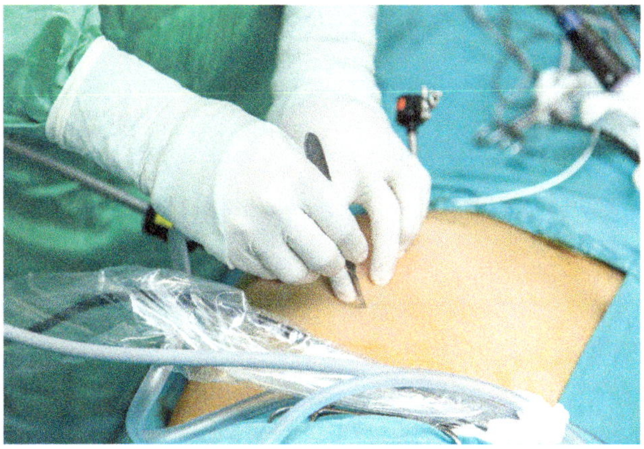

Figure 4.7 Laparoscopic Surgery Can Be Used for Gastrostomy Placement

If there is an existing gastrostomy tube, a transpyloric feeding tube can be placed through the previously placed PEG tube and placed endoscopically into the jejunum.[21]

Another way of performing this procedure is to place the tube directly into the small bowel. The technique is similar to the PEG method, except the guidewire and tube are placed endoscopically into the jejunum.[6,23,24]

Surgical Methods

If a patient is in a traumatic condition or is undergoing surgery, a surgical means of tube placement may be used. This can be done in an open tube procedure or with laparoscopy under general anesthesia (**Figure 4.7**). In **laparoscopy**, small ports are placed on the abdominal wall so that the peritoneal cavity can be accessed. Once a camera and second port are placed, the stomach is attached to the abdominal wall by use of small structures called "T-fasteners." A needle and wire can then be placed into the stomach lumen so that a gastrostomy tube can finally be placed.[23]

In the **open tube placement** technique, a small incision is made on the abdomen so that the gastrostomy tube can enter. Sutures are placed to fasten the stomach around the feeding tube, as well as to fasten the stomach to the top of the abdominal wall. Jejunostomy tubes can also be entered via open and laparoscopic techniques. A similar procedure is used to access the small bowel.[23]

Types of Enteral Tubes

Feeding tubes have developed over time to become more comfortable for the patient and experience less clogging and other malfunctions. Nasogastric tubes made of polyvinyl chloride are more rigid and allow simple access. They can also be used for gastric suctioning and administering medications. Currently, most nasoenteric tubes are composed of polyurethane or silicone.[25–27] Polyurethane tubes are more pliable than polyvinyl chloride tubes and cause less nasopharyngeal erosion, which gives greater comfort to the patient. The structure of these tubes also makes it more difficult for a patient to aspirate, mitigating feeding complications. Silicone tubes are also flexible, more so than polyurethane, and therefore more comfortable for the patient. Nasoenteric tubes are generally sized 8–12 Fr.[26] For PEG tube placements, polyurethane and silicone tubes can be used, although silicone tubes tend to be used more often. PEG tubes are generally sized 15–28 Fr in diameter.[26]

Gastric Versus Small Bowel Feeding

There are certain indications that might prompt a clinician to initiate gastric versus postpyloric feeding in a patient. Both types have advantages and disadvantages that will be discussed further in this section.

Gastric Feeding

If normal gastric function is presumed, then gastric feedings are generally used. One advantage of gastric feedings is that they are more physiologic. The stomach acts as a natural reservoir for nutrients, so gastric placement of the feeding tube more closely mimics how the body receives nutrients.[12] It also allows for intermittent and bolus feeds, which have both metabolic and lifestyle benefits. Bolus intragastric feeding more closely resembles how the GI tract functions physiologically, allowing contents to slowly empty into the small bowel.[12] The hydrochloric acid in the stomach also allows certain nutrients to be properly absorbed. Large-bore gastric tubes have less clogging than the small-bore tubes used in small bowel feeding.[28,29] In addition, there is more ease to gastric tube placement; there are usually fewer attempts to place the tube correctly, and it can be done at bedside.[28,29] This usually makes gastric feeding more cost-effective than small bowel feeding.[29] Lastly, the ease of bolus feedings has considerable lifestyle benefits. Incorporating bolus feedings on a routine schedule limits the amount of time the patient needs to be connected to a feeding pump, allowing more flexibility for the patient.

Certain disadvantages also exist for gastric feeding. There can be several procedure-related feeding interruptions or other forms of intolerance.[28] A commonly cited risk is **aspiration**, or the movement of liquid into the patient's lungs.[28–30] Aspiration risk with continuous nasogastric feeding can lead to nosocomial (hospital-acquired) pneumonia.[12,28–30] Those who are at risk of aspiration include patients who are neurologically impaired, have experienced severe trauma, have had a surgical operation, are heavily sedated, or have **gastroparesis** (delayed gastric emptying) due to a metabolic condition or operation.[28] In these cases, it may be more suitable to utilize small bowel feeding.[28,29]

Clinical Roundtable

Topic: Overcoming Barriers to Enteral Feeding

Background: One challenge to enteral feeding in a critical care setting is the need for interruption due to clinical interventions and procedures such as operating room visits, high-risk dressing changes, and extubation from a ventilator. Various strategies are employed to compensate for the energy and nutrient deficits associated with these procedures. Included among these are use of postpyloric feedings through the procedures, intermittent parenteral feedings during NPO phases, and volume-based feedings that increase the volume of feeding prior to and after procedures to assure an adequate amount of feedings. Each of these strategies is associated with some degree of risk related to intolerance of feedings, aspiration, infection (in the case of PN), or hyperglycemia.

Roundtable Discussion

Discuss the pros and cons of these approaches. Are there certain patient populations that might benefit more from one approach or another? How does placement of feeding tube and central venous catheter access affect your decision?

References

1. Holyk A, Belden V, Sirimaturos M, Chiles K, Fontenot N, Lista A, Broadway MK, Leon RS. Volume-based feeding enhances enteral delivery by maximizing the optimal rate of enteral feeding (FEED MORE). *JPEN*. 2020;44(6):1038-1046. doi:10.1002/jpen.1727.
2. Varon DE, Freitas G, Goel N, et al. Intraoperative feeding improves calorie and protein delivery in acute burn patients. *J Burn Care Res*. 2017;38(5):299-303. doi:10.1097/BCR.0000000000000514

CORE CONCEPT 3

Gastric feeding more closely mimics how the gastrointestinal tract physiologically functions, which offers a metabolic and lifestyle benefit.

Small Bowel Feeding

For small bowel feeding, placement can be in either the duodenum or jejunum. While duodenal placement allows for more volume and absorptive capacity, jejunal placement assures low aspiration risk (less likely for tube to be dislodged or pulled up to stomach). Duodenal or jejunal feeding may be preferred if a patient has gastroparesis or reflux, or is diagnosed with aspiration risk.[28,30] It may also accommodate issues with early satiety. For long-term small bowel feedings such as percutaneous endoscopic or surgically placed feeding tubes, the tube is placed in the jejunum.

Small bowel feedings afford an important advantage for patients who may have gastric complications or gastroparesis.[28] They decrease the risk of microaspiration, as well as of aspiration pneumonia.[28–30] Some studies demonstrate that small bowel feedings allow patients to achieve a goal rate of infusion that may have not been attained with gastric feedings, providing a means of adequate nutrition.[28] It has also been observed that small bowel feedings lead to decreased commencement of parenteral nutrition (PN). The benefit of being able to provide small bowel feedings through clinical procedures has contributed to this decreased reliance on PN. Postpyloric feedings are now often continued during clinical interventions requiring anesthesia, either at the bedside or in the operating room. Major advancements in practice have led in some cases to intraoperative feedings, where EN is continuously provided throughout an operation. This practice has proven to be safe and effective in minimizing the energy and protein deficits that normally take place during planned surgeries.[31]

There is an increased cost associated with using small bowel feedings, especially when using x-rays in fluoroscopy. Often, multiple attempts are needed to place the feeding tube correctly due to dislodgment of the feeding tube, and this can also be costly. Because it lacks holding capacity, the small intestine tends to be more sensitive to volume and osmotic load, so small bowel feedings can lead to symptoms similar to **dumping syndrome**, a condition that causes rapid gastric emptying.[12] In this condition, food and liquid move from the stomach to the small intestine too quickly, causing abdominal pain and diarrhea shortly after a meal or feeding. Another disadvantage to small bowel feedings is that bolus or large-volume intermittent feeding cannot be provided due to lack of a reservoir.

CORE CONCEPT 4

Small bowel feedings are recommended for patients with gastric complications, gastroparesis, or increased aspiration risk.

Formula Delivery Methods

There are several ways of delivering formula to ensure the patient is receiving adequate nutrition. Whether continuous, intermittent, or bolus feedings are used depends upon the location of the feeding tube, the patient's GI function and history of tolerance, and lifestyle considerations. Formula can be delivered to a patient via two systems. In a **closed tube feeding system**, a ready-to-use container or bag of formula is connected to the patient's feeding access.[25,32] In an **open tube feeding system**, formula from a can or package is poured into a separate container that is then attached to the patient's feeding access point.[25,32] A closed system product can safely be at room temperature for 24–48 hours, whereas an open system product should be at room temperature for no more than 4-8 hours, depending upon the formula hanging.[25,32] This is known as the **hang time**. Reconstituted formulas should hang for no more than 4 hours while sterile decanted formula has an 8-hour hang time (except for neonates).[25,32] Clinicians may also wish to limit hang time for certain high-risk populations, such as patients with burns or those who are immunocompromised. While closed tube feeding systems are preferred from an infection control standpoint, at times open tube feeding systems are used when modular components are needed to enhance protein or calories specific to the patient's requirements.

Continuous

Continuous feeding is a common delivery method used for hospitalized patients. This method provides a slow infusion of formula into the stomach or small intestine on an hourly basis, typically with a feeding pump (**Figure 4.8**). This method decreases risk for aspiration and gastric distention.[1] It tends to be the most easily tolerated because of its gradual delivery of formula, and it allows for greater nutrient uptake in patients who may have marginal absorptive capacity. Continuous feeding is often selected for patients with GI complications or severe trauma to assure better tolerance,

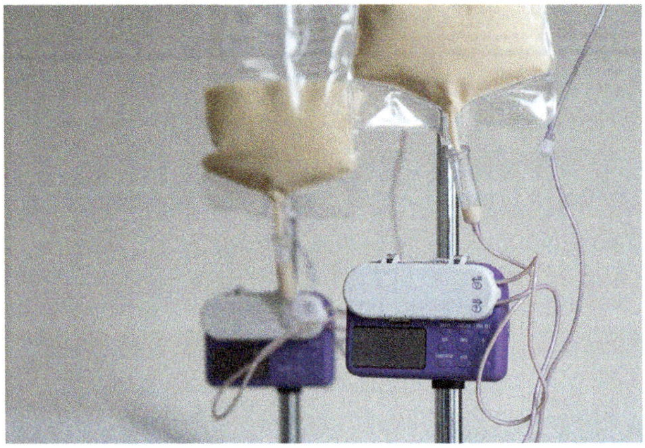

Figure 4.8 Continuous Delivery via an Enteral Feeding Pump Is the Most Common Form of Tube Feeding Administration in Hospitalized Patients

although this remains debated.[33] Despite a lack of evidence-based protocols for tube feeding advancement, conventional therapy consists of a moderate-to-low volume at initiation, followed by gradual advancement while continuously monitoring patient tolerance. Typically, continuous feeds begin at 20 mL/hour for adults. Once the patient demonstrates tolerance, the feeding rate advances incrementally. This rate increases by about 10–25 mL/hour every 4–24 hours until the goal rate is achieved.

Volume-Based Feeding

Interruption of enteral feeding, particularly in a critical care environment, is a common problem that can lead to underfeeding and malnutrition. Daily clinical interventions often require that continuous, rate-based feeds be stopped for reasons of safety, to accommodate therapeutic interventions, or elective bedside procedures. Also, drug–nutrient interactions may require that EN feeds are halted for several hours during the administration of certain medications.

It is typical that patients do not meet 100% of their goal requirement.[34] Volume-based feeding protocols can significantly improve calorie and protein intake in these instances. The basic premise is that delivery of feedings is based on a total volume as opposed to an hourly rate of continuous infusion. Typically, the nurse can adjust the hourly rate of delivery to accommodate interruption of feeding and provide a "catch-up" rate. Consideration must be given to patient tolerance of higher hourly volumes; however, these protocols have proven to be safe and effective.[34,35]

Here is an example of a volume-based feeding approach. A 50-kg female requiring 1800 calories is prescribed a 1 kcal/mL enteral formula. The total daily volume of feeding required is 1800 mL. The goal hourly rate for a continuous infusion would be 75 mL/hour to meet the patient's requirement. Assume the feedings must be held for 4 hours during medication administration. With 20 hours (vs. 24 hours) to receive full volume, the hourly rate can be adjusted temporarily to meet the goal volume: 1800 mL/20 hours = 90 mL/hour. A benefit of volume-based feeding is that the nurse can adjust the rate to ensure total daily volumes are met.

Intermittent

With **intermittent feeding**, formula is delivered over a 20- to 60-minute interval, 4–6 times per day.[1] The duration and timing of intervals depend upon the amount of formula needed to attain adequate nutrition. Intermittent feeding can be administered using an infusion pump or by using the gravity drip method. Intermittent feeding provides the benefit of cyclic elevation of insulin levels. The rise in insulin in response to feeding creates an anabolic environment that promotes protein synthesis and improved protein nutritional status.[36]

Bolus Feedings

In **bolus feedings**, a specific volume of formula is delivered over a short period of time a certain number of times per day.[1] An example feeding regimen would be rapid delivery of 240–480 mL of formula over approximately 15–30 minutes, 3–6 times per day.[1] Bolus feedings provide the benefit of mimicking normal eating.[1,12] Hormonal response to a feeding–fasting regimen is more anabolic than that observed with continuous feedings, resulting in increased amino acid and insulin levels and ultimately improved protein synthesis.[36] Often, a bolus regimen is preferable for stable patients because it does not rely on pumps and devices as much as the other methods, giving the patient an easier lifestyle (Figure 4.9).[1] While bolus feedings are less commonly used in patients who are critically ill due to presumed risk of aspiration pneumonia and issues with tolerance, studies do not consistently support this notion, even in high-risk patients. This method of feeding,

CORE CONCEPT 5

The feeding–fasting environment associated with bolus feeding induces a favorable hormonal and nutrient response that promotes protein synthesis and anabolism.

CASE STUDY REVISITED

A nasogastric feeding tube was successfully placed for enteral feedings. A nutrition consult is written for initiation of enteral feedings in 24 hours. Her estimated energy and protein requirements based on your nutrition standard of care for moderate stress are as follows:

Energy: 1755 kcal/day (Mifflin–St Jeor × 1.5 using admission weight)
Protein: 83 g protein/day (1.2 g/kg)

Questions

1. What formula would you recommend? (Choose from: Jevity 1.2, Peptamen 1.5, Vivonex RTF.)
2. Provide a recommendation for an EN formula type, including goal volume, method of delivery (continuous vs. bolus), and guidelines for initiation and advancement. What would the goal tube feed regimen provide (kcal, protein)?

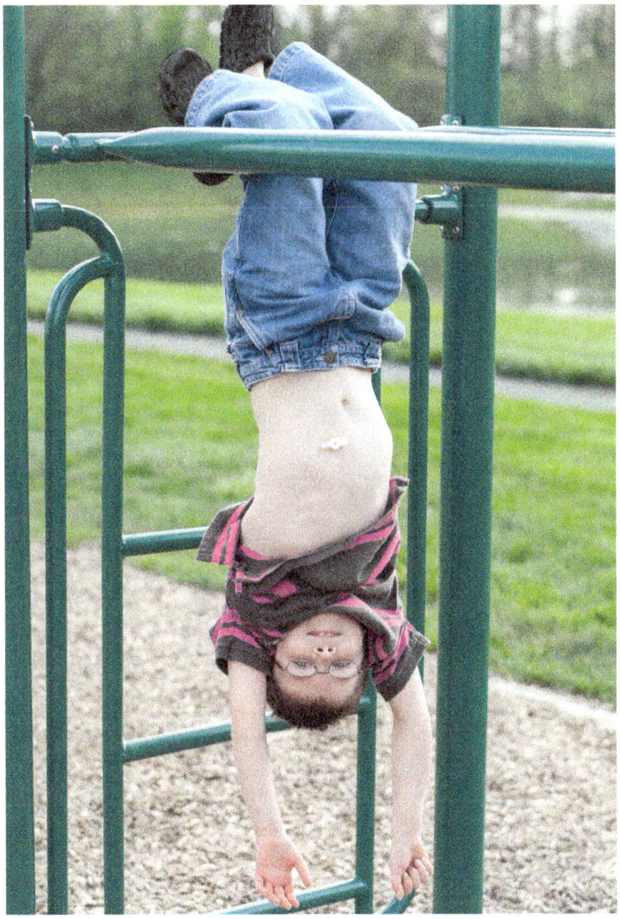

Figure 4.9 Bolus Tube Feedings Provide Lifestyle Benefit of Feeding from the Feeding Pump

when compared to continuous feeding in adult patients who are critically ill, is equally well tolerated with no difference in gastroesophageal reflux, aspiration, aspiration pneumonia, glycemic variability, or time to reach calorie goal.[33]

Enteral Formula Compositions

A clinician must determine a formula that will meet a patient's nutrient needs. Many different standard formulas exist that are strategic compilations of carbohydrate, fat, protein, fiber, prebiotics and probiotics, vitamins, minerals, and water. Formulas for individuals with impaired digestion, also known as "predigested," "semi-elemental," or "elemental" formulas, are available as well. Additionally, certain EN feedings are created for patients with specific diseases and conditions, such as diabetes, severe wounds, or complications with kidney, pulmonary, or liver function. Lastly, immune-enhancing feedings are available for the critically ill and patients with altered metabolism. **Table 4.1** displays various EN products categorized by composition and indication for use.

Tables 4.2 and **4.3** provide the nutrient composition of standard polymeric formulas and products used for patients with impaired digestion. The general nutritional content of these is similar; however, for those with impaired digestion, simpler or easier to digest forms of carbohydrate, protein, and fat are provided.

Carbohydrates

Carbohydrates are the primary energy source of enteral formulas. They generally comprise 40–90% of the formula.[37] Carbohydrate sources include monosaccharides such as glucose or fructose, and disaccharides including sucrose and maltose. Lactose is often omitted from enteral feeding products because it requires lactase, which can be insufficient in some

Table 4.1 Types of Tube Feeding Formulas for Adults

Formula	Indication	Examples
Standard	Normal gastrointestinal function and fluid needs, feeding well-tolerated	Osmolite Promote Nutren Replete
Standard with Fiber	Long-term need for tube feeding; diarrhea and/or constipation	Jevity Promote with fiber Nutren with fiber Replete with fiber
Standard-Nutrient Dense (high nitrogen or high calorie)	Increased wound healing	Osmolite 1.2, 1.5 Jevity 1.2, 1.5 Isosource 1.5 Nutren 1.5
Fluid-Restricted	Restricted fluid allowance	Two Cal HN Nutren 2.0
Peptide-Based (partially hydrolyzed whey protein)	Impaired digestion	Peptamen, Peptamen 1.5 w/Prebio Vital Vital 1.5
Amino Acid Based (100% free amino acids)	Impaired digestion	Vivonex T.E.N
Immune-Enhanced	State of stress or trauma	Impact, Oxepa, Pivot
Renal	Kidney dysfunction and restrictions of potassium, phosphorus, and fluid	Nepro, Suplena Novosource Renal
Diabetes	Moderate carbohydrate, fiber enhanced	Glucerna Glytrol Diabetisource
Pulmonary	Moderate-to-low carbohydrate, higher fat content	Pulmocare Nutren Pulmonary
Plant Based	Free of most common allergens (milk, eggs, fish, shellfish, peanuts, wheat, soybeans, sesame	Kate Farms Standard Kate Farms Peptide

Table 4.2 Nutrient Composition of Standard Adult Polymeric Enteral Formulations

Formula Name	Jevity Jevity 1.2 Jevity 1.5	Osmolite Osmolite 1.2 Osmolite 1.5	Promote Promote with Fiber	Nutren 1.0 with Fiber Nutren 1.5	Two Cal HN Nutren 2.0	Kate Farms (KF) Standard
Concentration (kcal/mL)	1.06 1.2 1.5	1.06 1.2 1.5	1.0 1.0	1.0 1.5	2.0 2.0	1.0
Protein g/1000 mL (% kcal)	44.3 (16.7) 55.5 (18.5) 63.8 (17)	44.3 (16.7) 55.5 (18.5) 62.7 (16.7)	62.5 (25) 62.5 (25)	40 (16) 68 (18)	83.5 (16.7) 48 (16)	49 (20)
Carbohydrate g/1000 mL (% kcal)	154.7 (58.3) 169.4 (56.4) 215.7 (57.5)	143.9 (54.3) 157.5 (52.5) 203.6 (54.3)	130 (52) 138.3 (55)	148 (54) 176 (47)	218.5 (43.2) 216 (43)	117 (47)

Formula Name	Jevity Jevity 1.2 Jevity 1.5	Osmolite Osmolite 1.2 Osmolite 1.5	Promote Promote with Fiber	Nutren 1.0 with Fiber Nutren 1.5	Two Cal HN Nutren 2.0	Kate Farms (KF) Standard
Fat g/1000 mL (% kcal)	34.7 (29) 39.3 (29) 49.8 (30)	34.7 (29) 39.3 (29) 49.1 (29)	26 (23) 28.2 (25)	34 (30) 60 (35)	90.5 (40.1) 92 (41)	37(33)
Sodium/ Potassium (mg/1000 mL)	930/1570 1350/1850 1330/2180	930/1570 1067/2274 1400/800	1000/1,980 1300/2100	880/1600 1300/2400	844/2110 1500/2100	800/1692
Calcium/ Phosphorus (mg/1000 mL)	910/760 1200/1200 1200/1200	760/760 1200/1200 1000/1000	1200/1200 1200/1200	800/800 1200/1200	1050/1050 1600/1400	1015/923
Vitamin D (IU/1000 mL)	305 400 400	305 400 400	400 400	400 640	415 800	862
Zinc/Copper (mg/1000 mL)	18/1.6 23/2.0 23/2.0	18/1.6 23/2.0 23/2.0	24/2 24/2	14/1.6 20/2	24/2.1 24/2.4	20/0.9
Selenium (mcg/1000 mL)	54 70 70	54 70 70	70 70	60 80	74 100	46
Osmolality (mOsm/kg H_2O)	300 450 525	244 360 525	405 410	340 530	710 780	400

Table 4.3 Nutrient Composition of Hydrolyzed and Monomeric Enteral Formulations

Formu la Name	Vivonex TEN	Vital	Peptamen	Peptamen 1.5 with Prebio	KF Peptide 1.5
Concentration (kcal/mL)	1.0	1.0	1.0	1.5	1.5
Protein g/1000 mL (% kcal)	38.3 (14)	40 (16)	40 (16)	68 (18)	74(20)
Carbohydrate g/1000 mL (% kcal)	206 (83)	130 (52)	128 (51)	184 (48)	138 (37)
Fat g/1000 mL (% kcal)	3 (3)	38.1 (34)	39.2 (33)	56 (34)	77 (46)
Sodium/Potassium (mg/1000 mL)	617/937	1050/1400	560/1500	880/2080	1077/2149
Calcium/Phosphorus (mg/1000 mL)	500/500	705/705	800/700	1000/1000	1077/923
Vitamin D (IU/1000 mL)	403	280	532	800	862
Zinc/Copper (mg/1000 mL)	11/1.0	21/1.4	24/2.0	22/3.2	18/1.5
Selenium (mcg/1000 mL)	37	56	50	100	58
Osmolality (mOsm/kg H_2O)	630	411	340	570	470

CASE STUDY REVISITED

After a few days, Laura has a difficult time reaching her goal volume tube feeding rate due to abdominal distention and multiple emesis throughout the day. Her EN is currently on hold due to poor tolerance. You are consulted for your recommendation.

Questions

1. What factors may be contributing to Laura's poor tolerance?
2. Assess Laura's original PES statements. Identify if each statement remains an active issue or if the PES statement has been resolved. If the PES statement remains an active issue, has improvement in the issue been noted? If the issue has been resolved, write a new PES statement.

patients, leading to poor tolerance and symptoms of cramping, bloating, and diarrhea.[37]

Other types of carbohydrates incorporated into formula include oligosaccharides and polysaccharides. Oligosaccharides are made of 2–10 glucose units. The most common oligosaccharide used in formula is maltodextrin, which is more soluble than starch and contributes less to the osmolality of the formula than glucose alone. Polysaccharides are made of more than 10 glucose units and include corn syrup solids and cornstarch.

Fats

Fats, or triglycerides, are composed of glycerol and fatty acids. They consist of chains of carbons with a carboxyl group at the end. The chain length influences the feeding tolerance, and the type of chain (such as monounsaturated fatty acids, saturated fatty acids, or polyunsaturated fatty acids) influences a patient's physiology.[37] Lipids are a secondary energy source in formula composition. Common sources of lipids in formulas include corn oil, safflower oil, and coconut oil.[37] In addition to providing energy, lipids are an impor tant component of enteral formulas because they carry fat-soluble vitamins and essential fatty acids that are important for physiologic function. Lipids are also isotonic, which helps lower the osmolality of the formula.

Often, a mixture of long-chain and medium-chain fatty acids is used in enteral formulations. Long-chain fatty acids are carbon chains of 14–24 units. These are cleared slowly from the bloodstream and are preferentially re-esterified and stored as triglycerides. Long-chain fatty acids require carnitine, which aids in the transport of long-chain fatty acids across the mitochondrial membrane for energy production. Long-chain fatty acids are also a source of essential fatty acids, such as linoleic and linolenic fatty acids.

For patients with impaired digestion, absorption, and transport of fats, medium-chain fatty acids can be added to the formula.[34] Medium-chain fatty acids are carbon chains of 6–12 units. Common sources include palm kernel oil and coconut oil. Medium-chain fatty acids are easier to digest because they are absorbed directly into the portal circulation and are not re-esterified into triglycerides. They do not require pancreatic enzymes or bile salts for absorption. They also do not require carnitine for transport across the mitochondrial membrane. Therefore, medium-chain fatty acids are a rapid energy source. However, because medium-chain fatty acids do not provide any essential fatty acids, some long-chain fatty acids are usually concurrently added to make sure the patient meets nutrient needs.[34]

PRACTICE POINT

Medium-chain fatty acids are absorbed directly into the portal system and are easier to digest; however, they do not provide essential fatty acids and so long-chain fatty acids should be provided as well.

Protein

Protein in enteral formulas can come in different forms, depending on what is indicated by the patient's need and medical condition. These forms of protein include intact proteins, hydrolyzed proteins, or free amino acids.[37] Intact proteins are large in size and have limited impact on the osmolality of a formula. They are the original, natural form of the protein, called an **isolate**.[37] Examples of intact proteins include soy isolates, casein or whey protein from milk, albumen from egg white, and pea protein. Intact proteins require normal levels of pancreatic enzymes for adequate digestion. For patients with GI dysfunction or malabsorption issues, semi-elemental or elemental formulations may be used. These include hydrolyzed proteins such as dipeptides, tripeptides, and free amino acids. These types of proteins are enzymatically broken down to smaller particles and increase the osmolality of the formula. The intestine can digest both smaller peptides and free amino acids because they use separate transport systems. Formulas may prefer smaller peptides because they are thought to more efficiently absorb nitrogen, but free amino acids and di- and tripeptides cause less trophic stimulation on the bowel than intact protein.

Vitamins and Minerals

Vitamins and minerals are vital components in enteral formulas. These micronutrients play an important role in the body as essential cofactors and coenzymes that are needed for metabolism and other physiologic functions. Formulas generally have 100% of the recommended dietary allowance (RDA) of each vitamin and mineral at specific volumes. Different metabolic stresses and disease states may require a higher or lower amount of certain micronutrients.

Fiber

Dietary fiber comes in soluble and insoluble forms and is added to some enteral formulas. Fiber is a plant polysaccharide that is indigestible by human digestive enzymes. The formulas that include fiber generally have about 4–14 g/L of total fiber.

Soluble fiber is viscous and found in legumes, oat bran, pectins, and gums. Anaerobic bacteria in the cecum rapidly ferment soluble fiber into short-chain fatty acids. Short-chain fatty acids offer the health benefits of maintaining colonic structure and function. This includes lowering the colonic pH to balance intestinal flora. It also enhances fluid and electrolyte absorption, which may help with diarrhea. Soluble fiber intake is also linked to lower serum cholesterol, as well as improved glucose tolerance. Soluble fiber is important to include in the enteral formulas of patients who have glucose intolerance, have had bowel surgery, or are undergoing antibiotic therapy.

Insoluble fiber is nonviscous and found in the cellulose of plant foods. Insoluble fiber is beneficial because it holds water. This increases bulk in fecal mass and allows softer stools, which helps prevent constipation and is recommended for those undergoing long-term feeding. Insoluble fiber may also be beneficial for patients with diverticulosis, which is when pouches accumulate in the colon.

Prebiotics and Probiotics

Some formulas also include prebiotics and probiotics to promote gut health; however, the benefit of these additions is still under debate. Because outcomes differ per patient and condition, it is currently difficult to make any broad recommendation for prebiotics and probiotics in formula.

Prebiotics are energy sources for the beneficial bacteria in the colon, commonly provided in EN formulas as fiber, fructo-oligosaccharides, and inulin. Soluble fiber can also be administered in modular form as well. Use of modular soluble fiber is helpful in patients with diarrhea. Furthermore, its fermentation to short-chain fatty acids in the colonocyte supports the microbiome while also generating an additional energy source. Prebiotics are generally included with probiotics so that microorganisms can flourish. **Probiotics** are ingested microorganisms thought to promote beneficial gut microflora and GI function, as well as compete against pathogenic bacteria. The numerous types of strains and their benefit across population types continue to be researched.[38]

Critical illness and sepsis often lead to dysbiosis, where there is a loss of commensal flora and abundance of pathogenic bacteria.[39] Use of probiotics in the patient with critical illness can improve GI health, protect against intestinal permeability, and modulate immune function.[40] Use of probiotics in certain ICU populations, including mechanically ventilated patients and those with traumatic brain injury and stroke, reduces GI complications, infection rates, and mortality.[41-44] Meta-analyses show a reduction in antibiotic-associated diarrhea with probiotic use, but the heterogeneity of the pooled data makes it difficult to draw conclusions to specific populations.[45] The data is either inconsistent or of low certainty with respect to outcome benefits related to ventilator days, ventilator- or hospital-associated pneumonia, or length of stay.[46,47] The risk of translocation and improper administration of probiotics resulting in blood infection is greater in this vulnerable population. Research is also needed to clarify which strands are most beneficial to humans, especially because the microbiota in the GI tract are so complex.[48]

PRACTICE POINT

Enteral feedings can provide a mixture of soluble and insoluble fiber. Advancement of fiber-containing feeds should take into consideration the total amount of fiber provided based on EN goal rate as well as history of gastrointestinal function to assure adequate tolerance.

CORE CONCEPT 6

Enteral nutrition formulas include carbohydrate, fat, protein, vitamins, minerals, and fiber adequate for meeting full nutrient requirements in most patients.

Disease-Specific Formulas

Certain health conditions require specific enteral formulations to ensure a patient meets their nutrient needs. Selection of enteral formula takes into account a patient's fluid limitations, electrolyte imbalances, increased nutrient requirement, decreased ability to receive nutrients due to disease or condition, and ease of digestion (**Table 4.4**).

Kidney Dysfunction

Patients with kidney dysfunction may require a formula that is more calorically dense and lower in phosphorus and potassium than standard polymeric formulas. Renal formulas should also assure protein of high biological value to include proportionately more essential amino acids. Patients who have stage 3 or 4 chronic kidney disease and are not yet on dialysis may need less protein in their formula. Amounts of potassium, phosphorus, and sodium are also reduced. When on dialysis or renal replacement therapy, formula composition is higher in protein to reflect increased protein losses associated with these therapies. Supplementation with enteral feedings designed for patients with kidney disease or essential amino acids is associated with improved markers of nutritional

Table 4.4 Disease-Specific Enteral Formulations

Formula Name	Suplena with Carb Steady	Nepro	Glucerna	Pulmocare
Concentration (kcal/mL)	1.8	1.8	1.0	1.5
Protein g/1000 mL (% kcal)	45 (10)	81 (18)	41.8 (17)	62.6 (17)
Carbohydrate g/1000 mL (% kcal)	200 (42)	161 (36)	95.6 (38)	105.7 (28)
Fat g/1000 mL (% kcal)	96 (48)	96 (48)	54.4 (49)	93.3 (56)
Sodium/Potassium (mg/1000 mL)	802/1139	1050/949	930/1570	1310/1960
Calcium/Phosphorus (mg/1000 mL)	1055/717	1050/717	705/705	1060/1060
Vitamin D (IU/1000 mL)	80	640	285	425
Zinc/Copper (mg/1000 mL)	27/2.1	13/1.8	16/1.5	24/2.2
Selenium (mcg/1000 mL)	76	74	50	74
Osmolality (mOsm/kg H_2O)	780	745	355	488
Description	Calorically dense, moderate carbohydrate, low protein for chronic kidney disease not on dialysis. Low sodium	Calorically dense, low protein for chronic kidney disease not on dialysis, low sodium, potassium	High protein, moderate carbohydrate, with fiber for better glucose control	Moderate fat, with increased medium-chain triglyceride for tolerance, antioxidant nutrients vit C, E, and beta carotene

status (as evidenced by body mass index, hand grip strength, and mid-arm circumference) as well as serum albumin and prealbumin.[49]

Pulmonary Dysfunction

Formulas for patients with pulmonary dysfunction have a modified carbohydrate-to-fat ratio to decrease carbohydrate intake. The rationale is that oxidation of carbohydrates results in greater carbon dioxide (CO_2) production than fat oxidation. In fact, studies confirm that use of a high-fat diet does result in reduced CO_2 production.[50] This is considered especially useful in patients with **hypercapnia** (CO_2 retention). Clinically, the use of a high-fat, low-carbohydrate formula in patients with chronic obstructive pulmonary disease may improve pulmonary function (forced expiratory volume in one second, minute ventilation, oxygen consumption, and CO_2 production) as well as arterial blood gases.[51,52] However, the strength of evidence is too low to make a recommendation on macronutrient distribution. Furthermore, a high fat intake can sometimes cause GI disturbances. Focus on avoiding overfeeding in total calories, regardless of the source (fat vs. carbohydrate), is considered best practice. Many formulas for patients with pulmonary dysfunction also incorporate immune-enhancing nutrients such as omega-3 fatty acids and antioxidants. Omega-3 fatty acids are anti-inflammatory and signal pathways that complement therapeutic efforts to maximize lung function. Use of omega-3 fatty acids in patients with acute respiratory distress is associated with improved lung injury scores, fewer days on mechanical ventilation, and reduced stays on the intensive care unit.[53] The role of antioxidants in fighting free radicals and reducing lung cell injury remains a primary research interest.

Liver Dysfunction

Patients with advanced liver disease often have ascites, or fluid accumulation in the abdomen, which may cause them to utilize nutrients inefficiently. Because of this condition, formulas for these patients are often calorically dense, providing a high calorie-to-nitrogen ratio. Protein composition in formulations designed for patients with liver failure includes a higher proportion of branched chain amino acids (BCAA) with lower amounts of aromatic amino acids in an attempt to minimize hepatic encephalopathy (a condition that is associated with liver disease). Levels of BCAA are often low in patients with liver disease due to their increased uptake in skeletal muscle to help detoxify and reduce ammonia.[54] While there is a lack of compelling evidence that nutritional support (enteral, parenteral, or oral) improves clinical outcomes in liver failure overall, use of BCAA-enhanced formulas during hepatic encephalopathy may be considered.[55]

Diabetes

Most patients with diabetes can be treated with standard polymeric formulas. Fiber-containing formulas slow gastric emptying and digestion of carbohydrates, which can improve glycemic control. For better glycemic control, diabetes-specific feedings, which are higher in fructose and monounsaturated fatty acids, can be used.[56] These formulas generally have a carbohydrate content of about 35%–40% of calories, approximately 10–15 g/L of soluble fiber, and fat (40–50% of calories). Because gastroparesis is common among patients with diabetes, diabetes-specific formulas, given their higher fat and soluble fiber, may be poorly tolerated; postpyloric feedings can be used in these instances.

Trauma/Wound Healing

Specialty formulations are available for use in patients with trauma or increased wound healing requirements. EN solutions that are high in protein and include arginine and glutamine, as well as micronutrients zinc and vitamin C, should enhance the process of wound healing due to their effects on protein anabolism (arginine and glutamine) and collagen synthesis (zinc and vitamin C). Pressure injury healing time decreases with use of these formulations.[57] Use of immune-enhancing formulas to promote wound healing in patients who are critically ill continues to be explored. These will be described in more detail in the "Immunonutrition" section of this chapter.

CORE CONCEPT 7

Disease-specific formulas that deviate from standard formulations can be used in many disease states to aid patients in meeting their nutritional needs.

Developing an EN Feeding and Hydration Plan

Table 4.5 provides a stepwise procedure for developing an EN feeding plan for a patient. The first step is selection of EN type. Based on the plethora of EN products, a clinician must evaluate what formula to select based on a patient's nutrient requirements;

Table 4.5 Step-Wise Process for Determination of Tube Feeding Volume and Delivery

Step 1	Choose the EN formula type based on condition. Examples: Standard, Condition (Impaired Digestion, Stress/Trauma), Disease-Specific	Example: 58-year-old male with head injury due to motorcycle accident with a nasogastric feeding tube EN Formula: Promote
Step 2	Determine the EN volume needed to meet the calorie goal.* 24-hour Calorie Goal/Formula Concentration (kcal/mL) = Total volume of EN needed over 24 hours *Consider: Stress level, malnourished vs. well nourished; clinical factors (intubated, sedated, sepsis); physical activity	Energy Goal: 2000 kcal Protein Goal: 130 g protein Promote (1.0 kcal/mL) = 2000 mL
Step 3	Calculate protein intake at that EN volume to assure protein is in the range of patient's goal. (Total EN volume/1000mL) × protein (g/L) = g protein/day OR (Total calorie intake at EN goal volume × % calories as protein/4 kcal/g = g protein/day	Promote has 62.5 g protein/1000 mL 2000mL/1000mL = 2.0L × 62.5 g = 125 g protein on this regimen Protein intake is sufficient
Step 4	If both calorie and protein needs are met, determine hourly rate: EN volume/24 = hourly rate * Rounding numbers is preferred to make daily calculations of input/output and order writing simplified If protein needs are not met, consider a nutrient-dense feeding with higher nitrogen or adding modular protein	Hourly EN = ~2000 mL/24 = 83.3 mL/hour Round up to 85 mL/hour
Step 5	Provide your TF type and hourly goal rate.	Promote @85 mL/hour
Step 6	Provide free water needed to meet hydration needs	Fluid needs: 2000 mL using 1mL/kcal. Promote @85 mL/hour provides 1734mL water Assume 85% free water content in 1 kcal/mL formula Additional free water needed: 2000 – 1734 = 266 mL (e.g., could give 45 mL water every 6 hours)
Step 7	Document what the TF will actually provide. Note: This may be a little different from your initially established goal, due to rounding and fine-tuning	This regimen provides 2040 kcal/128 g protein

clinical status, including fluid restrictions and electrolyte requirements; degree of metabolic stress; wound healing requirements; GI function; cost; and supporting evidence of benefit and risk of specific nutrient components provided, particularly in disease-specific and immune-enhancing feeds. **Figure 4.10** presents an algorithm for determining an optimal TF type.

An enteral formula often does not contain enough free water to meet a patient's total fluid needs. Once a formula, rate, and total volume are chosen to meet a patient's calorie and protein goals, recommendations for free water flushes must be provided to meet a patient's fluid requirement if they cannot take any fluids via oral intake.

Determining Fluid Requirement

There are many ways to determine a patient's fluid requirement. They can be energy-based or weight-based;

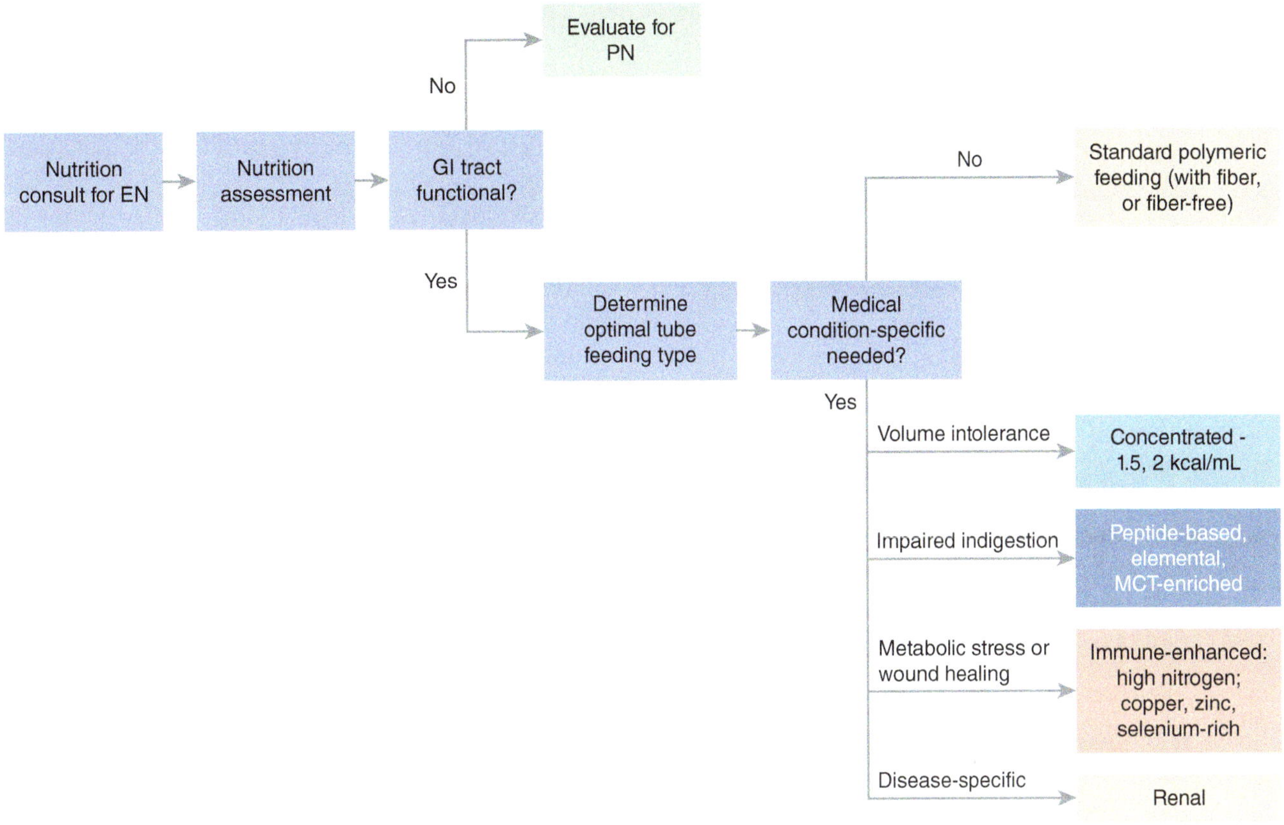

Figure 4.10 Algorithm for Determining Tube Feeding Type

however, to prevent dehydration, minimum requirement is usually 1500 mL/day unless there is a clinical need for fluid restriction.[58,59] Three common ways of calculating fluid requirement include[58,59]:

1. Energy based for adults:

   1 mL/calorie required

2. Body weight and age-based:

   Ages 18–55: 35 mL × kg body weight

   Ages 56–75: 30 mL × kg body weight

   Ages greater than 75: 25 mL × kg body weight

   Fluid restricted adults: <25 mL × kg body weight (such as patients with fluid overload, renal dysfunction, or cardiac diseases)

3. Holliday-Segar formula adjusted for age:

   Ages less than or equal to 50: 1500 mL for first 20 kg body weight + [20 mL × remaining body weight]

   Ages greater than 50: 1500 mL for first 20 kg body weight + [15 mL × remaining body weight]

Calculating Free Water Flushes

Once a patient's fluid requirement is determined, you can then calculate the amount of free water needed in addition to the chosen enteral formula to properly hydrate a patient. The steps to determine the free water needed to hydrate a patient include:

1. Calculate the fluid requirement using one of the equations above.
2. Determine the amount of free water the chosen enteral formula provides.
3. Subtract the free water calculated in Step 2 from the fluid requirement in Step 1. This is the amount of free water you must provide in addition to the formula.

Free water can be given via bolus in volumes of 30–250 mL in a gastrically placed tube and 30–150 mL in a small bowel placed tube for best tolerance. For continuous tube feeding, free water can be given in even spaced increments throughout the day. At a minimum, 30–60 mL must be given every 4–6 hours to keep the tube patent.[59] For cyclic tube feeds, 30–60 mL must be flushed before the cycle begins and when the cycle finishes to keep the tube patent; then, additional free water can be given throughout the day to meet hydration requirements as needed.[59,60] For bolus tube feeds, 30–60 mL water must be given both before and after the formula is bolused to keep the tube patent[59,60]; then, additional water may be given throughout the day to meet a patient's hydration needs as needed. It should also be noted that if a patient is receiving medications in liquid form or crushed tablet via their feeding tube, 30–60 mL water must be flushed prior to and after each medication is administered.[58–60]

It is important to give additional free water if excess losses are suspected such as from wounds, drains, vomiting, or diarrhea. It is also important to monitor signs of dehydration such as dark yellow urine, dry lips, poor skin turgor, or a patient's report of feeling thirsty.[58,59]

Complication Monitoring

Patients who are receiving TF must be monitored routinely, because complications can arise. Clinicians must check for signs of nausea and vomiting, obtain a baseline of the abdominal girth with routine subsequent monitoring, and keep track of stool patterns. Certain complications can be associated with enteral feeding, as well as illness or treatment side effects that a patient may be experiencing. These include nausea and vomiting, aspiration, abdominal distention, delayed gastric emptying, constipation,and diarrhea (**Table 4.6**).[60–65]

Reflux and Aspiration

Aspiration is a common complication associated with tube feeding. It occurs when a patient inhales a substance, such as water or tube feed, into the airway, which causes dyspnea and coughing. Prolonged aspiration is dangerous because it can lead to pneumonia.[62] Common practice to avoid aspiration includes elevating the head of bed above 30 degrees, providing continuous versus intermittent or bolus feedings, and switching to jejunal feedings. Continuous feedings generally are better tolerated in critically ill patients and contribute to earlier advancement to goal volume. However, their use has not been associated with reduced aspiration. Systematic reviews show that jejunal feedings can reduce the risk of reflux, aspiration, and pneumonia. Tolerance to EN volume advancement is not necessarily greater in jejunal versus gastric feedings. However, in patients at high risk for aspiration, jejunal feedings may be beneficial.[62,63] They offer the potential benefit of fewer interruptions for procedures versus gastric feedings.[62]

Nausea/Vomiting

Nausea and vomiting are common complications to enteral feeding and increase the risk of aspiration and pneumonia. There are many possible causes of nausea or vomiting. Both gastric retention and rapid infusion of hyperosmolar formula can cause nausea/vomiting. In these cases, a clinician must reduce the rate of feeding, but if the patient is vomiting, feeding should be held. The fat content of feeds also affects a patient's tolerance, with feedings that are lower in fat being generally better tolerated. The smell of the formula can affect the patient. Elemental formulas usually have a more unpleasant odor than polymeric formulas.[64]

Abdominal Distention

Abdominal distention is the accumulation of air or liquid in a patient's abdomen and can cause major discomfort to the patient. Abdominal distention can be diagnosed by observing an increase in abdominal girth (about 8–10 cm) and/or palpating the abdomen.[61] A patient's report of symptoms such as bloating and cramping can also indicate abdominal distention.[61] Rapid bolus or intermittent feeds of cold formula can cause abdominal distention. Using continuous and room-temperature feeds can treat this. Abdominal distention can also be caused by nutrient malabsorption, delayed gastric emptying, or the onset of a septic episode.

PRACTICE POINT

Baseline and daily measurement of abdominal girth is useful for monitoring feeding tolerance and onset of sepsis. Sudden increases in abdominal girth may indicate the onset of a septic episode.

Gastroparesis (Delayed Gastric Emptying)

Many factors can delay the emptying of gastric contents into the small bowel. Gastroparesis can be induced by trauma or be a result of a disease state such as cystic fibrosis or diabetes. It can also be caused by certain medications, such as opiates or paralytics. Feeding tolerance, feeding administration rate, and duodenogastric reflux may also contribute to delayed gastric emptying and aspiration risk; therefore, certain adjustments may be instituted.[66]

Historically, to mitigate the risk of gastroparesis, a clinician may check gastric residual volume (GRV) before initiating tube feeding, as well as every 4 hours after tube feeding. When monitoring **gastric**

residuals, gastric fluid is suctioned. The amount of fluid collected is measured over 24 hours. Normal GRVs range from 250 to 500 mL.[66,67] Anything greater than 600 mL may indicate delayed gastric emptying, which puts a patient at risk for aspiration. Controversy exists about whether checking gastric residuals is truly necessary,[66,67] and is out of practice in many centers. In current times, a common method of diagnosing gastroparesis is employing a gastric emptying study (GES).[68,69] This is a nuclear medicine study that can be tested using liquid or solid foods. The food of choice is labeled with nuclear material, so when the patient consumes it, the transit time through the digestive tract is measured. It is noninvasive and provides a quantitative measurement. It can also provide a way to grade the severity of gastroparesis.[68,69]

Continuous feeds may be preferred over intermittent or bolus feeds to normalize gastric emptying. A formula free of fiber and low in fat can also help. Prokinetic agents, such as metoclopramide and erythromycin, can mitigate delayed gastric emptying by increasing gastric motility.[14,16,17] Studies demonstrate that both individually and when combined, metoclopramide and erythromycin significantly decrease GRV. However, both medications have been associated with QT prolongation (a condition where the heart muscles take longer to contract and relax).[70]

Constipation

According to some reports, constipation is more frequent than diarrhea in patients receiving tube feeding.[71] Dehydration and lack of fiber are frequent causes of constipation. Enteral formulas with added fiber are associated with a lower incidence of constipation. Having adequate hydration in addition to the formula is important to prevent waste buildup. Immobility can also contribute to constipation, therefore ambulation when able is helpful for bowel regularity. Certain patient populations, such as those with developmental disabilities, are at risk for constipation. In these at-risk patients, it is important to have a proactive bowel regimen since hydration, fiber, and physical activity are not enough for regular bowel movements. Bowel regimens can include stool softeners or laxatives (such as docusate sodium, senna, polyethylene glycol, and bisacodyl). Sometimes, an enema may need to be considered if there is increased waste build-up.[64]

Diarrhea

Diarrhea is one of the most common complications with EN feeding. Although the definition may vary, diarrhea is defined as higher stool frequency (greater than 3–5 stools per day), volume of >500 mL/day for 2 consecutive days. In addition to frequency, stools are described as soft, liquid, or watery. Stool consistency may be soft but should not be watery.[55,63,64] Diarrhea is often managed by adjusting EN rate, formulation, or route of administration (gastric vs. duodenal). However, most causes of diarrhea are not incidental to tube feeding. Certain medications, especially those containing magnesium, phosphorus, and sorbitol, can be hyperosmolar, causing diarrhea. Diarrhea can also be due to bacterial growth.[55,63,64] Prolonged antibiotic use creates an imbalance in gut microflora and can result in antibiotic-associated diarrhea. Despite the fact that *Clostridium difficile*, a bacteria that causes diarrhea, is only one of the possible causes, a stool culture is often done to confirm antibiotic-induced diarrhea. Use of pre- and probiotics promotes proliferation and can restore the patient's microbiota to resolve diarrhea associated with harmful bacterial overgrowth.[40,41] However, as previously mentioned, use of probiotics runs the risk of bacteremia. Clinicians should decide whether the benefit outweighs the risk for any given population.[46,47]

If medications and infectious causes of diarrhea are ruled out, the EN formula can then be reviewed. Diarrhea can be caused by aspects directly related to tube feeding. Included among these are tube location, rapid feed infusion, hyperosmolar formula, carbohydrate malabsorption, or intolerance to fat in the formula. Continuous infusion at a low rate can help alleviate diarrhea. Provision of a hyperosmolar feeding into the jejunum can sometimes be improved by converting to gastric EN.[63] Consideration can be given to the type of EN formula as well. Patients experiencing diarrhea may benefit from the addition of soluble fiber, which also offers a prebiotic effect. In patients where malabsorption is present, use of semi-elemental or elemental formulas can be considered. Hyperosmolality will increase with more elemental formulas. These formulas provide a lower percent age of calories as fat and increased amounts of medium-chain triglycerides.

Patients can be exposed to bacterial growth on the tubing itself, leading to diarrhea. To prevent this, a closed tube feeding system can be used every 24–48

CORE CONCEPT 8

Patients must be monitored closely for complications related to enteral feeding or side effects to medical treatment. Feeding method and formula should be adjusted as needed.

CASE STUDY REVISITED

After 3 weeks, Laura is cleared for oral intake, gradually advancing from clear liquids to a blenderized diet. However, Laura currently feels full, and it is hard for her to eat more than a few bites at mealtimes. Her tube feeding continues at the goal rate and is well tolerated.

Questions

1. How might you adjust Laura's TF regimen to improve her oral intake?
2. Provide a possible tube feeding schedule to enhance oral intake.
3. Assess Laura's previous PES statements. Identify if each statement remains an active issue or if the PES statement has been resolved. If the PES statement remains an active issue, has improvement in the issue been noted? If the issue has been resolved, write a new PES statement.

hours. Tubing should be changed every 24 hours. In an open system, formula hang time should be limited to 4–8 hours.[25,32] Tube feeding containers and tubing should be flushed frequently. Sterile water must always be used for reconstitution.

Early Enteral Nutrition

Early enteral nutrition (EEN) generally refers to the initiation of EN within 24–48 hours of illness or a traumatic event. There are numerous clinical outcome benefits to EEN, including improved enteral tolerance, reduced time to meet energy and protein goals, reduced infectious complications, and reduced ICU and hospital lengths of stay.[72–76] The benefits of EEN apply to both adult and pediatric populations with disease states ranging from traumatic brain injury, abdominal trauma, postsurgical ICU, and acute pancreatitis.[77–80] Although it is intuitive that EN maintains gut integrity, EEN does so through increased **postprandial**

Table 4.6 Common Complications Encountered in Enteral Nutrition and Suggested Interventions

EN Complication	Risk Factors or Etiology	Interventions
Aspiration/Reflux	Mechanical Ventilation Age >70 years Neurological Impairment Supine	Continuous Feeding Prokinetic Agents Postpyloric Feeding Raise HOB Elevation
Constipation	Immobility Neurodevelopmental Disease Medications Calorically Dense Formula	Ambulation Insoluble Fiber Proactive Bowel Medication Regime Hydration—Add Free Water
Diarrhea	Hyperosmotic Feeding Antibiotic Use Infection or Sepsis Fever Prolonged Hospital Stay Jejunal Feedings	Hypoosmotic Feeding Pre and Probiotics Reduce Volume of Feeding Fiber-Containing Formula Gastric Feeding for Regulated Emptying
Nausea Vomiting/ Gastroparesis	Reflux Paralytic Ileus Mechanical Obstruction Diabetes	Prokinetic Agents Reduce Rate of Delivery Provide Brief Interruption of Feeds Low-Fat Formula Postpyloric Feeding

Data from Reintam Blaser A, Starkopf J, Alhazzani W, et al. Early enteral nutrition in critically ill patients: ESICM clinical practice guidelines. *Intensive Care Med.* 2017;43(3):380-398. doi:10.1007/s00134-016-4665-0

Table 4.7 Contraindications for Early Enteral Feeding

Hemodynamically unstable; uncontrolled shock
Uncontrolled hypoxemia, hypercapnia, or acidosis
Overt bowel ischemia
High-output fistula if EEN cannot be safely provided distal to fistula
Abdominal compartment syndrome
Upper gastrointestinal bleed
Large gastrointestinal aspirates (>500 mL/24 hours)

Data from Reintam Blaser A, Starkopf J, Alhazzani W, et al. Early enteral nutrition in critically ill patients: ESICM clinical practice guidelines. *Intensive Care Med.* 2017;43(3):380-398. doi:10.1007/s00134-016-4665-0

hyperemic response.[81,82] The presence of luminal nutrients promotes enterocyte function, microbial clearance, and maintenance of tight junctions. Enteral nutrients increase perfusion to the GI tract when cautiously delivered, which can be beneficial to gut integrity and prevention of ischemia.[83]

Although many benefits with EEN have been presented, EEN may not be indicated in certain scenarios (**Table 4.7**).[81–85] During hemodynamic instability, hypoperfusion of blood and oxygen to less vital organs, such as the GI tract, occurs. Patients in circulatory shock may also receive medications called "vasopressors" to improve blood flow to the vital organs, further diminishing GI perfusion. Overly aggressive feedings can increase GI oxygen needs beyond what can be met, inducing bowel ischemia. Monitoring vasopressor medication dosing can help guide the decision to resume feedings.[85] These findings underscore the delicate balance between promoting perfusion with judicious EEN and inducing GI ischemia through excessive nutrient provision. Current recommendations by ASPEN and the Society for Critical Care Medicine are to withhold EN until a patient becomes hemodynamically stable. Since clinical outcomes are similar between early PN and EEN, clinicians may choose PN if EEN is not feasible.[86,87]

Immunonutrition

Immunonutrition refers to the use of nutrients to alter or attenuate the inflammatory or immune response. This differs from conventional nutrition support therapy, where provision of nutrients is aimed at preventing deficiency or meeting requirements for increased utilization or losses. Nutrients such as the conditionally essential amino acids glutamine and arginine, omega-3 fatty acids, and antioxidants are considered to be beneficial in modulating inflammation and the course of disease. Today, numerous enteral formulations exist with these nutrients, either alone or in combination. These products are often used in patients with critical illness in an attempt to counteract the inflammatory response to stress, both at the systemic and cellular levels. Research into the role of these select nutrients is ongoing and inconclusive despite the plethora of immune-enhancing specialty formulas. Scientific evidence of the potential benefit of these products, as well as possible harm, is ongoing.

Gastrointestinal Tract as an Immune Organ

Traditionally, the GI tract is viewed for its primary role in digestion and absorption (**Figure 4.11**). However, a better understanding of its morphology, structure, and mediatory response to stress establishes the gut as having immunologic functions. First and foremost, the gut acts as a barrier to invasive organisms, preventing the spread of bacteria and toxins to other organs. This is accomplished through microbial, immunologic, and mechanical aspects of the gut. Increasing evidence confirms the role of the microbiome in immunology and health (**Figure 4.12**). Bacteria that are part of the normal intestinal flora inhibit colonization of invading bacteria, most basically by limiting the amount of space for bacteria to exist. Simply by virtue of their numbers, the normal GI bacteria can reduce the potential for bacterial invasion. In addition to space, the existing microbiome competes with foreign bacteria for nutrients, limiting the ability of pathogens to survive in the gut. This bacterial antagonism is essential for GI health and organ protection. Secondarily, the gut also contains immunologic factors, such as immunoglobulins that fight off foreign particles. Combined with the gut-associated lymphoid tissue (GALT), the gut is very effective at capturing and destroying invading bodies.[88]

From a mechanical perspective, the gut has a mucous gel layer, which prevents bacterial adhesion. Additionally, peristalsis protects against prolonged stasis, hindering the ability for bacteria to grow and multiply. The epithelial cell layer also plays a role in immunity by creating tight junctions and rearranging or shifting during desquamation, making it difficult for foreign bacteria to enter from the lumen. Rearrangement of

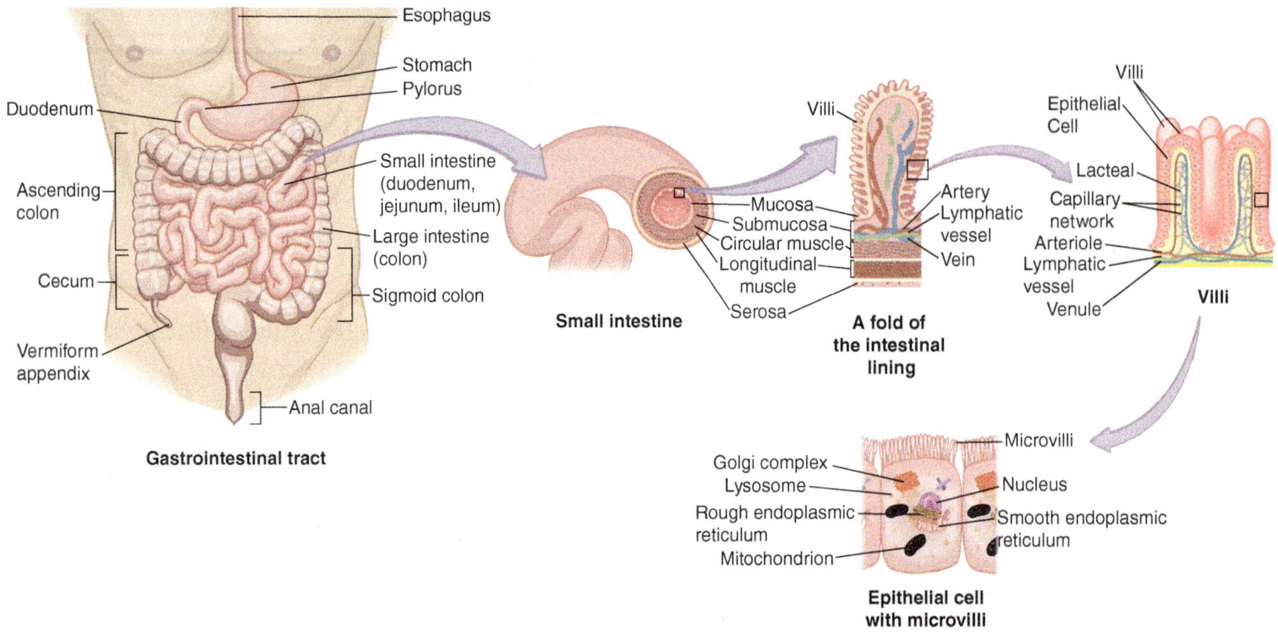

Figure 4.11 Morphology of the Intestinal Tract

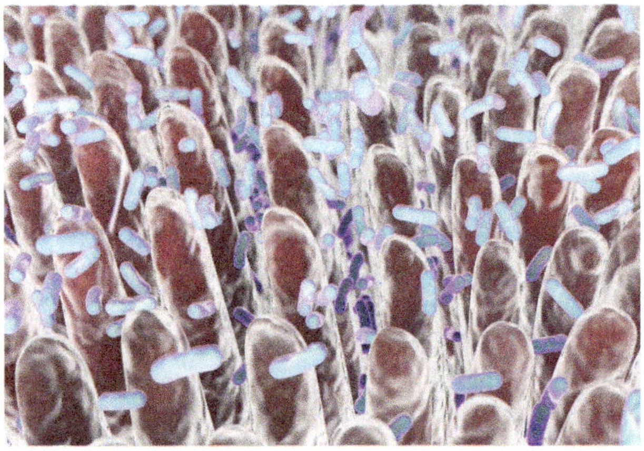

Figure 4.12 The Intestine Is Home to the Microbiome

tight junctions prevents intestinal permeability. This aspect of the gut, combined with GALT, may explain why bacterial translocation in humans rarely progresses to the bloodstream and other organs. Furthermore, the epithelial cells secrete cytokines that promote the synthesis of lymphocytes and immunity. By maintaining the epithelial layer and microbiome, EN facilitates the gut's immune function capacity.[88,89]

The Gut and Systemic Inflammatory Response System

The interaction between the gut and immunologic nutrients can be best understood in the context of the systemic inflammatory response. In systemic inflammatory response syndrome (SIRS), the intestine becomes a cytokine-generating organ due to ischemia (versus infection) as a result of certain conditions such as trauma, burns, obstructive GI injury, hemorrhagic shock, or sepsis. Select nutrients can serve as substrates that mediate this cytokine-induced response. As presented in **Figure 4.13**, various nutritional substrates can induce immune activity both at the cellular and systemic level. For example, omega-3 fatty acids act as a substrate that systemically promotes anti-inflammatory eicosanoids and cytokines, as well as modulates smooth vascular muscle tone. The result is increased dilation of the vessels, improved platelet function, and reduction of bronchoconstriction. Similarly, the amino acids glutamine and arginine participate in macrophage activity at the cell-mediated immunity level.[90–92] The optimal dose and route of provision of these nutrients remain unknown yet are imperative to achieving the beneficial aspects of these nutrients without posing harm. **Table 4.8** provides examples of immune-enhancing EN formulas.

Conditionally Essential Amino Acids

Stress-induced depletion of glutamine and arginine in blood and tissue pools has earned these amino acids the title of conditionally essential amino acids. While they can be synthesized within the body, during stress, synthesis does not meet their requirement.

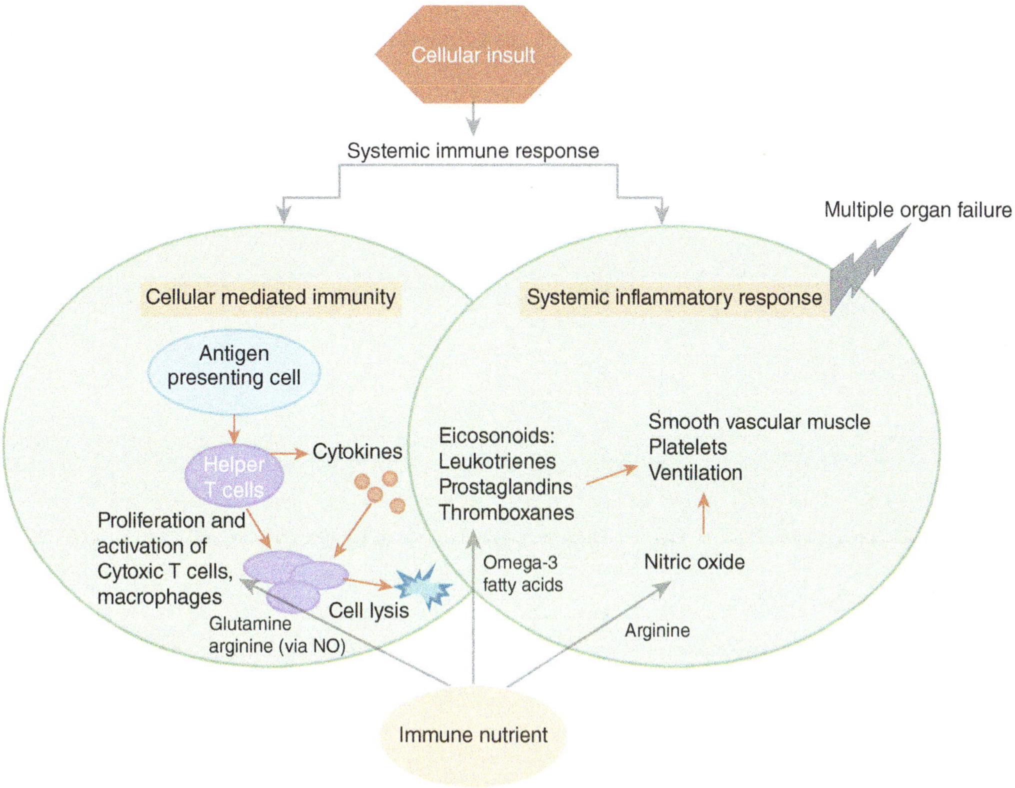

Figure 4.13 Immune Modulating Nutrients Act at Both the Cellular and Systemic Level

Data from Krauss H, Jablecka A, Sosnowski P, Bogdanski P. Influence of L-arginine on the nitric oxide concentration and level of oxidative stress during ischemia-reperfusion injury in a rat model. *J Clin Pharmacol Ther*. 2009;47(8):533-538.; Gadek JE, DeMichele SJ, Karlstad MD; Enteral Nutrition in ARDS Study Group. Effect of enteral feeding with eicosapentaenoic acid, gamma linolenic acid, and antioxidants in patients with acute respiratory distress syndrome. *Crit Care Med*. 1999;27(8):1409-1420.

Glutamine

Glutamine is a gluconeogenic amino acid that is synthesized in all tissues, with skeletal muscle as the major site. It is an important fuel source for rapidly dividing cells such as the gut epithelium, macrophages, lymphocytes, and fibroblasts. It contains two amine groups, making it a useful nitrogen shuttle to other organs. Glutamine also donates nitrogen to purines and pyrimidines for DNA synthesis. Because it is a precursor to glutathione, a potent antioxidant, glutamine helps protect cells from free radical damage.[91] Due to its properties, glutamine is used therapeutically in patients with GI disease and in patients with immune function disorders. It is also widely used among patients with metabolic stress, such as burn and trauma patients.

Arginine

Arginine plays a fundamental role in protein metabolism. As a precursor to insulin and growth hormone, it can play a major role in wound healing. Arginine is also a precursor to nitric oxide (NO), which provides cellular defense through the stimulus of increased lymphocyte activity, macrophage activation, and phagocytosis. NO is beneficial for tissue oxygenation because it reduces vascular tone, acting as a vasodilator.[90] Notably, uncontrolled production of NO can be damaging. Increased NO results in excessive inflammation, impaired cellular respiration, cytotoxicity, coagulation abnormalities, and worsening hemodynamic instability. NO is also a significant contributor in the ischemia reperfusion model, where a lack of oxygen and blood flow, followed by reperfusion of blood, generates powerful free radical substances such as peroxynitrate that can later cause tissue and microvascular damage.[93–95] Because NO can serve as both a precursor to free radical substances as well as a free radical scavenger, the need for the appropriate balance between adequate and excessive NO cannot be understated. These properties suggest caution when providing arginine in the diet. **Figure 4.14** outlines the impact of NO in the systemic immune response.

Omega-3 Fatty Acids

Many specialty products will now provide information on their omega-6 to omega-3 fatty acid ratio. While both are essential fatty acids, they have unique and

Table 4.8 Nutrient Composition of Immune-Enhancing Enteral Formulations

Formula Name	Impact	Perative	Pivot 1.5	Oxepa
Concentration (kcal/mL)	1.0	1.3	1.5	1.5
Protein g/1000 mL (% kcal)	56 (22)	66.7 (20.5)	93.8 (25)	62.7 (16.7)
Carbohydrate g/1000 mL (% kcal)	132 (53)	180.3 (53)	172.4 (46)	105.3 (28)
Fat g/1000 mL (% kcal)	28 (25)	35.2 (24)	50.8 (30)	93.8 (56)
Sodium/Potassium (mg/1000 mL)	960/1600	980/1640	1475/1983	1310/1960
Calcium/Phosphorus (mg/1000 mL)	800/800	840/840	1013/969	1060/1060
Vitamin D (IU/1000 mL)	532	332	1112	425
Zinc/Copper (mg/1000 mL)	15.2/1.7	18.8/1.68	31/2.2	24/2.2
Selenium (mcg/1000 mL)	100	60	78	74
Osmolality (mOsm/kg H_2O)	300	385	660	490
Description	Arginine 13 g/L Omega-3 3 g/L Low omega-3:6 ratio of 0.7:1 Nucleotides	Arginine 8 g/L scFOS Peptide based	Arginine 13 g/L Glutamine 7.6 g/L Omega-3 2.6 g/L scFOS Calorically dense Peptide based	EPA 4.6 g/L GLA 4 g/L Antioxidants C, E, beta-carotene

scFOS = short-chain fructo-oligosaccharide prebiotic soluble fiber; EPA = eicosapentaenoic acid; GLA = gamma-linolenic acid

contrasting properties due to the physiologic pathways they undergo. Omega-6 is a precursor to arachidonic acid and the eicosanoid 2 series, and substances such as prostaglandin 2, thromboxanes, and series 4 leukotrienes (**Figure 4.15**). These factors participate in proinflammatory activities such as vasoconstriction and platelet aggregation. Omega-3 fatty acids are anti-inflammatory, promoting vasodilation, inhibiting platelet aggregation, and competing with omega-6 production. Early clinical trials using omega-3 fatty acids were initially promising, with proven benefit in decreasing ventilator days and improving clinical outcome.[92,96,97]

Clinical Trials on Immunonutrition

Despite the mechanistic benefit of arginine, glutamine, omega-3 fatty acids, and antioxidants, recent clinical trials have not been able to demonstrate improved clinical outcomes with these immune-enhancing formulas, and in fact have raised the issue of adverse consequences.[98–100] What is known is that glutamine levels decline during critical illness. Low glutamine levels upon admission are associated with sepsis, higher severity of illness, polytrauma, and need for mechanical ventilation.[99] Noteworthy is the fact that high plasma glutamine levels were associated with liver failure and mortality, leading to a general consensus that glutamine should be avoided in patients with liver disease.[101,102] Glutamine supplementation has also been indicated to decrease inflammatory markers in a broad list of patient population types, including surgical, ICU, and those with COVID-19 in acute respiratory distress.[103–105] In patients with burn injury, glutamine supplementation has been associated with fewer infections, improved wound healing,

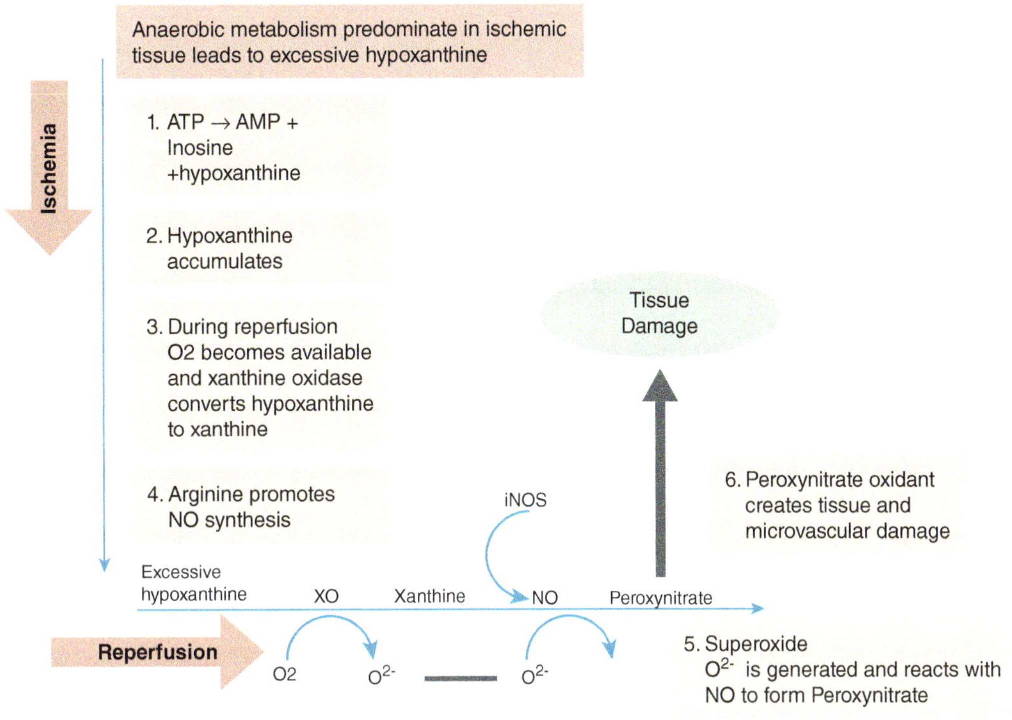

Figure 4.14 Nitric Oxide and the Ischemia-Reperfusion Model

Data from Yapca OE, Borekci B, Suleyman H. Ischemia-reperfusion damage. Eurasian J Med. 2013;45(2):126-127. doi:10.5152/eajm.2013.24; Beckman JS, Koppenol WH. Nitric oxide, superoxide, and peroxynitrite: the good, the bad, and ugly. Am J Physiol. 1996;271(5 Pt 1):C1424-C1437.

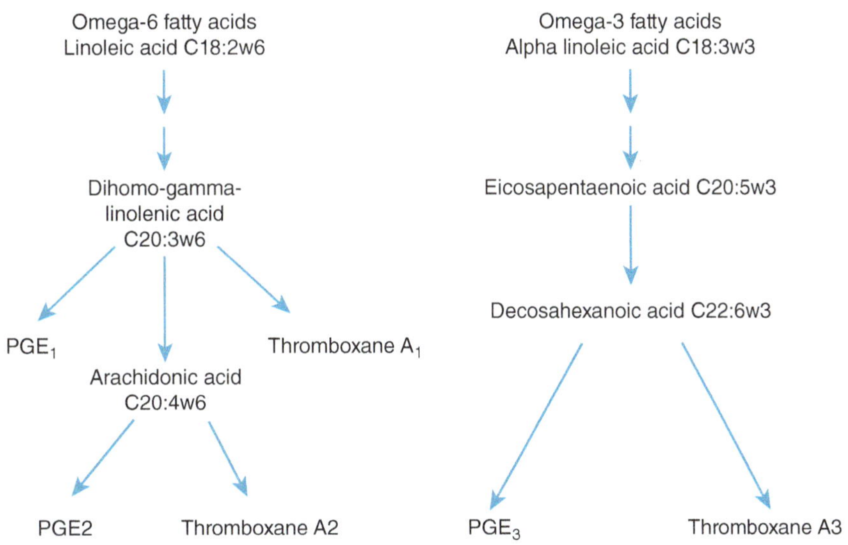

Figure 4.15 Omega-3 Versus 6 Fatty Acid Pathways

Data from Singer P, Theilla M, Fischer H, Gibstein L, Grozovski E, Cohen J. Benefit of an enteral diet enriched with eicosapentaenoic acid and gamma-linolenic acid in ventilated patients with acute lung injury. *Crit Care Med*. 2006;34(4):1033-1038.

and shorter hospital length of stay[106]; however, systematic reviews indicate that data is insufficient to recommend routine glutamine supplementation in patients with burn injury.[107,108]

Arginine has proven beneficial to patient outcomes across numerous clinical scenarios. Arginine supplementation has been demonstrated to optimize wound healing and has become routine practice in the treatment of pressure ulcers.[109] In the critically ill, arginine can reduce ICU length of stay, decrease complications, and lower infection rates.[110–112] The combination of arginine with fish oil and nucleotides is recommended for patients in the surgical ICU and those with traumatic brain injury, GI cancer, or head and neck cancer.[113]

Although initial studies with omega-3 fatty acids were promising, subsequent studies on omega-3 fatty

Clinical Controversy

Topic: Immunonutrition in Patients with Cancer Undergoing Surgery

Despite the interest in the use of immune-enhancing nutrients to improve clinical outcomes, clinical trials have questioned the value in patients with critical illness. In fact, some studies have found higher mortality in patients receiving immunonutrition than those receiving standard nutrition. The detrimental effects were most profound in patients with multiple organ failure. The consensus is that immune-enhancing enteral formulas may only be beneficial in certain populations.[85] The benefits of immunonutrition in people with cancer are currently being explored. Use of these special formulas perioperatively in patients with cancer has shown a reduction in infectious complications, hospital length of stay, and mortality. Yet, this remains controversial given variable results.[111,112]

Read the three studies in the reference list on immunonutrition in patients with cancer. Consider their findings and how study design, dosing, route of administration, and combination of nutrients may affect results. What is your opinion on use of immunonutrition in patients with cancer undergoing surgery?

References

1. Kavalukas S, McClave SA. Immunonutrition vs standard nutrition for patients with cancer. *Nutr Clin Pract*. 2023;38(4):924-931. doi:10.1002/ncp.10963
2. Lee SY, Lee J, Park HM, Kim CH, Kim HR. Impact of preoperative immunonutrition on the outcomes of colon cancer surgery: results from a randomized controlled trial. *Ann Surg*. 2023;277(3):381-386. doi:10.1097/SLA.0000000000005140
3. Li K, Xu Y, Hu Y, Liu Y, Chen X, Zhou Y. Effect of enteral immunonutrition on immune, inflammatory markers and nutritional status in gastric cancer patients undergoing gastrectomy: a randomized double-blinded controlled trial. *J Invest Surg*. 2020;33(10):950-959. doi:10.1080/08941939.2019.1569736

acid–enriched diets with antioxidants added demonstrated no clinical benefit in ventilator-free days or ICU days.[92,96,97] In fact, studies began to show a negative impact on mortality in groups getting omega-3 supplementation.[114,115] Following the COVID-19 pandemic, a renewed interest came in the potential benefit of omega-3 fatty acids.[116–118] Omega-3 fatty acids can reduce inflammation, ICU length of stay, and duration of ventilation.[118,119] Given the heterogeneity of populations studied, a recommendation for omega-3 supplementation in patients with critical illness cannot be made.[119]

Chapter Summary

Enteral nutrition is the preferred mode of feeding for most patients requiring nutrition support. Optimal outcome, however, depends on proper selection of feeding site, mode of delivery, and formula. Enteral feeding tube placement should take into consideration length of required support, gastric function, aspiration risk, and lifestyle needs of the patient. Formula selection is based on clinical and disease-related requirements of the patients. Over the last several decades, an abundance of specialized feeding products has become available. Choosing an appropriate formula can help support metabolic and disease-related needs in many patients. Disease- and condition-specific formulas are recognized for their unique nutrient characteristics, which can enhance provision of nitrogen and wound-healing nutrients. Differences in composition related to fiber, fluid, macronutrients, and micronutrients provide options to coincide with the medical management of the patient.

Key Terms

enteral nutrition (EN), percutaneous endoscopic gastrostomy (PEG) tube, immunonutrition, nasogastric tube, nasoenteric, oroenteric, nasoduodenal tube, nasojejunal tube, prokinetics, fluoroscopic tube placement, percutaneous endoscopic jejunostomy (PEJ), laparoscopy, open tube placement, aspiration, gastroparesis, dumping syndrome, closed tube feeding system, open tube feeding system, hang time, continuous feeding, intermittent feeding, bolus feeding, isolate, prebiotics, probiotics, hypercapnia, gastric residuals, early enteral nutrition (EEN), postprandial hyperemic response, arginine

References

1. Mueller CM, ed. *The ASPEN Adult Nutrition Support Core Curriculum*. 3rd ed. American Society for Parenteral and Enteral Nutrition; 2017.
2. Volkert D, Berner YN, Berry E, et al. ESPEN guideline on enteral nutrition: geriatrics. *J Clin Nutr.* 2006;25(2):330–360.
3. Mogensen KM, Malone A, Becker P, et al. and Malnutrition Committee of the American Society for Parenteral and Enteral Nutrition (ASPEN). Academy of Nutrition and Dietetics/American Society for Parenteral and Enteral Nutrition consensus malnutrition characteristics: usability and association with outcomes. *Nutr Clin Pract*. 2019;34(5):657–665.
4. Harkness L. The history of enteral nutrition therapy: from raw eggs and nasal tubes to purified amino acids and early postoperative jejunal delivery. *J Am Diet Assoc.* 2002;102(3):399–404.
5. Bechtold ML, Mir FA, Boumitri C, et al. Long-term nutrition: a clinician's guide to successful long-term enteral access in adults. *Nutr Clin Pract*. 2016;31(6):737–747. doi:10.1177/0884533616670103
6. Du G, Liu F, Ma X, et al. Comparison between percutaneous endoscopic gastrostomy and nasogastric feeding in 160 patients with swallowing disturbances: a two-year follow-up study. *Clin Intervent Aging*. 2022;17:1803–1810.
7. Bischoff SC, Austin P, Boeykens K, et al. ESPEN guideline on home enteral nutrition. *Clin Nutr.* 2020;39(1):5–22.
8. Reddick CA, Greaves JR, Flaherty JE, Callihan LE, Larimer CH, Allen SA. Choosing wisely: enteral feeding tube selection, placement, and considerations before and beyond the procedure room. *Nutr Clin Pract*. 2023;38:216–239. doi:10.1002/ncp.10959
9. Nunes G, Santos CA, Santos C, Fonseca J. Percutaneous endoscopic gastrostomy for nutritional support in dementia patients. *Aging Clin Exp Res*. 2016;28(5):983–989.
10. Shastri YM, Shirodkar M, Mallath MK. Endoscopic feeding tube placement in patients with cancer: a prospective clinical audit of 2055 procedures in 1866 patients. *Aliment Pharmacol Ther.* 2008;27(8):649–658.
11. Bloom L, Seckel M. Placement of nasogastric feeding tube and postinsertion care review. *AACN Adv Crit Care*. 2022;33(1):68–84.
12. Judd M. Confirming nasogastric tube placement in adults. *Nursing*. 2023;50(4):43–46.
13. Powers J, Brown B, Lyman B, et al. Development of a competency model for placement and verification of nasogastric and nasoenteric feeding tubes for adult hospitalized patients. *Nutr Clin Pract*. 2021;36:517–533.
14. Boeykens K, Holvoet T, Duysburgh I. Nasogastric tube insertion length measurement and tip verification in adults: a narrative review. *Crit Care*. 2023;27(1):317.
15. Haslam D, Fang J. Enteral access for nutrition in the intensive care unit. *Curr Opin Clin Nutr Metab Care*. 2006;9(2):155–159.
16. Hawk H, Valdivia H. Bedside methods for transpyloric feeding tube insertion in hospitalized children: a systematic review of randomized and non-randomized trials. *J Pedi Nurs*. 2021;60:238–246.
17. Ley D, Austin K, Wilson KA, Saha S. Tutorial on adult enteral tube feeding: Indications, placement, removal, complications, and ethics. *JPEN*. 2023;47(5):677–685.
18. Lord LM. Enteral access devices: types, function, care, and challenges. *Nutri Clin Pract*. 2018;33:16–38. doi:10.1002/ncp.10019
19. Bear DE, Champion A, Lei K, et al. Use of an electromagnetic device compared with chest x-ray to confirm nasogastric feeding tube position in critical care. *JPEN*. 2016;40:581–586.
20. Taylor S, Sayer K, Milne D, et al. Integrated realtime imaging system, 'IRIS', Kangaroo feeding tube: a guide to placement and image interpretation. *BMJ Open Gastro*. 2021;8:e000768. doi:10.1136/bmjgast-2021-000768
21. Wischmeyer PE, McMoon MM, Waldron NH, Dye EJ. Successful identification of anatomical markers and placement of feeding tubes in critically ill patients via camera-assisted technology with real-time video guidance. *JPEN*. 2019;43(1):118–125. doi:10.1002/jpen.1313
22. Kozin ED, Remenschneider AK, Cunnane ME, Deschler DG. Otolaryngologist-assisted fluoroscopic-guided nasogastric tube placement in the postoperative laryngectomy patient. *Laryngoscope*. 2014;124(4):916–920.
23. Rajan A, Wangrattanapranee P, Kessler J, Kidambi TD, Tabibian JH. Gastrostomy tubes: fundamentals, periprocedural considerations, and best practices. *World J Gastrointest Surg*. 2022;14(4):286–303. doi:10.4240/wjgs.v14.i4.286
24. Gkolfakis P, Arvanitakis M, Despott EJ, et al. Endoscopic management of enteral tubes in adult patients–Part 2: peri-and post-procedural management. European Society of Gastrointestinal Endoscopy (ESGE) Guideline. *Endoscopy.* 2021;53(02):178–195.
25. Bankhead R, Boullata J, Brantley S, et al. Enteral nutrition practice recommendations. *JPEN*. 2009;33(2):122–167.
26. Kwon RS, Banerjee S, Desilets D, et al. Enteral nutrition access devices. *Gastrointest Endosc*. 2010;72(2):236–248.
27. Metheny NA, Titler MG. Assessing placement of feeding tubes. *Am J Nurs*. 2001;101(5):36–45.
28. Schlein K. Gastric versus small bowel feeding in critically ill adults. *Nutr Clin Pract*. 2016;31(4):514–522.
29. Marik PE, Zaloga GP. Gastric versus post-pyloric feeding: a systematic review. *Crit Care*. 2003;7(3):R46–51.
30. Jiyong J, Tiancha H, Huiqin W, Jingfen J. Effect of gastric versus post-pyloric feeding on the incidence of pneumonia in critically ill patients: observations from traditional and Bayesian random-effects meta-analysis. *Clin Nutr*. 2013;32(1):8–15.
31. Varon DE1, Freitas G, Goel N, et al. Intraoperative feeding improves calorie and protein delivery in acute burn patients. *J Burn Care Res*. 2017;38(5):299–303. doi:10.1097/BCR.0000000000000514
32. Silva SMR, Silva de Assis MC, Rosane de Moraes Silveira C, Gomes M, Daniel de Mello E. Open versus closed enteral nutrition systems for critically ill adults: is there a difference? *Revista da Associação Médica Brasileira* (English Edition) 2012; 58(2): 229–233.
33. Abdelbaky AM, Elmasry WG, Awad AH. Bolus versus continuous enteral feeding for critically ill patients: a systematic review and meta-analysis. *Cureus*. 2024;16(2):e54136. doi:10.7759/cureus.54136.
34. Holyk A, Belden V, Sirimaturos M, et al. Volume-based feeding enhances enteral delivery by maximizing the optimal rate of enteral feeding (FEED MORE). *JPEN*. 2020;44(6):1038–1046. doi:10.1002/jpen.1727
35. Wang L, Wang Y, Li HX, et al. Optimizing enteral nutrition delivery by implementing volume-based feeding protocol for critically ill patients: an updated meta-analysis and systematic review. *Crit Care*. 2023;27(1):173. doi:10.1186/s13054-023-04439-0

36. Davis TA, Fiorotto ML, Suryawan A. Bolus versus continuous feeding to optimize anabolism in neonates. *Curr Opin Clin Nutr Metab Care.* 2015;18(1):102–108. doi:10.1097/MCO.0000000000000128
37. Cresci G, Lefton J, Esper DH. Enteral formulations. In: Mueller C, ed. *The A.S.P.E.N. Adult Nutrition Support Core Curriculum.* 2nd ed. American Society for Parenteral and Enteral Nutrition; 2012:186–203.
38. He P, Yu L, Tian F, Chen W, Zhang H, Zhai Q. Effects of probiotics on preterm infant gut microbiota across populations: a systematic review and meta-analysis. *Adv Nutr.* 2024;15(6):100233. doi:10.1016/j.advnut.2024.100233.
39. Batta VK, Rao SC, Patole SK. Bifidobacterium infantis as a probiotic in preterm infants: a systematic review and meta-analysis. *Pediatr Res* 2023;94:1887–1905. doi:10.1038/s41390-023-02716-w
40. Abenavoli L, Scarpellini E, Paravati MR, et al. Gut microbiota and critically ill patients: immunity and its modulation via probiotics and immunonutrition. *Nutrients.* 2023;15:3569. doi:10.3390/ nu15163569
41. Du T, Jing X, Song S, Lu S, et al. Therapeutic effect of enteral nutrition supplemented with probiotics in the treatment of severe craniocerebral injury: a systematic review and meta-analysis. *World Neurosurg.* 2020;139:e553–e571. doi:10.1016/j.wneu.2020.04.083.
42. Chen X, Hu Y, Yuan X, Yang J, Ka Li. Effect of early enteral nutrition combined with probiotics in patients with stroke: a meta-analysis of randomized controlled trials. *Eur J Clin Nutr.* 2022;76(4):592–603. doi:10.1038/s41430-021-00986-3
43. Lou J, Cui S, Huang N, et al. Efficacy of probiotics or synbiotics in critically ill patients: a systematic review and meta-analysis. *Clinical Nutrition ESPEN.* 2024;59:48–62. doi:10.1016/j.clnesp.2023.11.003
44. Panchal H, Athalye-Jape G, Rao S. et al. Growth and neurodevelopmental outcomes of probiotic supplemented preterm infants—a systematic review and meta-analysis. *Eur J Clin Nutr* 2023;77:855–871. doi:10.1038/s41430-023-01270-2
45. Hempel S, Newberry SJ, Maher AR, et al. Probiotics for the prevention and treatment of antibiotic-associated diarrhea: a systematic review and meta-analysis. *JAMA.* 2012;307(18):1959–1969. doi:10.1001/jama.2012.3507
46. Barraud D, Bollaert PE, Gibot S. Impact of the administration of probiotics on mortality in critically ill adult patients: a meta-analysis of randomized controlled trials. *Chest.* 2013;143(3):646–655.
47. Sharif S, Greer A, Skorupski, C, et al. Probiotics in critical illness: a systematic review and meta-analysis of randomized controlled trials. *Crit Care Med.* 2022; 50(8):1175–1186. doi:10.1097/CCM.0000000000005580
48. Naseri A, Seyedi-Sahebari S, Mahmoodpoor A, Sanaie S. Probiotics in critically ill patients: an umbrella review. *Indian J Crit Care Med.* 2022;26(3):339–360.
49. Kalantar-Zadeh K, Cano NJ, Budde K, et al. Diets and enteral supplements for improving outcomes in chronic kidney disease. *Nature Rev Nephrol.* 2011;7(7). doi:10.1038/nrneph.2011.60
50. Guerra BA, Pereira TG, Eckert IC, Bernardes S, Silva FM. Markers of respiratory function response to high-carbohydrate and high-fat intake in patients with lung diseases: a systematic review with meta-analysis of randomized clinical trials. *JPEN.* 2022 Sep;46(7):1522–1534. doi:10.1002/jpen.2385
51. Malmir H, Onvani S, Ardestani ME, Feizi A, Azadbakht L, Esmaillzadeh A. Adherence to low carbohydrate diet in relation to chronic obstructive pulmonary disease. *Front Nutr.* 2021;8:690880. doi:10.3389/fnut.2021.690880
52. Cai B, Zhu Y, Ma Yi, et al. Effect of supplementing a high-fat, low-carbohydrate enteral formula in COPD patients. *Nutrition.* 2003;19(3):229–232.
53. Hsieh MJ, Yang TM, Tsai YH. Nutritional supplementation in patients with chronic obstructive pulmonary disease. *J Formos Med Assoc.* 2016;115(8):595–601. doi:10.1016/j.jfma.2015.10.008
54. Koretz RL, Avenell A, Lipman TO. Nutrition support for liver disease. *Cochrane Database Syst Rev.* 2012;(5):CD008344. doi:10.1002/14651858.CD008344.pub2
55. Plauth M, Cabré E, Riggio O, et al. ESPEN Guidelines on enteral nutrition: liver disease. *Clin Nutr.* 2006;25(2):285–294.
56. Ojo O, Brooke J. Evaluation of the role of enteral nutrition in managing patients with diabetes: a systematic review. *Nutrients.* 2014;6(11):5142–5152. doi:10.3390/nu6115142
57. Ellinger S. Micronutrients, arginine, and glutamine: does supplementation provide an efficient tool for prevention and treatment of different kinds of wounds? *Adv Wound Care.* 2014;3(11):691–707. doi:10.1089/wound.2013.0482
58. Canada T, Lord L. Fluids, electrolytes, and acid-base disorders. In: Mueller C, ed. *The A.S.P.E.N. Adult Nutrition Support Core Curriculum.* 2nd ed. American Society for Parenteral and Enteral Nutrition 2017; 113–135.
59. Lord LM. Fluid needs in the older adult receiving tube feedings. *Nutr Clin Pract.* 2021;36(2):360–368. doi:10.1002/ncp.10634
60. Ley D, Austin K, Wilson KA, Saha S. Tutorial on adult enteral tube feeding: indications, placement, removal, complications, and ethics. *JPEN.* 2023;47(5);677–685. doi:10.1002/jpen.2510
61. Malone A, Seres D, Lord L. Complications of enteral nutrition. In: Mueller C, ed. *The A.S.P.E.N. Adult Nutrition Support Core Curriculum.* 2nd ed. American Society for Parenteral and Enteral Nutrition; 2012:219–231.
62. Tadlock MD, Hannon M, Davis K, et al. Nutritional support using enteral and parenteral methods. *Military Med.* 2018;183(2):153–160. doi:10.1093/milmed/usy074
63. Tatsumi, H. Enteral tolerance in critically ill patients. *J Intensive Care* 2019;7(3):1–10. doi:10.1186/s40560-019-0378-0
64. Bodoky G, Kent-Smith L. Basics in clinical nutrition: complications of enteral nutrition. *e-SPEN.* 2009;4:e209-e211.
65. Pancorbo-Hidalgo PL, García-Fernandez FP, Ramírez-Pérez C. Complications associated with enteral nutrition by nasogastric tube in an internal medicine unit. *J Clin Nurs.* 2001;10(4):482–490.
66. Montejo JC, Minambres E, Bordeje L, et al. Gastric residual volume during enteral nutrition in ICU patients: the REGANE study. *Intensive Care Med.* 2010;36(8):1386–1393.
67. Arabi YM, Casaer MP, Chapman M, et al. The intensive care medicine research agenda in nutrition and metabolism. *Intensive Care Med.* 2017. doi:10.1007/s00134-017-4711-6
68. MacLean J, El-Chammas K. Gastric emptying studies in pediatrics: Cincinnati children's hospital experience. *J Nuclear Med Tech.* 2024;52(1):40–45. doi:10.2967/jnmt.123.266857
69. Ashish Chogle, Saps M. Gastroparesis in children. *J Pedi Gastroenterol Nutr.* 2013;56(4):439–442. doi:10.1097/mpg.0b013e31827a789c
70. Rangoon V, Ukleja A. Gastroparesis in a hospital setting. *Nutr Clin Pract.* 2021;36(1):50–66.
71. Bittencourt AF, Martins JR, Logullo L, et al. Constipation is more frequent than diarrhea in patients fed exclusively

by enteral nutrition. *Nutr Clin Pract.* 2012;27:533–539. doi:10.1177/0884533612449488

72. Bistrian BR. The who, what, where, when, why, and how of early enteral feeding. *Am J Clin Nutr.* 2012;95(6):1303–1304.
73. Doig GS, Heighes PT, Simpson F, Sweetman EA. Early enteral nutrition reduces mortality in trauma patients requiring intensive care: a meta-analysis of randomized controlled trials. *Injury.* 2011;42:50–56.
74. Reintam Blaser A, Starkopf J, Alhazzani W, et al. Early enteral nutrition in critically ill patients: ESICM clinical practice guidelines. *Intensive Care Med.* 2017;43(3):380–398. doi:10.1007/s00134-016-4665-0
75. Liu Y, Zhao W, Chen W, et al. Effects of early enteral nutrition on immune function and prognosis of patients with sepsis on mechanical ventilation. *J Intensive Care Med.* 2020;35(10):1053–1061. doi:10.1177/0885066618809893
76. Tian F, Heighes PT, Allingstrup MJ, Doig GS. Early enteral nutrition provided within 24 hours of ICU admission: a meta-analysis of randomized controlled trials. *Crit Care Med.* 2018;46(7):1049–1056. doi:10.1097/CCM.0000000000003152
77. Li JY, Yu T, Chen GC, et al. Enteral nutrition within 48 hours of admission improves clinical outcomes of acute pancreatitis by reducing complications: a meta-analysis. *PLoS One.* 2013;8(6):e64926.
78. Mikhailov TA, Kuhn EM, Manzi J, et al. Early enteral nutrition is associated with lower mortality in critically ill children. *JPEN.* 2014;38(4):459–466.
79. Szabo FK, Fei L, Cruz LA, Abu-el-haija M. Early enteral nutrition and aggressive fluid resuscitation are associated with improved clinical outcomes in acute pancreatitis. *J Pediatr.* 2015;167(2):397–402.e1.
80. Liu J, Kong K, Tao Y, Cai W. Optimal timing for introducing enteral nutrition in the neonatal intensive care unit. *Asia Pac J Clin Nutr.* 2015;24(2):219–226.
81. Martindale RG, Warren M. Should enteral nutrition be started in the first week of critical illness? *Curr Opin Clin Nutr Metab Care.* 2015;18(2):202–206.
82. Ibrahim EH, Mehringer L, Prentice D, et al. Early versus late enteral feeding of mechanically ventilated patients: results of a clinical trial. *JPEN.* 2002;26(3):174–181.
83. Khalid I, Doshi P, Digiovine B. Early enteral nutrition and outcomes of critically ill patients treated with vasopressors and mechanical ventilation. *Am J Crit Care.* 2010;19(3):261–268.
84. Flordelís lasierra JL, Pérez-vela JL, Umezawa makikado LD, et al. Early enteral nutrition in patients with hemodynamic failure following cardiac surgery. *JPEN.* 2015;39(2):154–162.
85. Patel JJ, Rice T, Heyland DK. Safety and outcomes of early enteral nutrition in circulatory shock. *JPEN.* 2020;44:779–784. doi:10.1002/jpen.1793
86. McClave SA, Taylor BE, Martindale RG, et al. Guidelines for the provision and assessment of nutrition support therapy in the adult critically ill patient. *JPEN.* 2016;40:159–211. doi:10.1177/0148607115621863
87. Compher C, Bingham AL, McCall M, et al. Guidelines for the provision of nutrition support therapy in the adult critically ill patient: *JPEN.* 2022;46:12–41. doi:10.1002/jpen.2267
88. Hegazi RA, DeWitt T. Enteral nutrition and immune modulation of acute pancreatitis. *World J Gastroenterol.* 2014;20(43):16101–16105.
89. O'Hara AM, Shanahan F. The gut flora as a forgotten organ. *EMBO Reports.* 2006;7(7):688–693. doi:10.1038/sj.embor.740073
90. Krauss H, Jablecka A, Sosnowski P, Bogdanski P. Influence of L-arginine on the nitric oxide concentration and level of oxidative stress during ischemia-reperfusion injury in a rat model. *Int J Clin Pharmacol Ther.* 2009;47(8):533–538.
91. Smith RJ. Glutamine metabolism and its physiologic importance. *JPEN.* 1990;14(4 Suppl):40S–44S.
92. Gadek JE, DeMichele SJ, Karlstad MD. Enteral nutrition in ARDS study group. Effect of enteral feeding with eicosapentaenoic acid, gamma linolenic acid, and antioxidants in patients with acute respiratory distress syndrome. *Crit Care Med.* 1999;27(8):1409–1420.
93. Grootjans J, Lenaerts K, Derikx JPM, et al. Human intestinal ischemia-reperfusion–induced inflammation characterized: experiences from a new translational model. *Am J Pathol.* 2010;176(5):2283–2291. doi:10.2353/ajpath.2010.091069
94. Yapca OE, Borekci B, Suleyman H. Ischemia-reperfusion damage. *Eurasian J Med.* 2013;45(2):126–127. doi:10.5152/eajm.2013.24
95. Beckman JS, Koppenol WH. Nitric oxide, superoxide, and peroxynitrite: the good, the bad, and ugly. *Am J Physiol.* 1996;271(5):C1424–C1437.
96. Singer P, Theilla M, Fischer H, Gibstein L, Grozovski E, Cohen J. Benefit of an enteral diet enriched with eicosapentaenoic acid and gamma-linolenic acid in ventilated patients with acute lung injury. *Crit Care Med.* 2006;34(4):1033–1038.
97. Pontes-Arruda A, Aragao AM, Albequerque JD. Effects of enteral feeding with eicosapentaenoic acid, gamma-linolenic acid and antioxidants in mechanically ventilated patients with severe sepsis and septic shock. *Crit Care Med.* 2006;34(9):2325–2333.
98. van Zanten AR, Sztark F, Kaisers UX, et al. High-protein enteral nutrition enriched with immune-modulating nutrients vs standard high-protein enteral nutrition and nosocomial infections in the ICU: a randomized clinical trial. *JAMA.* 2014;6;312(5):514–524.
99. Heyland D, Muscedere J, Wischmeyer P, et al. A randomized trial of glutamine and antioxidants in critically ill patients. *N Engl J Med.* 2013;368(16):1489.
100. van Zanten ARH, Dhaliwal R, Garrel D, Heyland DH. Enteral glutamine supplementation in critically ill patients: a systematic review and meta-analysis. *Crit Care.* 2015;19:294–310.
101. Blaauw R, Nel DG, Schleicher GK. Plasma glutamine levels in relation to intensive care unit patient outcome. *Nutrients.* 2020; 12(2):402. doi:10.3390/nu12020402
102. Smedberg M, Helleberg J, Norberg Å, et al. Plasma glutamine status at intensive care unit admission: an independent risk factor for mortality in critical illness. *Crit Care.* 2021;25:240–245. doi:10.1186/s13054-021-03640-3
103. Gholamalizadeh M, Tabrizi R, Rezaei S, et al. Effect of glutamine supplementation on inflammatory markers in critically ill patients supported with enteral or parenteral feeding. *JPEN.* 2022;46:61–68. doi:10.1002/jpen.2217
104. Mohajeri M, Horriatkhah E, Mohajery R. The effect of glutamine supplementation on serum levels of some inflammatory factors, oxidative stress, and appetite in COVID-19 patients: a case–control study. *Inflammopharmacol* 2021;29,1769–1776. doi:10.1007/s10787-021-00881-0
105. Hasani M, Mansour A, Asayesh H, et al. Effect of glutamine supplementation on cardiometabolic risk factors and inflammatory markers: a systematic review and meta-analysis. *BMC Cardiovasc Disord.* 2021;21:190. doi:10.1186/s12872-021-01986-8

106. Al-Dorzi HM, Arabi YM. Nutrition support for critically ill patients. *JPEN*. 2021;45:S47–S59. doi:10.1002/jpen.2228
107. Tao W, Xu G, Zhou J, Luo Y, Li PS. Glutamine supplementation on burn patients: a systematic review and meta-analysis. *J Burn Care Res*. 2023;45(3):675–680.
108. Ortiz-Reyes L, Lee Z-Y, Chin Han Lew C, et al. The efficacy of glutamine supplementation in severe adult burn patients: a systematic review with trial sequential meta-analysis. *Crit Care Med*. 2023;51(8):1086–1095. doi:10.1097/CCM.0000000000005887
109. Cheshmeh S, Hojati N, Mohammadi A, et al. The use of oral and enteral tube-fed arginine supplementation in pressure injury care: a systematic review and meta-analysis. *Nurs Open*. 2022;9(6):2552–2561. doi:10.1002/nop2.974
110. Fiorentino G, Coppola A, Rizzo E, Annunziata A, Bernardo N, Lomarbid A. Effects of adding L-arginine orally to standard therapy in patients with COVID-19: a randomized, double-blind, placebo-controlled, parallel-group trial. Results of the first interim analysis et al. *eClinicalMedicine*. 2021;40:101125.
111. Martin ND, Schott LL, Miranowski MK, Desai AM, Lowen CC, Cao Z, et al. Exploring the impact of arginine-supplemented immunonutrition on length of stay in the intensive care unit: a retrospective cross-sectional analysis. *PLoS One*. 2024;19(4):e0302074.
112. García-Malpartida K, Aragón-Valera C, Botella-Romero F, Ocón-Bretón MJ, López-Gómez JJ. Effects of immunonutrition on cancer patients undergoing surgery: a scoping review. *Nutrients*. 2023;15(7):1776. doi:10.3390/nu15071776
113. Kavalukas S, McClave SA. Immunonutrition vs standard nutrition for patients with cancer. *Nutr Clin Pract*. 2023;38: 924–931.
114. Li C, Bo L, Liu W, Lu X, Jin F. Enteral immunomodulatory diet (omega-3 fatty acid, gamma-linolenic acid and antioxidant supplementation) for acute lung injury and acute respiratory distress syndrome: an updated systematic review and analysis. *Nutrients*. 2015;7:5572–5585.
115. Rice TW, Wheeler AP, Thompson BT, deBoiseblane BP, Steingrub J, Rock P. Enteral omega-3 fatty acid, gamma-linolenic acid, and antioxidant supplementation in acute lung injury. *JAMA*. 2011;306(14):1574–1582.
116. Doaei S, Gholami S, Rastgoo S, et al. The effect of omega-3 fatty acid supplementation on clinical and biochemical parameters of critically ill patients with COVID-19: a randomized clinical trial. *J Transl Med*. 2021;19:128. doi:10.1186/s12967-021-02795-5
117. Hathaway D, Pandav K, Patel M, et al. Omega 3 fatty acids and COVID-19: a comprehensive review. *Infect Chemother*. 2020;52(4):478–495. doi:10.3947/ic.2020.52.4.478
118. Taha AM, Shaarawy AS, Omar MM, et al. Effect of omega-3 fatty acids supplementation on serum level of C-reactive protein in patients with COVID-19: a systematic review and meta-analysis of randomized controlled trials. *J Transl Med*. 2022;20:401. doi:10.1186/s12967-022-03604-3
119. Koekkoek AC, Panteleon V, van Zanten, A current evidence on ω-3 fatty acids in enteral nutrition in the critically ill: a systematic review and meta-analysis. *Nutrition*. 2019;59:56–68.

CHAPTER 5

Parenteral Nutrition Therapy

Katie Fort
Kathy Prelack
Kelly Kane

CHAPTER OUTLINE

CORE CONCEPTS

1. Parenteral nutrition is a high-risk form of nutrition therapy that should only be used when clinically indicated. Enteral nutrition, if tolerated, is preferable to parenteral nutrition in patients who require nutrition support.
2. Venous access for parenteral nutrition is determined based on duration of therapy, desired concentration, solution type, and disease state/condition of the patient.
3. Candidates for parenteral nutrition must be fully evaluated for nutritional risk and nutritional status with adherence to standardized protocols for initiation of parenteral nutrition.
4. Parenteral nutrition is a hypertonic solution made up of, but not limited to, carbohydrate in the form of dextrose, crystalline amino acids, lipid emulsions, electrolytes, vitamins, minerals, and sterile water.
5. Many lipid emulsions are primarily composed of omega-6 fatty acids and should be provided judiciously given their role in inflammation.
6. Prescription of parenteral nutrition is based on energy and protein requirements with consideration of fluid specifications and substrate utilization of macronutrients.
7. Carbohydrate infusion from parenteral nutrition should not exceed 5 mg/kg/min in adults and children over the age of 2 years.
8. Intravenous lipid emulsion should not exceed 2.5 g/kg or 0.11 mg/kg/min.
9. Parenteral nutrition formulations are customizable to the specific needs of each patient.

10. Monitoring of anthropometric, clinical, and biochemical indices such as electrolytes, acid–base balance, serum glucose, and liver function tests is critical to ensure the safety of the patient.
11. Parenteral nutrition may be a long-term or even lifelong therapy for some patients.

LEARNING OBJECTIVES

1. Explain the history of parenteral nutrition therapy and its importance as a form of nutrition support therapy.
2. Identify the various methods of central and peripheral venous access.
3. Assess whether a patient is a candidate for parenteral nutrition by critically evaluating their disease state and biochemical parameters.
4. Identify the nutrition components and additions that commonly comprise parenteral nutrition.
5. Calculate a sample parenteral nutrition prescription/order.
6. Identify the anthropometric, biochemical, and physical examination components that constitute effective monitoring of parenteral nutrition patients.
7. Describe the potential mechanical and metabolic complications of parenteral nutrition and strategies to prevent and/or resolve them.

Introduction

Parenteral nutrition (PN) is a type of nutrition support that relies on the intravenous (IV) administration of nutrients to patients who are unable to take adequate nutrition orally or enterally. PN may be used as an addition to an oral diet and/or enteral nutrition (EN) to meet nutritional needs, as the sole source of nutrition during recovery from illness or injury of the gastrointestinal (GI) tract, or as a long-term life-sustaining therapy for patients who have compromised ability to enterally absorb nutrients.

PN is administered directly into the bloodstream via a catheter. Each PN formulation is customized to meet the individual needs of the patient and may contain carbohydrate, amino acids, lipids, vitamins, minerals, and sterile water. There are potentially serious metabolic and mechanical dangers associated with PN. For this reason, PN is only utilized when nutrition support is necessary and EN is inadequate and/or contraindicated.[1]

CORE CONCEPT 1

Parenteral nutrition is a high-risk form of nutrition therapy that should only be used when clinically indicated. Enteral nutrition, if tolerated, is preferable to parenteral nutrition in patients who require nutrition support.

Brief History of Parenteral Nutrition

Since the 17th century, intravenous nutrition has been of interest to the medical and nutrition communities as a means to improve nutrition status; however, it was not until the 1960s that it was successfully utilized in a human model.[2] The pioneers of PN, Dr. George Blackburn, Dr. Stanley Dudrick, Dr. Harry Vars, and Dr. Douglas Wilmore, were most interested in treating protein-energy malnutrition in patients who were either unable to use the GI tract or were experiencing failure to thrive despite sufficient oral consumption.[3]

Dr. Dudrick and his colleagues began their studies on the feasibility, efficacy, and safety of PN with a laboratory study. Six pedigreed beagle puppies were fed with PN for either 72, 100, 235, or 256 days after weaning from their mother at 8 weeks of age. The weight gain, skeletal growth, development, and activity of these puppies were compared to their orally fed littermates. At the end of the study period, the researchers found that each of the six intravenously fed puppies surpassed their controls in weight gain and matched them in skeletal growth, development, and activity. There were no significant differences between growth rates or weight gain between the experimental puppies.

The success of parenteral feeding with the beagles was encouraging for the researchers and prompted a clinical study in 30 human patients with chronic complicated GI disease. The parenteral solution provided to these patients was customized by a clinician daily to meet individual needs and compounded by a pharmacist with 20% glucose, 5% fibrin hydrolysate, electrolytes, trace minerals, and vitamins. The infusion was administered through a central catheter placed percutaneously into the superior vena cava for 10–200 days, depending on the patient. In this clinical study, positive nitrogen balance was achieved in all patients. As a result, patients experienced improvements

CASE STUDY INTRODUCTION

Alex is a 43-year-old male with a history of adenocarcinoma of the ileum and which has been in remission for 3 years. He now presents with intermittent abdominal cramping, abdominal distension, constipation, and loss of appetite and has not eaten for the past 4 days. The physician suspects that Alex's cancer treatment, including intensive radiation and two prior surgeries, has led to a small bowel obstruction. She orders a computerized tomography (CT) scan, which confirms that several intestinal adhesions have formed in the distal ileum, resulting in a complete bowel obstruction. Alex is scheduled for surgery in 5 days and is admitted to the hospital for management of his small bowel obstruction. Alex lives with his partner and 6-year-old daughter and works from home as a graphic designer.

Anthropometric Data:

Current weight: 64 kg
Usual body weight (UBW): 70 kg (6 months ago)
Height: 175 cm
Body mass index (BMI): 21 kg/m^2

Biochemical Data:

Sodium 133 (136–145 mEq/L)
Potassium 3.5 (3.5–5.0 mEq/L)
Chloride 109 (96–106 mEq/L)
Carbon dioxide 20 (22–31 mEq/L)
Blood urea nitrogen 5 (8–20 mg/dL)
Creatinine 0.6 (0.7–1.3 mg/dL)
Glucose 88 (70–139 mg/dL)
Glomerular filtration rate 99 mL/min/1.73 m^2
Calcium 8.7 (8.5–10.5 mg/dL)
Phosphorus 2.9 (2.5–4.5 mg/dL)
Magnesium 1.5 (1.5–2.7 mg/dL)
Albumin 3.5 (3.5–5.5 g/dL)
Hemoglobin 12.7 (14–18 g/dL)
Hematocrit 35% (40–50%)

Clinical Data:

Past Medical History: adenocarcinoma of the ileum s/p chemotherapy and radiation therapy
Medications: Imodium
Vital Signs: Blood pressure 110/77 mm Hg, Temperature 98.6°F
Nutrition-Focused Physical Exam: Patient appears pale with decreased muscle tone and skin turgor. Abdomen is distended with minimal bowel sounds.

Dietary Data:
Dietary History: Alex states that he has experienced intermittent abdominal cramping and poor appetite for the past several weeks. As a result, he has been skipping meals or eating half-sized portions of his usual intake. He has not eaten for the past 4 days due to worsening cramping.
Diet Prescription: NPO

Questions

1. What are Alex's nutritional risk factors?
2. Describe the possible pathophysiologic etiology associated with Alex's electrolyte abnormalities.
3. Write two Nutrition Diagnosis statements for Alex identifying the Problem/Etiology/Signs and Symptoms (PES) of Alex's active nutrition issues.
4. Identify the nutrition interventions you would like to initiate for Alex to address the problems identified in your PES statements.
5. What indicators should be included in your monitoring and evaluation plan? Why?

in wound healing, fistula closure, weight gain, and strength and activity.[4] These findings were groundbreaking, as the general consensus within the medical and nutrition communities during the 1960s was that feeding entirely by vein was not possible, practical, or affordable.

Despite its success in improving nutrition status of recipients, the research team encountered problems related to the preparation and administration of PN. Major challenges included formulating complete parenteral nutrient solutions, which did not exist at the time; concentrating **hypertonic** substrate components without precipitation; demonstrating utility and safety of long-term central venous catheterization; demonstrating efficacy and safety of long-term infusion of hypertonic nutrient solutions; maintaining **asepsis**, or the absence of bacteria throughout solution preparation and delivery; and anticipating, avoiding, and correcting metabolic imbalances or derangements.[2] Despite advances in medicine, many of these issues continue to be of concern with the preparation and administration of PN.

Parenteral Nutrition Administration

Venous Access

Depending on the type of venous access selected, PN may be referred to as **central PN (CPN)** or **peripheral PN (PPN)**. In CPN, venous access is acquired in a central vessel, namely the inferior or superior vena cava (SVC) or at the junction of the SVC and right atrium.[5] In PPN, access is obtained in a peripheral vessel, such as the vessels of the hand or forearm. Because catheters, also known as **"vascular access devices" (VADs)**, may be advanced some distance through the vasculature, the distinction between CPN and PPN is based solely on the location of the catheter tip. The location of the tip does not necessarily correspond with the site of **venipuncture** (the point where the catheter enters the vasculature) or the **exit site** (where the catheter exits the body).[5]

CORE CONCEPT 2

Venous access for parenteral nutrition is determined based on duration of therapy, desired concentration, solution type, and disease state/condition of the patient.

Figure 5.1 provides a basic algorithm for determining which form of access is appropriate for the patient.

Central Parenteral Nutrition

In CPN, the catheter tip is located in a large, high-flow vessel, typically the junction of the superior vena cava and right atrium. The vena cava and right atrium are sites of high blood flow that can quickly disperse PN solutions that might otherwise cause complications such as **thrombophlebitis**, or inflammation of a vein caused by a blood clot, and **extravasation**, or inadvertent administration or leakage of the PN into surrounding tissues instead of a vein.[5–7] The ideal tip location is the lower third of the superior vena cava or at the cavoatrial junction, as these locations are associated with the fewest mechanical and thrombotic complications.[7] The catheter tip should not be placed any deeper than this, as the risk of thrombotic complications increases when the catheter is inserted near the tricuspid valve or deeper.

The **VAD** may be centrally inserted, and the location of the catheter tip is advanced from the site of venipuncture and threaded through the vasculature

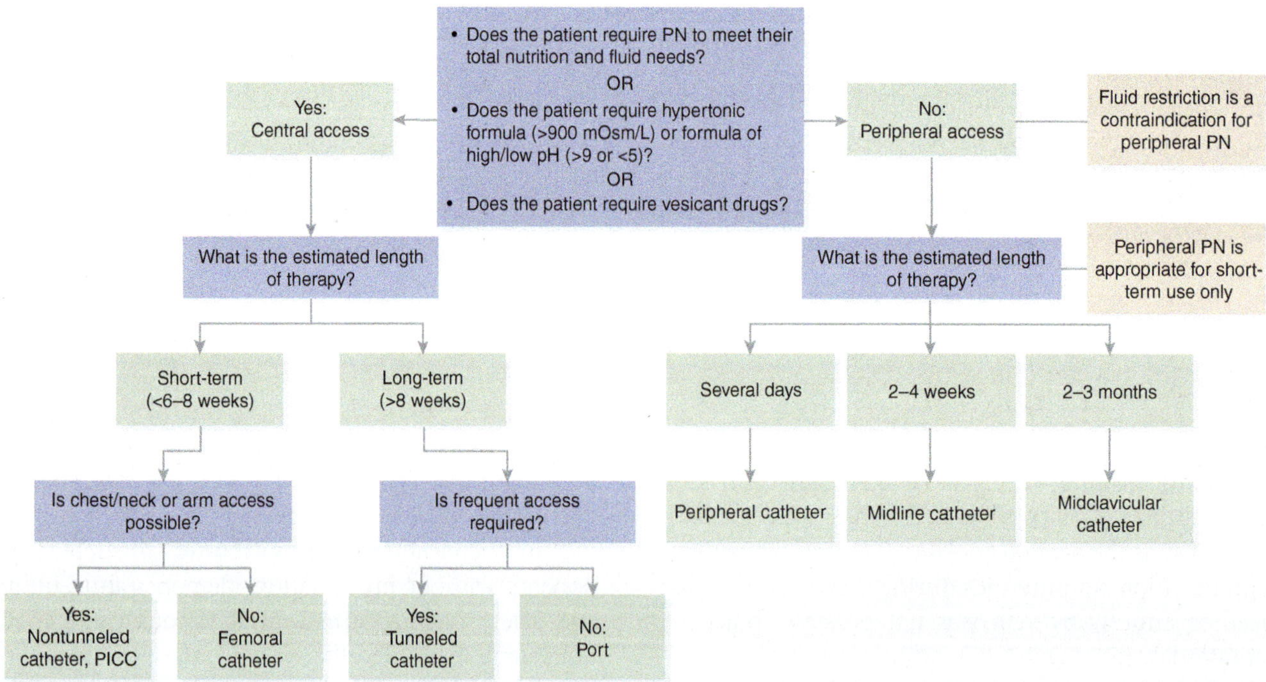

Figure 5.1 Determining Type of Intravenous Access

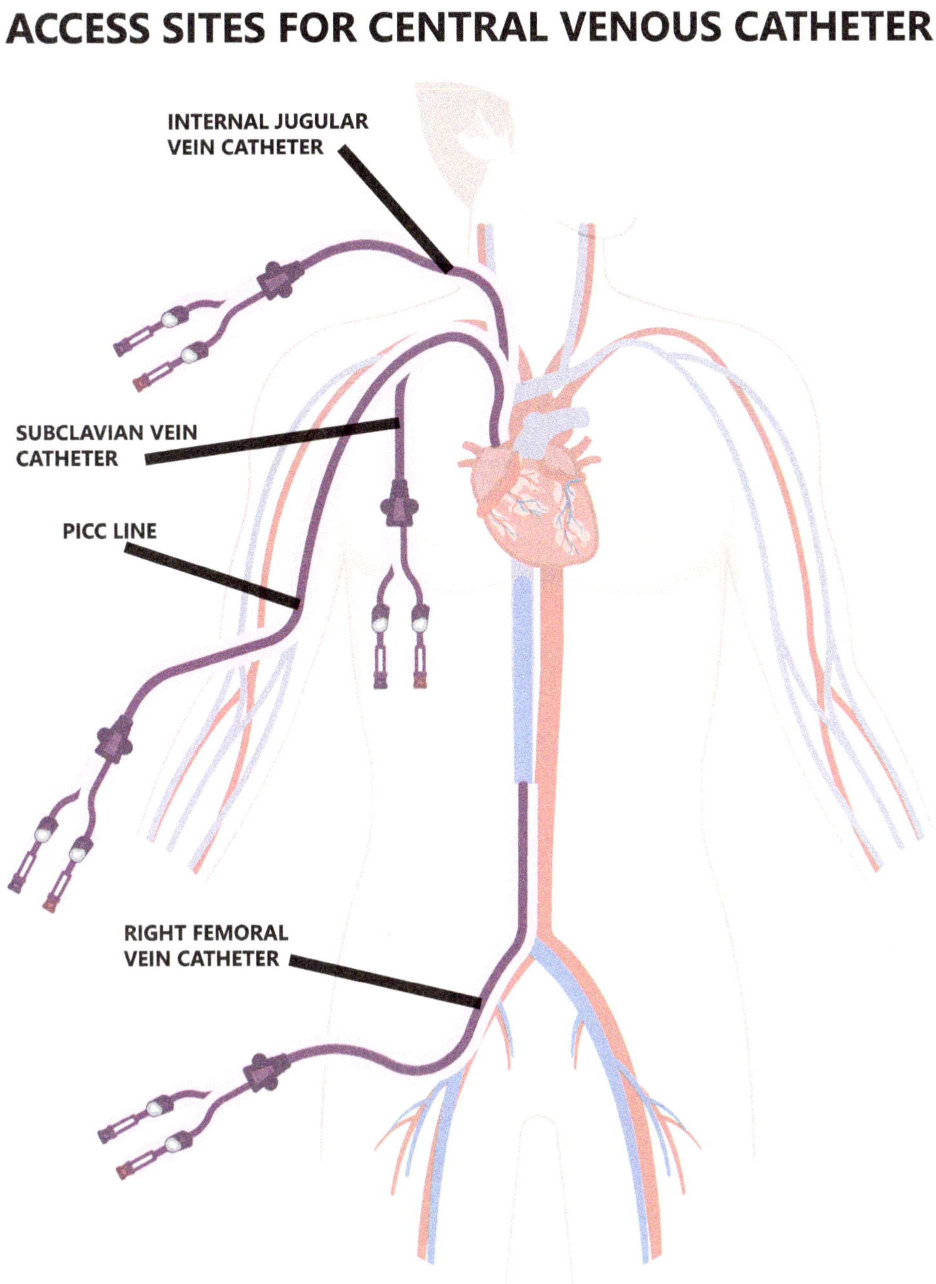

Figure 5.2 Access Sites for a Central Venous Catheter (CVC)

until the tip reaches the vena cava and/or right atrium.[5] There are two main types of central access: short-term and long-term **central venous catheters (CVCs)**. Short-term CVCs, often referred to as "non-tunneled catheters," vary by insertion site and may be inserted in the subclavian, internal or external jugular, or femoral veins. Catheter insertion into the femoral vein is associated with a higher risk of infection and thrombosis and is therefore not typically recommended for PN.[7] Alternately, short-term CVCs may be inserted in the arm via the cephalic or basilic vein. This form of access is considered a **peripherally inserted central catheter (PICC)**.[7] **Figures 5.2** and **5.3** show short-term CVCs.

Long-term central access seeks to separate the skin from the venous entry site to reduce infection risk. Long-term CVCs are often referred to as "tunneled catheters" as they are tunneled under the skin to the venous site, although the catheter exits through the skin. **Figure 5.4** displays a tunneled catheter.

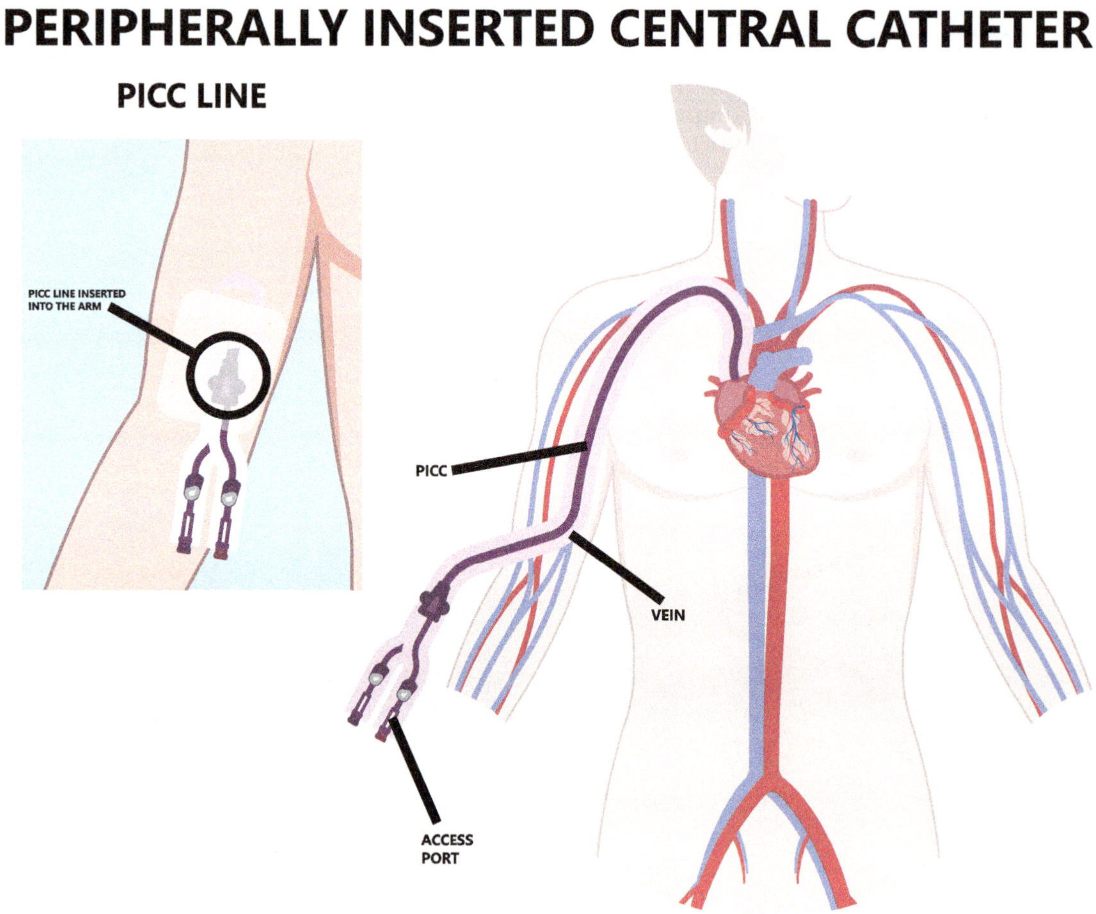

Figure 5.3 Peripherally Inserted Central Catheter (PICC) Line

Subcutaneously implanted ports are another form of long-term CVC, where an entrance port is a device that exists under the skin with a catheter connecting the device to the vein. Implantable ports are different from tunneled catheters in that there is no catheter exiting the skin, and access to the port requires puncturing the skin (**Figure 5.5** and **5.6**). Regardless of the entry site, the position of the tip should always be confirmed, whether through fluoroscopy or ultrasound during the procedure or through radiologic visualization after the procedure (**Figure 5.7**).[7]

There are advantages and disadvantages to both short-term and long-term CVCs. Short-term CVCs can typically be placed at the hospital bedside while long-term CVCs require surgical placement. Short-term CVCs, particularly those that are inserted through the subclavian, internal or external jugular, or femoral arteries, are more difficult to maintain sterile. Long-term CVCs are associated with lower infection risk and are preferred for use greater than 3 months.[7] **Table 5.1** describes various types of CVCs and their advantages and disadvantages.

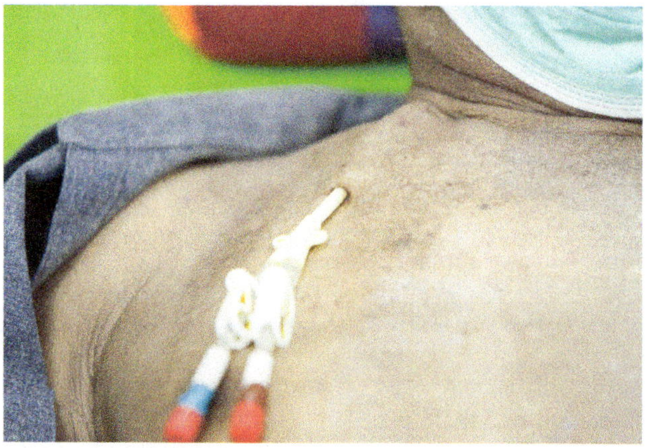

Figure 5.4 Tunneled Catheter Placement

CPN is usually the preferred form of access because it allows greater flexibility in the types of PN

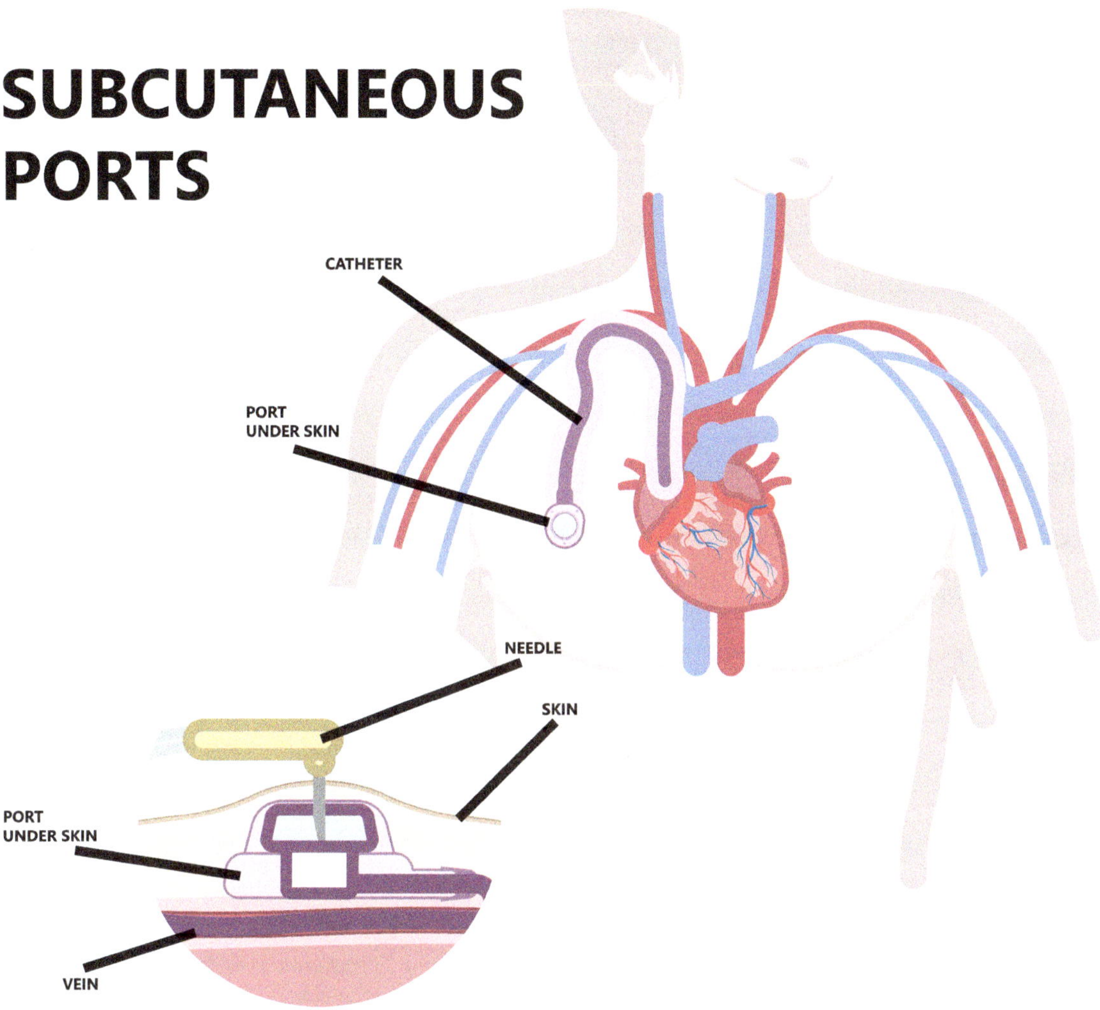

Figure 5.5 Subcutaneous Port

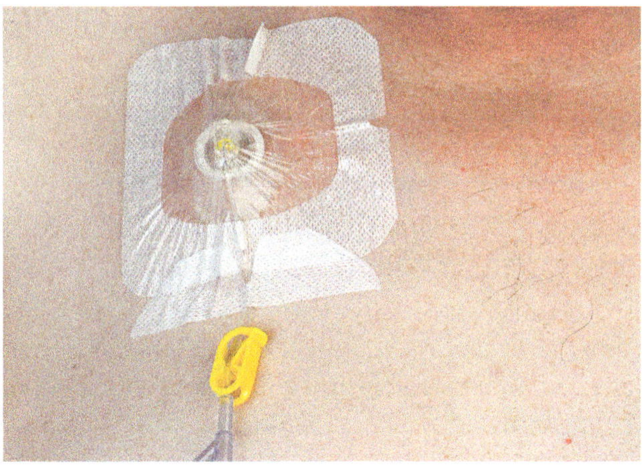

Figure 5.6 Patient with Central Venous Port

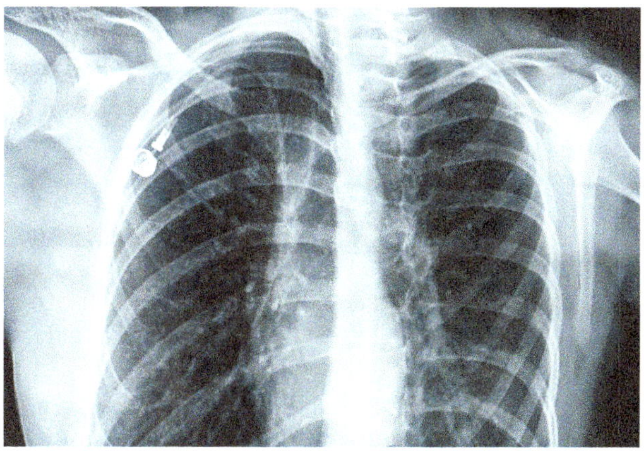

Figure 5.7 X-Ray Indicating Placement of Central Venous Port

infusions that can be administered.[5] Characteristics of PN formulas that would necessitate central access include the following:

- Hyperosmolarity (>900 mOsm/L due to concentration of dissolvable particles); osmolarity of PN is primarily due to glucose, amino acids, and electrolytes[7,8]
- High (>9) or low (<5) pH[7]
- Infusions containing vesicant drugs (can cause the vessels to become leaky)[5]

Table 5.1 Summary of Central Venous Catheters

Type of Central Venous Catheter	Description	Advantages	Disadvantages
Percutaneous nontunneled catheter	Typically used for short durations (days to weeks) in the acute care setting.	Less costly to place Easy to remove Can be exchanged over a guidewire	High risk of catheter-related infection Self-care can be difficult Requires sutures to secure in place Repair kits not readily available if catheter breaks
Peripherally inserted central catheter (PICC)	A type of percutaneous nontunneled catheter. Venipuncture occurs in a peripheral vein (e.g., basilic, cephalic, or brachial), but the tip is located in the vena cava. Can be used for weeks to months, including short-term home PN.	Low risk of placement-related complications Can be placed at bedside or radiology suite	Self-care can be difficult if placed in forearm Repair kits not readily available Cannot necessarily be used to sample blood
Tunneled catheter	The venipuncture site is removed from the catheter exit site, theoretically reducing the risk of infection. Appropriate for long-term use (months to years), including home PN.	Easier for self-care Dressings and sutures can be removed after 1 month Repair kits are available	Requires placement in operating room and a minor surgical procedure for removal
Implanted catheter	A subcutaneous port, usually placed in the chest. The port can be accessed 1000–2000 times and is ideal for patients who need infrequent IV therapy. Appropriate for long-term use, including home PN.	Easier to care for (only requires care when accessed and a monthly heparin flush) Is discrete, thus preserving body image Difficult to break Lowest rates of infection of all central venous access devices	Requires a needle to access Must be placed in operating room Requires surgical procedure for removal

Data from Tushar K. Parenteral access devices. In: Chan LN, ed. *The ASPEN Adult Nutrition Support Core Curriculum*. 4th ed. Silver Spring, MD: The American Society for Parenteral and Enteral Nutrition; 2025:435-465.

Peripheral Parenteral Nutrition

In peripheral access, the catheter tip is located outside of a central vessel.[7] Although central access is ideal, PPN may be selected because it is a safer and easier way to access the vasculature, particularly for short-term use.[5] PPN is typically used for a maximum of 2–6 weeks at a time, as the risk of dislocation and complications (e.g., **phlebitis** or inflammation of the vein) is more common than in CPN and the risk increases as dwell time increases.[5,7] An advantage of PPN is that there is evidence that it is associated with a lower risk of catheter-related infections, but this may be due to the shorter dwell time.[5]

Because PPN infuses into the smaller veins of the extremities, the PN formula cannot be as hypertonic as those formulas used in CPN. Formulas should be of low osmolarity, defined as <900 mOsm/L. There is evidence that formulas of higher osmolarity do not increase the risk of phlebitis in the short term, but these formulas may cause a burning sensation.[7,8] In clinical practice, routine use of PPN varies by institution.

Indications and Contraindications

When evaluating whether PN is an appropriate therapy for a patient, consider that PN carries a high risk

Table 5.2 Guidelines Support the Following as Reasonable Time Frames for the Initiation of PN

Adults	Well-nourished, stable	Initiate PN after 7 days
	Nutritionally-at-risk and unlikely to achieve desired oral or enteral intake	Initiate PN after 3–5 days
	Moderate or severe malnutrition and oral or enteral intake is not possible or adequate	Initiate PN as soon as feasible
Pediatric	Infant, child, or adolescent with a self-limited illness	Initiate PN after 7 days
	Child or adolescent unlikely to tolerate full oral or enteral intake for an extended period of time	Initiate PN within 4–5 days
	Infant unlikely to tolerate full oral or enteral intake for an extended period of time	Initiate PN within 1–3 days
Neonatal	Very low birth weight infant (<1500 grams)	Initiate PN promptly after birth

Data from Worthington P, Balint J, Bechtold M, et al. When is parenteral nutrition appropriate? *JPEN J Parenter Enteral Nutr*. 2017;41(3):324-377.

of serious complications. It is also a costly therapy, due to the expense of compounding, placing and maintaining VADs, monitoring laboratory values, and treating potential complications.[3] While PN has been demonstrated to improve markers of nutritional status, it does not consistently improve clinical outcomes.[3] PN is only indicated for a narrow range of circumstances and should generally not be considered a first line of therapy in nutrition support. For these reasons, the expected benefits of PN therapy should outweigh the risks.

Use of PN should not be based on medical diagnosis. Determining whether a patient is a candidate for PN requires a thorough nutrition assessment. Despite the preference for EN from a clinical perspective, there are circumstances in which PN is considered an appropriate nutrition intervention:

1. In adult patients: EN has been attempted (including trialing different tube placements) but has failed and/or EN is contraindicated due to a dysfunctional GI tract, such as short bowel syndrome, paralytic ileus, small bowel obstruction, mesenteric ischemia, enterocutaneous fistula distal to the feeding tube tip, high-output enterocutaneous fistula, and intestinal failure.[3,9]
2. In pediatric patients: EN has been attempted (including trialing different tube placements) but has failed and/or EN is contraindicated due to a dysfunctional GI tract, or when the nutrient needs to support growth are greater than that which can be provided through oral or enteral intake alone.
3. In neonates: In all critical care settings, regardless of diagnosis, when EN is unable to meet energy requirement for energy expenditure and growth.[9]

Table 5.3 Conditions in Which PN Should Be Used with Caution

Hemodynamic instability
Hyperglycemia: Glucose >300 mg/dL
Azotemia: BUN >100 mg/dL
Hyperosmolality: Serum osmolality >350 mOsm/kg
Hypernatremia: Na >150 mEq/L
Hypokalemia: K <3 mEq/L
Hyperchloremic metabolic acidosis: Cl >115 mEq/L
Hypophosphatemia: Phos <2 mg/dL

Data from Worthington P, Balint J, Bechtold M, et al. When is parenteral nutrition appropriate? *JPEN J Parenter Enteral Nutr*. 2017;41(3):324-377.

The timing of initiating PN is also an important consideration. **Table 5.2** presents current guidelines for timing of the initiation of PN.

In addition to assessing tolerance of EN, GI function, and disease state, it is also essential to assess whether the patient could tolerate PN. Patients must meet certain criteria in clinical status, including the ability to tolerate the quantities of fluid, carbohydrate, and protein required. PN should be used with caution or initiation delayed in cases of severe metabolic abnormalities. These conditions are outlined in **Table 5.3**.[3]

PRACTICE POINT

Severe hyperglycemia, azotemia, encephalopathy, and hyperosmolality, along with severe fluid and electrolyte imbalances are associated with poor tolerance of any type of nutrition support, whether it be EN or PN. These abnormalities should be corrected prior to starting nutrition support therapy.[3]

Clinical Controversy

Topic: Supplemental Parenteral Nutrition in the Intensive Care Unit

Malnutrition in the intensive care unit (ICU) is associated with increased postoperative complications, prolonged hospital stay, and increased mortality.[1] Protocols to enhance recovery after surgery (ERAS) recommend use of enteral nutrition immediately following surgery.[2] ASPEN states that either enteral or parenteral nutrition during the first week of ICU admission is acceptable given that, when energy provided is similar, there is no difference in clinical benefit or harm. These same guidelines, however, do not support the use of supplemental parenteral nutrition (SPN) during the first 7 days in patients who are unable to progress enterally. This recommendation is supported by several randomized, controlled trials showing clinical outcome benefit related to use of SPN in the ICU.[3] Although the strength of this recommendation is strong, there were discrepancies in approaches used and specific outcomes measured. One of these studies, conducted by Ridley et al., demonstrated that although SPN increased energy and protein delivery, there was no difference in clinical outcomes measured.[4] This is in contrast with a more recent study by Gao et al. demonstrating a reduction in nosocomial infections and days on antibiotics in patients receiving early SPN.[5]

Based on the two studies (references 4 and 5), provide how you might apply evidence-based findings and professional guidelines when providing nutrition support, and when you might determine that early SPN may be indicated. What are the strengths and weaknesses of each study in terms of their design and rigor? How might study population or clinical status impact your conclusion based on these studies?

References

1. Arends J, Baracos V, Bertz H, et al. ESPEN expert group recommendations for action against cancer-related malnutrition. *Clin Nutr*. 2017;36(5):1187–1196.
2. Weimann A, Braga M, Carli F, et al. ESPEN guideline: clinical nutrition in surgery. *Clin Nutr*. 2017;36(3):623–650.
3. Compher C, Bingham AL, McCall M, et al. Guidelines for the provision of nutrition support therapy in the adult critically ill patient: The American Society for Parenteral and Enteral Nutrition. *JPEN*. 2022;46:12–41.
4. Ridley EJ, Davies AR, Parke R, et al. Supplemental parenteral nutrition clinical investigators. Supplemental parenteral nutrition versus usual care in critically ill adults: a pilot randomized controlled study. *Crit Care*. 2018;22(1):12.
5. Gao X, Liu Y, Zhang L, et al. Effect of early vs late supplemental parenteral nutrition in patients undergoing abdominal surgery: a randomized clinical trial. *JAMA Surg*. 2022;157(5):384–393.

If PN is to be used, the next step is determining the venous access site and type of venous access device. In all patient populations, VAD selection should be individualized based on the risks and benefits of the device, clinical factors, and psychosocial considerations.[7,10–12] The smallest device with the fewest number of lumens necessary is preferred, although in patients with critical illness, it is often necessary to have multiple lumens to accommodate administration of medications and IV fluids, including PN. It is ideal if there is one lumen dedicated to PN administration. In patients who are acutely ill, a nontunneled or PICC line is generally appropriate, whereas a port would be reserved for extended need for access.[10] CPN is appropriate when PN is required for longer-term use (>2 weeks), peripheral venous access is inadequate, the patient has significant nutrient needs, or the patient is fluid restricted.[3] PPN may be considered if nutrition support is only needed for a short time frame (up to 2 weeks) if the patient is not a candidate for CPN.[3] PPN can provide partial or total nutrition, but because the PPN solution is less concentrated, a higher volume must be administered to provide total nutrition. For this reason, a patient who requires fluid restriction (e.g., due to kidney disease) would not be a candidate for PPN.[3] In general, patients receiving PPN should be able to tolerate 2–3 L of fluid per day. However, this can be useful to correct short-term nutrition deficits while avoiding need for a central line insertion.[11]

CORE CONCEPT 3

Candidates for parenteral nutrition must be fully evaluated for nutritional risk and nutritional status with adherence to standardized protocols for initiation of parenteral nutrition.

Parenteral Nutrition Formulations

Parenteral nutrition can be provided as either a ready-to-use (also known as “premixed” or “standardized”) PN solution, or as a custom compounded solution.

Ready-to-use PN products are sold in varying compositions, including those suitable for both peripheral and central administration. These products contain a set percentage of both carbohydrate and amino acids, with or without electrolyte additives. The amount of total nutrition delivered to the patient is controlled by the infusion rate and total volume delivered. Use of ready-to-use PN products varies by institution but is becoming increasingly more popular across the country. Custom PN solutions are individualized to each patient. The components that can be included in the solution are carbohydrate, amino acids, lipids, electrolytes, vitamins, trace minerals, sterile water, and a number of other specific additives.

Custom PN solutions can be compounded as either a 3-in-1 **total nutrient admixture (TNA)** (**Figure 5.8**) that contains all three macronutrients (dextrose, amino acids, and lipid) in one solution, or as a 2-in-1 formulation containing two macronutrients (dextrose and amino acids) in one solution with the option to provide an intravenous lipid emulsion (ILEs) as a separate infusion (**Figure 5.9**). When ILEs are infused as separate preparations from dextrose and amino acids, as with a 2-in-1 formulation, there is enhanced microbial growth potential because the pH of the ILE is biologically compatible with bacteria. For this reason, the Centers for Disease Control and Prevention recommends a 12-hour hang time limit for ILE. In contrast, a 3-in-1 TNA containing dextrose, amino acids, and lipid in the same container may be administered over 24 hours. The administration and hang time of 3-in-1 formulations is extended because bacterial growth is inhibited by the reduced pH (pH approximately 5.6–6) and the increased total osmolarity with the combination of all 3 substrates in one container.[13–15]

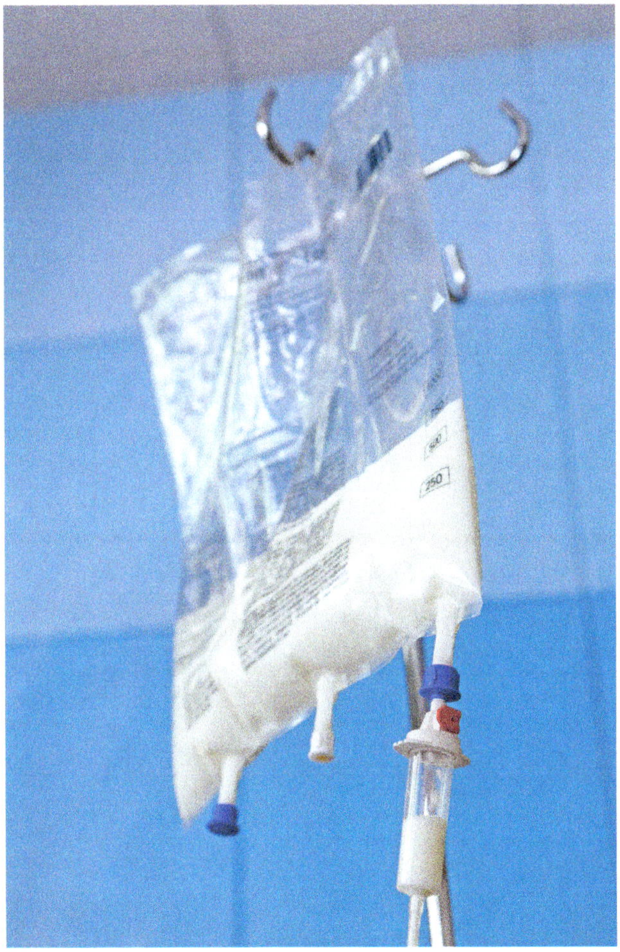

Figure 5.8 Example of a 3-in-1 TPN Solution Where Dextrose, Amino Acids, and Lipid Emulsion Are Combined

Given in the appropriate amounts, the IV administration of these components can maintain nutrition status and support life long-term without use of the GI tract.

CORE CONCEPT 4

Parenteral nutrition is a hypertonic solution made up of, but not limited to, carbohydrate in the form of dextrose, crystalline amino acids, lipid emulsions, electrolytes, vitamins, minerals, and sterile water.

Carbohydrate

As the primary energy source for the body, the carbohydrate component of PN is critical. Carbohydrate should always be included in PN because of its protein-sparing effect. The most commonly used carbohydrate substrate in PN formulas is dextrose monohydrate, the dextrorotatory form of glucose. In its hydrated

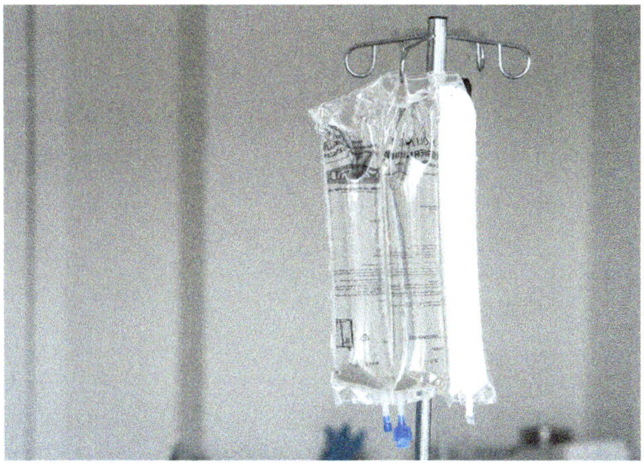

Figure 5.9 Example of a 2-in-1 TPN Solution Where Lipid Emulsions Are Provided Separately from Dextrose and Amino Acids

form, dextrose provides 3.4 kcal /g, not 4 kcal/g like dietary carbohydrates.[1,15]

Commercially, dextrose is available in multiple concentrations ranging from 5%–70%.[1] Because dextrose is an acidic molecule, the higher concentration solutions are more acidic. According to the United States Pharmacopeia (USP), dextrose solutions range from pH 3.5–6.5. Dextrose solutions greater than 10% concentration are typically reserved for central venous administration because the hypertonicity and acidity of the solution has the potential to cause thrombophlebitis in peripheral veins.[15]

Intravenous dextrose infusion can be challenging due to its effect on glycemic control. Infusing dextrose directly into the bloodstream raises serum glucose, which can lead to hyperglycemia if the body does not mount an appropriate metabolic response.[1] Protocolized monitoring of serum glucose and intervention to prevent both hyperglycemia and hypoglycemia must be implemented to avoid more serious complications.

The most common dextrose solution used in PN is 20% dextrose in water (D20W). This concentration supplies 200 grams of dextrose/L and 680 kcal/L. The mathematical process used to equate the grams of dextrose supplied per liter and the calories supplied per liter is demonstrated as follows:

$$\begin{aligned} 20\% \text{ dextrose} &= \frac{20 \text{ grams dextrose}}{100 \text{ mL}} \times \frac{1000 \text{ mL}}{1 \text{ L}} \\ &= \frac{200 \text{ grams dextrose}}{1 \text{ L}} \times 3.4 \frac{\text{kilocalories}}{\text{grams dextrose}} \\ &= 680 \text{ kilocalories} \end{aligned}$$

Table 5.4 displays different dextrose solutions available for use in PN, grams of dextrose per liter, kcal per liter, and peripheral versus central access requirement.

Amino Acids

A variety of illnesses and catabolic conditions can disturb the blood amino acid profile, promote a decrease in lean body mass, and increase body protein requirements. Mixed amino acid formulations that provide both essential and nonessential amino acids are a standard component of complete PN prescriptions to support cellular functions throughout the body.[15]

If oxidized for energy, crystalline amino acids supply 4 kcal/g. As with other PN components, amino acid solutions are available in different concentrations ranging from 3%–20%. All commercially available amino acid solutions for PN contain all nine essential amino acids in varying amounts between 38% and 57% of total amino acids. Standard solutions also provide some nonessential amino acids at about 43%–62% of total amino acids. Nitrogen content varies depending on the concentration of the solution and the amino acid profile.[15]

Specialty amino acid formulations are commercially available for use in certain disease states like kidney failure, hepatic encephalopathy, metabolic stress, trauma, thermal injury, and hypercatabolic states. These products are generally more costly than standard formulas and should only be used in patients who meet the intended indications and who are expected to benefit clinically from the specialty amino acid formula.[13] The American Society of Parenteral and Enteral Nutrition (ASPEN) has published guidelines for the use of these products in clinical practice.[15] **Table 5.5** provides more information on some of the standard and specialty crystalline amino acid solutions available for use in PN.[15–19]

Table 5.4 Dextrose Solutions

Solution	Grams of Dextrose per Liter (g/L)	Kilocalories per Liter (kcal/L)	Peripheral versus Central Administration
5% dextrose in water (D5W)	50	170	Peripheral or central
10% dextrose in water (D10W)	100	340	Peripheral or central
15% dextrose in water (D15W)	150	510	Central
20% dextrose in water (D20W)	200	680	Central
25% dextrose in water (D25W)	250	850	Central
30% dextrose in water (D30W)	300	1020	Central
40% dextrose in water (D40W)	400	1360	Central
50% dextrose in water (D50W)	500	1700	Central

Table 5.5 Commercially Available Crystalline Amino Acid Solutions

Brand Name, Manufacturer	Type/Indication	Stock Concentrations	Composition
Travasol, Baxter	Standard	3.5%, 4.25%, 5.5%, 8.5%, 10%	Essential amino acids + alanine, glycine, arginine, proline, serine, and tyrosine[16]
Clinisol, Baxter	Standard/fluid restriction	15%	Essential amino acids + alanine, arginine, proline, glutamic acid, serine, aspartic acid, and tyrosine[17]
ProSol, Baxter	Standard/fluid restriction	20%	Essential amino acids + alanine, glycine, arginine, proline, glutamic acid, serine, aspartic acid, and tyrosine[16]
Aminosyn II, Abbott	Standard	3.5%, 4.25%, 5%, 7%, 8.5%, 10%, 15%	Essential amino acids + alanine, glycine, arginine, proline, glutamic acid, serine, aspartic acid, tyrosine, and histidine[17]
FreAmine III, B. Braun	Standard	8.5%, 10%	Essential amino acids + alanine, glycine, arginine, proline, serine, histidine, and cysteine[19]
HepatAmine, B. Braun	Hepatic failure	8%	Essential amino acids + alanine, glycine, arginine, proline, serine, and histidine + branched chain amino acid enriched[19]
FreAmine HBC, B. Braun	Metabolic stress	6.9%	Essential amino acids + alanine, glycine, arginine, proline, serine, and histidine + branched chain amino acid enriched[19]
Aminosyn HBC, Abbott	Metabolic stress	7%	Essential amino acids + alanine, glycine, arginine, proline, serine, tyrosine, and histidine + branched chain amino acid enriched[17]
BranchAmin, Baxter	Metabolic stress	4%	Contains branched chain amino acids only (leucine, isoleucine, and valine)[15]
NephrAmine, B. Braun	Renal failure	5.4%	Contains essential amino acids only[15]
Aminosyn RF, Abbott	Renal failure	5.2%	Contains essential amino acids + arginine[19]
TrophAmine, B. Braun	Infants and young children	6%, 10%	Essential amino acids + alanine, glycine, arginine, proline, glutamic acid, serine, aspartic acid, tyrosine, taurine, and cysteine[16]

Lipids

The infusion of ILEs, also known as "injectable lipid emulsions," provides a high energy supply, contributes to the prevention of high glucose infusion rates, and is indispensable for supplying the body with essential fatty acids (EFAs).[20] In the United States, ILE components include an oil source, egg yolk phospholipid as an emulsifier, glycerin to render the formulation isotonic, and sodium hydroxide to adjust the final pH to a range of 6–9. Historically, the most common oil sources used in ILEs have been soybean oil and safflower oil, which contain long-chain triglycerides.[15] These oils were used because they are relatively inexpensive, abundant on the market, and effectively deliver nonglucose energy to the body. A disadvantage of soybean and safflower oils is their high levels of omega-6 fatty acid and low levels of omega-3 fatty acid, a ratio that is known to promote systemic inflammation. To address concerns associated with the soybean oil–based ILEs, alternative sources of fatty acids were and continue to be investigated.[15] In 2016, the Food and Drug Administration approved SMOFlipid™, which is comprised of four different oils: 30% soybean, 30% medium-chain triglycerides derived from coconut oil, 25% olive oil, and 15% fish

Table 5.6 Composition of Parenteral Lipid Emulsions

ILE, Manufacturer	Soybean Oil (%)	Coconut (Medium-Chain Triglyceride) Oil (%)	Olive Oil (%)	Fish Oil (%)
Intralipid, Fresenius Kabi	100	0	0	0
Lipofundin, B. Braun	50	50	0	0
SMOF Lipid™, Fresenius Kabi	30	30	25	15
Clinolipid (ClinOleic), Baxter	20	0	80	0
Omegaven, Fresenius Kabi	0	0	0	100

Data from Gura KM, Hise-Brown M, Brown JC. Lipids. In: Chan, LN ed. *ASPEN Adult Nutrition Support Core Curriculum*. 4th ed. Silver Spring, MD: The American Society for Parenteral and Enteral Nutrition; 2025:99–136.

oil. SMOFlipid, and others like it, have an improved omega-3:omega-6 ratio that may reduce inflammation as well as the risk of harmful changes to the liver, such as **parenteral nutrition-associated liver disease** or intestinal failure–associated liver disease (to be discussed later in this chapter), **hepatic steatosis**, and infection rates. This is particularly relevant for patients requiring long-term PN.[21,22] More research is needed in patients who are critically ill. Current ASPEN guidelines state that due to limited evidence, either soybean oil–based or mixed oil ILE can be provided, including during the first week of ICU admission.[23] **Table 5.6** presents the composition of commercially available ILE solutions.

ILEs are commercially available as 20% (2 kcal/mL) and 30% concentrations (2.9–3 kcal/mL, depending on the manufacturer); however, 30% ILE is not approved for direct IV administration. This high concentration is only approved for the compounding of a TNA. Previously, 10% ILE (1.1 kcal/mL) was commercially available; however, it is currently only available in premixed products or in products containing lipid emulsions such as propofol.[15]

In practice, lipid is not always provided in PN. Although institutions may have their own criteria, it is common to hold lipids when a patient is receiving propofol, which is a short-acting hypnotic sedative provided in a 10% lipid emulsion, or other medications delivered in a lipid emulsion. Lipids should also be withheld in patients who have an egg or soy allergy, or when they have hypertriglyceridemia prior to the initiation of lipid.[23]

Electrolytes

Parenteral solutions represent a significant portion, if not all, of total daily fluid and electrolyte intake.[1] Maintenance or therapeutic amounts of various electrolytes are added to PN formulations depending on the patient's individual requirements. Acetate and chloride do not have specific ranges for intake; rather, they are adjusted as needed to maintain acid–base balance.[24] Other electrolytes are available in various salt forms as outlined in **Table 5.7**. For administration in PN, calcium gluconate and magnesium sulfate are the preferred forms of these electrolytes compared to calcium chloride, calcium gluceptate, and magnesium chloride because they are less likely to produce **physiochemical incompatibility**, which are physical or chemical changes that can occur in PN leading to precipitation, color changes, or chemical degradation that can compromise the solution.[15]

Electrolytes are commercially available as individual salts and as combination products for ease in admixing. They are also pre-added to certain stock amino acid solutions or premixed PN formulations.[15]

CORE CONCEPT 5

Many lipid emulsions are composed of primarily omega-6 fatty acids and should be provided judiciously given their role in inflammation.

PRACTICE POINT

Parenteral nutrition formulas that are high in amino acids can contribute to a decrease in blood pH. To balance this effect, electrolytes in this situation can be provided as acetate.

Table 5.7 Commercially Available Parenteral Electrolyte Salts

	Chloride	Acetate	Phosphate	Sulfate	Gluconate	Gluceptate
Sodium	X	X	X	–	–	–
Potassium	X	X	X	–	–	–
Calcium	X	–	–	–	X	X
Magnesium	X	–	–	X	–	–

Data from American Society for Parenteral and Enteral Nutrition (ASPEN). *Appropriate dosing for parenteral nutrition: ASPEN recommendations*. Updated November 17, 2020. Accessed January 10, 2025. https://www.nutritioncare.org/PNdosing

Table 5.8 Composition of Adult Parenteral Multivitamin Products Available in the United States

Vitamin/Mineral	FDA requirement	MVI-12	MVI-13
Vitamin C (ascorbic acid)	200 mg	200 mg	200 mg
Vitamin B3 (niacin)	40 mg	40 mg	40 mg
Pantothenic acid (dexpanthenol)	15 mg	15 mg	15 mg
Vitamin E (dl-α-tocopherol acetate)	10 mg (10 USP units)	10 mg (10 USP units)	10 mg (10 USP units)
Vitamin B6 (pyridoxine)	6 mg	6 mg	6 mg
Vitamin B1 (thiamine)	6 mg	6 mg	6 mg
Vitamin B2 (riboflavin)	3.6 mg	3.6 mg	3.6 mg
Vitamin A (retinol)	1 mg (3300 USP units)	1 mg (3300 USP units)	1 mg (3300 USP units)
Folic acid	600 mcg	600 mcg	600 mcg
Vitamin K (phylloquinone)	150 mcg	0	150 mcg
Biotin	60 mcg	60 mcg	60 mcg
Vitamin D (ergocalciferol)	5 mcg (200 USP units)	5 mcg (200 USP units)	5 mcg (200 USP units)
Vitamin B12 (cyanocobalamin)	5 mcg	5 mcg	5 mcg

Data from: American Society for Parenteral and Enteral Nutrition (ASPEN). *Parenteral nutrition multivitamin product shortage considerations*. Accessed January 11, 2025. https://www.nutritioncare.org/Guidelines_and_Clinical_Resources/Product_Shortages/2021_Parenteral_Nutrition_Multivitamin_Product_Shortage_Considerations/

Multivitamins

In addition to macronutrients and electrolytes, patients receiving PN require vitamins to prevent deficiency and promote optimal health. Clinical practice guidelines include the justification, dosage, and route of delivery for inclusion of vitamins in patients receiving PN. Guideline adherence ensures optimum nutrition care and improves patient outcomes.

Commercially available vitamin products for PN supplementation include both single and multivitamin infusion products. In 2000, the Food and Drug Administration issued parenteral multivitamin dosing requirements. In accordance with these requirements, parenteral multivitamins include vitamin A, vitamin D, vitamin E, vitamin K, vitamin B1, vitamin B2, vitamin B6, vitamin B12, niacin, folic acid, pantothenic acid, biotin, and vitamin C. One parenteral multivitamin product is available without vitamin K for patients on warfarin anticoagulant therapy.[25] Composition of the standard parenteral multivitamin products available in the United States is included in **Table 5.8**.

Single vitamins are used when a patient requires more of a vitamin than a parenteral multivitamin provides. Currently, there are no single PN vitamin products available for biotin, pantothenic acid, riboflavin, vitamin A, vitamin D, or vitamin E.[15]

Trace Elements

The need for trace elements in long-term PN was realized when patients began to develop deficiency symptoms that were alleviated through trace element supplementation. Some of the deficiencies that developed were copper, zinc, manganese, selenium, chromium, and molybdenum.[26] Of these, copper, zinc, manganese, selenium, and chromium are the most commonly supplemented trace elements in PN formulations. These trace minerals are available in both individual form and various trace element combinations at concentrations safe for use in neonates, pediatrics, and adults.[15] The American Medical Association and ASPEN have published recommendations for daily parenteral doses of selenium, zinc, copper, manganese, and chromium, as presented in **Table 5.9**.[15]

Other trace elements that are less commonly used in PN but are still available are molybdenum, iodine,

Table 5.9 Trace Element Deficiencies Associated with Long-Term Parenteral Nutrition

Trace Element	Deficiency Symptoms	ASPEN Recommendation
Copper	Sensory ataxia Lower extremity spasticity Paresthesias in extremities Hypochromic microcytic anemia Leukopenia Neutropenia Hypercholesterolemia Decreased ceruloplasmin Reduced erythrocyte copper to zinc ratio Increased erythrocyte turnover Abnormal electrocardiographic patterns Myeloneuropathy	0.3–0.5 mg/day
Zinc	Inadequate growth Acrodermatitis Hypogonadism Impaired night vision Anorexia Diarrhea Alterations in taste and smell Alopecia Impaired epithelialization and wound healing Impaired immune function	2.5–5 mg/day
Manganese	Poor reproductive performance Congenital abnormalities in offspring Abnormal bone/cartilage formation Ataxia Growth retardation Defects in lipid/carbohydrate metabolism	60–100 mcg/day
Selenium	Oxidative injury Increased susceptibility to mercury poisoning Altered thyroid hormone metabolism Increased plasma glutathione levels Keshan disease	20–60 mcg/day
Chromium	Weight loss Hyperglycemia refractory to insulin Glycosuria Elevated plasma free fatty acids Peripheral neuropathy Hyperlipidemia	10–15 mcg/day

Trace Element	Deficiency Symptoms	ASPEN Recommendation
Molybdenum	Tachycardia Tachypnea Visual/mental changes Elevated methionine Headache Lethargy Nausea Vomiting	None
Iron	Microcytic hypochromic anemia Tachycardia Poor capillary refilling Fatigue Sleepiness Headache Anorexia Nausea Pallor Impaired ability to maintain body temperature in cold environments Increased lead absorption Koilonychia Glossitis	None

Data from McKeever L. Trace Elements and Other Compounds. In: Chan, LN ed. *ASPEN Adult Nutrition Support Core Curriculum*. 4th ed. Silver Spring, MD: The American Society for Parenteral and Enteral Nutrition; 2025:231–254.

and iron. Iron dextran is the only iron product approved for addition to PN. This product should only be added to 2-in-1 dextrose–amino acid formulations as opposed to PN formulas that contain lipid, like a 3-in-1 TNA, because ILEs are disrupted by iron.[15] If iron dextran is administered, a strict protocol should be followed, and the patient should be closely monitored as anaphylaxis is a potential side effect. Nonetheless, iron is still an essential part of most long-term PN regimens and is necessary to prevent deficiency.[27]

Other Additives

Insulin

The development of hyperglycemia during inpatient PN therapy has been independently associated with higher rates of mortality and hospital complications. These observations indicate that prevention and correction of hyperglycemia through modification of nutrient composition or by insulin administration should be strongly considered during PN therapy.[28] Insulin can be administered through subcutaneous injection, IV infusion, as a direct additive into the PN solution, or any combination of these. The most common initial regimen for insulin in PN is 1 unit of regular insulin per 10 grams of dextrose. A target blood glucose range for hospitalized patients receiving PN is 140–180 mg/dL.[29,30] The regimen may increase to 1.5 units of regular insulin per 10 grams of dextrose.[31] It is critical to use hospital- or unit-specific protocols for insulin infusions that include careful monitoring blood glucose to allow for proper intervention of both high and low levels.

Medications

Addition of certain medications into PN solutions is generally not advised due to potential for the formation of precipitates, adverse reactions, and disturbances in acid–base balance.[15,24] Medication compatibility with PN often depends on the hydrophilicity or hydrophobicity of the drug/medication and the formulation of the PN solution. Lipid-based (hydrophobic) medications are more likely to be compatible with ILE or TNA, while water-based medications (hydrophilic) are more likely to be compatible with a 2-in-1 dextrose-amino acid solutions.[15] Under current practice standards, pharmacists can admix certain medications into PN solutions; however, medication should never be added after the solution leaves the pharmacy or compounding center (Figure 5.10).[32]

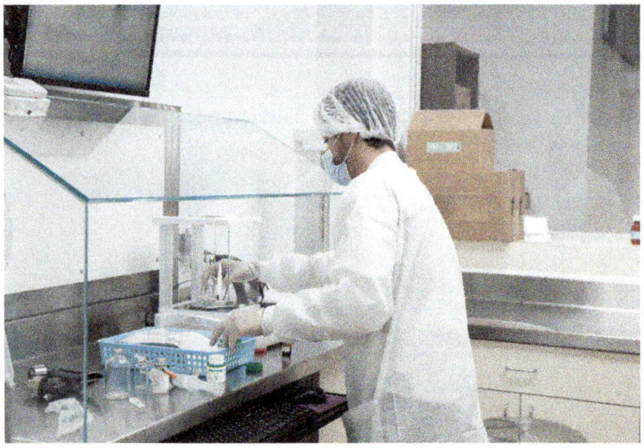

Figure 5.10 Pharmacist Compounding Medications for IV Solution Under Sterile Conditions

PRACTICE POINT

When in doubt about compatibility or safety of a medication or parenteral nutrition additive, seek evidence in existing literature and consult the pharmacist responsible for admixing parenteral solutions at your institution.

Initiation and Progression of Parenteral Nutrition

As previously stated in this chapter, PN is a type of nutrition support that is typically individualized to the needs of the patient. This customization requires knowledge of each of the component parts that compose PN and use of basic mathematics. Calculating the PN prescription and completing the order form appropriately is often the most intimidating aspect of PN for clinical trainees and novice clinicians. **Table 5.10** provides a method to calculate a PN prescription. An example of this method is provided in **Table 5.11**.

Safety Check of Macronutrient Infusion Rates to Avoid Overfeeding

Due to risk of complications, there are maximum daily doses and/or infusion rates set for both lipid and carbohydrate. Dosing for ILE varies slightly based on lipid source. For patients who are critically ill, the recommended dose is <1 gram/kg for soybean oil, and

Clinical Roundtable

Topic: PN Component Shortages: An Ethical Challenge

Background: PN component shortages have been consistently impacting hospitals and home infusion companies. Every parenteral nutrition component has been in short supply at some point, including ILE, amino acids, vitamins, electrolyte additives, and sterile water.[1] Shortages arise due to issues in the manufacturing process. Because producing PN components and other drugs is a highly controlled process for safety and sterility, there are a limited number of production lines that can meet these requirements. When a problem arises at one of these locations, pharmaceutical companies are responsible for notifying the Food and Drug Administration if a decrease in supply is projected.

Currently, there is no mandatory timeframe to resolve the manufacturing issue. Because the PN drug market is not a particularly profitable one, there is little incentive for pharmaceutical companies to resolve shortages quickly. These shortages pose a significant risk for patients who rely on PN as their sole source of nutrition. If a component is in short supply, clinicians are forced to administer a lower dose, prioritize which patients receive the component, or omit the component entirely. Various deficiencies have been reported as a result of this ongoing issue.[1]

In response to ongoing drug shortages, ASPEN created the Parenteral Nutrition Product Shortage Committee as a subcommittee of the Clinical Practice Committee. This group continually disseminates information on current and expected component and drug shortages.[1] They have also developed and published a set of recommendations for managing shortages. The recommendations provide strategies for rationing and conserving products so that drugs and PN components are available for the most critical patients.

Roundtable Discussion

Consider a scenario in which there was a PN component shortage at your institution.

1. How would you prioritize which patients would continue to receive PN and which patients would not?
2. What strategies could you use to ensure that as many patients as possible receive adequate nutrition despite the shortage?

References

1. ASPEN. Parenteral nutrition multivitamin product shortage considerations. Updated October 9, 2024. Accessed January 11, 2025. https://www.nutritioncare.org/Guidelines_and_Clinical_Resources/Product_Shortages/2021_Parenteral_Nutrition_Multivitamin_Product_Shortage_Considerations

Table 5.10 Parenteral Nutrition Formula Calculation Method

Determine energy requirements	■ Use the standard method utilized by your institution including but not limited to: • Indirect calorimetry • Harris–Benedict equation • Mifflin–St Jeor predictive equation • Penn State predictive equation • Estimation using kcal/kg
Determine protein requirements and calories from protein	Protein stress factor based on disease state or severity of disease = protein requirement (grams) $$\text{Protein (grams)} \times 4\frac{\text{kcal}}{\text{gram}} = \text{kcal from protein}$$
Determine ILE requirements	Does the patient need to receive lipids? No: • If patient is receiving propofol/clevidipine **or** • If patient has hypertriglyceridemia (TG >300 mg/dL) **or** • If patient has egg or soy allergy Yes: If above conditions do not apply and/or if the patient has essential fatty acid deficiency
	If yes: Total energy requirement (kcal) × % energy from lipid = lipid requirement (kcal) *energy from lipid is typically 30% or less and should not exceed 60% kcal from lipid
Calculate kcal remaining for dextrose	Total energy requirement – [(protein kcal) + (lipid kcal)] = dextrose kcal
Calculate grams of dextrose	$$\text{Dextrose (kcal)} \div 3.4\frac{\text{kcal}}{\text{gram}} = \text{dextrose (grams)}$$
Determine desired total volume	Is the patient fluid restricted? If yes: Aim for 1 L volume of PN or less per day If no: Use predictive equation for fluid: $$x \text{ fluid in } \left(\frac{\text{mL}}{\text{kg}}\right) \times \text{weight (kg)} = \text{fluid requirement (mL)}$$ x is the factor being used to calculate fluid. Typical factors for maintenance fluid needs are listed below: If fluid losses are expected or the nutrition care plan includes home PN, be sure to provide at least maintenance fluid needs. Young adults: 35 mL/kg body weight Adults: 30 mL/kg body weight Older Adults: 25 mL/kg body weight
Calculate component concentration/volume	Protein (concentration): $$\text{protein requirement (grams)} \div \text{desired volume of parental nutrition (mL)} \times 1000\frac{\text{mL}}{\text{L}}$$ $$= \text{concentration of amino acid solution}\frac{\text{grams AA}}{\text{L}}$$ $$\div 100 \rightarrow \text{percent AA\%}$$ Round to the nearest available amino acid concentration

(continues)

Table 5.10 Parenteral Nutrition Formula Calculation Method *(continued)*

	Lipid (volume and grams): lipid requirement (kcal) ÷ ILE concentration $\frac{\text{kcal}}{\text{mL}}$ = lipid requirement (mL) lipid volume (mL) × ILE concentration $\frac{\text{kcal}}{\text{mL}} \times \frac{\text{1 gram ILE}}{\text{10 kcal}}$ = lipid grams (grams) ILE volume is considered anhydrous, and some may prefer to exclude ILE volume from total fluid volume when providing maintenance fluid requirements. kcal/gram ILE fat = 10 kcal $\left(\frac{\text{as opposed to 9 kcal}}{\text{gram}}\right)$
	Dextrose (concentration): dextrose requirement (grams) ÷ desired volume of parental nutrition (mL) × 1000 $\frac{\text{mL}}{\text{L}}$ = concentration of dextrose solution $\frac{\text{gram}}{\text{L}}$ grams dextrose/L ÷ 100 → percent dextrose% Round to the nearest available dextrose concentration
Determine goal rate	Total volume (mL) ÷ 24 hours/day = goal rate (mL/hour)
Final answer	The PN prescription can be ordered per day or per liter. Per day: Total grams of dextrose per day, total grams of amino acids per day, and total grams of lipid per day = ______ kcal/day, __________ grams protein/day Per liter: D (percent concentration of dextrose) AA (percent concentration of amino acid) with (concentration of ILE) ILE at (goal rate) mL/hour = ______ kcal/day, ______ gram protein/day

*Note if ILE is provided as part of a 2:1 mixture, volume is run over 12 hours. If a 3-in-1 mixture is used, ILE volume is included as part of total volume and will run over 24 hours along with dextrose and amino acids

Table 5.11 Parenteral Nutrition Formula Calculation Method: A Sample Calculation

70-year-old male
178 cm, 91 kg
Trauma, hypermetabolic, intubated, sedated, 8 days NPO
All labs within normal limits
Propofol: 20 mL/hour, Maintenance fluid requirement: 25 mL/kg
The hospital utilizes 2-in-1 PN formulations and 20% ILE

Determine energy requirements	Penn State Equation = 2650 kcal/day
Determine protein requirements and calories from protein	Protein stress factor based on disease state or severity of illness × weight in kg = protein requirement $\left(\frac{\text{gram}}{\text{kg}}\right)$ $1.4 \frac{\text{g}}{\text{kg}} \times 91$ kg = 127 grams protein/day Protein requirement = 127 grams/day 127 Protein (grams) × 4 $\frac{\text{kcal}}{\text{gram}}$ = 508 kcal from protein

Determine ILE requirements	Does the patient need to receive IV lipids? No: ■ If patient is receiving propofol **or** ■ If patient has hypertriglyceridemia (TG >300 mg/dL) **or** ■ If patient has egg or soy allergy **or** Yes: If above conditions do not apply and/or if the patient has essential fatty acid deficiency No, the patient is receiving propofol at 20 mL/hour. To calculate calories from propofol which is based on 10% ILE: $$\frac{20\text{ mL}}{\text{hour}} \times \frac{24\text{ hours}}{\text{day}} = \frac{480\text{ mL}}{\text{day}}$$ $$480\text{ mL} \times \frac{1.1\text{ kcal}}{\text{mL}} = 528\text{ kcal}$$ This is supplying the patient with 528 kcal/day from lipids. If the patient was not receiving propofol, triglycerides were within normal limits, and their goal was set at 20% of total calories, their requirement would be 530 kcal. This is calculated with the following equation: $$\text{total energy requirement (kcal} \times \%\text{ energy from lipid} = \text{lipid requirement (kcal)}$$ $$2650\text{ kcal} \times 20\%\text{ energy from lipid} = 530\text{ (kcal)}$$ After 14 days of NPO status, if no other lipid source is provided, the patient should be given essential fatty acids at a minimum of 2–4% of total kcal to prevent essential fatty acid deficiency.
Calculate kcal remaining for dextrose	$$\text{Total energy requirement (kcal)} - (\text{protein (kcal)} + \text{lipid (kcal)}) = \text{dextrose (kcal)}$$ $$2650\text{ kcal} - (508\text{ kcal} + 528\text{ kcal}) = 1614\text{ kcal}$$ $$\text{kcal remaining for dextrose} = 1614$$
Calculate grams of dextrose	$$\text{Dextrose (kcal)} \div 3.4\frac{\text{kcal}}{\text{gram}} = \text{dextrose (g)}$$ $$1614\text{ kcal} \div 3.4\frac{\text{kcal}}{\text{gram}} = 475\text{ grams}$$ 475 grams of dextrose/day
Determine desired total volume	$$\times\text{ fluid} = \frac{\text{mL}}{\text{kg}} \times \text{weight (kg)} = \text{fluid requirement (mL)}$$ $$25\left(\frac{\text{mL}}{\text{kg}}\right) \times 91\text{ (kg)} = 2275\text{ mL/day}$$ This patient is not on a fluid restriction, so the predictive equation for adults was used. The desired volume of both the patient's maintenance fluid and parenteral nutrition is 2275 mL/day.
Calculate component concentrations/volume	Protein (concentration): $$(\text{Protein requirement (grams)} \div \text{desired volume of parental nutrition (mL)}) \times 1000$$ $$= \text{concentration of amino acid solution } \frac{\text{gram AA}}{\text{L}}$$ $$(127\text{ (g)} \div 2275\text{ (mL)}) \times 1000 = 55.8\text{ grams/L}$$ $$\text{gram AA/L} \div 100 \rightarrow \text{percent AA\%}$$ $$55.8\text{ grams} \div 100 = 5.6\%\text{ amino acid (rounded)}$$

(continues)

Table 5.11 Parenteral Nutrition Formula Calculation Method: A Sample Calculation *(continued)*

	Lipid (volume): No ILE required. Sufficient lipid coming from propofol at 20 mL/hour. If the patient was not receiving propofol and required 530 kcal from ILE, the volume of 20% ILE needed to meet their lipid requirement would be calculated as follows: $530 \text{ kcal} \div 2 \frac{\text{kcal}}{\text{mL ILE}} = 265 \text{ mL ILE at 20\% concentration}$ $265 \text{ mL} \times 2 \frac{\text{kcal}}{\text{mL}} \times \frac{1\text{g ILE}}{10 \text{ kcal}} = 53 \text{ grams lipid}$
	Dextrose (concentration): [dextrose requirement (gram) ÷ desired volume of parental nutrition (mL)] × 1000 mL = concentration of dextrose solution $[475 \text{ (grams)} \div 2275 \text{ (mL)}] \times 1000 = 209 \frac{\text{grams dextrose}}{\text{L}}$ grams dextrose/L ÷ 100 → percent dextrose% = 209 grams/L ÷ 100 = 20% dextrose (rounded)
Calculate total amount of fluid, calories, grams dextrose, protein	Per day: 475 grams dextrose/day, 127 grams AA/day with propofol at 20 mL/hour = 2603 kcal/day, 127 grams protein/day Per liter: D20AA5.6 at 95 mL/hour with propofol at 20 mL/hour = 2280 mL 456 grams CHO × 3.4 kcal/gram = 1550 kcal 126 grams protein/day × 4 kcal/gram = 504 kcal 480 mL of 10% propofol = 528 kcal Total kcal 1550 + 504 + 528 = 2582 kcal Note that when ordering per liter, numbers tend to be rounded leading to slight difference in calculated calories and protein
Final Order	D20AA5.6 at 95 mL/hour with propofol at 20 mL/hour = 2582 kcal/day, 126 grams protein/day

CORE CONCEPT 6

Prescription of parenteral nutrition is based on energy and protein requirements with consideration of fluid specifications and substrate utilization of macronutrients.

1–2 grams/kg when using mixed oils. ILE dose should not exceed 2.5 grams/kg or 0.11 gram/kg/hour regardless of lipid source or patient status. ILE should not exceed 60% of calories regardless of source of lipid.[15,23,24]

The maximum glucose infusion rate (GIR) is 4–5 mg/kg/min in stable adult patients, and <4 mg/kg/min in critically ill or injured adult patients. These rates differ in neonatal and pediatric patients.[24,33] A GIR of 5 mg/kg/min refers to the maximum oxidation rate of glucose once it enters the cell. It is important not to exceed the GIR as the glucose is no longer efficiently utilized. This leads to excess glucose going to nonoxidative pathways that can lead to hepatic steatosis, a complication of PN. Note that despite euglycemia, or normal blood glucose levels, exceeding the GIR can still lead to steatosis.[33]

To calculate the glucose infusion rate, convert carbohydrate requirement in grams to milligrams by multiplying by 1000. Then, divide the requirement in milligrams by the weight of the patient in kilograms. Lastly, divide this number by the infusion time in minutes (1440 minutes for a 24-hour infusion, 720 minutes for a 12-hour infusion) to give the infusion rate of milligrams per kilogram of body weight per minute (**Table 5.12**). If the glucose infusion rate is calculated to be greater than the maximum infusion rate, it is highly recommended that the PN formula be adjusted to reduce the risk of PN-associated adverse events.

Table 5.12 Calculating Glucose Infusion Rate

Carbohydrate (dextrose) requirement (gram) $\times 1000 \frac{\text{mg}}{\text{1 gram}}$ = dextrose requirement (mg)

Dextrose requirement (mg) ÷ body weight (kg) = Glucose infusion $\left(\frac{\text{mg}}{\text{kg body weight}}\right)$

Glucose Infusion $\left(\frac{\text{mg}}{\text{kg}} \div 1440 \text{ minutes} = \text{body weight} \div \frac{\text{1440 minutes}}{\text{24-hours}} = \text{day}\right)$

Glucose Infusion Rate (GIR) $\frac{\text{mg}}{\text{kg body weight}}$ minute

Convenience Equation: gram dextrose/body weight in kg/1.44

Example: 70-year-old male

178 cm, 91 kg

PN Order: D20AA5.6 at 95 mL/hour

Volume of PN: 95 mL/hour × 24 hours = 2280
Dextrose grams 2280 (20% solution) = 456 grams of dextrose
GIR = 456 grams/91 kg/1.44 = 3.47 = ~3.5
GIR = 3.5 mg/kg/min

Note: GIR should be reported with every PN Order.

CORE CONCEPT 7

Carbohydrate infusion from parenteral nutrition should not exceed 5 mg/kg/min in adults and children over the age of 2 years.

CORE CONCEPT 8

Intravenous lipid emulsion should not exceed 2.5 grams/kg or 0.11 mg/kg/min

Electrolyte Requirements

It is common that electrolytes are ordered in milliequivalents instead of milliliters in PN solutions. The standard daily electrolyte requirements in milliequivalents are listed in **Table 5.13**, although electrolyte levels should be monitored regularly and adjusted as needed. Each component of a PN solution contributes to its osmolarity, which ultimately determines into which type of vein (central versus peripheral) the solution can be infused. Refer to **Table 5.14** for one method to calculate osmolarity.

Table 5.13 Daily Electrolyte Requirements

Electrolyte	Daily Parenteral Requirement
Sodium	1–2 mEq/kg
Potassium	1–2 mEq/kg
Chloride	As needed to maintain acid-base balance
Acetate	As needed to maintain acid-base balance
Calcium	10–15 mEq
Magnesium	8–20 mEq
Phosphate	20–40 mmol

Data from ASPEN. Appropriate dosing for parenteral nutrition: ASPEN recommendations. Updated November 17, 2020. Accessed January 10, 2025. http://www.nutritioncare.org/PNDosing

Vitamin and Trace Element Requirements

Typically, the adult dose of multivitamin is 10 mL/day and multiple trace element is 5 mL/day. If a patient has needs beyond what is provided in the standard multivitamin and trace element solutions, additional

CASE STUDY REVISITED

You determine that PN is justified for Alex and are asked to provide Alex's PN prescription.

Questions

1. Is the provision of lipid as a component of Alex's PN indicated? Justify your answer.
2. Calculate a PN prescription for Alex assuming Alex requires 1920 kcal and 85 grams protein. Calculate the glucose infusion rate of your prescription. Does the glucose infusion rate of your prescription follow safe protocol?

CORE CONCEPT 9

Parenteral nutrition formulations are customizable to the specific needs of each patient or patient population.

Table 5.14 **Osmolarity Calculation**

1. Multiply grams of dextrose per liter by 5
2. Multiply grams of amino acids per liter by 10
3. Multiply total mEq per liter of electrolytes (calcium, magnesium, potassium, and sodium) by 2
4. Add numbers 1–3 to calculate total osmolarity in mOsm/L

Data from Gasser R, Parekh N. Parenteral nutrition: macronutrient composition and requirements. Support Line. 2005;27(6):6-12.; Cober M, ed. *ASPEN Parenteral Nutrition Workbook*. 2nd ed. Silver Spring, MD: American Society for Parenteral and Enteral Nutrition; 2022.

may be provided in single-nutrient form. This may add to the total volume of PN provided.[15,24]

Progression of PN

Before initiating PN, ensure that the patient has stable vital signs and normal fluid and electrolyte balance. Refer to Table 5.3 for details on clinical scenarios in which PN should be used with caution. Any imbalances should be corrected and addressed prior to PN initiation.[3] Shortly after the initiation of PN is a common time for patients to experience metabolic disturbances, so it is critical for the patient to be monitored closely during this time to reduce the risk of complications.

For patients previously on insulin or hypoglycemic agents, or those with a fasting glucose ≥200 mg/dL, dextrose should be limited to approximately 100–150 grams on the first day of PN.[30] However, if a patient's blood glucose exceeds 300 mg/dL, PN should be withheld until glycemic control improves.

Tapering of PN is dependent on patient population and may vary according to hospital protocols. When necessary, slow advancement of PN formulations can begin with a reduced nutrient content, approximately 50% of energy needs, and then advanced gradually over 2–3 days to minimize risks of metabolic complications.[3,34,35] Patients at risk of developing refeeding syndrome should progress at a slower rate, over 3–4 days.[36]

Patients who are critically ill require special considerations for advancement of PN as they are at greater risk for hyperglycemia and insulin resistance. In addition, among some patients with critical illness, excessive energy intake is associated with greater risk of infectious morbidity, increased duration of mechanical ventilation, and increased length of stay.[29] Energy from calorie-containing medications, such as those compounded in 5% dextrose and those based in a lipid emulsion, such as propofol that is provided in a 10% lipid emulsion and clevidipine that is provided in a 20% lipid emulsion, should be considered to avoid calorie overfeeding.

Administration of PN may be through **continuous infusion** (over 24 hours) or **cyclical infusion** (<24 hours/day). PN is generally initiated as a continuous infusion. The infusion time may be shortened to a cyclic regimen once the patient is tolerating their goal PN formulation, especially if the patient is ambulatory, as this allows freedom from the pump.

Transitional Feeding

Use of the GI tract is ideal when possible, and so patients may be transitioned from PN to EN or oral intake under careful supervision. Among the critically ill, once a patient is stabilized on PN, EN should be periodically trialed. If transitioning to EN, begin at a slow rate with a formula appropriate to the patient's needs to assess tolerance. As the volume of EN received increases, the amount of energy provided by PN should decrease accordingly to prevent overfeeding. However, PN should not be terminated until

≥60% of target calories are provided enterally.[37] As with initiating PN, terminating PN should be done gradually to prevent hypoglycemia.[35]

Transitioning from PN to oral intake is a less predictable process than transitioning from PN to EN due to variations in patients' appetite and motivation to eat. Oral intake should account for approximately 75% of the patient's calorie needs before discontinuing PN. For patients who cannot meet this goal, PN may continue to provide supplementary nutrition.

CORE CONCEPT 10

Monitoring of anthropometric, clinical, and biochemical indices such as electrolytes, acid–base balance, serum glucose, and liver function tests is critical to ensure the safety of the patient.

Parenteral Nutrition Monitoring

Parenteral nutrition is a costly therapy that requires regular clinical monitoring and diligent care of the patient to support a good outcome. Nutritional monitoring is needed to determine efficiency of the solution being administered, to discover and prevent complications, and to document changes in the clinical course. Monitoring should preferably be carried out by a nutrition support team, which monitors efficiency and sufficiency of PN with regard to specific endpoints defined by the patient's underlying illness, clinical status, the facilities available in the institution caring for the patient, and patient requests.[10,37,38]

Anthropometrics

Weight monitoring of patients receiving PN is vital. Steep, short-term increases and decreases in body weight may indicate changes in fluid status such as dehydration or edema. Intake and output can give further insight into suspected changes in fluid status.

Vital Signs

Vital signs include temperature, blood pressure, pulse, and respiration rate. Temperature is important to monitor in patients receiving PN because fever is an indicator of infection and increases energy requirements. This may change the course of clinical care and PN requirements.

Blood pressure is important to monitor because it reflects hemodynamic stability or instability. If a patient is hemodynamically unstable, they may not be able to tolerate PN and require a medical intervention to correct the issue.

Heart rate is important to monitor because many electrolyte imbalances, a common occurrence in patients receiving PN, present with changes in pulse and arrhythmias when severe enough.

In patients receiving PN, respiratory quotient is more useful information than respiration rate. The respiratory quotient is the ratio of carbon dioxide eliminated to oxygen consumed. Measurement of respiratory quotient in patients receiving PN is important in the prevention of fat accumulation in the liver and alleviation of potential respiratory distress secondary to excess glucose. Respiratory quotient should ideally be maintained between 0.7 and 1.0 to avoid metabolic disturbances.[39]

Biochemistry

Biochemical monitoring of electrolyte balance, blood glucose, kidney function, iron studies, liver function, and vitamin and trace element levels is important for both acute and long-term PN. Biochemical markers should be measured and analyzed on a defined, regular basis since attention to and adjustment of biochemical trends can reveal and prevent complications related to PN. **Table 5.15** contains a sample monitoring schedule for anthropometric measurements, vital signs, and biochemical markers.

Nutrition-Focused Physical Exam

Nutrition-focused physical exam (NFPE) of patients on PN is a necessary component of monitoring. Physical signs to evaluate in an NFPE, their etiology, and PN implications are further described in **Table 5.16**.

Central Venous Access Complications and Their Management

Patients receiving PN are at risk for a wide variety of **catheter-related complications (CRCs)**, beginning at the time of catheter placement. These complications may be mechanical (infectious or noninfectious) or metabolic in nature. Risk of CRCs is impacted by the type of catheter used, the team's procedural experience, the duration of PN therapy, the quality of catheter care, and the patient's underlying disease state.[40] Some complications may be relatively

Table 5.15 Suggested Parenteral Nutrition Monitoring Schedule (*May Vary between Institutions*)

Parameter	Initiation Period	Stable Period	Long-Term
Vital signs	3–4×/day	Daily	As needed
Weight	Daily	2×/week	Weekly
Intake and output	Daily	Daily	As needed
Blood glucose	Every 6 hours	Daily	Monthly
Sodium	Daily	Weekly	Monthly
Potassium	Daily	Weekly	Monthly
Chloride	Daily	Weekly	Monthly
Bicarbonate	Daily	Weekly	Monthly
Blood urea nitrogen	Daily	Weekly	Monthly
Creatinine	Daily	Weekly	Monthly
Calcium	Daily	Weekly	Monthly
Magnesium	Daily	Weekly	Monthly
Phosphorus	Daily	Weekly	Monthly
Complete blood count with differential	Weekly	Weekly	Monthly
Liver function tests (ALT and AST)	Weekly	Weekly	Monthly
Triglycerides	Weekly	Weekly	Monthly
Prothrombin time	Weekly	Monthly	4×/year
Prealbumin	Weekly	Monthly	4×/year
Trace element levels	N/A	N/A	4×/year

Data from Kumpf VJ. Complications of parenteral nutrition. In: Chan LN, ed. *ASPEN Adult Nutrition Support Core Curriculum*. 4th ed. Silver Spring, MD: The American Society for Parenteral and Enteral Nutrition; 2025:467-486.

Table 5.16 Nutrition-Focused Physical Exam in Monitoring Patients on Parenteral Nutrition

Physical Sign	Etiology	Parenteral Nutrition Implication
"Tenting" of skin Dry mucosa Poor skin turgor Sunken eyes Decreased urine output	Dehydration	Increase fluid provided through PN if not on restriction
Edema (pitting or abdominal) Dilution per laboratory values Weight gain	Overhydration	Decrease fluid provided through PN by transitioning to more-concentrated solution
Inflammation at the catheter site (swollen, red, or hot to the touch)	Potential infection	Appropriate medical intervention and patient education on proper catheter-site care if applicable
Signs of nutrient deficiency in sites with high cell turnover (hair, skin, mouth, tongue)	Nutrient deficiency	Test to confirm and add to PN prescription to compensate
Changes in clinical status such as intubation/sedation		May require changes to PN prescription

Data from Canada TW, Lord LM. Fluid, electrolytes, and acid-base disorders. In: Chan LN, ed. *ASPEN Adult Nutrition Support Core Curriculum*. 4th ed. Silver Spring, MD: The American Society for Parenteral and Enteral Nutrition; 2025:159-191.; Pogatshnik C, Hamilton C. Nutrition-focused physical examination: skin, nails, hair, eyes, and oral cavity. *Support Line*. 2011;33(2):7-13.

manageable, while others are more serious. For these reasons, careful monitoring by a skilled team is essential. The prevention of many CRCs is possible with strict adherence to evidence-based protocols.[38,41]

Catheter-Related Mechanical Complications

Mechanical complications are related to the insertion of and care for the catheter and can be classified as either infectious or noninfectious. Some complications may develop at the time of catheterization or soon after (e.g., pneumothorax, arterial puncture, air embolism), while others develop over time (e.g., occlusion, infection).[42]

Certain types of venous access devices and their method of securement (e.g., sutures versus suture-less) are associated with more or less frequent occurrence of complications. PICCs and implantable ports are associated with a particularly low rate of mechanical complications, whereas nontunneled catheters are associated with a higher rate of bloodstream infections and symptomatic venous thrombosis.[41] The method of catheter placement also impacts risk of complications. Using ultrasound-guided catheterization can significantly reduce complications such as pneumothorax and catheter-related thrombosis compared to "blind" catheterization that relies on anatomical landmarks.[41,43]

Noninfectious Mechanical Complications

Noninfectious mechanical complications include pneumothorax, arterial puncture, embolism, occlusion, and venous thrombosis. In general, these complications are rare, occurring in 1–4% of central catheter placements when access is established by an experienced operator, and potential complications can be identified early on by radiologic and clinical exam.[40]

Pneumothorax

Catheterization carries the risk of **pneumothorax**, a puncture in the pleura of the lung leading to air accumulation in the pleural space, resulting in a collapsed lung.[44] Depending on the severity of the pneumothorax, the patient may require a chest tube while the air leak seals. PICCs carry a lower risk of pneumothorax, although they are more likely to be malpositioned.[40]

Arterial Puncture

In general, the veins used for PN are large and easy for an experienced operator to access. Accidental arterial puncture can occur resulting in complications such as temporary occlusion, pseudoaneurysm, and hematoma. Factors that contribute to the risk of arterial puncture include darkly pigmented skin and anatomical variations such as thoracic outlet syndrome.[44]

Occlusion

A **catheter occlusion** is the most common type of noninfectious mechanical complication and is defined as the inability to infuse, flush, and/or aspirate on the venous access device.[5,45] Occlusions can be caused by the precipitation of minerals, medications, and lipids, which then obstruct the catheter. Symptoms include neck vein distension, edema, tingling/pain in the arm and neck, a tight feeling in the throat, and prominent veins of the anterior chest.[5] Occlusions may be cleared via repeated saline flushes.[40] Failing this, flushing with other solutions such as thrombolytics, sodium bicarbonate, hydrochloric acid, and sodium hydroxide can be used. If the catheter cannot be cleared, it may need to be replaced.

Catheter-related venous thrombosis (CRVT) may occur when catheterization damages the vessel wall, activating the coagulation of platelets and fibrin and resulting in a thrombus.[5] This process can begin within minutes of catheter placement. The risk of thrombus development is influenced by the catheter tip location, catheter material, type of PN formula, and length of catheter duration. The major risks of venous thrombosis are the potential for **thrombotic occlusion** (the cannulated vessel is blocked) and **thromboembolism** (the thrombus breaks free and blocks an artery).[5,40] The symptoms of thrombotic occlusion are similar to a catheter occlusion (edema, neck vein distension, tingling of the arm and neck). If the catheter is still functional (i.e., not fully occluded), there is evidence that the catheter should be left in situ rather than removed. Removing the catheter could dislodge any thromboses in contact with the catheter and result in thromboembolism.[46] Thrombolytics injected into the catheter may be used to treat this complication. Currently, there is no universally accepted strategy to prevent CRVT. Commonly used strategies include the use of heparin and heparin-bonded catheters.[40]

Embolism

Embolisms are a rare occurrence in which material becomes lodged in an artery, resulting in significant morbidity and mortality.[47] In PN, various types of embolism are possible, including thromboembolism, **catheter embolism**, and **air embolism**.[40]

Catheter embolisms can occur if the catheter becomes damaged, and a piece of the equipment breaks free. Air embolisms can occur when there is a connection between the air and the cannulated vessel.[47] The pressure gradient drives air into the bloodstream, halting blood flow. Depending on the location of the blockage, embolisms may affect the cardiovascular, pulmonary, and neurological systems.

Phlebitis

Phlebitis, or inflammation of the vein, is a relatively common complication in PN and is more common in PICC lines than other forms of access.[40] Inflammation at the exit site often raises suspicion of a bloodstream infection. However, in phlebitis, the inflammation is due to physical or chemical irritation from the catheter as opposed to infection.[40] Unless the exit site is overtly inflamed, and particularly if the patient has a fever, the appearance of the site is not a reliable indicator of catheter-related bloodstream infection.[48]

Infectious Complications

Catheter-related infections may be local or systemic. Local infections include infections of the exit site, tunnel, and port-pocket. They are usually treated by removing the catheter or port and administering a course of systemic antibiotics.[44] An exit-site infection in a tunneled catheter may not necessitate removal of the catheter, rather, frequent dressing changes coupled with a course of antibiotics should be provided.

Conversely, **catheter-related bloodstream infection (CRBSI)**, also called **central line-associated bloodstream infection (CLABSI)**, is a systemic infection and is one of the most serious complications of PN. Not only does it contribute to increased costs per patient, but CRBSI also increases hospital length of stay and mortality risk.[49] CRBSI may lead to **sepsis**, a condition in which the body's normal inflammatory response to infection is amplified. Sepsis can lead to organ dysfunction, hypotension, and death.[50]

CRBSI is characterized by fever, chills, and increased white blood cell count, and the diagnosis is confirmed through positive blood cultures drawn from the catheter lumen(s) and peripherally.[43] Increased bacterial growth in blood drawn from the catheter indicates CRBSI. CRBSI is commonly caused by *Candida* or yeast species, Gram-positive bacteria (including *Staphylococcus aureus*, *Staphylococcus epidermis*, and *Enterococcus*), and Gram-negative bacteria (including *Pseudomonas*, *Serratia marcescens*, *Klebsiella pneumoniae*, and *Escherichia coli*).[44]

CRBSI is first treated by administering broad-spectrum antibiotics through the catheter to avoid catheter removal.[44] However, it is necessary to remove the infected catheter if the patient continues to deteriorate or if blood cultures remain positive.[40,44]

Use of "care bundles" for the insertion and maintenance of central venous access devices, improvements in central venous access device care, and tighter glycemic control have reduced infection rates over time, curtailing one of the most common and serious adverse events associated with PN administration.[51] Prevention of CRBSI requires following strict guidelines at every point from choosing the appropriate venous access device to caring for the exit site. **Table 5.17** contains evidence-based strategies for preventing CRBSI.

Table 5.17 Points at Which Catheter-Related Bloodstream Infection Can Be Prevented

Time Point	Strategies to Prevent CRBSI
Device selection	For long-term PN, use tunneled and implanted catheters Antimicrobial-coated catheters are effective for short-term PN Use single-lumen catheters unless the patient requires multiple ports If using multiple lumens, one lumen should be reserved exclusively for PN
Catheterization procedure	Use ultrasound-guided venipuncture Take maximal barrier precautions during insertion: cap, mask, disposable gown, gloves, and large drape
PN administration and site care	Enforce a strict hand washing policy Use 2% chlorhexidine as skin antiseptic Appropriately dress the exit site Disinfect hubs, stopcocks, and needle-free connectors Regularly change administration sets Use antibiotic-lock or ethanol-lock: catheter lumen is filled with antibiotic solution or ethanol when not in use

Data from Tushar K. Parenteral access devices. In: Chan LN, ed. *ASPEN Adult Nutrition Support Core Curriculum*. 4th ed. Silver Spring, MD: The American Society for Parenteral and Enteral Nutrition; 2025:435-465.; Pittiruti M, Hamilton H, Biffi R, MacFie J, Pertkiewicz M; ESPEN. ESPEN guidelines on parenteral nutrition: central venous catheters (access, care, diagnosis and therapy of complications). *Clin Nutr*. 2009;28(4):365-377.; Hamilton C. Vascular access. In: Charney P, Malone AM, eds. *ADA Pocket Guide to Parenteral Nutrition*. Chicago, IL: Academy of Nutrition and Dietetics; 2007:33-51.

CASE STUDY REVISITED

Alex has been on PN for 2 weeks. Below are his weight and his most recent metabolic panel:

Anthropometric Data:

Weight: 68 kg
Admission weight: 64 kg

Biochemical Data:

Sodium 133 (136–145 mEq/L)
Potassium 3.7 (3.5–5.0 mEq/L)
Chloride 99 (96–106 mEq/L)
Carbon dioxide 22 (22–31 mEq/L)
Blood urea nitrogen 8 (8–20 mg/dL)
Creatinine 0.4 (0.7–1.3 mg/dL)
Glucose 180 (70–139 mg/dL)
Aspartate transaminase (AST) 110 (10–40 U/L)
Alanine transaminase (ALT) 99 (28–33 IU/L)
Alkaline phosphatase (ALP) 130 (30–120 U/L)
Direct (conjugated) bilirubin 3.0 (0–0.3 mg/dL)
Total bilirubin 1.9 (0.3–0.9 mg/dL)
Calcium 9 (8.5–10.5 mg/dL)
Phosphorus 3.4 (2.5–4.5 mg/dL)
Magnesium 1.5 (1.5–2.7 mg/dL)
Albumin 3.0 (3.5–5.5 g/dL)

Questions

1. What is your interpretation of Alex's weight?
2. What biochemical labs are concerning?
3. How might you alter the PN composition or prescription? Provide specific changes to the initial PN prescription if necessary.
4. Are there other options you might consider for feeding Alex?

Metabolic Complications

Hyper- and Hypoglycemia

It is normal for blood glucose to rise after initiating PN. However, endogenous insulin secretion should bring glucose back to a normal range. Hyperglycemia is the most common metabolic complication of PN. Prolonged, uncontrolled hyperglycemia can lead to nonketotic dehydration, coma, and death.[38] It is usually caused by excessive dextrose infusion, although it can also be a result of the stress response in patients with acute illness or sepsis. These patients are known to develop insulin resistance, suppressed insulin secretion, and increased gluconeogenesis and glycogenolysis.[36] Patients with diabetes, acute pancreatitis, or on corticosteroid medication are also at risk of hyperglycemia. To prevent hyperglycemia, ensure that dextrose is not infused faster than the recommended glucose infusion rate for the patient population. However, note that hyperglycemia can exist despite GIR being within the recommended range. In addition, identify other potential sources of dextrose or changes in medications (e.g., corticosteroids). Hyperglycemia is treated with insulin, which can be administered subcutaneously, intravenously, or added to the PN formula itself.[31]

Patients receiving PN are typically secreting higher-than-normal levels of insulin due to the high concentration of dextrose in the formula. Abruptly stopping PN infusion can therefore result in reactive hypoglycemia within 15–60 minutes. A blood glucose level <70 mg/dL would suggest hypoglycemia.[52] This complication can be prevented by slowly tapering PN over 1–2 hours or by infusing half of the infusion rate. If a rapid discontinuation of PN is needed, a 10% dextrose immediately after PN cessation is recommended.[38] The safest way to provide and manage insulin therapy is through standardized protocols.

Electrolyte Abnormalities

As discussed in the "Parenteral Nutrition Formulation" section, the electrolyte content added to PN is customizable to the patient's needs. Biochemical monitoring should be performed regularly to assess whether a patient requires more or less of particular electrolytes.

When initiating PN, severe electrolyte disturbances may be indicative of refeeding syndrome, especially in patients with malnutrition. Refeeding syndrome is characterized by a decrease in any 1, 2, or 3 of serum phosphorus, potassium, and/or magnesium; decreases range in severity between mild (10–20%), moderate (20–30%), and severe (>30%) in addition to disturbances in glucose metabolism, fluid, and sodium balance, and thiamine deficiency.[53] Advancing PN gradually over several days and supplementing electrolytes can help to prevent severe electrolyte abnormalities due to refeeding syndrome.

Electrolyte abnormalities may also result in acid–base disturbances. Arterial blood normally has a pH range of 7.35–7.45, and this range should be closely monitored to ensure optimal organ function.[54] Many factors can contribute to disturbances in a patient's acid–base balance, including components of the PN formula. Treatment of acid–base disturbances should address the underlying cause. Acidosis (arterial pH <7.35) may be corrected by decreasing the amount of chloride provided or by providing bicarbonate in the form of acetate (a bicarbonate precursor).[54] Bicarbonate itself should not be added to the PN formula, as it is unstable. Alkalosis (arterial pH >7.45) may be corrected by decreasing the amount of acetate salts provided or replacing any potassium and magnesium deficits.[54]

Hyper- and Hypovolemia

Patients may receive all their fluid intake from PN alone, but some may also be consuming fluids orally or enterally. For these patients, assess whether there have been any changes in oral intake. Hypervolemia, or fluid overload, is likely due to excessive PN or IV fluid infusion.[55] Symptoms include weight gain, edema, and shortness of breath. Manage hypervolemia by maintaining or decreasing PN volume, unless fluid overload is severe, in which case PN may need to be discontinued temporarily.

Hypovolemia, or a deficit in the extracellular fluid, can occur in a variety of ways, including significant GI losses, fever, or diuresis.[55,56] Symptoms include weight loss, decreased urine output, decreased urinary sodium concentration (<15 mEq/L), low blood pressure, muscle cramps, weakness, dizziness, thirst, and dry mouth.[54,55] Hypovolemia may or may not be accompanied by an electrolyte deficit. Repletion with IV fluids should take into consideration whether any electrolytes must also be repleted.[55]

Overfeeding

Dr. Jonathan Rhoads, one of the founders of PN, originally described this form of nutrition support as "hyperalimentation" (overfeeding).[57] It was initially believed that malnourished or hypermetabolic patients should be fed much more than their required nutrient needs to stimulate an anabolic response. However, it is now recognized that overfeeding increases the risk of complications, particularly bloodstream infections.[58] Other complications associated with overfeeding include hyperglycemia, hyperlipidemia, hypertriglyceridemia, hypercapnia, and liver dysfunction. Overfeeding is more common in the ICU setting because patients who are critically ill and/or septic may not metabolize glucose and lipids normally, and excess glucose and lipids increase metabolic stress and exacerbate the storage impairments associated with insulin resistance.[59]

Essential Fatty Acid Deficiency

Linoleic acid, an omega-6 fatty acid, and alpha-linolenic acid, an omega-3 fatty acid, are considered EFAs because they cannot be synthesized by humans.[60] EFA deficiency can develop in infants and children receiving fat-free PN within a few days, and in adults receiving fat-free PN within 2 weeks.[38,60,61] Clinical signs of essential fatty acid deficiency include hepatomegaly, thrombocytopenia, impaired wound healing, hair loss, and dry, desquamated skin.[60] In order to prevent EFA deficiency in patients receiving fat-free PN, 2–4% and 0.25–0.05% of calories from linoleic and alpha-linolenic acid, respectively, must be administered.[61] **Table 5.18** contains more information on the amount of EFA required to prevent deficiency.

Hepatobiliary Complications

There are essentially three types of hepatobiliary disorders associated with PN therapy: **hepatic steatosis**, **cholestasis**, and **cholelithiasis**.[62] These complications can happen without the use of PN; however, when attributable to the usage of PN, these complications are referred to as "PN-associated liver disease" (PNALD) or "intestinal failure–associated liver disease" (IFALD). A wide range of IFALD prevalence has been reported between 4.3% and 65% depending on criteria used.[63]

Hepatic steatosis is the accumulation of fat in the liver. Although the development of hepatic steatosis is thought to be multifactorial, the use of soybean lipid emulsions is believed to be one of the largest

CASE STUDY REVISITED

Shortly after surgery, Alex remains on PN, but you believe that he is ready for trial oral feeding. A liquid diet is ordered, which he appears to tolerate well, and his PN is tapered. Two days later, Alex develops a fever, abdominal distention, and diarrhea. A CT scan reveals an enterocolonic fistula between the distal ileum and ascending colon. The surgeon determines that Alex will require further surgery to repair the fistula but advises waiting 3–6 months to allow the densest peritoneal adhesions to resolve. Until then, Alex will need to remain NPO and continue receiving PN. After another week in the hospital, Alex's fever, distention, and diarrhea have resolved and he is ready to be discharged on home PN.

Questions

1. What questions would you ask to determine whether Alex would be able to independently manage home PN?
2. Describe three common complications associated with long-term PN. What symptoms and lab values would you monitor?
3. Assess Alex's previous PES statements. Identify if each statement remains an active issue or if the PES statement has been resolved. If the PES statement remains an active issue, has improvement in the issue been noted? If the issue has been resolved, write a new PES statement.

Table 5.18 Amount of Linoleic Acid Required to Prevent Essential Fatty Acid Deficiency During Different Stages of the Life Cycle

Preterm infants	0.25 gram/kg/day
Term infants and older children	0.1 gram/kg/day
Adults	2–4% of total calorie intake

Data from Gramlich L, Ireton-Jones C, Miles JM, Morrison M, Pontes-Arruda A. Essential fatty acid requirements and intravenous lipid emulsions. *JPEN J Parenter Enteral Nutr*. 2019;43: 697-707. doi:10.1002/jpen.1537; ESPEN. Guidelines of pediatric parenteral nutrition 4. Lipids. *J Pediatr Gastroenterol Nutr*. 2005;41(2):S19-S27.

contributing factors. Although the lipid particles in parenteral soybean oil emulsion mimic the size and structure of chylomicrons, they primarily contain omega-6 fatty acids and triglycerides and are devoid of cholesterol or protein. With reduced cholesterol, lipolysis is limited and the liver is prone to the accumulation of lipid particles. Although steatosis is reversible, it can advance to more serious stages of liver disease, and eventually to cirrhosis, if not appropriately managed.[64]

Cholestasis is a condition of reduced bile flow. This can be caused by any impairment between hepatocytes, which produce bile, and the duodenum, the site where bile is incorporated into the GI tract. When bile flow is stopped, the pigment bilirubin escapes into the bloodstream and accumulates. For this reason, the primary indicator of cholestasis is a serum conjugated bilirubin >2 mg/dL. IFALD is initially characterized by cholestasis but can progress to fibrosis and cirrhosis with continued exposure to PN.[65,66]

Cholelithiasis is the presence of gallstones or gallbladder sludge. Gallstones can develop in patients receiving PN due to gallbladder stasis, or inactivity of the gallbladder. When the gallbladder is not stimulated to secrete stored bile, the bile begins to form sludge, which may turn into gallstones.[67]

When a patient receiving PN develops hepatobiliary complications, it is necessary to rule out all treatable causes and minimize other risk factors. All potential hepatotoxic medications and herbal supplements should be eliminated. Modifications to the PN regimen that may be helpful include reduction of calories, reduction of ILE dose to <1 gram/kg/day, replacement of an omega-6 lipid source with an omega-3 containing lipid source, supplementation of taurine in the infant, and use of cyclic infusion. Initiation of even small amounts of EN and use of ursodiol may be beneficial in stimulating bile flow. In the patient receiving long-term PN with severe and progressive liver disease, intestinal or liver transplantation may be the only remaining treatment option.[62] **Table 5.19** provides examples of interventions for managing PN-associated liver disease.

Home Parenteral Nutrition

Indications and Access

Home parenteral nutrition (HPN) is becoming an increasingly common therapy. By most recent estimates, over 25,000 patients are on HPN.[68]

Table 5.19 Interventions for Managing Parenteral Nutrition–Associated Liver Disease

Rule out Non-PN Etiologies	Modifications to PN	Enteral Nutrition	Pharmacologic Therapy
Medication hepatotoxicity	Reduce calories from dextrose	Maximize oral intake	Increase bile flow (ursodeoxycholic acid)
Herbal supplements	Decrease ILE to <1 gram/kg/day	Provide low-dose enteral tube feeding	
Hepatitis	Provide balanced intake from dextrose and ILE	Treat bacterial overgrowth	
Biliary obstruction	Cycle PN Feeds		

Data from Kumpf VJ. Complications of parenteral nutrition. In: Chan LN, ed. *ASPEN Adult Nutrition Support Core Curriculum*. 4th ed. Silver Spring, MD: The American Society for Parenteral and Enteral Nutrition; 2025:467-486.

The indications for HPN are similar to those for hospitalized patients. These patients have long-term (≥2 weeks) intestinal failure, cannot meet their nutritional needs through the enteral route alone, and can be treated outside of the acute care setting.[3,69] HPN is not recommended for patients with terminal illness who have a short life expectancy; however, it may be considered in order to prevent an earlier death due to malnutrition in patients with cancer if it will increase their life expectancy beyond 1–3 months, even if not undergoing treatment.[70] ASPEN provides guidelines related to the ethical issues of nutrition support in end of life.[71]

Because hospitalization is no longer necessary, indications for HPN involve further considerations. Is the patient, family, or caregiver capable of administering PN? Is the home environment safe for PN? Will the patient's insurance cover HPN-related costs?

PRACTICE POINT

In the United States, the federal-level health insurance program Medicare will only cover HPN-related costs if it is documented that the patient's GI tract is nonfunctional, the condition is "permanent" (i.e., at least 90 days of therapy are needed), and the patient cannot tolerate EN.

In terms of type of venous access indicated for HPN, current guidelines recommend tunneled catheters or implanted ports.[68–70,72] As discussed earlier in this chapter, CRBSIs are one of the most common complications associated with catheters. PICCs carry a lower risk of CRBSI in the hospital setting, but this has not yet been demonstrated definitively in the home setting.[73] In addition, placement of PICCs does not have the potential for some of the serious mechanical complications associated with tunneled catheters, including pneumothorax and accidental arterial puncture.[73] Recent studies have assessed the feasibility of PICCs for HPN and have found that, overall, PICCs are associated with the same incidence of complications as traditional forms of access.

HPN is usually administered on a cyclic schedule. The infusion rate is controlled by an automatic pump that gradually increases the rate over the first 30 minutes, administers the total volume over 12–15 hours, then gradually tapers over the last 30 minutes.[69] Many patients choose to infuse overnight to allow freedom from the pump for daytime activities. Since the downside of nighttime infusion is frequent urination, some patients may choose daytime infusion to ensure a better night's sleep.[74]

Once it has been established that a patient will return home on PN, it is essential to involve an interprofessional team to assist in the transition. This team may include a physician, specialized nurse, dietitian, and pharmacist. In reality, this is challenging, and few patients with HPN in the United States receive care from interprofessional nutrition support teams due to healthcare-cost restraints.[75] A psychologist and/or social worker may also be needed, depending on how HPN affects the patient's personal and social life. The primary goals of patient/caregiver education are to promote the patient's independence, improve their quality of life, and make living with HPN as normal as possible.[75]

HPN is a complex therapy that requires intensive education and training. Patients and caregivers must learn how to administer the PN formula, care for the IV site, and identify and address complications. Several factors can affect a patient's level of success in managing HPN. These include health literacy (performing basic reading and math skills in a healthcare environment), socioeconomic status, knowledge of the English language (or dominant language), and age (older than 65 years is associated with poorer health literacy).[76]

It can be difficult to assess a patient on HPN's quality of life as it is affected both by HPN itself and the underlying disease state. Quality of life (QOL) is defined as "enjoying life" and "being able to do what you want to do when you want to do it."[77,78] Assessments of HPN patients' QOL have found that the poorest QOL is experienced during the first year, particularly if the patient was previously well.[55] QOL tends to improve with time. Strong self-esteem, spousal and family support, and financial security are associated with improved quality of life.[55,79]

Factors that negatively contribute to QOL include frequent catheter-related infections; the inability to work and loss of income (although some patients can continue to work); decreased social interactions; lack of energy and stamina; the inconvenience of the catheter, tubing, and pump; and the rigidity of the infusion schedule.[55,77]

Transitioning to HPN can be an intense, stressful experience. Patients will have different attitudes in how they approach this new phase of their life. The infusion schedule can be particularly challenging. Some patients may be able to maintain a relatively spontaneous lifestyle and learn to adjust their infusion schedule accordingly, while others may feel burdened by a strict infusion schedule. Successful patients will acknowledge that their lives have changed but will learn to redefine their "new normal." It can be helpful for patients to focus on what they can still do while on HPN, rather than what they cannot do.[77]

Prognosis of HPN

Retrospective cohort studies have found that the 5-year survival rate for patients on HPN ranges from 58% to 83%.[79] Because there are a wide variety of conditions that may necessitate HPN, the most influential and variable effect on survival rate is the underlying disease state.[79] For example, patients with cancer may have an expected survival of several months, whereas patients with Crohn's disease can expect to measure survival in decades. In the overwhelming majority of cases, death of a patient on HPN is due to the underlying disease and not a complication of HPN, particularly for patients on HPN for <1 year. As the length of HPN use increases, so does the risk of serious complications such as sepsis, liver failure, and thrombosis. Among patients on long-term HPN, complications account for 15–20% of deaths.[79] Additional factors that influence the prognosis of patients on HPN include the following[55]:

- Age (better prognosis among younger patients)
- Experience of supervising clinician
- Use of narcotics (associated with increased incidence of sepsis)
- Peer-support and education programs (associated with decreased incidence of sepsis)

While some patients will remain on lifelong HPN, others may be able to transition off HPN to an oral diet. Depending on the length and type of bowel that remains intact, patients with short bowel syndrome may undergo a process known as "adaptation." If the colon remains intact, absorption improves over 1–3 years, and with dietary counseling, patients may be able to reduce PN or transition off of PN entirely. Intestinal adaptation is further discussed in Chapter 11, *Nutritional Management of Gastrointestinal Malabsorption*.

CORE CONCEPT 11

Parenteral nutrition may be a long-term or even lifelong therapy for some patients.

Chapter Summary

Parenteral nutrition is a life-sustaining therapy for individuals with a nonfunctional GI tract who cannot consume adequate nutrition through oral intake or enteral nutrition. It may be used to sustain patients before they are able to resume oral or enteral intake, whereas for those who have permanent GI dysfunction, it may be used for decades. PN is a highly complex therapy that requires careful calculation of nutrient needs, strict hygienic practices when administering PN and caring for the catheter site, and constant monitoring for complications. An experienced, interprofessional team is ideal for managing PN.

Key Terms

parenteral nutrition (PN), hypertonic, asepsis, central PN (CPN), peripheral PN (PPN), vascular access device (VAD), venipuncture, exit site, thrombophlebitis, extravasation, central venous catheter (CVC), peripherally inserted central catheter (PICC), phlebitis, parenteral nutrition–associated liver disease (PNALD), hepatic steatosis, total nutrient admixture (TNA), physiochemical incompatibility, continuous infusion, cyclical infusion, catheter-related complication (CRC), pneumothorax, catheter occlusion, catheter-related venous thrombosis (CRVT), thrombotic occlusion, thromboembolism, catheter embolism, air embolism, catheter-related bloodstream infection (CRBSI), central line–associated bloodstream infection (CLABSI), sepsis, cholestasis, cholelithiasis, home parenteral nutrition (HPN), vascular access devices (VAD)

Acknowledgments

The authors acknowledge Grace Ling for contributions to the previous version of this chapter.

References

1. American Society for Parenteral and Enteral Nutrition. What is Parenteral Nutrition? Accessed January 9, 2025. https://www.nutritioncare.org/About_Clinical_NutritionWhat_Is_Parenteral_Nutrition
2. Dudrick SJ. History of parenteral nutrition. *J Am Coll Nutr.* 2009;28(3):243–251.
3. Mirtallo JM, Mulherin DW. Overview of parenteral nutrition. In: Chan LN, ed. *ASPEN Adult Nutrition Support Core Curriculum.* 4th ed. The American Society for Parenteral and Enteral Nutrition; 2025:387–402.
4. Dudrick SJ, Wilmore DW, Vars HM, Rhoads JE. Long-term total parenteral nutrition with growth, development, and positive nitrogen balance. *Surgery.* 1968;64(1):134–142.
5. Tushar KT. Parenteral nutrition access devices. In: Chan LN, ed. *ASPEN Adult Nutrition Support Core Curriculum.* 4th ed. The American Society for Parenteral and Enteral Nutrition; 2025:435–465.
6. Derenski K, Catlin J, Allen L. Parenteral nutrition basics for the clinician caring for the adult patient. *Nutr Clin Pract.* 2016;31(5):578–595.
7. Pittiruti M, Hamilton H, Biffi R, MacFie J, Pertkiewicz M, ESPEN. ESPEN guidelines on parenteral nutrition: central venous catheters (access, care, diagnosis and therapy of complications). *Clin Nutr.* 2009;28(4):365–377.
8. Boullata JI, Mirtallo JM, Sacks GS, et al. Parenteral nutrition compatibility and stability: a comprehensive review. *JPEN.* 2022;46(2):273–299.
9. Worthington P, Balint J, Bechtold M, et al. When is parenteral nutrition appropriate? *JPEN.* 2017;41(3):324–377.
10. Massouh A, Kwan SW, Fidelman N, et al. ACR appropriateness criteria® central venous access device and site selection. *J Am Coll Radiol.* 2023;20(5):S3–19.
11. Bidgood E, Huang J, Murphy E, Prentice R, Hede B, Russell D. Peripheral parenteral nutrition: a retrospective observational study to evaluate utility and complications. *Nutr Clin Pract.* 2025;40(4):942–949. doi:10.1002/ncp.11237
12. Centers for Disease Control and Prevention. Guidelines for the Prevention of Intravascular Catheter-Related Infections. Updated February 28, 2024. Accessed January 10, 2025. https://www.cdc.gov/infection-control/hcp/intravascular-catheter-related-infections/summary-recommendations.html.
13. O'Grady NP, Alexander M, Burns LA, et al. Healthcare Infection Control Practices Advisory Committee (HICPAC). Guidelines for the prevention of intravascular catheter-related infections. *Clin Infect Dis.* 2011;52(9):e162–193. doi:10.1093/cid/cir257
14. McCowan KC, Ling PR. Carbohydrates. In: Chan LN, ed. *ASPEN Adult Nutrition Support Core Curriculum.* 4th ed. The American Society for Parenteral and Enteral Nutrition; 2025:79–98.
15. Patel R, Mowatt-Larssen C. Parenteral nutrition formulations. In: Chan LN, ed. *ASPEN Adult Nutrition Support Core Curriculum.* 4th ed. The American Society for Parenteral and Enteral Nutrition; 2025:403–432.
16. Yarandi SS, Zhao VM, Hebbar G, Ziegler TR. Amino acid composition in parenteral nutrition: what is the evidence? *Curr Opin Clin Nutr Metab Care.* 2011;14(1):75–82.
17. 15% Clinisol [package insert]. Baxter Healthcare Corporation; 2018. Accessed January 11, 2025. https://www.baxterpi.com/pi-pdf/Clinisol_PI.pdf
18. Aminosyn II with Electrolytes [package insert]. Hospira, Inc.; 2008. Accessed January 11, 2025. https://labeling.pfizer.com/ShowLabeling.aspx?id=4333
19. Friedman M. *Absorption and Utilization of Amino Acids.* Vol 2. CRC Press; 1989.
20. Mundi MS, Nystrom EM, Hurley DL, McMahon MM. Management of parenteral nutrition in hospitalized adult patients. *JPEN.* 2017;41:535–549. doi:10.1177/0148607116667060
21. Haines K, Grisel B, Gorenshtein L, Wischmeyer PE. Lipid emulsions in parenteral nutrition: does it matter? *Curr Opin Crit Care.* 2023;29(4):293–299.
22. Rochling FA. Intravenous lipid emulsions in the prevention and treatment of liver disease in intestinal failure. *Nutrients.* 2021;13(3):895.
23. Mirtallo JM, Ayers P, Boullata J, et al. ASPEN Lipid Injectable Emulsion Safety Recommendations, Part 1: Background and adult considerations. *Nutr Clin Pract.* 2020;35:769–782. doi:10.1002/ncp.1049625.
24. ASPEN. Appropriate dosing for parenteral nutrition: ASPEN recommendations. Updated November 17, 2020. Accessed January 10, 2025. http://www.nutritioncare.org/PNDosing
25. ASPEN. Parenteral nutrition multivitamin product shortage considerations. Updated October 9, 2024. Accessed January 11, 2025. https://www.nutritioncare.org/Guidelines_and_Clinical_Resources/Product_Shortages/2021_Parenteral_Nutrition_Multivitamin_Product_Shortage_Considerations

26. Itokawa Y. Trace elements in long-term total parenteral nutrition. *Nihon Rinsho Jpn J Clin Med.* 1996;54(1):172–178.
27. Rampton D, Folkersen J, Fishbane S, et al. Hypersensitivity reactions to intravenous iron: guidance for risk minimization and management. *Haematologica.* 2014;99(11):1671–1676.
28. Mirtallo J, Canada T, Johnson D, et al. Safe practices for parenteral nutrition. *JPEN.* 2004;28(6):S39–70.
29. Compher C, Bingham AL, McCall M, et al. Guidelines for the provision of nutrition support therapy in the adult critically ill patient: the American Society for Parenteral and Enteral Nutrition. *JPEN.* 2022;46:12–41. doi:10.1002/jpen.2267
30. Tucker AM, Derenski K, Walker R. Diabetes mellitus. In: Chan LN, ed. *ASPEN Adult Nutrition Support Core Curriculum.* 4th ed. The American Society for Parenteral and Enteral Nutrition; 2025:577–615.
31. McCulloch A, Bansiya V, Woodward JM. Addition of insulin to parenteral nutrition for control of hyperglycemia. *JPEN.* 2018;42:846–854. doi:10.1177/0148607117722750
32. Hadaway LC. Administering parenteral nutrition with other I.V. drugs. *Nursing.* 2005;35(2):26.
33. Burke JF, Wolfe RR, Mullany CJ, Mathews DE, Bier DM. Glucose requirements following burn injury. Parameters of optimal glucose infusion and possible hepatic and respiratory abnormalities following excessive glucose intake. *Ann Surg.* 1979;190(3):274–285.
34. ASPEN. ASPEN Parenteral Nutrition Care Pathway. Accessed January 12, 2025. https://www.nutritioncare.org/SmartPN_Pathway.aspx
35. Al-Zubeidi D, Davis MB, Rahhal R. Prevention of complications for hospitalized patients receiving parenteral nutrition: a narrative review. *Nutr Clin Prac.* 2024;39(5):1037–1053.
36. de Vargas Cony K, de Magalhaes Francesconi CF. An unexpectedly high incidence of refeeding syndrome in patients with total parenteral nutrition in a reference university hospital. *Clin Nutr.* 2021; 40:3702–3707.
37. McClave SA, Taylor BE, Martindale RG, et al. Guidelines for the provision and assessment of nutrition support therapy in the adult critically ill patient. *JPEN.* 2016;40:159–211. doi:10.1177/0148607115621863
38. Kumpf VJ. Complications of parenteral nutrition. In: Chan LN, ed. *ASPEN Adult Nutrition Support Core Curriculum.* 4th ed. The American Society for Parenteral and Enteral Nutrition; 2025:467–486.
39. Berger MM, De Waele E, Gramlich L, et al. How to interpret and apply the results of indirect calorimetry studies: A case-based tutorial. *Clin Nutr ESPEN.* 2024;63:856–869.
40. Ghabril MS, Aranda-Michel J, Scolapio JS. Metabolic and catheter complications of parenteral nutrition. *Curr Gastroenteroly Rep.* 2004;6:327–334.
41. Cotogni P, Barbero C, Garrino C, et al. Peripherally inserted central catheters in non-hospitalized cancer patients: 5-year results of a prospective study. *Support Care Cancer.* 2015;23(2):403–409.
42. Ukleja A, Romano MM. Complications of parenteral nutrition. *Gastroenterol Clin N A.* 2007;36:23–46.
43. Cavanna L, Civardi G, Vallisa D, et al. Ultrasound-guided central venous catheterization in cancer patients improves the success rate of cannulation and reduces mechanical complications: a prospective observational study of 1,978 consecutive catheterizations. *World J Surg Oncol.* 2010;8:91.
44. Hamilton C. Vascular access. In: Charney P, Malone AM, eds. *ADA Pocket Guide to Parenteral Nutrition*: Academy of Nutrition and Dietetics; 2007:33–51.
45. Brandt CF, Tribler S, Hvistendahl M, et al. Home parenteral nutrition in adult patients with chronic intestinal failure: catheter-related complications over 4 decades at the main Danish Tertiary Referral Center. *JPEN.* 2017;41(7):1178–1187.
46. Lirk P, Keller C, Colvin J, et al. Unintentional arterial puncture during cephalic vein cannulation: case report and anatomical study. *Br J Anaesth.* 2004;92(5):740–742.
47. McCarthy CJ, Behravesh S, Naidu SG, Oklu R. Air embolism: practical tips for prevention and treatment. *J Clin Med.* 2016;5(11):93.
48. Safdar N, Maki DG. Inflammation at the insertion site is not predictive of catheter-related bloodstream infection with short-term, noncuffed central venous catheters. *Crit Care Med.* 2002;30(12):2632–2635.
49. Fonseca G, Burgermaster M, Larson E, Seres DS. The relationship between parenteral nutrition and central line–associated bloodstream infections: 2009–2014. *JPEN.* 2017:1–5.
50. Moriyama K, Ando T, Kotani M, et al. Risk factors associated with increased incidences of catheter-related bloodstream infection. *Medicine.* 2022;101(42):e31160.
51. ASPEN. Parenteral Nutrition Resources. Dispelling PN myths in practice. Updated September 11, 2023. Accessed January 12, 2025. https://www.nutritioncare.org/uploadedFiles/Documents/Guidelines_and_Clinical_Resources/PN_Resources/PN-Myths-Practice-Tool.pdf
52. Olveira G, Tapia MJ, Ocon J, et al. Hypoglycemia in noncritically ill patients receiving total parenteral nutrition: a multicenter study. *Nutrition.* 2015;31(1):58–63.
53. da Silva JSV, Seres DS, Sabino K, et al. ASPEN consensus recommendations for refeeding syndrome. *Nutr Clin Pract.* 2020;35:178–195. doi:10.1002/ncp.10474
54. Ayers P, Warrington L. Diagnosis and treatment of simple acid-base disorders. *Nutr Clin Prac.* 2008;23(2):122–127.
55. Howard L. Home parenteral nutrition: survival, cost, and quality of life. *Gastroenterology.* 2006;130(2):S52–S59.
56. Rhoda KM, Porter MJ, Quintini C. Fluid and electrolyte management. *JPEN.* 2011;35(6):675–685.
57. Vinnars E WD. History of parenteral nutrition. *JPEN.* 2003;27(3):225–231.
58. Jeejeebhoy KN. Total parenteral nutrition: potion or poison? *Am J Clin Nutr.* 2001;74:160–163.
59. Griffiths RD. Too much of a good thing: the curse of overfeeding. *Crit Care.* 2007;11(6):176.
60. Gramlich L, Ireton-Jones C, Miles JM, Morrison M, Pontes-Arruda A. Essential fatty acid requirements and intravenous lipid emulsions. *JPEN.* 2019;43:697–707. doi:10.1002/jpen.1537
61. ESPEN. Guidelines of Pediatric Parenteral Nutrition 4. Lipids. *J Ped Gastroenterol Nutr.* 2005;41(2):S19–S27.
62. Kumpf VJ. Parenteral nutrition-associated liver disease in adult and pediatric patients. *Nutr Clin Pract.* 2006;21(3):279–290.
63. Tabone T, Mooney P, Donnellan C. Intestinal failure–associated liver disease: current challenges in screening, diagnosis, and parenteral nutrition considerations. *Nutr Clin Pract.* 2024;39(5):1003–1025.
64. Nandivada P, Carlson SJ, Chang MI, Cowan E, Gura KM, Puder M. Treatment of parenteral nutrition-associated liver disease: the role of lipid emulsions. *Adv Nutr.* 2013;4:711–717.
65. Cholestasis. Merckmanuals.com. Updated January 2023. Accessed January 12, 2025. https://www.merckmanuals.com/home/liver-and-gallbladder-disorders/manifestations-of-liver-disease/liver-failure

66. Guglielmi FW, Regano N, Mazzuoli S, et al. Cholestasis induced by total parenteral nutrition. *Clin Liver Dis*. 2008;12(1):97–110, viii. doi:10.1016/j.cld.2007.11.004
67. Cholelithiasis. Merckmanuals.com. Updated August 2023. Accessed January 12, 2025. https://www.merckmanuals.com/professional/hepatic-and-biliary-disorders/gallbladder-and-bile-duct-disorders/overview-of-biliary-function
68. Bering J, DiBaise JK. Home parenteral and enteral nutrition. *Nutrients*. 2022; 14(13):2558. doi:10.3390/nu14132558
69. Wanten G, Calder PC, Forbes A. Managing adult patients who need home parenteral nutrition. *BMJ*. 2011;342:d1447.
70. Kumpf VJ, Tillman EM. Home parenteral nutrition: safe transition from hospital to home. *Nutr Clin Prac*. 2012; 27(6):749–757.
71. Schwartz DB, Barrocas A, Annetta MG, et al. Ethical aspects of artificially administered nutrition and hydration: an ASPEN position paper. *Nutr Clin Pract*. 2021;36(2):254–267.
72. Pironi L, Boeykens K, Bozzetti F, et al. ESPEN practical guideline: home parenteral nutrition. *Clin Nutr*. 2023;42(3): 411–430.
73. Botella-Carretero JI, Carrero C, Guerra E, et al. Role of peripherally inserted central catheters in home parenteral nutrition: a 5-year prospective study. *JPEN*. 2013;37(4):544–549.
74. Dashti HS, Rhyner JJ, Mogensen KM, et al. Infusion timing and sleep habits of adults receiving home parenteral and enteral nutrition: a patient-oriented survey study. *JPEN*. 2023;47(1):130–139.
75. Kumpf VJ. Challenges and obstacles of long-term home parenteral nutrition. *Nutr Clin Pract*. 2019;34(2):196–203.
76. Gifford H, DeLegge M, Epperson LA. Education methods and techniques for training home parenteral nutrition patients. *Nutr Clin Prac*. 2010;25(5):443–450.
77. Winkler MF, Hagan E, Wetle T, Smith C, O'Sullivan Maillet J, Touger-Decker R. An exploration of quality of life and the experience of living with home parenteral nutrition. *JPEN*. 2010;34(4):395–407.
78. Winkler MF, Machan JT, Xue Z, Compher C. Home parenteral nutrition patient-reported outcome questionnaire: sensitive to quality of life differences among chronic and prolonged acute intestinal failure patients. *JPEN*. 2021;45(7):1475–1483.
79. Dibb M, Soop M, Teubner A, et al. Survival and nutritional dependence on home parenteral nutrition: three decades of experience from a single referral centre. *Clin Nutr*. 2017;36(2):570–576.

SECTION 2

Medical Nutrition Therapy in Disease States

CHAPTER 6

Nutrition in Critical Illness

Maggie Dylewski Begis
Kathy Prelack

CHAPTER OUTLINE

CORE CONCEPTS

1. The physiologic response to critical illness is characterized by hypermetabolism, protein catabolism, and hyperglycemia.
2. The SCCM and ASPEN published evidence-based guidelines to assist with the nutritional assessment and treatment of patients who are critically ill.
3. Due to the catabolic characteristics of critical illness, malnutrition can develop quickly in the intensive care unit.
4. Screening tools exist for identifying malnutrition risk among patients with critical illness.
5. Accurate height and weight measurements are needed to determine baseline and ongoing nutritional status.
6. Hyperglycemia is common among patients in the ICU. Maintaining blood glucose levels between 140 and 200 mg/dL decreases morbidity and mortality.
7. Biochemical assessment of protein nutritional status is not accurate during critical illness.
8. The nutrition-focused physical exam assists with identifying signs of malnutrition, including muscle and fat wasting.
9. It is important to collect and analyze calorie and protein intake regularly to ensure patients are receiving adequate energy and protein to support recovery.
10. Energy and protein requirements are increased during critical illness.
11. Enteral nutrition is the gold standard of nutrition support in the intensive care unit.

LEARNING OBJECTIVES

1. Describe the characteristics of the stress response associated with critical illness, including hypermetabolism, protein catabolism, and hyperglycemia.
2. List the elements included in a comprehensive nutritional assessment of a patient who is critically ill.
3. Calculate energy and protein needs of patients who are critically ill.
4. Establish an appropriate nutrition treatment plan for patients with critical illness.
5. Determine the appropriate timing and route of nutrition support during critical illness.

Introduction

The term "critical illness" includes a variety of different disease states, such as trauma, burns, organ failure, and sepsis. Although the severity of illness can vary, most patients present with catabolic stress and are at increased risk for significant morbidity and mortality. Optimal and appropriate nutrition support delivery is vital to the survival and outcome of patients who are critically ill.

CASE STUDY INTRODUCTION

Manuel is a 73-year-old male admitted to the ICU with major trauma after falling from a ladder earlier in the day. He is currently hemodynamically stable but in respiratory failure requiring mechanical ventilation. He has a central venous catheter and a nasogastric feeding tube in place. A nutrition consult was initiated to assess Manuel's nutritional status and provide nutrition support recommendations. The following clinical information was collected upon admission.

Anthropometric Data:

Weight: 109 kg
Height: 179 cm
Body mass index (BMI): 33.4 kg/m^2

Weight History
Usual weight: 107 kg

Biochemical Data:

Sodium 137 (136–145 mEq/L)
Potassium 3.4 (3.5–5.0 mEq/L)
Chloride 99 (96–106 mEq/L)
Carbon dioxide 28 (22–31 mEq/L)
Blood urea nitrogen 20 (8–20 mg/dL)
Creatinine 1.3 (0.7–1.3 mg/dL)
Blood glucose 220 (70–139 mg/dL)

Calcium 7.0 (8.5–10.5 mg/dL)
Phosphorus 2.3 (2.5–4.5 mg/dL)
Magnesium 1.2 (1.5–2.7 mg/dL)
Albumin 1.3 (3.5–5.5 g/dL)

Clinical Data:

Past Medical History: HTN, Type 2 DM, Hyperlipidemia, CAD, CHF
Medications: Ace inhibitor, fenofibrate, hydrochlorothiazide, metformin, SGLT2 inhibitor, statin
Vital Signs: Blood pressure 195/85 mm Hg, Temperature 99.1°F, Heart rate 89 beats/min
Nutrition-Focused Physical Exam: Acanthosis nigricans on neck, large abdominal girth, edematous knees and ankles. No apparent signs of muscle or fat wasting.

Disease severity scores:
APACHE II: 20
SOFA: 8

Dietary Data:

Dietary History: Unknown
Diet Prescription: NPO

Questions

1. What are Manuel's nutritional risk factors?
2. Describe the hypermetabolic state associated with major trauma and its impact on nutritional status; How might Manuel's past medical history impact his nutrition plan?
3. Write two Nutrition Diagnosis statements for Manuel identifying the Problem/Etiology/Signs and Symptoms (PES) of Manuel's active nutrition issues.
4. Identify the nutrition interventions you would like to initiate for Manuel to address the problems identified in your PES statements. Include estimated requirements and specific recommendations for nutrition therapy.
5. What indices should be included in your monitoring and evaluation plan? Why?

Pathophysiology of the Catabolic Response Associated with Critical Illness

The **catabolic stress response** associated with critical illness is characterized by significant alterations in physiology, immune function, and metabolism. Driven by inflammatory mediators, life-threatening changes in all major organ systems occur, often requiring intensive care management. Physiologic changes in cardiac function and circulatory hemodynamics are foremost in the response to injury, requiring fluid resuscitation and restoration of vascular integrity.[1] The inflammatory response that ensues calls upon a network of immune and endocrine mediators that work both locally and systemically to ultimately ensure survival. This comes at a metabolic cost, which includes increased energy expenditure, increased protein catabolism, and impaired glucose utilization.

Increased resting energy expenditure, or **hypermetabolism**, persists throughout the disease process, necessitating the need for aggressive nutritional support.[2] The need for **acute-phase reactants** and proteins for wound healing draws upon the skeletal muscle for necessary amino acids. This leads to **catabolism** or breakdown of skeletal muscle. The extent of hypermetabolism and catabolism depends on the type and severity of illness. The pathophysiology of the response to critical illness and its general management are provided in **Table 6.1**.

The shock (ebb) phase starts immediately after injury and continues for 24–72 hours.[1,2] During this time, capillary integrity is compromised, causing fluid to shift from the plasma into the interstitial space. This often results in edema, particularly in patients with severe trauma or burns. Additional fluid may be lost through wounds. The redistribution and loss of fluid leads to hypovolemia, hypotension, and reduced tissue perfusion. Inadequate blood flow to tissues may advance to organ failure. Aggressive fluid resuscitation is required to replete plasma volume and reduce the risk of organ failure. The ebb phase is also characterized by a reduction in oxygen consumption, metabolic rate, and body temperature.[1,2]

The hyperdynamic or flow phase is characterized by a shift in cardiac dynamics, restoration of vascular fluid, and a full-blown systemic inflammatory response, which ultimately leads to hypermetabolism and muscle protein catabolism. This stage may persist for several months, depending on the degree of injury. Immune cells, in response to tissue injury, inflammation, or infection, release proinflammatory **cytokines**, such as interleukin-1, interleukin-6, and tumor necrosis factor.[2,3]

Throughout the flow stage, the body is working diligently to mobilize glucose and protein to support energy requirements, wound healing, and immune function. Oxygen consumption increases to support ATP-consuming metabolic pathways, including

Table 6.1 Characteristics of the Physiologic Response to Critical Illness

Primary Systems Affected	Etiology	Treatment Goals
Shock (Ebb) Phase		
Cardiac and Circulatory Tachycardia Decreased cardiac output	Myocardial depression	Fluid resuscitation/repletion of intravascular volume to maintain tissue perfusion and minimize ischemia
Hypovolemic Shock Loss of intravascular volume Hypotension Decreased tissue perfusion Oxygen consumption	Increased vascular permeability due to release of cytokines Increased systemic vascular resistance	Airway management and ventilatory support
Lungs/Pulmonary Pulmonary edema Bronchospasm Acute respiratory distress syndrome	Inhalation injury or increased vascular permeability and edema	Restore tissue perfusion
Kidneys Decreased urine output	Decreased glomerular filtration, elevated aldosterone and ADH	

(continues)

Table 6.1 Characteristics of the Physiologic Response to Critical Illness *(continued)*

Primary Systems Affected	Etiology	Treatment Goals
Hyperdynamic, Hypermetabolic (Flow) Phase		
Cardiac and Circulatory Tachycardia Increased oxygen saturation Increased oxygen consumption Increased carbon dioxide production	Cardiac dysfunction, metabolic stress, oxidative stress	Pharmacologic management including blockade of sympathetic nervous system
Lungs/Pulmonary Pulmonary edema Bronchospasm Acute respiratory distress syndrome	Resorption of edema Continued respiratory distress due to inhalation injury or inflammatory mediators released with cell damage	Supportive care, mechanical ventilation
Liver and Skeletal Muscle Altered metabolic function Fatty liver Fat recycling Increased gluconeogenesis Decreased coagulation Increased amino acid release Muscle wasting	Endocrine-mediated release of catabolic hormones: glucagon, cortisol, epinephrine, norepinephrine	Nutritional support and pharmacological modulation of increased energy expenditure and protein breakdown

Data from Bittner EA, Shank E, Woodson L, Martyn JAJ. Acute and perioperative care of the burn-injured patient. *Anesthesiology*. 2015;122(2):448-464. doi:10.1097/ALN.0000000000000559; Simsek T, Simsek HU, Canturk NZ. Response to trauma and metabolic changes: posttraumatic metabolism. *Ulus Cerrahi Derg*. 2014;30(3):153–159. doi:10.5152/UCD.2014.2653

Table 6.2 Endocrine and Metabolic Response to Critical Illness

Endocrine Response	Alterations in Macronutrient Metabolism	Metabolic Consequence
Glucagon	Gluconeogenesis Glycogenolysis	Hyperglycemia
Cortisol	Gluconeogenesis Glycogneolysis Proteolysis	Hyperglycemia Hypertriglyceridemia Muscle wasting
Epinephrine	Gluconeogenesis Lipolysis Insulin resistance	Hyperglycemia Hypertriglyceridemia Muscle wasting
Norepinephrine	Gluconeogenesis Lipolysis	Hyperglycemia Hypertriglyceridemia

protein synthesis and hepatic gluconeogenesis. Alterations in macronutrient metabolism mediated by **catecholamines** (epinephrine and norepinephrine), glucagon, and cortisol persist throughout the course of injury and result in muscle wasting and hyperglycemia (**Table 6.2**).[4–6]

Substrates required for gluconeogenesis, including glycerol, alanine, and lactate, are provided by adipose tissue lipolysis, hepatic glycogenolysis via the Cori cycle, and gluconeogenesis via the alanine cycles[5,7–9] (**Figure 6.1**). Glutamine is also released from muscle to provide fuel to the immune system and enterocytes. Although rates of lipolysis are increased, fatty acids are not efficiently utilized during critical illness and thus are primarily reesterified within adipose tissue.[10]

The catabolic nature of critical illness persists despite the administration of nutrition, which, under normal physiologic conditions, would abate catabolic pathways such as proteolysis, lipolysis, and gluconeogenesis. Instead, these metabolic adaptations contribute to a state of hyperglycemia and muscle wasting. Stress hyperglycemia is further aggravated by insulin resistance, which is common during critical illness. In healthy individuals, glucose produced from gluconeogenesis or glycogenolysis is taken up by insulin-

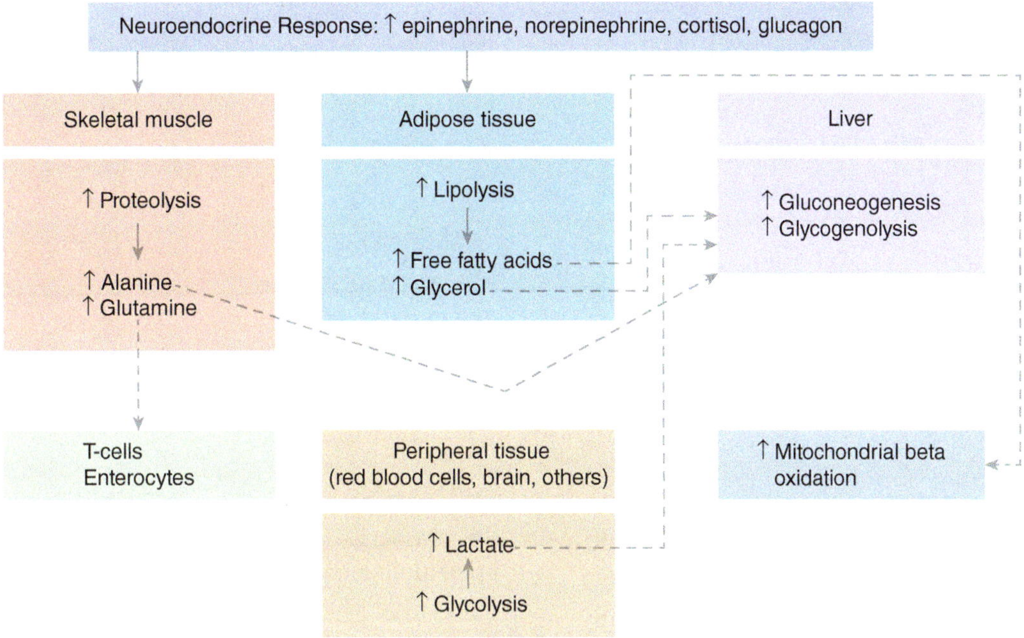

Figure 6.1 Inflammatory Mediated Alterations of Intermediary Metabolism within the Muscle, Liver, and Adipose Tissue

Table 6.3 Morbidity and Mortality Associated with Lean Body Mass Catabolism

Loss of Lean Body Mass	Associated Morbidity	Associated Mortality Rate
10%	Reduced immune function Increased risk of infection	10%
20%	Decreased wound healing	30%
30%	Pressure sores	50%
40%	Increased risk for pneumonia	100%

Data from Demling RH, Seigne P. Metabolic management of patients with severe burns. *World J Surg*. 2000;24(6):673-680. doi:10.1007/s002689910109

independent organs (such as the brain or red blood cells) or by insulin-dependent organs (such as muscle or liver) to be used for energy production. In critical illness, insulin resistance decreases glucose clearance and contributes to hyperglycemia.[11,12] Increased proteolysis, which provides alanine for gluconeogenesis, also depletes muscle protein and leads to muscle wasting. Loss of lean body mass is highly correlated to morbidity and mortality (**Table 6.3**).[13,14]

CORE CONCEPT 1

The physiologic response to critical illness is characterized by hypermetabolism, protein catabolism, and hyperglycemia.

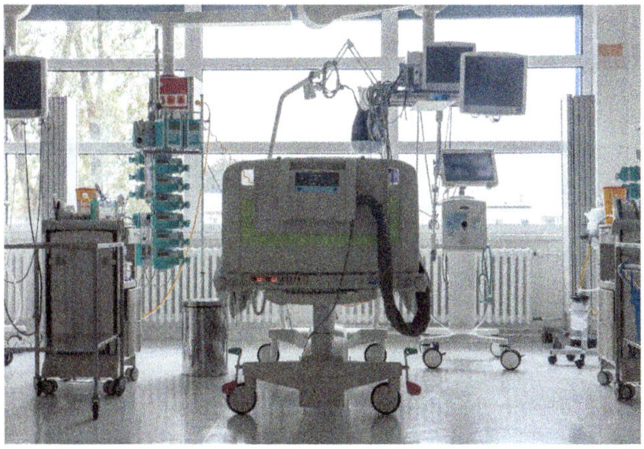

Figure 6.2 Intensive Care Unit with Monitors and Mechanical Ventilator

Medical Treatment/ Clinical Course

Most patients who are critically ill are managed in the intensive care unit (ICU). The heterogeneity of patients in the ICU is vast and may include those with or without mechanical ventilation (**Figure 6.2**), trauma, sepsis, obesity, malnutrition, and/or surgical requirements.

Patients may be young or old and have a variety of comorbidities. Thus, the clinical course depends on the diagnosis. The treatment of critical illness is highly interprofessional and includes input from physicians, nurses, occupational and physical therapists, respiratory therapists, dietitians, speech-language pathologists, social workers, and psychologists. Clinicians must work as a team to create treatment plans that support optimal patient outcomes.

Nutritional Management

The nutritional management of patients in the ICU is complex and dynamic. Assessment and treatment plans may differ among disease states, and the patient's past medical history must be carefully considered. Several professional societies have published guidelines to direct the medical nutrition therapy of patients with critical illness. These include:

1. Guidelines for the Provision and Assessment of Nutrition Support Therapy in the Adult Critically Ill Patient: Society of Critical Care Medicine and American Society for Parenteral and Enteral Nutrition (SCCM/ASPEN 2016)[15]
2. Guidelines for the Provision of Nutrition Support Therapy in the Adult Critically Ill Patient: American Society for Parenteral and Enteral Nutrition (ASPEN 2021)[16]
3. The European Society for Clinical Nutrition and Metabolism (ESPEN) Practical and Partially Revised Guideline: Clinical Nutrition in the Intensive Care Unit (ESPEN 2023)[17]

These tools provide the foundation for nutrition assessment, diagnosis, treatment, and monitoring in the ICU. In addition to guidelines and evidence-based recommendations, clinicians are also encouraged to use their clinical judgment when providing medical nutrition therapy.

CORE CONCEPT 2

The SCCM and ASPEN published evidence-based guidelines to assist with the nutritional assessment and treatment of patients who are critically ill.

Malnutrition, both preexisting and hospital acquired, must routinely be assessed. Nutritional status can quickly deteriorate in the ICU due to the metabolic stress associated with critical illness coupled with potential intolerance to nutrition support or frequent cessation of nutrition support for medical procedures.[18–20] A joint statement from the Academy of Nutrition and Dietetics (AND) and ASPEN provides recommendations for assessing and diagnosing malnutrition among patients who are critically ill, also known as the "AND/ASPEN Indicators to Diagnose Malnutrition (AAIM criteria)."[21]

CORE CONCEPT 3

Due to the catabolic characteristics of critical illness, malnutrition can develop quickly in the intensive care unit.

PRACTICE POINT

Clinicians may use the AAIM criteria coupled with current evidence-based recommendations and good clinical judgment to assess, diagnose, treat, and monitor nutritional status in the intensive care unit.

Nutrition Assessment

Nutrition Screen

The Joint Commission mandates that all patients admitted to the hospital be screened for nutritional risk within 24 hours of admission.[22] Nutritional risk of patients in the ICU may be identified using a screening tool that captures characteristics of both nutritional status and disease severity. This combination allows for identification of current malnutrition and the risk of transitioning to a malnourished state while in the hospital.[23] It is particularly important to identify patients at risk for malnutrition so that the medical team can accurately prioritize nutrition support.

The Nutritional Risk Screening (NRS)[24] and the Nutrition Risk in the Critically Ill (NUTRIC)[25,26] score are both appropriate tools for assessing nutritional risk of the adult patient in the ICU and are supported by the 2016 SCCM/ASPEN Guidelines.[15] Using the NRS, risk is determined by adding the impaired nutritional status score to the severity of disease score (Risk = score >3; High risk = score ≥ 5).

The NUTRIC tool was developed by including the following risk factors: age, disease severity, organ failure, IL-6 (as a marker of inflammation), comorbidities, days from admission to intensive care, percent oral intake in the past week, percent weight loss in the past 3 months, and body mass index (BMI) in a model and assigning a point value to them based on their association with 28-day mortality. Interestingly, all variables were significant except for indicators of preexisting nutritional status. In other words, percent oral intake, percent weight loss, and BMI were not considered to be significant risk factors and are not included in this tool. A NUTRIC score of ≥5 is suggested as high risk and warrants aggressive nutritional support.[25] The tool was recently modified from its original version by eliminating IL-6, and was subsequently validated in a separate data set. There was a strong association found between nutritional adequacy and high NUTRIC scores and 28-day mortality. The lower the NUTRIC score, the less impact nutritional intake had on 28-day mortality.[26]

Table 6.4 demonstrates examples of nutrition risk screening tools used in the critically ill. Alternatively, the 2023 ESPEN guidelines[17] suggest a more practical approach to determining nutrition risk. Under these guidelines, all patients who remain in the ICU for greater than 48 hours are assumed to be at risk for malnutrition and should be evaluated for medical nutrition therapy.

It is important to note that regardless of the type of malnutrition screening tool, patients who are initially identified as well-nourished should be routinely reassessed, as nutrition status may rapidly decline in the ICU.

CORE CONCEPT 4

Screening tools exist for identifying malnutrition risk among patients with critical illness.

Table 6.4 Nutrition Risk Screening Tools Available to Use in Patients with Critical Illness

Screening Tool	Description	Indicators of Nutritional Status	Additional Non-Nutritional Risk Indicators
Nutrition Risk Screening Tool (NRS)	Developed by ESPEN for use in acute care setting Requires a two-step process	Unintentional weight loss or BMI Reduced food intake	Disease severity based on acute or chronic condition Age
Nutrition Risk in Critically Ill (NUTRIC)	Developed for use in critically ill patients. Relies only on indicators of acute pathophysiology and comorbidities	None	Acute physiology as measured by APACHE II and SOFA scores Age Number of comorbidities Days in ICU Inflammatory markers (if available)
Malnutrition Universal Screening Tool	Developed by the British Association for Parenteral and Enteral Nutrition Considered for use in all hospitalized patients Involves a five-step process	BMI Unplanned weight loss	Acute illness in the setting of little or no nutritional intake for ≥5 days
Malnutrition Screening Tool	Developed based on general medical and surgical inpatients Two-question tool that requires no measurements or additional calculations	Recent appetite Nutritional intake Unintentional weight loss	None
Prognostic and Inflammatory and Nutritional Index	Originally designed for critically ill patients Now used in patients with cancer, surgery, liver diseases, trauma, burns Includes four biomarkers	None	Albumin Transthyretin C-reactive protein Alpha-acid glycoprotein

Data from Serón-Arbeloa C, Labarta-Monzón L, Puzo-Foncillas J, Mallor-Bonet T, Lafita-López A, Bueno-Vidales N, Montoro-Huguet M. Malnutrition Screening and Assessment. *Nutrients*. 2022; 14(12):2392. https://doi.org/10.3390/nu14122392

Anthropometrics

Important anthropometric measurements in the ICU include height, weight, BMI, and weight history.[27] A patient's current BMI and recent weight change are considered when evaluating baseline nutritional status. Accurate height and weight measurements will also help the medical team determine energy requirements and appropriate rates for nutrition support and weight-based medications.

Repeated measurements throughout the continuum of care are essential for diagnosing hospital-acquired malnutrition. **Table 6.5** features characteristics associated with adult malnutrition according to the guidelines of AND/ASPEN.[21]

Obtaining accurate height and weight measurements in the ICU may be difficult, as most patients are bed bound and sedated. Estimated height and weight may be inaccurate,[28] and standardized evidence-based methods are not currently available. Clinicians may use bed scales and patient lifts to obtain weight (**Figure 6.3**) and tape measures to determine recumbent height,[29] but should be mindful of possible measurement errors.[30] Frequent measurements will improve accuracy and confidence in the measurements.

Table 6.5 Indicators of Malnutrition During Acute Illness

	Malnutrition*	
	Moderate	**Severe**
Energy intake	<75% of energy needs for >7 days	≤50% of energy needs for ≥5 days
Weight loss	1–2% over 1 week 5% over 1 month 7.5% over 3 months	>2% over 1 week >5% over 1 month >7.5% over 3 months
Loss of subcutaneous fat	Mild	Moderate
Muscle loss	Mild	Moderate
Edema	Mild	Moderate/Severe
Reduced grip strength	N/A	Reduced

* Having two or more of these characteristics supports a malnutrition diagnosis.
Data from White JV, Guenter P, Jensen G, et al. Consensus statement of the Academy of Nutrition and Dietetics/American Society for Parenteral and Enteral Nutrition: characteristics recommended for the identification and documentation of adult malnutrition (undernutrition). *J Acad Nutr Diet*. 2012;112(5):730-738. doi:10.1016/j.jand.2012.03.012.

Anthropometric measurements are often influenced by medical factors, such as hydration status. If a patient requires aggressive fluid resuscitation or has visual evidence of edema or ascites, clinicians should use a dry or usual body weight.[15] A dry weight is obtained in the absence of excess fluid, and usual body weight may be collected from a knowledgeable family member.

CORE CONCEPT 5

Accurate height and weight measurements are needed to determine baseline and ongoing nutritional status.

Biochemical Assessment

Laboratory data, relevant to the nutritional care of the patient, varies among critical care diagnoses and may change throughout the hospital course. Monitoring glucose, electrolytes, acid–base balance, and liver and kidney function is often necessary.

Table 6.6 includes biochemical markers typically monitored during the acute phase of critical illness. Frequency of measurements may vary and is influenced by preexisting comorbidities and degree of injury.

PRACTICE POINT

Monitoring of electrolytes, including phosphorus and magnesium, before and during initiation of nutrition support is important, as initiation of feeds may result in cellular shifts. Low levels should be repleted despite advancement of feedings.

Many patients in the ICU will have hyperglycemia, characterized by elevated blood glucose levels, due to the acute-phase response. Blood glucose control is critical in the ICU, as hyperglycemia among

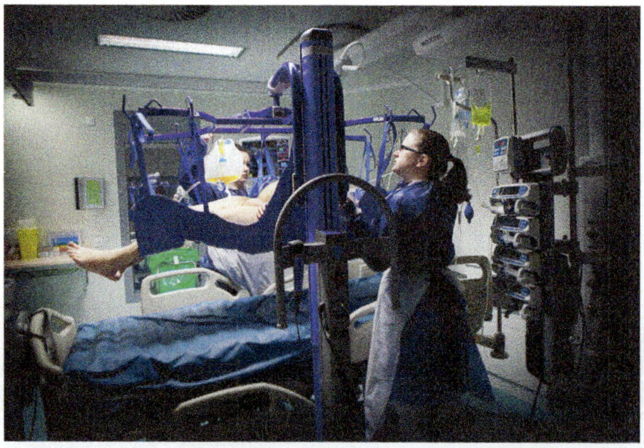

Figure 6.3 Patient Being Weighed in an ICU Hospital Bed

Table 6.6 Biochemical Monitoring of Patients with Critical Illness

Biochemical Marker	Frequency
Electrolytes	2–4 times per day
Phosphorus	2–4 times per day
Magnesium	2–4 times per day
Glucose	2–4 times per day
Liver function tests	Weekly
Blood urea nitrogen/ creatinine	Weekly
Triglycerides	Weekly
Serum lipase	Weekly
Urinary urea nitrogen	Weekly

Data from McClave SA, Taylor BE, Martindale RG, et al. Guidelines for the provision and assessment of nutrition support therapy in the adult critically ill patient: Society of Critical Care Medicine (SCCM) and American Society for Parenteral and Enteral Nutrition (A.S.P.E.N.). *JPEN J Parenter Enteral Nutr.* 2016;40(2):159-211. doi: 10.1177/0148607115621863.

patients increases mortality and infection rates.[31–33] Current guidelines from the SCCM recommend keeping blood glucose levels between 140 and 200 mg/dL[31] (**Table 6.7**). Insulin protocols should maintain blood glucose levels within this range, while preventing episodes of hypoglycemia (blood glucose ≤70 mg/dL).[31]

PRACTICE POINT

Protocols or algorithms should be used when using insulin therapy for safety and efficacy.

CORE CONCEPT 6

Hyperglycemia is common among patients in the ICU. Maintaining blood glucose levels between 140 and 200 mg/dL decreases morbidity and mortality.

Current SCCM/ASPEN guidelines do not support the use of serum proteins (albumin, prealbumin, retinol-binding protein, transferrin) to assess protein status during critical illness.[15,34–36] Decreases in these acute-phase proteins most likely reflect reprioritization of protein synthesis in the liver and are not related to nutritional status in this setting.[15,37]

In some situations, obtaining urinary urea nitrogen from a 24-hour urine collection and calculating nitrogen balance may be useful for assessing the adequacy of dietary protein intake.[38] Clinicians should aim for a nitrogen balance of +2 g/day. A considerably

Table 6.7 General Guidelines for Blood Glucose Monitoring in the ICU

- Maintain blood glucose between 140 and 200 mg/dL.
- Choose continuous intravenous (IV) insulin infusion over subcutaneous intermittent insulin provision.
- For patients receiving IV insulin, blood glucose should be monitored at least every hour.
- Insulin is a high-risk medication. Standardized protocols are needed to reduce medication errors.

Data from Honarmand K, Sirimaturos M, Hirshberg EL, et al. Society of Critical Care Medicine guidelines on glycemic control for critically ill children and adults 2024. *Crit Care Med.* 2024;52(4):e161–e181. doi:10.1097/CCM.0000000000006174

negative nitrogen balance indicates that dietary protein intake is insufficient to meet metabolic demands. Nitrogen balance studies may be unreliable if the patient has kidney failure or significant protein losses via wounds, drains, or dialysate.[38,39] Refer to Chapter 2 *Biochemical Assessment* for an example of a nitrogen balance calculation.

Assessment of micronutrient status in the ICU may also be inaccurate due to potential alterations in absorption, transport, metabolism, and excretion.[40,41] Thus, interpretation of blood micronutrient levels among this population should be interpreted with caution.

PRACTICE POINT

Nitrogen balance is a useful way to determine protein adequacy. In patients who have open wounds, it is important to account for increased protein losses in the wound.

CORE CONCEPT 7

Biochemical assessment of protein nutritional status is not accurate during critical illness.

Nutrition-Focused Physical Exam

A head-to-toe inspection of the patient will evaluate a variety of characteristics that are essential for the nutrition assessment of a patient who is critically ill (**Figure 6.4**). Elements of the nutrition-focused physical exam (NFPE) include the following:

- Overall appearance
- Skin (open wounds, decubitus ulcers, evidence of micronutrient deficiency)
- Muscle and fat wasting
- Fluid accumulation

- Assistive feeding devices (gastric tubes, enteral tubes)
- Peripheral and central catheters
- Ostomies

The NFPE is used, along with other assessment tools, to identify existing malnutrition or changes in nutritional status. If a patient is identified as having two or more of the criteria listed in Table 6.5, a diagnosis of malnutrition is indicated.[21]

Completing an NFPE may be challenging in patients who require extensive wound dressings, such as with multiple-trauma or burn injury. A thorough inspection of the patient should be completed when the dressings are removed, such as during daily dressing changes or during an operative procedure.

CORE CONCEPT 8

The NFPE assists with identifying signs of malnutrition, including muscle and fat wasting.

Dietary Assessment

In the absence of reliable biochemical markers, evaluation of dietary intake is one of the only methods to determine adequate energy and protein intake. If possible, a complete dietary history should be obtained upon admission either from the patient or a reliable family member. In addition to documenting food preferences, usual dietary patterns may be used to assess baseline nutritional status.

Ongoing documentation of nutrient intake while in the ICU is critical to assessing adequate oral intake

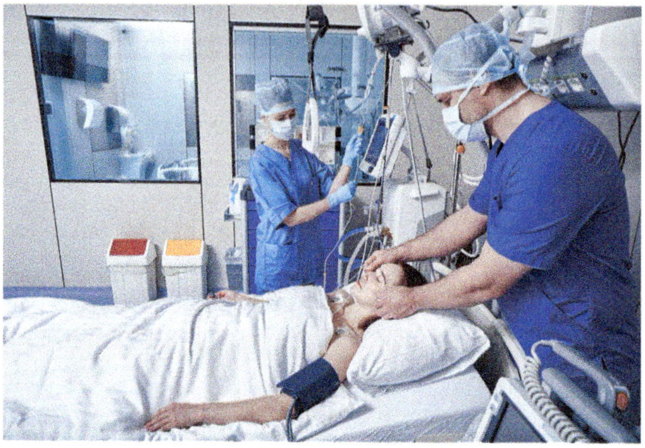

Figure 6.4 Performing an NFPE in a Critically Ill Patient

or provision of nutrition support. Daily calorie/protein counts are useful for documenting macronutrient deficits. It is important to remember that some medications contain calories (propofol, dextrose) and should be included in the dietary intake totals.

Sufficient protein intake is especially important for patients in the ICU, as it is the primary macronutrient responsible for wound healing, immune function, and lean body mass preservation.[15]

PRACTICE POINT

Dietary energy and protein deficits should be calculated daily and communicated with the medical team on a regular basis.

Specific micronutrient requirements during critical illness have not been established and most likely

Clinical Roundtable

Micronutrient Supplementation During Critical Illness

Background: Many aspects of critical illness, particularly burn injury, intuitively increase micronutrient requirements. Antioxidant nutrients may be useful in fighting free radicals. Selenium, zinc, and copper are important for wound healing and infection control. The acute-phase response associated with critical illness and catabolic stress alters micronutrient status. Many nutrients are lost through wounds and urine. In addition, certain nutrients such as zinc and selenium depend on specific protein carriers to be transported to organs and wound tissue. These protein carriers may be downregulated during stress. In addition, because nutrients work in systems and/or can be antagonistic to one another, single nutrient supplementation may affect the status of other nutrients. Specific recommendations for micronutrient supplementation during critical illness are not available.

Roundtable Discussion

1. How do you assess micronutrient status?
2. How would you prevent deficiency and toxicity?
3. Which nutrients, if any, would you recommend providing to patients in addition to the amount they receive via nutrition support?
4. What might you monitor?
5. How well do enteral feeding products meet micronutrient requirements during illness?

Reference

1. de Man AME, Amrein K, Casaer MP, et al. LLL 44-4: micronutrients in acute disease and critical illness. *Clin Nutr ESPEN*. 2024;61:437–446. doi:10.1016/j.clnesp.2024.04.011

differ across diagnoses. It is important to ensure that all patients are receiving at least the Dietary Reference Intake (DRI) for all essential micronutrients.

CORE CONCEPT 9

It is important to collect and analyze calorie and protein intake regularly to ensure patients are receiving adequate energy and protein to support recovery.

Determining Energy Needs

The best way to estimate energy requirements in the ICU is by using indirect calorimetry (IC).[17] Measurements should be repeated in timely intervals, ideally more than once a week, to account for the dynamic features of critical illness, including changes in metabolic stress, wound healing, medications, and treatment plans.[15,42]

If IC is unavailable and the patient is intubated, resting energy expenditure (REE) may be calculated by obtaining VCO_2 measurements from the ventilator ($REE = VCO_2 \times 8.19$).[17] This method is less accurate than IC, but more accurate than predictive equations.[43,44]

Predictive equations are inaccurate and should only be used if IC and VCO_2 are not available. These equations tend to be particularly erroneous among patients with obesity or who are underweight.[45–48] Several predictive equations are supported by professional organizations when IC is not available (**Table 6.8**). Most of these are simple weight-based equations that do not require additional activity or stress factors.

Permissive underfeeding (<60% estimated needs) is recommended during the first 3 days of acute illness to reduce the risk of complications associated with overfeeding. Low-dose enteral nutrition (EN) during this time has not been associated with negative outcomes or mortality when compared to a standard goal bed approach.[17,49] If predictive equations are used to determine energy needs, permissive underfeeding may be extended through days 7–10.[16,17] Subsequently, energy intake may be increased to meet 80–100% of estimated energy requirements.[17]

Regardless of the method chosen, the clinician should refer to guidelines and utilize clinical judgment when deciding the precise range for energy needs. Patients should be monitored closely, and goals should be adjusted if signs of under- or overfeeding are observed.

Table 6.8 Estimating Energy Requirements for Patients with Critical Illness

	Equation	Source of Recommendation
ICU patients	12–25 kcal/kg in the first 7–10 days of ICU stay	2021 ASPEN
ICU patients	25–30 kcal/kg/day	SCCM/ASPEN
ICU patients	20–25 kcal/kg/day For patients with obesity, use the adjusted body weight weight + 0.25 × (actual weight − ideal body weight)	2023 ESPEN
ICU patients with obesity BMI 30–50 kg/m^2 BMI >50 kg/m^2	11–14 kcal/kg/day (use actual body weight) 22–25 kcal/kg (use ideal body weight) 16–20 kcal/kg (use actual body weight)	SCCM/ASPEN ESPEN
Mechanically ventilated	PSU 2003b RMR = MSJ (0.96) + VE (31) + Tmax (167) - 6212	AND EAL[27]
Mechanically ventilated with obesity <60 years	PSU 2003b RMR = MSJ (0.96) + VE (31) + Tmax (167) - 6212	AND EAL[27]
>60 years	PSU 2010 RMR = MSJ (0.71) + VE (64) + Tmax (85) - 3085	

PSU: Penn State University
RMR: Resting metabolic rate
MSJ: Mifflin-St Jeor equation
RMR males = 10 × weight (kg) + 6.25 × height (cm) - 5 × age (years) + 5
RMR females = 10 × weight (kg) + 6.25 × height (cm) - 5 × age (years) - 161
VE: minute ventilation (L/min)
AND - Academy for Nutrition and Dietetics
EAL - Evidence Analysis Library
Tmax: maximum temperature in Celsius
Data from Academy of Nutrition and Dietetics. Critical illness guidelines. Updated 2012. Accessed January 12, 2026. http://www.andeal.org/topic.cfm?menu=5302; McClave SA, Taylor BE, Martindale RG, et al. Guidelines for the provision and assessment of nutrition support therapy in the adult critically ill patient: Society of Critical Care Medicine (SCCM) and American Society for Parenteral and Enteral Nutrition (ASPEN). *JPEN J Parenter Enteral Nutr.* 2016;40(2):159-211. doi:10.1177/0148607115621863

Clinical Controversy

Topic: Permissive Underfeeding versus Standard Feeding in Critically Ill Patients

When rounding with the medical team on the ICU, the medical team questions the use of a hypocaloric feeding for a patient who is critically ill. You are asked whether the patient might have a better outcome when fed at 60% to 70% of the energy goal. You reply that you will review the literature and return with your recommendation.

Optimal provision of calorie targets in patients who are metabolically stressed remains elusive. While consensus exists on the negative impact of overfeeding, the use of permissive underfeeding continues to be debated. A study by Sun et al. found that compared to low energy or full energy feeds, moderate energy reduction (approximating 60% of energy goal) improved intestinal barrier function, inflammatory markers, and nutritional status without significant feeding intolerances. Conversely, Powierza et al. showed a lower incidence of hospital mortality in patients who achieved their full energy goals early versus late in their hospitalization. Using the two journal papers described, critically review study design, research findings, and conclusions. Based on the evidence, what is your recommendation for feeding your patient? Provide a persuasive argument and rationale for your decision.

References

1. Sun JK, Nie S, Chen YM, Zhou J, Wang X, Zhou SM, Mu XW. Effects of permissive hypocaloric vs standard enteral feeding on gastrointestinal function and outcomes in sepsis. *World J Gastroenterol*. 2021;27(29):4900-4912. doi:10.3748/wjg.v27.i29.4900.
2. Powierza CS, Doyle MM, Wasden K, et al. Early goal enteral nutrition associated with decreased in-hospital death in mechanically ventilated critically ill adults: a retrospective cohort study. *BMJ Open Respir Res*. 2024;11:e001962. doi:10.1136/bmjresp-2023-001962.

PRACTICE POINT

Clinicians should be mindful of fluid accumulation when utilizing predictive equations. To prevent overestimation of energy requirements, equations should include the patient's dry weight.

Calculating Protein Needs

For all patients who are critically ill, adequate protein is required to maintain lean body mass and support immune function. In some subsets of critical illness, protein is also needed to support wound healing. Protein requirements typically range from 1.2 to 2.0 g/kg actual body weight[15–17] and may be higher among patients with burn injury, trauma, or those on dialysis[8] (**Table 6.9**). Of note, it is not recommended to restrict protein during renal insufficiency or liver failure.[15]

CORE CONCEPT 10

Energy and protein requirements are increased during critical illness.

Nutrition Intervention

Treatment options should be individualized and established using the data collected during the nutrition assessment. Nutritional risk and severity of disease will be significant factors when determining the appropriate nutrition intervention. Adequate provision of nutrition support will impact patient outcomes including infection rates and length of stay.[50–52]

Table 6.9 Daily Protein Requirements for Patients with Critical Illness

ICU patient	1.2–2.0 g/kg
Patients with obesity in the ICU BMI 30–40 kg/m^2 BMI >40 kg/m^2	 2 g/kg using ideal body weight up to 2.5 g/kg ideal body weight
Hemodialysis or continuous renal replacement therapy	Up to 2.5 g/kg
Burns	1.5–2 g/kg

Data from McClave SA, Taylor BE, Martindale RG, et al. Guidelines for the provision and assessment of nutrition support therapy in the adult critically ill patient: Society of Critical Care Medicine (SCCM) and American Society for Parenteral and Enteral Nutrition (ASPEN). *JPEN J Parenter Enteral Nutr*. 2016;40(2):159-211. doi: 10.1177/0148607115621863

Nutrition Support

Most patients who are critically ill require EN and/or parenteral nutrition (PN) support to meet the metabolic demands of the illness. Professional organizations, including ASPEN[15,16] and ESPEN,[17] provide evidence-based guidelines for the provision of nutrition support (**Table 6.10**). These guidelines are similar but do provide several distinct recommendations based on their interpretation of the available literature. Clinicians must

Table 6.10 Comparison of ASPEN and ESPEN Nutrition Support Guidelines

Type of Nutrition Support	
ASPEN	■ EN or PN is acceptable during the first week of critical illness. (2021) ■ Avoid supplementing EN with PN until day 7. (2021)
ESPEN	■ EN is the preferred route. ■ Continuous EN feedings are preferred. ■ If EN is contraindicated and the patient is severely malnourished, PN may be initiated within 3–7 days of ICU admission. ■ If EN is not tolerated or contraindicated, PN should be initiated within 3–7 days.
Dose	
ASPEN	■ Provide 12–25 kcal/kg/day for the first 7–10 days of ICU admission. (2021)
ESPEN	■ Hypocaloric feedings (<70% of estimated needs) should be provided for the first 3–5 days. ■ If predictive equations are used to determine energy needs, hypocaloric nutrition may be extended through days 7–10.
Timing of Nutrition Support	
ASPEN	■ Initiate EN within 24–48 hours of ICU admission. (2016)
ESPEN	■ Initiate EN within 24–48 hours of ICU admission. ■ EN or PN should not be advanced to goal rate until 3–7 days.
Location of EN Device	
ASPEN	■ Most patients should be fed into the stomach. ■ When the risk for aspiration is high or if patients are not able to tolerate gastric feedings, jejunal feedings may be considered. (2016)
ESPEN	■ Most patients should be fed into the stomach. ■ When the risk for aspiration is high or if patients are not able to tolerate gastric feedings, jejunal feedings may be considered.
Composition of EN	
ASPEN	■ A standard, isotonic (1–1.5 kcal/mL) polymeric formula is appropriate for most patients. (2016) ■ Special additives (eicosapentaenoic acid, docosahexaenoic acid, glutamine, nucleic acids, omega-3 fish oils) are not indicated for most patients.
ESPEN	■ Special additives (glutamine, omega-3 fish oils) are not indicated for most patients.
Composition of PN	
ASPEN	■ Intravenous lipids, 100% soybean oil or mixed oil emulsions, may be included in PN.
ESPEN	■ Glucose infusion rate should not exceed 5 mg/kg/min. ■ Intravenous lipids should be included, but should not exceed 1.5 g lipids/kg/day. ■ Intravenous lipids may include fish oil doses of 0.1–0.2 g/kg/day. ■ Trace elements and vitamins should be provided daily.

Data from McClave SA, Taylor BE, Martindale RG, et al. Guidelines for the provision and assessment of nutrition support therapy in the adult critically ill patient: Society of Critical Care Medicine (SCCM) and American Society for Parenteral and Enteral Nutrition (ASPEN). *JPEN J Parenter Enteral Nutr.* 2016;40(2):159–211. doi: 10.1177/0148607115621863

use clinical judgment when deciding which guidelines are the most relevant to their specific patients.

The exact amount, route, and timing of nutrition support continues to be studied and debated. Collectively, current guidelines support starting nutrition support early and judiciously to prevent a prolonged nutritional deficit.[15–17]

To avoid overfeeding, nutrition support should be advanced slowly, and goal rates should not be achieved until 3–7 days post admission.[17] Clinicians should monitor complications, such as hyperglycemia, respiratory acidosis, or hypertriglyceridemia, closely and reduce the amount of nutrition support accordingly.

CASE STUDY REVISITED

Manuel's tube feedings (TFs) were initiated and gradually advanced to the goal rate by day 7. It is reported that Manuel is having increasing loose stools and diarrhea since initiating feedings. At rounds, the team asks if you have any recommendations to improve patient tolerance.

Anthropometric Data:

Current weight: 111 kg
Admission weight: 109 kg
Height: 179 cm

Biochemical Data:

Sodium 133 (136–145 mEq/L)
Potassium 4.2 (3.5–5.0 mEq/L)
Chloride 114 (96–106 mEq/L)
Carbon dioxide 19 (22–31 mEq/L)
Blood urea nitrogen 21 (8–20 mg/dL)
Creatinine 1.0 (0.7–1.3 mg/dL)
Blood glucose 175 mg/dL (70–139 mg/dL)
Calcium 7.0 (8.5–10.5 mg/dL)
Phosphorus 2.8 (2.5–4.5 mg/dL)
Magnesium 1.2 (1.5–2.7 mg/dL)
Albumin 1.5 (3.5–5.5 g/dL)

Clinical Data:

Past Medical History: HTN, Type 2 DM, Hyperlipidemia, CAD, CHF
Medications: cefepime, fenofibrate, hydrochlorothiazide, imipenem, insulin, lasix, levofloxacin, magnesium gluconate, potassium phosphate
Vital Signs: Blood pressure 168/80 mm Hg, Temperature 99°F, Heart rate 77 beats/min
Nutrition-Focused Physical Exams: Patient remains edematous
Disease severity Scores: APACHE II: 20; SOFA: 8

Dietary Data:

Dietary History: Mean Intake × 7 days = 85% of goal via TF
Diet Prescription: TF per RD recommendations

Questions

1. What are the possible causes of Manuel's diarrhea?
2. What is your intervention?
3. Write one PES statement for Manuel identifying Manuel's active nutrition problem.
4. How will you monitor efficacy of your intervention?

CORE CONCEPT 11

Enteral nutrition is the gold standard of nutrition support in the intensive care unit.

Enteral Nutrition Support

It is well known that EN is the preferred long-term method of nutrition support, as it maintains gut integrity and blunts the hypermetabolic response.[17,53–55] Patients who receive timely EN have lower mortality and infection rates compared to those who receive delayed EN.[15]

In most cases, specialty formulas (disease-specific, organ-specific, immune-modulating, elemental, semi-elemental) are not indicated for patients in the ICU. A standard, high-protein, polymeric (whole protein), 1–1.5 kcal/mL EN formula is sufficient to meet macro- and micronutrient requirements.[15]

Formulas with immune-modulating components (eicosapentaenoic acid, docosahexaenoic acid, glutamine, nucleic acid) and anti-inflammatory lipids (omega-3 fatty acids) do not provide additional benefit.[15,17] Thus, these specialty formulas, which are often more expensive than standard formulas, are not necessary. The few exceptions to this recommendation are listed in **Table 6.11**.

The addition of fermentable soluble fiber is recommended for all patients in the ICU who are hemodynamically stable, especially among patients with diarrhea.[15]

Table 6.11 Appropriate Use of Enteral Nutrition Formulas for Patients with Critical Illness

Condition	Suggested Formula Type
Most critically ill patients	High protein, polymeric
Acute respiratory failure	Fluid-restricted, energy dense (1.5–2 kcal/mL)
Renal failure	High protein, polymeric If needed, formula low in phosphorus, potassium
Traumatic brain injury	Immune-modulating (with arginine)
Postoperative surgical ICU patients	Immune-modulating
Critically ill patients with persistent diarrhea due to malabsorption	Semi-elemental

Data from McClave SA, Taylor BE, Martindale RG, et al. Guidelines for the provision and assessment of nutrition support therapy in the adult critically ill patient: Society of Critical Care Medicine (SCCM) and American Society for Parenteral and Enteral Nutrition (ASPEN). *JPEN J Parenter Enteral Nutr.* 2016;40(2):159–211. doi: 10.1177/0148607115621863.

Loose bowel movements that progress to diarrhea are common among patients who require aggressive antibiotic therapy or hypertonic medications, such as sodium chloride.

Soluble fiber supports bowel health by producing short-chain fatty acids and functioning as a prebiotic. **Short-chain fatty acids**, products of soluble fiber fermentation in the colon, are fuel for colonocytes and promote water and electrolyte absorption.[56] As a prebiotic, soluble fiber stimulates the growth of healthy bacteria, including *Bifidobacteria* and *Lactobacillus*, in the colon.[57] For patients with diarrhea, the enhanced water absorption via the colon is especially beneficial for decreasing loose stools. The SSCM/ASPEN guidelines recommend providing a total of 10–20 g of

PRACTICE POINT

For patients who are frequently going to the operating room or who have their feedings held for medical procedures, feeding volume can be upwardly adjusted to compensate for interruption of feedings. An example of how to provide volume-based feedings is provided in Chapter 4, *Enteral Nutrition Therapy*.

CASE STUDY REVISITED

On day 12 of admission, Manuel becomes septic and hemodynamically unstable requiring vasopressor support. His respiratory status continues to decline. His abdominal girth is significantly increased since yesterday. His TFs have been stopped. You are asked to provide your recommendation for nutrition support.

Anthropometric Data:

Current weight: 110 kg
Admission weight: 109 kg
Height: 179 cm

Biochemical Data:

Sodium 137 (136–145 mEq/L)
Potassium 4.2 (3.5–5.0 mEq/L)
Chloride 111 (96–106 mEq/L)
Carbon dioxide 39 (22–31 mEq/L)
Blood urea nitrogen 22 (8–20 mg/dL)
Creatinine 1.1 (0.7–1.3 mg/dL)
Blood glucose 275 mg/dL (70–139 mg/dL)
Calcium 7.9 (8.5–10.5 mg/dL)
Phosphorus 2.8 (2.5–4.5 mg/dL)
Magnesium 1.2 (1.5–2.7 mg/dL)
Albumin 1.5 (3.5–5.5 g/dL)

Arterial Blood Gas:

pH 7.31 (7.35–7.45)
PaCO2 50 (35–45 mm Hg)
PaO2 90 (80–100 mm Hg)
HCO3 29 (22–26 mEq/L)

Clinical Data:

Past Medical History: HTN, Type 2 DM, Hyperlipidemia, CAD, CHF

Medications: dopamine, epinephrine, fenofibrate, hydrochlorothiazide, imipenem, insulin, lasix, levofloxacin, magnesium gluconate, potassium phosphate

Vital Signs: Blood pressure 128/55 mm Hg, Temperature 99.9°F, Heart rate 77 beats/min, mean arterial blood pressure 48 (<50 mm Hg)

Questions

1. What do the guidelines recommend regarding nutrition support given Manuel's clinical description?
2. What labs are concerning? What labs might you check before initiating your nutrition plan?
3. Assess Manuel's original PES statements. Identify if each statement remains an active issue or if the PES statement has been resolved. If the PES statement remains an active issue, has improvement in the issue been noted? If the issue has been resolved, write a new PES statement.
4. Provide your nutrition support intervention for Manuel. Include estimated requirements and specific recommendations for nutrition therapy.

fiber/day to all patients in the ICU.[15,58] Ideally, this dose would be provided in intervals throughout the day or added to the EN to provide a continuous infusion.

Full-strength EN formulas may be started at 10–40 mL/hour and advanced as tolerated (typically, 10–20 mL every 8–12 hours).[39,59] Volume-based feeding regimens may also be useful in the ICU, especially if patients require frequent breaks in EN due to medical procedures. The goal of this type of feeding protocol is to meet the daily volume of EN (instead of focusing on a specific hourly rate), which often requires fluctuating the rate of EN to account for periods when EN has been held.[15,60]

Parenteral Nutrition Support

If EN is contraindicated, PN is an acceptable alternative during the first week of admission.

Additionally, if a patient is only able to tolerate small volumes of EN, supplemental PN may be introduced to help meet energy and protein goals.[16]

Judicial utilization and monitoring of PN is critical to prevent complications of overfeeding. Hypocaloric (≤20 kcal/kg/day or up to 80% of estimated kcal needs) PN regimens that supply adequate amounts of protein (≥1.2 g/kg/day) reduce the risk of complications, such as hyperglycemia and infection, during the first week of admission.[15,61,62] PN may be increased thereafter, as tolerated by the patient.[15] Glucose infusion rates should not exceed glucose oxidation capacity (5 mg/kg/min).[17]

Intravenous lipid injectable emulsion (ILE) may be added to PN at the time of initiation. All types of ILE available in the United States, including 100% soybean oil, mixed oil, and those containing fish oil, are safe and effective calorie sources for patients in the ICU. The addition of ILE may help meet energy goals while decreasing the need for excess dextrose provision. When PN is the only source of nutrition for more than 10 days, ILE should be included with the PN to prevent essential fatty acid deficiency. When using ILE, serum triglycerides should be obtained at baseline and monitored to assess for hypertriglyceridemia.[16]

Supplements

Vitamins/Minerals. All patients who are critically ill should receive at least the DRI for all essential micronutrients. This can easily be accomplished in patients receiving EN, as most commercial EN products provide 100% or more of the DRI for all essential micronutrients. If PN is required, clinicians should ensure that micronutrient provision is adequate.

Specific guidelines for micronutrient supplementation during critical illness are not well established. It is clear that high doses of antioxidant supplements (>10 times the DRI) are not recommended unless a specific deficiency has been identified.[17]

Dosing, route of administration, and specific micronutrient combinations differ among clinicians who specialize in critical illness, and micronutrient requirements most likely vary among disease states. Thus, provision of micronutrients should be individualized and closely monitored to prevent deficiency and toxicity.

Glutamine. Glutamine is an amino acid that is a component of protein and thus included in standard EN products. Additional glutamine supplementation is not indicated for most patients in the ICU, although it may be beneficial for individuals with large (>20% body surface area) burn injury or trauma, as it has been demonstrated to decrease rates of infectious morbidity and mortality.[17] Current guidelines recommend providing supplemental enteral glutamine to these patient populations once EN is initiated. For patients with burns, the dose is 0.3–0.5 g/kg/day glutamine for 10–15 days. Among patients with trauma, it is recommended to provide 0.2–0.3 g/kg/day glutamine for 5 days or up to 15 days for patients with delayed wound healing.[17]

Disease-Specific Considerations

Trauma and Burn Injury

Patients with severe trauma are particularly susceptible to persistent hypermetabolism and lean body mass depletion. Burn injury, one of the most severe forms of trauma, may increase the metabolic rate by 40-80% and remain elevated for at least 1-year postinjury.[63–66] Despite aggressive treatment strategies, a loss of up to 25% of total body mass may occur following a large burn injury.[67,68]

The protein requirement of patients with trauma is particularly high (1.5–2 g/kg/day) and may even exceed 2.5 g/kg/day to improve nitrogen balance. Wound healing and nitrogen balance studies should be followed closely and correlated with protein intake as appropriate.

Continuous nutrition support must provide an optimal provision of protein to promote protein synthesis and reduce lean body mass catabolism. As discussed earlier, it is also recommended that patients with burn injuries exceeding 20% body surface area should receive 0.3–0.5 g/kg/day of enteral glutamine for 10–15 days.[69]

Sepsis

Systemic inflammatory response syndrome and sepsis are potential complications of critical illness. **Systemic inflammatory response syndrome (SIRS)** describes an inflammatory response that occurs throughout the body in response to infection, inflammation, trauma, and burns. In general, **sepsis** is defined as a systemic infection that leads to SIRS (**Table 6.12**).[70] If organ failure is present, it is considered severe sepsis.

Hemodynamic instability, a condition associated with sepsis and characterized by hypotension, is a contraindication of EN[15] as it may interfere with the utility of the gastrointestinal tract. A substantial drop in blood pressure will reduce perfusion to the gut tissue and thus decrease peristalsis. Under these conditions, an ileus (lack of intestinal peristalsis) may develop, which may directly interfere with EN therapy. Providing EN to patients with advanced hemodynamic instability may result in ischemia/reperfusion injuries and, in severe cases, the development of ischemic bowel.

Table 6.12 Criteria for Diagnosing Systemic Inflammatory Response Syndrome (SIRS)

A diagnosis of SIRS requires two or more of the following clinical outcomes:

- Heart rate: >90 beats/min
- Respiratory rate: >20 breaths/min
- Temperature: >38°C or <36°C
- White blood cell count: >12,000/mm^3, <4000/mm^3, or >10% bandemia

Data from Bone RC, Sprung CL, Sibbald WJ. Definitions for sepsis and organ failure. *Crit Care Med.* 1992;20(6):724–726.

EN should be stopped if mean arterial blood pressure is <50 mm Hg or if the patient requires aggressive use of vasopressor medications (norepinephrine, phenylephrine, epinephrine, dopamine) to maintain blood pressure.[15] Low-dose EN (20–50% of TEE) may be introduced once the symptoms of hemodynamic instability start to subside.[17] If EN cannot be used, PN should be provided.[17]

PRACTICE POINT

In patients who are exhibiting signs of sepsis, provision of enteral feedings should be carefully evaluated. It may be necessary to hold feedings or delay initiation until the patient is hemodynamically stable.

Obesity and Underlying Comorbidities

Similar to rates in the general population, obesity is a common comorbidity of patients admitted to the ICU.[71,72] Despite a larger body mass, patients with obesity also experience significant hypermetabolism and protein catabolism.[73] Specific guidelines for detecting malnutrition among patients with obesity do not exist. Clinicians should closely monitor changes in weight, muscle mass, fat mass, and signs of micronutrient deficiencies.[73] The ratio of lean body mass to fat mass will differ among patients with obesity. Therefore, IC is the preferred method for measuring energy expenditure. If IC is not available, energy needs may be calculated using one of the suggested predictive equations.[73]

While guidelines vary over the appropriate weight to use (actual, ideal, or adjusted) when estimating energy requirement, the overall objective is to avoid overfeeding of calories and, in some cases, underfeed. This also helps prevent volume overload and hyperglycemia. A high-protein, hypocaloric diet will help maintain lean body mass and promote the breakdown of adipose tissue.[15] Patients should receive at least 1.3 g/kg of protein, calculated using adjusted body weight.[17] ASPEN guidelines[16] recommend using 11–14 kcal/kg actual body weight/day for patients with BMI 30–50 kg/m^2 and 22–25 kcal/kg ideal body weight/day for patients with BMI >50 kg/m^2. ASPEN guidelines[16] also recommend that protein be provided at 2.0 g/kg ideal body weight/day for patients with BMI of 30–40 kg/m^2 and up to 2.5 g/kg ideal body weight/day for patients with BMI ≥40 kg/m^2. Protein intake of 2–2.5 g/kg ideal body weight has also been suggested in hypocaloric diets providing less than 20 kcal/kg of adjusted body weight.[74]

Patients with obesity may have difficulty with fuel utilization as obesity is often linked to insulin resistance and altered lipid metabolism. Screening for preexisting comorbidities such as hypertension, diabetes, and cardiac disease should be included as part of a nutritional assessment. Biochemical parameters including glucose, HbA1C, triglycerides, and liver enzymes and inflammatory markers such as CRP should be determined prior to initiating nutrition therapy.[15] Nutrition support for these patients must be a judicious balance of providing metabolic support without aggravating pathophysiology associated with these conditions.

Hypocaloric feeding is often used to provide a lower calorie-to-protein ratio in patients with obesity. This differs from permissive underfeeding, which is recommended during the first 3–7 days of critical illness with or without obesity.[15–17]

Acute Respiratory Distress Syndrome in COVID-19

The COVID-19 pandemic presented many unique challenges within the ICU setting, including for the provision of nutrition therapy. Up to 10% of patients with COVID-19 develop acute respiratory distress syndrome (ARDS) requiring urgent respiratory support.[74–76] Age is the strongest risk factor for severity of outcome, with risk of death 340 times as great in those aged 85 years and older compared with 18-to-29-year-olds (**Figure 6.5**). Risk of severe outcome is also increased with certain underlying conditions such as obesity, diabetes with complications, and anxiety-related disorders. Furthermore, as the number of underlying conditions increases, so does the risk of death. **Figure 6.5** shows COVID-19 death risk ratio based on age and underlying medical conditions.[77–79]

A significant portion of patients (34.6%) with COVID-19 in the ICU are at risk for malnutrition.[75] Identification of malnutrition risk using any number of validated screening tools, such as NUTRIC, Prognostic Nutritional Index (PNI), and Malnutrition Universal Screening Tool (MUST), has been demonstrated to predict mortality in patients with acute illness. All patients with COVID-19 should be screened upon admission to the ICU with a nutritional assessment and diagnosis made for malnutrition accordingly.[76,80–82,21]

The nutritional consequences of COVID-19 are similar to those in critical illness. Severe respiratory illness results in a profound inflammatory state, with increased energy expenditure related to hypermetabolism as well as the work of ventilation. Energy expenditure in patients with severe respiratory illness progressively increases over time. Because IC is not always feasible or safe in patients with COVID-19, energy needs are usually assessed empirically. Predictive equations tend to underestimate energy needs in this population, with the exception of the Penn State equation, which was found to be most accurate.[83] Similar to other patients in the ICU, low-dose EN during the first week of illness is recommended. Feeding should be initiated to provide 15–20 kcal/kg (or 70–80% of total energy goal).[84] Gradual advancement toward a final goal of 25 or 30 kcal/kg for patients who are underweight is recommended. A protein target of at least 1.3 g/kg is suggested.[75]

The timing of EN is considered extremely important. Early EN within 24–36 hours of admission or 12 hours of mechanical intubation is recommended.[16,75,84] Provision of early EN has been associated with shorter ICU and hospital length of stay, decreased days on mechanical ventilation, and decreased mortality.[84–86] Gastric tube feedings are suggested as they are more physiological, require minimal expertise, and facilitate early initiation of EN. Caution, however, is needed particularly in patients who are hemodynamically unstable, at risk for refeeding syndrome, or with gastrointestinal intolerance. For patients who cannot tolerate EN, PN should be provided, including during the first week of care. Interestingly, this corresponds with more recent ASPEN guidelines that state that low-dose intake of either EN or PN during the first week of care results in similar outcomes.[21,75,84]

One of the barriers to EN provision is the need for patients to be in the prone position to improve oxygenation. Among the lessons learned during the COVID-19 pandemic is that gastric feeding while in

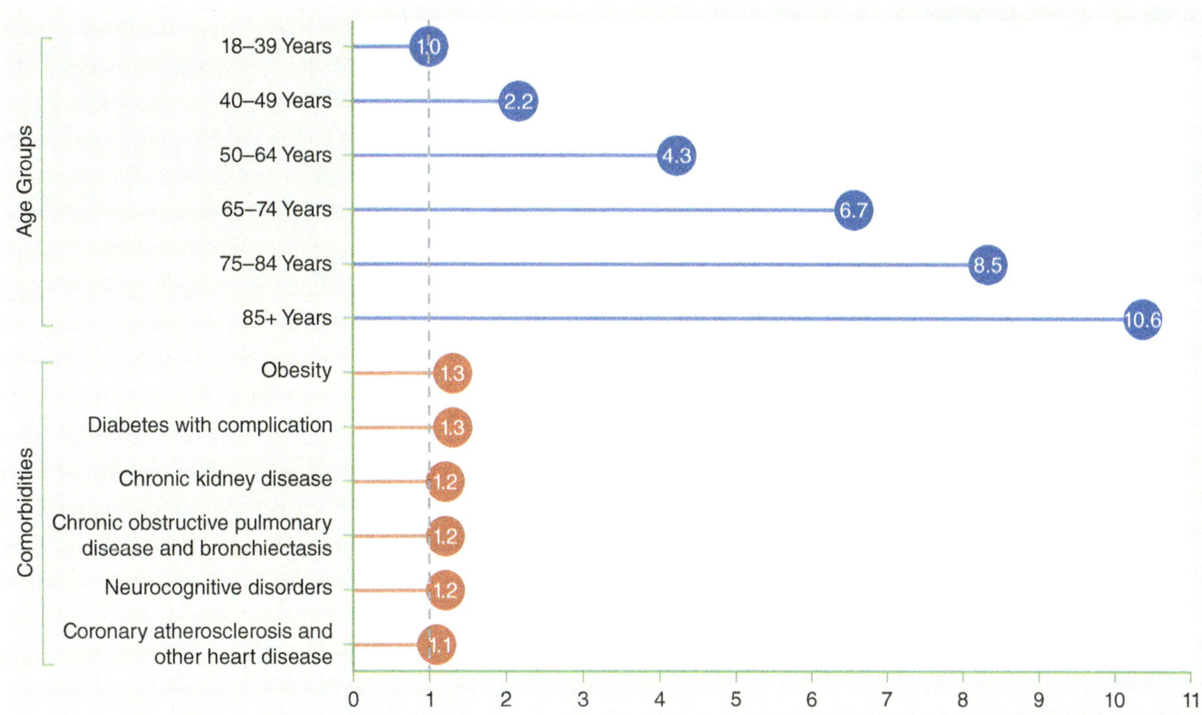

Figure 6.5 COVID-19 Death Ratio According to Age and Comorbid Conditions

Data from Kompaniyets L, Pennington AF, Goodman AB, Rosenblum HG, Belay B, Ko JY, et al. Underlying medical conditions and severe illness among 540,667 adults hospitalized with COVID-19, March 2020–March 2021. *Prev Chronic Dis*. 2021. Accessed January 12, 2026. https://www.cdc.gov/pcd/issues/2021/21_0123.htm; Pennington AF, Kompaniyets L, Summers AD, Danielson ML, Goodman AB, Chevinsky JR, et al. Risk of clinical severity by age and race/ethnicity among adults hospitalized for COVID-19—United States, March–September 2020. *Open Forum Infect Dis*. 2021;8(2):ofaa638. doi:10.1093/ofid/ofaa638

the prone position is generally well tolerated. When feedings are provided in the prone position, the head of the bed should be elevated to at least 10–30 degrees to minimize the risk of aspiration, facial swelling, and intraabdominal hypertension.[85–91]

Standard polymeric formulas are appropriate in this patient population. Emphasis on provision of omega-3 fatty acid–containing formulas has been made given the potential benefit on respiratory function; however, there is little evidence to support this in COVID-19-associated ARDS.[75,84] In patients requiring PN, use of soy-based lipids should generally be avoided due to their proinflammatory nature, especially given that lipid emulsions that include olive oil, MCT, and/or fish oil are now widely available. Hypertriglyceridemia is common during COVID-19 due to hemolymphophagocytic histiocytosis (HLH), which occurs as part of an inflammatory response to a cytokine storm that can occur in patients with COVID-19. Serum triglyceride levels can be further exacerbated by use of propofol. Therefore, baseline triglyceride levels should always be obtained and monitored throughout the course of PN therapy when ILE is provided, regardless of the fat source.[75,84] As the patient recovers and is extubated, screening for postextubation swallowing disorder, particularly in older patients, is needed. Dysphagia may last up to 21 days following extubation. Loss of skeletal muscle mass due to hypercatabolism and prolonged illness is also likely. Patients may continue to need supplemental nutrition in combination with physical therapy during their rehabilitation phase of care.[75]

Extracorporeal Membrane Oxygenation

Extracorporeal membrane oxygenation (ECMO) is a form of mechanical circulatory support used in patients with cardiopulmonary failure (**Figure 6.6**). Use of this life-saving approach has increased in ICUs following the COVID-19 pandemic. In ECMO, blood is pumped out of the body into a machine that removes carbon dioxide and adds oxygen to the blood supply. It essentially does the work of the heart and lungs in patients with acute or chronic cardiac or respiratory illness. Patients requiring ECMO undergo systemic inflammation and release of cytokines resulting in a hypermetabolic state. Duration of therapy can last for days to weeks making nutrition support essential to prevent significant protein catabolism.[92,93] Many patients are

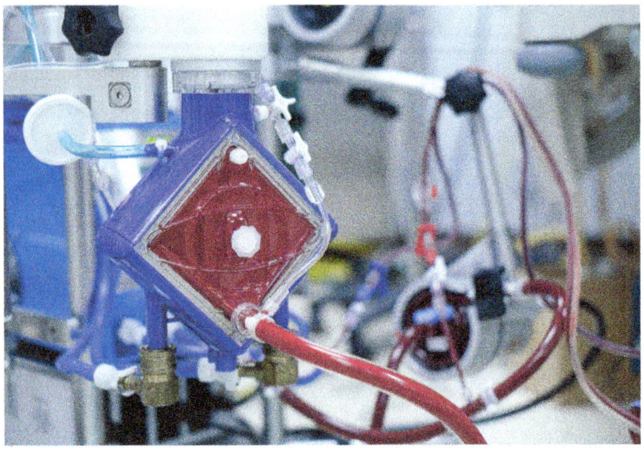

Figure 6.6 Extracorporeal Membrane Oxygenation Therapy In extracorporeal membrane oxygenation (ECMO), blood is pumped outside of the body to a heart-lung machine. The machine removes carbon dioxide and sends oxygen-rich blood back to the body. Blood flows from the right side of the heart to the heart-lung machine. It's then rewarmed and sent back to the body

hemodynamically unstable and on vasopressor support. Other perceived barriers include sedation and poor gastric motility. However, EN is the preferred choice of nutrition support in patients receiving ECMO. Furthermore, early EN within 48 hours using a hypocaloric dose (~500 calories) has been proven safe, well tolerated, and associated with improved outcomes.[94] A gradual increase in energy intake by 10% of target per day or to reach ~95% of goal over the first week is associated with decreased hospital mortality.[94,95]

Monitoring and Evaluation

Indicators to assess nutritional status and nutritional adequacy are lacking during critical illness. Measures of weight are useful to trend with consideration given to fluid status, applied dressings, and medical apparatus at the time of measurement. These should be recorded along with the weight measurement for proper interpretation. Loss of lean body mass often goes undetected in patients with fluid edema or obesity. Measures of mid-arm, calf, and thigh circumference are useful for measuring the decline in muscle mass within 3 days of initial assessment.[96] Ultrasonography as a tool for assessing muscle mass has the ability to measure short-term changes in quadricep muscles (**Figure 6.7**).[96–98] Measures of quadricep muscle layer thickness (QMLT) have been demonstrated to decrease with reduced energy and protein intake as well as days on mechanical ventilation. Reduction in QMLT was also associated with increased 28-day mortality.[97]

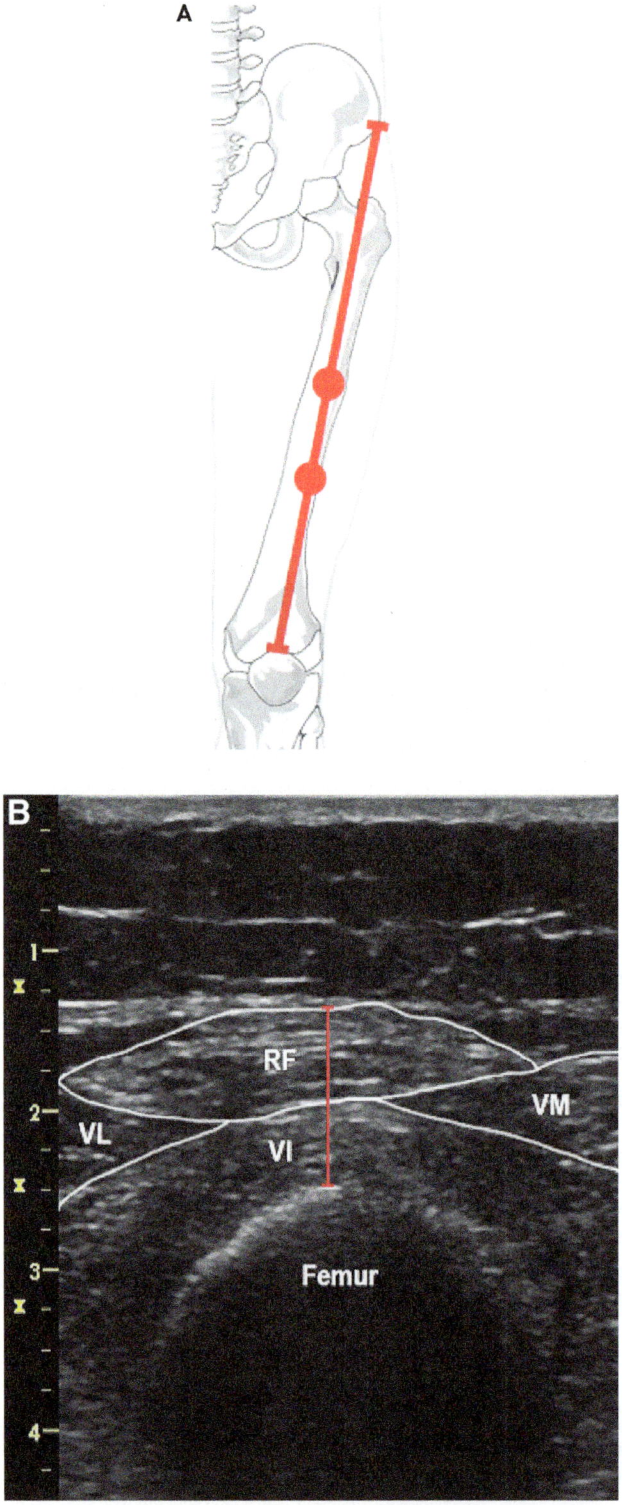

Figure 6.7 Ultrasound assessment of the quadriceps femoris muscle thickness. **A.** Anatomical diagram locating the "midpoint" and the "two-thirds" measurement sites. From Wikimedia Commons. **B.** Transverse ultrasound section made by linear probe at the midpoint site. RF: rectus femoris; VL: vastus lateralis; VM: vastus medialis; VI: vastus intermedius

Downregulation of visceral proteins makes serum albumin and prealbumin insensitive to changes in nutritional status during the early stage of acute care. Trending measures of CRP along with prealbumin can be used to interpret the role of inflammation. Higher serum prealbumin levels are associated with improved wound healing.[99]

One of the most practical ways of monitoring nutritional adequacy is by monitoring actual intake via nutrition support. Evaluating and reporting on the percent of energy and protein targets met routinely is an effective way to identify obstacles to intake and correct them.[100] Protein breakdown as indicated by urinary urea nitrogen as well as formal nitrogen balance studies to guide protein intake should be used. Other outcome measures such as wound healing and muscle strength and pulmonary function can contribute to overall assessment.

Chapter Summary

Patients with critical illness have heightened protein and energy requirements due to the hypermetabolic and catabolic physiologic response. Comprehensive, ongoing nutrition assessments are essential to identify patients at risk for malnutrition. An interdisciplinary team approach is required for the development and implementation of successful treatment plans to optimize recovery, survival, and outcome measures.

Key Terms

catabolic stress response, hypermetabolism, acute phase reactants, catabolism, catecholamines, cytokines, systemic inflammatory response syndrome (SIRS), sepsis, hemodynamic instability, short-chain fatty acids

References

1. Nielson CB, Duethman NC, Howard JM, Moncure M, Wood, JG. Burns: pathophysiology of systemic complications and current management. *J Burn Care Res*. 2017;38(1):e469–e489.
2. Bittner EA, Shank E, Woodson L, Martyn JAJ. Acute and perioperative care of the burn-injured patient. *Anesthesiology*. 2015;122(2):448–464. doi:10.1097/ALN.0000000000000559
3. Simsek T, Simsek HU, Canturk NZ. Response to trauma and metabolic changes: posttraumatic metabolism. *Ulus Cerrahi Derg*. 2014;30(3):153–159. doi:10.5152/UCD.2014.2653
4. Harrison T. Sixth national burn seminar. Adrenaline and noradrenaline excretion following burns. *J Trauma*. 1967;7(1):137–140.
5. McCowen KC, Malhotra A, Bistrian BR. Stress-induced hyperglycemia. *Crit Care Clin*. 2001;17(1):107–124.
6. Jeschke MG, Chinkes DL, Finnerty CC, et al. Pathophysiologic response to severe burn injury. *Ann Surg*. 2008;248(3):387–401. doi:10.1097/SLA.0b013e3181856241
7. Robinson LE, van Soeren MH. Insulin resistance and hyperglycemia in critical illness: role of insulin in glycemic control. *AACN Clin Issues*. 2004;15(1):45–62.
8. Wilmore DW, Mason AD Jr, Pruitt BA Jr. Insulin response to glucose in hypermetabolic burn patients. *Ann Surg*. 1976;183(3):314–320.
9. Tredget EE, Yu YM. The metabolic effects of thermal injury. *World J Surg*. 1992;16(1):68–79.
10. Wolfe RR, Herndon DN, Peters EJ, Jahoor F, Desai MH, Holland OB. Regulation of lipolysis in severely burned children. *Ann Surg*. 1987;206(2):214–221.
11. Little RA, Henderson A, Frayn KN, Galasko CS, White RH. The disposal of intravenous glucose studied using glucose and insulin clamp techniques in sepsis and trauma in man. *Acta Anaesthesiol Belg*. 1987;38(4):275–279.
12. Black PR, Brooks DC, Bessey PQ, Wolfe RR, Wilmore DW. Mechanisms of insulin resistance following injury. *Ann Surg*. 1982;196(4):420–435.
13. Demling RH, Seigne P. Metabolic management of patients with severe burns. *World J Surg*. 2000;24(6):673–680. doi:10.1007/s002689910109
14. Pollack SV. Wound healing: a review. III. Nutritional factors affecting wound healing. *J Dermatol Surg Oncol*. 1979;5(8):615–619.
15. McClave SA, Taylor BE, Martindale RG, et al. Guidelines for the provision and assessment of nutrition support therapy in the adult critically ill patient: Society of Critical Care Medicine (SCCM) and American Society for Parenteral and Enteral Nutrition (A.S.P.E.N.). *JPEN*. 2016;40(2):159–211. doi:10.1177/0148607115621863
16. Compher C, Bingham AL, McCall M, et al. Guidelines for the provision of nutrition support therapy in the adult critically ill patient: The American Society for Parenteral and Enteral Nutrition. *JPEN*. 2022;46(1):12–41. doi:10.1002/jpen.2267. [Published correction appears in *JPEN*. 2022;46(6):1458-1459. doi:10.1002/jpen.2419]
17. Singer P, Blaser AR, Berger MM, et al. ESPEN practical and partially revised guideline: clinical nutrition in the intensive care unit. *Clin Nutr*. 2023;42(9):1671–1689. doi:10.1016/j.clnu.2023.07.011
18. Jensen GL, Bistrian B, Roubenoff R, Heimburger DC. Malnutrition syndromes: a conundrum vs continuum. *JPEN*. 2009;33(6):710–716. doi:10.1177/0148607109344724
19. Jensen GL, Mirtallo J, Compher C, et al. Adult starvation and disease-related malnutrition: a proposal for etiology-based diagnosis in the clinical practice setting from the international consensus guideline committee. *JPEN*. 2010;34(2):156–159. doi:10.1177/0148607110361910

20. Jensen GL, Wheeler D. A new approach to defining and diagnosing malnutrition in adult critical illness. *Curr Opin Crit Care.* 2012;18(2):206–211. doi:10.1097/MCC.0b013e328351683a
21. White JV, Guenter P, Jensen G, et al. Consensus statement of the Academy of Nutrition and Dietetics/American Society for Parenteral and Enteral Nutrition: characteristics recommended for the identification and documentation of adult malnutrition (undernutrition). *J Acad Nutr Diet.* 2012;112(5):730–738. doi:10.1016/j.jand.2012.03.012
22. Standard FAQ Detail. The Joint Commission. Accessed November 25, 2024. https://www.jointcommission.org/standards_information/jcfaqdetails.aspx?StandardsFaqId=872&ProgramId=46
23. Kondrup J, Allison SP, Elia M, et al. ESPEN guidelines for nutrition screening 2002. *Clin Nutr.* 2003;22(4):415–421.
24. Kondrup J, Rasmussen HH, Hamberg O, Stanga Z, Ad Hoc ESPEN Working Group. Nutritional risk screening (NRS 2002): a new method based on an analysis of controlled clinical trials. *Clin Nutr*. 2003;22(3):321–336.
25. Heyland DK, Dhaliwal R, Jiang X, Day AG. Identifying critically ill patients who benefit the most from nutrition therapy: the development and initial validation of a novel risk assessment tool. *Crit Care.* 2011;15(6):R268. doi:10.1186/cc10546
26. Rahman A, Hasan RM, Agarwala R, Martin C, Day AG, Heyland DK. Identifying critically ill patients who will benefit most from nutritional therapy: further validation of the "modified NUTRIC" nutritional risk assessment tool. *Clin Nutr*. 2016;35(1):158–162. doi:10.1016/j.clnu.2015.01.015
27. Academy of Nutrition and Dietetics. Critical illness guidelines. Updated 2012. Accessed November 25, 2024. http://www.andeal.org/topic.cfm?menu=5302
28. Bloomfield R, Steel E, MacLennan G, Noble DW. Accuracy of weight and height estimation in an intensive care unit: implications for clinical practice and research. *Crit Care Med.* 2006;34(8):2153–2157. doi:10.1097/01.CCM.0000229145.04482.93
29. Dennis DM, Hunt EE, Budgeon CA. Measuring height in recumbent critical care patients. *Am J Crit Care*. 2015;24(1):41–47. doi:10.4037/ajcc2015761
30. Freitag E, Edgecombe G, Baldwin I, Cottier B, Heland M. Determination of body weight and height measurement for critically ill patients admitted to the intensive care unit: a quality improvement project. *Aust Crit Care*. 2010;23(4):197–207. doi:10.1016/j.aucc.2010.04.003
31. Honarmand K, Sirimaturos M, Hirshberg EL, et al. Society of Critical Care Medicine Guidelines on Glycemic Control for Critically Ill Children and Adults 2024. *Crit Care Med.* 2024;52(4):e161–e181. doi:10.1097/CCM.0000000000006174
32. Falciglia M, Freyberg RW, Almenoff PL, D'Alessio DA, Render ML. Hyperglycemia-related mortality in critically ill patients varies with admission diagnosis. *Crit Care Med.* 2009;37(12):3001–3009. doi:10.1097/CCM.0b013e3181b083f7
33. Bagshaw SM, Egi M, George C, Bellomo R, Australia New Zealand Intensive Care Society Database Management Committee. Early blood glucose control and mortality in critically ill patients in Australia. *Crit Care Med.* 2009;37(2):463–470. doi:10.1097/CCM.0b013e318194b097
34. Raguso CA, Dupertuis YM, Pichard C. The role of visceral proteins in the nutritional assessment of intensive care unit patients. *Curr Opin Clin Nutr Metab Care*. 2003;6(2):211–216. doi:10.1097/01.mco.0000058592.27240.95
35. Stroud M. Protein and the critically ill; do we know what to give? *Proc Nutr Soc*. 2007;66(3):378–383.
36. Academy of Nutrition and Dietetics. Does serum albumin correlate with weight loss in four models of prolonged protein-energy restriction: Anorexia nervosa, non-malabsorptive gastric partitioning bariatric surgery, calorie-restricted diets or starvation. Accessed November 25, 2017. http://www.andeal.org/topic.cfm?cat=4302&evidence_summary_id=251043&highlight=albumin&home=1
37. Davis CJ, Sowa D, Keim KS, Kinnare K, Peterson S. The use of prealbumin and C-reactive protein for monitoring nutrition support in adult patients receiving enteral nutrition in an urban medical center. *JPEN*. 2012;36(2):197–204. doi:10.1177/0148607111413896
38. Young L, Kearns L, Schoepfel S, Clark N. Protein. In: Mueller CM, ed. *The A.S.P.E.N. Adult Nutrition Support Core Curriculum*. 2nd ed. American Society for Parenteral and Enteral Nutrition; 2012:83–97.
39. Collier BR, Cherry-Bukowiek JR, Mills ME. Trauma, surgery, and burns. In: Mueller CM, ed. *The A.S.P.E.N. Adult Nutrition Support Core Curriculum*. 2nd ed. Silver Spring, MD: American Society for Parenteral and Enteral Nutrition; 2012:392–411.
40. Visser J, Labadarios D, Blaauw R. Micronutrient supplementation for critically ill adults: a systematic review and meta-analysis. *Nutrition*. 2011;27(7-8):745–758. doi:10.1016/j.nut.2010.12.009
41. Berger MM, Shenkin A. Update on clinical micronutrient supplementation studies in the critically ill. *Curr Opin Clin Nutr Metab Care*. 2006;9(6):711–716. doi:10.1097/01.mco.0000247466.41661.ba
42. McClave SA, Martindale RG, Kiraly L. The use of indirect calorimetry in the intensive care unit. *Curr Opin Clin Nutr Metab Care*. 2013;16(2):202–208. doi:10.1097/MCO.0b013e32835dbc54
43. Stapel SN, de Grooth HJ, Alimohamad H, et al. Ventilator-derived carbon dioxide production to assess energy expenditure in critically ill patients: proof of concept. *Crit Care*. 2015;19:370. doi:10.1186/s13054-015-1087-2
44. Oshima T, Graf S, Heidegger CP, Genton L, Pugin J, Pichard C. Can calculation of energy expenditure based on CO_2 measurements replace indirect calorimetry. *Crit Care*. 2017;21(1):13. doi:10.1186/s13054-016-1595-8. [published correction appears in *Crit Care*. 2017;21(1):95. doi:10.1186/s13054-017-1650-0]
45. Anderegg BA, Worrall C, Barbour E, Simpson KN, Delegge M. Comparison of resting energy expenditure prediction methods with measured resting energy expenditure in obese, hospitalized adults. *JPEN*. 2009;33(2):168–175. doi:10.1177/0148607108327192
46. Frankenfield DC, Ashcraft CM, Galvan DA. Prediction of resting metabolic rate in critically ill patients at the extremes of body mass index. *JPEN*. 2013;37(3):361–367. doi:10.1177/0148607112457423
47. Frankenfield DC, Ashcraft CM. Estimating energy needs in nutrition support patients. *JPEN*. 2011;35(5):563–570. doi:10.1177/0148607111415859
48. Kross EK, Sena M, Schmidt K, Stapleton RD. A comparison of predictive equations of energy expenditure and measured energy expenditure in critically ill patients. *J Crit Care*. 2012;27(3):321.e5–321.12. doi:10.1016/j.jcrc.2011.07.084
49. Sun JK, Nie S, Chen YM, et al. Effects of permissive hypocaloric vs standard enteral feeding on gastrointestinal

function and outcomes in sepsis. *World J Gastroenterol.* 2021;27(29):4900–4912. doi:10.3748/wjg.v27.i29.4900

50. Heyland DK, Schroter-Noppe D, Drover JW, et al. Nutrition support in the critical care setting: current practice in Canadian ICUs—opportunities for improvement? *JPEN.* 2003;27(1):74–83. doi:10.1177/014860710302700174
51. Kreymann KG, Berger MM, Deutz NE, et al. ESPEN guidelines on enteral nutrition: intensive care. *Clin Nutr.* 2006;25(2):210–223.
52. McClave SA, Heyland DK. The physiologic response and associated clinical benefits from provision of early enteral nutrition. *Nutr Clin Pract.* 2009;24(3):305–315. doi:10.1177/0884533609335176
53. Kang W, Kudsk KA. Is there evidence that the gut contributes to mucosal immunity in humans? *JPEN.* 2007;31(3):246–258.
54. Windsor AC, Kanwar S, Li AG, et al. Compared with parenteral nutrition, enteral feeding attenuates the acute phase response and improves disease severity in acute pancreatitis. *Gut.* 1998;42(3):431–435.
55. Ammori BJ. Importance of the early increase in intestinal permeability in critically ill patients. *Eur J Surg.* 2002;168(11):660–661; author reply 662.
56. Wong JM, de Souza R, Kendall CW, Emam A, Jenkins DJ. Colonic health: fermentation and short chain fatty acids. *J Clin Gastroenterol.* 2006;40(3):235–243.
57. Silk DB, Walters ER, Duncan HD, Green CJ. The effect of a polymeric enteral formula supplemented with a mixture of six fibres on normal human bowel function and colonic motility. *Clin Nutr.* 2001;20(1):49–58. doi:10.1054/clnu.2000.0359
58. Homann HH, Kemen M, Fuessenich C, Senkal M, Zumtobel V. Reduction in diarrhea incidence by soluble fiber in patients receiving total or supplemental enteral nutrition. *JPEN.* 1994;18(6):486–490. doi:10.1177/0148607194018006486
59. Bankhead R, Boullata J, Brantley S, et al. Enteral nutrition practice recommendations. *JPEN.* 2009;33(2):122–167. doi:10.1177/0148607108330314
60. Heyland DK, Murch L, Cahill N, et al. Enhanced protein-energy provision via the enteral route feeding protocol in critically ill patients: results of a cluster randomized trial. *Crit Care Med.* 2013;41(12):2743–2753. doi:10.1097/CCM.0b013e31829efef5
61. McCowen KC, Friel C, Sternberg J, et al. Hypocaloric total parenteral nutrition: effectiveness in prevention of hyperglycemia and infectious complications–a randomized clinical trial. *Crit Care Med.* 2000;28(11):3606–3611.
62. Ahrens CL, Barletta JF, Kanji S, et al. Effect of low-calorie parenteral nutrition on the incidence and severity of hyperglycemia in surgical patients: a randomized, controlled trial. *Crit Care Med.* 2005;33(11):2507–2512.
63. Finnerty CC, Mabvuure NT, Ali A, Kozar RA, Herndon DN. The surgically induced stress response. *JPEN.* 2013;37(5 Suppl):21S–29S. doi:10.1177/0148607113496117
64. Hart DW, Wolf SE, Mlcak R, et al. Persistence of muscle catabolism after severe burn. *Surgery.* 2000;128(2):312–319.
65. Jeschke MG, Gauglitz GG, Kulp GA, et al. Long-term persistance of the pathophysiologic response to severe burn injury. *PLoS One.* 2011;6(7):e21245. doi:10.1371/journal.pone.0021245
66. Porter C, Herndon DN, Borsheim E, et al. Uncoupled skeletal muscle mitochondria contribute to hypermetabolism in severely burned adults. *Am J Physiol Endocrinol Metab.* 2014;307(5):E462–467. doi:10.1152/ajpendo.00206.2014
67. Newsome TW, Mason AD Jr, Pruitt BA Jr. Weight loss following thermal injury. *Ann Surg.* 1973;178(2):215–217.
68. Porter C, Tompkins RG, Finnerty CC, Sidossis LS, Suman OE, Herndon DN. The metabolic stress response to burn trauma: current understanding and therapies. *Lancet.* 2016;388(10052):1417–1426.
69. Rousseau AF, Pantet O, Heyland DK. Nutrition after severe burn injury. *Curr Opin Clin Nutr Metab Care.* 2023;26(2):99–104. doi:10.1097/MCO.0000000000000904
70. Bone RC, Sprung CL, Sibbald WJ. Definitions for sepsis and organ failure. *Crit Care Med.* 1992;20(6):724–726.
71. Alexopoulos AS, Fayfman M, Zhao L, et al. Impact of obesity on hospital complications and mortality in hospitalized patients with hyperglycemia and diabetes. *BMJ Open Diabetes Res Care.* 2016;4(1):e000200. doi:10.1136/bmjdrc-2016-000200
72. Abhyankar S, Leishear K, Callaghan FM, Demner-Fushman D, McDonald CJ. Lower short- and long-term mortality associated with overweight and obesity in a large cohort study of adult intensive care unit patients. *Crit Care.* 2012;16(6):R235. doi:10.1186/cc11903
73. Dickerson RN, Andromalos L, Brown JC, et al. Obesity and critical care nutrition: current practice gaps and directions for future research. *Crit Care.* 2022;26(1):283. doi:10.1186/s13054-022-04148-0 [Published correction appears in *Crit Care.* 2023;27(1):177. doi:10.1186/s13054-023-04456-z]
74. Dickerson RN. Hypocaloric, high-protein nutrition therapy for critically ill patients with obesity. *Nutr Clin Pract.* 2014;29:786–791. doi:10.1177/0884533614542439
75. Barazzoni R, Bischoff SC, Breda J, et al. ESPEN expert statements and practical guidance for nutritional management of individuals with SARS-CoV-2 infection. *Clin Nutr.* 2020;39(6):1631–1638. doi:10.1016/j.clnu.2020.03.022
76. Bell J, Heyer N, Greenstein A, Fragkos K, Baxter-Derrington C, Mehta S. A retrospective analysis of malnutrition risk, nutritional support and outcomes in COVID-19 patients. *Clin Nutr ESPEN.* 2022;50:196–206. doi:10.1016/j.clnesp.2022.05.017
77. Centers for Disease Control and Prevention. Underlying Conditions and the Higher Risk for Severe COVID-19. Updated July 30, 2024. Accessed January 4, 2025. https://www.cdc.gov/covid/hcp/clinical-care/underlying-conditions.html
78. Kompaniyets L, Pennington AF, Goodman AB, Rosenblum HG, Belay B, Ko JY, et al. Underlying medical conditions and severe illness among 540,667 adults hospitalized with COVID-19, March 2020–March 2021. *Prevent Chronic Dis.* 2021;18. https://www.cdc.gov/pcd/issues/2021/21_0123.htm
79. Pennington AF, Kompaniyets L, Summers AD, et al. Risk of clinical severity by age and race/ethnicity among adults hospitalized for COVID-19—United States, March–September 2020. *Open Forum Infect Dis.* 2021;8(2). doi:10.1093/ofid/ofaa638
80. Kasapoglu US, Gok A, Delen LA, Ozer AB. Comparison of nutritional risk status assessment tools in predicting 30-day survival in critically ill COVID-19 pneumonia patients. *Ann Saudi Med.* 2022;42(4):236–245. doi:10.5144/0256-4947.2022.236
81. Bodolea C, Nemes A, Avram L, et al. Nutritional risk assessment scores effectively predict mortality in critically ill patients with severe COVID-19. *Nutrients.* 2022;14(10):2105. doi:10.3390/nu14102105
82. Cederholm T, Jensen GL, Correia MITD, et al. GLIM criteria for the diagnosis of malnutrition - a consensus report from the global clinical nutrition community. *Clin Nutr.* 2019;38:1–9. doi:10.1016/j.clnu.2018.08.002

83. Burslem R, Gottesman K, Newkirk M, Ziegler J. Energy requirements for critically ill patients with COVID-19. *Nutr Clin Pract.* 2022;37(3):594–604.
84. Martindale R, Patel JJ, Taylor B, Arabi YM, Warren M, McClave SA. Nutrition therapy in critically ill patients with coronavirus disease 2019. *JPEN.* 2020 Sep;44(7):1174–1184. doi:10.1002/jpen.1930
85. Haines KS, Parker V, Ohnuma T, et al. Role of early enteral nutrition in mechanically ventilated COVID-19 patients. *Crit Care Explor.* 2022;4(4):e0683. doi:10.1097/CCE.0000000000000683
86. Ojo O, Ojo OO, Feng Q, et al. The effects of enteral nutrition in critically ill patients with COVID-19: a systematic review and meta-analysis. *Nutrients.* 2022;14(5):1120. doi:10.3390/nu14051120
87. Alves de Paula J, Rabito EI, Justino SR, et al. Administration of enteral nutrition and gastrointestinal complications in COVID-19 critical patients in prone position. *Clin Nutr Open Sci.* 2022;45:80–90. doi:10.1016/j.nutos.2022.08.003
88. Louzon PR, Ochogbu O, Rascon L, Moore S, Ali F. Tolerance of enteral nutrition during prone therapy in a COVID-19 cohort. *Intensive Crit Care Nurs.* 2023;74:103338. doi:10.1016/j.iccn.2022.103338
89. Powers J, Richardson J, Rechter J. Innovative strategy to improve enteral nutrition in prone positioning with patients with COVID-19. *Nutr Clin Pract.* 2023;38(3):602–608. doi:10.1002/ncp.10946
90. Pérez-Cruz E, Ortiz-Gutiérrez S, Castañón-González JA, Luna-Camacho Y, Garduño-López J. Effectiveness and tolerance of enteral nutrition in critically ill patients with COVID-19. *Br J Nutr.* 2024;132(11):1446–1453. doi:10.1017/S0007114524002666
91. Hinkelmann JV, de Oliveira NA, Marcato DF, et al. Nutritional support protocol for patients with COVID-19. *Clin Nutr ESPEN.* 2022;49:544–550. doi:10.1016/j.clnesp.2022.03.002
92. Dresen E, Naidoo O, Hill A, et al. Medical nutrition therapy in patients receiving ECMO: evidence-based guidance for clinical practice. *JPEN.* 2023;47(2):220–235. doi:10.1002/jpen.2467
93. Stoppe C. Goetzenich A, Whitman G, Ohkuma R, Brown T, Hatzakorzian R, et al. Role of nutrition support in adult cardiac surgery: a consensus statement from an International Multidisciplinary Expert Group on Nutrition in Cardiac Surgery. *Crit Care.* 2017;21(1):131.
94. Kim S, Jeong SK, Hwang J, Kim JH, Shin JS, Shin HF. Early enteral nutrition and factors related to in-hospital mortality in people on extracorporeal membrane oxygenation. *Nutrition.* 2021;89:111222.
95. Lu GY, Xu H, Li J-H, Chen J-K, Ning YG. Safety and outcome of early enteral nutrition in patients receiving extracorporeal membrane oxygenation. *Clin Nutr.* 2023; 42:1711–1714.
96. Rodrigues CN, Ribeiro Henrique J, Ferreira ÁRS, Correia MITD. Ultrasonography and other nutrition assessment methods to monitor the nutrition status of critically ill patients. *JPEN.* 2021;45:982–990. doi:10.1002/jpen.1966.
97. Lopes MLG, Cidade JP, Sousa D, et al. Ultrasound assessment of muscle mass in critically ill patients: a correlation with nutritional support and clinical outcomes, *J Crit Care.* 2024;85:154938.
98. Dresen E, Weißbrich C, Fimmers R, Putensen C, Stehle P. Medical high-protein nutrition therapy and loss of muscle mass in adult ICU patients: a randomized controlled trial. *Clin Nutr.* 2021;40(4):1562–1570.
99. Vanaclocha N, Miranda Gómez L, Pérez Del Caz MD, Vanaclocha Vanaclocha V, Miranda Alonso FJ. Higher serum prealbumin levels are associated with higher graft take and wound healing in adult burn patients: A prospective observational trial. *Burns.* 2024 May;50(4):903–912. doi:10.1016/j.burns.2023.12.015. Epub 2024 Jan 4. PMID: 38302393.
100. Matejovic M, Huet O, Dams K, et al. Medical nutrition therapy and clinical outcomes in critically ill adults: a European multinational, prospective observational cohort study (EuroPN). *Crit Care.* 2022;26:143–157. doi:10.1186/s13054-022-03997-z

CHAPTER 7

Weight and Health

Jillian Reece
Caroline MacDonald

CHAPTER OUTLINE

CORE CONCEPTS

1. Excess weight can be a risk factor for a variety of health conditions including type 2 diabetes, hyperlipidemia, hypertension, heart disease, stroke, certain cancers, metabolic dysfunction–associated steatotic liver disease, sleep apnea, gallbladder disease, respiratory problems, arthritis, and depression.
2. The etiology of obesity is complex and includes many interacting factors including genetics, environmental, social, biological, and developmental factors.
3. Body weight is regulated by a complex network of systems and signaling pathways that become dysregulated with excess weight and chronic positive energy balance.
4. Body weight is regulated by metabolic, neuroendocrine, and autonomic systems in the body including signals released from adipose, gastrointestinal, and endocrine tissues that are integrated by the liver and central nervous system.
5. Approaches to weight management include individual and comprehensive lifestyle intervention, pharmacotherapy, and metabolic and bariatric surgery.
6. Stigma exists among individuals with obesity and public frameworks such as Health at Every Size® (HAES®) aim to create a more weight inclusive health environment by reducing weight bias and promoting body acceptance.

LEARNING OBJECTIVES

1. Describe the magnitude and etiology of weight and obesity.
2. Explain how obesity is defined and classified.
3. Identify the pathophysiology of weight and obesity.
4. Discuss the signaling pathways and hormones involved in body weight regulation.
5. Assess nutrition status and develop a nutrition care plan for individuals with obesity.
6. List the characteristics used to define metabolic syndrome.
7. Identify the disease states associated with obesity and their pathophysiology.
8. Describe three non-surgical nutrition interventions for weight loss.
9. Identify three types of medications used for treatment of weight management.
10. Classify three metabolic and bariatric surgery procedure types.
11. List the recommended micronutrient supplementation for a patient post metabolic and bariatric surgery.
12. Describe the diet progression following Roux-en-Y gastric bypass or sleeve gastrectomy.

Introduction

Weight is a sensitive topic when it comes to health. Simply defined as the relative mass or quantity of a body, it is a physical characteristic that all individuals possess but a subject matter that not everyone views in the same way. Traditional approaches to weight and health emphasize the impact that excess weight can have on the body and strategies to employ to lower body mass index (BMI) into a socially constructed and medically acceptable range. Yet, this view and approach to weight has not reduced the rate of weight-related issues observed in society today. Newer paradigms such as Health at Every Size® (HAES®) challenge this framework citing the need for a more weight-inclusive approach to medicine and one that removes weight from the conversation by focusing instead on healthy lifestyle behaviors for all. However, does this encourage individuals to ignore increasing weight and discount potential health issues that may come with living in a larger body? Weight is a complex topic and one that will continue to stem polarizing conversations among individuals and medical professionals. This chapter aims to address weight from both traditional and modern frameworks with the goal of increasing clinical knowledge about the role that weight and obesity play in health.

Overweight and **obesity** are medical conditions to describe excess body fat stores for a given height in an individual. The World Health Organization (WHO) uses **body mass index (BMI)** (weight in kg/height in m^2) to classify stages of overweight and obesity, and the perceived health risk of an individual. A BMI of 25–29.9 kg/m^2 is defined as overweight and a BMI ≥ 30 kg/m^2 is defined as obese.[1] Pediatric overweight and obesity is defined as the 85th–95th percentile and greater than the 95th percentile, respectively, using BMI-for-age scales.[2] (See Chapter 22, *Nutritional Management of Pediatric Obesity*, for more information on pediatric overweight and obesity.) Obesity is a potential risk factor for a variety of health conditions including type 2 diabetes mellitus (T2DM), hyperlipidemia, hypertension (HTN), heart disease, stroke, certain cancers, metabolic dysfunction–associated steatotic liver disease (MASLD, previously known as "nonalcoholic fatty liver disease"), obstructive sleep apnea (OSA), gallbladder disease, respiratory problems, arthritis, and depression.[3] Higher classes of obesity are associated with increased all-cause mortality, primarily from cardiovascular disease, T2DM, and certain cancers.[3] Additionally, individuals with obesity may experience social stigmatization, discrimination, and report a decreased quality of life greatly impacting their mental well-being.[4] Over the last decade, the estimated annual medical cost of obesity has increased to $173 billion. Annual medical expenses for individuals with obesity are higher than those with a lower BMI by an estimated $1861.[5] If current trends continue, obesity-related healthcare costs in the United States will continue to rise. Nutrition interventions in the prevention and treatment of obesity are important initiatives in addressing this population trend.

When discussing weight management, weight sensitivity and inclusivity should be at the forefront of assessing and providing nutrition care. Weight is an anthropometric measurement and assessment of health risk, not a measurement of overall health, value, or ability. Registered dietitians (RDs) are responsible for providing medical nutrition therapy in a respectful, psychologically safe, and empowering way. When providing evidence-based weight management nutrition therapy, it is important to understand external and internal weight biases and weight-related prejudices and how they may influence health care as well as the systems in which we live.

Weight management and weight loss are not synonymous. The role of the RD is to entrust patients to prosper through nutrition and food including taking part in weight management services, health-seeking activities, preventative services, including mental and physical health services, and creating support systems for future challenges. Weight management, healthy weight loss approaches, mindful eating, and lifestyle counseling approaches such as those from HAES® can coincide with providing other traditional evidence-based care for patients while facilitating healthier relationships between patients, their bodies, and their health. Intuitive and mindful eating can strengthen body positivity and motivate patients to understand their internal hunger signals. Healthy eating strategies such as portion awareness, integration of intuitive eating and mindful practices, and lifestyle changes can help patients meet their goals while promoting both body positivity and healthy weight loss approaches.[6]

The medical community is responsible for providing care with this understanding in order to welcome patients of all sizes, optimize health, and reduce barriers to patient care.[7] Therapy implemented within these weight-inclusive environments should be patient-centered to enhance benefit and decrease harm for the patient, culture, and healthcare system. RDs can facilitate care and champion for weight inclusive environments and human-centered communication to increase benefit and reduce harm for all.[7]

CORE CONCEPT 1

Obesity is a risk factor for a variety of health conditions, including diabetes, hyperlipidemia, hypertension, heart disease, stroke, certain cancers, metabolic dysfunction–associated steatotic liver disease, sleep apnea, gallbladder disease, respiratory problems, arthritis, and depression.

Prevalence

According to the Centers for Disease Control and Prevention (CDC), more than one-third (41.9%) of adults and approximately 19.7% of children in the United States have obesity.[2,5] Trends show that obesity prevalence increased from 30.5% to 41.9% in the last two decades despite a period of minimal change among adults or children from 2007–2008 to 2011–2012.[5,8] The most recent estimates of obesity prevalence in the United States are based on the 2021 National Health and Nutrition Examination Survey.[9] Within these trends, there are observed differences between age groups, sex, ethnicity, race, U.S. location, and socioeconomic status. Women may be more likely to have obesity (42.1%) when compared to men (41.6%).[9] Sexual and gender underrepresented groups may be at increased risk compared to their straight and gender-conforming counterparts.[10] Middle-aged adults rank in the highest risk category compared to young adults (20–39 years of age) and older adults (age 60 and older).[5] Non-Hispanic Black adults have the highest age-adjusted rates of obesity (49.9%) compared with Hispanic adults (45.6%), non-Hispanic White adults (41.4%) and non-Hispanic Asian adults (16.1%).[5] Geographically, U.S. obesity prevalence is currently highest in the South (35.6%), followed by the Midwest (35.8%), Northeast (30.5%), and the West (29.5%)[11] (**Figures 7.1-7.3**). There are also varying rates of obesity based on education level and socioeconomic status. In 2020, the USDA reported that 14.8% of households with children are food insecure.[12] The odds of children in food insecure homes having obesity are 5 times higher than children in food secure homes.[13] The prevalence of obesity is inversely correlated with adult education level. Adults with a college degree are less likely to have obesity (27.2%) compared to adults with some college education (35.9%) and adults with a high school diploma only (37.6%).[11] However, despite having a degree, highly educated non-Hispanic White males are less likely to have obesity when compared to highly educated non-Hispanic Black males.[10]

Classification of Obesity: Is Obesity a Disease?

In June 2013, the American Medical Association (AMA) adopted a policy that recognizes obesity as a disease due to its chronic, relapsing, and multifactorial characteristics. While many major health organizations agree, it has sparked much debate in the medical community as some experts question the definition of disease and feel that labeling obesity this way could increase weight stigma further perpetuating the issue. Despite this, obesity is associated with other chronic diseases such as cancers and heart disease and a range of medical interventions are available for treatment and prevention. BMI is used as a simple, noninvasive way to predict an individual's risk for disease; however, it does not come without disadvantages. BMI does not directly measure

CASE STUDY INTRODUCTION

Allison is a 30-year-old Black female presenting to the nutrition clinic with concerns about her weight. She shares that she is seeking weight loss to improve her T2DM as well as sleep and doing so she feels is likely to improve her energy levels. She noticed herself gaining weight as a child and throughout her adult years, and her weight further increased especially during college. After college, she was diagnosed with T2DM, and her asthma worsened resulting in more frequent use of prednisolone and the start of insulin. Her mother also struggles with weight, and Allison says T2DM runs in her family on her mother's side, but she is unsure about her father's family history. Currently, Allison is single and lives alone. She works full time in sales and spends most of her day at a desk. Occasionally, she will walk for 10–15 minutes on her lunch break but otherwise states that she is too busy for exercise. She eats out 4–5 times per week and states that cooking for one person can be difficult. Additionally, the nearest grocery store is about 20 miles away, making it difficult to shop more than 2 times per month.

Anthropometric Data:

Weight: 95 kg
Height: 158 cm
BMI: 38 kg/m^2

Weight History:

Usual body weight: 95 kg
Highest adult weight: 110 kg 4 years ago
Lowest adult weight: 91 kg 8 years ago

Biochemical Data:

Fasting Blood Glucose: 150 mg/dL (70–99 mg/dL)
Hemoglobin A1c: 8.0% (4.3–5.6%)
Low-Density Lipoprotein (LDL-C): 119 mg/dL (Desirable: <100 mg/dL)
High-Density Lipoprotein (HDL-C): 38 mg/dL (Desirable: >40 mg/dL)
Triglycerides: 175 mg/dL (Desirable: <150 mg/dL)
25 (OH) Vitamin D: 17 ng/mL (20–100 ng/mL)

Clinical Data:

Past Medical History: T2DM, asthma, obesity
Medications: glargine insulin 20 units at bedtime, glipizide at breakfast and dinner, glucophage at breakfast and dinner, prednisolone
Vital Signs: Blood pressure 132/85 mm Hg, Temperature 98.2°F, Heart rate 82 beats/min
Nutrition-Focused Physical Exam: Excess weight visible with notable central adiposity. No visible muscle wasting but no significant tone noted, either. Mild ankle edema. Darkened skin consistent with acanthosis nigricans observed on back of neck.

Diet History:

Eating 3 meals per day and 1–2 snacks. Portions reportedly large on days when lunches are too light, particularly at dinner. A typical takeout meal could be chicken alfredo pasta with a side of broccoli and a dessert. When cooking at home, she tries to prepare lower carbohydrate meals with a protein source, brown rice, fruit, and a vegetable. Recently, she is reporting persistent hunger despite daily intake of around 2200 calories/day. She is logging her food daily via a written journal.

Questions

1. What factors may have contributed to weight gain for Allison?
2. In what ways is her past medical history affecting her weight and energy level?
3. What are the important considerations when determining the appropriate nutrition intervention for Allison?
4. What changes to her diet might you discuss with Allison?
5. What is your interpretation of Allison's laboratory values?
6. Write 2 Problem/Etiology/Signs and Symptoms (PES) statements for Allison.
7. Identify the nutrition interventions you would like to initiate for Allison to address the problems identified in your PES statements.
8. What indices are included in your monitoring and evaluation plan? Why?

body fat stores or muscle mass. As a result, some individuals may be classified as having "obesity" due to an elevated BMI without having excess body fat. Factors that contribute to disease risk but are not captured by BMI measurements include body fat distribution, such as visceral versus subcutaneous fat, ethnicity, age, fitness level, and smoking status. The diagnosis of obesity must be individualized since health risks vary by ethnicity.

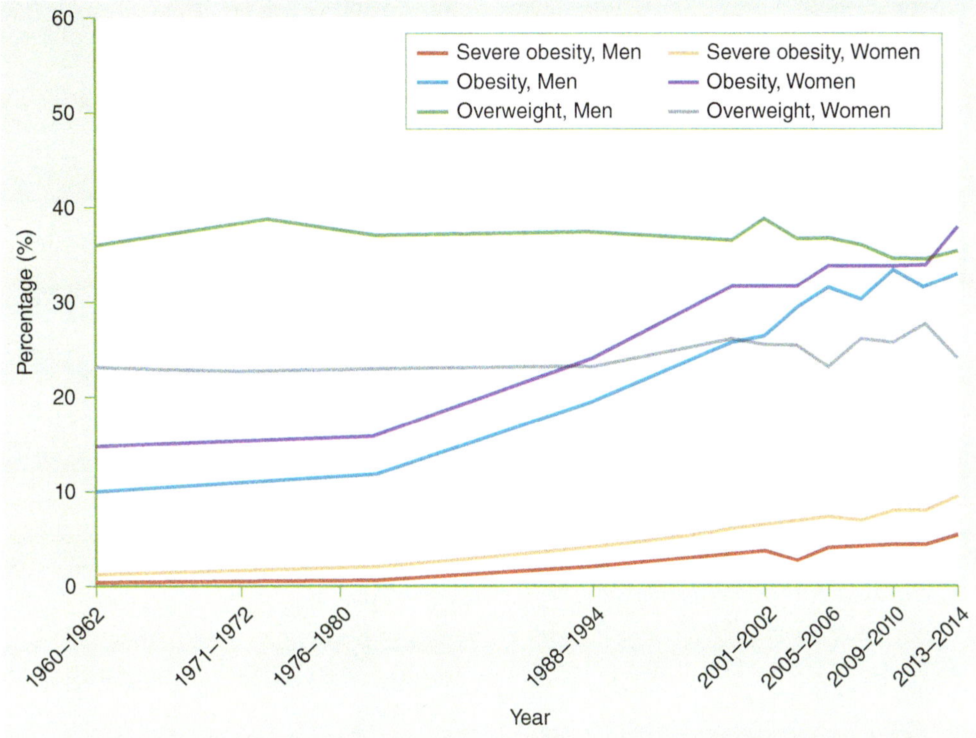

Figure 7.1 Age-Adjusted Trends in Overweight, Obesity, and Severe Obesity Among Men and Women Aged 20–74: United States, 1960–2018

Reproduced from Fryar CD, Carroll MD, Afful J. Prevalence of overweight, obesity, and severe obesity among adults aged 20 and over: United States, 1960–1962 through 2017–2018. *NCHS Health E-Stats*. National Center for Health Statistics; 2020. Accessed January 12, 2026. https://www.cdc.gov/nchs/data/hestat/obesity-adult-17-18/obesity-adult.htm

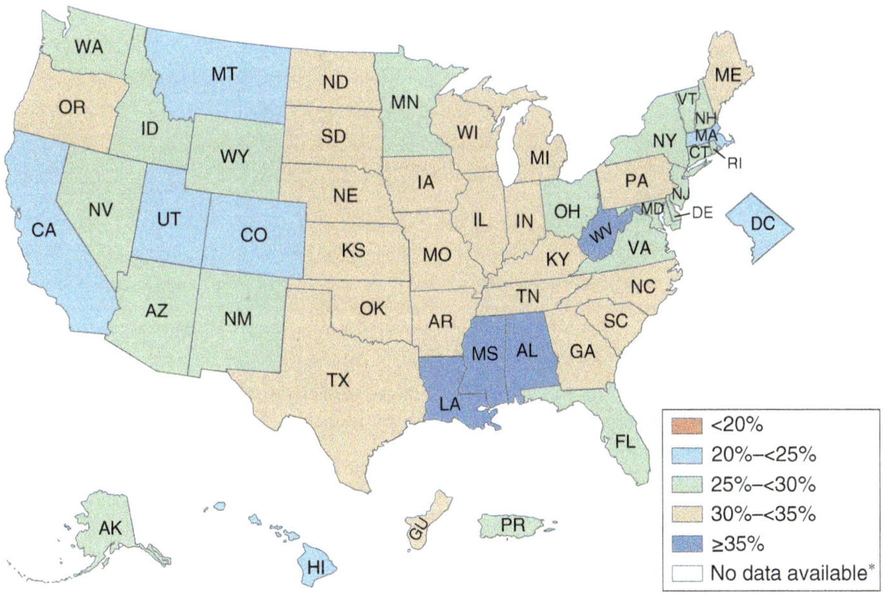

Figure 7.2 Prevalence of Self-Reported Obesity Among U.S. Adults by State and Territory, Behavioral Risk Factor Surveillance System, 2023

Reproduced from Centers for Disease Control and Prevention. *Adult obesity prevalence maps*. U.S. Department of Health and Human Services; 2023. Accessed January 12, 2026. https://www.cdc.gov/obesity/data-and-statistics/adult-obesity-prevalence-maps.html

For example, T2DM risk starts to increase at a BMI of 23 kg/m^2 for East Asian individuals (e.g., individuals from China, Japan, Korea), while disease risk may be lower in the Black American and White population with the same BMI. Black Americans tend to have higher muscle mass compared to other racial and ethnic groups.[14] Asian Americans have a higher prevalence of visceral fact compared to other populations

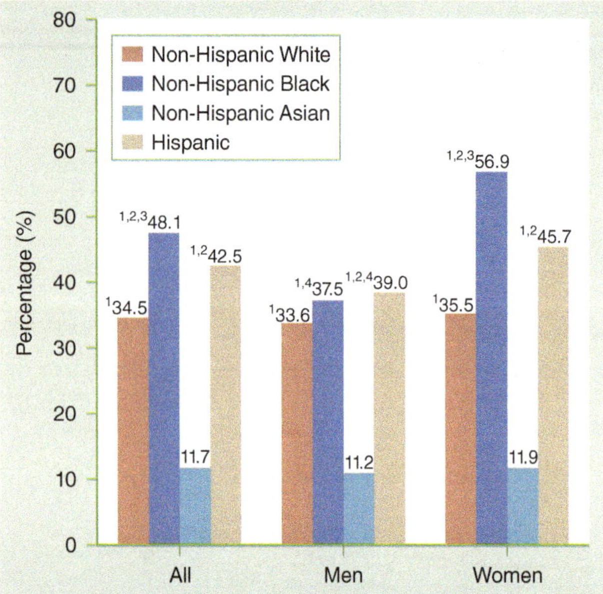

Figure 7.3 Age-Adjusted Prevalence of Obesity Among Adults Aged 20 and Over, by Sex and Race and Hispanic Origin: United States, 2017–2018

Reproduced from Hales CM, Carroll MD, Fryar CD, Ogden CL. Prevalence of obesity and severe obesity among adults: United States, 2017–2018. NCHS Data Brief. 2020;(360):1-8. National Center for Health Statistics. Accessed January 12, 2026. https://www.cdc.gov/nchs/products/databriefs/db360.htm

Table 7.1 Classification of Obesity Using Body Mass Index

BMI (kg/m^2)	Classification
<18.5	Underweight
18.5–24.9	Healthy weight
25.0–29.9	Overweight
30.0–34.9	Obesity Class 1
35.0–39.9	Obesity Class 2
≥40.0	Obesity Class 3 or Severe Obesity

Data from U.S. Department of Health and Human Services; National Heart, Lung, and Blood Institute. Body mass index table. Accessed January 12, 2026. https://www.nhlbi.nih.gov/health/educational/lose_wt/BMI/bmi_dis.htm

and may exhibit different body composition patterns at lower BMIs, making them more susceptible to health risks with visceral fat at "healthier" BMI's.[15] Despite the demonstrated shortcomings of BMI measurements, some studies suggest that it correlates well with morbidity and mortality for the general population.[16] **Table 7.1** lists the cutoff ranges used to determine overweight and obesity.

PRACTICE POINT

Body composition should be considered when using BMI to classify obesity in individuals who present as highly muscular.

Causes and Contributions to the Obesity Epidemic

The etiology of obesity is complex and includes many interacting factors.[17]

Genetic Factors

Changes in the genotype of humans occur too slowly to explain the rapid rise in obesity over recent decades; however, the variation of weight regulation among individuals in the same environment suggests that genetics play a role. A systematic review of 12 studies including 8179 monozygotic and 9977 dizygotic twin pairs in addition to individual participant data for 629 monozygotic and 594 dizygotic pairs from four twin registries assessed the genetic influence of BMI.[18] Results suggest that the heritability of BMI ranged from 61% to 80% for both male and female subjects and was high across all age categories. The number of known markers and chromosome regions associated with obesity is greater than 250.[19] Numerous genes are involved in obesity; however, there has been a major focus on two in particular: the ob gene and the β-adrenoreceptor gene. The ob gene produces leptin, a hormone involved in energy regulation, and the β-adrenoreceptor gene is one of many genes involved in regulation of resting metabolic rate and fat oxidation in humans. It was thought that mutations of these genes were involved in weight gain; although, one particular gene is not likely to be the major contributor of obesity, but rather several polygenic factors in combination with other determinants.[20] Although only a small number of rare, single genetic abnormalities that cause obesity have been identified, the area of epigenetics examines the relationship by which obesity-predisposing genes interact with the environment and may influence an individual's response to treatment.[21]

Environmental Factors

In addition to genetics, there are strong environmental influences on obesity. The food environment has shifted over the years to promote overeating through increased availability of inexpensive, calorie-dense foods, such as fast-food restaurants, convenience stores, and vending machines. Not only has the availability of processed foods high in calories, fat, and sugar increased over time, but portion sizes have increased dramatically as well.[22,23] While fast-paced life in the United States may leave many individuals turning to high calorie, convenience foods by choice, others may be limited by their geographical location. "Food deserts," described as areas where limited access to fresh and affordable foods exists, occur within the United States, making it difficult for certain individuals to eat an optimal diet for health and disease prevention.[24]

Decreased involvement in physical activity for both children and adults is another contributing factor to obesity. According to a report by the CDC, only 1 in 4 individuals meet the 2018 Physical Activity Guidelines for Americans, which includes cardiovascular and muscle strengthening exercise.[25] Generally, there has been a significant decrease in activities of daily of living over the past three or four decades due to many environmental factors.[17] The energy that individuals use to spend in these activities has now been replaced by technology, such as purchasing groceries online from home instead of grocery shopping, using remote controls for television, placing a call or text on a cell phone versus delivering a message in person, visiting drive-through restaurants in place of our own food preparation, and more time spent on computers.

Another contributing factor to excess weight is the use of weight-promoting medications. Many commonly used medications are associated with weight gain, including psychotropic medications, steroid hormones, contraceptives, diabetes medications, antihypertensives, antihistamines, and protease inhibitors.[17] **Table 7.2** identifies several medications that promote weight gain. In some instances, alternative medications that do not have an impact on weight may be available to treat the same condition. When visiting a primary care physician or specialist who is prescribing medication, individuals should discuss in detail any potential side effects associated with its use.

Sleep deprivation may also be contributing to the rise in obesity. Americans now sleep less than they did a few decades ago. Mechanisms that may explain the relationship between sleep loss and weight include both metabolic and endocrine changes within the body. These include a decrease in glucose tolerance and insulin sensitivity, increased concentrations of stress hormones such as cortisol, which occur later in the day, increased levels of ghrelin, and decreased levels of leptin. Cumulatively, these factors can contribute to increased appetite, which may result in overeating and potentially weight gain in some individuals.[26]

Social Factors

Social determinants of health, defined by the WHO as conditions in which individuals are born, grow, live, work, and age, may also pose a risk for obesity due to health disparities that they create. Shaped by the distribution of money, power, and resources at national and local levels, this includes demographic characteristics, education level, socioeconomic status, and perceived social and cultural norms.[27] Examples include safe housing, access to nutritious food and food security, equitable job opportunities, and language.[23] Specifically, the interactions that individuals have with others, as described by their social network, can have a powerful influence on weight. A study examining 12,067 people from the Framingham Heart Study between 1971 and 2003 found that an individual's chance of developing obesity increased by 57% if a friend also had obesity. Additionally, among adult siblings, the risk of obesity increased by 40% if one sibling had obesity. Similar trends are observed with married couples; if one spouse had obesity, the likelihood that the other would develop obesity increased by 37%.[28]

Biological Factors

Recent research has examined the influence of intestinal microbiota on obesity showing a potential link between alterations in the gut microbiome and weight gain. The human gastrointestinal (GI) tract is host to trillions of live bacteria that have metabolic interactions with each other and the human host, influencing human nutrition and metabolism.[29] Gut microbiota synthesize essential B vitamins, vitamin K, and harvest energy from the diet that is used to produce short-chain fatty acids that provide an energy source for cells in the colon and liver. The role of gut microbiota on body weight regulation originated from studies using mice models in which transplantation of intestinal microbiota from mice with obesity to lean mice led to a 60% increase in body fat content and development of insulin resistance despite reduced food intake.[30] One mechanism by which obesity may be related to these changes in gut microbiota is the varying absorption of energy from dietary intake depending on the composition of the microbiota. Research suggests that mice with obesity absorb more energy (kilocalories) from dietary carbohydrate than conventional mice who lack obesity. While there is less data in humans, association studies

Table 7.2 Medications That Promote Weight Gain

Class	Drugs	Comments
Tricyclic antidepressants (TCAs)	Amitriptyline, nortriptyline, clomipramine, doxepin, imipramine, trimipramine, desipramine, dosulepine	Amytriptyline and imipramine have the greatest effect on weight gain; notriptyline and desipramine have the smallest
Monoamine oxidase inhibitors (MAOIs)	Phenelzine, moclobemide	Weight gain is less intense than with TCAs
Selective serotonin reuptake inhibitors (SSRIs)	Paroxetine, citalopram, sertraline, fluoxetine	
Phenothiazines	Chlorpromazine	
Tetracyclic antidepressants	Mirtazapine	
Antipsychotics	*Typical:* Haloperidol, Perphenazine *Atypical:* Clozapine, olanzapine, risperidone, amisulpiride	Clozapine may increase appetite
Antimanics	Lithium	
Anticonvulsants	Valproic acid, gabapentin, carbamazepine	Valproic acid and carbamazepine may increase appetite
Antidiabetic agents	Insulin *Meglitinides*: repaglinide, nateglinide *Sulonylureas*: glyburide *Thiazolidinediones*: rosiglitazone, ploglitaxone	Insulin increases deposition of adipose tissue
Alpha-adrenergic blockers	Prazosin, doxazosin, terazosin	
Antihypertensives	*Beta blockers*: Propranolol, atenolol, metoprolol, acebutolol *Calcium channel blockers*: Nisoldipine	
Alpha-adrenergic agonists	Methyldopa, clonidine	
Anabolic steroids	Oxandrolone	
Steroid	*Corticosteroids:* Prednisone, methylprednisone *Contraceptives*: Nexplanon *Synthetic progestins:* Medroxyprogesterone, norethindrone *Chemotherapy:* Tamoxifen, arimidex	Indirectly promote weight gain by stimulating appetite; increase truncal fat (adipose) tissue deposits
Antihistamines	Meclizine, diphenhydramine, fexofenadine, cetirizine	Indirectly promote weight gain by stimulating appetite
Antineoplastic agents	Megatrol	Indirectly promote weight gain by stimulating appetite

Data from Motylev A. The operating room pharmacist and bariatric surgery. US Pharm. 2008;33(12):HS19-HS27. Accessed January 12, 2026. https://www.uspharmacist.com/article/the-operating-room-pharmacist-and-bariatric-surgery

indicate that humans with obesity have reduced microbial diversity and alterations in the genes involved in metabolic pathways compared to lean individuals. Similarly to mice, increased efficiency of energy absorption from food in individuals with obesity compared to lean counterparts is one possible mechanism explaining the link between gut microbiota and obesity.[31] The best current evidence supports the hypothesis that dietary factors induce changes in microbiota that support an obese phenotype through multiple mechanisms.

Developmental Factors

Early life determinants including in utero factors and the impact of breastfeeding have been studied. Research suggests that children with obesity are more likely to retain excess weight as adults; therefore, further studies involving this population are essential. While the direct causes of obesity are not well understood, breastfeeding may play a protective role early in life. Human milk is often lower in calories, fat, and protein and contains satiety hormones such as leptin compared to infant formulas.[32] This balance may trigger less of an insulin response in the infant and protect against increased fat accumulation and excessive weight gain.[33] Further studies examining the duration of breastfeeding during infancy and obesity suggest an inverse relationship; the longer an infant is breastfed, the lower the risk for overweight and obesity extending through childhood (<1 month compared to >6 months).[34] Despite the large number of studies in support of an inverse correlation between breastfeeding and obesity, further research is needed to examine its impact on weight and disease risk later in life.[35,36]

The numerous causes and influences of obesity continue to be a highly researched topic, and it is essential for healthcare professionals to be aware of the complexity of this condition. Additional factors that may contribute to weight not mentioned but worth considering include endocrine disruption due to environmental exposure, political influences on weight, variations in ethnicities, and impact of increasing gravida age, infection, and inflammation.[17] The nutrition assessment for individuals with obesity should include a comprehensive evaluation that identifies the potential contributors to weight and ultimately supports an individualized approach to care.

CORE CONCEPT 2

The etiology of obesity is complex and includes many interacting factors including genetics, environmental, social, biological, and developmental factors.

Hormonal Factors

Body weight is regulated by metabolic, neuroendocrine, and autonomic systems as well as a complex network of signals released from adipose, endocrine, and GI tissues that are integrated by the liver and central nervous system (CNS). When the body experiences a slight change in energy intake or energy loss, these systems work together to maintain a state of weight equilibrium. As the systems become overtaxed, such as that with repeated overfeeding and a positive energy balance, weight gain can result. The term "adaptive thermogenesis" has been used to explain why individuals who have tried to achieve a state of negative energy balance tend to regain lost weight over time (with an 80–90% return rate to pre-weight loss levels of body fat). The effect is observed in both lean and individuals with obesity.[37] There is variability among individuals regarding the degree of weight gain when exposed to an adipogenic environment, which can be explained in part by genetic influences that reflect individual metabolic responses to increased energy intake or decreased expenditure.[37]

Understanding the interplay between GI hormones and the CNS and how these factors regulate appetite and food intake is essential to obesity management. The hypothalamus in the brain plays a central role in energy balance and weight regulation. It receives both peripheral signals (GI tract, pancreas, adipocytes) and central signals that communicate how much energy from food is needed by the body in the short term and how much energy is available in the body for long-term use. The arcuate nucleus (ARC) region within the hypothalamus contains hormone receptors with two regions predominantly responsible for integrating these signals: the pro-opiomelanocortin (POMC) neurons, which aim to suppress appetite, and the neuropeptide Y (NPY) and agouti-related peptide (AgRP) neurons, which aim to stimulate appetite (**Figure 7.4**).[38] The hypothalamus manages input from the cortex and hedonic pathways, which is activated by the sight, smell, and social aspects of food. When these signals reach the regions in the hypothalamus, changes in their activity and release of neuropeptides influence eating behavior, meal patterns, and energy expenditure.[39]

Orexigenic Hormone

Ghrelin is the only **orexigenic**, or appetite-inducing, GI hormone. It is short acting and secreted in the fundus of the stomach, in small quantities in other parts of the GI tract, in the pancreas, and

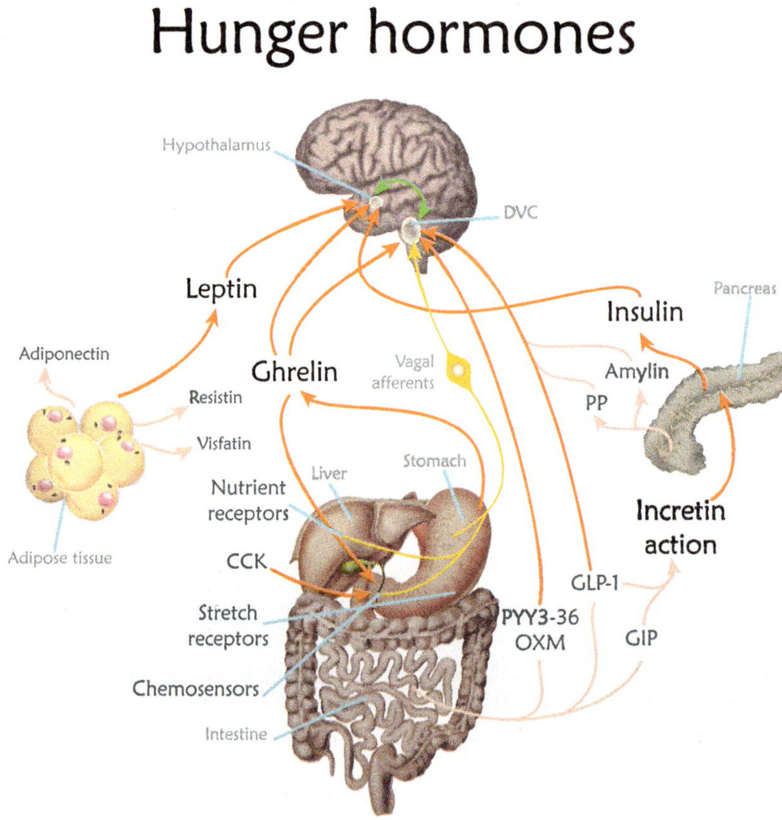

Figure 7.4 Selected Pathways Involved in Body Weight Regulation

in ghrelin-neurons in the hypothalamus. Ghrelin levels are at their peak preprandially, which helps to stimulate food intake, and at their lowest postprandially to signal the end of eating. The release of ghrelin increases GI motility and decreases insulin secretion. The exact mechanism of action of ghrelin remains unclear. Ghrelin may reach the hypothalamus via the bloodstream or inhibit activity of the vagus nerve and reduce activity of neurotransmitters in the brain, which then reduces the discharge of neurotransmitters. Afferent neurons contain ghrelin receptors. This may lead to the local release of ghrelin in the hypothalamus, which stimulates appetite by increasing activity of orexigenic neurons in the ARC. Ghrelin concentrations in the body appear to be inversely related to BMI and may be inadequately suppressed in obesity. Following a period of energy restriction or weight reduction, ghrelin levels will rise to stimulate appetite and assist the body in returning to its original weight. An exception to this relationship is observed with the sleeve gastrectomy, a metabolic and bariatric surgical procedure that removes the fundus of the stomach and thus reduces ghrelin secretion.[40]

> **CORE CONCEPT 3**
>
> Body weight is regulated by a complex network of systems and signaling pathways that become dysregulated with obesity and chronic positive energy balance.

Anorexigenic Hormones

Leptin

Leptin is a hormone produced by white adipose tissue that relays the status of body fat storage to the brain via the bloodstream and affects both energy intake and expenditure. Leptin inhibits appetite by decreasing the activity of orexigenic (NPY and AgRP) neurons and increasing the activity of the **anorexigenic** (POMC) neurons in the hypothalamus, leading to a loss of appetite. In a state of energy balance, leptin circulates at levels proportional to body fat. During periods of weight gain and when **adipose** tissue increases, leptin levels will rise. Conversely, leptin will fall in a state of negative energy balance or weight loss. In individuals with obesity, there is suspected "leptin resistance" or impairment in the leptin signaling pathways that results in higher-than-expected leptin levels (for adipose tissue) and a reduced sense of satiety by the brain, which may lead to increased energy intake and weight gain. This concept is like that of insulin resistance observed in T2DM. If an individual with obesity attempts to lose weight and reduce adipose tissue, leptin levels will fall, although the body remains in a leptin resistant state and will attempt to regain lost adipose tissue over time. Impairments in this signaling pathway are partially responsible for why it is so difficult for many individuals with obesity to lose weight and keep it off.

The effects of white fat versus brown fat in the body are an ongoing and important area of research. There is evidence to support that in rodents, leptin increases energy expenditure through thermogenesis in brown adipose tissue due to increased sympathetic activation.[41] The loss of brown adipose tissue function in rodents is linked to metabolic dysfunction and obesity,[42] and abnormalities in the sympathetic nervous system have been observed in leptin-deficient adults.[43] Much is still unknown about how brown adipose tissue behaves in adults; however, its ability to burn calories likely means that it plays a key role in weight management for some individuals.

Insulin

Insulin works in tandem with leptin and has an orexigenic effect on the ARC in the hypothalamus. Insulin is produced and secreted by the beta (β) cells of the pancreas in response to ingestion and breakdown of carbohydrate to glucose, and later absorption of glucose into the bloodstream. Insulin assists glucose into various cells in the body for energy, where it can be used or stored for later use. Individuals with obesity are at risk for insulin resistance, which occurs when cells such as those in muscle, fat, and the liver become less responsive to insulin. The β cells in the pancreas continue to produce insulin to lower blood glucose levels and eventually are not able to keep up with the body's demand, resulting in inflammation, development of T2DM, and other chronic health conditions.[44]

Islet Amyloid Polypeptide (Amylin)

Islet amyloid polypeptide (IAPP) or amylin is co-secreted with insulin by the β cells of the pancreas and acts on receptors in the brain via the bloodstream. Amylin works to promote satiety by slowing gastric emptying, assisting with secretion of gastric acids, and preventing postprandial spikes in blood sugar. Amylin also enhances the effects of cholecystokinin.[45]

Cholecystokinin

Cholecystokinin (CCK) is secreted by cells in the intestine and stimulates bile production by the liver, influences release of bile from the gallbladder, stimulates release of enzyme from the pancreas, and through the control of the gastric sphincter, decreases the rate of gastric emptying. CCK stimulates the vagus nerve, which affects the neurotransmitters in the brain and provides a message of satiety. CCK may also stimulate short-term satiety by influencing release of leptin.[46] If an individual with obesity attempts to lose weight, CCK levels will fall, resulting in decreased feelings of satiety.

Peptide YY (PYY)

Like CKK, peptide YY (PYY) acts as a satiety messenger and produces an anorexigenic effect via the ARC. It is stimulated by food entering the gut, and high-protein meals may result in prolonged effects of PYY. Peptide YY also delays gastric emptying and inhibits gastric acid secretion.[47] Levels of this hormone are decreased in obesity, leading to lower satiety.

Incretins (GLP-1 and GIP)

Glucagon-like peptide-1 (GLP-1) and glucose-dependent insulinotropic polypeptide (GIP) are two incretin hormones that are released by the intestine in response to carbohydrate and fat intake and stimulate release of insulin from the pancreatic β cells. GLP-1 suppresses glucagon secretion from pancreatic alpha α cells, which results in delaying gastric emptying and suppressing appetite (**Figure 7.5**), while GIP works with insulin to promote energy storage in adipose tissue. There is a decreased functionality of GLP-1 hormones resulting in a blunted effect on satiation.[48]

CORE CONCEPT 4

Body weight is regulated by metabolic, neuroendocrine, and autonomic systems in the body, including signals released from adipose, gastrointestinal, and endocrine tissues that are integrated by the liver and central nervous system.

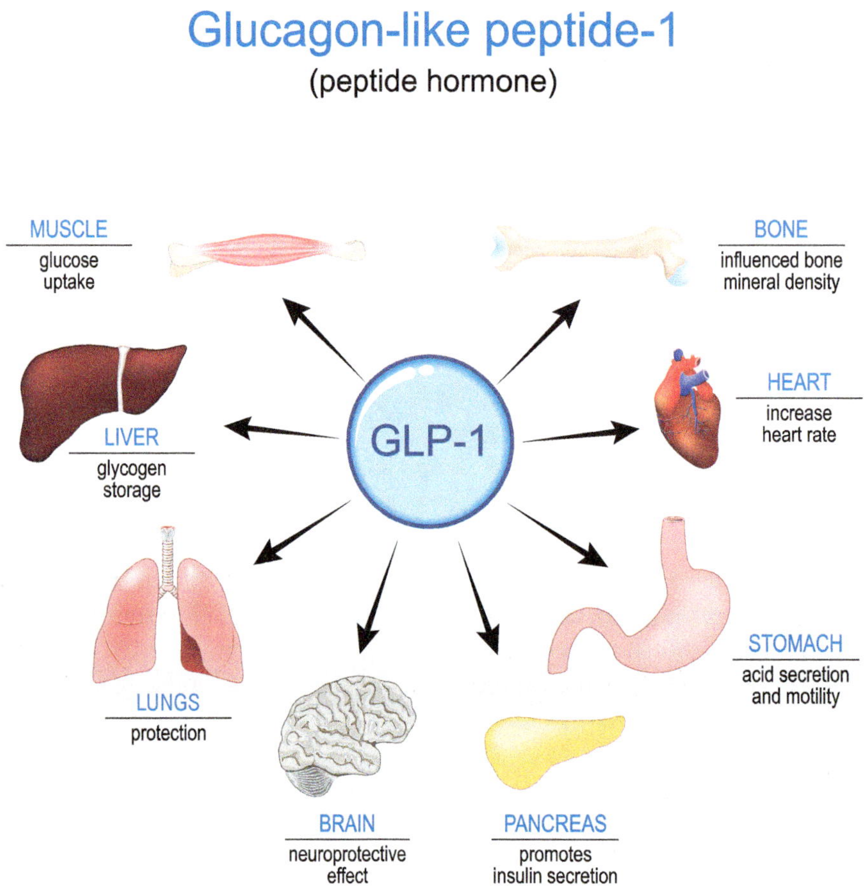

Figure 7.5 Glucagon-Like Peptide-1 Appetite Regulation

Alterations in Body Composition in Obesity

Body weight includes fat mass and fat-free mass (FFM). Fat mass includes fat from all sources of the body including adipose tissue, brain, and skeleton, while FFM is devoid of fat and includes water, protein, and mineral components. Individuals with obesity tend to have a higher percentage of body fat compared with the normal-weight individual; however, there are always exceptions.[49]

Fat in the body is categorized as "essential" or "storage." Essential body fat is present in the nerve tissues, bone marrow, and organs, and is needed for normal physiological functioning. In males, 2–3% of body fat is considered essential compared to 5–12% for females, which is higher due to childbearing and hormonal functions. Lean body mass (LBM) is FFM combined with essential fat. Storage fat, or "nonessential" fat, represents an energy reserve in the subcutaneous adipose tissue or visceral fat. The optimal amount of total body fat, which includes essential plus storage fat, is 21–36% in females, and 8–25% in males. These ranges vary depending on age and ethnicity.[50]

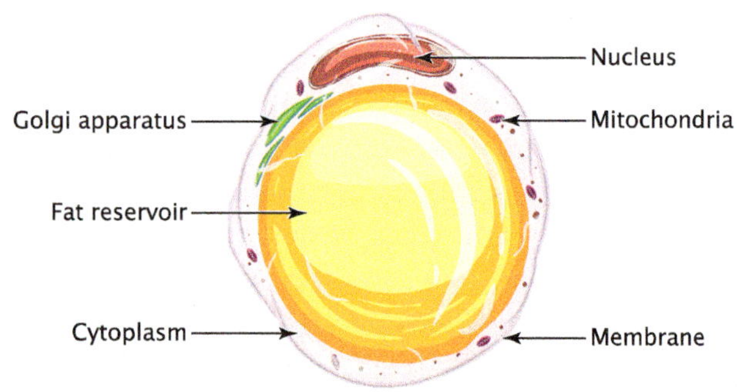

Figure 7.6 Adipocyte Structure

Adipocytes are connective tissue cells that can synthesize and store fat (**Figure 7.6**). The function of white adipocytes is to store energy, while the function of brown adipocytes is to dissipate energy in a heat-producing process called "thermogenesis." Adipocytes play a role in maintaining proper energy balance by mobilizing sources of energy that are hormonally stimulated, and storing calories in lipid form, as triacylglycerols. When fat stores are mobilized, non-esterified fatty acids are released into the bloodstream. Adipose tissue grows by two mechanisms: hyperplasia (cell number increase) and hypertrophy (cell size increase). Weight gain may result in hyperplasia, hypertrophy, or a combination. The enlargement of these adipocytes through increased fat storage may play a key role in weight gain in adults through the enlargement of the fat depots.[51] Genetics and diet may affect contributions of these two mechanisms to the growth of adipose tissue in obesity.[52] Evidence suggests that adipocyte population growth starts at a young age, and in people with early-onset obesity, involves a more significant increase in adipocyte number leading to a larger number of adipocytes when reaching adulthood. While the population of adipocytes increases throughout childhood and adolescence, it is tightly regulated during adulthood. Changes in fat mass in adults are likely the result of changes in adipocyte size as opposed to an increase in adipocyte number, and adipocyte populations are not influenced by energy balance.[53]

While large amounts of adipose tissue can negatively impact health risk, the distribution in the body also plays a significant role. A larger waist circumference (WC) is associated with increased metabolic complications such as of T2DM, dyslipidemia, HTN, coronary heart disease, stroke, and early mortality.[4] An android distribution of fat, greater fat located around the abdomen, also sometimes referred to as an "apple" figure, conveys greater risk of developing cardiovascular disease, HTN, and T2DM. This type of fat distribution is more commonly observed in males. A gynecoid distribution of fat, greater fat located around the hips also referred to as a "pear" figure, does not increase the risk of developing medical complications, and is more commonly observed among females.[4]

Nutrition Assessment in Obesity

A nutrition assessment completed by an RD is a crucial component of the Nutrition Care Process and Model (NCPM), and the first step in evaluating an individual's current nutritional patterns and dietary history. The nutrition assessment is defined as a method for observing, obtaining, analyzing, and interpreting necessary data to identify nutrition-related problems and to develop a plan. Data is gathered from the medical record, individual interview, measurements, observation, and other healthcare providers or specialists involved in the individual's care. There are several areas for the RD to assess to evaluate obesity and formulate an appropriate plan with the interprofessional team.

Anthropometric Assessment

Anthropometric assessment should include accurate height and weight, BMI, and may include a waist-to-hip ratio (WHR) and/or WC, and measurement of body composition, if attainable.

Body Mass Index

BMI is the most used anthropometric measurement when screening for obesity. As previously stated, a major limitation of BMI is that it fails to distinguish between lean mass and fat mass.[54] The current definition of obesity is based solely on BMI, although excess body fat has been linked with a variety of metabolic issues.[55] There have been numerous studies to measure the accuracy of BMI in determining body adiposity and metabolic risks, and the results vary significantly. Direct methods to accurately measure body fat such as dual energy X-ray absorptiometry (DXA), magnetic resonance imaging (MRI), and computed tomography (CT) analysis are rarely used in clinical practice due to high cost and impracticality. There are also indirect methods such as air-displacement plethysmography (ADP), bioelectrical impedance (BIA), hydrostatic weighing, skinfold thickness, WC, and WHR. Despite its limitations, BMI is used extensively in epidemiological studies and is incorporated regularly in clinical practice due to its practicality and simplicity. In addition to BMI, determination of individual energy needs through calculation of resting energy expenditure (REE) can help guide nutrition education and prescriptions.

Waist Circumference

WC is another screening tool for individuals with overweight and obesity.[3] Cardiometabolic risk, morbidity, and mortality increase with a larger WC starting at 88 cm for females or greater than 102 cm for males.[3]

Waist-to-Hip Ratio

WHR is the comparison of WC to that of the hips. A WHR above 1.0 for males and above 0.8 for females is suggestive of increased health risk.[4] Data is lacking on appropriate cutoffs for WHRs for predicting risk of mortality in ethnic and population groups.[51]

Weight History

Weight history should include the highest and lowest adult weights, patterns of weight changes throughout life, contributors to significant shifts, a family weight history, and any attempts at changing weight through lifestyle change or medical intervention.

Biochemical Assessment

Laboratory values are important indicators of potential comorbidity related to obesity. Biochemical assessment could include a lipid profile, measure of hyperglycemia, and iron status among other measures. Laboratory values can provide information on potential deficiencies, such as low vitamin D, which is commonly observed with obesity.

Clinical Assessment

A thorough clinical assessment is necessary to identify any medical or psychosocial issues, histories, or past or current therapies that may impact food and nutrient ingestion and absorption.

Medical and Psychosocial History

Medical and psychosocial history includes current and past medical conditions and obesity-related comorbidities, medications, past surgical history, and family medical history. For individuals who may benefit from metabolic and bariatric surgery (MBS), a thorough evaluation by a mental health provider is required. Note that if a patient is undergoing mental health treatment, asking permission from the patient to contact their provider may be of great value when considering medical nutrition therapy recommendations. Any history of eating disorders should be noted. A psychologist may evaluate history of binge eating, bulimia, or other specified feeding or eating disorders, current/past psychiatric diagnosis, alcohol/tobacco/drug use, self-care challenges, stress management, and coping mechanisms.

Nutrition-Focused Physical Exam

A nutrition-focused physical examination can also provide valuable information in the assessment of obesity by identifying an individual's fat, muscle, fluid, and micronutrient status as well as markers of inflammation, chronic disease, and nutrient deficiencies. An exam specific to obesity can include assessment of total and regional adiposity, presence of lean mass or muscle loss, hydration status, skin hyperpigmentation, numbness or tingling in extremities, and presence or absence of edema and/or wounds.

Dietary Assessment

Dietary assessment is important to identify nutrient intake, variety, and patterns to assess for inadequate, excessive, or imbalanced intake. It is possible for an individual to have both excess weight and malnutrition, and therefore monitoring of both deficiencies and toxicities is key.

Dietary History

A comprehensive nutrition evaluation for overweight and obesity should document previous attempts at weight change including structured medical programs, commercial programs, previous RD visits for health management, self-directed approaches to weight loss, weight-loss medications, and any weight-loss surgery. Working with the individual to identify which method(s) were most effective and sustainable may help to guide future recommendations for management.

Nutrition Patterns

Current intake (24-hour recall or food frequency questionnaire) of food/fluid, timing of meals and snacks, portion sizes, hunger and satiety levels, eating patterns such as frequency of meals out or sugar sweetened beverage consumption, vitamin/mineral supplements, dietary supplements (i.e., protein supplements, fish oil, herbal supplements, etc.), and food allergies and intolerances are important to assess and evaluate as a component of the comprehensive nutrition assessment.

Other Considerations

Physical Activity

Individuals should be evaluated for current activity level, which includes their activities of daily living, time spent in sedentary activities, type and amount of time spent in planned activities such as structured exercise, and any barriers to activity. Addressing barriers that inhibit movement and determining what activities are most enjoyable are key to understanding an individual's ability and desire to engage in movement. Aiding the individual in creating realistic movement goals can encourage more consistent and enjoyable activity patterns.

Sleep Patterns

Assessing an individual's sleep patterns may give clues as to its impact on physical, mental, and emotional functioning. A short duration of sleep (<7 hours for

CASE STUDY REVISITED

Allison is eager to try to improve her weight and health through lifestyle management. Today, she brought a food log and says she is interested in additional forms of self-monitoring. She reports that she has a sedentary lifestyle and spends most of her workdays at her desk. Her hobbies include reading and watching TV due to stress, low energy, and fatigue. You request more detailed information about her diet, and she shares the following:

Breakfast (6 am): two 12 oz cups of coffee with fat-free half and half and artificial sweetener
Lunch (11:30 am): Tuna sandwich on whole wheat bread, 2 cups of strawberries, 1 can soda
Snack (3 pm): 1 cup of grapes, 3 chocolate chip cookies, and a small coffee with half and half and artificial sweetener
Dinner at home (7 pm): Salad with romaine lettuce, carrots, tomatoes, and blue cheese salad dressing, baked chicken breast, 1/2 baked sweet potato with margarine and sour cream, water
Bedtime snack (10 pm): 6 crackers with peanut butter and 8 oz fat-free milk

Questions

1. What do you estimate Allison's energy needs to be to support weight loss?
2. Based on her most recent dietary recall, what are two topics you might address with Allison to lower her calorie intake?
3. What is your interpretation of Allison's motivation and readiness to change?

adults), frequent night wakings, and conditions such as sleep apnea (OSA) have the potential to negatively impact health.[56] Assess if the individual might be snoring, gasping for breath while sleeping, waking with a headache, or experiencing daytime somnolence as these are possible symptoms of OSA. If the individual displays one or more of these symptoms, they may need referral to their primary care or sleep medicine physician for a further work-up.

Readiness/Motivation

Motivations or reasons for intervention; readiness to make behavioral changes; willingness to adhere to a health prescription; expected time, frequency, and duration of follow-up; and expectations regarding any weight change should be included in the assessment.

Support System

The individual's support system (including friends, family, case workers, support animals, etc.) and relationship to the individual should be evaluated. It is important to consider other individuals involved in cooking, grocery shopping, and daily activities, because they may influence an individual's food choices or activity patterns.

Cultural and Socioeconomic Factors

Cultural factors include dietary restrictions, food/activity customs, and other practices that influence food choice and eating behavior. Socioeconomic status and the ability to access recommended foods or supplements should be evaluated. Additionally, health disparities adversely affect certain populations, and this should be acknowledged when assessing health risk.

Other

Assessment of obesity should also address any potential barriers to weight loss, including low literary skills, poor vision or hearing, language barriers, and/or learning disabilities.

PRACTICE POINT

The nutrition assessment of individuals with obesity should include collection of anthropometric measurements, past medical and psychosocial history, diet and weight history, nutrition, physical activity, sleep patterns, biochemical assessment, cultural factors, support systems, and readiness to change.

Assessment of Energy Requirement

The most practical way to estimate resting metabolic rate (RMR) in the clinical setting is by using predictive equations using anthropometric data. These equations were developed from both indirect and direct calorimetry measures, although they still have varying margins of error. Of the most commonly used

Table 7.3 Assessment of Resting Energy Expenditure (REE)

Use the **Mifflin–St Jeor** equation to estimate REE (kcal/day):
Women: RMR = (9.99 × actual weight [kg]) + (6.25 × height [cm]) − (4.92 × age [years]) − 161
Men: RMR = (9.99 × actual weight [kg]) + (6.25 × height [cm]) − (4.92 × age [years]) + 5
TEE = REE × AF (study or population-specific activity factor)
Multiply the REE by an activity factor of 1.3 for sedentary individuals.

Data from Academy of Nutrition and Dietetics. Weight management: overweight and obesity (2021): comparative standards. Nutrition Care Manual®. Accessed April 26, 2025. https://www.nutritioncaremanual.org/topic.cfm?ncm_category_id=1&lv1=272986&lv2=275050&lv3=275058&ncm_toc_id=275058&ncm_heading=Nutrition%20Care

equations (Mifflin–St Jeor, Harris–Benedict, Cunningham, Owen, and World Health Organization/Food and Agriculture Organization/United Nations University [WHO/FAO/UNU]), the Mifflin–St Jeor has the least margin of error and is believed to estimate RMR within as little as 10% of individuals who are of normal weight and those with obesity.[57,58] Since there is no direct measurement of body stores, there are limitations when generalized to certain age and ethnic groups. In some cases, indirect calorimetry may be a more appropriate measure when the clinician deems that a predictive method fails in a clinically relevant way. The recommendation for using the Mifflin–St Jeor as the preferred equation to predict RMR is for healthy individuals (**Table 7.3**) and other equations may be more appropriate for various disease states.[57]

PRACTICE POINT

The Mifflin–St Jeor is the best predictive equation for estimating energy needs for healthy individuals and individuals with obesity.

Pathophysiology Associated with Obesity

Obesity meets standards of a medical disease, including a known etiology, recognized signs and symptoms, and a range of structural and functional changes that culminate in pathologic consequences. Excess adipose tissue produces excess free fatty acids (FFAs), tumor necrosis factor-alpha (TNF-α), interleukin-6 (IL-6), leptin, and plasminogen activator inhibitor-1. This production is associated with hyperinsulinemia, hyperglycemia, insulin resistance, development of T2DM, endothelial damage, and the onset and progression of atherosclerotic lesions.[59]

Weight-Related Comorbidities

Obesity increases the risk of several conditions, including cardiovascular disease, T2DM, coronary heart disease (CHD), OSA, gastroesophageal reflux disease (GERD), HTN, arthritis, and certain cancers, among others (**Figure 7.7**).

Cardiovascular System

Obesity is also strongly associated with HTN and cardiovascular conditions such as CHD, heart failure, atrial fibrillation, and sudden cardiac death.[5,60] Obesity-related HTN is caused by activation of the sympathetic nervous system and activation of the renin-angiotensin system, among other irregularities. Other factors that affect obesity-related HTN are hyperinsulinemia, structural changes in the kidney, and various adipokines (hormones) such as leptin.[61] These factors may contribute to sodium reabsorption and fluid retention, resulting in HTN. Numerous studies suggest that obesity-related HTN is associated with an increased risk of kidney insufficiency.[62]

Obesity may impact cardiovascular disease through its effect on its risk factors such as HTN, inflammatory markers, glucose intolerance, and dyslipidemia.[63] Increased levels of C-reactive protein (CRP) and leptin are associated with cardiovascular events.[64] In addition, several variations in cardiac function and structure may occur with excess adipose tissue, and individuals with obesity have higher cardiac workload and cardiac output.[65] Although obesity is associated with cardiovascular diseases, it is well documented that individuals with obesity who have heart disease have improved prognosis when compared to lean or underweight individuals,often referred to as the obesity paradox.[60]

Metabolic/Endocrine System

Currently 11.6% or approximately 38.4 million Americans are living with T2DM, an estimate that is up from 8.3% a few years ago.[66] By 2050, diabetes prevalence is predicted to rise to 21%.[66,67] T2DM accounts for 90–95% of all diabetes diagnoses in the United States.[66] The precursor to T2DM is insulin resistance, which results from gradual dysfunction of pancreatic islet β-cells and the inability to effectively move glucose out of the bloodstream into various cells in the body. This eventually leads low β-cell mass, impaired

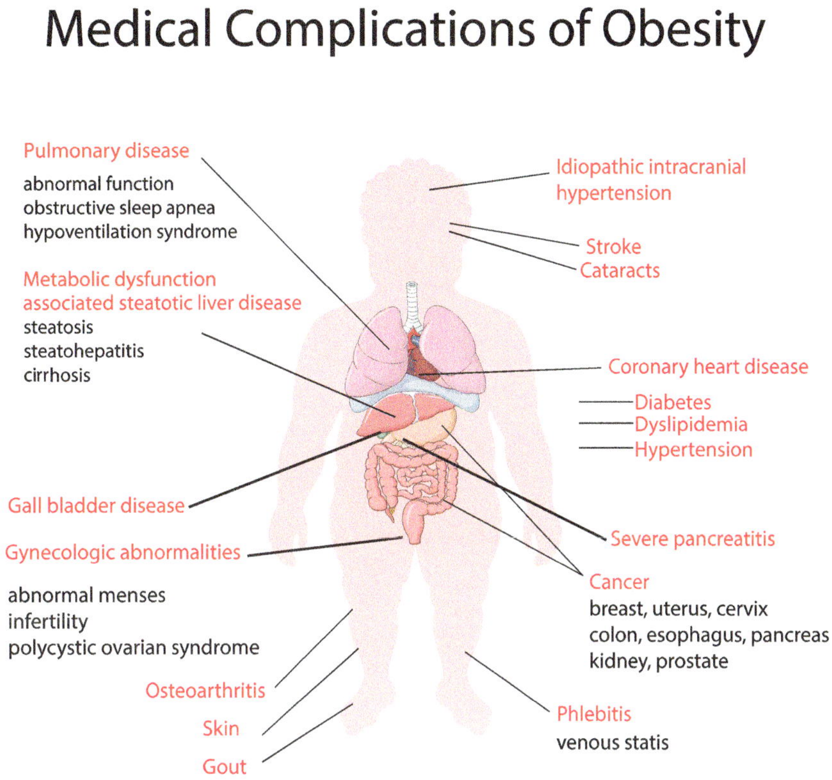

Figure 7.7 Medical Complications of Obesity

incretin response, and inadequate suppression of glucagon production. The lack of glucagon suppression leads to inadequate uptake, storage, and clearance of glucose as well as elevated production of glucose by the liver resulting in significant hyperglycemia. Once the body is no longer able to properly manage blood glucose levels effectively, T2DM results and can progress to an insulin-dependent state if not effectively treated.

Factors contributing to T2DM are both environmental and genetic. While the relationship of insulin resistance and pancreatic cell dysfunction is believed to be important in the development and progression of T2DM, the precise mechanisms are unclear. Adipose tissue likely plays a key role in the development of disease given that the majority of individuals have excess central and visceral (intra-abdominal) adiposity. Although corporal adipose tissue also poses a risk, it is generally thought that an accumulation of central visceral fat is an independent risk for T2DM, despite the degree of obesity. Since not all individuals with obesity develop hyperglycemia, an underlying abnormality of the β-cell must coexist with excess adipose tissue to promote T2DM.[68]

Proinflammatory molecules produced by adipose tissue have been associated with the development of metabolic disease such as T2DM.[69] Excess adipose tissue releases higher amounts of glycerol, nonesterified fatty acids, hormones, proinflammatory cytokines, and other factors that are involved with the development of insulin resistance. Chronic increase in fatty acids reduces the usage of glucose as a source of energy, and impairs β-cell function, acting in conjunction with insulin resistance to worsen hyperglycemia. Moderate weight reduction (7–10% of total body weight) can improve glycemic control and reduce diabetes risk.

The term "metabolic syndrome" is used to define a combination of cardiovascular risk factors that may be present in individuals with obesity. These include dyslipidemia, HTN, insulin resistance, abdominal adiposity, and a proinflammatory and prothrombotic state. Diagnostic criteria for metabolic syndrome differ by organization (Adult Treatment Panel III,[70] WHO, American Association of Clinical Endocrinologists) due to differences among human populations, although the most common measures are included in **Table 7.4**. A diagnosis of metabolic syndrome is made when an individual exhibits 3 of the 5 qualifying characteristics.[71] Research suggests that there is strong evidence to support an association among metabolic syndrome, T2DM, and cardiovascular disease, requiring close medical monitoring in order to optimize treatment.[3] Elevations in the proinflammatory marker

Table 7.4 ATP III Clinical Identification of Metabolic Syndrome

Risk Factor Criteria	Level
Waist circumference: Males	≥102 cm (≥40 in)
Waist circumference: Females	≥88 cm (≥35 in)
HDL-C: Males	<40 mg/dL
HDL-C: Females	<50 mg/dL
Triglyceride	≥150 mg/dL
Blood pressure	≥130/85 mm Hg
Fasting blood sugar	≥110 mg/dL

Data from Om Murti A. Table 2: ATP. Accessed January 12, 2026. http://www.jcpcarchives.org/userfiles/table-2-atp.jpg

CRP may be a strong predictor of future cardiovascular disease events with or without a firm diagnosis of metabolic syndrome; however, it is not used as diagnostic criteria.[72]

Gastrointestinal System

Gastroesophageal Reflux Disease

Obesity and particularly central adiposity are associated with increased risk of developing GERD. Once present, the severity of GERD symptoms can increase in severity with weight gain. Obesity is a risk factor for more serious conditions including development of Barrett's esophagus and adenocarcinoma of the esophagus related to increased acid exposure to the esophagus.[73,74] There are several mechanisms by which obesity may contribute to GERD, although the exact relationship is not clearly defined. One commonly described pathway is increased abdominal pressure associated with a larger WC that may cause the lower esophageal sphincter to relax and allow acidic gastric contents to come in contact with the esophageal mucosa. Adipocytokines released from visceral fat including IL-6 and TNF-α may also increase symptoms of GERD and play a role in consequent carcinogenesis.[75] Some research suggests that weight loss decreases symptoms of GERD, although once erosions are present, it is unclear if weight reduction would have beneficial effects. Improvement in GERD symptoms has also been observed in individuals following Roux-en-Y gastric bypass (RYGB) surgery with near complete cessation of acid production.[73]

Steatohepatitis

Overweight and obesity are implicated as a primary cause in the development of metabolic dysfunction–associated steatotic liver disease (MASLD), a form of steatohepatitis in which excess fat builds up in the liver without significant alcohol consumption.[76,77] Liver cells, or hepatocytes, only contain small amounts of storage lipids. In MASLD, these cells contain greater than normal amounts of triglycerides. Some individuals with MASLD have liver cell injury and inflammation in addition to excessive fat (>5%),[77] causing a more severe condition termed "metabolic dysfunction–associated steatohepatitis" (MASH). MASLD does not lead to increased short-term mortality or morbidity, although progression to MASH dramatically increases risk of cirrhosis, liver failure, and hepatocellular carcinoma (HCC).[76] The reported rates of disease progression from MASLD to MASH and ultimately to cirrhosis, liver failure, and HCC vary greatly depending on disease definitions, populations studied, and the diagnostic methods used. Globally, the prevalence of MASLD is increasing along with rates of obesity. It is estimated that 32% of adults have MASLD and 20–30% of these cases will progress to MASH.[78,79]

The pathogenesis of MASLD is not entirely understood.[76] Experts agree that MASLD begins with excess energy intake mediated by important genetic and environmental factors. Central obesity, glucose intolerance, T2DM, dyslipidemia, HTN, and other features of metabolic syndrome are associated with MASLD. Insulin resistance, oxidative stress, and cytokines are considered important contributing factors to the pathogenesis of MASLD.[75] These factors contribute to a proinflammatory cascade in the body that is mediated by various proteins and immune factors hypothesized to contribute to the development of MASLD/MASH. The presence of hyperinsulinemia and hyperglycemia drives hepatic lipogenesis, which may cause insulin resistance in peripheral sites such as muscle and adipose tissue. This progression is mediated by inflammatory factors like TNF-α and IL-6, which also may arise from stressed and inflamed adipose tissue. Once insulin resistance is systemic, FFAs released from adipose tissue circulate continuously and likely cause the hepatic lipid accumulation and injury (lipotoxicity). Genetic factors that drive consumption of calorie dense foods and those that affect lipid storage are likely to also play an important role and MASLD/MASH pathogenesis. It is difficult to determine the relationship between steatosis and insulin resistance as both states can potentiate the other and which arises first remains unclear. Refer to Chapter 13, *Nutrition in Liver Disease*, for more information on nutritional therapy for MASLD/MASH.

Immune System

Overweight and obesity are implicated in about 4-8% of all cancer cases.[80] According to the World Cancer Research Fund (WCRF) and American Institute for Cancer Research (AICR), obesity is a risk factor for cancers of the mouth, esophagus, stomach, gallbladder, kidney, pancreas, liver, colon, rectum, prostate, endometrium, ovaries, and breast (postmenopausal).[81] The American Cancer Society also suggests that overweight and obesity are associated with increased mortality from liver cancer, pancreatic cancer, non-Hodgkin's lymphoma, and myeloma.[80] The mechanisms by which obesity increases cancer risk are being studied and vary by type of cancer. Obesity and metabolic syndrome are associated with chronic low-grade inflammation, which is thought to play a central role. CRP level, which is a marker of inflammation, may be correlated with increased cancer risk.[81] Adipocytes release inflammatory markers that have been associated with poor prognosis from cancer.[78] Fat tissue also produces and releases hormones, adipokines, and cytokines such as leptin, adiponectin, TNF-α, and IL-6 that may play a role in cancer development. Leptin has been studied as a mediator in cancer development via its role in increasing inflammatory pathways, while adiponectin may have anticancer effects through decreasing inflammatory actions within the body.[81] Insulin and insulin-like growth factor (IGF)-1 may also be important factors contributing to cancer development. Observational studies have linked increased cancer mortality with T2DM and obesity, which may be due to increased insulin and/or elevated IGF-1 in these individuals.[82] Understanding the pathways that may link obesity with increased cancer risk is helpful in determining therapeutic targets; however, preventing overweight and obesity remains the number one priority

Musculoskeletal System

Obesity is associated with several musculoskeletal conditions including osteoarthritis (OA), low back pain, diffuse idiopathic skeletal hyperostosis, gait disturbance, fibromyalgia, rheumatoid arthritis, osteoporosis, gout, and soft tissue conditions such as plantar fasciitis.[83] These conditions can lead to physical consequences including chronic pain, disability, and impaired quality of life, as well as the societal burden of increasing direct and indirect healthcare costs. According to the CDC, 31% of adults with obesity have arthritis compared to 16% of adults without obesity.[84] Researchers are beginning to identify potential mechanisms by which obesity increases musculoskeletal conditions, particularly for osteoarthritis. Studies suggest that weight loss is important for preventing and managing knee osteoarthritis as individuals with obesity and knee OA have elevated cartilage turnover biomarkers. Inflammatory cytokines released from adipose tissue may also play a role in the development of musculoskeletal conditions.[85] Other studies have shown that MBS reduces symptoms of OA and can reduce knee pain, although more research is needed in this area.[86]

Respiratory System

Obstructive sleep apnea (OSA) is a medical condition characterized by ongoing episodes of complete obstruction (apnea) or partial obstruction (hypopnea) of the upper airway. OSA leads to poor sleep and intermittent hypoxia during sleep.[87] It is estimated that 50–60% of individuals with obesity and metabolic syndrome have OSA.[88] Recent studies show that individuals with OSA were 6–9 times more likely to have metabolic syndrome compared to those without OSA. Obesity is a significant risk factor for OSA as it may be associated with enlargement of soft tissue structures within and around the airway, resulting in pharyngeal airway narrowing. In addition, increased abdominal adipose tissue and recumbent posture may reduce lung volume. This can further narrow the airway due to the decrease in pharyngeal wall tension and longitudinal tracheal traction forces.[89] There is evidence that markers of cardiovascular risk, such as systemic inflammation, elevated CRP, sympathetic activation, and endothelial dysfunction, are increased in individuals with obesity with OSA compared to those with obesity without OSA. OSA may also increase the risk of developing HTN, dysrhythmias, myocardial infarction, stroke, pulmonary hypertension, heart failure, and overall mortality.[90] Continuous positive airway pressure (CPAP) treatment can improve pathophysiological changes associated with OSA, including lowering blood pressure and increased insulin sensitivity. Modest weight loss will improve OSA as well as metabolic and cardiovascular risk.

Nutrition Interventions in Obesity

Weight management requires a lifelong commitment to lifestyle behaviors such as sustainable eating patterns and daily physical activity in order to maintain energy balance within the body.[91] If attempting to lose weight, realistic targets should be set by the individual; sustained weight loss of even 3–5% is likely to lead to clinically significant health improvements, including reductions in triglycerides, blood glucose, HbA1c and the risk of developing T2DM. Greater metabolic health improvements are typically noticed as weight loss increases.[3]

Comprehensive Lifestyle Intervention

Comprehensive lifestyle programs utilize dietary counseling, physical activity, and behavior modification to encourage weight loss, and those lasting at least 6 months are often most effective (**Figure 7.8**).[3] Individuals who enter a comprehensive lifestyle program should be ready to commit to behavioral changes such as self-monitoring of dietary behaviors and physical activity, be free of any untreated major depressive symptoms, and enter at a stable juncture in their lives.[92] Intensive Behavior Therapy (IBT) programs, which include 14 or more sessions led by a trained interventionist, such as an RD, are often most effective.[3] Programs may be conducted in an individual or group setting, and in person or via electronic setting (internet or phone). In some cases, programs conducted via telecommunications technology prove to be more convenient for the individual and/or the provider due to timing, location, and cost of travel. Since the start of the COVID-19 pandemic, the use of telehealth for visits is more widely utilized; however, the debate remains as to whether virtual programs encourage as much weight loss as traditional face-to-face programs.[3,93]

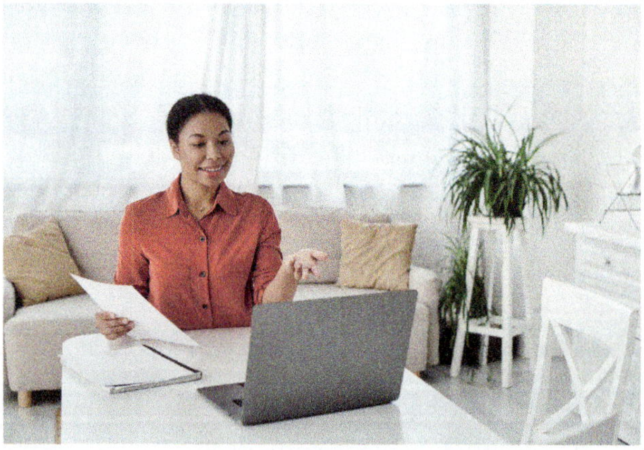

Figure 7.8 Comprehensive Lifestyle Interventions Facilitated by a Dietitian Can Promote Weight Loss

Dietary

Nutrition prescriptions in a comprehensive lifestyle program should focus first on calorie reduction (versus macronutrient content, processing of foods, etc.) as this will encourage the greatest amount of weight change. This could include specific calorie prescriptions (usually 1200–1500 kcal/day for females and 1500–1800 kcal/day for males, adjusted based on body weight and physical activity), or a standard caloric reduction (500–1000 calories) taken from an individual's estimated energy needs using predictive equations.[3] A number of dietary approaches that restrict certain types of food or nutrients have been approved for weight loss when used in the setting of calorie reduction. These include a high-protein diet, low-fat and low-carbohydrate diets, the DASH diet, and the Mediterranean-style diet, among others.[68] Many of the foods consumed with these approaches are typically low in energy density (e.g., fruits, vegetables, whole grains, and lean protein) and aim to support an estimated weight loss of about 1–2 lb (approximately 0.5–1 kg) per week.[91] Federal guidelines further encourage balanced macronutrient intake for optimal health (<30% fat, <10% saturated fat, 15% protein, and the remainder from carbohydrate) and should be considered when formulating dietary prescriptions together with the individual. Within a reduced-calorie eating plan, few studies have examined the impact of specific dietary patterns on weight loss. The use of single-serve, portion-controlled meals, reduction in sugar-sweetened beverage intake, and consumption of more calories earlier in the day instead of at night may suggest a positive association with weight loss and should be discussed with the individual as part of a reduced-calorie eating plan.[94] While often encouraged, there is limited evidence to support that the sole consumption of breakfast and/or fruits and vegetables (specifically), reduction of fast food intake, or increase in eating frequency will result in significant weight loss.[92] However, these patterns combined with additional efforts aimed at weight loss (i.e., calorie reduction, behavioral changes, and physical activity) have been shown to have a cumulative positive effect.[93,95] Further research is needed in these areas to determine the optimal dietary pattern for weight loss. Ultimately, the best prescription for the individual is one that is realistic and sustainable for their lifestyle.

Individuals seeking a more structured and specific meal prescription may benefit from the use of meal replacements. Meal replacements are typically defined as portion controlled, micronutrient-fortified entrees, shakes, and bars, and provide a convenient tool to reduce calories, manage portions, and

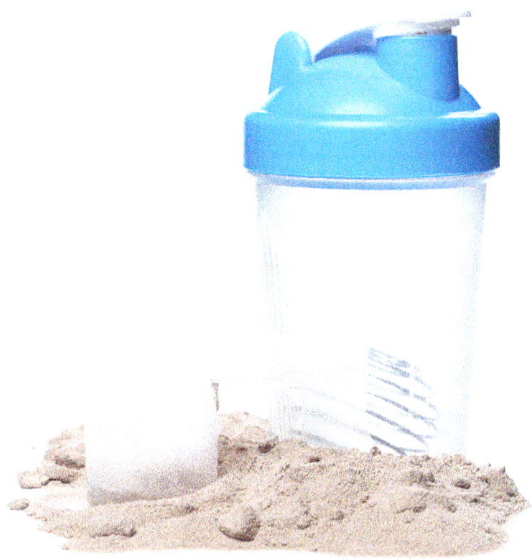

Figure 7.9 Meal Replacement Plans Often Include Protein Shakes

simplify meal preparation (**Figure 7.9**). Research has shown that the use of meal replacements leads to greater weight loss than a prescribed diet with the same number of calories where individuals are left to select their own foods.[96] Meal replacements are often used as part of low-calorie diet (LCD) and very low-calorie diet (VLCD) eating plans that prescribe highly specific food choices and calorie levels. An LCD usually consists of 800–1600 calories/day and may offer a partial or full meal replacement plan while a VLCD consists of <800 calories/day and usually consists of liquid shakes only.[92] Given the significant calorie reduction of a VLCD plan, this approach requires close medical monitoring and is best delivered by a trained interventionist. This is due to rapid weight loss and the potential for health complications.[3] A VLCD will produce the greatest amount of weight loss; however, it is less frequently used as an intervention compared to an LCD. Research from randomized-controlled trials suggests that both an LCD and VLCD plan result in similar weight loss at 1 year.[92,93] Meal replacements are often used for weight loss prior to **metabolic and bariatric surgery**. The Clinical Controversy in this chapter explores the evidence around this practice.[97,98]

Behavior

Behavior modification interventions should focus on habits that will encourage weight loss including self-monitoring of food intake (such as paper or electronic records), physical activity (such as activity meters, step counters), and weight; goal setting; stress reduction techniques; stimulus control; and sustainable approaches to problem solving via cognitive restructuring. Self-monitoring in the form of food journals or records is associated with greater weight loss when compared to not self-monitoring.[93] Many new tools have emerged over the years to track intake and physical activity, including phone-based apps and online programs that allow individuals to search specific foods and track total calorie and nutrient intake. These programs have many advantages, although individuals should be aware of potential challenges when interpreting data such as user error, under- or overestimation of portion sizes, and preloaded program data that may be inaccurate such as the number of calories in a certain food.

Cognitive approaches involved in behavior change focus on building skills and habits that will promote long-term weight maintenance. Cognitive behavior therapy (CBT) aims to help individuals examine the role that their thought process plays in behavior and can help to identify cognitive distortions such as "all-or-nothing thinking" that are commonly observed in humans and in weight loss therapy.[95] Use of motivational interviewing techniques by a provider encourages collaboration with the individual rather than control and aims to enhance motivation and self-efficacy to ultimately drive behavior change.[92] Current research suggests that no one behavior change strategy is best for weight loss and that a combination can be used in effective treatment.[92]

Behavior interventions can be offered in a variety of settings including clinical, community, commercial, and electronic. Intensive behavioral therapy (IBT) programs are often offered in the academic and clinic setting and involve a medical interprofessional team consisting of a physician, physician's assistant, behavioral provider, and RD. While these programs can be very effective (i.e., Diabetes Prevention Program [DPP]), they may also be expensive and difficult for some individuals to access.[99] In one study where a version of the DPP was adopted at a YMCA community setting, participants lost 6% of their starting weight compared to 2% in the control group and paid a fraction of the cost of an IBT program.[99] Commercial weight loss programs such as Weight Watchers™, Jenny Craig™, and Nutrisystem™ are widely available and utilize a variety of behavior strategies such as prepackaged meals, dietary counseling, group support, and self-monitoring. Emerging evidence also supports the use of electronically delivered interventions (such as telephone- or internet-based) when in-person visits are not possible. These types of programs are effective for weight loss, although generally less is observed than with in-person visits.[3]

⚠ Clinical Controversy

Weight Loss Before Metabolic and Bariatric Surgery
Patients undergoing metabolic and bariatric surgery (MBS) are often encouraged to lose weight prior to their procedure. Some literature suggests that weight loss may improve surgical outcomes such as operating times, re-operation rate, risk of infection, and overall patient safety. Following a nutrition plan such as a very low-calorie diet (VLCD) preoperatively via meal replacements or a standard food diet can help to achieve this weight loss. However, there is much debate as to whether preoperative weight loss improves outcomes significantly enough to warrant it. Recent research suggests that preoperative weight loss serves as an unnecessary barrier to a population that is having difficulty managing weight to begin with and does not predict postoperative weight loss.

Questions

1. Based upon the studies referenced, how might you apply evidence-based findings when deciding how to discuss weight loss before MBS?
2. Discuss the potential risks and benefits of providing a VLCD.
3. What factors might you consider when deciding on the best approach with the patient?

References

1. Schouten et al. Comparison of preoperative diets before bariatric surgery: a randomized, single blinded, non-inferiority trial. *Obes Surg*. 2016;26:1743–1749.
2. Bettini S, Belligoli A, Fabris R, Busetto L. Diet approach before and after bariatric surgery. *Rev Endocr Metab Disord*. 2020;21(3):297–306.

CASE STUDY REVISITED

Allison has participated in a behavioral weight management program for 6 months but found that this form of lifestyle intervention did not result in significant weight loss, significant biochemical change, or improvements in body composition.

Anthropometric Data:

Weight: 94 kg
Height: 158 cm
BMI: 38 kg/m^2

Biochemical Data:

Fasting Blood Glucose: 152 mg/dL (70–99 mg/dL)
Hemoglobin A1c: 7.9% (4.3–5.6%)

Questions

1. Following lifestyle intervention, what other treatment options are available to Allison?
2. What are potential advantages and disadvantages of these interventions?

Physical Activity

Regular physical activity can help some individuals lose weight, although it is more effective at maintaining weight or preventing weight regain following a loss (**Figure 7.10**).[100] Research suggests that caloric restriction is more effective at achieving weight loss compared to physical activity on its own, although increasing physical activity is an important part of health maintenance. When prescribed adjunct to calorie reduction, exercise may result in an additional 1–3% of weight loss.[9] Individuals should be encouraged to participate in at least 150 minutes of moderately intense physical activity (e.g., walking) per week with an additional 2 days of strength training to achieve health benefits and prevent weight gain.[94,101]

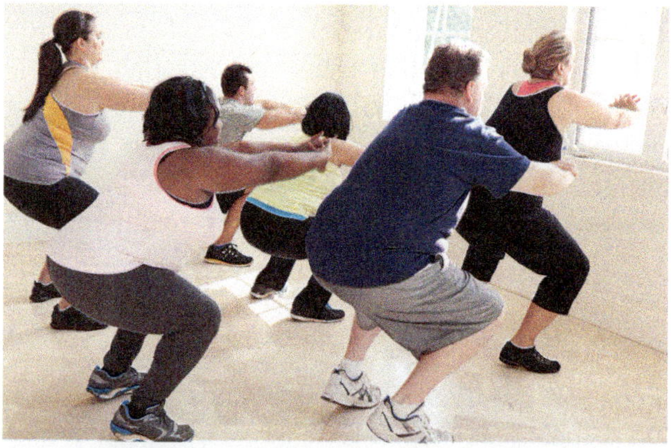

Figure 7.10 Regular Physical Activity Can Help Individuals Lose Weight, Maintain Weight Loss, and Prevent Weight Regain

More clinically significant weight loss is observed in individuals with overweight and obesity when a level of >250 minutes/week is achieved.[94] Individuals who are sedentary should be encouraged to gradually increase their physical activity and participate in activity that is both sustainable and enjoyable.

Results from the largest U.S. weight loss study (Look AHEAD) show successful long-term weight loss maintenance following an intensive lifestyle intervention (>1 year comprehensive program).[102] This study found that participants in the lifestyle intervention program maintained more than half of their weight loss after 8 years and almost 40% of those who lost ≥10% of initial weight after the first year maintained the loss by the eighth year. This study shows meaningful results given its long duration and high retention rate and participants likely achieved positive outcomes due to the intensive and comprehensive nature of the intervention.

Experts have proposed several recommendations for long-term weight loss maintenance. These include regular follow-up contact every other week (or monthly if biweekly is not possible) for 1 year with a trained interventionist (such as an RD) in either a group or individual setting.[103,104] Individuals should follow a reduced-calorie diet necessary to maintain their lower body weight. Physical activity, as mentioned previously, is also an essential component of long-term weight management. Individuals should aim to participate in 200–300 minutes/week of moderately vigorous aerobic activity. Occasional use of food records and/or activity monitoring tools may be beneficial. In addition, individuals should weigh themselves twice per week or daily and participate in a behavior-change program that provides feedback on setback prevention and problem solving.[103,105]

PRACTICE POINT

For health benefits, individuals should participate in at least 150 minutes/week of moderately vigorous physical activity with additional recommended strength training. For weight loss and maintenance, individuals should be instructed to participate in 200–300 minutes/week of moderately vigorous aerobic activity.

PRACTICE POINT

When creating a lifestyle program for weight management, aim for 14 or more sessions over a 6-month period led by a trained interventionist, such as an RD.

Pharmacotherapy

The use of medications to assist in weight loss is appropriate for those with a BMI ≥30 kg/m^2 or those with a BMI ≥27 kg/m^2 with a comorbid condition (e.g., HTN or T2DM) (**Figures 7.11A** and **7.11B**). Any individual being treated with medications for overweight or obesity should also participate in lifestyle modification through diet and exercise to maximize efforts.[3,106] In 2012, the FDA approved two drugs for the treatment of overweight and obesity, marketed as Belviq (Lorcaserin), which has since been removed due to cancer risk, and Qsymia (Phentermine/Topiramate).

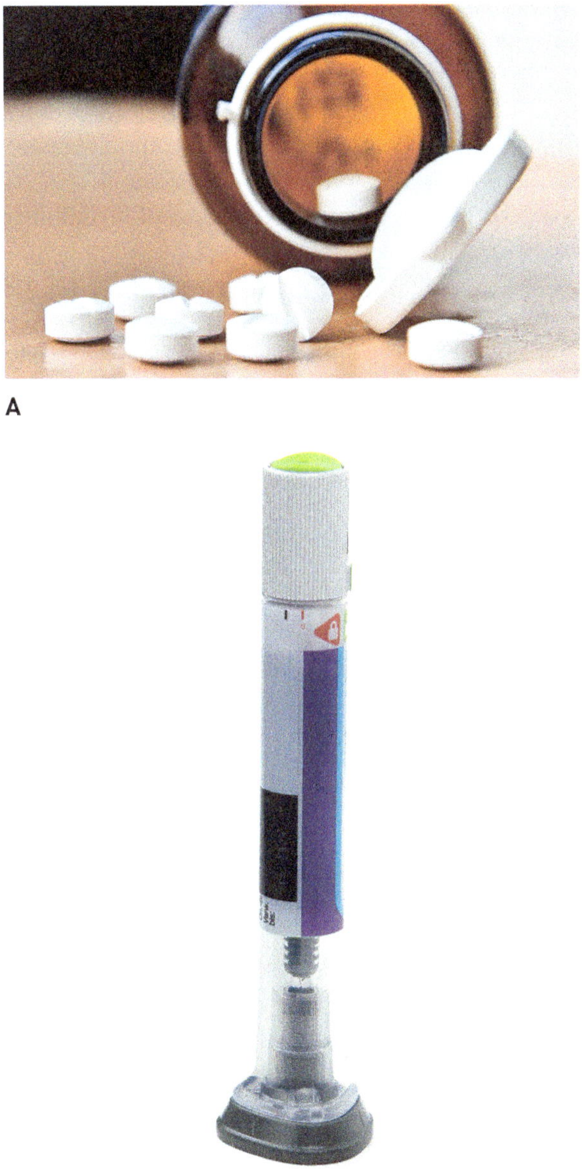

A

B

Figure 7.11 Pharmacotherapy for Weight Loss Can Be Used for Individuals with a BMI ≥30 or Those with a BMI ≥27 with a Comorbid Condition. **A.** Pharmacotherapy as oral medications **B.** Pharmacotherapy as an injectable pen

At the time, these were the first drugs approved for long-term weight management in 13 years.[107] Since then, several other medications have been approved by the FDA including Wegovy (Semaglutide), a subcutaneous, injectable medication that improves satiety by mimicking the actions of the hormone GLP-1, and Zepbound (Tirzepatide), an injectable medication that both mimics GLP-1 and serves as a GIP inhibitor. Clinical trials involving medication for weight management have demonstrated weight loss in the 5–22.5% range, with greater losses attributed to newer, injectable medications. Physicians may occasionally prescribe medications, such as metformin, for reasons other than weight loss, which can result in weight loss as a side effect. The use of medications in this way is deemed "off label" use. Medications for the treatment of overweight and obesity will be most effective with long-term use, when combined with lifestyle modifications, and when used under medical supervision.[106] A list of commonly prescribed FDA-approved weight loss medications are described in **Table 7.5**.

CORE CONCEPT 5

Approaches to obesity management include individual and comprehensive lifestyle intervention, pharmacotherapy, and metabolic and bariatric surgery.

Metabolic and Bariatric Surgery

The rise in obesity has led to an increased number of MBS procedures over the years. Over half a million operations were performed in 2021 worldwide[108] with 262,893 in the United States.[109] For the past 30 years, the guidelines proposed by the National Institutes of Health Consensus Statement on Gastrointestinal Surgery for Severe Obesity[110] served as standards for insurance coverage and obesity care. These guidelines proposed that MBS be considered for individuals with a BMI >35 kg/m^2 with significant comorbidities or for those with a BMI >40 kg/m^2 with or without comorbidities[110] (**Table 7.6**). In 2022, the American Society for Metabolic and Bariatric Surgery (ASMBS) and the International Federation for the Surgery of Obesity and Metabolic Disorders (IFSO) proposed new standards based on updated research, advocating to lower the BMI criteria for MBS.[111] MBS is widely considered the most effective long-term treatment for obesity and lowering the BMI criteria would increase access to care.[111]

Procedure Type

There are several types of MBS procedures that support weight loss and work through different mechanisms. These include restrictive, malabsorptive, or both restrictive and malabsorptive procedures.

CASE STUDY REVISITED

One year later, Allison noticed a further increase in her weight, and she is seeking a more effective intervention to improve her weight and T2DM. She shares that she tried a GLP-1 agonist medication and lost 15 lb (6.8 kg) but does not want to take a medication for the rest of her life. Meal replacements and very low-calorie diets also did not yield long-term weight loss results.

Anthropometric Data:

Weight: 104.5 kg
Height: 158 cm
BMI: 42 kg/m^2

Clinical Data:

Allison has newly diagnosed obstructive sleep apnea.

Biochemical Data:

Fasting Blood Glucose: 165 mg/dL (70–99 mg/dL)

HbA1c: 9.4% (4.3–5.6%)

Questions

1. Assess Allison's PES statement(s) from her initial RD encounter. Identify if each statement remains an active issue or if the PES statement has been resolved. If the PES statement remains an active issue, is it being addressed and/or has improvement in the issue been noted? If the issue has been resolved, write a new PES statement.
2. Having tried lifestyle intervention and pharmacotherapy with limited long-term changes in her weight, T2DM, and OSA, what are Allison's options for improvement in comorbidity?
3. How does Allison's anthropometric, biochemical, and clinical data guide this decision?

Table 7.5 FDA-Approved Weight Loss Medications

Medication Name	Brand Name	Mechanism of Action	Contraindications
Phentermine	Adipex, Suprenza	Releases norepinephrine	Heart disease, uncontrolled HTN, pregnancy, breastfeeding, hyperthyroidism, substance use disorder, use of monoamine oxidase inhibitors (MAOIs)
Diethylproprion	Tenuate	Releases norepinephrine	Same as phentermine
Phendimetrazine	Bontril	Releases norepinephrine	Same as phentermine
Benzphentamine	Didrex	Releases norepinephrine	Same as phentermine
Orlistat	Alli, Xenical	Inhibits pancreatic and gastric lipases	Pregnancy, breastfeeding, use of levothyroxine or warfarin, malabsorption syndrome, use of seizure drugs
Phentermine/ Topiramate	Qsymia	Releases norepinephrine, modulates gamma-aminobutyric acid	Pregnancy, breastfeeding, hyperthyroidism, use of MAOIs, glaucoma
Naltrexone/ bupropion	Contrave	Opioid antagonist; inhibits dopamine and norepinephrine uptake	Uncontrolled HTN, seizures, use of MAOIs, anorexia, bulimia, opioid/alcohol use disorder
Setmelanotide	Imcivree	Melanocortin 4 (MCR) agonist	Lack of ultra-rare genetic disease: proopiomelanocortin (POMC), proprotein convertase subtilisin/kexin type 1 (PCSK1), leptin receptor (LEPR) deficiencies; pregnancy
Liraglutide	Saxenda	Activates GLP-1	Medullary thyroid carcinoma history, multiple endocrine neoplasia type 2 history, pancreatitis history
Semaglutide	Wegovy	Activates GLP-1	Medullary thyroid carcinoma history, multiple endocrine neoplasia type 2 history, pancreatitis, pregnancy
Tirzepatide	Zepbound	Activates GLP-1, Inhibits GIP	Medullary thyroid carcinoma history, multiple endocrine neoplasia type 2 history, pancreatitis, pregnancy

Data from National Institute of Diabetes and Digestive and Kidney Diseases. Prescription medications to treat overweight and obesity. Accessed January 12, 2026. https://www.niddk.nih.gov/health-information/weight-management/prescription-medications-treat-overweight-obesity

Table 7.6 Inclusion and Exclusion Criteria for Consideration of Metabolic and Bariatric Surgery

	1991 NIH Guidelines	2022 ASMBS/IFSO Guidelines
Guidelines Comparison	Class 2 obesity: BMI >35 kg/m^2 with comorbid conditions: ■ HTN ■ T2DM ■ OSA ■ Coronary artery disease OR Class 3 obesity: BMI >40 kg/m^2 with or without comorbidity	Class 2 obesity: BMI >35 kg/m^2 OR Class 1 obesity: BMI 30–34.9 kg/m^2 with comorbid conditions: ■ HTN ■ T2DM ■ OSA Coronary artery disease
Inclusion Criteria	■ Absence of medical contraindications ■ Little results with nonsurgical weight loss ■ Well-informed, adherent, motivated patient	
Antineoplastic agents	■ Uncontrolled, severe psychiatric illness ■ Reversible endocrine or other disorders that can cause obesity ■ Current substance use disorder	

Data from Eisenberg D, Shikora SA, Aarts E, et al. 2022 American Society for Metabolic and Bariatric Surgery (ASMBS) and International Federation for the Surgery of Obesity and Metabolic Disorders (IFSO): indications for metabolic and bariatric surgery. *Surg Obes Relat Dis*. 2022;18(12):1345-1356. doi:10.1016/j.soard.2022.08.013.

CASE STUDY REVISITED

After evaluation by an RD, physician, and psychologist, the interprofessional team recommends metabolic and bariatric surgery for Allison. Allison agrees that this may be the best approach given her elevated BMI, related health conditions, and previous attempts at significant and long-term weight loss. She is referred for a surgical evaluation.

Questions

1. What are advantages and disadvantages of metabolic and bariatric surgery?
2. Which surgery would have the greatest likelihood of improving Allison's T2DM?

1. Restrictive procedures
    - **Laparoscopic adjustable gastric band (LAGB)**

Adjustable Gastric Band (Lap Band)

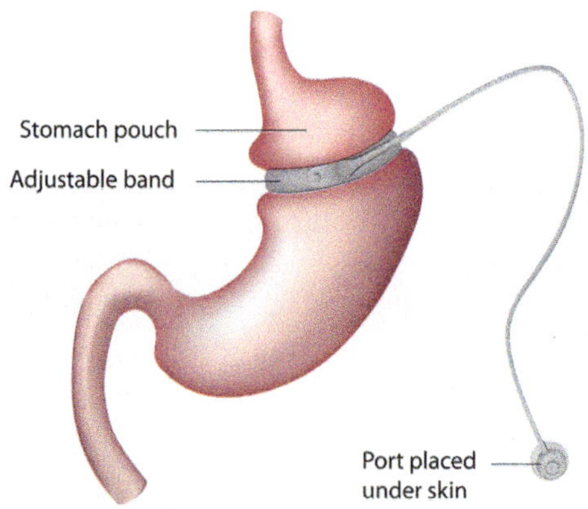

© Alila Medical Media/Shutterstock

2. Restrictive and malabsorptive (combination):
    - **Sleeve gastrectomy (SG)** (mostly restrictive)
    - **Roux-en-Y gastric bypass (RYGB)**

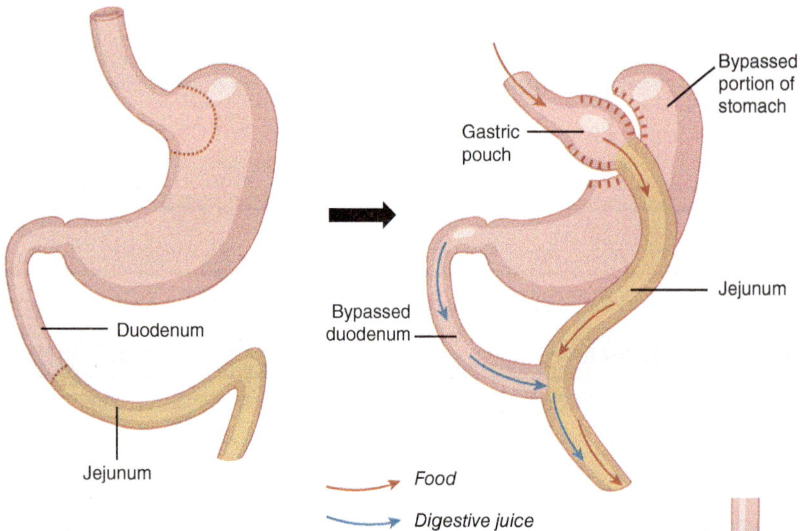

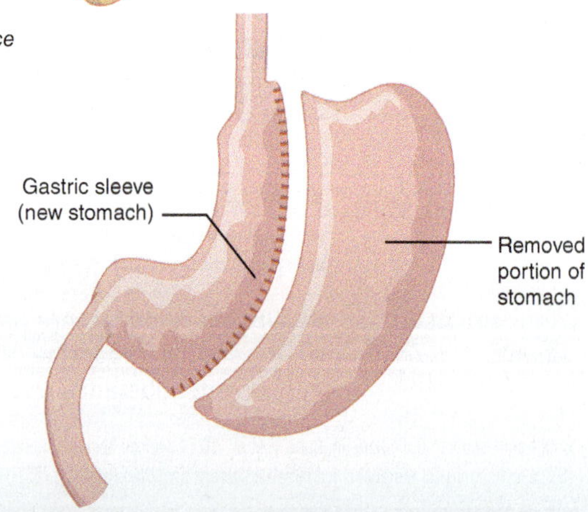

3. Malabsorptive procedures:
    - Biliopancreatic diversion (BPD)
    - BPD with duodenal switch (BPD/DS)

Restrictive Procedures

Laparoscopic Adjustable Gastric Banding (LAGB). The LAGB was first utilized in the United States in 2001.[112] It works by physically restricting the stomach, decreasing the overall transit time of food leading to early sense of satiety and decreased intake.[112] A small pouch is created by placing a hollow, silicone band around the top part of the stomach. The band is then tethered to a tubing connected to a port that is placed just underneath the skin. Approximately 6 weeks after placement, the band is inflated by injection of a small amount of saline into the port. These saline injections are called "fills" or "adjustments" and are completed over a period of 6–8 weeks until the right amount of restriction is achieved to reduce the size of the individual's intake. The LAGB requires regular medical follow-up for band adjustment at which time counseling sessions with the RD and behavioral health provider should also be offered. Following band placement, discussion topics could include intuitive and nutrient dense eating, slow eating, thorough chewing, and limiting of foods that could potentially risk obstruction. Soft, high-calorie foods and beverages (i.e., sodas, juices, chips, ice cream, etc.) can more easily pass through the restricted outlet, although can also lead to excess caloric intake. Individuals opting for a LAGB should be aware of this side effect.

Many individuals are initially attracted to the LAGB due to its less invasive and potentially reversible nature when compared to other MBS procedures. Average total weight loss (TWL) with the band is estimated to be about 20% within 1–2 year postsurgery and 14% at 10-years postsurgery.[113] In 2008, the LAGB accounted for over 90% of outpatient metabolic and bariatric procedures in the United States, although numbers have fallen dramatically.[109,114] The potential long-term complications associated with the band include band slippage, erosion, infection, and scar tissue formation, which have led to reports of a reoperation rate of up to 60%.[115] Additionally, inadequate weight loss is the most reported basis for reoperation.[3,116] Many surgeons are converting the LAGB to the SG or RYGB and, more recently, surgeons are choosing to perform the SG.

Combination Procedures

Sleeve Gastrectomy (SG). The SG was initially used as a first step approach to the biliopancreatic diversion-duodenal switch (BPD/DS) procedure as individuals with severe obesity are at high risk for surgical complications. Following the start of SG procedures, research demonstrated effective weight loss, making this its own standalone procedure. The SG involves a left partial gastrectomy, which removes about 80% of the stomach including the fundus and greater curvature. The remaining gastric pouch resembles the shape of a banana or sleeve. While the SG was initially thought to induce weight loss primarily through restriction, research shows that there are resulting gut hormonal changes and metabolic influences including the reduction of ghrelin and increase in satiety hormones such as GLP-1. This leads to improvement in blood sugar control, increased satiety, and reduced hunger.[112]

In 2013, the SG surpassed the RYGB as the most utilized procedure in the United States and its numbers continue to climb.[109] This is due to its significant weight loss results with reduced postsurgical complications compared to the RYGB.[112] The average TWL following the SG is around 25%.[117] While there is limited long-term data on micronutrient deficiencies after SG, short-term studies have shown that there may be some risk involved. The current recommendations for daily vitamin and mineral supplementation are essentially the same as those for RYGB. Long-term (greater than 5–10 years) outcome data is needed to fully assess its efficacy.

Roux-en-y Gastric Bypass (RYGB). The RYGB is considered a combination procedure involving both restriction and malabsorption and is widely accepted as the "gold standard" in metabolic and bariatric surgery. Although all the mechanisms by which the RYGB influences the weight regulatory system are not fully understood, there is strong evidence of changes in neural and hormonal pathways that favor durable and significant weight loss and improvement in obesity-related comorbid conditions. In the RYGB, a small gastric pouch is created in the upper portion of the stomach by dividing and reattaching the stomach and the distal jejunum. The remaining stomach, duodenum, and proximal jejunum are bypassed, and the remaining stomach aids in digestion by producing enzymes that will eventually mix with food in the jejunum. The accelerated passage of undigested nutrients directly into the jejunum activates chemoreceptors that decrease hunger and that stimulate satiety.[118] Changes in GLP-1 and PYY have been well studied. More recent data supports that there may be specific effects of RYGB surgery on the microbiota that influence on weight loss.[119] These combined factors may contribute to the long-term effectiveness of the RYGB and other combination procedures, with excess weight loss of 60–80%.[119] Improvement or remission

Table 7.7 Morbidity Outcomes: Percentage of Patients Who Achieved Comorbidity Remission or Significant Improvement at 1-Year Post Surgery

	Metabolic and Bariatric Surgery Type		
Condition	Roux-en-Y gastric bypass (RYGB)	Sleeve Gastrectomy (SG)	Laparoscopic Adjustable Gastric Banding (LAGB)
Type 2 diabetes	83%	55%	44%
Hypertension	79%	68%	44%
Hyperlipidemia	66%	35%	33%
Sleep apnea	66%	62%	38%
Gastroesophageal reflux	70%	55%	64%

Data from a longitudinal data collection system including 109 hospitals and 28,616 patients. Modified from Hutter MM, Schirmer BD, Jones DB, et al. *Ann Surg*. 2011;254(3):410-422.

of obesity-related comorbidities such as T2DM have been well documented, often occurring independent of weight loss and is usually seen within days of surgery (**Table 7.7**). Risks for complications (14.6%) include infection, bleeding, stricture, obstruction, and dehydration.[120] The mortality rate is relatively low at around 0.1%.[120] Since major parts of the stomach, the entire duodenum, and proximal jejunum are bypassed, individuals are at risk for micronutrient deficiencies such as vitamin B12, iron, zinc, thiamine, calcium, and vitamin D, among others. Individuals need to consent to lifelong vitamin and mineral supplementation to ensure optimal body functioning.

Comorbidity Outcomes

The RYGB has the greatest documented improvement in comorbidities as compared to the SG and the LAGB. The 30-day postoperative complication rate is slightly higher (5.6 vs. 5.9) for the RYGB compared to the SG, while weight loss and improvement of comorbidities is higher with the RYGB.[121] Reports of T2DM remission post metabolic and bariatric surgery vary significantly. In a recent randomized controlled trial conducted by Shauer et al.,[122] there was 45% full remission at 1 year in patients post RYGB.

The changes that occur due to the manipulation of the stomach and/or digestive tract have been a field of investigation for the past decade, particularly related to gut hormones (**Table 7.8**). The mechanisms are not fully known, although the durability of weight loss is most likely due to changes in the physiological regulation of body weight. The Swedish Obese Subjects (SOS) study showed that patients who had MBS who maintained a loss of 15–25% of initial weight 10 years later had a 29% reduction in all-cause mortality, when compared with a control group that was matched on 18 characteristics. The major reductions in mortality resulted from decreases in cardiovascular and cancer-related deaths. Due to its metabolic impact on the body and the durability of weight loss for patients post MBS it is considered one of the most effective therapies for obesity management.

There is no standardization of diet stages, but **Table 7.9** outlines diet advancement protocols providing adequate fluid, protein, and fiber intake, as well as proper texture progression for individuals who undergo MBS.

Micronutrient Concerns

Following MBS, individuals need additional supplementation for vitamins and minerals compared to individuals who have not undergone surgery. There are several micronutrients that can become deficient based on the type of surgery performed. Across all procedures, the most common are vitamin B12, iron, zinc, folate, copper, thiamine, calcium, and vitamin D. Recommendations for dosages and frequency of vitamins and minerals are established by the ASMBS. These are described in **Tables 7.10** and **7.11**.

PRACTICE POINT

Following MBS, individuals will need to take additional vitamin and mineral supplements to prevent deficiencies in vitamin B12, iron, zinc, folate, copper, thiamine, calcium, and vitamin D.

Table 7.8 Gut Hormones and Mechanisms of Weight Loss After Metabolic and Bariatric Surgery

Gut Hormone/Mechanism	Roux-en-Y Gastric Bypass (RYGB) Postprandial	Sleeve Gastrectomy (SG) Postprandial	Laparoscopic Adjustable Gastric Banding (LAGB)
GLP-1 ■ Slows gastric emptying ■ Inhibits glucagon secretion ■ Acts synergistically with PYY: satiety and inhibits food intake ■ Augments the insulin response to nutrients	Increased	Increased	No effect
PYY ■ Shown to induce satiety and reduce food intake ■ Inhibitory effect on GI mobility	Increased	Increased	No effect
Ghrelin ■ Produced from the fundus of the stomach and the proximal intestine ■ Only known orexigenic gut hormone ■ Primary source is the gastric mucosa ■ Nutrient exposure to the small intestine is sufficient for food-induced ghrelin suppression in humans; therefore, gastric nutrient exposure is not necessary for suppression	Inconclusive	Decreased	Ghrelin has been shown to increase in response to caloric restriction after LAGB as seen in low-calorie dieting; this may be the reason for less weight loss and more hunger in patients post-LAGB

Data from Stefater MA, Wilson-Perez HE, Chambers AP, et al. *Endocr Rev*. 2013;33(4):595-622.; Pournaras DJ, le Roux CW. *World J Surg*. 2009;33:1983-1988.; Ochner CN, Gibson C, Shanik N, et al. *Int J Obes*. 2011;36:153-166.

Table 7.9 Diet Stage Progression Following Metabolic and Bariatric Surgery

LAGB, RYGB, SG Diet Stage	Duration of Intervention	Food/Fluid Stage	Diet Guidelines	Supplements
Stage I	1/2 day	Water	Take sips of water and ice chips only	
Stage II	1/2–1 day	Clear Liquids ■ Low-sugar or artificially sweetened liquids ■ Salty/savory fluids ■ Solid liquids such as sugar-free popsicles ■ Less than 25 grams sugar per serving in full liquids ■ Protein-rich liquids (15–30 grams protein per serving)	Minimum 48–64 oz total fluids per day: 24–32 oz or more ounce clear liquids; plus 24–32 oz any combination of full liquids: Low-fat or fat-free milk mixed with: ■ Whey or soy protein powder (limit 20 g protein per serving) ■ Lactose-free milk or soy milk mix with soy protein powder ■ Light yogurt, blended ■ Plain yogurt	Begin supplementation: ■ Chewable multivitamin with minerals, 2×/day ■ Chewable or liquid 1200–1500 mg/day calcium citrate with vitamin D

(continues)

Table 7.9 Diet Stage Progression Following Metabolic and Bariatric Surgery (continued)

LAGB, RYGB, SG Diet Stage	Duration of Intervention	Food/Fluid Stage	Diet Guidelines	Supplements
Stage III:	2 weeks	Full liquids with soft, moist, and/or semi-solid protein sources as tolerated Stage III protein sources: Protein shakes, milk and soy milk, low-sugar yogurts, low-fat cottage cheese, sugar-free pudding, bone broth, Egg whites	Protein food choices are encouraged 3–6 times per day; patients may only be able to tolerate a few tbsp at each meal/snack. Mindful, slow eating is essential. Patients should not drink with meals and wait 30 minutes after each meal before resuming fluids	Daily supplements essential
Stage IV:	4 weeks	High-protein, low-fat, low-sugar solids Stage IV foods: Stage III foods plus eggs, ground meats, lean poultry, soft, moist fish, (add gravy, bouillon, light mayo, low-fat/low-sugar condiments to moisten) cooked beans and bean soups, tbsp of all-natural nut/seed butters Advance diet as tolerated. If protein foods are well tolerated and meet protein needs, can add well-cooked, soft vegetables; and soft and/or peeled fruit. Protein first	High-protein, low-fat, low-sugar solids Stage IV foods: Stage III foods plus eggs, ground meats, lean poultry, soft, moist fish, (add gravy, bouillon, light mayo, low-fat/low-sugar condiments to moisten) cooked beans and bean soups, tbsp of all-natural nut/seed butters Advance diet as tolerated. If protein foods are well tolerated and meet protein needs, can add well-cooked, soft vegetables; and soft and/or peeled fruit.	Daily supplements essential
Stage V:	Long-term	Continue to consume protein with some fruit or vegetable at each meal; some people tolerate salads 1 month to 6 weeks postop	**AVOID** rice, bread, and pasta until comfortably consuming adequate protein per day and fruits/vegetables. Aim for high fiber, complex sources in small portion. Focus on small frequent meals that include a lean protein source, added fiber from fruit or vegetables, and small amounts of starch once tolerating it. Continue to take daily vitamin/mineral supplements. Starches and grains can be gradually introduced once consistently meeting protein and fluid targets and weight stabilizes. Long-term nutrition and energy needs based on height, weight, age, and activity level.	Daily supplements essential Nutritional labs should be drawn 3, 6, 12 months and annually indefinitely for RYGB and SG and at 1, 2, and 12 months for LAGB** Bone density test at baseline and every 2 years

*Roux-en-Y gastric bypass (RYGB)

**Laparoscopic adjustable gastric banding (LAGB)

***There is no standardization of diet stages, but the above diet advancement protocol provides adequate fluid, protein, and fiber intake, as well as proper texture progression.

****Similar nutrition guidelines and dietary advancements are recommended for various MBS procedures.

Data from Majumdar MC, Isom KA; Weight Management Dietetic Practice Group. *Pocket Guide to Bariatric Surgery*. 3rd ed. Academy of Nutrition and Dietetics; 2021.

Clinical Roundtable

Topic: Benefits and Risks of GLP-1 Receptor Agonist Medications

Background: GLP-1 receptor agonist medications (GLP-1s) have been utilized for the treatment of T2DM since 2005 and work to effectively lower HbA1c. When initially prescribed, weight loss was a common side effect, but historically not the primary reason for use. More recently, the FDA approved liraglutide, semaglutide, and tirzepatide for the treatment of obesity, and research suggests that some individuals can lose more than 20% of their total body weight when taking the medication regularly. As a result, the demand for GLP-1s has quickly increased. The health benefits of GLP-1s extend beyond weight loss and blood glucose management; however, studies show that weekly use reduces the incidence of death from cardiovascular disease, heart attacks, and strokes in individuals with existing disease when compared to a placebo. This result was observed in individuals without T2DM, suggesting the GLP-1s may possibly have a role in reducing risk for cardiovascular disease. However, there have been reports of adverse GI side effects including nausea, vomiting, and abdominal pain, leading the FDA to list delayed gastric emptying on the semaglutide label. There has also been rare reports of pulmonary aspiration when GLP-1s were provided during the perioperative period.

Roundtable Discussion:

1. Should GLP-1 receptor agonist medications such as semaglutide be used in patients "off label" for significant cardiovascular disease?
2. What factors would you consider when recommending this type of treatment?
3. How might using this medication impact an individual's nutritional intake?
4. How might a clinician weigh the risks and benefits of GLP-1 receptor agonist medications?

References

1. Jastreboff AM, Aronne LJ, Ahmad NN, et al. Tirzepatide once weekly for the treatment of obesity. *N Engl J Med*. 2022;387(3):205–216. doi:10.1056/NEJMoa2206038
2. Lincoff AM, Brown-Frandsen K, Colhoun HM,et al. Semaglutide and cardiovascular outcomes in obesity without diabetes. *N Engl J Med*. 2023;389(24):2221–2232.
3. Gallagher A. FDA adds delayed gastric emptying as adverse event on semaglutide label. *Pharmacy Times*. November 12, 2024. Accessed December 1, 2024. https://www.pharmacytimes.com/view/fda-event-on-semaglutide-label
4. Kindel TL, Wang AY, Wadhwa A, et al. Multi-society clinical practice guidance for the safe use of glucagon-like peptide-1 receptor agonists in the perioperative period. *Surg Endosc*. 2025;39(1):180–183. doi:10.1007/s00464-024-11263-2

CASE STUDY REVISITED

Immediately following Allison's surgery, you are consulted to review Allison's dietary progression following the procedure.

Questions

1. What concerns might you have regarding Allison's nutritional status?
2. What are her short-term nutrition goals?
3. What are her long-term nutrition goals?
4. Which biochemical parameters would you monitor postoperatively?

Monitoring and Evaluation

Monitoring patients with obesity would include tracking weight and BMI to assess for weight loss or gain. Monitoring would also include evaluating oral intake, including portion sizes, timing of meals and snacks, self-monitoring and physical activity behaviors, medications, and sleep schedule. RDs should check biochemical measures including HbA1c, iron studies, and vitamin D. For those post MBS, it is critical to check supplement adherence. Finally, assessing barriers to weight loss efforts, ways to manage relapses,

Table 7.10 Potential Vitamin/Mineral Deficiencies After Metabolic and Bariatric Surgery

Vitamin/Mineral	Markers	Deficiency Prevalence Postprocedure	Repletion
Iron	Fe Ferritin TIBC	3 months to 10 years 14% LAGB <18% SG 20–25% RYGB 13–62% BPD 8–50% DS	150–300 mg 2–3×/day iron infusion
Vitamin B12	Serum B12 (cobalamin) MMA	2–5 years <20% RYGB 4–20% SG	1000 mcg orally/day 1000 mcg IM/month
Thiamine	Serum B1	<1–49%, depending on surgery May occur with IV hydration, vomiting	100 mg orally 2–3×/day 200 mg IV 3×/day 200 mg IM 1×/day
Folic acid	RBC folate	Reported in up to 65% patients	1000 mcg orally/day
Calcium	Serum Ca Phosphorous Alk Phos PTH Bone density	N/A	1500–2000 mg/day for LAGB, SG, RYGB 1800–2400 mg/day for BPD/DS
Vitamin D	25-OH Vitamin D PTH Alk Phos	Up to 100% of patients	2000–6000 IU/day 50,000 IU D2 1–2×/week for 5–8 weeks, recheck
Vitamin A **Vitamin E** **Vitamin K**	Plasma retinol Plasma alpha tocopherol Prothrombin time	Within 4 years 70% RYGB, BPD/DS Deficiencies uncommon	10,000–25,000 IU/day for 1–2 weeks 100–400 IU/day + 1–2 mg/day orally
Zinc	Plasma zinc	34% LAGB 19% SG 40% RYGB up to 70% BP/DS	Insufficient evidence to recommend dose
Copper	Serum copper Ceruloplasmin	As high as 10–20% RYGB 90% BPD/DS	3–8 mg/day oral copper gluconate or sulfate 2–4 mg/day IV copper for 6 days for severe deficiency

Data from Parrott J, et al. American Society for Metabolic and Bariatric Surgery integrated health nutritional guidelines for the surgical weight loss patient 2016 update: micronutrients. *Surg Obes Relat Dis*. 2017;13(5):727-741.

problem-solving strategies, patterns relating to eating out, and support systems is important to optimize success in weight loss efforts and quality of life.

Emerging Treatment Options

Many new treatment options for severe obesity have emerged over the past several years due to the relapsing nature of the condition and the need for less invasive procedures/treatments. These include electrical stimulation systems such as the Maestro Rechargeable System™, gastric emptying systems including the Aspire Assist™, and a variety of gastric balloon systems. Specifically, the Orbera™ intragastric balloon was approved by the FDA in August 2015.[123] This device is a system that uses a gastric balloon to occupy space in the stomach (**Figure 7.12**). Once the balloon is in place, it is filled with 400–700 mL of saline to occupy the stomach and assist in reducing food intake. The balloon is only intended for temporary use

Table 7.11 Current Standard for Vitamin Mineral Supplementation After Metabolic and Bariatric Surgery*

Supplement	Dosage
Multivitamin First month, chewable 2×/day	100–200% daily value
Calcium citrate with Vitamin D (Citrate preferred) Divided doses for maximum absorption	1200–1500 mg/day 400–800 IU of vitamin D
Vitamin D	3000 IU daily
Elemental iron contained in multivitamin; additional as indicated (not to be taken with calcium)	18–27 mg/day elemental 40–65 mg/day for menstruating females
Vitamin B12	350–500 mcg/day orally/—sublingual/nasal or 1000 mcg IM

*Patients with preoperative or postoperative biochemical deficiency states are treated beyond these recommendations.

Data from Mechanick JI, Youdim A, Jones DB, et al. Clinical practice guidelines for the perioperative nutritional, metabolic, and nonsurgical support of the bariatric surgery patient—2013 update: cosponsored by the American Association of Clinical Endocrinologists, The Obesity Society, and the American Society for Metabolic & Bariatric Surgery. *Endocr Pract*. 2013;19(2):337-372. doi:10.4158/EP12437.GL

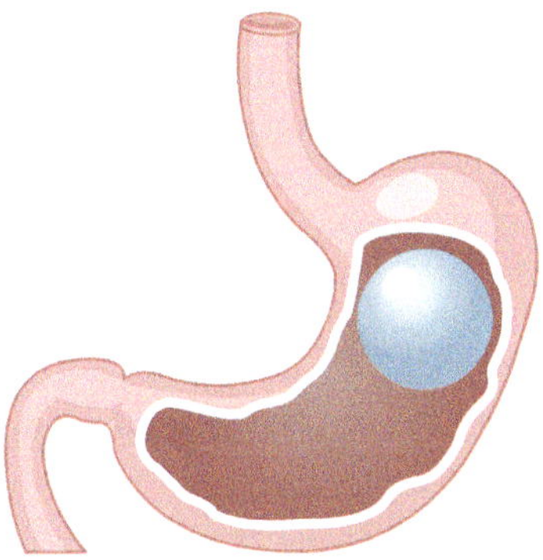

Figure 7.12 Intragastric Balloon

and should be removed after 6 months. It is approved for adults with a BMI of 30–40 kg/m^2.

A meta-analysis of the Orbera™ intragastric balloon found an average of 32.1% excess weight loss of 32.1% after 6 months with improvements in blood pressure, fasting glucose, and lipid profile.[124] Significant improvements in HbA1c have been observed among patients with T2DM who have used Orbera™. However, more research is needed on long-term weight maintenance after the intragastric balloon. Nutrition guidelines following placement of the intragastric balloon have also not yet been established by the ASMBS. In general, the RD should work closely with the patient to ensure that they are following a nutrient-dense meal plan and meeting micronutrient needs. This procedure is considered investigational and therefore not yet covered, and the cost may be prohibitive for many individuals. Other endoscopic procedures are currently under investigation and aim to bridge the gap between medication and metabolic and bariatric surgery by providing effective, but less invasive, methods for weight loss.

Chapter Summary

The topic of weight in health is complex. Obesity is a medical term used to describe a state where excess body mass exists and its connotation comes with an unfortunate level of stigma for individuals with this condition. Obesity involves a variety of interacting genetic, environmental, social, biological, and developmental factors and is a risk factor for several health conditions including T2DM, hyperlipidemia, HTN, heart disease, stroke, certain cancers, MASLD, OSA, gallbladder disease, respiratory problems, arthritis, and depression. Due to its high prevalence rate in the United States, it remains a significant health concern for Americans. Many approaches exist to address the condition. The cornerstone of weight management is facilitating change through a comprehensive lifestyle program that includes diet, physical activity, and behavior modification. All lifestyle interventions should be individualized. Adjunct approaches include pharmacological treatments that can augment lifestyle programs and metabolic and bariatric surgery that can elicit metabolic improvement yielding durable results. Despite these advanced therapies, continued treatment and ongoing support are necessary to maintain optimal health.

Key Terms

obesity, body mass index (BMI), ghrelin, leptin, orexigenic, anorexigenic, adipose, metabolic and bariatric surgery, laparoscopic adjustable gastric band (LAGB), sleeve gastrectomy (SG), Roux-en-Y gastric bypass (RYGB)

References

1. World Health Organization. Obesity and Overweight. Accessed February 19, 2024. https://www.who.int/news-room/fact-sheets/detail/obesity-and-overweight
2. Centers for Disease Control and Prevention. Childhood Overweight and Obesity. Accessed February 19, 2024. https://www.cdc.gov/obesity/childhood/index.html
3. Jensen MD, Ryan DH, Apovian CM, et al. 2013 AHA/ACC/TOS Guideline for the Management of Overweight and Obesity in Adults: a report of the American College of Cardiology/American Heart Association Task Force on Practice Guidelines and The Obesity Society. *J Am Coll Cardiol*. 2013;129(25_Suppl_2). doi: 10.1161/01.cir.0000437739.71477.ee
4. National Heart, Lung, and Blood Institute Obesity Education Initiative Expert Panel on the Identification, Evaluation, and Treatment of Obesity in Adults (US). Clinical Guidelines on the Identification, Evaluation, and Treatment of Overweight and Obesity in Adults: The Evidence Report. *Obes Res*. 1998;6(Suppl_2):51S–209S.
5. Centers for Disease Control and Prevention. Adult Obesity Facts. Updated May 14, 2024. Accessed November 30, 2024. https://www.cdc.gov/obesity/adult-obesity facts/?CDC_AAref_Val=https://www.cdc.gov/obesity/data/adult.html
6. Young L, Stollman L. One size does not fit all: how mindful eating and healthy weight-loss strategies can coexist. *FNCE® 2021 Sessions*. 2021. Accessed August 1, 2024. https://www.eatrightstore.org/cpe-opportunities/fnce-2021-sessions/one-size-does-not-fit-all-how-mindful-eating-and-healthy-weight-loss-strategies-can-coexist
7. Tewksbury C, Nwankwo R, Peterson J. Academy of Nutrition and Dietetics: Revised 2022 Standards of Practice and Standards of Professional Performance for Registered Dietitian Nutritionists (Competent, Proficient, and Expert) in Adult Weight Management. *J Acad Nutr Diet*. 2022;122(10):1940–1954.e45. doi:10.1016/j.jand.2022.06.008
8. Flegal KM, Kruszon-Moran D, Carroll MD, Fryar CD, Ogden CL. Trends in obesity among adults in the United States, 2005 to 2014. *JAMA*. 2016;315(21):2284–2291.
9. Stierman B, Afful J, Carroll MD, et al. NCHS National Health Statistics Reports. National Health and Nutrition Examination Survey 2017–March 2020 Prepandemic Data Files - Development of Files and Prevalence Estimates for Selected Health Outcomes. no. 158. September 14, 2021. Accessed November 30, 2024. https://stacks.cdc.gov/view/cdc/106273
10. Anekwe CV, Jarrell AR, Townsend MJ, Gaudier GI, Hiserodt JM, Stanford FC. Socioeconomics of obesity. *Curr Obes Rep*. 2020;9(3):272–279.
11. Centers for Disease Control and Prevention. Obesity Prevalence Maps. Updated September 12, 2024. Accessed November 30, 2024. https://www.cdc.gov/obesity/data-and-statistics/adult-obesity-prevalence-maps.html?CDC_AAref_Val=https://www.cdc.gov/obesity/data/prevalence-maps.html
12. Coleman-Jenson A, Rabbitt MP, Gregory CA, Singh A. USDA Economic Research Service. Household Food Security in the United States in 2020. Accessed November 30, 2024. https://www.ers.usda.gov/webdocs/publications/102076/err-298.pdf
13. Browne NT, Cuda SE. Nutritional and activity recommendations for the child with normal weight, overweight, and obesity with consideration of food insecurity: an Obesity Medical Association (OMA) clinical practice statement 2022. *Obes Pillars*. 2022;2:100012.
14. Figueroa AJ, Hsieh Y, Wiggins B, et al. Racial differences in skeletal muscle mass and quality in older adults: the role of physical activity. *J Aging Phys Act*. 2020;28(3):435–444.
15. Park YW, Goran MI, Pomeroy J, et al. Visceral fat accumulation in Asian American populations: implications for obesity-related health risks. *Obesity*. 2018;26(6):1046–1054.
16. Tsai AG, Wadden TA. In the clinic obesity. *Ann Intern Med*. 2013;159(5):ITC3-1.
17. Wright SM, Aronne LJ. Causes of obesity. *Abdom Imaging*. 2012;37(5):730–732.
18. Nan C, Guo B, Warner C, Zeegers M. Heritability of body mass index in pre-adolescence, young adulthood and late adulthood. *Eur J Epidemiol*. 2012;27(4):247–253.
19. Perusse L, Chagnon YC, Weisnagel SJ, et al. The human obesity gene map: the 2000 update. *Obes Res*. 2001;9:135–169.
20. Shuldiner AR, Sabra M. TRp64Arg 3-adrenoceptor; when does a candidate gene become a disease-susceptibility gene? *Obes Res*. 2001;9;806.
21. Choquet H, Meyre D. Molecular basis of obesity: current status and future prospects. *Curr Genomics*. 2011;12(3):154–168.
22. Ledikwe JH, Ello-Martin JA, Rolls BJ. Portion sizes and the obesity epidemic. *J Nutr*. 2005;135(4):905–909.
23. Healthy People 2030. US Department of Health and Human Services. Office of Disease Prevention and Health Promotion. Accessed September 9, 2024. https://health.gov/healthypeople/priority-areas/social-determinants-health
24. Beaulac J, Kristjansson E, Cummins S. A systematic review of food deserts, 1966-2007. *Prev Chronic Dis* 2009;6(3):A105.
25. Centers for Disease Control and Prevention. Physical Activity Among Adults Aged 18 and Over: United States, 2020. Accessed February 18, 2024. https://www.cdc.gov/nchs/data/databriefs/db443.pdf
26. Leproult R, Van Cauter E. Role of sleep and sleep loss in hormonal release and metabolism. *Endocr Dev*. 2010;17:11–21.
27. World Health Organization: Social Determinants of Health. Accessed May 5, 2024. https://www.who.int/health-topics/social-determinants-of-health#tab=tab_1
28. Christakis NA, Fowler JH. The spread of obesity in a large social network over 32 years. *N Engl J Med*. 2007;357(4):370–379.
29. Ramakrishna BS. Role of the gut microbiota in human nutrition and metabolism. *J Gastroenterol Hepatol*. 2013;28 Suppl 4:9–17.
30. Bäckhed F, Ding H, Wang T, et al. The gut microbiota as an environmental factor that regulates fat storage. *Proc Natl Acad Sci U S A*. 2004;101(44):15718–15723.
31. Yan J, Liu L, Zhu Y, et al. The association between breastfeeding and childhood obesity: a meta-analysis. *BMC Public Health*. 2014;14:1267.

32. Hediger ML, Overpeck MD, Kuczmarski RJ, Ruan WJ. Association between infant breastfeeding and overweight in young children. *J Am Med Assoc*. 2001;285:2453–2460.
33. Wang L, Collins C, Ratliff M, et al. Breastfeeding reduces childhood obesity risks. *Childhood Obes*. 2017;13(3): 197–204. doi:10.1089/chi.2016.0210
34. Monasta L, Batty GD, Cattaneo A, et al. Early-life determinants of overweight and obesity: a review of systematic reviews. *Obes Rev*. 2010;11(10):695–708.
35. Casazza K, Fontaine KR, Astrup A, et al. Myths, presumptions, and facts about obesity. *N Engl J Med*. 2013;368(5):446–454.
36. Rosenbaum M, Leibel RL. Adaptive thermogenesis in humans. *Int J Obes*. 2010;34 Suppl 1:S47–55.
37. Sumithran P, Proietto J. The defence of body weight: a physiological basis for weight regain after weight loss. *Clin Sci (Lond)* 2013 Feb;124(4):231–241.
38. Perry B, Wang Y. Appetite regulation and weight control: the role of gut hormones. *Nutr Diabetes*. 2012;2:e26.
39. Klok MD, Jakobsdottir S, Drent ML. The role of leptin and ghrelin in the regulation of food intake and body weight in humans: a review. *Obes Rev*. 2007;8:21–34.
40. Rahmouni K, Morgan DA. Hypothalamic arcuate nucleus mediates the sympathetic and arterial pressure responses to leptin. *Hypertension*. 2007;49:647–652.
41. Lowell BB, S-Susulic V, Hamann A, et al. Development of obesity in transgenic mice after genetic ablation of brown adipose tissue. *Nature*. 1993;366:740–742.
42. Ozata M, Ozdemir IC, Licinio J. Human leptin deficiency caused by a missense mutation: multiple endocrine defects, decreased sympathetic tone, and immune system dysfunction indicate new targets for leptin action, greater central than peripheral resistance to the effects of leptin, and spontaneous correction of leptin-mediated defects. *J Clin Endocrinol Meta*. 1999;84:3686–3695.
43. National Institute of Diabetes and Digestive and Kidney Diseases. Pre-diabetes and insulin resistance. Accessed May 5, 2024. https://www.niddk.nih.gov/health-information/diabetes/overview/what-is-diabetes/prediabetes-insulin-resistance
44. Lutz TA. The role of amylin in the control of energy homeostasis. *Am J Physiol Regul Integr Comp Physiol*. 2010;298(6): R1475–R1484.
45. Dockray GJ. Cholecystokinin and gut-brain signaling. *Regulatory Peptides*. 2009;155:6–10.
46. Parker SML, Balasubramanian A. Y2 receptors in health and disease. *Br J Pharmacology*. 2008;153:420–431.
47. Lean MEJ, Malkova D. Altered gut and adipose tissue hormones in overweight and obese individuals: cause or consequence? *Int J Obes*. 2016;40(4):622–632.
48. Deurenberg P, Yap M. The assessment of obesity: methods for measuring body fat and global prevalence of obesity. *Baillieres Best Pract Res Clin Endocrinol Metab*. 1999;13(1):1–11.
49. Gallagher D, Heymsfield SB, Heo M, et al. Healthy percentage body fat ranges: an approach for developing guidelines based on body mass index. *Am J Clin Nutr*. 2000; 72(3):694–701.
50. Lear SA, James PT, Ko GT, Kumanyika S. Appropriateness of waist circumference and waist-to-hip ratio cutoffs for different ethnic groups. *Eur J Clin Nutr*. 2010 Jan;64(1):42–61.
51. Jo J, Gavrilova O, Pack S, et al. Hypertrophy and/or hyperplasia: dynamics of adipose tissue growth. *PLoS Comput Biol*. 2009;5(3):e1000324.
52. Spalding KL, Arner E, Westermark PO, et al. Dynamics of fat cell turnover in humans. *Nature*. 2008;453:783–787.
53. Kontogianni MD, Panagiotakos DB, Skopouli FN. Does body mass index reflect adequately the body fat content in perimenopausal women? *Maturitas*. 2005;51:307–313.
54. Romero-Corral A, Somers VK, Sierra-Johnson J, et al. Normal weight obesity: a risk factor for cardiometabolic dysregulation and cardiovascular mortality. *Eur Heart J*; 2010;31(6):737–746.
55. World Health Organization. Waist Circumference and Waist–Hip Ratio: Report of a WHO Expert Consultation. Accessed November 30, 2024. https://iris.who.int/bitstream/handle/10665/44583/9789241501491_eng.pdf?sequence=1
56. Watson NF, Badr MS, Belenky G, et al. Recommended amount of sleep for a healthy adult: a joint consensus statement of the American Academy of Sleep Medicine and Sleep Research Society. *Sleep*. 2015;38(6):843–844.
57. Namazi N, Aliasgharzadeh S, Mahdavi R, et al. Accuracy of the common predictive equations for estimating resting energy expenditure among normal and overweight girl university students. *J Am Coll Nutr*. 2016;35(2):136–142.
58. Aronne LJ, Nelinson DS, Lillo J. Obesity as a disease state: a new paradigm for diagnosis and treatment. *Clin Cornerstone*. 2009;9(4):9–25.
59. Lavie CJ, Milani RV, Artham SM. The obesity paradox, weight loss, and coronary disease. *Am J Med*. 2009;122(12):1106–1114se.
60. Ne R. Obesity-related hypertension. *Ochsner J*. 2009;9(3): 133–136.
61. Hall JE. Pathophysiology of obesity hypertension. *Curr Hypertens Rep*. 2000;2(2):139–147.
62. Poirier P, Giles T, Bray G, et al. Obesity and cardiovascular disease: pathophysiology, evaluation, and effect of weight loss. An update of the 1997 American Heart Association Scientific Statement on Obesity and Heart Disease from the Obesity Committee of the Council on Nutrition, Physical Activity, and Metabolism. *Circulation*. 2006;113:898–918.
63. Romero-Corral A, Sierra-Johnson J, Lopez-Jimenez F, et al. Relationships between leptin and C-reactive protein with cardiovascular disease in the adult general population. *Nat Clin Pract Cardiovasc Med*. 2008;5(7):418–425.
64. Poirier P, Martin J, Marceau P, et al. Impact of bariatric surgery on cardiac structure, function and clinical manifestations in morbid obesity. *Expert Rev Cardiovasc Ther*. 2004;2:193–201.
65. Centers for Disease Control and Prevention. National Diabetes Statistics Report. Updated May 15, 2024. Accessed November 30, 2024. https://www.cdc.gov/diabetes/data/statistics-report/index.html
66. Garvey WT, Mechanick JI, Brett EM, et al. American Association of Clinical Endocrinologists and American College of Endocrinology Comprehensive Clinical Practice Guidelines for Medical Care of Patients with Obesity. *Endocrine Practice*: 2016; 22 Supplement (3):1–203.
67. Kahn SE, Hull RL, Utzschneider KM. Mechanisms linking obesity to insulin resistance and type 2 diabetes. *Nature*. 2006;444:840–846.
68. Hajer GR, van Haeften TW, Visseren FL. Adipose tissue dysfunction in obesity, diabetes, and vascular diseases. *Eur Heart J*. 2008;29:2959–2971.
69. Third report of the National Cholesterol Education Program (NCEP) expert panel on detection, evaluation, and treatment of high blood cholesterol in adults (Adult Treatment Panel III). Final report. *Circulation*. 2002;106:3143–3421.
70. Grundy SM, Brewer HB, Cleeman JI, et al. Definition of metabolic syndrome: report of the National Heart, Lung, and Blood Institute/American Heart Association conference on scientific issues related to definition. *Circulation*. 2004;109(3):433–438.
71. Kaur J. A comprehensive review on metabolic syndrome. *Cardiol Res Pract*. 2014;2014:943162.

72. Anand G, Katz PO. Gastroesophageal reflux disease and obesity. *Gastroenterol Clin North Am.* 2010;39(1):39–46.
73. Ayazi S, Hagen JA, Chan LS. Obesity and gastroesophageal reflux: quantifying the association between body mass index, esophageal acid exposure, and lower esophageal sphincter status in a large series of patients with reflux symptoms. *J Gastrointest Surg.* 2009;13(8):1440–1447.
74. Emerenziani S, Rescio MP, Guarino MP, et al. Gastro-esophageal reflux disease and obesity, where is the link? *World J Gastroenterol.* 2013;19(39):6536–6539.
75. Fabbrini E, Sullivan S, Klein S. Obesity and nonalcoholic fatty liver disease: biochemical, metabolic, and clinical implications. *Hepatology.* 2010;51(2):679–689.
76. World Gastroenterology Organisation. Nonalcoholic Fatty Liver Disease and Nonalcoholic Steatohepatitis. Updated June 2012. Accessed February 26, 2024. https://www.worldgastroenterology.org/guidelines/nafld-nash/nafld-nash-english
77. American Liver Foundation. NASH Definition & Prevalence. Updated January 18, 2024. Accessed February 26, 2024. https://liverfoundation.org/liver-diseases/fatty-liver-disease/nonalcoholic-steatohepatitis-nash/nash-definition-prevalence/
78. Teng ML, Ng CH, Huang DQ, et al. Global incidence and prevalence of nonalcoholic fatty liver disease. *Clin Mol Hepatol.* 2023 Feb;29(Suppl):S32–S42.
79. Fernando DH, Forbes JM, Angus PW, Herath CB. Development and progression of non-alcoholic fatty liver disease: the role of advanced glycation end products. *Int J Mol Sci.* 2019;20(20):5037.
80. Wolin KY, Carson K, Colditz GA. Obesity and cancer. *Oncologist.* 2010;15(6):556–565.
81. World Cancer Research Fund/American Institute for Cancer Research. Food, Nutrition, Physical Activity, and the Prevention of Cancer: a global perspective, 2007. Accessed February 2, 2014. http://www.dietandcancerreport.org/cancer_resource_center/downloads/Second_Expert_Report_full.pdf
82. Vucenik I, Stains JP. Obesity and cancer risk: evidence, mechanisms, and recommendations. *Ann NY Acad Sci.* 2012;1271:37–43.
83. van Kruijsdijk RC, van der Wall E, Visseren FL. Obesity and cancer: the role of dysfunctional adipose tissue. *Cancer Epidemiol Biomarkers Prev.* 2009;18(10):2569–2578.
84. Gallagher EJ, LeRoith D. Minireview: IGF, insulin, and cancer. *Endocrinology.* 2011;152(7):2546–2551.
85. Anandacoomarasamy A, Caterson I, Sambrook P, et al. The impact of obesity on the musculoskeletal system. *Int J Obes.* 2008:(32):211–222.
86. Rishi L, Bhandari M, Kumar R. Can bariatric surgery delay the need for knee replacement in morbidly obese osteoarthritis patients. *J Minim Access Surg.* 2018;14(1):13–17. doi:10.4103/jmas.JMAS_129_16
87. Anandacoomarasamy A, Fransen M, March L. Obesity and the musculoskeletal system. *Curr Opin Rheumatol.* 2009;21(1):71–77.
88. Hooper MM, Stellato TA, Hallowell PT, et al. Musculoskeletal findings in obese subjects before and after weight loss following bariatric surgery. *Int J Obes.* 2007;31(1):114–120.
89. Sleep-related breathing disorders in adults: recommendations for syndrome definition and measurement techniques in clinical research. The Report of an American Academy of Sleep Medicine Task Force. *Sleep.* 1990; 22(5):667–689.
90. Drager LF, Lopes HF, Maki-Nunes C, et al. The impact of obstructive sleep apnea on metabolic and inflammatory markers in consecutive patients with metabolic syndrome. *PLoS One.* 2010;5:12065.
91. Isono S. Obesity and obstructive sleep apnea: mechanisms for increased collapsibility of the passive pharyngeal airway. *Respirology.* 2012;17:32–42.
92. Partinen M, Jamieson A, Guilleminault C. Long-term outcome for obstructive sleep apnea syndrome patients. Mortality. *Chest.* 1988;94:1200–1204.
93. Pi-Sunyer X, Blackburn G, Brancati FL, et al. Reduction in weight and cardiovascular disease risk factors in individuals with type 2 diabetes: one-year results of the look AHEAD trial. *Diabetes Care.* 2007;30(6):1374–1383.
94. Raynor HA, Champagne CM. Position of The Academy of Nutrition and Dietetics: Interventions for the Treatment of Overweight and Obesity in Adults. *J Acad Nutr Diet.* 2016;116(2):339–340.
95. Thomas JG, Bond DS, Phelan S, Hill JO, Wing RR. Weight-loss maintenance for 10 years in the National Weight Control Registry. *Am J Prev Med.* 2014;46(1):17–23.
96. Astbury NM, Piernas C, Hartmann-Boyce J, Lapworth S, Aveyard P, Jebb SA. A systematic review and meta-analysis of the effectiveness of meal replacements for weight loss. *Obes Rev.* 2019;20(4):569–587.
97. Bettini S, Belligoli A, Fabris R, Busetto L. Diet approach before and after bariatric surgery. *Rev Endocr Metab Disord.* 2020;21(3):297–306.
98. Schouten R, van der Kaaden I, van't Hof G, et al. Comparison of preoperative diets before bariatric surgery: a randomized, single blinded, non-inferiority trial. *Obes Surg.* 2016:26:1743–1749.
99. Baer HJ, Rozenblum R, De La Cruz BA, et al. Effect of an online weight management program integrated with population health management on weight change: a randomized clinical trial. *JAMA.* 2020;324(17):1737–1746.
100. Swift DL, Johannsen NM, Lavie CJ, Earnest CP, Church TS. The role of exercise and physical activity in weight loss and maintenance. *Prog Cardiovasc Dis.* 2014;56(4):441–447.
101. Physical Activity Guidelines Advisory Committee. *Physical Activity Guidelines Advisory Committee Report, 2008.* U.S. Department of Health and Human Services; 2008. Accessed November 30, 2024. https://odphp.health.gov/our-work/nutrition-physical-activity/physical-activity-guidelines/previous-guidelines/2008-physical-activity-guidelines/advisory-report
102. Look AHEAD Research Group. Eight-year weight losses with an intensive lifestyle intervention: the look AHEAD study. *Obesity.* 2014;22(1):5–13.
103. Tsai AG, Wadden TA. The evolution of very-low-calorie diets: an update and meta-analysis. *Obesity.* 2006;14(8):1283–1293.
104. Hall KD, Kahan S. Maintenance of lost weight and long-term management of obesity. *Med Clin North Am.* 2018;102(1):183–197.
105. Hernández-Reyes A, Cámara-Martos F, Vidal Á, Molina-Luque R, Moreno-Rojas R. Effects of self-weighing during weight loss treatment: a 6-month randomized controlled trial. *Front Psychol.* 2020;11:397.
106. UpToDate. Obesity in adults: Drug therapy. Accessed March 13, 2024. https://www.uptodate.com/contents/obesity-in-adults-drug-therapy
107. U.S. Food and Drug Administration. Medications target long-term weight control. Updated July 17, 2012. Accessed May 5, 2024. https://web.archive.org/web/20160303045620/http://www.fda.gov/forconsumers/consumerupdates/ucm312380.htm

108. Angrisani L, Santonicola A, Iovino P, et al. IFSO Worldwide Survey 2020–2021: current trends for bariatric and metabolic procedures. *Obes Surg.* 2024;34:1075–1085. doi:10.1007/s11695-024-07118-3
109. American Society for Metabolic and Bariatric Surgery. Estimate of Bariatric Surgery Number, 2011–2022. Accessed March 13, 2024. https://asmbs.org/resources/estimate-of-bariatric-surgery-numbers
110. Gastrointestinal surgery for severe obesity: National Institutes of Health Consensus Development Conference statement. *Am J Clin Nutr.* 1992;55(2):615S–619S.
111. Eisenberg D, Shikora SA, Aarts E, et al. 2022 American Society for Metabolic and Bariatric Surgery (ASMBS) and International Federation for the Surgery of Obesity and Metabolic Disorders (IFSO): indications for metabolic and bariatric surgery. *Surg Obes Relat Dis.* 2022;18(12):1345–1356. doi:10.1016/j.soard.2022.08.013
112. American Society for Metabolic and Bariatric Surgery. Bariatric surgery procedures. Updated May 2021. Accessed March 17, 2024. https://asmbs.org/patients/bariatric-surgery-procedures
113. Abraham A, Ikramuddin S, Jahansouz C, et al. Trends in bariatric surgery: procedure selection, revisional surgeries, and readmissions. *Obes Surg.* 2016; 26:1371.
114. Sjöström L, Narbo K, Sjöström CD, et al. Effects of bariatric surgery on mortality in Swedish obese subjects. *N Engl J Med.* 2007;357(8):741–752.
115. Himpens J, Cadiere GB, Bazi M, et al. Long-term outcomes of laparoscopic adjustable gastric banding. *Arch Surg.* 2011;146(7):802–807.
116. American Society for Metabolic and Bariatric Surgery. Story of Obesity Surgery. Accessed March 17, 2024. https://asmbs.org/resources/story-of-obesity-surgery
117. Stenberg E, Bruze G, Sundström J, et al. Comparison of sleeve gastrectomy vs intensive lifestyle modification in patients with a BMI of 30 to less than 35. *JAMA Netw Open.* 2022;5(7):e2223927.
118. Moran TH. Cholecystokinin and satiety: current perspectives. *Nutrition.* 2000;16:858–865.
119. American Society for Metabolic and Bariatric Surgery. Metabolic and Bariatric Surgery. Accessed May 5, 2024. https://asmbs.org/resources/metabolic-and-bariatric-surgery
120. Liou AP, Paziuk M, Luevano JM, et al. Conserved shifts in the gut microbiota due to gastric bypass reduce host weight and adiposity. *Sci Transl Med.* 2013;5(178):178ra41.
121. Hutter MH, Schirmer BD, Jones DB, et al. First report from the American College of Surgeons Bariatric Surgery Center Network, Laparoscopic sleeve gastrectomy has morbidity and effectiveness positioned between the band and the bypass. *Ann Surg.* 2011;254(3):410–422.
122. Schauer PR, Kashyap SR, Wolski K, et al. Bariatric surgery versus intensive medical therapy in obese patients with diabetes. *N Engl J Med.* 2012;366(17):1567–1576.
123. U.S. Food and Drug Administration. Premarket Approval (PMA). Updated November 25, 2024. Accessed November 30, 2024. https://www.accessdata.fda.gov/scripts/cdrh/cfdocs/cfpma/pma.cfm?id=p140008
124. Imaz I, Martínez-Cervell C, García-Alvarez EE, et al. Safety and effectiveness of the intragastric balloon for obesity. A meta-analysis. *Obes Surg.* 2008;18:841–846.

CHAPTER 8

Nutrition in Diabetes Mellitus

Alexa Cosgrove

CHAPTER OUTLINE

CORE CONCEPTS

1. Diabetes is a lifelong, chronic disease, in which patient self-management is key.
2. While relative or absolute insulin deficiency is the major defining characteristic of diabetes, diabetes is a host of metabolically differentiated diseases.
3. Type 1 diabetes is an autoimmune disease brought about by the interaction of genetics and environmental triggers, resulting in a near or complete pancreatic β cell failure.
4. Type 2 diabetes results from relative insulin deficiency triggered by insulin resistance at the cellular level, coupled with a reduction in insulin production in the β cells.
5. Insulin resistance is exacerbated by obesity.
6. During exercise, in the presence of elevated circulating insulin, glycogenolysis is blunted and insulin-enhanced muscle glucose uptake augmented, leaving the individual at risk for hypoglycemia.
7. Improvements in glycemic control stimulated by physical activity are generally due to reductions in insulin resistance in skeletal muscle.
8. For every 1% decrease in blood glucose levels, there is a corresponding reduction in the risk of complications related to diabetes of approximately 21%.
9. Although diet and exercise remain the cornerstones of diabetes management, all people diagnosed with type 1 diabetes will require insulin as a lifelong treatment modality.
10. The most common and serious side effect of insulin therapy is hypoglycemia.

LEARNING OBJECTIVES

1. Identify the magnitude and etiology of the diabetes epidemic today.
2. Describe the pathophysiology of the different types of diabetes.
3. Assess nutritional status and formulate a nutrition care plan for people with type 1 diabetes.
4. Describe methods of meal planning for people with diabetes.
5. Identify nutrition interventions for nephropathy, neuropathy, and cardiovascular disease.
6. Specify the classes of diabetes medications and their mechanism of action.
7. State the benefits of exercise and the exercise recommendations for people with diabetes.
8. Determine optimal enteral and parenteral feeding practices for blood glucose control.

Introduction: Incidence and Scope

In ancient Greece, diabetes mellitus (commonly known as diabetes) was known as the sweet urine disease because the taste of urine of people with the condition was honey tinged. Even then, "physicians" knew this sweetness was a sign of poor health. Today, we know that diabetes encompasses a large group of metabolic conditions, all stemming from the body's inability to produce or use sufficient insulin to transfer glucose in the bloodstream into cells to be converted into energy or stored as fat for later use. Alterations in insulin action affect the metabolism of protein and fat in addition to glucose and, if left untreated, can damage a wide range of organs from the heart to the oral mucosa to the kidneys.

In the United States today, 38.4 million people have diabetes and 97.6 million have prediabetes, a condition of abnormal blood glucose metabolism that is not as severe as diabetes.[1] Of those, at least 8.7 million are not aware they have diabetes. The diabetes epidemic is expected to grow more ominous over the next several decades. By the year 2060, it is estimated that 60.6 million people will have diabetes.[2] Diabetes is now a worldwide epidemic, with China and India leading in diabetes prevalence.[3]

Diabetes is a major drain on economic resources. It is the seventh leading cause of death and a major cause of heart disease and stroke.[4] In 2022, the United States spent over $413 billion in total costs related to diagnosed diabetes.[1] This includes medical costs associated with the diagnosis and treatment of the disease and its complications, but also indirect costs such as lost wages, missed days of work, and unemployment.[1]

The face of diabetes has changed markedly over the past 20 years. Type 2 diabetes mellitus (T2DM) is no longer a disease relegated to older adults, but now younger ages are susceptible. There has been a 6.8% annual increase in the diagnosis of T2DM in children and adolescents ages 6–18 years in the years 2011–2019.[5] Most youth diagnosed with T2DM are overweight, sedentary, and have a strong family history of diabetes.

Caring for patients with diabetes is a challenge in both outpatient and inpatient settings. Because diabetes is a lifelong, chronic disease in which self-management by the patient is key, this chapter will focus on assessment and treatment options for the ambulatory patient, while reviewing key concepts for the management of glucose control in the inpatient setting.

CORE CONCEPT 1

Diabetes is a lifelong, chronic disease in which patient self-management is key.

Pathophysiology of Diabetes

Although the major defining characteristics of relative or absolute insulin deficiency are commonalities, diabetes is not a single disease; rather, it is a host of metabolically differentiated diseases under one rubric. The majority of people diagnosed with diabetes have T2DM, which accounts for between 90% and 95% of all instances of diabetes.[6] Type 1 diabetes mellitus (T1DM), gestational diabetes, latent autoimmune diabetes in adults (LADA), drug-induced diabetes, diabetes related to specific genetic variations, and maturity-onset diabetes of the young (MODY) account for the remaining cases of diabetes.

CORE CONCEPT 2

While relative or absolute insulin deficiency is the major defining characteristic of diabetes, diabetes is a host of metabolically differentiated diseases.

Type 1 Diabetes

T1DM is an autoimmune disease brought about by the interaction of genetics and environmental triggers. T1DM incidence rates rise from infancy and peak during puberty (ages 10–14 years).[7] The highest reported incidents occur in Northern Europe, Australia/New Zealand, and North America for ages 0-14 years.[7] The hallmark of T1DM is pancreatic beta cell (β cell) destruction in which antibodies to insulin attack the insulin-producing β cells in the pancreas, destroying most or all insulin-secreting capacity. When diagnosed in childhood or teenage years, β cell destruction usually occurs rapidly, while patients diagnosed as adults may have a much longer period of β cell decline. Studies of 50-year medalists (people with T1DM who have lived with diabetes for 50 years) at Joslin Diabetes Center show the preservation of some insulin-producing capacity in those people who have avoided many of the acute and chronic complications of T1DM.[8] Although clinical symptoms usually have a rapid onset, autoantibodies to the islet cells are often present months to years before the onset of clinical indicators and are helpful in distinguishing among

CASE STUDY INTRODUCTION

Joseph is a 19-year-old male patient presenting to the emergency department with vomiting and abdominal pain. He describes a 1-month history of polyuria and polydipsia, accompanied by an approximately 15-pound weight loss over the last 3 months and blurred vision.

Anthropometric Data:

Height: 178 cm
Weight: 95 kg
BMI: 30.1 kg/m^2

Last Primary Care Visit (6 months ago)
Height: 178 cm
Weight: 102 kg

Biochemical Data:

Sodium 131 (136–145 mEq/L)
Potassium 4.0 (3.5–5.0 mEq/L)
Chloride 100 (96–106 mEq/L)
Carbon dioxide 10 (22–31 mEq/L)
Blood urea nitrogen 30 (8–20 mg/dL)
Creatinine 1.5 (0.7–1.3 mg/dL)
Glucose 466 (70–139 mg/dL)

Magnesium 1.1 (1.5–2.7 mg/dL)
Calcium 8.8 (8.5–10.5 mg/dL)
Phosphorus 3.7 (2.5–4.5 mg/dL)
Osmolarity 299 (275–295 mOsm/kg)
pH 7.29 (7.35–7.45)
β-hydroxybutyrate 3 mmol/L H (none)
Urine Acetone +2H (none)

Clinical Data

Past Medical History: None
Family History: Biological father with type 2 diabetes, grandfather died of kidney disease, age 35; no family history of type 1 diabetes
Medications: None

Vital Signs: Blood pressure 130/80 mm Hg
Nutrition-Focused Physical Exam: Patient appears pale, fatigued, and a fruity odor is present in his breath, Kussmaul breathing

Dietary Data:

Dietary History: Patient normally eats a regular diet. Typically has good appetite except for most recently with vomiting and abdominal cramping.

Questions

1. What are Joseph's nutritional risk factors?
2. Describe the possible pathophysiologic etiology associated with Joseph's symptoms and electrolyte abnormalities?
3. Write two Nutrition Diagnosis statements for Joseph identifying the Problem/Etiology/Signs and Symptoms (PES) of Joseph's active nutrition issues.
4. Identify the nutrition interventions you would like to initiate for Joseph to address the problems identified in your PES statements.
5. What should be included in your monitoring and evaluation plan? Why?

diabetes types. Ninety percent of people with T1DM have at least one islet cell or endogenous insulin autoantibody present at diagnosis. These include islet cell autoantibodies, glutamic acid decarboxylase autoantibodies, insulinoma-associated-2 autoantibodies, insulin antibodies, and zinc transporter autoantibodies.[9]

CORE CONCEPT 3

Type 1 diabetes is an autoimmune disease brought about by the interaction of genetics and environmental triggers, resulting in a near or complete pancreatic β cell failure.

Common presenting symptoms of T1DM include **polyphagia** (hunger), **polyuria** (frequent urination), **polydipsia** (excessive thirst), and weight loss. Severe insulin deficiency precipitates **hyperglycemia** (the increase of glucose in the blood) and cellular energy deprivation. Under circumstances of **euglycemia** (normal blood glucose levels), virtually 100% of glucose that is presented to the kidneys is reabsorbed in the proximal renal tubules.[10] When the renal threshold for glucose is exceeded, glucose is diverted into the urine. To maintain the required fluid volume to produce adequate urine for glucose excretion, the renin-aldosterone system is activated, stimulating the thirst mechanism and perpetuating the cycle of unquenchable thirst and frequent urination. Inability to access glucose triggers both increased appetite and a shift to fat metabolism with production of the ketone bodies: **acetone**, **acetoacetic acid**, and **β-hydroxybutyric acid**. Normally, the acidic hydrogen ions are buffered by bicarbonate. However, the large quantity of acid produced by metabolism of ketone bodies soon depletes the supply of bicarbonate, and metabolic acidosis occurs. Left untreated, **diabetic ketoacidosis (DKA)** ensues, a condition where excessive ketone bodies cause the blood pH to drop to dangerous levels and can quickly lead to death. Patients often present with depleted sodium levels secondary to fluid shifts caused by severe hyperglycemia. Insulin deficiency and acidosis will cause potassium to shift to the extracellular space. DKA typically develops quickly and within a few hours.[11] Many patients in DKA present with nausea, vomiting, and a fruity odor to their breath from the buildup of ketones. In severe DKA, patients may have **Kussmaul's respirations**, abnormally deep breathing associated with metabolic acidosis. Diagnostic criteria for DKA are listed in **Table 8.1**.[11]

Initial treatment for ketoacidosis includes intravenous insulin administration, correction of the metabolic acidosis and electrolyte abnormalities, and

Table 8.1 Diagnostic Criteria of Diabetic Ketoacidosis (DKA) and Hyperglycemic Hyperosmolar State (HHS)

	Mild DKA	Moderate DKA	Severe DKA	HHS
Plasma glucose (mg/dL [mmol/L])	>250 (13.9)	>250	>250	>600 (33.3)
Arterial pH	7.25–7.30	7.00–7.24	<7.00	>7.30
Serum bicarbonate (mEq/L)	15–18	10 to <15	<10	>15
Urine ketones	Positive	Positive	Positive	Small
Serum ketones	Positive	Positive	Positive	Small
β-hydroxybutyrate	High	High	High	Normal or elevated
Effective serum osmolality (mOsm/kg)*	Variable	Variable	Variable	>320
Anion gap**	>10	>12	>12	Variable
Alteration in sensoria or mental obtundation	Alert	Alert/drowsy	Stupor/coma	Stupor/coma

*Effective serum osmolality = 2 × measured Na (mEq/L) + (glucose [mg/dL] + 18)
**Anion gap = $Na^+ - (Cl^- + HCO3^-$ [mEq/L])
Data from Gosmanov AR, Gosmanova EO, Kitabchi AE. Hyperglycemic crises: diabetic ketoacidosis and hyperglycemic hyperosmolar state. In: Feingold KR, Anawalt B, Blackman MR, et al, eds. *Endotext*. MDText.com, Inc.; 2021. Accessed January 12, 2026. https://www.ncbi.nlm.nih.gov/books/NBK279052/

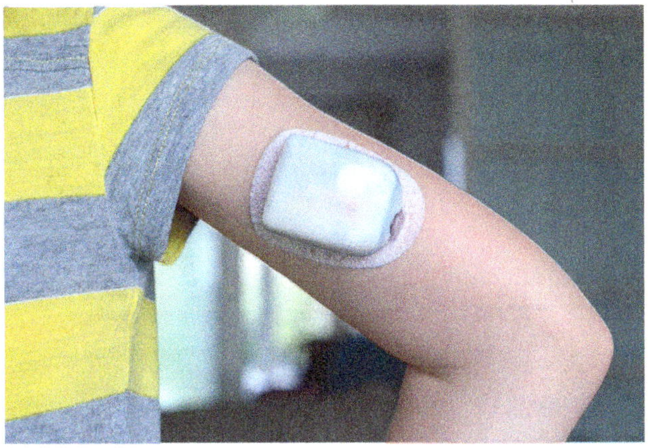

Figure 8.1 Example of a Tubeless Insulin Pump Device

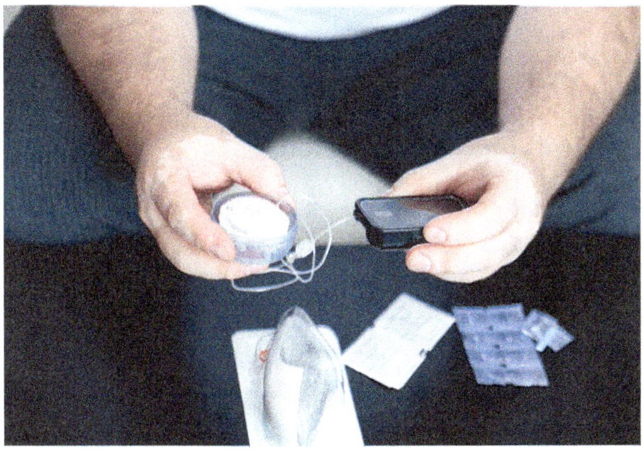

Figure 8.2 Example of a Tubed Insulin Pump Device

PRACTICE POINT

Common presenting symptoms of T1DM include polyphagia (hunger), polyuria (frequent urination), polydipsia (excessive thirst), and weight loss.

repletion of fluids. When stable, patients are started on subcutaneous insulin. For many, the reduction of glucose levels and the correction of metabolic parameters temporarily restore glucose homeostasis. This period of limited exogenous insulin is known as the "honeymoon phase." Lasting up to a year, the honeymoon phase eventually ends with an increasing need for exogenous insulin until complete insulin coverage is required for both basal and bolus insulin either by injection or through an insulin pump. **Figures 8.1** and **8.2** show examples of a tubeless insulin pump and tubed insulin pump, respectively. **Figure 8.3** displays an example of an insulin injection pen.

Prediabetes

Prediabetes is classified by blood glucose levels that are elevated above what is normal, but not elevated enough to be classified as diabetes. Prediabetes increases the risk of developing T2DM and cardiovascular disease (CVD).[12] Prediabetes is indicated by an HbA1c level of 5.7–6.4%, a fasting blood glucose of 100–125 mg/dL, or an oral glucose tolerance test 2-hour blood glucose of 140–199 mg/dL. A diagnosis of prediabetes does not necessarily mean T2DM will develop, but modifications in lifestyle behavior may aid in delaying or preventing its onset.[12,13]

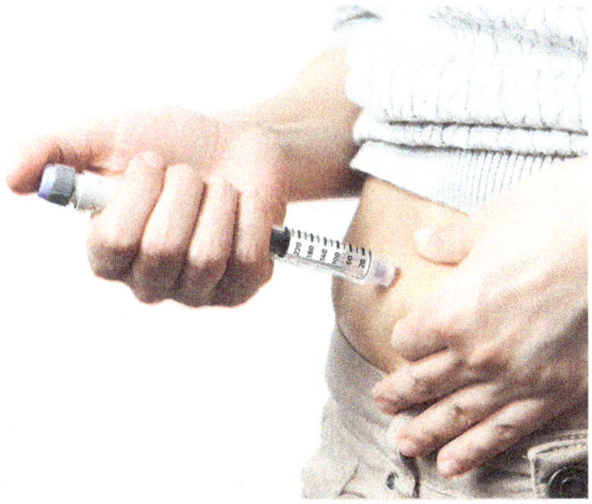

Figure 8.3 Injection of Insulin into the Abdominal Area

Type 2 Diabetes

Unlike T1DM, in which complete or near complete β cell failure occurs, T2DM results from relative insulin deficiency triggered by insulin resistance at the cellular level, coupled with a reduction of insulin production in the β cells. Reduction in β cell mass may be due to apoptosis (cell death) without compensatory regeneration. A number of causal factors, including prolonged exposure to elevated glucose levels (glucotoxicity) and fatty acid concentrations (lipotoxicity), infiltration of proinflammatory cytokines, and deposition of islet cell amyloid, have been postulated to explain the damage to the β cells.[14–16]

Insulin resistance is triggered by insulin receptor defects in target cells, with environmental factors such as obesity and lack of physical activity contributing to its development, as presented in **Figure 8.4**.[17]

T2DM is not an autoimmune disease, but it has a large genetic component. Family history, in addition to lifestyle factors, plays a major role in its development.

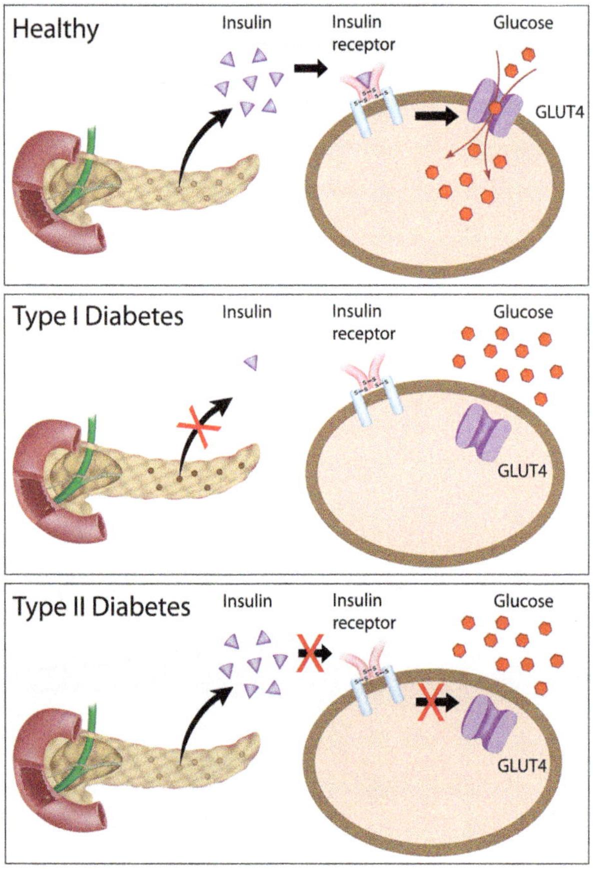

Figure 8.4 Insulin Receptor Defects

Risk factors include older age, family history, hypertension, dyslipidemia, obesity, lack of physical activity, ethnicity, polycystic ovarian disease, and history of gestational diabetes.[18]

CORE CONCEPT 4

T2DM results from relative insulin deficiency triggered by insulin resistance at the cellular level, coupled with a reduction in insulin production in the β cells.

The onset of T2DM is usually insidious, occurring over a number of years. Many people are unaware they have it until a routine physical examination brings the condition to light. Initially, insulin resistance of the muscle and liver cells stimulates the pancreas to produce more insulin and normal glucose levels are maintained. In many cases, people in the early stages (prediagnostic) of T2DM will hypersecrete insulin in compensation for insulin resistance.[16]

Insulin resistance is often exacerbated by obesity. Metabolic defects contributing to hyperglycemia include excess hepatic glucose secretion mediated by the loss of insulin's effects on suppressing **glycogenolysis** (breakdown of glycogen stores for glucose) and **gluconeogenesis** (synthesis of glucose from non-carbohydrate sources, usually amino acids). High circulating levels of free fatty acids increase insulin resistance and further impair pancreatic insulin secretion in adults and children.[19,20]

CORE CONCEPT 5

Insulin resistance is exacerbated by obesity.

As the disease progresses, the pancreas's ability to meet the demand for insulin is overcome and diabetes ensues. The loss of postprandial euglycemia occurs, followed by the inability to maintain fasting glucose levels in target range. Insulin secretory capacity is diminished due to the impairment of two incretin hormones—gastric inhibitory polypeptide (glucose-dependent insulinotropic polypeptide) and glucagon-like peptide-1 (GLP-1)—which normally stimulate up to 50% of postprandial insulin secretion, as well as the loss of β cell mass.[21]

By the time diabetes is diagnosed, islet cell function is reduced to approximately 50% of normal.[16,22] Insulin is secreted in two phases. After eating, there is an initial release of preformed insulin stored in the granules in the β cells. The first phase of insulin secretion occurs within 2 minutes of eating and lasts between 10 and 15 minutes. It is responsible for muscle cell glucose disposal, suppresses glucose production by the liver, and maintains normal blood glucose levels. The second phase, which may last 1–2 hours, is derived from newly formed insulin released in oscillating pulses. In T2DM, the phase 1 response is destroyed and the phase 2 response is diminished, causing the insulin response time to a mixed meal to be delayed.[22]

PRACTICE POINT

By the time diabetes is diagnosed, islet cell function is reduced to approximately 50% of normal.

A third contributor to T2DM is the increase in hepatic glucose output due to greater gluconeogenesis driven by hepatic insulin resistance. The hormonal picture is one of high levels of glucagon and cortisol with even smaller amounts of insulin.

Treatment of T2DM focuses on its various metabolic defects and the degree of hyperglycemia present at the time of diagnosis. People may begin treatment with lifestyle measures and/or oral medications, but over time there is a diminution in β cell mass, leading to the need for eventual insulin administration.

National Diabetes Prevention Program

The National Diabetes Prevention Program (National DPP) aims to prevent and/or delay the onset of T2DM in adults that are at high risk. Prediabetes often progresses to T2DM if active intervention through lifestyle changes is not incorporated. The National DPP has implemented a Centers for Disease Control and Prevention (CDC)-recognized lifestyle change program that focuses on lifestyle modifications for people with prediabetes or at increased risk of developing T2DM. Participants in this change program learn about healthy eating and nutrient-dense foods, incorporating physical activity into daily life, managing stress, and learning to manage eating out and making healthful decisions in other social situations. People with prediabetes enrolled in this change program can decrease their risk of developing T2DM by 58% within the first year of participation.[23–26]

Double Diabetes

Double diabetes (DD), also known as hybrid diabetes, demonstrates features of both T1DM and T2DM. Common symptoms of DD include obesity, insulin resistance, type of latent autoimmune diabetes in youth (LADY), and autoantibodies. Additional research is needed to develop more individualized treatment regimens for these cases.[26]

Gestational Diabetes

Gestational diabetes mellitus (GDM) is defined as any degree of abnormal glucose tolerance with first appearance or recognition during pregnancy.[27,28] Pregnancies complicated by glucose intolerance are on the rise in the United States due to the explosion of obesity and sedentary behavior, with higher rates among ethnic communities and those of limited economic resources. Current prevalence estimates vary widely between 5% and 9% of all pregnancies, depending on the groups surveyed.[29] Pregnancy distorts the normal hormonal milieu toward one of insulin resistance and decreased insulin output. During the first trimester, insulin secretion increases, fostering the accumulation of adipose tissue. In the later stages of pregnancy, insulin resistance and lipolysis develop. Late gestation is characterized by a several-fold increase in circulating postprandial free fatty acid levels, which further reduces insulin activity and stimulates liver glycogenolysis, increasing insulin resistance. Several pregnancy hormones facilitate this process. Human placental lactogen increases up to 30-fold throughout pregnancy, and human placental growth hormone increases 6- to 8-fold during gestation, replacing normal pituitary growth hormone in the maternal circulation.[30]

Although glucose levels are usually not as elevated as those with overt diabetes, GDM carries significant risks for the mother and the fetus. GDM increases the mother's risk for preeclampsia and cesarean section delivery. Infants born to mothers with uncontrolled GDM are at risk for excessive weight gain, shoulder dystocia, post-delivery hypoglycemia, and respiratory distress syndrome. Neonatal hypoglycemia, jaundice, polycythemia, and hypocalcemia may complicate infant delivery. Females also face the possibility of developing obesity and T2DM later in life.[28,31] Any degree of maternal hyperglycemia is injurious to the fetus.[32] Alterations in glucose metabolism are a continuum, which has made choosing an ideal screening paradigm so difficult. The International Association of Diabetes and Pregnancy Study groups published their recommendation on the Diagnosis and Classification of Hyperglycemia in Pregnancy in March 2010 after reviewing the results of the Hyperglycemia and Adverse Pregnancy Outcome study (HAPO).[33] They recommend a single method of screening for GDM. This method employs a 2-hour oral glucose tolerance test (OGTT) using a 75-g glucose solution. Blood glucose measurements are drawn fasting and at 1 hour and 2 hours after drinking the sweetened beverage. Diagnostic cutoffs for the diagnosis of GDM using both methods are listed in **Table 8.2**.[28]

Some females with overt diabetes would be misdiagnosed following this guideline. Therefore, the American Diabetes Association (ADA) recommends that females with risk factors for diabetes should be screened during their first prenatal visit.[28] However, the American College of Obstetricians and Gynecologists and the U.S. Preventive Services Task Force have deemed current research to be insufficient, and justify the continuation of previous screening criteria involving a two-step approach, in which all females are screened using a 50-g glucose solution. Those whose blood glucose levels exceed 140 mg/dL 1 hour after ingesting the beverage go on to take a 100-g OGTT, where blood glucose levels are tested two times over a

Table 8.2 Screening and Diagnostic Criteria for Gestational Diabetes

Two-Step Approach *	One-Step Approach*
Prescreen with 50-g GLT between 24- and 28-weeks gestation. Screening threshold ≥140 mg/dL.	Screen with 2-hour OGTT using 75-g glucose between 24- and 28-weeks gestation. One value exceeding the defined threshold is diagnostic for GDM: ▪ Fasting: ≥92 mg/dL (5.1 mmol/L) ▪ 1 hour: ≥180 mg/dL (10.0 mmol/L) ▪ 2 hours: ≥153 mg/dL (8.5 mmol/L)
3-hour OGTT using 100-g glucose	
Two values exceeding the defined threshold are diagnostic or GDM.	

*Should be performed in the morning after an overnight fast of at least 8 hours.
GDM, gestational diabetes mellitus; GLT, glucose load test; OGTT, oral glucose tolerance test.
Data from American Diabetes Association. Diagnosis and classification of diabetes. Sec. 2. In: *Standards of Care in Diabetes 2024. Diabetes Care.* 2024;47(Suppl 1):S20-S42, Table 2.7.

3-hour period. There must be two abnormal glucose readings for a GDM diagnosis.[34,35]

Latent Autoimmune Diabetes in Adults (LADA)

Latent Autoimmune Diabetes in Adults (LADA) is an autoimmune disease that is a slow progressive form of diabetes and shares features of both T1DM and T2DM.[36,37] LADA is similar to T1DM in that antibodies to islet β cells are present, but immune destruction occurs at a much slower rate than compared to a classic T1DM case. Most patients will present with insulin resistance that causes hyperglycemia that is not as extreme as someone with T1DM, which leads to a misdiagnosis and management of T2DM. LADA shares the trait of autoimmunity with T1DM, and mimics the metabolic derangements demonstrated in cases of T2DM. An endocrinologist at the Joslin Diabetes Center in Boston estimates that as many as 10% of patients who are diagnosed with T2DM might actually have LADA.[38] Diagnostic criteria for LADA include age greater than 30 years, positive autoantibodies to islet β cells, and insulin independence for at least the initial 6 months of diagnosis. Treatment and management of LADA may include medical nutrition therapy, exercise recommendations, and insulin therapy. There is not much data on the use of sulfonylureas, metformin, thiazolidinediones, and dipeptidyl peptidase 4 inhibitors in patients with LADA. The goals of treatment are to obtain glycemic control and to prevent and/or delay complications related to diabetes.[36]

Drug-Induced Diabetes (DID)

Common medications or classes of medications may interfere with glucose homeostasis and can increase the risk for developing hyperglycemia. Prolonged hyperglycemia related to medication use will lead to a subsequent diagnosis of diabetes. Drug-induced diabetes (DID) is a type of diabetes that results from the use of medication. These medication classes that are associated with hyperglycemia or diabetes include steroids, antipsychotics, antiretrovirals, chemotherapy, transplant immunosuppressants, thiazide diuretics, lipid-lowering agents, and β-blockers, which may cause increased insulin resistance, increased hepatic glucose production, decreased insulin secretion, glucose intolerance, and autoimmune destruction of pancreatic β cells.[39] High doses of glucocorticosteroids over a short period of time may result in severe acute, but reversible hyperglycemia, whereas low doses for an extended period of time may result in diabetes. DID may be reversible with cessation of the medication; however, it may be irreversible depending on medication, dosage, duration, patient's age, body weight, and family history. Treatment of DID is similar to that of other types of diabetes, focusing on healthy lifestyle habits and escalating to metformin or insulin when and if necessary.[40]

Maturity-Onset Diabetes of the Young (MODY)

Maturity-Onset Diabetes of the Young (MODY) is a monogenic form of diabetes where pancreatic autoantibodies are not present, rather β cell dysfunction causes impaired insulin secretion.[41] MODY is an autosomal dominant disease that has a strong family history and is inherited, and patients generally have heterozygous mutations.[41,42] There are at least 14 known MODY mutations that vary based on age of onset, response to treatment, and presence of C-peptide.[41–43] MODY accounts for about 1–5% of diabetes cases, but it is estimated to be higher due to misdiagnosis for T1DM or T2DM.[41,42] Diagnostic criteria for MODY include age of onset in a family member of 25 years of age, at least two consecutive generations of diabetes in the family, no β cell autoantibodies, persistent endogenous insulin production as evidenced by C-peptide levels >200 pmol/L, and lack of need for insulin therapy.[41–43] It may also be diagnosed through genetic testing.[41] Treatment and management of MODY varies on the gene mutation, but may include dietary and lifestyle behavior changes and the use of sulfonylureas, GLP-1 agonists, and in metformin, and in some cases will require insulin therapy.[41–43]

Screening, Risk Factors, and Diagnosis of Diabetes

Diabetes Screening and Risk Factors

In 2011, the CDC undertook a study to determine when and if large-scale screenings for T2DM were warranted. It was determined that the yield of diabetes diagnoses from community-based screenings is poor and does not represent a good use of resources, and that identification of persons with diabetes should be accomplished in the clinical setting. In 2022, the U.S. Preventive Service Task Force (USPSTF) and the ADA updated their screening guidelines and recommended screening for prediabetes and T2DM starting at age 35, compared to previous guidelines of age 45.[44] Currently, it is recommended that screening for prediabetes and risk of future diabetes should be done for all individuals 35 years of age and older, asymptomatic adults who are overweight or obese with a body mass index (BMI) ≥25 (≥23 in Asian Americans), and adults having one or more risk risks as defined in **Table 8.3**.[28]

Screening for T1DM has increased traction, as 90% of new cases of T1DM do not have a family history.[45] There are new therapies available that can delay or prevent the onset of T1DM. Previously, screening programs were targeted at identifying individuals with a family member who has T1DM. The screening tests look for positive autoantibodies.

Diagnostic Criteria and Staging

Prediabetes and diabetes are diagnosed by clinical presentation or with a variety of blood tests (**Table 8.4**).[12,28] Fasting glucose and oral glucose tolerance tests have been used for many years. In 2010, the hemoglobin A1c test (A1c or HbA1c), also known as "glycohemoglobin test," was added to these other well-established methods of diagnosing diabetes. The A1c test is based on the attachment of glucose to hemoglobin, the protein in red blood cells. Since the average lifespan of a red blood cell is about 3 months, A1c reflects the 2–3-month average blood glucose level, reported as a percentage. The A1c is often the easiest test for patients to complete because it can be accomplished without fasting. The ADA recommends using the term estimated average glucose, or eAG, alongside reports on A1c results. Conversion of A1c percentage to eAG is depicted in **Table 8.5**.[46,47]

Table 8.3 Risk Factors Indicating the Need to Screen for Diabetes and Prediabetes

Risk Factor Category	Indicators
Biological and physiological factors	≥35 years of age
Family history	First-degree relative with diabetes
Medical history	Cardiovascular disease, polycystic ovary syndrome, females diagnosed with GDM, HIV, exposure to high-risk medicines, and history of pancreatitis
Biochemical indices	HbA1c ≥ 5.7% (≥39 mmol/mol), IGT* or IFG**, high-density lipoprotein cholesterol ≤35 mg/dL (≤0.9 mmol/L) or triglycerides ≥250 mg/dL (≥2.8 mmol/L)
Clinical conditions	Hypertension (HTN): ≥130/80 mm/Hg, factors associated with insulin resistance (acanthosis nigricans, severe obesity), physical inactivity
Race and ethnicity	High-risk race and ethnicity: African American, Latino, Native American, Asian American, Pacific Islander

GDM, gestational diabetes mellitus; IGT, impaired glucose tolerance; IFG, impaired fasting glucose.

*IGT is higher than normal glucose level 2 hours after an oral glucose tolerance test (140–199 mg/dL). A result in that range is consistent with prediabetes.

**IFG is a higher than normal fasting glucose level (100–125 mg/dL). A result in that range is consistent with prediabetes.

Data from American Diabetes Association. Diagnosis and classification of diabetes. Sec. 2. In: *Standards of Care in Diabetes 2024. Diabetes Care.* 2024;47(Suppl 1):S20-S42, Table 2.4.

Table 8.4 Diagnostic Criteria for Prediabetes and Diabetes Compared to Normal Lab Values

	Normal	Prediabetes	Diabetes
Hemoglobin A1c	<5.7%	5.7–6.4%	≥6.5%
Fasting plasma glucose	<100 mg/dL	100–125 mg/dL	≥126 mg/dL
Postprandial glucose	<140 mg/dL	140–199 mg/dL	≥200 mg/dL
Oral glucose tolerance test	<140 mg/dL	140–199 mg/dL	≥200 mg/dL
Random plasma glucose	<140 mg/dL	140–199 mg/dL	≥200 mg/dL

Data from American Diabetes Association. Diagnosis and classification of diabetes. Sec. 2. In: *Standards of Care in Diabetes 2024. Diabetes Care.* 2024;47(Suppl 1):S20-S42, Tables 2.1 and 2.2.

Table 8.5 HbA1c and Estimate Average Glucose (eAG)

HbA1c	eAG	
%	mg/dL	mmol
5.5	111	6.2
6	126	7.0
6.5	140	7.8
7	154	8.6
7.5	169	9.4
8	183	10.1
8.5	197	10.9
9	212	11.8
9.5	226	12.6
10	240	13.4

Data from American Diabetes Association. eAG/A1C conversion calculator. Accessed January 12, 2026. https://professional.diabetes.org/glucose_calc

In T1DM, the progression of the disease that accompanies β cell failure is well characterized. The ADA provides staging for T1DM (**Table 8.6**). At least two autoimmune antibodies are persistently present well before the onset of symptoms or an increase in biochemical indices such as glucose and A1c, making these indices useful predictors of diabetes and hyperglycemia. During stage 1, despite the presence of these antibodies, euglycemia exists. As β cell failure progresses into stage 2, impaired glucose tolerance and fasting glucose levels become evident without clinical manifestations until the patient progresses into stage 3.[28,46]

Nutrition Requirements in Diabetes

Nutritional requirements for people with diabetes are similar to those of the general healthy population. There is not one optimal macronutrient composition of the diet for people with diabetes.[48] A variety of dietary patterns can result in adequate glycemic control. The Mediterranean diet, a vegetarian or vegan diet, a very low to moderate-carbohydrate diet, and a low glycemic index diet have been demonstrated to be effective in promoting glycemic control.[48–50] Low-carbohydrate diets have an advantage in producing a more favorable cardiac profile, improving triglyceride levels, and diminishing the reduction in high-density lipoprotein (HDL) levels that occur with weight loss.[51] A Mediterranean-style eating pattern is effective in achieving glycemic control and improves CVD risk factors, including blood pressure and lipids, without the need for weight loss.[48,52,53] All three macronutrients—carbohydrates, protein, and fat—impact blood glucose levels by different mechanisms (**Figure 8.5**).[54]

Carbohydrates

The amount of carbohydrate consumed and available insulin are the most important factors in determining postprandial blood glucose levels.[48] Carbohydrate modification was the cornerstone of nutrition intervention prior to the discovery of insulin. An early treatment modality for diabetes was the near elimination of carbohydrate-containing foods from the diet. Although effective in lowering blood glucose levels, this approach ignored the role of carbohydrate as the body's main source of energy and needed vitamins, minerals, fiber, and phyto substances. Diets overly restricted in carbohydrate can cause ketosis

Table 8.6 Criteria for Staging of Type 1 Diabetes

Stages	Clinical Characteristics and Diagnostic Criteria	Laboratory Indices
1	Presence of autoimmunity Presymptomatic Euglycemia	Presence of two or more autoantibodies Normal FPG and PPG
2	Autoimmunity Dysglycemia (increased fasting glucose and impaired glucose tolerance) Presymptomatic	Presence of multiple autoantibodies FPG: 100–125 mg/dL PPG: 140–199 mg/dL HgA1c 5.7–6.4% or ≥10% increase in A1c
3	Autoimmunity New-onset hyperglycemia Symptomatic	Meets standard diabetes screening criteria as described in Table 8.4.

FPG, fasting plasma glucose; PPG, postprandial plasma glucose
Data from American Diabetes Association. Diagnosis and classification of diabetes. Sec. 2. In: *Standards of Care in Diabetes 2024. Diabetes Care.* 2024;47(Suppl 1):S20-S42, Table 2.3.

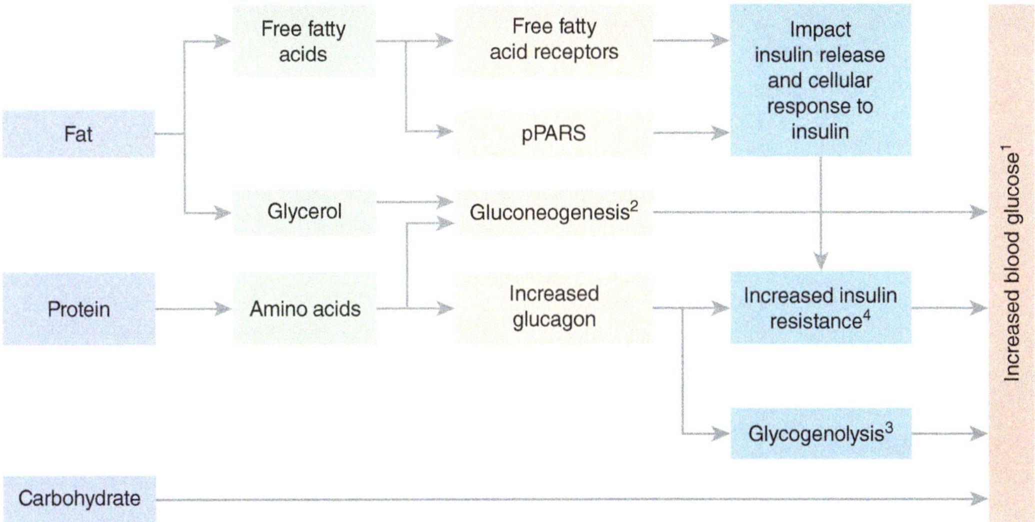

Figure 8.5 Mechanism of Macronutrients Impact on Blood Glucose
Data from American Diabetes Association. eAG/A1C conversion calculator. Accessed January 12, 2026. https://professional.diabetes.org/glucose_calc

and dehydration, which is a serious concern, particularly in older adults. Low-carbohydrate diets are often constipating due to their lack of fiber and, because of what many perceive as a lack of palatability, can be difficult to follow long-term.

PRACTICE POINT

The amount of carbohydrate consumed and available insulin are the most important factors in determining postprandial blood glucose levels.

Neither the ADA nor the Academy of Nutrition and Dietetics (AND) specifies a particular amount of carbohydrate to be used in the diets of people with diabetes. Both organizations recommend that the percentage of carbohydrate in the diet be individualized to the needs and preferences of the individual with diabetes. Joslin Diabetes Center, in its Clinical Nutrition Guideline of Overweight and Obese Adults with Type 2 Diabetes, Prediabetes, or a High Risk for Developing Type 2 Diabetes, recommends that carbohydrate should be restricted to between 40% and 45% of calories to reduce excess glycemic excursions.[55]

PRACTICE POINT

The percentage of carbohydrates in the diet should be individualized to the needs and preferences of the individual with diabetes.

Carbohydrate foods consist of grains, legumes, milk and yogurts, fruit, and starchy and non-starchy vegetables. Non-starchy vegetables, unless consumed in large quantities, provide little carbohydrate and in practical terms are often considered "free foods" in the diet. The brain and nervous system have an obligatory requirement for glucose, and the Dietary Guidelines for Americans 2020–2025 recommends a minimum intake of 130 grams of carbohydrate per day to supply the brain, nervous system, and red blood cells with glucose without reliance on gluconeogenesis from other fuel sources.[56]

Glycemic Index

The type of carbohydrate consumed is secondary to the total quantity eaten in affecting glycemic response. However, the digestibility of different carbohydrate sources affects blood glucose excursions differently. The **glycemic index (GI)** describes the quantity and rate at which different carbohydrate foods influence blood glucose response. Fifty grams of carbohydrate-containing foods are ranked according to how much they raise glucose levels in comparison to either 50 grams of glucose or 50 grams of white bread. Foods are ranked in comparison to the ranking of glucose: low glycemic foods are designated as less than or equal to 55, intermediate GI foods have a designation of between 56 and 69, and those greater than or equal to 70 are considered to have a high GI.[57]

Many variables affect the GI of a food, including but not limited to, fat, fiber, acidity level, the form in which it is consumed (solid, liquid), processing, and cooking by altering how quickly a food is digested. In general, those foods that contain greater amounts of fat and fiber have a lower GI. Although the GI can be a valuable tool for people with diabetes to refine their metabolic control, its use is not without certain caveats. Fat plays such a seminal role in determining the GI of a food; some foods, such as candy bars, often have far lower GI rankings than more nutrient-dense foods, such as skim milk, yet the latter is a better choice from a nutrition standpoint.

Glycemic Load

The GI of a food is the same no matter how much carbohydrate is consumed. The **glycemic load (GL)** attempts to reconcile the digestibility rate of foods with the amount of carbohydrate they contain. The GL is calculated by multiplying the GI ranking of the food by the number of grams of carbohydrate in a serving and then dividing by 100. A GL of 10 or less is low, 11–19 is medium, and greater than 20 is high.[58] For example, the GI of a white bagel is 72; the GL of a 5-oz bagel is 51, and that of a 2.5-oz bagel is 25. There are approximately 75 grams of carbohydrate in a 5-oz bagel versus 35 grams of carbohydrate in a 2.5-oz bagel, and so:

$$72\ (\text{GI}) \times 75\ (\text{g of carbohydrate}) = 5400/100$$

$$= 54\ \text{GL (5-oz bagel)}$$

$$72\ (\text{GI}) \times 35\ (\text{g of carbohydrate}) = 2520/100$$

$$= 25\ \text{GL (2.5-oz bagel)}$$

It is important to remember that the GI and GL are based on individual foods, but that people eat mixed meals. The GI and GL of a mixed meal will be the average of all carbohydrate foods consumed. Foods that are primarily protein and fat do not have a GI. The GI is often an adjunct tool that people with diabetes can use in addition to carbohydrate regulation. The response of glucose levels to the same quantity of different GI foods can be ascertained by checking blood glucose both before and 2–3 hours after eating. Refer to **Table 8.7** for a sample of the GI and GL of a variety of foods.

There can be significant variability in the GI among the same foods due to differences in growing conditions, brand, and variety, as well as a wide range of responses to the same food in different individuals. Patients often need to take a trial-and-error approach to how specific foods will influence their glycemic control by checking their blood glucose after meals. They can make more informed decisions about behaviors around certain foods such as pairing with protein, fat, or fiber-based foods or physical activity after a meal to also help with the food's effect on blood glucose levels.

Consistency in the timing and amount of carbohydrate eaten at meals has been shown to improve glycemic control in people with T1DM and T2DM who use oral hypoglycemic medications or fixed or sliding scale insulin regimens.[59,60] Greater flexibility in carbohydrate intake and improved glycemic control have also been demonstrated in people who match their insulin doses to the amount of carbohydrate they eat at meals.[61,62]

Fiber

Fiber is defined as the indigestible part of plant products. Dietary fiber can be divided into two types: soluble and insoluble. From a practical standpoint, fiber

Table 8.7 Glycemic Index and Glycemic Load of Selected Foods

Food	Serving Size	Carbohydrates (grams)	Glycemic Index	Glycemic Load
Bread and tortillas				
Bread, pumpernickel	1 slice	11	46	5
Bread, white or wheat	1 slice	13	68	9
Bread, whole wheat	1 slice	14	73	10
Tortilla, corn	1 (small)	24	52	12
Tortilla, wheat	1 (small)	26	30	8
Cereals				
Cheerios	1 cup	20	74	15
Cream of Wheat	1 cup	26	66	17
Oatmeal	1 cup	23	75	17
Special K	1 cup	21	69	14
Crackers/snacks				
Popcorn	2 tbsp	11	72	8
Pretzels	8 pretzels	19	83	16
Rice cakes	3 cakes	21	82	17
Grains				
Barley	1 cup	42	25	11
Couscous	1 cup	35	65	23
Quinoa	1/2 cup	17	53	9
Rice, brown	1 cup	48	50	24
Spaghetti, whole grain	1 cup	44	32	14
Starchy vegetables				
Corn, canned	1/3 cup	15	46	7
Corn, boiled	1 large ear	33	60	20
Potato	3/4 cup	21	57	12
Sweet potato	1/2 cup	26	48	13
Fruit				
Apple	1 (medium)	15	40	6
Apricot, dried	6	25	32	8
Banana, ripe	1 (medium)	24	51	12
Cherries	12	13	22	3
Grapes	15	18	43	8
Figs, dried	3	26	61	16
Kiwi	2 (small)	12	53	6

(continues)

Table 8.7 Glycemic Index and Glycemic Load of Selected Foods *(continued)*

Food	Serving Size	Carbohydrates (grams)	Glycemic Index	Glycemic Load
Mango	1/2	17	51	8
Orange	1 (medium)	9	48	4
Papaya	1/2 cup	8	60	5
Peach	1 (medium)	7	28	2
Pear	1 (medium)	13	33	29
Pineapple	1/2 cup	13	59	7
Plum	1 (large)	14	24	3
Prunes	6	33	29	10
Raisins	1/4 cup	44	64	28
Strawberries	1/2 cup	3	40	1
Watermelon	1/2 cup	6	72	4
Dairy				
Non-fat milk	1 cup	13	32	4
Non-fat yogurt	6.5 ounces	14	24	3
Soy yogurt	6.5 ounces	26	50	13
Vegetables				
Carrots, boiled	1/2 cup	5	41	2
Carrots, raw	1/2 cup	16	16	3
Tomato juice	12 oz-can	11	33	4
Plant proteins				
Baked beans	1/2 cup	15	48	7
Black beans	1/2 cup	23	30	7
Chickpeas	1/2 cup	24	36	9
Green peas	1/2 cup	6	51	3
Hummus	2 tbsp	5	6	0
Kidney beans	1/2 cup	24	23	6
Lentils	1/2 cup	15	22	3
Lima beans	1/2 cup	30	32	10
Pinto beans	1/2 cup	26	39	10
Split peas	1/2 cup	19	32	6

Data from Atkinson FS, Brand-Miller JC, Foster-Powell K, Buyken AE, Goletske J. International tables of glycemic index and glycemic load values: 2021. *Am J Clin Nutr.* 2021;114(5):1625-1632.

has no caloric value, although metabolism by bacteria in the colon can contribute to energy requirements. Insoluble fiber provides bulk to the stool and reduces gastrointestinal transit time, which can alleviate constipation. Soluble fiber can lower cholesterol levels by two mechanisms. One is by binding to cholesterol and decreasing its absorption in the intestine. The second mechanism involves reducing enterohepatic recirculation of bile acids. Soluble fiber binds to cholesterol and bile acids in the intestine and promotes their excretion in the feces. The removal of bile acids leads to a decrease in the amount of bile acids in the recirculated bile acid pool. The liver must then produce additional bile acids to compensate for this loss. Since cholesterol is necessary to make bile acids, this deficit in the bile acid pool leads to a decrease in intracellular cholesterol stores, which in turn increases catabolism of low-density lipoprotein (LDL). Soluble fiber also slows gastric emptying, and dietary fiber intake above the 24 g/day recommended by the ADA improves glycemic control, decreases hyperinsulinemia, and lowers plasma lipid concentrations.[63-66] Recommendations for fiber intake are between 25 g/day for adult females and 38 g/day for adult males, or 14 g of fiber/1000 cal.[67] Actual fiber intakes for Americans are significantly below recommendations, in the range of 8–10 g/1000 cal/day. It is estimated that only 7% of adults meet the fiber recommendations.[68] Refer to **Table 8.8** for examples of foods that are high in fiber.

There is a large area of research that supports the effect of beans on glycemic control. One study found that glucose concentrations 90 minutes after a meal were significantly lower for meals that contained beans.[69] Beans are a great source of not only fiber, but also plant-based protein, which can be a great option for people with diabetes who follow vegetarian or vegan diets. Overall, it is important to encourage people with diabetes to choose carbohydrates from vegetables, fruits, whole grains, legumes, and low-fat dairy products over those that contain added- sugars, fats, and sodium, such as sugar-sweetened beverages, bakery products, or frozen desserts.

Table 8.8 Sources of Soluble and Insoluble Fiber

Soluble Fiber Sources	Insoluble Fiber Sources
Apples	Potatoes
Barley	Nuts
Beans	Wheat bran
Carrots	Whole-wheat flour
Citrus fruits	Berries
Oats	Cauliflower
Peas	Green beans

Data from Cleveland Clinic. What's the difference between soluble and insoluble fiber? Accessed January 12, 2026. https://health.clevelandclinic.org/whats-the-difference-between-soluble-and-insoluble-fiber

Sucrose and Other Nutritive Sweeteners

The time is long past when sucrose was a forbidden component in the diet of persons with diabetes. It has been well established that sucrose and other caloric sweeteners do not increase glycemic response any more than equivalent amounts of starch.[70] In fact, as foods containing sucrose may also have appreciable amounts of fat, the rise in glucose levels from these foods compared to equivalent amounts of carbohydrate from pure monosaccharides may be attenuated. However, caloric sweeteners such as sucrose, fructose, honey, corn syrup, and molasses contain 4 cal/g, the same as most dietary carbohydrates. Many foods containing a significant amount of sucrose or other caloric sweeteners are high in calories and fat and lacking in micronutrients. Therefore, sucrose-containing foods should not replace calories supplied from foods from the major food groups in the diet. Substitution of fructose for glucose, which does have a lower GI, does not appear to provide any dietary advantage. When consumed in excessive quantities, fructose can exacerbate hypertriglyceridemia or lead to further deterioration in glucose levels in those with poor metabolic control since fructose is converted to glucose when insulin is lacking.[71]

PRACTICE POINT

Sucrose can be incorporated as a part of the diet in persons with diabetes.

Protein

Protein has a limited impact on glycemic response. In people with T2DM, protein causes an increase in insulin response without a corresponding rise in blood glucose levels.[72] It has been hypothesized that higher protein diets may be beneficial for glycemic control in T2DM.[73] Several studies have found a role of higher protein diets (30–40% of total energy) in the reduction of A1c and the improvement of lipid levels.[74–76] Increasing protein intake may help promote satiety, which can aid in calorie reduction in people who desire weight loss.[73] Other research has started to compare the effects of animal-based versus plant-based proteins on obesity and T2DM.[73]

The influence of protein on insulin response and glucose excursions in people with T1DM is less clear-cut, but the impact of dietary protein to increase postprandial glucose excursions has been recognized.[76–80] Protein has a delayed and prolonged impact on blood glucose levels in people with T1DM.[80–83] As presented in Figure 8.5, amino acids are converted to glucose through gluconeogenesis, and glucagon, cortisol, growth hormone, IGF-1, and ghrelin increase insulin resistance; therefore, there may be a subsequent increase in blood glucose levels.[82] People without diabetes will experience a significant postprandial insulin response that is required for amino acid uptake, whereas people with diabetes have increased blood glucose levels and increased insulin requirements.[77,84] One study showed that the addition of ≥28 grams of protein to a mixed meal or consuming ≥75 grams of protein alone will likely result in significant and sustained postprandial hyperglycemia about 2–3 hours post-meal and may continue beyond 5 hours post-meal.[77] Some studies have found that increased protein in the diet will lead to a range of 30–50% increase in insulin dose needs.[77,79,82,85-87] Contrastingly, a randomized controlled trial of additional bolus insulin for protein did not show improvement in glycemic control or time in range in patients with well-controlled T1DM.[88]

The Institute of Medicine recommends a usual protein intake of 10–35% of daily energy (1.0–1.5 g/kg body weight/day).[89,90] Note that the ADA takes no position on the optimal amount of protein in the diet of people with diabetes other than to recommend that it be individualized to meet patient needs.[89,90] On the other hand, the Joslin Diabetes Center believes that the evidence for higher protein intakes for people with T2DM who are overweight is convincing and recommends that protein make up between 20% and 30% of calories (~1.2 g/kg body weight/day).[91]

Fat

The acceptable macronutrient range for fat set by the Institute of Medicine, and recommended by AND, is between 20% and 35% of calories, although no tolerable upper intake level is provided.[89] The 2020 Dietary Guidelines recommend limiting saturated fat to less than 10% of calories per day.[56]

Excess saturated fat has been linked to insulin resistance and metabolic syndrome.[92–94] Dietary fat consumed alone or as part of a mixed meal slows gastric emptying times and, when eaten in large enough quantities, increases insulin requirements.[77] Similar to dietary protein, dietary fat can have a delayed and prolonged impact on postprandial blood glucose levels, even with additional insulin.[77,82] Studies have investigated the amount of additional insulin required for fat and they ranged between 32% and 124%, with some reports of participants requiring no additional insulin.[82,87,95,96] Conversely, moderate amounts of healthy dietary fat may help prevent rapid spikes in blood glucose associated with a large carbohydrate intake. As displayed in Figure 8.5, dietary fat impacts blood glucose levels through gluconeogenesis, action of fatty acids, fat's effect on other hormones like GLP-1, GIP, and ghrelin, and on gastric emptying, which increases insulin resistance.[77,82] Most studies agree that dietary fat should be included in the calculations for insulin dosing, but do not provide a clinical guideline for calculating these doses.[97–99] An individualized approach for people using fast-acting insulin at meal times to adjust insulin doses and change insulin delivery times and methods, including split doses or extended bolus, when dietary fat makes up a substantial portion of the meal in order to maintain glycemic control, is recommended.[82,84]

People with diabetes are at 2–4 times the risk of CVD compared to the people without diabetes, and the risk increases as glycemic control worsens.[100] CVD strikes at a younger age and puts those with diabetes at the same risk of CVD as those without diabetes who have preexisting cardiovascular damage.[101] Reduction in saturated and trans fats is associated with both an improvement in lipid profile and better glycemic control. A Mediterranean dietary pattern, which is lower in total carbohydrate and higher in monounsaturated fatty acids, may be beneficial in controlling cardiac risk factors, as well as glycemic control even in the absence of weight reduction in persons with T2DM.[48,52,53] Omega-3 fatty acids help reduce triglyceride levels and cardiac arrhythmias, although there may be an accompanying rise in LDL cholesterol when supplements are used.[102] The recommendation for people with diabetes, as well as the general public, is to eat food high in long-chain omega-3 fatty acids such as fatty fish, nuts, and seeds.[103] Despite the improvement in lipid profiles, results of trials looking at the outcome of supplementing eicosapentaenoic and docosahexaenoic fatty acids have not demonstrated a decrease in the rate of cardiovascular events.[48,103–105]

At 9 cal/g, fat provides more than double the caloric density of protein and carbohydrate. Therefore, when weight loss is a goal, persons with diabetes may need to moderate total fat intake as part of a calorie-reduced meal plan.

There have been some hypotheses about food sequencing or the order that foods are eaten in (i.e., protein and fat before carbohydrate to slow digestion) and the impact on blood glucose, but there has not been data to support this.

Non-Nutritive Sweeteners

Although caloric sweeteners are permitted as part of a food plan for persons with diabetes, the calorie and carbohydrate load associated with their use has encouraged the development of alternative, low-calorie sweeteners. Non-nutritive sweeteners, also known as "artificial sweeteners," are often hundreds of times sweeter than their counterparts and require the use of only extremely small amounts to mirror the sweetness of sugar. They provide few, if any, calories or carbohydrates. All non-nutritive sweeteners on the market in the United States have undergone premarket safety testing or have been granted GRAS (generally regarded as safe) status by the Food and Drug Administration (FDA). Use of each of the sweeteners is permitted during pregnancy, although some healthcare providers discourage the consumption of saccharin because it crosses the placenta. In 2023, the International Agency for Research on Cancer, World Health Organization, Food and Agriculture Organization, and Joint Expert Committee of Food Additives (JECFA) classified aspartame as a possible carcinogen to humans. JECFA established an acceptable daily intake (ADI) of 0–40 mg/kg body weight, which is far below the doses at which potential effects have been described.[106]

There have been a number of epidemiological studies linking use of non-nutritive sweeteners, especially in diet sodas, to an increase in caloric intake and weight gain.[107] Several theories have been postulated as to the mechanism of the phenomenon, including that consumption of liquids containing sweetness, but no calories, stimulates appetite receptors in the brain.[108] At present there is inadequate evidence to support or refute these propositions. Currently, the ADA states that non-nutritive sweeteners can be used to reduce overall caloric intake associated with caloric sweeteners, presuming that intake does not compensate by consuming other caloric foods.[103] For all non-nutritive sweeteners, the FDA determines an acceptable daily limit (ADL) of intake (**Table 8.9**). The ADL includes a 100-fold safety factor and generally exceeds the average intake of these sweeteners by people with diabetes.[103,106–109]

Alcohol

Moderate intake of alcoholic beverages has little effect on glycemic control, and there is a body of evidence that suggests that it may improve CVD risk and overall glycemic control.[110,111] Alcohol is digested and absorbed in the body without the need for insulin. It interferes with gluconeogenesis and blunts the hormonal counter-regulatory response to **hypoglycemia** (undesirably low blood sugar, less than 70 mg/dL). The liver requires approximately an hour to process an ounce of alcohol. During this time, it effectively suspends its role in glucose replenishment; therefore, alcohol can induce hypoglycemia in people with diabetes who take insulin or oral insulin secretagogues. This may be undesirable because the body's response to alcohol in someone with diabetes can be quite complex. Many alcoholic beverages contain significant amounts of carbohydrate; a piña colada, for example, has approximately 30 grams of carbohydrate. Depending on the number and type of alcoholic beverages consumed, balancing the need for insulin to metabolize the carbohydrate against the glucose-lowering effects of alcohol can be difficult. Counseling patients to limit and/or avoid alcoholic beverages with higher carbohydrate content is often advisable. Consuming alcohol with foods that contain carbohydrates can help prevent delayed hypoglycemia.

Although moderate alcohol consumption may bestow some metabolic benefits, intemperate intake is discouraged. Excess alcohol consumption (greater than three drinks a day) has been associated with both hyperglycemia and hypertension.[110,111] Alcohol is a source of non-nutritive calories, providing 7 calories per gram. Excess consumption of alcohol can displace the intake of nutrient-dense food in the diet and promote weight gain.

Persons with diabetes who choose to drink should be counseled to do so in moderation: no more than one alcoholic beverage per day for females and no more than two alcoholic beverages per day for males. One alcoholic beverage is defined as 1.5 ounces of distilled spirits, 12 ounces of beer, or 5 ounces of wine. To reduce the risk of hypoglycemia, those persons taking insulin or oral secretagogues should be advised to eat carbohydrate-containing foods along with their alcoholic beverages. The Joslin Diabetes Center

Table 8.9 Non-Nutritive Sweeteners

Generic Name	Brand Name	Sweetness Compared to Sucrose (Number of Times Sweeter)	ADI (mg/kg/day)	Number of 12-oz Soda Cans = to ADI for 150-lb (68-kg) Person	Number of Table-top Sweetener Packets = to ADI for 150-lb (68-kg) Person	Cooking and Baking Conversion for 1/2 cup Granular White Sugar	Heat Stable
Acesulfame-K	Sweet One Sunett	200	15	25	20	6 packets	Yes
Aspartame	Equal NutraSweet	200	40	14-17	68	1/2 cup	No
Neotame	Newtame	7000–13,000	2	N/A ND	200	0.125 cup	Yes
Saccharin	Sweet'N Low Sweet Twin	300	5	42	9	1/2 cup	Yes
Sucralose	Splenda	600	15	15	30	1/4 cup Splenda Sugar Blend	Yes
Stevia	Truvia PureVia Sweet Leaf	200–300	4	16	30	12 packets	Yes
Luo Han Guo	Nectresse Monk Fruit in Raw PureLo	150	ND	ND	ND	12 packets	Yes

ADI, acceptable daily intake. ADI calculation is determined by dividing X mg/kg by 100, which X = daily dose that showed no effect.

ND - No Data Note: Beverages, sauces, puddings, and frozen desserts are better sweetened with non-nutritive sweeteners than cakes and cookies, which depend on sugar for moistness and tenderness as well as sweetness. Generally, no more than half the amount of sugar called for in the recipe should be replaced with artificial non-nutritive sweeteners.

Data from American Heart Association, American Diabetes Association. Nonnutritive sweeteners: current use and health perspectives. *Diabetes Care*. 2012;35(8):1798-1808.; U.S. Food and Drug Administration. Additional information about high-intensity sweeteners permitted for use in food in the United States. Accessed January 12, 2026. https://www.fda.gov/Food/IngredientsPackagingLabeling/FoodAdditivesIngredients/ucm397725.htm; University of Illinois Extension. Can you cook and bake with artificial sweeteners? Updated June 2014. Accessed January 12, 2026. http://extension.illinois.edu/diabetes2/subsection.cfm?SubSectionID=34

recommends adjustments in insulin dosing plans after 2 or more drinks for females and 3–4 drinks for males. It is important to take into account the type and amount of alcohol being consumed, the time period alcohol is being consumed, what type of food is being eaten, and what/if there was engagement in physical activity that day.[112] People using insulin pumps for administration may choose to decrease basal insulin delivery, also known as a "temporary basal rate," or use an activity or exercise feature to increase target blood glucose levels during periods of time with alcohol consumption and for 8–12 hours following to prevent hypoglycemia.

PRACTICE POINT

Alcohol can induce hypoglycemia in people with diabetes who take insulin or oral insulin secretagogues.

Caffeine

There is some speculation that caffeine may have an impact on blood glucose levels and how the body uses insulin, but there are no large clinical trials or reviews of this topic.

Micronutrients

There is no evidence that suggests that people with diabetes who eat a balanced diet have micronutrient needs in excess of the general public. Although both chromium and magnesium play pivotal roles in glucose metabolism, and supplementation for those individuals who are deficient in these nutrients is beneficial in restoring euglycemia, increasing intake in those with adequate reserves has not been proven efficacious.[113–117] Other studies have supported the use of additional supplementation of coenzyme Q10, vitamins B1, B9, C, D, E, K, and zinc for glycemic control in people with T2DM.[109,113] There are also studies that show the clinical benefit of supplementing omega-3 and omega-6 fatty acids, not only for glycemic control, but CVD markers as well.[114–117] Individuals who are infirm, older adults, pregnant individuals, and those who eat vegan or very low-calorie diets may require supplementation of specific nutrients.

There has been interest in the connection between vitamin D and insulin resistance. Vitamin D is associated with glucose-induced insulin secretion. Many people with and without diabetes are vitamin D deficient, specifically if they live in climates far from the equator. The incidence of T1DM increases the farther people live from the equator.[117] An association between vitamin D deficiency and T1DM has been hypothesized, but further research is warranted.[118] Some studies report an association between low levels of vitamin D and an increased risk of developing T2DM.[116] The Recommended Dietary Allowance for vitamin D for children and adults ages 1–70 years is 600 IU/day; for people older than 70 years, the requirement increases to 800 IU; for infants under the age of 12 months, the requirement is 400 IU.[119] As vitamin D is poorly distributed in the food supply and sunscreen is ubiquitously used, recommending a vitamin D supplement to people with diabetes, especially older adults, may be appropriate.

Herbal and Dietary Supplements

A variety of dietary supplements, such as bitter melon, fenugreek, ginseng, milk thistle, and various Chinese herbal medicines, may have effects on glucose metabolism and insulin resistance. However, there are currently no large-scale, double-blind clinical trials for herbal or dietary supplements that have proven a consistent, reproducible effect on diabetes control. There is some evidence that the use of berberine may have a beneficial effect on glycemic control, insulin resistance, and lipid metabolism in people with T2DM. Probiotic supplementation may have favorable effects on glycemic control in people with GDM, T1DM, and T2DM.[120–122] Resveratrol is a polyphenol that has been hypothesized to have potential benefits on glycemic control in people with T2DM.[123] Myo-inositol and d-chiro-inositol have gained some attention with its potential to lower blood glucose levels by improving insulin sensitivity; most of the data supports use in people with T2DM.[124,125] One study discusses the benefits of myo-inositol supplementation and its impact not only on people with T2DM, but insulin resistance, metabolic syndrome, T1DM, GDM, and polycystic ovarian syndrome (PCOS).[125] People who take insulin or insulin secretagogues should consult their healthcare providers before taking any herbal or dietary supplements to avoid any unwanted side effects.[119]

Cinnamon

Cinnamon is the familiar spice used to give flavor to everything from French toast to Middle-Eastern poultry dishes. There are two types of cinnamon. Ceylon, which is native to Sri Lanka, and Cassia, is the type commonly found in the United States. Cassia cinnamon contains coumarin, a compound that can be toxic to the liver if consumed in high doses. Cinnamon's use in diabetes control has been controversial for some time. It purportedly helps improve glycemic control by reducing insulin resistance. However, a 2022 systematic review looking at the effects of cinnamon on glucose control, regardless of type used, has demonstrated inconsistent results and emphasizes the need for dose–response relationship to be explored.[126]

A meta-analysis, which compared the results of 24 randomized controlled trials, found that cinnamon was helpful in lowering both fasting glucose and hemoglobin A1c.[127] The compound cinnamaldehyde, found in cinnamon, is thought to be responsible for its insulin-stimulating action.[128] Cinnamon is generally considered safe in usual amounts consumed and therefore could be suggested as a dietary measure with minimal cost and safety concern to patients who want to use a dietary adjunct to their medications. Patients who want to give cinnamon a try in relatively high doses may want to opt for the Ceylon version.

Medical Nutrition Therapy for Diabetes

Lifestyle intervention, including nutrition therapy, remains a foundational element in the management of diabetes. The ADA guidelines encourage self-management education and support for individuals with diabetes. The clinician should facilitate the development of knowledge and skills for ongoing self-management to improve clinical outcomes and quality of life for their patients. Education should be patient centered and responsive to individualized needs and preferences. The overarching goals of nutrition management in adults with diabetes are to:

1. improve over health, HgA1C, blood pressure and lipid profile.
2. achieve and maintain body weight goals; and

CASE STUDY REVISITED

One week later, Joseph returns to the outpatient clinic for medical nutrition therapy with a registered dietitian. As instructed at discharge, he keeps a record of his blood glucose levels and diet recall for the past 24 hours. His anthropometrics and insulin regimen are also provided below.

Anthropometric Data:

Height: 178 cm
Weight: 100 kg
BMI: 31.6 kg/m^2

Biochemical Data:

Record blood glucose levels previous 24 hours
8 am: 290 (upon awakening/before breakfast)
11 am: 166 (before lunch)
2 pm: 170 (midday check, before snack)
4 pm: 188 (before dinner)
10 pm: 199 (before bed)

Clinical Data:

Past Medical History: Type 1 diabetes (new onset).

Medications:
Medications: Insulin degludec (Tresiba): 28 units at bedtime
Vital Signs: Blood pressure 117/60 mm Hg
Nutrition-Focused Physical Exam: Patient appears to have good skin tone, no signs of muscle wasting or fat loss.
Insulin lispro (Humalog) matching insulin to carbohydrate intake

Dietary Data:

Dietary History: At home, Joseph has college classes at various times throughout the week. Every day is different with regard to meal times due to his scattered class schedule. Joseph is a good student and is involved in his college's football team. Joseph expresses some hesitation and stress related to management of glycemia and football.

Typical Diet Recall:

8–10 am: Breakfast: bacon, egg, and cheese sandwich, chocolate milk
Sometimes mid-morning snack if he has 8 am class and early breakfast: granola bar
12–1 pm: Lunch: deli sandwich or wrap
3–4 pm: Snack: chips and soda
6–7 pm: Dinner: spaghetti and meatballs and side salad
9–10 pm: Evening snack: ice cream
Physical activity: Plays on college football team (practice 4×/week; games on Saturday)

Questions

1. What is your assessment of Joseph's current glycemic control?
2. What additional questions might you ask to assess Joseph's understanding of the relationship between insulin and carbohydrate intake?
3. Are you able to resolve any PES statements? Do you need to add any new PES statements?
4. What is the appropriate meal plan for Joseph?

3. delay and prevent complications of diabetes. Evidence based healthy meal patterns that incorporate individual nutrition needs based on personal and cultural preferences should be used. Key factors emphasized in these meal patterns include:
   - Selecting more non-starchy vegetables and lean proteins, including milk
   - Choosing high quality carbohydrate foods such as whole grains, fruits
   - Choosing more legumes, peas, lentils
   - Minimizing added sugars and refined grains
   - Minimizing saturated fat and sodium
   - Choosing whole and minimally processed foods
   - Emphasizing foods to help meet dietary fiber requirements.

Table 8.10 Recommended Nutrition Visits for Diabetes Diagnosis

Initial Encounters		Follow-Up Encounters	
Number	Duration	Number	Duration
3–6	45–90 minutes	Once yearly	Unspecified

Data from Franz MJ, MacLeod J, Evert A, et al; Academy of Nutrition and Dietetics. Academy of Nutrition and Dietetics evidence-based practice guidelines. *J Acad Nutr Diet.* 2017;117:1659-1679.

Goals for nutrition therapy in pediatric diabetes as defined by the American Academy of Pediatrics should balance blood glucose goals with avoiding hypoglycemia and should promote a healthy lipid profile and blood pressure.[129]

Medical nutrition therapy (MNT) is effective and recommended for all people with diabetes.[103] Studies have found that MNT can reduce A1c by a decrease of 0.3–2.0% and 1.0–1.9% in T2DM and T1DM patients, respectively.[130,131] Patients benefit most when MNT is provided shortly after diagnosis. **Table 8.10** presents the Academy of Nutrition and Dietetics Evidence-based Practice Guideline for recommended nutrition visits.[130]

The initial encounters with a patient generally will focus on nutrition assessment as well as establishing a good rapport, which will continue throughout several sessions. The nutrition assessment may also take several sessions in order to collect all of the essential data that provide the basis for nutrition interventions. Follow-up is important to evaluate the efficacy of intervention and establish new goals, with adjustment of nutrition therapy accordingly.

Nutrition Assessment

Nutrition assessment relies upon the usual data elements obtained through anthropometric measures, including waist circumference, weight and calculated BMI, biochemical analysis, clinical assessment, and diet history. Diet history and assessment of food intake should be comprehensive, with attention to meal patterns, meal preparation, food shopping habits, and cultural values and beliefs of the patient. At this time, social and economic stressors should be assessed as well as knowledge and skill level, willingness for change, and barriers to dietary adherence. Diet recall and food records are used to evaluate overall energy intake and macronutrient distribution. Weight history and physical activity (frequency and intensity) are determined. Hydration habits and levels should be evaluated. Sleep patterns and quality of sleep should also be assessed, as these can impact glycemic control. Clinical data, including biochemical indices related to glucose control and cardiac risk factors such as lipid profile and blood pressure, are obtained. Medications and their impact on glycemia are determined. Nutrition planning should coincide with glycemic goals, medical comorbidities, and patients' preferences and ability to adhere to recommendations.[130] Self-monitoring of blood glucose is important to overall glycemic control. As overweight and obesity is an overwhelming component of T2DM—nearly half of all people with T2DM also have obesity—a focus on modest weight loss, which includes an evaluation of calories consumed, is important.[132]

Nutrition Intervention

Meal Planning

The best meal plan for a particular person is the one that they are willing to use. Determination of the appropriate method to employ is derived from a thorough nutrition assessment. As much as is feasible, the dietary regimen should be adjusted to fit the individual's preferences and lifestyle, not the other way around.[103]

PRACTICE POINT

Individuality in meal planning is necessary to assure willingness to comply.

A variety of meal planning methods, ranging from the simplistic to those requiring the use of mathematical calculations, are available. Regardless of which method is employed, a basic focus on food/food groups as opposed to nutrients is usually a more effective teaching tool when instructing patients. For patients who take insulin and are on a fixed insulin dose, consistency in carbohydrate intake with respect to time and amount is helpful in maintaining blood glucose control. Patients on a flexible insulin dosing regimen may be prescribed carbohydrate counting to maximize glycemic control.[103] Patients taking oral agents that cause the pancreas to secrete insulin, such as sulfonylureas, also benefit from having fixed meal periods with standardized amounts of carbohydrate at each meal. As a starting point or for persons with low literacy or understanding, simple messages focusing on the content of the U.S. Dietary Guidelines may be appropriate.[56] Guidelines should direct at increasing consumption of nutrient-dense carbohydrates that are high in fiber, which include fruits and vegetables, legumes, and whole grains. In addition, reducing excess sodium and added sugars, and aiming for consistency in carbohydrate intake and meal timing can be employed.[103]

Plate Method

The "plate method," a visual rendering of the appropriate amounts of the major food groups to eat at each meal, has the benefits of incorporating all food groups, not only those with carbohydrates. It is easy to understand, is reproducible in almost any dining situation, and enforces a basic method of portion control. **Figure 8.6** depicts the Diabetes Plate Method. Patients are instructed to divide their plate into three sections by bifurcating the plate and then bifurcating one of the halves again. The largest section, one-half of the plate, is filled with non-starchy vegetables, and the other two sections are made up of protein and starchy foods, respectively. A glass of water or a zero-calorie drink accompanies the plate.[133] The ADA on their website includes a step-by-step method to assemble a healthy plate: https://professional.diabetes.org/sites/dpro/files/2023-12/plan_your_plate.pdf

Exchange Method

Meal plans based on an exchange or substitution list have been used over several decades. With this approach, foods that have similar calorie and macronutrient content are grouped together. Food groups include dairy, fat, fruits, vegetables, meats/proteins, and starches. Patients are prescribed a certain number of servings from each food group for each meal and snack. These food choice plans provide structure for the type and amount of food allowed at each meal but provide patients latitude in selecting the particular food(s) that will fill each group. This type of planning tool is often beneficial for those who desire weight loss, because the total number of food groups assigned per day is based on a particular calorie level. **Table 8.11** provides a meal plan based on the exchange method for a 1800-calorie diet.

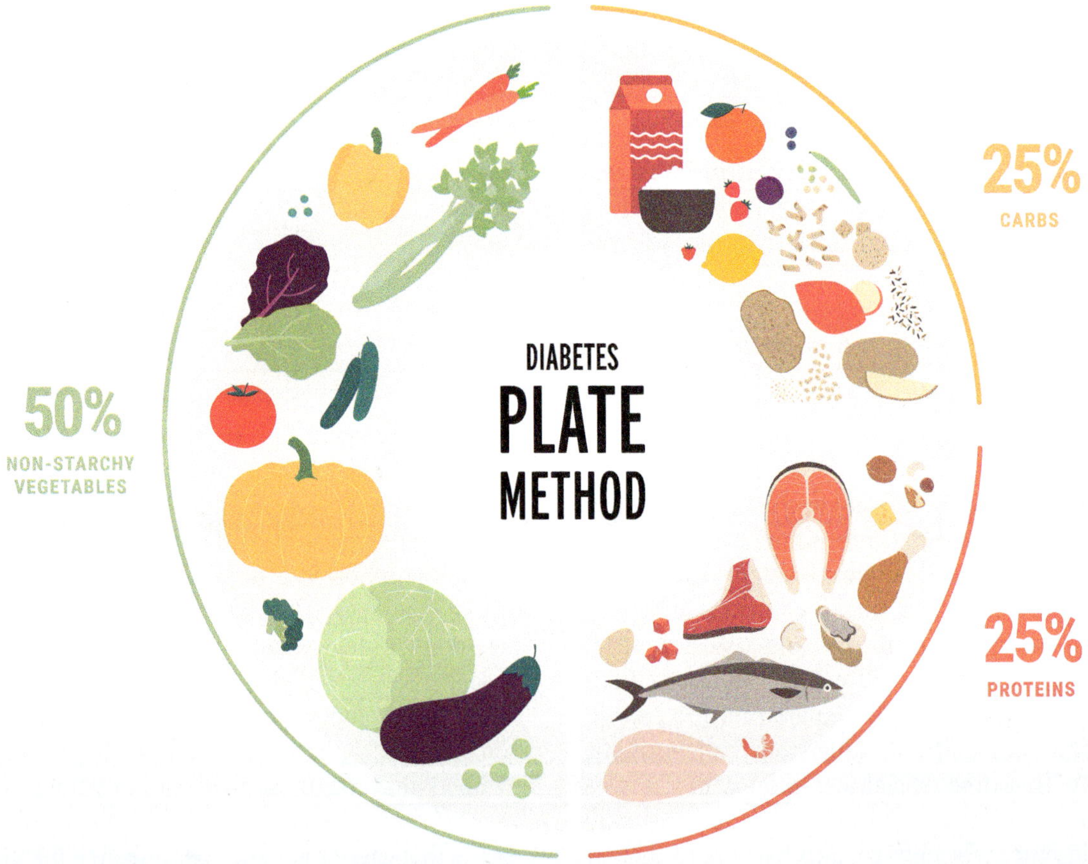
50%
NON-STARCHY VEGETABLES
DIABETES
PLATE
METHOD
25%
CARBS
25%
PROTEINS

Figure 8.6 Diabetes Plate Method

Table 8.11 Recommended Servings for a 1800-Calorie Plan

Meal	Food Group					
	Meat and Meat Substitutes	Starch	Fruit	Milk (Skim)	Fats	Non-Starchy Vegetables
Breakfast	1	1	1	1	2	
Lunch	2	2			2	2
Dinner	6	3		1	2	2
Snack 1			1		2	
Snack 2		1		1		
Totals	8	7	2	3	7	4

Nutrient distribution: 1,805 calories; 191 grams carbohydrate (42%); 115 grams protein (25%); 66 grams fat (33%)
Sample Menu

Breakfast	Lunch	Dinner	
1 scrambled egg 1 slice whole grain toast 1 1/4 cups strawberries 1 teaspoon soft spread 1 cup low-fat milk	1 small salad (1 cup mixed greens; 1 cup mixed cucumber, tomato, peppers) 2 tablespoons dressing 1 cup of lean meat-based chili with 1/4 cup of low-fat cheddar cheese topping	6 oz of broiled halibut 1 cup of garlic roasted Brussel sprouts 1 medium sweet potato 2 teaspoons soft spread 1 8 oz cup of non-fat-sugar-free yogurt	
	Snack 1 1 small apple with 20 almonds	**Snack 2** 8 oz of low-fat milk 1/2 whole grain English muffin with 1 teaspoon low-sugar jam	

Data from National Institutes of Health. Food exchange lists. https://www.nhlbi.nih.gov/health/educational/lose_wt/eat/fd_exch.htm

Basic Carbohydrate-Counting Method

Meal plans based on carbohydrate counting have become a popular and flexible method of meal planning. Basic carbohydrate counting involves adding up the total amount of carbohydrate, regardless of its source, to be eaten at a meal either in choices or in grams. When counting carbohydrates, it is important to acknowledge the portion size of all food items being eaten. Any packaged foods will have a food label with the portion size and total carbohydrate, which creates ease when eating packaged foods. For produce or other nonpackaged foods that do not come with a food label, it is important to have reference pages either online or in a book to refer to when carbohydrate counting. Some patients find it helpful to use a food scale for more accurate carbohydrate counting. One carbohydrate choice provides 15 grams of carbohydrate. Patients are provided a goal amount of carbohydrate to aim for at a meal; for example, a person with T2DM may have 45–60 grams of carbohydrate to use at dinner. Basic carbohydrate counting allows for consistency in meal carbohydrate intake, but does not teach healthy eating guidelines or how to choose healthier carbohydrate selections. Combining the use of basic carbohydrate counting with the glycemic index can assist people with diabetes in selecting those carbohydrates that are digested slowly and will have less impact on blood glucose levels. The ADA recommends protein and fat gram counting for better glycemic control in some individuals.[103]

PRACTICE POINT

Basic carbohydrate counting involves adding up the total amount of carbohydrate, regardless of its source, to be eaten at a meal either in choices or in grams.

CASE STUDY REVISITED

One month later, Joseph comes in for a nutrition visit. Your assessment of his knowledge indicates that he has improved his understanding of carbohydrate counting and his blood glucose levels are relatively well managed. Joseph has been highly motivated and would like to further control his glucose. With the help of the nurse practitioner, he recently started using the method of matching insulin to carbohydrate to dose his insulin.

Questions

1. Based on Joseph's most recent weight data, what is his total daily dose?
2. Calculate Joseph's insulin-to-carbohydrate ratio based on the total daily dose.
3. Calculate Joseph's correction based on the total daily dose.
4. Based on the ICR and CF you calculated, how many units of insulin should Joseph take if his blood glucose pre-meal is 280 mg/dL and he is planning to eat 72 grams of carbohydrate?
5. If Joseph requires 2500 kcal daily, use the carbohydrate-counting method to calculate a meal plan and insulin regimen for Joseph.

Advanced Carbohydrate Counting or Matching Insulin to Carbohydrate Method

Those people who use multiple daily injections of insulin or wear an insulin pump may use an advanced method of carbohydrate counting known as "matching insulin to carbohydrate." The amount of insulin given at a meal is a combination of the insulin units needed for both the carbohydrate content of the meal and the amount required to reduce the blood glucose into the target range. In this method, the **insulin-to-carbohydrate ratio (ICR)** defines the amount of carbohydrate processed by one unit of insulin. The **correction factor (CF)**, also known as the "sensitivity factor," defines the number of points one unit of insulin will lower the blood glucose.

A variety of equations exist for determining ICR and CF. In general, they include variations of adding together all the insulin given on an average day, including both basal and bolus insulin (the total daily dose [TDD]), and dividing a constant or a multiple of body weight in pounds by the TDD to arrive at the ICR and CF. Davidson et al.[134] advocated the 1700 rule for correcting insulin and using 2.8 times the weight in pounds divided by the TDD to establish the ICR. Researchers have used data derived from continuous glucose monitoring and continuous subcutaneous insulin infusion (CSII) to attempt to refine dosing guidelines.[135] In practice, 450–500 divided by the TDD is used to determine the ICR and 1500–2000 divided by the TDD for the CF. The larger the numerator, the greater the margin of safety. In addition, patients are provided a target or goal blood glucose number. This can range from 100 to 150 mg/dL depending on the patient's age, state of health, blood glucose control, and the frequency of and sensitivity to hypoglycemic reactions. Using this method (450 for the carbohydrate factor and 1500 for the correction factor), assuming the TDD is 100, the ICR would be 4.5 (round up to 5), and the CF 15. For a meal containing 50 grams of carbohydrate in which the pre-meal glucose value is 250 mg/dL and the goal glucose is 100 mg/dL, the patient will take 20 units of insulin.

Example:

Determination of Insulin-to-Carbohydrate ratio (ICR):

- Total daily dose of insulin (TDD): 100 units
- Divide 450 by TDD: 450/100 = 4.5 (round up to 5)
- ICR is 1:5 (1 unit of insulin: 5 grams carbohydrate)

Determination of Correction Factor (CF):

- Divide 1500 by TDD: 1500/100 = 15
- Correction Factor (CF) = 15 (1 unit of insulin brings glucose down by ~ 15 mg/dL)

Determination of Total Bolus Insulin Dose:

Current glucose = 250 mg/dL

Goal glucose = 100 mg/dL

Meal contains 50 grams of carbohydrates; how much total insulin is required?

How much insulin is needed to cover the meal?

With an ICR of 1:5, 1 unit of insulin is needed to process 5 grams of carbohydrate. How much would be needed to cover 50 grams of carbohydrate?

1 unit insulin/5 g carbohydrate
X units insulin/50 g carbohydrate

X = 10 units insulin

How much insulin is needed to lower the glucose?

Current glucose − goal glucose = amount of glucose needs to be lowered

250 mg/dL − 100 mg/dL = 150 mg/dL

The glucose needs to be lowered by 150 mg/dL

With a CF of 15, 1 unit of insulin will lower the glucose by 15 mg/dL.

1 unit insulin/15   X units insulin/150

X = 10 units insulin

Total bolus insulin needs: 10 units + 10 units = 20 units of insulin total

Insulin ratios can also be determined if patients have kept food and blood glucose records. The correction factor can be ascertained if the pre- and post-glucose values are available and if the number of units of insulin given is known. (To calculate the CF, subtract the post-glucose number from the pre-glucose value and divide by the units of insulin injected.) For example, if 5 units of insulin were given to reduce the blood glucose by 100 points, the correction factor is 20. The initial calculation should be viewed as a jumping off point that will need further refinements through trial and error.

CF = (post-glucose value − pre-glucose value)/units of insulin administered

Example: (200 mg/dL − 100 mg/dL)/5 units = 20

Correction Factor = 20

PRACTICE POINT

The total daily dose (TDD) is determined by adding together all the insulin given on an average day, including both basal and bolus insulin. The ICR is determined by dividing 450–500 by the TDD. The correction factor (CF) is calculated by dividing 1500–2000 by the TDD.

Matching insulin to carbohydrate allows for flexibility in meal planning. Meals do not have to be eaten at fixed times, nor does the amount of carbohydrate need to remain consistent. Although often used together at mealtimes, the CF can be used independently of the ICR to bring the blood glucose levels down at times when they are elevated between meals or overnight. Patients may have one carbohydrate ratio for the day or their ratio may vary depending on the meal or time of day. Insulin sensitivity changes throughout the day and is also affected by the amount of dietary fat consumed. Some people will have a smaller carbohydrate ratio at dinner because their dinner meal is often higher in fat than their breakfast or lunch meals. Often, patients will also have an alternate correction factor that they use during the night when they are more sensitive to insulin. Some people may experience a natural rise in blood glucose in the early morning hours, also known as the "dawn phenomenon," and may experience more insulin resistance during this time.

PRACTICE POINT

Matching insulin to carbohydrate allows flexibility in meal planning.

In addition to glycemic control, nutrition interventions for people with diabetes should account for risk reduction strategies for CVD, hypertension, and excess weight where applicable. Eating patterns such as the Dietary Approaches to Stop Hypertension (DASH) diet, the Mediterranean diet, and a plant-based diet have been found effective in improving glycemic control and ameliorating CVD risk factors.[103] For those individuals desiring weight reduction, a meal plan designed to produce a calorie deficit and lifestyle modification may be most appropriate.[103] Examples of usual amounts of carbohydrate recommended for females and males with T2DM are listed in **Table 8.12**.

Calculations for Basal Insulin or Long-Acting Insulin

Many patients with diabetes who use mealtime insulin will also use a long-acting insulin to help blood sugars

Table 8.12 Recommended Amounts of Carbohydrate per Meal for People with Type 2 Diabetes

	Males	Females
Active	60–75 grams	45–60 grams
Sedentary	45–60 grams	30–45 grams
For weight loss	45–60 grams	30–45 grams

Data from American Diabetes Association. Carbohydrate counting and diabetes. Accessed January 12, 2026. https://diabetes.org/food-nutrition/understanding-carbs/carb-counting-and-diabetes

stay in range between meals and overnight. People with T1DM will always need basal insulin.[136] Basal insulin is typically calculated by dividing weight in pounds by 4 to get the TDD, which is then divided by 2, as 50% should be basal insulin and the other 50% should be bolus insulin.[137]

For example:

Total Daily Insulin = weight in pounds/4 OR weight in kilograms × 0.55

If a patient weighs 200 lb…

TDD = 200 lb / 4 = 50 units

Basal insulin = TDD/2

50 units/2 = **25 units of basal insulin**

Nutrition Monitoring and Evaluation

Guidelines for monitoring the efficacy of nutrition care will vary according to individual needs and intervention strategies used. Evaluation of glycemic control will often include self-monitoring of glucose either by fingerstick, or a continuous glucose monitor (to be discussed below). Monitoring of fasting blood glucose, frequency of being within target ranges, and routine HbA1c levels should be included. Hypoglycemia and contributing risk factors should be assessed including exercise and alcohol intake. Analysis of dietary intake for overall energy balance as well as macronutrient distribution should be completed at each visit. It is equally important to assess patient knowledge and understanding of their prescribed diet as well as any challenges with their current regimen and adjust accordingly. Routine measures of weight, blood pressure, and biochemical indices to screen for cardiac and renal complications should also be included. Specific target ranges and parameters to monitor based on patient needs are described in more detail in the following sections.

Exercise

Exercise and physical activity are key components in the self-management guidelines for people with diabetes. Exercise improves cardiovascular health, sleep, and bone density; contributes to weight loss; and improves glucose control.

PRACTICE POINT

Exercise and physical activity are key components in the self-management guidelines for people with diabetes.

Type 1 Diabetes

The normal response to moderate exercise in those without diabetes is a reduction in insulin output and increase in glucagon secretion that results in glycogenolysis and gluconeogenesis.[138,139] In the presence of elevated circulating insulin, glycogenolysis is blunted and insulin-enhanced muscle glucose uptake is augmented, leaving the individual at risk for hypoglycemia. In addition, counter-regulatory mechanisms (catecholamines, growth hormone, and cortisol) present in healthy individuals that help prevent hypoglycemia during exercise may be curtailed by repeated episodes of low blood glucose in the person with T1DM.[140] Prolonged insulin

CASE STUDY REVISITED

Follow-up visit: Now that football season is in full swing, Joseph finds himself at times light-headed and anxious. His blood glucose levels have been running on the low side, particularly on days of football practice. He asks whether he should be adjusting his insulin or carbohydrate intake in any way.

Questions

1. What physiological explanations are there for Joseph's change in glycemic state? How does exercise alter Joseph's insulin requirements?
2. What signs and symptoms will you instruct Joseph to monitor for following exercise?
3. Describe your diet education plan for exercise management.
4. Based on the ICR and the CF you calculated, how many units of insulin should Joseph take prior to eating dinner if his blood glucose pre-meal is 280 mg/dL and his goal glucose is 145 mg/dL. He is planning to eat 72 grams of carbohydrate.

sensitivity following moderate to vigorous exercise, with long-duration, can induce hypoglycemia up to 24–48 hours after exercise in people with T1DM.[140–142] It is important to note that different types of activity and exercises will have different impacts on blood glucose levels, and no all activity will cause decreases in blood glucose levels.

CORE CONCEPT 6

During exercise, in the presence of elevated circulating insulin, glycogenolysis is blunted and insulin-enhanced muscle glucose uptake is augmented, leaving the individual at risk for hypoglycemia.

Although hypoglycemia is the most prevalent complication of exercise for people with T1DM, strenuous exercise, such as resistance training, can induce hyperglycemia and, in individuals whose diabetes is poorly controlled, diabetic ketoacidosis.[139] High-intensity exercise stimulates an increase in catecholamine levels, changing the balance between glucose generation and disposal toward greater glucose release. As endogenous insulin supplementation is not available, glucose levels increase temporarily, but generally decline within 1–2 hours; this is also known as an "adrenaline high."[143] In those persons with elevated blood glucose levels and ketone production, absolute insulin deficiency enhances additional ketone production and the risk of ketoacidosis.

Exercise provides many of the same benefits to people with T1DM as experienced by the general public and people with T2DM. However, the ability of exercise, specifically related to the type of exercise, to improve A1c values is not well established.[143,144] This is likely because although increased physical activity improves insulin sensitivity and reduces the total quantity of insulin administered,[144] exercise can induce both hypoglycemia and hyperglycemia.

Type 2 Diabetes

Improvement in glycemic control stimulated by physical activity is generally due to reductions in insulin resistance in skeletal muscle. Glucose uptake into skeletal muscle can increase dramatically in people with T2DM.[145–148] Insulin-dependent glucose uptake into muscle is accomplished through the translocation of glucose transporter protein type 4 (GLUT4), which is impaired in T2DM.[145,147] Exercise increases GLUT4 abundance and blood glucose transport, improving glycemic control.[145] Hypoglycemia in people not taking insulin or insulin secretagogues is usually rare, as the decline in endogenous plasma insulin level exceeds the transport of glucose into the muscle cells. Reduction of glucose levels may continue up to 72 hours post-exercise.[142]

CORE CONCEPT 7

Improvements in glycemic control stimulated by physical activity are generally due to reductions in insulin resistance in skeletal muscle.

The ADA and the WHO recommend that adults with diabetes perform at least 150 min/week of moderate-intensity aerobic physical activity or at least 75 min/week of vigorous-intensity aerobic physical activity, with no more than two consecutive days without exercise.[149,150] In the absence of contraindications, adults with T2DM should be encouraged to perform resistance training at least twice per week.[149] In children and adolescents, and in those for whom weight loss is a priority, 60 minutes or more per day of physical activity may be required.[103,151]

In individuals with T2DM performing moderate exercise, glucose transport by muscle usually rises more than hepatic glucose production, causing blood glucose levels to decline.[152] There is a compensatory reduction in plasma insulin levels, making the risk of exercise-induced hypoglycemia in anyone not taking insulin or insulin secretagogues quite minimal, even with prolonged activity.[152] These improvements in insulin action can last between 24 and 72 hours. The benefits of moderate exercise persist whether the activity is accomplished all at once or is divided into multiple sessions throughout the day.[153] Prevention and management of hypoglycemia during exercise requires coordination between reducing available insulin levels and increasing blood glucose levels with carbohydrate intake. In those individuals who are not taking insulin or insulin secretagogues, increases in carbohydrate consumption are not needed and, in the case of those with T2DM and overweight or obesity, not recommended. People who control their diabetes with an insulin pump or multiple daily injections of insulin can reduce bolus and/or basal insulin to help prevent hypoglycemia. If exercise is completed postprandially, reduction of pre-meal bolus dose between 25% and 75% of the usual dose is recommended.[154] Alternatively or additionally, depending on the duration and intensity of exercise, pump basal rates can be reduced by 20–50% 1–2 hours before exercise, and basal rates can be reduced or suspended during exercise.[154,155]

CASE STUDY REVISITED

At his routine nutrition counseling visit, Joseph is doing remarkably well. His blood glucose levels have ranged in the 150s. He is interested in knowing what the ideal glucose target range is for himself. He would like to maintain tight control. He also wants to know how often he should be monitoring his blood sugars.

Questions

1. What is the ideal glucose target range for Joseph?
2. What are the risks of tight glycemic control?
3. How often should Joseph be monitoring his glucose?
4. Do you think Joseph is a good candidate for a continuous glucose monitor? Explain.

Some insulin pump systems on the market have an activity or exercise mode feature that will make the adjustments to basal automatically for the user.

Carbohydrate Adjustment

The amount of carbohydrate necessary to prevent hypoglycemia is dependent on the intensity and duration of exercise. All exercise and activity should be delayed if blood glucose is <70 mg/dL. **Table 8.13** provides general guidelines for carbohydrate adjustment in exercise.

Glycemic Targets and Self-Monitoring of Blood Glucose

Self-monitoring of blood glucose (SMBG) is an important tool for both patients and providers to determine appropriate meal and correction medication doses for those on insulin, to assess the efficacy of the treatment regimens, and to identify patients' response to hyperglycemia and hypoglycemia. The frequency and timing of SMBG is related to the individual's medication regimen, their level of control, and the information being sought. Both the ADA and the American Association of Clinical Endocrinologists endorse the practice of individuals with diabetes, who take insulin multiple times per day, checking their blood glucose on a regular basis. The ADA is more prescriptive, stating that SMBG in those using multiple-dose injection insulin or an insulin pump should be performed prior to meals, at bedtime, prior to exercise, driving, occasionally postprandial, and whenever low blood glucose levels are suspected. In children with T1DM, more frequent self-monitoring is associated with lower A1c levels.[156,157]

The benefit of SMBG stems from maintaining better glycemic control. Lower A1c levels are associated with reduced microvascular complications and neuropathy and decreased cardiovascular events. However, the clinician should carefully consider the patient's risk for hypoglycemia and whether a lower glycemic target outweighs that risk. Patients who have a longer life expectancy and few comorbidities are ideal candidates, assuming that hypoglycemia is not a persistent obstacle. **Table 8.14** lists the targets suggested by the ADA for blood glucose monitoring.[156,158]

Fingerstick Blood Glucose Monitoring

People with diabetes should be properly trained on the use of blood glucose monitors, also known as "glucometers," even if they use a continuous glucose monitor. Historically, before continuous glucose monitors existed, fingerstick blood glucose monitoring was the standard of care for all people with diabetes, especially those using insulin.[158] These devices measure blood glucose levels from capillary blood. To check fingerstick blood glucose levels, wash hands thoroughly and insert a test strip into the glucometer. Once the glucometer turns on, use a lancing device on the side of the fingertip to get a drop of blood. Touch and hold the edge of the test strip in the drop of blood and wait for the results to appear on the glucometer screen.[159] For people not on insulin or insulin secretagogues, blood glucose monitoring has not demonstrated significant reductions in A1c levels, but may be helpful when altering lifestyle plans.[158] Fingerstick blood glucose

Table 8.13 Exercise and Carbohydrate Adjustment

Duration and Intensity	Blood Glucose Levels	Carbohydrate Adjustment
30 minutes or less low intensity*	<100 mg/dL	5–10 g
Leisurely walk, playing in the yard	100–200 mg/dL	No need for extra carbohydrate
	>200 mg/dL	No need for extra carbohydrate
30–60 minutes, moderate intensity*	<100 mg/dL	20–30 g
Brisk walking, bike riding, jogging	100–180 mg/dL	10–20 g
	180–300 mg/dL	No need for extra carbohydrate
	≥300 mg/dL	Test for ketones; if present, avoid exercise. Exercise with caution if no ketones and keep well hydrated.
30–60 minutes, high intensity*	<100 mg/dL	15–25 g
Soccer, field hockey, running	100–180 mg/dL	15–25 g
	180–300 mg/dL	No need for extra carbohydrate
>60 minutes, moderate intensity*	<100 mg/dL	20–30 g in the first hour, then additional 20–30 g/hour of activity
	100–180 mg/dL	10–20 g in the first hour, then additional 10–20 g/hour of activity
	180–300 mg/dL	No need for extra carbohydrate in the first hour, then 5–10 g/hour of activity

*For all types of exercise: if blood glucose is <70 mg/dL, exercise should be delayed until blood glucose is >70 mg/dL and give additional carbohydrates based on type and duration of exercise.
Data from Children's Mercy. Physical activity and carbohydrate counting: FAQ and terms. Accessed September 29, 2024. https://www.childrensmercy.org/contentassets/2442be4b1cc34304a9fcd953051568fa/physicalactivity-carb-counting-faq-terms.pdf

Table 8.14 Glycemic Targets for Insulin-Dependent Diabetes

Glycemic Target Category	HbA1c	Mean Fasting Plasma Glucose	Indicated Population
Stringent	<6.5%	122 112–127	Long life expectancy, short-duration diabetes, type 2 diabetes treated with lifestyle or metformin, pregnant females*
Reasonable	<7%	126 (100–152)	Non-pregnant adults
Flexible	<7.5%	152 (143–162)	Children (all age groups); in setting goals, long-term benefits must be weighed against the risk of hypoglycemia
Less Stringent	<8%	183 (147–217)	History of hypoglycemia, limited life expectancy, extensive comorbidities or vascular complications, difficulty achieving goals due to lifestyle management

*During later pregnancy, in the second and third trimesters, an A1c of <6% may be desirable if hypoglycemia is absent.
Data from American Diabetes Association. Glycemic goals and hypoglycemia. Chapter 6. In: *Standards of Care in Diabetes—2024. Diabetes Care.* 2024;47(Suppl 1):S111.https://diabetesjournals.org/care/article/47/Supplement_1/S111/153951/6-Glycemic-Goals-and-Hypoglycemia-Standards-of. Accessed January 12, 2026.

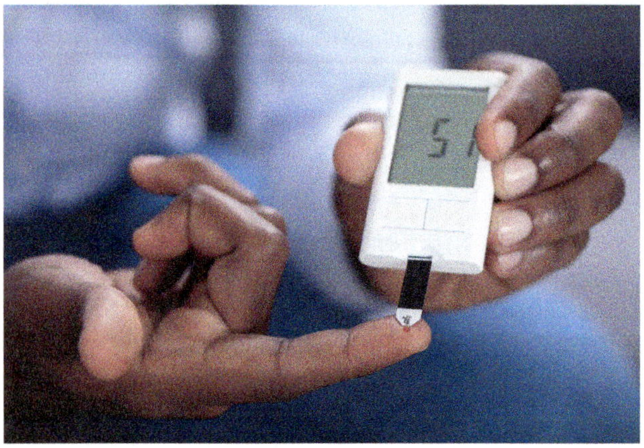

Figure 8.7 Demonstration of Blood Glucose Monitoring

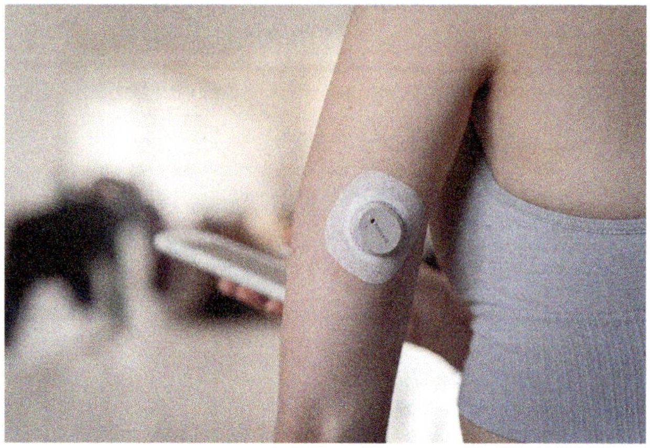

Figure 8.8 Demonstration of Continuous Glucose Monitoring

monitoring provides blood glucose data at one point in time, but does not give data on trends or what happens in between fingerstick tests. A photo demonstration of blood glucose monitoring by fingerstick is displayed in **Figure 8.7**.

Continuous Blood Glucose Monitoring

Continuous glucose monitors (CGMs) measure interstitial glucose, which correlates with plasma glucose. CGMs provide glucose data continuously for periods of time allowing people with diabetes to identify trends in their blood glucose values. There are two types of CGM devices that are used: real-time CGM (rtCGM) and intermittently scanned CGM (isCGM).[157] People with diabetes who are on insulin and capable of using a CGM should be offered their choice of device. These devices typically have a 10-to-14-day wear. Improvements in A1c levels and episodes of hypoglycemia when wearing a CGM have been demonstrated. CGM data provides reports on time in range (TIR), average blood glucose, glycemic variability, and ambulatory glucose profile (AGP). The ADA sets a goal of at least 70% TIR, which is blood glucose levels between 70 and 180 mg/dL. TIR correlates well with A1c. Time below range is categorized as blood glucose levels below 70 mg/dL, and time above range is any blood glucose level above 180 mg/dL. Some CGM reports provide a glycemic management index (GMI), which is an estimation of a person's A1c level based on their average glucose levels over a period of time.[159] A study by the University of Washington Diabetes Care Center analyzed CGM data from 641 patients with diabetes and compared A1c test results with GMI reports. They found that 11% of patients had a <0.1% difference, 50% of patients had differences of greater than or equal to 0.5%, and 22% of patients had differences greater than or equal to 1%.[160] Despite the benefits of CGMs, there can be a lag in data if glucose levels are rising or falling rapidly, so it is important for people with diabetes to have access to a glucometer. In addition, there may be times that the CGM is not providing accurate readings and may require calibrations. Most CGM companies emphasize the importance of understanding one's body and how it is always better to double-check with a fingerstick. Some people experience skin reactions, irritation, or allergy to the adhesive tape of CGMs.[157,158] A photo of a CGM is provided in **Figure 8.8**. **Figure 8.9** depicts a CGM report including average blood glucose, glycemic variability, TIR, AGP, and GMI.

For SMBG to become a routine part of people's treatment plans, patients must be educated on its purpose and use. Too often, patients check their blood glucose without understanding the importance or meaning of the numbers and SMBG becomes an exercise in busy work.

For many patients controlled on oral agents or taking one injection of basal insulin a day, checking once or twice per day is usually sufficient to extrapolate their control level. Bedtime and fasting numbers can be used to titrate the dose of basal insulin. SMBG can also help identify glucose patterns related to the quantity and types of food ingested. Paired tests, in which the patient checks blood glucose levels both prior to and 2–3 hours after a

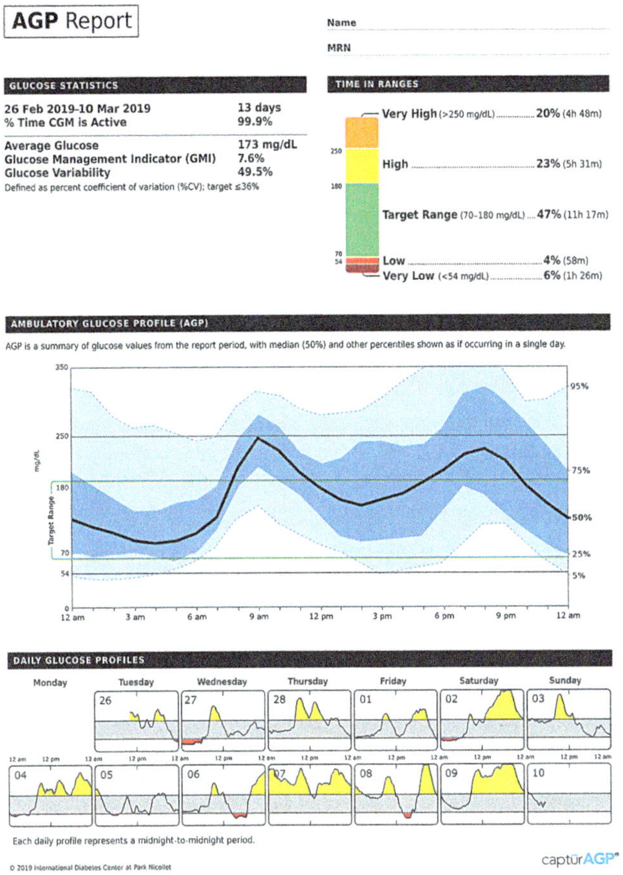

Figure 8.9 Example of Ambulatory Glucose Profile Report

Credit shared by RH - © 2025 International Diabetes Center, Minneapolis, MN. Used with permission. Visit AGPreport.org for more information.

meal, are useful to help determine whether changes in food choices and/or medication are indicated.

Acute and Chronic Complications of Diabetes

Acute Complications

The acute complications of diabetes are hyperglycemia and hypoglycemia. The causes of hyperglycemia and hypoglycemia are listed in **Table 8.15**, while the symptoms of both complications are presented in **Figure 8.10**. Hyperglycemia and hypoglycemia occur when there is a mismatch between the amount of insulin present in the blood and the available glucose concentration. Excessive glucose in relation to insulin results in hyperglycemia, while elevated levels of insulin in the absence of sufficient glucose predispose to hypoglycemia. A comparison of hyperglycemia and hypoglycemia can be found in **Table 8.16**.

Table 8.15 Causes of Hyperglycemia and Hypoglycemia

Hypoglycemia Causes	Hyperglycemia Causes
Excessive diabetes medicine	Insufficient diabetes medicine
Inadequate carbohydrate	Excessive carbohydrate
Exercise	Exercise
Alcohol	Steroids
Illness resulting in suboptimal intake	Some psychiatric medications
	Critical illness and metabolic stress

Data from InformedHealth.org [Internet]. Cologne, Germany: Institute for Quality and Efficiency in Health Care (IQWiG); 2006-. Type 2 diabetes: learn more – hyperglycemia and hypoglycemia in type 2 diabetes. Updated December 18, 2023. Accessed January 12, 2026. https://www.ncbi.nlm.nih.gov/books/NBK279510/

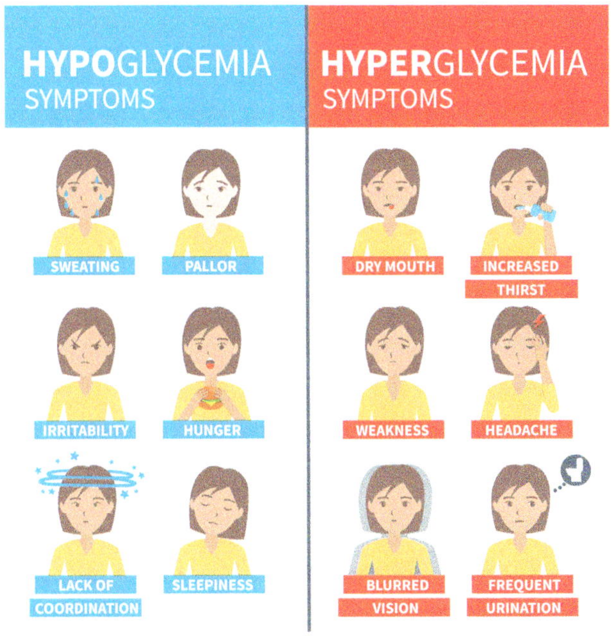

Figure 8.10 Symptoms of Hypo- and Hyperglycemia

© Irina Strelnikova/Shutterstock

Hyperglycemia may be defined as a blood glucose level above 130 mg/dL after an 8-hour fast and a glucose level greater than 180 mg/dL 2 hours postprandially. Excessive carbohydrate intake, illness, certain medications such as corticosteroids, limited activity, strength training, and skipping insulin or oral hypoglycemics can all lead to hyperglycemia. Persistent hyperglycemia in the face of insulin deficiency can

Table 8.16 **Distinguishing Symptomology of Hypoglycemia Versus Hyperglycemia**

Symptoms of Hypoglycemia	Symptoms of Hyperglycemia
Adrenergic	Increased thirst
Sweating	Dry mouth or skin
Shakiness	Fatigue
Rapid heartbeat	Blurred vision
Anxiety	Increased infections
Hunger	Frequent urination
Weakness	Headache
Tingling around the mouth	
Neurologic symptoms	
Headache	
Double vision	
Lack of coordination	
Confusion	
Seizures	
Inappropriate behavior	

Data from InformedHealth.org [Internet]. Cologne, Germany: Institute for Quality and Efficiency in Health Care (IQWiG); 2006-. Type 2 diabetes: learn more – hyperglycemia and hypoglycemia in type 2 diabetes. Updated December 18, 2023. Accessed January 12, 2026. https://www.ncbi.nlm.nih.gov/books/NBK279510/

Table 8.17 **Classification of Hypoglycemia Level**

Level	Classification	Threshold
1	Glucose alert level	≤70 mg/dL
2	Clinically significant hypoglycemia	<54 mg/dL
3	Severe hypoglycemia	Not established*

*Severe hypoglycemia does not have a specific threshold, but can be defined as hypoglycemia that results in severe cognitive impairment that requires medical intervention.
Data from Davis HA, Spanakis EK, Cryer PE, et al. Hypoglycemia during therapy of diabetes. Table 1. Classification of hypoglycemia in diabetes. In: Feingold KR, Ahmed SF, Anawalt B, et al., eds. *Endotext* [Internet]. South Dartmouth, MA: MDText.com, Inc.; 2000-. Updated July 7, 2024. Accessed January 12, 2026. https://www.ncbi.nlm.nih.gov/books/NBK279100/table/hypoglycm-thrpy-diab.T.classification_of/

Table 8.18 **Treatment of Hypoglycemia**

3–4 glucose tabs
1 tbsp honey or sugar
4 oz juice
6 oz regular soda
8 jelly beans
8 oz skim milk

Data from American Diabetes Association. Signs, symptoms, and treatment for hypoglycemia (low blood sugar). Accessed January 12, 2026. https://diabetes.org/living-with-diabetes/hypoglycemia-low-blood-glucose/symptoms-treatment

precipitate dehydration, ketone formation, and ketoacidosis in persons with T1DM and susceptible individuals with T2DM. People with T2DM can also develop hyperosmolar hyperglycemic nonketotic coma (HHNC). Persons with T2DM who develop HHNC usually are older adults with several comorbidities and have a diminished thirst sensation. Treatment for hyperglycemia is additional insulin, sugar-free fluids, and/or exercise.

The ADA recognizes a blood glucose level below 70 mg/dL as consistent with hypoglycemia in those with diabetes.[156] Mild hypoglycemia can be disorienting to the person and often frightening to bystanders, while severe hypoglycemia can lead to serious consequences such as motor vehicle accidents and falls. The symptoms of hypoglycemia are divided into those that are derived from the autonomic nervous system, such as sweating and palpitations, and those that are due to the brain's glucose deprivation. Initial neuroglycopenic (shortage of glucose in the brain) symptoms may include difficulty concentrating and the inability to perform simple mathematical computations. As hypoglycemia worsens, deterioration in the ability to think clearly, slurred speech, confusion, irrational behaviors, lethargy, seizures, and loss of consciousness can occur. **Table 8.17** provides the classification for level of hypoglycemia, from alert levels 1 (minor) to 3 (severe). Severe hypoglycemia does not have a specific threshold but can be defined as hypoglycemia that results in severe cognitive impairment that requires medical intervention.

Symptoms of hypoglycemia can also occur even if the blood glucose level is above 70 mg/dL. This often happens if the glucose level falls rapidly from a higher value to a much lower value. When those whose blood glucose is in poor control have their glucose levels brought into the normal range rapidly, they may also experience the symptoms for hypoglycemia due to the release of epinephrine.

The treatment for low blood glucose is carbohydrate, which is described in more detail in **Table 8.18**. All carbohydrates will eventually raise glucose levels, but carbohydrates that contain excess fiber or fat

Clinical Roundtable

Topic: Type 1 Diabetes and Celiac Disease

Background: Type 1 diabetes and celiac disease are both autoimmune diseases that have clinical and genetic overlap. Approximately 6% of people with type 1 diabetes develop celiac disease. Studies emphasize the importance of early screening for celiac disease within the first year of type 1 diabetes diagnosis, then again at 2 years and 5 years after diagnosis. The recommendations regarding the frequency of screening after 5 years of diagnosis are not clear. There are no data supporting that a gluten-free diet can prevent the development of celiac disease in patients with type 1 diabetes. This presents clinicians with the need to establish practice guidelines for screening and further research on prevention or delaying the onset of celiac disease.

Roundtable Discussion

1. What might you suggest as best practice for monitoring these patients?
2. Should all patients be screened for celiac disease after 5 years of diagnosis or only if celiac disease is suspected from lab results, family history, or unexplained frequent hypoglycemia? Explain.
3. What other criteria might you put in place to be most efficient in identifying new cases of celiac disease in patients with type 1 diabetes?

References

1. Flores Monar GV, Islam H, Puttagunta SM, et al. Association between type 1 diabetes mellitus and celiac disease: autoimmune disorders with a shared genetic background. *Cureus*. 2022:14(3):e22912.
2. Hatun Ş, Dalgıç B, Gökşen D, Aydoğdu, S, et al. Recommendations for clinical decision-making in children with type 1 diabetes and celiac disease: type 1 diabetes and celiac disease joint working group report. *J Clin Res Ped Endocrinol*. 2022;14(1):1–9.

should be avoided because they will slow digestion, and in turn delay blood glucose from rising. Use of the "15/15" rule is recommended in clinical practice. Specifically, it is recommended for patients to eat 15 grams of carbohydrate and wait 15 minutes. For glucose levels of 50–70 mg/dL, consuming 15 grams of carbohydrate, such as 4 ounces of juice, 6 ounces of regular soda, or 3–4 glucose tabs, will usually bring glucose levels back to target range. Blood glucose levels less than 50 mg/dL often require at least 30 grams of carbohydrate to return blood glucose values back to the target range. After waiting 15 minutes, blood glucose should be rechecked to make sure levels have risen above 80 mg/dL. Protein increases insulin response without raising blood glucose, so protein-containing foods should not be used to treat hypoglycemia. Additional treatment is required if glucose levels have not reached targets. Severe hypoglycemia that produces unconsciousness or seizing may require the use of glucagon, either by intramuscular injection or nasal actuation spray. Glucagon raises blood glucose by releasing glucose stored in the liver. It can also induce nausea and vomiting, requiring that the person be placed on their side to avoid aspiration.

Chronic Complications

Uncontrolled diabetes leads to a host of microvascular, macrovascular, and neurological complications. Both the Diabetes Control and Complication Trial (DCCT) and the United Kingdom Prospective Diabetes Study support the role of intensive control of glucose in reducing the risk of complications.[161,162] For every 1% decrease in blood glucose levels, there is a corresponding reduction in the risk of complications related to diabetes of approximately 21%.[163] Chronic complications of diabetes are outlined in **Figure 8.11**. **Figure 8.12** is a graph from the DCCT depicting the relative risk and progression of diabetes complications by mean A1c.

CORE CONCEPT 8

For every 1% decrease in blood glucose levels, there is a corresponding reduction in the risk of complications related to diabetes of approximately 21%.

Psychological Complications

Diabetes distress, sometimes referred to as "diabetes burnout," is defined as the intense stress related to the experience of living with diabetes. Patients with diabetes often have negative psychological effects from the constant worry of daily medications management, dietary specifications, and blood glucose monitoring, as well as the long-term concern of disease progression. Data on diabetes distress estimates a prevalence of 18–45% in those with diabetes. To make matters

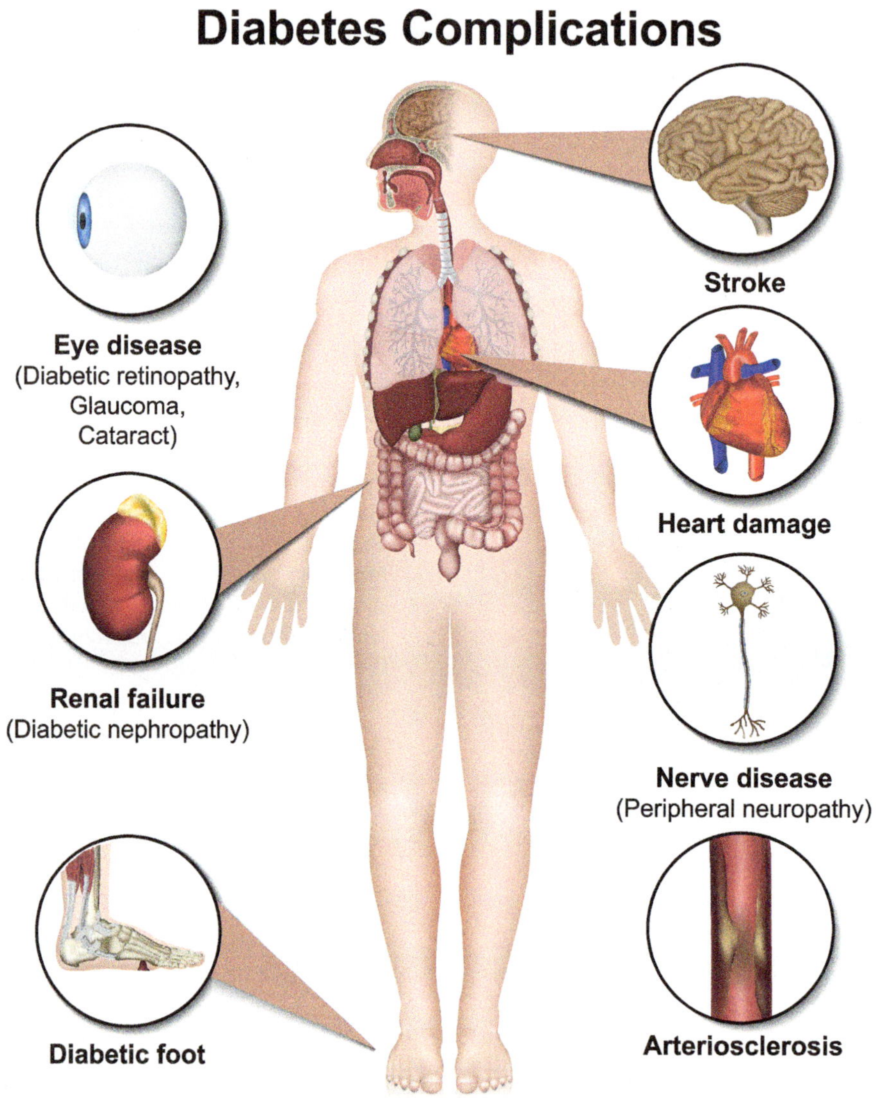

Figure 8.11 Chronic Complications of Diabetes

worse, those with diabetes distress are more likely to have higher A1c levels, nutritionally inadequate diets, lower exercise levels, and lower self-efficacy. The ADA recommends provision of additional specific diabetes education to address any areas of concern for the patient, followed by referral to a mental health specialist who is ideally familiar with diabetes management.[103]

Diabulimia refers to anyone with insulin-dependent diabetes who omits or restricts their insulin. ED-DM refers to anyone with comorbid diabetes and an eating disorder, regardless of type. The *Diagnostic and Statistical Manual of Mental Disorders* does not recognize any diabetes-specific diagnoses, but it does acknowledge insulin restriction/omission as a purging behavior. People with diabetes have a higher risk of developing an eating disorder with intense focus on food, labels, weight, blood glucose, A1c, and control for diabetes management. Warning signs and symptoms may include increasing neglect or secrecy of diabetes management, avoiding diabetes-related appointments, fear of hypo- and hyperglycemia, fear that insulin causes weight gain, anger about having diabetes, avoidance of medications, extreme increase or decrease in diet, extreme anxiety about body image, restricting certain foods or food groups to lower insulin doses, avoiding eating with family or in public, discomfort testing blood glucose and administering insulin in front of others, excessive exercise habits, increased sleep, withdrawal from friends and family, depression or anxiety, infrequently filled prescriptions, overly strict food rules, and obsession with food, weight, or calories. The National Eating

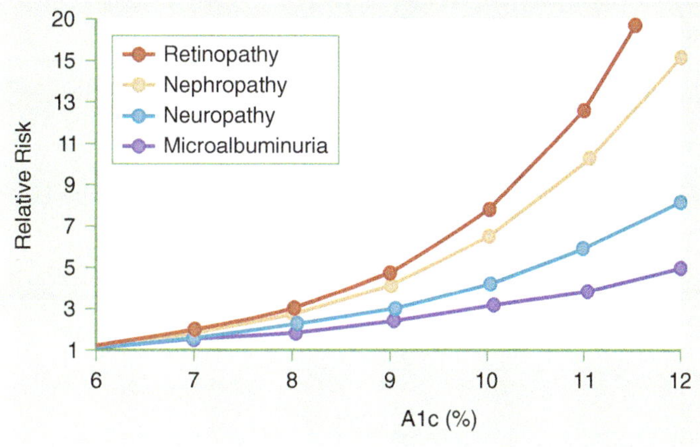

Figure 8.12 Diabetes Control and Complications Trial

Modified from Skyler JS. Diabetic complications: the importance of glucose control. Endocrinol Metab Clin North Am. 1996;25(2):243-254. doi:10.1016/s0889-8529(05)70323-6. PMID: 879969

Disorder Association recommendations include the importance of seeing an interdisciplinary team (endocrinologist, dietitian, diabetes educator, psychiatrist), "good enough" diabetes care over "perfect," and acknowledgment that eating disorders are serious mental health disorders and cannot be treated by reinforcing diabetes education.[164]

PRACTICE POINT

Dietary interventions include limiting saturated fat to <7% of calories, minimizing or eliminating artificial trans fat, increasing fiber intake, and including 2 grams of plant stanols and sterols, and omega-3 fatty acids in the form of fatty fish or plant sources.

Macrovascular Complications

Macrovascular complications include heart disease, stroke, and peripheral vascular disease. Unlike the impressive reductions in the risk of microvascular damage with intensive glycemic control, intensive control of blood glucose does not completely reduce the risk of developing macrovascular complications in persons with diabetes. One of the defining features of CVD is endothelial dysfunction. Insulin resistance and hyperglycemia contribute to endothelial dysfunction, which diminishes the normal anti-atherogenic properties of the endothelial cells.[165] Endothelial dysfunction is often present in people with prediabetes and metabolic syndrome and is an independent risk factor for CVD. Persons with diabetes often have independent CVD risk factors such as hypertension and dyslipidemia in addition to diabetes. Target blood pressure for people with diabetes is less than 130 mm Hg systolic and less than 80 mm Hg diastolic.[166] Guidelines for lipid control do not recommend target levels for LDL and HDL cholesterol.[167] Rather, a target percentage reduction is based on the patient's age and initial LDL starting level. Lifestyle modification is recommended for everyone, but statins are suggested for those with diabetes who are older than 40 years of age. Uncontrolled hyperglycemia can lead to severely elevated triglyceride levels because of its suppressive effects on the hormone lipoprotein lipase. Lowering A1c is often effective in bringing triglycerides back into the target range. For those patients with both CVD and diabetes, use of liraglutide (GLP-1 receptor antagonist) and empagliflozin (SGLT-2 inhibitor) is now recommended as treatment following the results of two large-scale clinical trials.[168]

The ADA recommends lifestyle intervention for those persons with blood pressure greater than 120/80 mm Hg; those whose blood pressure exceeds 130/80 mm Hg should be managed with lifestyle and pharmacological interventions.[169] **Table 8.19** provides an overview of blood pressure classification in adults. The 2017 ADA Standard of Medical Care in Diabetes has expanded to provide four options of blood pressure–reducing medications to treat those with both hypertension and diabetes. These medications include ACE inhibitors, thiazide-like diuretics, angiotensin receptor blockers, and dihydropyridine calcium channel blockers.[170] Studies have demonstrated positive effects on lipid parameters and blood pressure of diets that limit saturated fat, trans fat, cholesterol, and sodium intake.[171,172] In addition, Mediterranean diets

Table 8.19 Blood Pressure Classification in Adults

	American College of Cardiology/American Heart Association 2017 Guideline for High Blood Pressure Levels in Adults		
Category	**Systolic (mm Hg)****		**Diastolic (mm Hg)****
Normal	Less than 120	And	Less than 80
Elevated	120–129	And	Less than 80
Hypertension Stage 1	130–139	Or	80–89 or higher
Hypertension Stage 2	≥140	Or	≥90

*For adults ages 18 and older who are not on medicine for high blood pressure and do not have a short-term serious illness.

**If systolic and diastolic pressures fall into different categories, overall status is the higher category.

Data from Whelton PK, Carey RM, Aronow WS, et al; American College of Cardiology/American Heart Association. 2017 Guideline for the prevention, detection, evaluation, and management of high blood pressure in adults: a report of the American College of Cardiology/American Heart Association Task Force on Clinical Practice Guidelines. *Hypertension*. 2018;71:e13–e115.

have demonstrated promise in helping those with diabetes lower cardiac risk.[173] The DASH diet, which promotes a diet low in sodium (<1500 mg/day) and saturated fat (6% of calories) but high in potassium (4700 mg), has been proven effective in lowering blood pressure.[174]

Microvascular Complications

Nephropathy. In the United States, diabetes is the leading cause of end-stage kidney disease.[1] It is estimated that 35–50% of new cases of end-stage kidney disease are due to diabetic **nephropathy** (damage to the kidneys due to diabetes).[175] Approximately one-third of people with T1DM will develop nephropathy within 20 years of being diagnosed with diabetes. Although far fewer people with T2DM will develop end-stage nephropathy, the sheer number of people who have T2DM means that the burden of treating those who will need dialysis could become overwhelming.[1] The Kidney Disease Outcomes Quality Initiative (KDOQI) guidelines divide kidney disease into five stages, which are further discussed in Table 8.20. The loss of glomerular filtration rate (GFR) and the recommended nutrition intervention per stage of kidney disease are given in **Tables 8.20** and **8.21**.[176,177] In the initial stages, the concentrating ability of the kidneys is not affected and blood urea nitrogen (BUN) and creatinine are normal. Often, microalbuminuria is the first indication that the kidneys are functioning abnormally. **Microalbuminuria** is defined as greater than 30 mg but less than 300 mg of albumin in the urine daily. Overt proteinuria correlates closely with a more rapid rate of progression to end-stage kidney disease.[178] Lifestyle interventions concentrate on controlling hyperglycemia and blood pressure. Dyslipidemia is often a concurrent finding in those with diabetes and kidney disease and is a major risk factor for CVD. Control of lipid levels through dietary modification along with appropriate medications has become a more pressing concern as more evidence has accumulated linking dyslipidemia of diabetic kidney disease to increased morbidity and mortality. People with diabetes in the early stages of kidney disease can often continue to follow the same healthful dietary patterns suggested for controlling diabetes and other chronic diseases such as a Mediterranean or DASH diet, both low in saturated fat, added sodium, and sugars and plentiful in fruits and vegetables.[179]

In the past, aggressive protein restriction was thought to preserve kidney function and extend the time prior to the onset of dialysis. Secondary analyses of the data from the Modification in Diet in Renal Disease, the larger multicenter study to address the relationship between protein intake and kidney function, indicated that protein restriction does have a role in slowing diabetic and non-diabetic kidney disease.[180] However, the results of newer studies evaluating whether protein restriction prevents decline in albumin excretion rate (AER) and in GFR have been mixed.[181,182] Although clinical trials have demonstrated a reduction in AER, reducing protein has not been as effective in preventing the decline in GFR, and extremely low levels of dietary protein can lead to malnutrition. Plant-based protein sources may be encouraged for early-stage kidney disease as they contain less saturated fat and provide a better fiber source than animal proteins. Even though evidence supporting protein restriction remains limited, clinical guidelines developed by the major kidney and diabetes organizations often still call for protein modifications for people with diabetes and kidney

Table 8.20 Stages of Chronic Kidney Disease

Stage	GFR	Description	Symptoms	Action for Individuals with DM
1	90 or greater	Normal kidney function with structural or urine abnormalities	None usually	Observation Healthy lifestyle Testing of blood and parameters, control of blood pressure and blood glucose
2	60–89	Mild CKD	None usually	Observation Healthy lifestyle Testing of blood and parameters, control of blood pressure and blood glucose
3a	45–59	Moderate CKD	Possible fatigue, fluid retention, anemia, high blood pressure	Control of blood pressure and blood glucose. More frequent estimation of creatinine, HbA1c, and urinary protein
3b	30–44	Moderate CKD	Possible fatigue, fluid retention, anemia, high blood pressure	Control of blood pressure and blood glucose. More frequent estimation of creatinine, HbA1c, and urinary protein
4	15–29	Severe CKD	Development of bone disease, high blood pressure, anemia, cardiac disease, possible uremia, hyperkalemia, and hyperphosphatemia	Planning for end-stage disease. Control of blood pressure and blood parameters. Three-month estimation of creatinine, HbA1c, urinary protein, potassium, and phosphorus
5	<15	End-stage CKD	Uremia if not on dialysis	Dialysis

CKD, chronic kidney disease; GFR, glomerular filtration rate; KDOQI, Kidney Disease Outcomes Quality Initiative.
Data from UK Kidney Association; KDOQI. Clinical practice guidelines and clinical practice recommendations for diabetes and chronic kidney disease. *Kidney Int Suppl*. 2020;10(1):1-115.

disease. The 2012 Kidney Disease Improving Global Outcomes Practice Guideline for the Evaluation and Management of Chronic Kidney Disease suggests 0.8 g/kg/day of protein in adults with diabetes and GFR <30 mL/min/1.73 m^2 and avoidance of intake >1.3 g/kg in adults with chronic kidney disease at risk of progression.[179] AND nutrition guidelines suggest an intake of 0.6–0.8 g/kg body weight with at least 50% coming from high biological value protein sources particularly in patients with diabetes.[183] The ADA has moved to a more liberal approach suggesting patients maintain usual levels of dietary protein intake.[184]

As damage to the kidneys continues, their ability to remove waste products is diminished and dietary modifications of minerals, potassium and phosphorus, in addition to sodium, are required. Persons with diabetes taking angiotensin-converting enzyme inhibitors or angiotensin receptor blockers may be predisposed to higher potassium levels and need modification of these nutrients sooner than is customarily required. When patients reach Stage 5 (GFR <15 mL/min/1.73 m^2), the kidneys can no longer eliminate waste products effectively without mechanical intervention. Hemodialysis or peritoneal dialysis (PD) is initiated. In addition to modifications in minerals and macronutrients, patients on dialysis must restrict fluid and the patient using PD must take into account the glucose absorbed

Table 8.21 Nutrition Recommendations for Diabetes and Chronic Kidney Disease

Nutrient	Chronic Kidney Disease Stage	Recommendation
Protein	1–4	0.8 g/kg/day
Phosphorus	1–2	1.7 g/day
	3–4	0.8–1.0 g/kg/day
Potassium	1–2	>4 g/day
	3–4	2.4 g/day
Sodium	1–4	<2.3 g/day

Data from National Kidney Foundation. KDOQI clinical practice guidelines and clinical practice recommendations for diabetes and chronic kidney disease: 2012 update. *Am J Kidney Dis*. 2012;60(5):850-886.

from the dialysis solution when calculating carbohydrate and energy needs. Blood glucose levels should be monitored closely when patients start or change dialysis solutions.

Retinopathy. Diabetes is the leading cause of new cases of blindness in adults ages 20-70 years.[185] After 20 years of diabetes, most people will have some evidence of diabetic eye disease. There are four stages of **retinopathy**, but retinopathy can be broadly divided into two major categories: nonproliferative and proliferative retinopathy. In nonproliferative retinopathy, high blood glucose causes the lining of blood vessels in the retina to thicken and leak. Leakage of blood and fluid into the center of the retina, called "macular edema," can result in loss of central vision. In proliferative retinopathy, new, fragile cells grow on the surface of the retina, obscuring vision. If left untreated, proliferative retinopathy can cause blindness. Because of the pressure exerted on the retina by scar tissue, advanced proliferative retinopathy may also lead to retinal detachment. The manifestations of diabetic retinopathy are presented in **Figure 8.13**.

Retinopathy cannot be cured, but it can be treated with laser photocoagulation and vitrectomy surgery. Diabetic eye disease does not usually cause vision loss until it is well advanced. Quitting smoking and controlling blood glucose levels, cholesterol levels, and blood pressure are key to preventing and slowing the progression of retinopathy.[186] People with diabetes are also at higher risk of eye conditions that affect people without diabetes, such as cataracts and age-related macular degeneration. The Age-Related Eye Disease Study (AREDS), conducted in 2001, found that daily high doses of vitamins C and E, β-carotene, and the minerals zinc and copper can help slow the progression to advanced AMD. In 2006, a second, 5-year study, called "AREDS2," determined that the AREDS formulation with the addition of lutein and zeaxanthin and the removal of β-carotene, reduced the risk of AMD.[187,188]

Dental Disease. Blood glucose control and optimal dental care are important in maintaining good oral health and euglycemia. High glucose levels in the oral mucosa are associated with increased levels of bacteria and the development of periodontal disease.[189] People with high glucose levels often have dry mouth due to reduction in saliva output. Lack of saliva, which provides both a chemical and mechanical barrier to bacterial infection, can hasten the development of sores and tooth decay. Uncontrolled periodontal disease increases cytokine production, worsening insulin resistance and destabilizing glucose control. Poor oral health, which can lead to discomfort and pain when chewing and swallowing, may impinge on adequate consumption of nutrients, contributing both to malnutrition and glycemic deterioration.[190]

Neuropathy. Diabetic **neuropathy** is caused by elevated glucose levels, which damage the nerves throughout the body. There are four types of diabetic neuropathy: peripheral neuropathy, autonomic neuropathy, radiculoplexus neuropathy (diabetic amyotrophy), and mononeuropathy. The most common type is peripheral neuropathy, which affects nerves in the extremities, the feet, legs, hands, and arms. **Figure 8.14** demonstrates a diabetic foot check, which

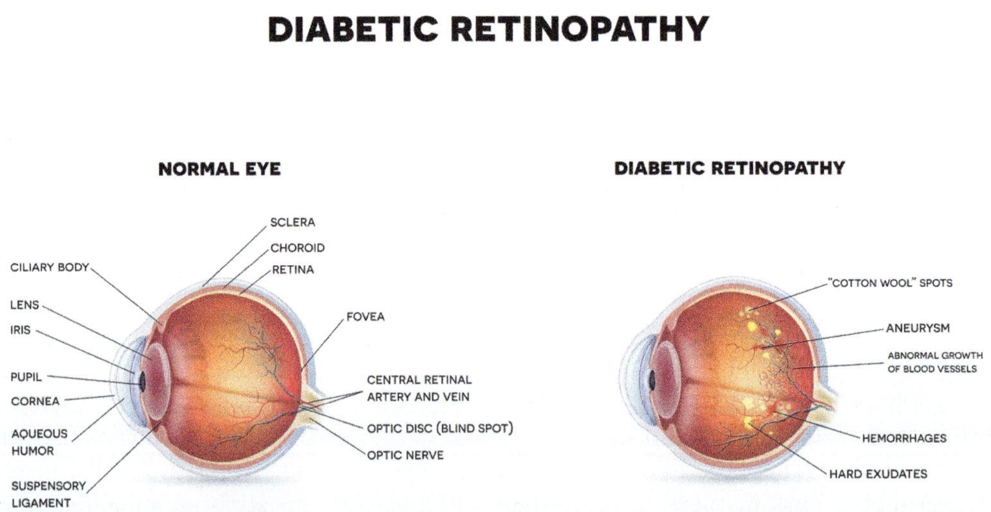

Figure 8.13 Manifestations of Diabetic Retinopathy

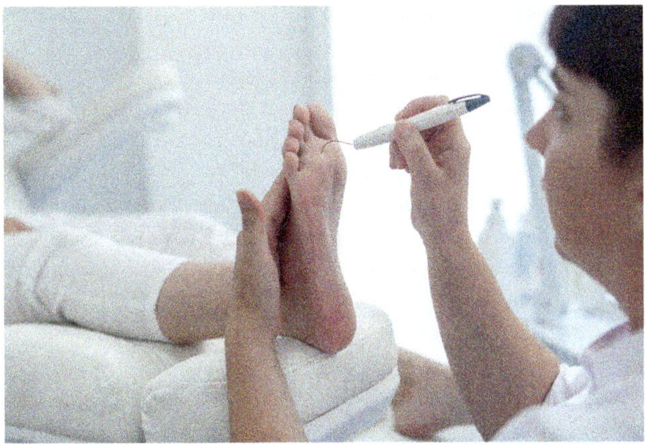

Figure 8.14 Demonstration of Diabetic Foot Check

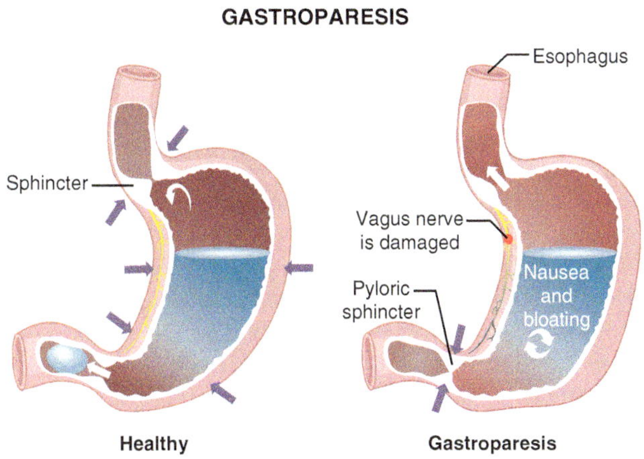

Figure 8.15 Delayed Gastric Emptying

is helpful to determine any abnormalities in patients with neuropathy who may not otherwise feel or notice the condition. Symptoms include tingling or burning, loss of ability to feel pain or sensation in the affected limb, muscle weakness, and foot abnormalities. Although incurable, there are a variety of medications available to treat peripheral neuropathies.

Many gastrointestinal problems, including constipation, diarrhea, bloating, and heartburn, arising from diabetes are the result of autonomic neuropathy. One of the most difficult to treat diabetic complications is **gastroparesis**. Gastroparesis is present in approximately 4.8% of individuals with T1DM, 1% of people with T2DM, and 0.1% of people without diabetes.[191] Delayed gastric emptying is present in 30–50% of individuals with long-standing, complicated diabetes.[192]

In gastroparesis, the nerves enervating the gastrointestinal tract are affected, and there is delayed gastric emptying in the absence of mechanical gastric outlet obstruction. Figure 8.15 illustrates the damaged vagus nerve and its effect on delayed gastric emptying. Gastroparesis compromises the delivery of food to the small intestine in a consistent manner. People with gastroparesis may experience early satiety, nausea and vomiting, bloating, abdominal pain, and constipation. The focus of treatment is on the control of symptoms, although the severity of symptoms does not correlate well with the degree of nerve damage, and the prevention or alleviation of malnutrition.[193] Both soluble fiber and fat can slow the pace of digestion; therefore, diets for gastroparesis are low in both of these nutrients.[77,193] Small, frequent feedings are preferred over larger meals to prevent bloating and early satiety. Liquids, which empty faster than solids from the stomach, are usually better tolerated, and patients with more severe symptoms may find a completely liquid diet easier to digest. Early satiety, nausea, and vomiting can lead to poor intake and malnutrition, so patients with severe symptoms and unintentional weight loss of 5–10% of their usual body weight within 3–6 months may need to be managed wholly on enteral, or in rare cases, parenteral, nutrition.[193] Monitoring of weight status is essential in gastroparesis.

In addition to adjustments in food intake, gastroparesis often requires modifications to timing and type of medications. In patients taking insulin or insulin secretagogues, delayed gastric emptying can cause hypoglycemia. Changing the timing of insulin administration to 30 minutes after meals for those taking injections, or using an insulin pump to deliver an extended bolus, in which a portion of the insulin dose is given prior to the meal and the remainder is given over a set time period, has been demonstrated to improve glycemic control.[194] Semaglutide, a GLP-1 receptor agonist, is a medication that is frequently used in the treatment of T2DM and sometimes T1DM. If a patient has gastroparesis or has experienced bloating, nausea, abdominal pain, and discomfort in the abdomen, its use is contraindicated.[195]

Medical Treatment of Diabetes

Although diet and exercise remain the cornerstone of diabetes management, all people diagnosed with T1DM diabetes will require insulin as a lifelong treatment modality. Most of those with T2DM will also find the need for pharmacological intervention. T2DM is a chronic disease whose natural history includes the slow, progressive loss of β cell function.

Clinical Controversy

Glucagon-like peptide 1 (GLP-1) receptor agonists were initially approved to improve metabolic control in patients with diabetes. Recently, the use of GLP-1 in people who do not have diabetes has been increasing and shortages have occurred. There are various findings on the use of GLP-1 in patients without diabetes. Moll et al. reported that, despite several harm outcomes, achieving a 10% weight loss outweighs the cumulative harms, which include cholelithiasis, constipation, diarrhea, alopecia, hypoglycemia, skin reactions, and vomiting for both patients with and without diabetes. Singh et al. reported that patients without diabetes treated with GLP-1 not only had a weight reduction, but reduced major adverse cardiovascular events, all cause death, myocardial infarction, and revascularization. Xu et al. noted that there is no long-term safety data on the use of GLP-1 in patients without diabetes; however, cardiovascular outcome trials support the safety of GLP-1 in the long term for patients with diabetes, with no increase in hypoglycemia or pancreatitis. Liu et al. provided strong support for the use of GLP-1 for weight loss in patients without diabetes, with low-to-moderate risk of adverse effects. Similarly to Xu et al., they acknowledged the lack of long-term data on this topic.

Questions

1. What are the advantages and disadvantages of GLP-1 use in people without diabetes?
2. After evaluating the evidence presented in these papers, how would you advise patients without diabetes for weight loss?
3. What factors about your patient should you consider before recommending a GLP-1 to their management plan?

References

1. Moll H, Frey E, Gerber P, et al. GLP-1 receptor agonists for weight reduction in people living with obesity but without diabetes: a living benefit-harm modelling study. *EClinicalMedicine*. 2024;73;102661.
2. Xu D, Nair A, Sigston C, et al. Potential roles of glucagon-like peptide 1 receptor agonists (GLP-1 RAs) in nondiabetic populations. *Cardiovasc Ther*. 2022;6820377.
3. Liu Y, Ruan B, Jiang H, et al. The weight-loss effect of GLP-1RAs glucagon-like peptide-1 receptor agonists in non-diabetic individuals with overweight or obesity: a systematic review with meta-analysis and trial sequential analysis of randomized controlled trials. Am J Clin Nutr. 2023;118(3):614–626.
4. Singh S, Garg A, Tantry US, Bliden K, Gurbel PA, Gulati, M. Safety and efficacy of glucagon-like peptide-1 receptor agonists on cardiovascular events in overweight or obese non-diabetic patients. *Curr Prob Card*. 2024;49(3):102403.

CASE STUDY REVISITED

During the 6-month follow-up, Joseph's insulin needs have continued to increase with insulin resistance. He has gained 5 kg, now weighing 105 kg. His endocrinologist introduced the idea of using other diabetes medicines alongside insulin.

Questions

1. What diabetes medications do you think would help Joseph?
2. Write an updated Nutrition Diagnosis/PES statement for Joseph
3. Identify the nutrition intervention you would like to initiate for Joseph. Would you recommend lifestyle changes, in addition to medication? Explain.
4. What indices will you monitor, including frequency?

CORE CONCEPT 9

Although diet and exercise remain the cornerstone of diabetes management, all people diagnosed with type 1 diabetes will require insulin as a lifelong treatment modality.

PRACTICE POINT

The role of drug therapy for type 2 diabetes is to "achieve clinical and biochemical targets with as few adverse consequences as possible."

The American Association of Clinical Endocrinologists defines the role of drug therapy for T2DM to "achieve clinical and biochemical targets with as few adverse consequences as possible."[196] Currently available hypoglycemic agents provide the same glucose-lowering capacity, decreasing A1c between 0.5% and 2%.[197] Decisions about which agent to use are made based on the appropriate level of glucose intolerance, the patient's weight and comorbidities, convenience, and patient preference.

The landscape for medications for patients with T2DM has changed significantly in the last 30 years. Whereas in the early 1990s there were only two choices of oral medications available in the United States, the sulfonylureas and the biguanides, there are now 11 categories of drugs, often with several choices among each category. As our understanding of diabetes as a disease affecting multiple organ systems has grown, so have the diverse avenues of pharmacological management multiplied.

New medications are continually being developed. As a practicing professional in the field of nutrition, familiarity with the different classes of drugs, understanding how they function, their side effects and contraindications, and how they interact with food intake is vital. **Table 8.22** reviews currently available oral and injectable non-insulin medications.[198,199]

These medications are typically used in patients with T2DM, although patients with T1DM may use some of these medications in combination with insulin to reduce insulin resistance and insulin requirements. There are several clinical trials and meta-analyses to show the efficacy and safety of these drugs in addition to insulin therapy in people with T1DM. Metformin has an insulin-sensitizing effect and can reduce insulin dose requirements.[200,201] Sodium glucose transporter 2 inhibitor (SGLT-2i), GLP-1 receptor agonist, and pramlintide reduce A1c and insulin dosage requirements without increasing the risk for hypoglycemia or ketoacidosis. A-glucosidase inhibitors assisted in A1c reduction without subsequent hypoglycemia. Thiazolidinediones and dipeptidyl peptidase 4 inhibitor (DPP-4i) are safe for use, but did not significantly impact A1c or insulin dose requirements.[201] Sulfonylureas, meglitinides, bile acid sequestrants, and dopamine-2-agonists are not approved or indicated for use in people with T1DM. Insulin can lead to weight gain, so being able to reduce the amount required can assist with weight management in people with T1DM.

Insulin is the one drug that is appropriate for use in all types of diabetes. Previously derived from pork or beef pancreas, all insulin currently in use in the United States is made in the laboratory from recombinant DNA. Insulins are categorized based on their strength, onset of action, peak action, and duration of action. Most insulins in the United States are U-100, which means that there are 100 units of insulin dissolved in 1 mL of liquid; however, U-500, which is five times as strong, is available for those people who are severely insulin resistant. **Table 8.23** reviews the characteristics of available insulins.[202] **Figure 8.16** describes the insulin action time for various insulins.

Most insulins can be divided into two major categories: those that are used as basal insulin and those used for bolus therapy. Basal insulins are long-acting insulins (24–42 hours) that provide insulin replacement throughout the day and help reduce excess glucose secretion from the liver. They are usually given as either one or two injections in the morning and either at dinner or bedtime. Bolus (short-acting or fast-acting) insulin is used to cover the blood glucose excursions following meals and to correct or reduce blood glucose elevations due to a mismatch between available insulin and glucose levels such as can occur with the dawn effect (rise in blood glucose in the early morning caused by release of counter-regulatory hormones).

Premixed insulins are combinations of analogs of long-acting insulin and fast-acting insulin. These preparations do not achieve tight glucose control provided by basal and bolus insulin taken separately, but they are more convenient to use because they generally do not require patients to take insulin injections in the middle of the day. The most common side effect of insulin is hypoglycemia, although in rare instances, people can be allergic to either insulin or the ingredients added to the insulin to maintain a balanced pH and delay bacterial growth.

In 2015, a rapid-acting inhaled insulin called "Afrezza" became available in the United States for adults with T1DM or T2DM who required bolus insulin at meals. Inhaled insulin's start time is about 12–15 minutes, with its peak at 30 minutes and duration lasting no longer than 3 hours.[203] INHALE-3, a randomized controlled trial comparing the efficacy of inhaled insulin, found improvements in A1c and helped to pave the way for an alternative approach to diabetes management.[204]

CORE CONCEPT 10

The most common and serious side effect of insulin therapy is hypoglycemia.

Table 8.22 Oral and Injectable Non-Insulin Medications

Class	Product	Primary Mechanism of Action	Advantages	Side Effects	Dose	Cost	A1C Reduction
Biguanides	Metformin	Reduction in hepatic glucose production	No hypoglycemia Reduction in CVD episodes Long history of safe use	Gastrointestinal distress (diarrhea, gas, cramping) B12 deficiency Lactic acidosis (rare) Cannot be used in significant CKD	500–2500 mg	Low	1–2%
Sulfonylurea (second generation)	Glyburide Glipizide Glimepiride	Increases insulin secretion	Long history of use Possible decrease in microvascular risk	Hypoglycemia, enhanced in older adults Weight gain Loses effectiveness over time Blunts myocardial ischemic pre-conditioning	Glyburide 1.25–20 mg Glipizide 5–15 mg Glimepiride 1–8 mg	Low	1–1.5%
Meglitinides	Repaglinide Nateglinide	Increase insulin secretion	Dosing flexibility Decrease postprandial glucose excursions	Hypoglycemia Weight gain Blunts myocardial ischemic pre-conditioning	Repaglinide 0.5–4 mg Nateglinide 60–540 mg	Moderate	0.5–1.0%
Thiazolidine-diones	Pioglitazone Rosiglitaz	Increase peripheral glucose uptake by enhancing insulin action Decrease hepatic glucose output	No hypoglycemia Efficacy Acceptable in renal insufficiency Well tolerated Once-daily dosing	Weight gain (can be significant) Fluid gains Decrease triglycerides (TGs) Increase HDL-C Fracture risk is doubled	Pioglitazone 15–45 mg taken once daily without regard to meals Rosiglitaz 4–8 mg once daily without regard to meals	Low	1–1.5%
α-Glycosidase inhibitors	Acarbose Miglitol	Slows intestinal carbohydrate digestion/absorption	No hypoglycemia Decreased postprandial glucose excursions Decreased CVD events Weight neutral	Modest A1C reduction Major dose-related gastrointestinal intolerance (10-35%) Compliance issues (must be taken with first bite of meal)	25–150 mg/day Acarbose must be taken with the first bite of a meal	Moderate	0.5–1%
DPP-4-inhibitors	Sitagliptin Vildagliptin Saxagliptin Linagliptin Alogliptin	Increase insulin secretion (glucose dependent) Decrease glucagon secretion (glucose dependent)	No hypoglycemia Well tolerated No weight gain Fewer safety concerns than with the glitazones Once daily dosing	A1C reduction somewhat less than metformin, sulfonylureas, and glitazones Long-term efficacy and safety unknown Pancreatitis Expensive	Linagliptin 5 mg once daily Saxagliptin 5 mg once daily Sitagliptin 100 mg once daily	High	0.5–1.0%

Bile acid sequestrants	Colesevelam	Decreased hepatic glucose production Increase incretin levels	No hypoglycemia Decrease LCL-C	Modest A1C reduction Constipation Increase TGs May decrease absorption of other medications	1875 mg (three tablets) orally twice a day with meals or 3750 mg (six tablets) orally once a day with a meal	High	0.5%
Dopamine-2 agonists	Bromocriptine	Modulates hypothalamic regulation of metabolism Increases insulin sensitivity	No hypoglycemia Decreased CVD events	Modest A1C reduction Dizziness Nausea Fatigue Rhinitis	0.8–4.8 mg once daily within 2 hours of waking	High	0.5%
SGLT2 inhibitors	Canagliflozin Dapagliflozin Empagliflozin	Blocks glucose reabsorption by the kidney, increasing glucosuria	No hypoglycemia Weight reduction Decreased blood pressure	Genitourinary infections Polyuria Volume depletion Increased LDL-C	Canagliflozin 100–300 mg Dapagliflozin 5–10 mg Empagliflozin 10–25 mg	High	0.7–1.0%
GLP-1 receptor agonists	Exenatide Exenatide extended release Liraglutide Albiglutide Lixisenatide Dulaglutide Semaglutide Tirzepatide	Increase insulin secretion (glucose dependent) Slow gastric emptying Decrease glucagon secretion	No hypoglycemia Weight reduction Decreased postprandial glucose excursions	Long-term efficacy unknown Long-term safety unknown (possible link to thyroid cancer) In pancreatitis: caution if GFR <50 Must be injected Major dose-related gastrointestinal intolerance	Exenatide is injected twice daily 0–60 min before breakfast and supper, 5–10 mcg SC BID Liraglutide is injected once daily without regard to mealtimes, 0.6 mg SC 1.8 mg/day Semaglutide 0.25–2.4 mg	High	0.8–1.8%
Amyline mimetics	Pramlintide	Decrease glucagon secretion Increase satiety Slow gastric emptying	Decreased postprandial glucose excursions Weight reduction	Modest A1C reduction Gastrointestinal side effects (nausea & vomiting) Injectable Frequent dosing schedule	15–120 mcg given with meals	High	0.5–0.7%

SC, subcutaneous.

Data from Inzucchi SE, Bergenstal RM, Buse JB. Management of hyperglycemia in type 2 diabetes, 2015: a patient-centered approach: update to a position statement of the American Diabetes Association and the European Association for the Study of Diabetes. *Diabetes Care*. 2015;38(1):140-149.; Davies MJ, Aroda VR, Collins BS, et al. Management of hyperglycemia in type 2 diabetes, 2022: a consensus report by the American Diabetes Association and the European Association for the Study of Diabetes. *Diabetes Care*. 2022;45(11):2753-2786.

Table 8.23 Insulin Action Times

Category	Insulin	Start Time	Peak	Durations
Rapid-acting	Lispro, Aspart, Glulisine	15–30 minutes	30–180 minutes	2–5 hours
Ultra-rapid-acting	Fiasp	5 minutes	30 minutes	3–5 hours
Short-acting	Regular (R)	30–60 minutes	2–4 hours	5–8 hours
Intermediate-acting	NPH	2–4 hours	4–10 hours	8–16 hours
Long-acting	Detemir, Glargine, Degludec	0.5–6 hours	6–12 hours	24–42 hours
Pre-mixed NPH (intermediate-acting) and regular (short-acting)	70% NPH and 30% Regular	30–60 minutes	Varies	10–16 hours
	50% NPH and 50% Regular	30–60 minutes	Varies	10–16 hours
Pre-mixed insulin lispro protamine suspension (intermediate-acting) and insulin lispro (rapid-acting)	75% lispro protamine and 25% lispro	10–15 minutes	Varies	10–16 hours
	50% lispro protamine and 50% lispro	10–15 minutes	Varies	10–16 hours
Pre-mixed insulin aspart protamine suspension (intermediate-acting) and insulin aspart (rapid-acting)	70% aspart protamine and 30% aspart	5–15 minutes	Varies	10–16 hours

Data from Yau M, Sperling MA. Treatment of diabetes mellitus in children and adolescents. In: Feingold KR, Anawalt B, Blackman MR, et al., eds. *Endotext* [Internet]. MDText.com, Inc.; 2021. Accessed January 12, 2026. https://www.ncbi.nlm.nih.gov/books/NBK279087/

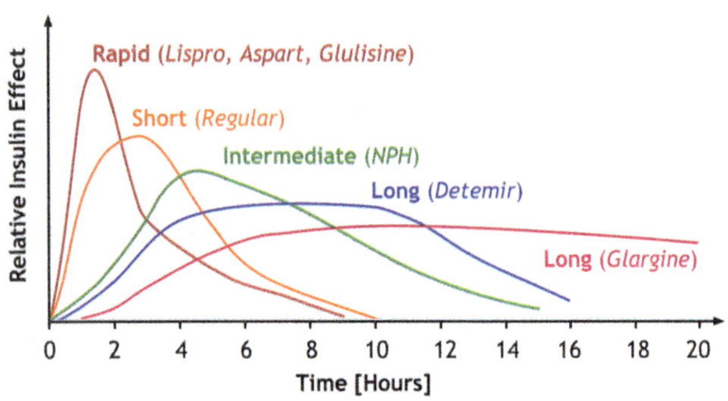

Figure 8.16 Insulin Action Times

Courtesy of Michał Komornicza. https://creativecommons.org/licenses/by/3.0/deed.en

There are a variety of insulin delivery devices on the market, including vial and syringe, insulin pens, insulin pumps, and hybrid pen/pumps. Insulin pumps are the most complicated to use but provide the most precise simulation of normal insulin delivery in the body. To use a vial and syringe, patients are instructed to pull air into the syringe using the plunger to the amount of units needed. The syringe needle is then placed at the top of the vial and all of the air is pushed in and the vial flipped upside down, then the insulin is pulled back to the number of units required for a dosage. A small amount of insulin is then dispensed into a napkin to ensure that the needle works and the injection is administered. Insulin pens either come with whole- or half-unit increments. Patients are instructed to screw a pen needle onto the insulin pen. The pen is then dialed to two units and dispensed into a napkin to ensure that the needle works. Then, the pen is dialed to the required number of units and the insulin is injected. Last, insulin pumps, also known as "continuous subcutaneous insulin infusion" (CSII), continuously deliver insulin over a 24-hour period as basal insulin and have a personal diabetes manager (PDM) or controller to allow the user to administer bolus insulin based on programmed settings in the insulin pump. Ideal sites for insulin administration are sites with a layer of fatty tissue: back of the arms, lower abdomen, upper buttocks, and thighs. In addition, it is important to rotate insulin administration sites to prevent scar tissue buildup. Certified Diabetes

Care and Education Specialists can provide education on all insulin delivery types, but to initiate an insulin, they must be a Certified Pump Trainer for the specific insulin pump they are training patients on.

A newer innovation is closed-loop systems or automated insulin delivery (AID) systems. These insulin pumps require the user to wear both an insulin pump and a compatible/integrated CGM. The CGM and insulin pump create a metabolic algorithm and over time learn patterns of the user and will adjust basal insulin delivery as total daily dose increases or decreases over time. In addition, these systems can increase, decrease, or pause basal insulin delivery based on the blood glucose data from the CGM and where the algorithm predicts blood glucose will be in 30–60 minutes. Regardless of the AID system used, as there are a few different types on the market, they have demonstrated improvements in A1c, TIR, and quality of life. AIDs still require interaction from the user to enter carbohydrate-counting information for meal bolus delivery, but it takes some of the burden of diabetes management off of their shoulders.[205]

People with T1DM are usually initiated on a basal–bolus insulin regimen. Those with T2DM whose disease has progressed beyond the control of oral agents usually begin with one injection of basal per day. As their β cells continue to fail, they may require coverage of meals with prandial insulin. Prandial insulin can be dosed in a variety of ways, from fixed dose and sliding scale to the use of ratios. Patients using a fixed dose regimen will take the same amount of insulin at meals regardless of the blood glucose level or the amount of carbohydrate eaten. Those using a sliding scale will vary their amount of insulin based on their preprandial glucose level, while those using matching insulin to carbohydrate titrate their dose based on both their preprandial glucose level and the amount of carbohydrate they intend to consume.

Nutritional management is key to effective insulin use. The proper timing of insulin doses can affect how well the postprandial elevation in glucose is controlled. Regular insulin should be taken 30 minutes before meals, whereas food must be taken within 15 minutes of taking fast-acting insulin. Consistency of carbohydrate intake is seminal to avoiding erratic blood glucose patterns in those using fixed-dose or sliding-scale insulin regimens. Both the glycemic index of the meal and its fat content will determine when it is best to administer insulin. For example, a breakfast of a highly processed cereal may require that fast-acting insulin be given up to 30 minutes before the meal to match the rapid rise in blood glucose caused by the easily digested carbohydrate. On the other hand, for a meal of fettuccine alfredo, splitting the total insulin between two doses given at the beginning of the meal and 2 hours later can help to adjust insulin delivery so that it coincides with the delay in glucose appearance in the bloodstream caused by the meal's high fat content.

Metabolic and Bariatric Surgery

An interesting approach to treatment of T2DM is bariatric and metabolic surgery (MBS). MBS may cause drastic effects on those with diabetes, including improved glycemic control and reduced CVD risk. Randomized controlled trials have demonstrated diabetes remission in 30–63% of patients with follow-up of 1–5 years; however, 35–50% of patients have recurrence with an estimated remission period of 8.3 years following Roux-en-Y gastric bypass.[206] The high cost and long-term concerns of MBS, such as dumping syndrome, lifelong need of vitamin and mineral supplements, and postprandial hypoglycemia, are of concern if considering this treatment option. The 2021 recommendations for metabolic surgery in diabetes are listed in **Table 8.24**, provided that the patient is assessed for mental health and ability to follow nutrition and lifestyle recommendations postsurgery. **Table 8.25** describes the common procedures endorsed by the American Society for Metabolic and Bariatric Surgery.[207] Refer to Chapter 7, *Weight and Health*, for more information on nutritional therapy for MBS.

Table 8.24 Indications for Metabolic Surgery in Adults with Type 2 Diabetes

BMI Cutoff	Indication
≥40 kg/m^2 (≥35 kg/m^2 if Asian American)	Regardless of level of glycemic control or medication use
35–39.9 kg/m^2 (32.5–37.5 mg/m^2 if Asian American)	If hyperglycemia is inadequately controlled despite optimal medical therapy and lifestyle changes
30.0–34.9 kg/m^2 (27.5–32.4 kg/m^2 if Asian American)	If hyperglycemia is inadequately controlled despite optimal medical therapy through oral and/or injectable medication (including insulin)

Data from American Diabetes Association. Obesity management for the treatment of type 2 diabetes. Sec. 8. In: *Standards of Care in Diabetes 2021. Diabetes Care.* 2021;47(Suppl 1):S145-S157.

Table 8.25 Metabolic and Bariatric Surgery Procedures

	Procedure	How It Works	Advantages	Disadvantages
Sleeve Gastrectomy	1. The stomach is freed from organs around it. 2. Surgical staplers are used to remove 80% of the stomach.	Smaller stomach holds less food and liquid help to reduce the amount (and calories) that are consumed. The portion of the stomach that produces the most of the "hunger hormone", is removed, so it decreases hunger, increases fullness, and allows the body to reach and maintain a healthy weight and glycemic control.	Simple and short surgery Can be performed in patients with high-risk medical conditions May be performed as the first step for patients with severe obesity May be used as a bridge to gastric bypass or SADI-S procedures Effective weight loss and improved of obesity-related conditions	Nonreversible procedure May worsen or cause new onset reflux and heartburn Less impact on metabolism compared to RYGB
Roux-en-Y Gastric Bypass (RYGB)	1. The stomach is divided into a small top portion (pouch) and the larger part of the stomach is bypassed and no longer stores or digests food. 2. The small intestine is divided and connected to the small pouch to allow food to pass. The small bowel segment, which empties the bypassed or larger stomach, is connected into the small bowel, resulting in a bowel connection resembling the shape of the letter Y. 3. The stomach acids and digestive enzymes from the bypassed stomach and first portion of the small intestine will mix with food that is eaten.	The stomach pouch is smaller and holds less food, which means fewer calories are consumed. The food does not come in contact with the first portion of the small bowel, which results in decreased absorption. The modification of the food course through the GI tract decreases hunger, increases fullness, and allows the body to reach and maintain a healthy weight.	Improved diabetes control Improved acid reflux and heartburn Reliable and long-lasting weight loss Effective for remission of obesity-associated conditions Refined and standardized technique	More complex compared to sleeve gastrectomy or AGB More vitamin and mineral deficiencies, then sleeve gastrectomy or AGB Risk for small bowel complications and obstruction Risk of developing ulcers, especially with use of NSAIDs or tobacco May cause dumping syndrome

Adjustable Gastric Band (AGB)	1. A silicone device is placed and secured around the top part of the stomach creating a small pouch about the band.	The feeling of fullness depends on the size of the opening between the pouch and the rest of the stomach. Food goes through the stomach normally but is limited by the smaller opening of the band.	Lowest rate of complications No division of the stomach or intestines Patients can go home on the day of surgery The band can be removed if needed Lowest risk for vitamin and mineral deficiencies	The band may need several adjustments and monthly office visits during the first year Slower and less weight loss than other procedures Risk of band movement (slippage) or damage to the stomach over time (erosion) Requires a foreign implant to remain in the body High rate of re-operations May result in swallowing problems or enlargement of the esophagus
Biliopancreatic Diversion with Duodenal Switch (BPD/DS)	1. A tube-shaped stomach pouch is created. 2. The first portion of the small intestine is separated from the stomach. 3. A part of the small intestine is connected to the outlet of the pouch, so when a patient eats, the food goes through the sleeve pouch and into the latter part of the small intestine.	The smaller stomach allows patients to eat less food. The food stream bypasses roughly 75% of the small intestine. There is a significant decrease in the absorption of calories and nutrients. Reduces hunger, increases fullness, and improves glycemic control.	Best results for improving obesity Affects bowel hormones to cause less hunger and more fullness after eating Most effective procedure for treatment of type 2 diabetes	Higher complication rates than other procedures Highest malabsorption and greater possibility of vitamin and micronutrient deficiencies Reflux and heartburn can develop or get worse Risk of looser and more frequent bowel movements More complex surgery
Single Anastomosis Duodeno-Ileal Bypass with Sleeve Gastrectomy (SADI-S)	1. A smaller tube-shaped stomach is made. 2. The first part of the small intestine is divided after the stomach. 3. A loop of intestine is measured several feet from its end and connected to the stomach.	When a patient eats, food goes through the pouch and directly into the latter portion of the small intestine. The food mixes with digestive juices from the first part of the small intestine. This allows for enough absorption of vitamins and minerals. This surgery offers good weight loss along with less hunger, more fullness, and diabetes improvement.	Highly effective for long-term weight loss and remission of type 2 diabetes Simpler and faster to perform than AGB or BPD-DS Excellent option for patients who have already had a sleeve gastrectomy	Vitamins and minerals are not absorbed as well as in the sleeve gastrectomy or AGB Newer procedure with small amount of outcome data Potential to worsen or develop new onset acid reflux Risk of looser and more frequent bowel movements

GI, gastrointestinal.
Data from American Society for Metabolic and Bariatric Surgery. Bariatric surgery procedures. Accessed January 12, 2026. https://asmbs.org/patients/bariatric-surgery-procedures/

CASE STUDY REVISITED

Joseph suffered a football injury and is planning to come to the hospital for repair of a torn meniscus. Based on the complexity of his injury, he will need open surgery, thus requiring him to stay in the hospital. He is expected to have nothing by mouth after midnight prior to the surgery, which is scheduled early in the morning.

Questions

1. How must Joseph's diet and insulin regimen be altered?
2. What is your recommendation to the inpatient medical team regarding an appropriate glycemic target?
3. What laboratory indices should be drawn upon Joseph's admission?
4. What triggers for hypoglycemia should be monitored?

The intragastric balloon procedure has been introduced to serve as a noninvasive tool to induce weight loss. An air-filled balloon is placed into the stomach to restrict space and promote the feeling of satiety.[208] Advantages of this procedure include it being reversible and noninvasive. Despite the ease of this procedure, there are little long-term data on its outcomes.

Hospitalization and Illness in Patients with Diabetes

As a patient with diabetes ages, hospitalization is common. Factors to consider include new management of insulin based on changes in nutritional intake or clinical status, monitoring of blood glucose levels, and awareness of risk factors that can alter glycemia. Control of hyperglycemia and hypoglycemia is an important consideration for patients in the hospital setting. While both are associated with adverse outcomes (increased mortality in hospitalized patients), hypoglycemia is difficult to detect and acutely dangerous.[209] Previously, tight control of glucose levels below a target of 110 mg/dL was recommended for patients in the hospital setting.[210] However, studies have either failed to show benefit or have concluded that too-intensive treatment of elevated glucose levels leads to higher rates of mortality.[211] The American Society for Parenteral and Enteral Nutrition, in its clinical guidelines for nutrition support of adult patients with hyperglycemia, the American Association of Clinical Endocrinologists, and the ADA Consensus Statement recommend a goal range of blood glucose between 140 and 180 mg/dL.[212, 213]

Noncritical Patients with Diabetes Admitted to the Hospital

For planned admissions, a baseline A1c should be measured (if none in the past 3 months). In addition, the patient's home regimen, ability to self-manage, and overall knowledge and behavior should be assessed ideally prior to admission. For patients requiring insulin who are noncritically ill, a basal insulin dose should be given along with bolus correction if necessary. Studies indicate that this basal–bolus method is associated with fewer complications than a sliding scale. Typical insulin dosing may change from the patient's usual regimen if their nutritional intake declines or while they are ill.

A protocol for monitoring and prevention of hypoglycemia should be in place. Awareness of triggering events for hyperglycemia such as emesis, change in steroid medication, interruption of intake, or alteration in meal schedule is necessary. For patients with poor intake, a fasting-acting insulin given immediately after the patient eats, or based on carbohydrate counting, can be effective. Once a patient's appetite improves, insulin injections should align with meals and in accordance with point of care testing of blood glucose.[213]

Management of Patients with Diabetes Requiring Nutrition Support

Enteral Nutrition

Enteral nutrition is the preferred method of feeding for all patients with a functioning gastrointestinal tract, including in the ICU setting.[214] Some common formulas and their nutrient content are listed in **Table 8.26**.

Both regular and diabetes-specific enteral feeding formulations have been used in patients who are not able to tolerate oral feedings. Diabetes-specific formulations are lower in total carbohydrate and higher in total fat (and sometimes protein). Micronutrient composition is similar to standard enteral feedings.

Table 8.26 Nutrient Content of Formulas Derived from Manufacturers' Websites

Formula	Density (calories/mL)	Protein (%)	Carbs (%)	Fat (%)	Fiber (g)	Carb Source	Meets RDA (mL)
Glucerna 1.0	1.0	16.7	34.2	49	14.4	Corn maltodextrin, fructose, short-chain fructooligosaccharides	1420
Glucerna 1.2	1.2	20	35	45	16	Corn maltodextrin, fructose	1250
Glucerna 1.5	1.5	22	33	45	17	Corn maltodextrin, fructose, short-chain fructooligosaccharides	1000
Diabetissource AC	1.2	20	36	44	15.2	Pureed fruits and vegetables	1250
Glytrol	1.0	18	40	42	15.2	Modified cornstarch	1500

Data from Abbott Nutrition. Glucerna Original Shake. Accessed January 12, 2026. https://www.abbottnutrition.com/our-products/glucerna-original-shake; Nestlé Medical Hub. Therapeutic areas: diabetes. Accessed January 12, 2026. https://www.nestlemedicalhub.com/therapeutic-areas/diabetes?therapeutic_area=products-section; AccuCare. Nutren Glytrol hyperglycemia formula, Nestlé enteral nutrition. Accessed January 12, 2026. https://www.accucare-inc.com/product/nutren-glytrol-hyperglycemia-formula-nestle-enteral-nutrition#:~:text=Ideal%20for%20the%20nutritional%20management,8.45%20fl%20oz

The carbohydrate sources in these formulas (e.g., isomaltulose and sucromalt) often have a low GI. Diabetes-specific formulations may also contain appreciable amounts of fiber, and many provide fat in the form of monounsaturated and omega-3 fatty acids. Both the fiber, and fat content of these formulas slow gastric emptying, thereby blunting excessive glucose rise. Studies have found a benefit in glycemia control as well as a diminution in the amount of insulin required to maintain euglycemia when these feedings are used.[215] However, the latest iteration of the American Society for Enteral and Parenteral Nutrition Clinical Guidelines: Nutrition Support of Adult Patients with Hyperglycemia does not endorse diabetes-specific formulations over standard formulas for use in hospitalized patients with hyperglycemia.[212] Comorbidities such as kidney disease and gastroparesis may exclude the use of these feedings due to electrolyte imbalances and the need to limit fat and fiber content.

Outside of critical care units, subcutaneous insulin administration is a more common method of insulin delivery. Scheduled subcutaneous insulin should consist of basal, meal, and corrections components (with the latter two being administered before meals). In patients receiving continuous enteral infusion, half the total daily dose of insulin can be given as basal insulin with the rest provided as regular or short-acting provided four to six times per day. Prolonged use of sliding scale insulin as the sole method of glucose control is discouraged.[216]

In stable patients, either in the hospital, nursing home, or at home, a basal–bolus approach to insulin therapy similar to that used for oral feeding, can be instituted. Basal insulin doses can be given with either long-acting insulin once per day or intermediate-acting insulin twice a day. Short-acting or rapid-acting insulin, in conjunction with food, can be provided to account for glucose excursions following nutrient intake.

Parenteral Nutrition (PN)

Parenteral nutrition is administered in those patients who are malnourished or at risk for malnutrition whose gastrointestinal tract is compromised. Hyperglycemia is a frequent finding in patients both with and without diabetes.[217] The stress of illness, especially infection, promotes insulin resistance. In addition, dextrose supplied intravenously circumvents the normal incretin response, adding to the hyperglycemic milieu. As many patients receiving PN are malnourished, reduction in muscle mass also contributes to insulin resistance.

PN solutions should provide adequate carbohydrate to spare protein for tissue synthesis while avoiding hyperglycemia. Carbohydrate is usually initially limited to 1.5–2 mg/kg of body weight per minute to avoid hyperglycemia.[218] This translates into 100–150 grams of carbohydrate given over 24 hours. Once glycemic control has been established and electrolytes stabilized, the dextrose in the PN can be advanced to a maximum of 4 mg/kg/min.[219] Patients in the ICU on PN can be maintained on 80% of calculated energy requirements to avoid insulin resistance.[214] For patients with obesity, calorie intake should be kept at 60–70% of estimated needs.[220] However, in patients fed hypocaloric solutions, an increase in the protein content to 2 g/kg body weight may be indicated to aid in protein sparing.[221] Although higher levels in PN may displace carbohydrate calories and may decrease the risk of hyperglycemia, normalization in blood glucose levels may also be achieved by decreasing the fat content of the PN. High circulating levels of fatty acids and muscle fat content increase insulin resistance and may induce immunosuppression. For this reason, lipid emulsions above 1.3 g/kg/day are not recommended.[222]

Most patients with diabetes require insulin to control hyperglycemia while on PN. Until the PN dose is established, intravenous infusion of insulin is preferred. This allows immediate titration of the insulin dose without having to wait until the next bag of PN is hung.[215] Once the dextrose in the PN is advanced to goal, insulin can be added to the bag of PN. When intravenous insulin is not possible, insulin can be added to the PN. One method of determining a starting insulin dose is to provide 0.05–0.1 units of regular insulin per gram of dextrose in the PN. Breakthrough hyperglycemia is controlled by subcutaneous insulin injection, and one-half to two-thirds of the amount of subcutaneous insulin used that day is added to the next day's PN formulation. This procedure continues until blood glucose levels are stabilized.

Chapter Summary

Diabetes is a complex disease that can only be managed through the support of medical, psychological, and nutritional interventions. Patients with all types of diabetes require support from the care team to increase self-efficacy and take charge in management of this disease. The acute complications of diabetes, hypoglycemia, and hyperglycemia must be managed daily in both the inpatient and outpatient settings. More threatening in the long term are the chronic complications of diabetes, which may be minimized or avoided through a daily pharmacological and lifestyle regimen. As the research continues to grow on the best practices for diabetes management, clinicians must strive to ensure that patients have the best comprehensive care and follow the most up-to-date recommendations to feel better and live longer.

Key Terms

Polyuria, polydipsia, polyphagia, acetone, acetoacetic acid, β-hydroxybutyric acid, hyperglycemia, diabetic ketoacidosis (DKA), Kussmaul's respirations, euglycemia, gluconeogenesis, glycogenolysis, insulin resistance, prediabetes, gestational diabetes mellitus (GDM), glycemic index (GI), glycemic load (GL), hypoglycemia, insulin-to-carbohydrate ratio (ICR), correction factor (CF), diabetes distress, nephropathy, retinopathy, neuropathy, gastroparesis, microalbuminuria

Acknowledgments

The author acknowledges Nora Saul for contributions to the previous version of this chapter.

References

1. Centers for Disease Control and Prevention. *National Diabetes Statistic Report*. May 15, 2023. Accessed January 7, 2025. https://www.cdc.gov/diabetes/php/data-research/
2. Lin J, Thompson TJ, Cheng YJ, et al. Projection of the future diabetes burden in the United States through 2060. *Popul Health Metr*. 2018;16(1):9. doi:10.1186/s12963-018-0166-4
3. Magliano DJ, Boyko EJ, IDF Diabetes Atlas 10th edition scientific committee. Table 3.4, Top 10 countries or territories for number of adults (20–79 years) with diabetes in 2021 and 2045. In: *IDF Diabetes Atlas*. 10th ed. International Diabetes Federation; 2021.
4. Centers for Disease Control and Prevention. *Leading Causes of Death Reports, 1981-2018*. Accessed January 7, 2025. https://www.cdc.gov/injury/wisqars/leadingcauses.html
5. Centers for Disease Control and Prevention. *Youth-onset diabetes: Incidence and trends*. In: *National Diabetes Statistics Report*. May 15, 2023. Accessed January 7, 2025. https://www.cdc.gov/diabetes/data-research/research/trends-new-diabetes-cases-young-people.html
6. Pinhas-Hamiel O, Zeitler P. Type 2 diabetes in children and adolescents: a focus on diagnosis and treatment. In: Feingold KR, Anawalt B, Blackman MR, et al. eds. *Endotext*. MDText.com, Inc.; 2023.
7. Gomber A, Ward ZJ, Ross C, et al. Variation in the incidence of type 1 diabetes mellitus in children and adolescents by world region and country income group: a scoping review. *PLOS Globl Public Health*. 2022;2(11):e0001099. doi:10.1371/journal.pgph.0001099/
8. Keenan HA, Sun JK, Levine J, et al. Residual insulin production and pancreatic β-cell turnover after 50 years of diabetes: Joslin Medalist Study. *Diabetes*. 2010;59(11):2846–2853. doi:10.2337/db10-0676

9. Banday MZ, Sameer AS, Nissar S. Pathophysiology of diabetes: an overview. *Avicenna J Med.* 2020;10(4):174–188. doi:10.4103/ajm.ajm_53_20
10. Fernandes R. The controversial role of glucose in the diabetic kidney. *Porto Biomed J.* 2021;6(1):e113. doi:10.1097/j.pbj.0000000000000113
11. Gosmanov AR, Gosmanova EO, Kitabchi AE. Hyperglycemic Crises: Diabetic Ketoacidosis and Hyperglycemic Hyperosmolar State. In: Feingold KR, Anawalt B, Blackman MR, et al., eds. *Endotext.* MDText.com, Inc.; 2021.
12. American Diabetes Association. Diagnosis. *Diabetes.org.* Accessed September 28, 2024. https://diabetes.org/about-diabetes/diagnosis
13. American Diabetes Association. Prediabetes. *Diabetes.org.* Accessed September 28, 2024. https://diabetes.org/about-diabetes/prediabetes
14. Dludla PV, Mabhida SE, Ziqubu K, et al. Pancreatic β-cell dysfunction in type 2 diabetes: implications of inflammation and oxidative stress. *World J Diabetes.* 2023;14(3):130–146. doi:10.4239/wjd.v14.i3.130.
15. Wang J, Wang H. Oxidative stress in pancreatic beta cell regeneration. *Oxid Med Cell Longev.* 2017;1930261. doi:10.1155/2017/1930261
16. Wajchenberg BL. β-cell failure in diabetes and preservation by clinical treatment. *Endocr Rev* 2007;28(2):187–218. doi:10.1210/er.2006-0038
17. National Institute of Diabetes and Digestive and Kidney Diseases. Prediabetes & insulin resistance. *National Institute of Diabetes and Digestive and Kidney Diseases.* Accessed September 28, 2024. https://www.niddk.nih.gov/health-information/diabetes/overview/what-is-diabetes/prediabetes-insulin-resistance
18. National Institute of Diabetes and Digestive and Kidney Diseases. Risk factors for type 2 diabetes. *National Institute of Diabetes and Digestive and Kidney Diseases.* Accessed January 7, 2025. https://www.niddk.nih.gov/health-information/diabetes/overview/risk-factors-type-2-diabetes
19. Kim JY, Bacha F, Tfayli H, Michaliszyn SF, Yousuf S, Arslanian S. Adipose tissue insulin resistance in youth on the spectrum from normal weight to obese and from normal glucose tolerance to impaired glucose tolerance to type 2 diabetes. *Diabetes Care.* 2019;42(2):265–272. doi:10.2337/dc18-1178
20. Sobczak ISA, Blindauer CA, Stewart AJ. Changes in plasma free fatty acids associated with type-2 diabetes. *Nutrients.* 2019;11(9):2022. doi:10.3390/nu11092022
21. Boer GA, Holst JJ. Incretin hormones and type 2 diabetes-mechanistic insights and therapeutic approaches. *Biology.* 2020;9(12):473. doi:10.3390/biology9120473
22. Gerich JE. Is reduced first-phase insulin release the earliest detectable abnormality in individuals destined to develop type 2 diabetes? *Diabetes.* 2002;51(suppl_1): S117–S121. doi:10.2337/diabetes.51.2007.S117
23. American Diabetes Association. National Diabetes Prevention Program. *American Diabetes Association.* Accessed September 28, 2024. https://professional.diabetes.org/clinical-support/national-diabetes-prevention-program
24. Centers for Disease Control and Prevention. Lifestyle change program details. *Centers for Disease Control and Prevention.* Accessed September 28, 2024. https://www.cdc.gov/diabetes-prevention/lifestyle-change-program/lifestyle-change-program-details.html
25. Los Angeles County Department of Public Health. National Diabetes Prevention Program. *Los Angeles County Department of Public Health.* Accessed September 28, 2024. http://publichealth.lacounty.gov/diabetes/prevention/nationaldpp.htm
26. Khawandanah J. Double or hybrid diabetes: a systematic review on disease prevalence, characteristics and risk factors. *Nutri Diabetes.* 2019;9(1):33. doi:10.1038/s41387-019-0101-1
27. ElSayed NA, Aleppo G, Aroda VR, et al. 2. Classification and Diagnosis of Diabetes: Standards of Care in Diabetes-2023. *Diabetes Care.* 2023;46(Suppl 1):S19–S40. doi: 10.2337/dc23-S002 [Erratum in: *Diabetes Care.* 2023;46(5):1106. doi: 10.2337/dc23-er05. Erratum in: *Diabetes Care.* 2023; 46(9):1715. doi: 10.2337/dc23-ad08]
28. American Diabetes Association Professional Practice Committee. 2. Diagnosis and Classification of Diabetes: Standards of Care in Diabetes-2024. *Diabetes Care.* 2024 Jan 1;47(Suppl 1): S20–S42. doi: 10.2337/dc24-S002. PMID: 38078589; PMCID: PMC10725812.
29. Centers for Disease Control and Prevention. *Gestational diabetes and postpartum depression.* Accessed September 29, 2024. https://www.cdc.gov/diabetes/about/gestational-diabetes-postpartum-depression.html.
30. Barbour LA, McCurdy CE, Hernandez TL, Kirwan JP, Catalano PM, Friedman JE. Cellular mechanisms for insulin resistance in normal pregnancy and gestational diabetes. *Diabetes Care.* 2007;30(Supplement_2):S112–S119. doi:10.2337/dc07-s202
31. ElSayed NA, Aleppo G, Aroda VR, et al. Management of diabetes in pregnancy: standards of care in diabetes—2023. *Diabetes Care.* 2023;46(Suppl_1):S254–S266. doi:10.2337/dc23-S015
32. Metzger BE, Coustan DR, Trimble ER. Hyperglycemia and adverse pregnancy outcomes. *Clinical Chemistry.* 2019;65(7):937–938. doi:10.1373/clinchem.2019.303990
33. International Association of Diabetes and Pregnancy Study Groups Consensus Panel, Metzger BE, Gabbe SG, et al. International association of diabetes and pregnancy study groups recommendations on the diagnosis and classification of hyperglycemia in pregnancy. *Diabetes Care.* 2010;33(3): 676–682. doi:10.2337/dc09-1848
34. US Preventive Services Task Force. Screening for gestational diabetes: US Preventive Services Task Force recommendation statement. *JAMA.* 2021;326(6):531–538. doi:10.1001/jama.2021.11922
35. ACOG Clinical Practice Update: Screening for Gestational and Pregestational Diabetes in Pregnancy and Postpartum. *Obstetr Gynecol.* 2024;144(1):e20–e23.
36. Rajkumar V, Levine SN. Latent autoimmune diabetes. In: *StatPearls.* StatPearls Publishing; 2024.
37. Buzzetti R, Tuomi T, Mauricio D, et al. Management of latent autoimmune diabetes in adults: a consensus statement from an international expert panel. *Diabetes.* 2020;69(10): 2037–2047. doi:10.2337/dbi20-0017
38. KFF Health News. Diabetes misdiagnosis: How Black women are often misdiagnosed with type 2 diabetes when they actually have LADA. *KFF Health News.* September 26, 2024. Accessed January 7, 2024. https://kffhealthnews.org/news/article/diabetes-misdiagnosis-type-2-lada-black-women/
39. LaPreze J, Robinson A. Detecting and managing drug-induced diabetes. *US Pharm.* 2021;46(11):18–30. https://www.uspharmacist.com/article/detecting-and-managing-druginduced-diabetes
40. Fève B, Scheen AJ. When therapeutic drugs lead to diabetes. *Diabetologia,* 2022;65(4):751–762. doi:10.1007/s00125-022-05666-w
41. Hoffman LS, Fox TJ, Anastasopoulou C, et al. Maturity onset diabetes in the young. In: *StatPearls.* StatPearls Publishing; 2023.

42. Kant R, Davis A, Verma V. Maturity-onset diabetes of the young: rapid evidence review. *Am Fam Physician*. 2022;105(2):162–167.
43. Naylor R, Knight Johnson A, del Gaudio D. Maturity-onset diabetes of the young overview. In: Adam MP, Feldman J, Mirzaa GM, et al., eds. *GeneReviews*. University of Washington, Seattle; 2018. https://www.ncbi.nlm.nih.gov/books/NBK500456/
44. Ali MK, Imperatore G, Benoit SR, et al. Impact of changes in diabetes screening guidelines on testing eligibility and potential yield among adults without diagnosed diabetes in the United States. *Diabetes Res Clin Pract*. 2023;197:110572. doi:10.1016/j.diabres.2023.110572
45. Sims EK, Besser REJ, Dayan C, et al. Screening for type 1 diabetes in the general population: a status report and perspective. *Diabetes*. 2022;71(4):610–623. doi:10.2337/dbi20-0054
46. American Diabetes Association Professional Practice Committee. Diagnosis and classification of diabetes: standards of care in diabetes—2024. *Diabetes Care*, 2024;47(Suppl 1): S20–S42. doi:10.2337/dc24-S002
47. American Diabetes Association. *Glucose calculator*. Accessed September 29, 2024. https://professional.diabetes.org/glucose_calc
48. Evert AB, Dennison M, Gardner CD, et al. Nutrition therapy for adults with diabetes or prediabetes: a consensus report. *Diabetes Care*. 2019;42(5):731–754. doi:10.2337/dci19-0014.
49. Jing T, Zhang S, Bai M, et al. Effect of dietary approaches on glycemic control in patients with type 2 diabetes: a systematic review with network meta-analysis of randomized trials. *Nutrients*. 2023;15(14):3156. doi:10.3390/nu15143156
50. Quarta A, Guarino M, Tripodi R, Giannini C, Chiarelli F, Blasetti A. Diet and glycemic index in children with type 1 diabetes. *Nutrients*. 2023;15(16):3507. doi:10.3390/nu15163507
51. Dong T, Guo M, Zhang P, Sun G, Chen B. The effects of low-carbohydrate diets on cardiovascular risk factors: a meta-analysis. *PloS One*. 2020;15(1):e0225348. doi:10.1371/journal.pone.0225348
52. Martínez-González MA, Gea A, Ruiz-Canela M. The Mediterranean diet and cardiovascular health. *Circ Res*. 2019;124(5): d779–798. doi:10.1161/CIRCRESAHA.118.313348.
53. Martín-Peláez S, Fito M, Castaner O. Mediterranean diet effects on type 2 diabetes prevention, disease progression, and related mechanisms. A review. *Nutrients*. 2020;12(8):2236. doi:10.3390/nu12082236
54. Smart CEM, King BR, Lopez PE. Insulin dosing for fat and protein: Is it time? *Diabetes Care* 2020;43(1):13–15. doi:10.2337/dci19-0039
55. Hamdy O, Ganda OP, Maryniuk M, Gabbay RA, Members of the Joslin Clinical Oversight Committee. CHAPTER 2. Clinical nutrition guideline for overweight and obese adults with type 2 diabetes (T2D) or prediabetes, or those at high risk for developing T2D. *Am J Managed Care*. 2018;24 (7 Spec No.):SP226–SP231.
56. U.S. Department of Health and Human Services & U.S. Department of Agriculture. *Dietary Guidelines for Americans, 2020-2025*. Accessed January 7, 2025. https://www.dietaryguidelines.gov/sites/default/files/2020-12/Dietary_Guidelines_for_Americans_2020-2025.pdf
57. Atkinson FS, Brand-Miller JC, Foster-Powell K, Buyken AE, Goletzke J. International tables of glycemic index and glycemic load values 2021: a systematic review. *Am J Clin Nutr*. 2021;114(5):1625–1632. doi:10.1093/ajcn/nqab233
58. Lu ZQ, Yan J. Ch 27. Dietary carbohydrate and age-related cataract. In VR Preedy (Ed.), *Handbook of Nutrition, Diet and the Eye*. Academic Press; 2014:271–277.
59. Gómez-Ruiz RP, Cabello-Hernández AI, Gómez-Pérez FJ, Gómez-Sámano MÁ. Meal frequency strategies for the management of type 2 diabetes subjects: a systematic review. *PloS One*. 2024;19(2):e0298531. doi:10.1371/journal.pone.0298531
60. Cristello Sarteau A, Mayer-Davis E. Too much dietary flexibility may hinder, not help: could more specific targets for daily food intake distribution promote glycemic management among youth with type 1 diabetes? *Nutrients*. 2022;14(4):824. doi:10.3390/nu14040824
61. Petrovski G, Campbell J, Pasha M, et al. Twelve-month follow-up from a randomized controlled trial of simplified meal announcement versus precise carbohydrate counting in adolescents with type 1 diabetes using the MiniMed™ 780G advanced hybrid closed-loop system. *Diabetes Technol Ther*. 2024;26(S3):76–83. doi:10.1089/dia.2023.0429
62. Centenaro A, do Nascimento C, Beretta MV, da Costa Rodrigues T. Carbohydrate counting as a strategy to optimize glycemic control in type 1 diabetes mellitus. *Arch Endocrinol Metab*. 2023;67(3):385-394. doi:10.20945/2359-3997000000596
63. Basu A, Hooyman A, Richardson LA, Alman AC, Snell-Bergeon JK. Longitudinal associations of dietary fiber intake with glycated hemoglobin and estimated insulin sensitivity in adults with and without type 1 diabetes. *Nutrients*. 2023;15(21):4620. doi:10.3390/nu15214620
64. Giuntini EB, Sardá FAH, de Menezes EW. The effects of soluble dietary fibers on glycemic response: an overview and futures perspectives. *Foods*. 2022;11(23):3934. doi:10.3390/foods11233934
65. Reynolds AN, Akerman AP, Mann J. Dietary fibre and whole grains in diabetes management: systematic review and meta-analyses. *PLoS Med*. 2020;17(3):e1003053. doi:10.1371/journal.pmed.1003053.
66. DeAngelis AM, Berde CB. The role of pharmacogenetics in the treatment of diabetes. *Biomarkers Cancer*. 2017;9:39–48. doi:10.1016/j.bcdf.2017.07.005
67. American Dietetic Association. Position of the American Dietetic Association: health implications of dietary fiber. *J Am Dietet Assoc*. 2008;108(10):1716–1731. doi:10.1016/j.jada.2008.08.007
68. American Society of Nutrition. Most Americans are not getting enough fiber in our diets. June 9, 2021. Accessed January 7, 2025. https://nutrition.org/most-americans-are-not-getting-enough-fiber-in-our-diets/
69. Thomas DJ, Shafiee M, Nosworthy MG, Lane G, Ramdath DD, Vatanparast H. Unveiling the evidence for the use of pulses in managing type 2 diabetes mellitus: a scoping review. *Nutrients*. 2023;15(19):4222. doi:10.3390/nu15194222
70. Cozma AI, Sievenpiper JL. The role of fructose, sucrose and high-fructose corn syrup in diabetes. *Europ Endocrinol*. 2014;10(1):51–60. doi:10.17925/EE.2014.10.01.51
71. Dugic A, Kryk M, Mellenthin C, et al. Fructose-induced severe hypertriglyceridemia and diabetes mellitus: a cautionary tale. *Endocrinol Diabet MetabolCase Reports*. 2021;21-0110. doi:10.1530/EDM-21-0110
72. Yanagisawa Y. How dietary amino acids and high protein diets influence insulin secretion. *Physiologi Rep*. 2023;11(2): e15577. doi:10.14814/phy2.15577
73. Anjom-Shoae J, Feinle-Bisset C, Horowitz M. Impacts of dietary animal and plant protein on weight and glycemic control in health, obesity and type 2 diabetes: friend or foe? *Front Endocrinol*. 2024;15:1412182. doi:10.3389/fendo.2024.1412182
74. Malaeb S, Bakker C, Chow LS, Bantle AE. High-protein diets for treatment of type 2 diabetes mellitus: a systematic review. *Adv Nutr*. 2019;10(4):621–633. doi:10.1093/advances/nmz002

75. Tettamanzi F, Bagnardi V, Louca P, et al. High protein diet is more effective in improving insulin resistance and glycemic variability compared to a Mediterranean diet-a cross-over controlled inpatient dietary study. *Nutrients.* 2021;13(12):4380. doi:10.3390/nu13124380
76. Zhao WT, Luo YM, Zhang Y, Zhou Y, Zhao TT. High protein diet is of benefit for patients with type 2 diabetes: an updated meta-analysis. *Medicine.* 2018;97(46):e13149. doi:10.1097/MD.0000000000013149
77. Paterson M, Bell KJ, O'Connell SM, Smart CE, Shafat A, King B. The role of dietary protein and fat in glycaemic control in type 1 diabetes: implications for intensive diabetes management. *Curr Diabet Rep.*2015;15(9):61. doi:10.1007/s11892-015-0630-5
78. Abdou M, Hafez MH, Anwar GM, et al. Effect of high protein and fat diet on postprandial blood glucose levels in children and adolescents with type 1 diabetes in Cairo, Egypt. *Diabet Metabol Syndrome.* 2021;15(1):7–12. doi:10.1016/j.dsx.2020.11.020
79. Paterson MA, Smart CE, Rafferty J, et al. A 30% increased insulin dose is necessary to control postprandial hyperglycemia for high protein meals in individuals with type 1 diabetes using insulin pump therapy. *Diabetes.* 2019;68(Suppl_1):330-OR. doi:10.2337/db19-330-OR
80. Paterson MA, Smart CE, Lopez PE, et al. Influence of dietary protein on postprandial blood glucose levels in individuals with Type 1 diabetes mellitus using intensive insulin therapy. *Diabetic Med.* 2016;33(5):592–598. doi:10.1111/dme.13011
81. Delahanty LM, Weinstock RS. *Type 1 diabetes and diet: Beyond the basics.* February 3, 2023. Accessed September 29, 2024. https://www.uptodate.com/contents/type-1-diabetes-and-diet-beyond-the-basics/print
82. Smart CEM, King BR, Lopez PE. Insulin dosing for fat and protein: Is it time? *Diabetes Care.* 2020;43(1):13–15. doi:10.2337/dci19-0039
83. Paterson MA, Smart CEM, Lopez PE, et al. Increasing the protein quantity in a meal results in dose-dependent effects on postprandial glucose levels in individuals with Type 1 diabetes mellitus. *Diabetic Med.* 2017;34(6):851–854. doi:10.1111/dme.13347
84. Evert AB. Factors beyond carbohydrate to consider when determining meantime insulin doses: protein, fat, timing, and technology. *Diabetes Spectrum.* 2020;33(2):149–155. doi:10.2337/ds20-0004
85. Smart CE, Evans M, O'Connell SM, et al. Both dietary protein and fat increase postprandial glucose excursions in children with type 1 diabetes, and the effect is additive. *Diabetes Care.* 2013;36(12):3897–3902. doi:10.2337/dc13-1195
86. Evans M, Smart CEM, Paramalingam, N, et al. Dietary protein affects both the dose and pattern of insulin delivery required to achieve postprandial euglycaemia in Type 1 diabetes: a randomized trial. *Diabetic Med.* 2019;36(4):499–504. doi:10.1111/dme.13875
87. Keating B, Smart CEM, Harray AJ, et al. Additional insulin is required in both the early and late postprandial periods for meals high in protein and fat: a randomized trial. *J Clin Endocrinol Metabol.* 2021;106(9):e3611–e3618. doi:10.1210/clinem/dgab318
88. Hall RM, Marshall HJ, Parry-Strong A, Corley B, Krebs JD. A randomized controlled trial of additional bolus insulin using an insulin-to-protein ratio compared with insulin-to-carbohydrate ratio alone in people with type 1 diabetes following a carbohydrate-restricted diet. *J Diabetes Complications.* 2024;38(7):108778. doi:10.1016/j.jdiacomp.2024.108778
89. Reynolds A, Mitri J. Dietary advice for individuals with diabetes. In: Feingold KR, Anawalt B, Blackman MR, et al., eds. *Endotext.* MDText.com, Inc; 2024.
90. ElSayed NA, Aleppo G, Aroda VR, et al. Facilitating positive health behaviors and well-being to improve health outcomes: Standards of care in diabetes—2023. *Diabetes Care.* 2023;46(Suppl_1):S68–S96. doi:10.2337/dc23-S005
91. Campbell AP, Rains TM. Dietary protein is important in the practical management of prediabetes and type 2 diabetes. *J Nutr.* 2015;145(1):164S–169S. doi:10.3945/jn.114.194878
92. Lytrivi M, Gomes Da Silveira Cauduro C, Kibanda J, Kristanto P, Paesmans M, Cnop M. Impact of saturated compared with unsaturated dietary fat on insulin sensitivity, pancreatic β-cell function and glucose tolerance: a systematic review and meta-analysis of randomized, controlled trials. *Am J Clin Nutr.* 2023;118(4):739–753. doi:10.1016/j.ajcnut.2023.07.018
93. Sears B, Perry M. The role of fatty acids in insulin resistance. *Lipid Health Dis.* 2015;14:121. doi:10.1186/s12944-015-0123-1
94. von Frankenberg AD, Marina A, Song X, Callahan HS, Kratz M, Utzschneider KMA. High-fat, high-saturated fat diet decreases insulin sensitivity without changing intra-abdominal fat in weight-stable overweight and obese adults. *Eur J Nutr.* 2017;56(1):431–443. doi:10.1007/s00394-015-1108-6
95. Bell KJ, Toschi E, Steil GM, Wolpert HA. Optimized mealtime insulin dosing for fat and protein in type 1 diabetes: application of a model-based approach to derive insulin doses for open-loop diabetes management. *Diabetes Care.* 2016;39(9):1631–1634. doi:10.2337/dc15-2855
96. Smith TA, Marlow AA, King BR, Smart CE. Insulin strategies for dietary fat and protein in type 1 diabetes: a systematic review. *Diabetic Med.* 2021;38(11):e14641. doi:10.1111/dme.14641
97. Al Balwi R, Al Madani W, Al Ghamdi A. Efficacy of insulin dosing algorithms for high-fat high-protein mixed meals to control postprandial glycemic excursions in people living with type 1 diabetes: a systematic review and meta-analysis. *Pediatr Diabetes.* 2022;23(8):1635–1646. doi:10.1111/pedi.13436
98. Bell KJ, Fio CZ, Twigg S, et al. Amount and type of dietary fat, postprandial glycemia, and insulin requirements in type 1 diabetes: a randomized within-subject trial. *Diabetes Care.* 2020;43(1):59–66. doi:10.2337/dc19-0687
99. Furthner D, Lukas A, Schneider AM, et al. The role of protein and fat intake on insulin therapy in glycaemic control of paediatric type 1 diabetes: a systematic review and research gaps. *Nutrients.* 2021;13(10):3558. doi:10.3390/nu13103558
100. Smith TA, Marlow AA, King BR, Smart CE. Insulin strategies for dietary fat and protein in type 1 diabetes: a systematic review. *Diabetic Med.* 2021;38(11):e14641. doi:10.1111/dme.14641
101. National Institute of Diabetes and Digestive and Kidney Diseases. Heart disease and stroke. Accessed September 29, 2024. https://www.niddk.nih.gov/health-information/diabetes/overview/preventing-problems/heart-disease-stroke
102. Oelrich B, Dewell A, Gardner CD. Effect of fish oil supplementation on serum triglycerides, LDL cholesterol and LDL subfractions in hypertriglyceridemic adults. *Nutr Metabol Cardiovasc Dis.* 2013;23(4):350–357. doi:10.1016/j.numecd.2011.06.003
103. American Diabetes Association. Lifestyle management: Standards of medical care in diabetes—2019. Diabetes Care. 2019;42(Suppl 1):S46-S60. doi:10.2337/dc19-S005

104. American Diabetes Association Professional Practice Committee. 5. Facilitating positive health behaviors and well-being to improve health outcomes: Standards of care in diabetes—2024. *Diabetes Care.* 2024; 47(Suppl 1): S77–S110. doi:10.2337/dc24-S005
105. ORIGIN Trial Investigators, Bosch J, Gerstein HC, Dagenais GR, et al. n-3 fatty acids and cardiovascular outcomes in patients with dysglycemia. *New Engl J Med.* 2012;367(4): 309–318. doi:10.1056/NEJMoa1203859
106. World Health Organization. Aspartame hazard and risk assessment results released. July 14, 2023. Accessed January 7, 2025. https://www.who.int/news/item/14-07-2023-aspartame-hazard-and-risk-assessment-results-released
107. Sylvetsky AC, Rother KI. Nonnutritive sweeteners in weight management and chronic disease: a review. *Obesity (Silver Spring, Md.).* 2018;26(4):635–640. doi:10.1002/oby.22139
108. Gardner C, Wylie-Rosett J, Gidding SS, et al. Nonnutritive sweeteners: current use and health perspectives: a scientific statement from the American Heart Association and the American Diabetes Association. *Circulation.* 2012;126(4): 509–519. doi:10.1161/CIR.0b013e31825c42ee
109. U.S. Food and Drug Administration. High-intensity sweeteners. May 19, 2014. Accessed January 7, 2025. https://www.fda.gov/food/food-additives-petitions/high-intensity-sweeteners
110. Steiner JL, Crowell KT, Lang CH. Impact of alcohol on glycemic control and insulin action. *Biomolecules.* 2015;5(4):2223–2246. doi:10.3390/biom5042223
111. Schrieks IC, Heil ALJ, Hendriks HFJ, Mukamal KJ, Beulens JWJ. The effect of alcohol consumption on insulin sensitivity and glycemic status: a systematic review and meta-analysis of intervention studies. *Diabetes Care.* 2015;38(4):723–732. doi:10.2337/dc14-1556
112. Joslin Diabetes Center. Drinking with type 1: Four tips for making it safe. December 29, 2020. Accessed January 7, 2025. https://joslin.org/news-stories/all-news-stories/education/2020/12/drinking-type-1-four-tips-making-it
113. Asbaghi O, Fatemeh N, Mahnaz RK, et al. Effects of chromium supplementation on glycemic control in patients with type 2 diabetes: a systematic review and meta-analysis of randomized controlled trials. *Pharmacol Res.* 2020;161:105098. doi:10.1016/j.phrs.2020.105098
114. Kim Y, Oh YK, Lee J, Kim E. Could nutrient supplements provide additional glycemic control in diabetes management? A systematic review and meta-analysis of randomized controlled trials of as an add-on nutritional supplementation therapy. *Arch Pharmacol Res.* 2022;45(3):185–204. doi:10.1007/s12272-022-01374-6
115. ELDerawi WA, Naser IA, Taleb MH, Abutair AS. The effects of oral magnesium supplementation on glycemic response among type 2 diabetes patients. *Nutrients.* 2018;11(1):44. doi:10.3390/nu11010044
116. National Institutes of Health. National Center for Complementary and Integrative Health. Diabetes and dietary supplements: What you need to know. Updated November 2023. Accessed January 7, 2025. https://www.nccih.nih.gov/health/diabetes-and-dietary-supplements-what-you-need-to-know
117. Xiao Y, Zhang Q, Liao X, Elbelt U, Weylandt KH. The effects of omega-3 fatty acids in type 2 diabetes: a systematic review and meta-analysis. *Prostaglandins Leukot Essent Fatty Acids.* 2022;182:102456. doi:10.1016/j.plefa.2022.102456
118. Miller KM, Hart PH, de Klerk NH, Davis EA, Lucas RM. Are low sun exposure and/or vitamin D risk factors for type 1 diabetes?. *Photochem Photobiol Sci.* 2017;16(3):381–398. doi:10.1039/c6pp00294c
119. National Institutes of Health. Office of Dietary Supplements. Vitamin D: Fact sheet for health professionals. Updated July 26, 2024. Accessed January 7, 2025. https://ods.od.nih.gov/factsheets/VitaminD-HealthProfessional/
120. Li G, Feng H, Mao XL, et al. The effects of probiotics supplementation on glycaemic control among adults with type 2 diabetes mellitus: a systematic review and meta-analysis of randomised clinical trials. *J Translation Med.* 2023; 21(1):442. doi:10.1186/s12967-023-04306-0
121. Yefet E, Bar L, Izhaki I, et al. Effects of probiotics on glycemic control and metabolic parameters in gestational diabetes mellitus: systematic review and meta-analysis. *Nutrients.* 2023;15(7):1633. doi:10.3390/nu15071633
122. Baroni I, Fabrizi D, Luciani M, et al. Probiotics and synbiotics for glycemic control in diabetes: a systematic review and meta-analysis of randomized controlled trials. *Clin Nutr.* 2024;43(4):1041–1061. doi:10.1016/j.clnu.2024.03.006
123. Abdelhaleem IA, Brakat AM, Adayel HM, Asla MM, Rizk MA, Aboalfetoh AY. The effects of resveratrol on glycemic control and cardiometabolic parameters in patients with T2DM: a systematic review and meta-analysis. *Medicina Clinica.* 2022;158(12):576–585. doi:10.1016/j.medcli.2021.06.028
124. Pintaudi B, Di Vieste G, Bonomo. The effectiveness of myo-inositol and D-chiro inositol treatment in type 2 diabetes. *Int J Endocrinol.* 2016;9132052. doi:10.1155/2016/9132052
125. DiNicolantonio JJ, O'Keefe J. Myo-inositol for insulin resistance, metabolic syndrome, polycystic ovary syndrome and gestational diabetes. *Open Heart.* 2022;9(1):e001989. doi:10.1136/openhrt-2022-001989
126. Silva ML, Bernardo MA, Singh J, de Mesquita MF. Cinnamon as a complementary therapeutic approach for dysglycemia and dyslipidemia control in type 2 diabetes mellitus and its molecular mechanism of action: a review. *Nutrients.* 2022;14(13):2773. doi:10.3390/nu14132773
127. Moridpour AH, Kavyani Z, Khosravi S, et al. The effect of cinnamon supplementation on glycemic control in patients with type 2 diabetes mellitus: an updated systematic review and dose-response meta-analysis of randomized controlled trials. *Phytother Res.* 2024;38(1):117–130. doi:10.1002/ptr.8026
128. Shang C, Lin H, Fang X, et al. Beneficial effects of cinnamon and its extracts in the management of cardiovascular diseases and diabetes. *Food Function.* 2021;12(24):12194–12220. doi:10.1039/d1fo01935j
129. American Academy of Pediatrics. Nutrition therapy for children and adolescents. In: *Pediatric Nutrition: A Handbook for Health Care Professionals* (6th ed.). AAP; 2020.
130. Evert AB, Dennison M, Gardner CD, et al. Nutrition therapy for adults with diabetes or prediabetes: a consensus report. *Diabetes Care.* 2019;42(5):731–754. doi:10.2337/dci19-0014
131. Blonde L, Umpierrez GE, Reddy SS, et al. American Association of Clinical Endocrinology Clinical Practice Guideline: Developing a Diabetes Mellitus Comprehensive Care Plan-2022 Update. *Endocrine Pract.* 2022;28(10):923–1049. doi:10.1016/j.eprac.2022.08.002

132. Cameron NA, Petito LC, McCabe M, et al. Quantifying the sex-race/ethnicity-specific burden of obesity on incident diabetes mellitus in the United States, 2001 to 2016: MESA and NHANES. *J Am Heart Assoc.* 2021;10(4):e018799. doi:10.1161/JAHA.120.018799
133. American Diabetes Association. Diabetes Food Hub. *What is the diabetes plate method?* February 20, 2020. Accessed January 7, 2025. https://diabetesfoodhub.org/blog/what-diabetes-plate
134. Davidson PC, Hebblewhite HR, Bode BW, et al. Statistically based CSII parameters: correction factor, (CR (1700 rule), carbohydrate-to-insulin ratio, CIR (2.8 rule), and basal-to-bolus ratio. *Diabetes Technol Ther.* 2003;3:237.
135. King AB, Kuroda A, Matsuhisa M, Hobbs T. A review of insulin-dosing formulas for continuous subcutaneous insulin infusion (CSII) for adults with type 1 diabetes. *Curr Diabetes Rep.* 2016;16(9):83. doi:10.1007/s11892-016-0772-0
136. Rushakoff RJ. Inpatient Diabetes Management. In: Feingold KR, Anawalt B, Blackman MR, et al., eds. *Endotext.* MDText.com, Inc.; 2019.
137. UCSF Diabetes Care. *Calculating insulin dose.* Accessed January 7, 2025. https://dtc.ucsf.edu/types-of-diabetes/type2/treatment-of-type-2-diabetes/medications-and-therapies/type-2-insulin-rx/calculating-insulin-dose/
138. Trefts E, Williams AS, Wasserman DH. Exercise and the regulation of hepatic metabolism. *Prog Mol Biol Trans Sci.* 2015;135:203–225. doi:10.1016/bs.pmbts.2015.07.010
139. Chu L, Hamilton J, Riddell MC. Clinical management of the physically active patient with type 1 diabetes. *Physic Sports Med.* 2011;39(2):64–77. doi:10.3810/psm.2011.05.1896
140. Sprague JE, Arbeláez AM. Glucose counterregulatory responses to hypoglycemia. *Pediatric Endocrinology Reviews: PER* 2011;9(1):463–475.
141. Scheiner G. Dealing with "D'OH", *Delayed onset hypoglycemia: A new understanding of a common problem.* Integrated Diabetes Services. Accessed January 7, 2025. https://integrateddiabetes.com/Articles/exer/delayed%20onset%20hypoglycemia%20article.pdf
142. Adams OP. The impact of brief high-intensity exercise on blood glucose levels. *Diabetes, Metabolic Syndrome and Obesity: Targets and Therapy.* 2013;6:113–122. doi:10.2147/DMSO.S29222
143. Adolfsson P, Taplin CE, Zaharieva DP, et al. ISPAD Clinical Practice Consensus Guidelines 2022: Exercise in children and adolescents with diabetes. *Pediatr Diabetes.* 2022;23(8):1341–1372. doi:10.1111/pedi.13452
144. Colberg SR, Sigal RJ, Yardley JE, et al. Physical activity/exercise and diabetes: a position statement of the American Diabetes Association. *Diabetes Care.* 2016;39(11):2065–2079. doi:10.2337/dc16-1728
145. Evans PL, McMillin SL, Weyrauch LA, Witczak CA. Regulation of skeletal muscle glucose transport and glucose metabolism by exercise training. *Nutrients.* 2019;11(10):2432. doi:10.3390/nu11102432
146. Olson AL, Humphries K. Recent advances in understanding glucose transport and glucose disposal. *F1000Research.* 2020; 9:F1000 Faculty Rev-639. doi:10.12688/f1000research.22237.1
147. Hulett NA, Scalzo RL, Reusch JEB. Glucose uptake by skeletal muscle within the contexts of type 2 diabetes and exercise: an integrated approach. *Nutrients.* 2022;14(3):647. doi:10.3390/nu14030647
148. Merz KE, Thurmond DC. Role of skeletal muscle in insulin resistance and glucose uptake. *Compr Physiol.* 2020;10(3):785–809. doi:10.1002/cphy.c190029
149. Zhang C, Yang J. Personalizing physical activity for glucose control among individuals with type 2 diabetes: are we there yet? *Diabetes Care.* 2024; 47(2):196–198. doi:10.2337/dci23-0063
150. American Diabetes Association. Weekly Exercise Targets. Accessed January 7, 2025. https://diabetes.org/health-wellness/fitness/weekly-exercise-targets#:~:text=Spread%20it%20out&text=Each%20breakdown%20will%20have%20
151. Kanaley JA, Colberg SR, Corcoran MH, et al. Exercise/physical activity in individuals with type 2 diabetes: a consensus statement from the American College of Sports Medicine. *Med Sci Sports Exerc.* 2022;54(2):353–368. doi:10.1249/MSS.0000000000002800
152. Colberg SR, Sigal RJ, Fernhall B, et al. Exercise and type 2 diabetes: The American College of Sports Medicine and the American Diabetes Association: joint position statement. *Diabetes Care.* 2010;33(12):e147–e167. doi:10.2337/dc10-9990
153. Shiau K, Tsao TH, Yang CB. Effects of single versus multiple bouts of resistance training on maximal strength and anaerobic performance. *J Hum Kinet.* 2018; 62:231–240. doi:10.1515/hukin-2017-0122
154. Phillip M, Nimri R, Bergenstal RM, et al. Consensus recommendations for the use of automated insulin delivery technologies in clinical practice. *Endocrine Rev.* 2023;44(2):254–280. doi:10.1210/endrev/bnac022
155. Zaharieva DP, Riddell MC. Insulin management strategies for exercise in diabetes. *Can J Diabetes.* 2017;41(5):507–516. doi:10.1016/j.jcjd.2017.07.004
156. American Diabetes Association Professional Practice Committee. 6. Glycemic Targets: Standards of Medical Care in Diabetes-2022. *Diabetes Care.* 2022;45(Suppl 1):S83–S96. doi:10.2337/dc22-S006
157. American Diabetes Association Professional Practice Committee. 7. Diabetes Technology: Standards of Care in Diabetes-2024. *Diabetes Care.* 2024;47(Suppl 1):S126–S144. doi:10.2337/dc24-S007
158. American Diabetes Association Professional Practice Committee. 6. Glycemic Goals and Hypoglycemia: Standards of Care in Diabetes-2024. *Diabetes Care.* 2024;47(Suppl 1):S111–S125. doi:10.2337/dc24-S006
159. Selvin E. The glucose management indicator: time to change course? *Diabetes Care.* 2024;47(6):906–914. doi:10.2337/dci23-0086
160. Perlman JE, Gooley TA, McNulty B, Meyers J, Hirsch IB. HbA1c and glucose management indicator discordance: a real-world analysis. *Diabetes Technol Therapeut.* 2021;23(4):253–258. doi:10.1089/dia.2020.0501
161. Diabetes Control and Complications Trial (DCCT): results of feasibility study. The DCCT Research Group. *Diabetes Care.* 1987;10(1):1–19. doi:10.2337/diacare.10.1.1
162. King P, Peacock I, Donnelly R. The UK prospective diabetes study (UKPDS): clinical and therapeutic implications for type 2 diabetes. *Br J Clin Pharmacol.* 1999;48(5):643–648. doi:10.1046/j.1365-2125.1999.00092.x
163. Stratton IM, Adler AI, Neil HA, et al. Association of glycaemia with macrovascular and microvascular complications of type 2 diabetes (UKPDS 35): prospective observational study. *BMJ (Clinical Research ed.).* 2000;321(7258):405–412. doi:10.1136/bmj.321.7258.405

164. National Eating Disorders Association. Eating disorders and diabetes. Accessed January 7, 2025. https://www.nationaleatingdisorders.org/eating-disorders-and-diabetes/
165. Rask-Madsen C, King G. Mechanisms of disease: endothelial dysfunction in insulin resistance and diabetes. *Nature Rev Endocrinol.* 2007;3(1):46–56. doi:10.1038/ncpendmet0366
166. Whelton PK, Carey RM, Aronow WS, et al. 2017 ACC/AHA/AAPA/ABC/ACPM/AGS/APhA/ASH/ASPC/NMA/PCNA Guideline for the Prevention, Detection, Evaluation, and Management of High Blood Pressure in Adults: Executive Summary: a report of the American College of Cardiology/American Heart Association Task Force on Clinical Practice Guidelines. *Hypertension.* 2018;71(6):1269–1324. doi:10.1161/HYP.0000000000000066
167. Grundy SM, Stone NJ, Bailey AL, et al. AHA/ACC/AACVPR/AAPA/ABC/ACPM/ADA/AGS/APhA/ASPC/NLA/PCNA Guideline on the Management of Blood Cholesterol: Executive Summary: a report of the American College of Cardiology/American Heart Association Task Force on Clinical Practice Guidelines. *J Am Coll Cardiol.* 2019;73(24):3168–3209. doi:10.1016/j.jacc.2018.11.002
168. American Diabetes Association Professional Practice Committee. 9. Pharmacologic approaches to glycemic treatment: standards of care in diabetes—2024. *Diabetes Care.* 2024;47(Suppl 1):S158–S178. doi:10.2337/dc24-S009
169. American Diabetes Association Professional Practice Committee. 10. Cardiovascular disease and risk management: Standards of care in diabetes—2024. *Diabetes Care.* 2024;47(Suppl 1):S179–S218. doi:10.2337/dc24-S010
170. de Boer IH, Bangalore S, Benetos A, et al. Diabetes and hypertension: a position statement by the American Diabetes Association. *Diabetes Care.* 2017;40(9):1273–1284. doi:10.2337/dci17-0026
171. Feingold KR. The effect of diet on cardiovascular disease and lipid and lipoprotein levels. In: Feingold KR, Anawalt B, Blackman MR, et al., eds. *Endotext.* MDText.com, Inc.; 2024.
172. Diab A, Dastmalchi LN, Gulati M, Michos ED. A heart-healthy diet for cardiovascular disease prevention: where are we now? *Vascular Health and Risk Management.* 2023;19:237–253. doi:10.2147/VHRM.S379874
173. Zheng X, Zhang W, Wan X, et al. The effects of Mediterranean diet on cardiovascular risk factors, glycemic control and weight loss in patients with type 2 diabetes: a meta-analysis. *BMC Nutrition.* 2024;10(1):59. doi:10.1186/s40795-024-00836-y
174. National Heart, Lung, and Blood Institute. *DASH Eating Plan.* Updated December 29, 2023. National Institutes of Health. Accessed January 7, 2025. https://www.nhlbi.nih.gov/education/dash-eating-plan
175. United States Renal Data System. 2023 Annual Report. *Chronic kidney disease: 1. CKD in the general population.* National Institute of Diabetes and Digestive and Kidney Diseases. Accessed January 7, 2025. https://usrds-adr.niddk.nih.gov/2023/chronic-kidney-disease/1-ckd-in-the-general-population
176. UK Kidney Association. *UK ECKD guide: Chronic kidney disease stages.* UK Kidney Association. Accessed January 7, 2025. https://ukkidney.org/health-professionals/information-resources/uk-eckd-guide#ckd-stages
177. Ko GJ, Kalantar-Zadeh K, Goldstein-Fuchs J, Rhee CM. Dietary approaches in the management of diabetic patients with kidney disease. *Nutrients.* 2017;9(8):824. doi:10.3390/nu9080824
178. Go AS, Yang J, Tan TC, et al. Contemporary rates and predictors of fast progression of chronic kidney disease in adults with and without diabetes mellitus. *BMC Nephrology.* 2018;19:146. doi:10.1186/s12882-018-0942-1
179. National Kidney Foundation. KDOQI Clinical Practice Guideline for Diabetes and CKD: 2012 Update. *Am J Kid Dis.* 2012;60(5):850–886. doi:10.1053/j.ajkd.2012.07.005
180. Pedrini MT, Levey AS, Lau J, et al. The effect of dietary protein restriction on the progression of diabetic and nondiabetic renal diseases: a meta-analysis. 1996. In: *Database of Abstracts of Reviews of Effects (DARE): Quality-assessed Reviews.* Centre for Reviews and Dissemination (UK); 1995.
181. Zhu HG, Jiang ZS, Gong PY, et al. Efficacy of low-protein diet for diabetic nephropathy: a systematic review of randomized controlled trials. *Lipid Health Dis.* 2018;17(1):141. doi:10.1186/s12944-018-0791-8
182. Jiang S, Fang J, Li W. Protein restriction for diabetic kidney disease. *Cochrane Database Syst Rev.* 2023;1(1):CD014906. doi:10.1002/14651858.CD014906.pub2
183. Beto JA, Ramirez WE, Bansal VK. Medical nutrition therapy in adults with chronic kidney disease: integrating evidence and consensus into practice for the generalist registered dietitian nutritionist. *J Acad Nutr Diet.* 2014;114(7):1077–1087. doi:10.1016/j.jand.2013.12.009
184. Evert AB, Boucher JL, Cypress M, et al. Nutrition therapy recommendations for the management of adults with diabetes. *Diabetes Care.* 2014;37(Suppl 1):S120–S143. doi:10.2337/dc14-S120
185. Kropp M, Golubnitschaja O, Mazurakova A, et al. Diabetic retinopathy as the leading cause of blindness and early predictor of cascading complications-risks and mitigation. *EPMA J.* 2023;14(1):21–42. doi:10.1007/s13167-023-00314-8
186. Centers for Disease Control and Prevention. *Diabetes and vision loss.* May 15, 2024. Accessed January 7, 2025. https://www.cdc.gov/diabetes/diabetes-complications/diabetes-and-vision-loss.html
187. Vitale S, Agrón E, Clemons TE, et al. Association of 2-year progression along the AREDS AMD scale and development of late age-related macular degeneration or loss of visual acuity: AREDS Report 41. *JAMA Ophthalmol.* 2020;138(6):610–617. doi:10.1001/jamaophthalmol.2020.0824
188. Chew EY, Clemons TE, Agrón E, et al. Long-term outcomes of adding Lutein/Zeaxanthin and ω-3 fatty acids to the AREDS supplements on age-related macular degeneration progression: AREDS2 Report 28. *JAMA Ophthalmol.* 2022;140(7):692–698. doi:10.1001/jamaophthalmol.2022.1640
189. Păunică I, Giurgiu M, Dumitriu AS, et al. The bidirectional relationship between periodontal disease and diabetes mellitus-a review. *Diagnostics.* 2023;13(4):681. doi:10.3390/diagnostics13040681
190. Kossioni AE. The association of poor oral health parameters with malnutrition in older adults: a review considering the potential implications for cognitive impairment. *Nutrients* 2018;10(11):1709. doi:10.3390/nu10111709
191. Aswath GS, Foris LA, Ashwath AK, et al. Diabetic Gastroparesis. In: *StatPearls.* StatPearls Publishing; 2023.
192. Jalleh RJ, Jones KL, Rayner CK, et al. Normal and disordered gastric emptying in diabetes: recent insights into (patho)physiology, management, and impact on glycaemic control. *Diabetologia.* 2020;65:1981–1993. doi:10.1007/s00125-022-05796-1

193. Wang Z, Song QZ, Jiang JX, Wu XH, Chen JQ. Nutritional therapy for gastroparesis. *J Nutr Oncol.* 2023;8(1):25–30. doi:10.1097/JN9.0000000000000005
194. Young CF, Moussa M, Shubrook JH. Diabetic gastroparesis: a review. *Diabetes Spectrum.* 2020;33(3):290–297. doi:10.2337/ds19-0062
195. Chaudhry A, Gabriel B, Noor J, Jawad S, Challa SR. Tendency of semaglutide to induce gastroparesis: a case report. *Cureus.* 2024;16(1):e52564. doi:10.7759/cureus.52564
196. Handelsman Y, Bloomgarden ZT, Grunberger G, et al. American Association of Clinical Endocrinologists and American College of Endocrinology – clinical practice guidelines for developing a diabetes mellitus comprehensive care plan – 2015. Endocr Pract. 2015;21(Suppl 1):1-87. doi:10.4158/ep15672.glsuppl.
197. Blonde L, Umpierrez GE, Reddy SS, et al. American Association of Clinical Endocrinology Clinical Practice Guideline: Developing a Diabetes Mellitus Comprehensive Care Plan-2022 Update. *Endocrine Practice.* 2022;28(10):923–1049. doi:10.1016/j.eprac.2022.08.002
198. Inzucchi SE, Bergenstal RM, Buse JB, et al. Management of hyperglycemia in type 2 diabetes, 2015: a patient-centered approach: update to a position statement of the American Diabetes Association and the European Association for the Study of Diabetes. *Diabetes Care.* 2015;38(1):140–149. doi:10.2337/dc14-2441
199. Davies MJ, Aroda VR, Collins BS, et al. Management of hyperglycemia in type 2 diabetes, 2022: A consensus report by the American Diabetes Association (ADA) and the European Association for the Study of Diabetes (EASD). *Diabetes Care.* 2022;45(11):2753–2786. doi:10.2337/dci22-0034
200. Beysel S, Unsal IO, Kizilgul M, Caliskan M, Ucan B, Cakal E. The effects of metformin in type 1 diabetes mellitus. *BMC Endocrine Disorders.* 2018;18(1):1. doi:10.1186/s12902-017-0228-9
201. Cai X, Lin C, Yang W, Nie L, Ji L. Non-insulin antidiabetes treatment in type 1 diabetes mellitus: a systematic review and meta-analysis. *Diabetes Metabol J.* 2021;45(3):312–325. doi:10.4093/dmj.2020.0171
202. Yau M, Sperling MA. Treatment of diabetes mellitus in children and adolescents. In: Feingold KR, Anawalt B, Blackman MR, et al., eds. *Endotext.* MDText.com, Inc.; 2021.
203. American Diabetes Association. *Insulin Basics for Diabetes.* Accessed January 7, 2025. https://diabetes.org/health-wellness/medication/insulin-basics
204. American Diabetes Association. *Study shows promising results for inhaled insulin treatment in type 1 diabetes.* June 22, 2024. Accessed January 7, 2025. https://diabetes.org/newsroom/press-releases/study-shows-promising-results-inhaled-insulin-treatment-type-1-diabetes.
205. Sherr JL, Heinemann L, Fleming GA, et al. Automated insulin delivery: benefits, challenges, and recommendations. A consensus report of the Joint Diabetes Technology Working Group of the European Association for the Study of Diabetes and the American Diabetes Association. *Diabetes Care.* 2022;45(12):3058–3074. doi:10.2337/dci22-0018
206. American Diabetes Association. 8. Obesity management for the treatment of type 2 diabetes: standards of medical care in diabetes—2021. *Diabetes Care.* 2021;44(Suppl 1): S100–S110. doi:10.2337/dc21-S008
207. American Society for Metabolic and Bariatric Surgery. Public Education Committee. *Bariatric surgery procedures.* Updated May 2021. Accessed January 7, 2025. https://asmbs.org/patients/bariatric-surgery-procedures/
208. Crossan K, Sheer AJ. Intragastric balloon. In: *StatPearls.* StatPearls Publishing; 2023.
209. Fernandez CJ, Rajgopal RK, Pappachan JM. Hypoglycaemia associated with critical illness and hormone deficiencies: a narrative review. *J Lab Precision Med.* 2021;6(0). doi:10.21037/jlpm-2020-ash-01
210. Kodner C, Anderson L, Pohlgeers K. Glucose management in hospitalized patients. *Am Fam Physician.* 2017;96(10): 648–654. https://www.aafp.org/pubs/afp/issues/2017/1115/p648.html
211. Dhatariya K, Corsino L, Umpierrez GE. Management of diabetes and hyperglycemia in hospitalized patients. In Feingold KR, Anawalt B, Blackman MR, et al. eds. *Endotext.* MDText.com, Inc.; 2024.
212. McMahon MM, Nystrom E, Braunschweig C, Miles J, Compher, C. A.S.P.E.N. clinical guidelines. Nutrition support of adult patients with hyperglycemia. *JPEN.* 2013;37(1):23–36. doi:10.1177/0148607112452001
213. American Diabetes Association Professional Practice Committee. 16. Diabetes care in the hospital: standards of care in diabetes—2024. *Diabetes Care.* 2024;47(Suppl 1): S295–S306. doi:10.2337/dc24-S016
214. McClave SA, Taylor BE, Martindale RG, et al. Guidelines for the provision and assessment of nutrition support therapy in the adult critically ill patient. JPEN. 2016;40(2):159–211. doi:10.1177/0148607115621863
215. Polavarapu P, Pachigolla S, Drincic A. Glycemic management of hospitalized patients receiving nutrition support. *Diabetes Spectrum.* 2022;35(4):427–439. doi:10.2337/dsi22-0010
216. Gosmanov AR, Mendez CE, Umpierrez GE. Challenges and strategies for inpatient diabetes management in older adults. *Diabetes Spectrum.* 2020;33(3):227–235. doi:10.2337/ds20-0008
217. Olveira G, Tapia MJ, Ocón J, et al. Parenteral nutrition–associated hyperglycemia in non–critically ill inpatients increases the risk of in-hospital mortality (multicenter study). *Diabetes Care.* 2013;36(5):1061–1066. doi:10.2337/dc12-1379
218. Via MA, Mechanick JI. Inpatient enteral and parenteral [corrected] nutrition for patients with diabetes. *Curr Diabetes Rep.* 2011;11(2):99–105. doi:10.1007/s11892-010-0168-5
219. Gosmanov AR, Umpierrez GE. Management of hyperglycemia during enteral and parenteral nutrition therapy. *Curr Diabetes Rep.* 2013;13(1):155–162. doi:10.1007/s11892-012-0335-y
220. Vest MT, Newell E, Shapero M, et al. Energy balance in obese, mechanically ventilated intensive care unit patients. *Nutrition.* 2019;66:48–53. doi:10.1016/j.nut.2019.02.021
221. Stolarski AE, Young L, Weinberg J, et al. Early metabolic support for critically ill trauma patients: a prospective randomized controlled trial. *J Trauma Acute Care Surg.* 2022;92(2):255–265. doi:10.1097/TA.0000000000003453
222. Adolph M, Heller AR, Koch T, et al. Lipid emulsions - guidelines on parenteral nutrition, Chapter 6. *Ger Med Sci.* 2009;7:Doc22. doi:10.3205/000081

CHAPTER 9

Nutrition in Cardiovascular Disease and Heart Failure

Xuemeng Chen

CHAPTER OUTLINE

CORE CONCEPTS

1. Promoting a healthy lifestyle throughout life is the most important way to prevent ASCVD before considering pharmacological treatments.
2. Exposure to stressors such as high serum cholesterol, hyperglycemia and toxins, weakens the endothelial lining, triggering an inflammatory cascade that results in oxidized LDL-C and formation of foam cells.

3. Many artherosclerotic cardiovascular disease risk factors are modifiable and can be prevented or improved with early intervention; these include dyslipidemia, diabetes mellitus, hypertension, obesity/overweight, physical inactivity, diet, and tobacco use/secondhand smoke. Nonmodifiable risk factors include male sex, older age, and race.
4. Dyslipidemia refers to alterations in the normal transport of lipids and lipoproteins that contribute to major ASCVD risk. Modifiable risk factors for dyslipidemia include tobacco use/secondhand smoke, diet choices of high saturated fat/trans fat intake, excess energy, inadequate fiber intake, added sugar intake, overweight/obesity, physical inactivity, hypertension, and diabetes mellitus.
5. Hypertriglyceridemia refers to elevated fasting serum triglyceride levels (>150 mg/dL) occurring within dyslipidemia or as an independent lipid metabolism disorder. Modifiable risk factors for hypertriglyceridemia are similar to dyslipidemia but have some marked characteristics in dietary choices including excess simple sugar intake, a low-fat and high-refined carbohydrate diet, and excess alcohol consumption.
6. Nutrition intervention for hypertension includes sodium restriction which lowers blood pressure in a dose-response manner.
7. An elevated body mass index categorized as overweight or obese increases cardiovascular morbidity and mortality risk.
8. Type 2 diabetes mellitus (DM) increases risk for cardiovascular disease development by 2- to 3-fold, as both conditions have many overlapping risk factors of overweight/obesity, dyslipidemia, hyperglycemia, hypertension, suboptimal dietary choices, and physical inactivity.
9. Heart failure (HF) refers to the heart's inability to provide the body with adequate oxygenated blood due to symptomatic structural or functional impairment of ventricular filling or ejection of blood. HF can result in fatigue, dyspnea, fluid retention, lack of appetite, nausea, malnutrition, and death.
10. Cardiac cachexia is an uncontrollable loss of weight that includes muscle, fat, and eventually bone loss. It is associated with a 20–40% mortality rate annually. The condition is not reversible with nutrition intervention, but adequate nutrition may diminish negative outcomes.
11. Cardiac rehabilitation as a secondary prevention includes physician-prescribed aerobic exercise training, cardiac lifestyle risk factor modification including nutrition counseling on a heart-healthy diet, weight and diabetes management, tobacco cessation, psychosocial support and outcomes assessment.

LEARNING OBJECTIVES

1. Explain the normal function of the cardiovascular system.
2. Describe the pathophysiology of cardiovascular disease and common related conditions.
3. Discuss the significance of cardiovascular disease prevention specifically atherosclerotic cardiovascular disease and the most recent American Heart Association and American College of Cardiology guidelines.
4. Develop evidence-based nutrition interventions for individuals with disorders of lipid metabolism, hypertension, and/or heart failure.
5. Identify nutrition-related implications of medications used in the treatment of cardiovascular disease and heart failure.
6. Recognize the significance of obesity and malnutrition in cardiovascular disease and heart failure progression and related outcomes.
7. Determine when it is appropriate to initiate nutrition support in the cardiovascular disease and heart failure populations and explain the best method for providing nutrition support and monitoring outcomes.
8. Discuss a comprehensive secondary cardiovascular disease prevention method, cardiac rehabilitation services, its qualification criteria, outcomes, barriers, potential solutions, and the RD's role in a cardiac rehabilitation program.

Introduction

Heart disease includes a range of conditions that affect the heart such as heart blood vessel disease, heart failure (HF), cardiomyopathy, arrhythmias, heart valve disease, and congenital heart defects. **Cardiovascular disease (CVD)** encompasses several conditions affecting the heart and blood vessels.[1,2] **Atherosclerosis**, the hardening and narrowing of arteries due to cholesterol deposits or plaques, can lead to blood vessel blockages,[2] is the major underlying cause of CVD, and remains the leading cause of morbidity and mortality globally resulting in over 17.9 million deaths per year.[1–4] CVD that is mainly atherosclerosis in origin is referred to as **atherosclerotic cardiovascular disease (ASCVD)**.[5] Atherosclerotic plaques can erode or rupture causing blood clots as thromboses/emboli and a closure of the blood vessel, resulting in myocardial infarction (MI or heart attack), stroke, extremity ischemia, and death.[1,2]

CVD is the leading cause of disability and mortality in the United States for most racial and ethnic groups, and close to 5% of adults have at least one type of CVD, with 1 out of 5 deaths due to CVD.[3,6,7] Coronary artery disease, the most common subset of ASCVD, singularly causes about 20% of deaths among adults in the United States and costs over $230 billion per year when considering cost of health care, medications, and lost productivity.[3,7] Globally, CVD causes 17.9 million deaths per year, representing 30% of all deaths.[8] Uncontrolled ASCVD risk factors and suboptimal implementation of prevention and intervention strategies contribute to most of the CVD cost. Promoting a healthy lifestyle throughout life is the most important way to prevent ASCVD before considering pharmacological treatments.[4,5,8]

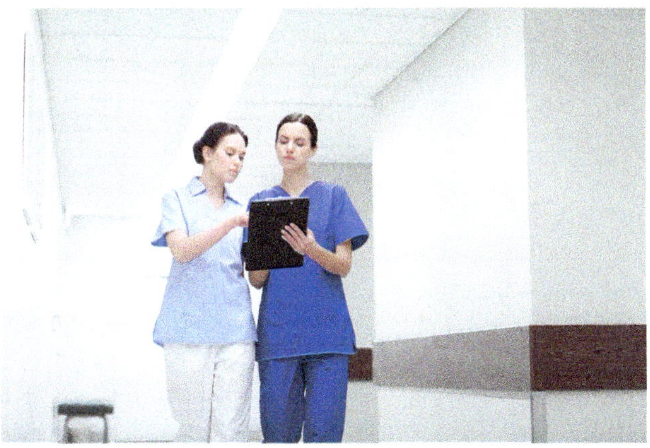
© Af Ground Picture/Shutterstock

CORE CONCEPT 1

Promoting a healthy lifestyle throughout life is the most important way to prevent ASCVD before considering pharmacological treatments.

Cardiac Physiology in Health and Disease

The cardiovascular system is responsible for the transport of oxygen-rich blood and nutrients throughout the body, and for the removal of carbon dioxide and waste products. Its vital role is to maintain interstitial homeostasis.[9] The cardiovascular system is composed of the heart and blood vessels. The heart is made up of three layers: the epicardium (outer layer), **myocardium** (middle layer), and endocardium (inner layer). The heart is divided into four chambers. The top chambers are the right and left atria, and the bottom chambers are the right and left ventricles. Under normal conditions, the right atrium collects oxygen-poor blood delivered from two large veins, the superior vena cava and the inferior vena cava. Blood flows down from the right atrium to the right ventricle through the tricuspid valve. The blood is then pumped from the right ventricle through the pulmonary valve and pulmonary artery to the lungs to become oxygenated. Oxygen-rich blood is delivered from pulmonary veins to the left atrium and flows to the left ventricle through the mitral valve. From the left ventricle, blood is pumped through the aortic valve and the aorta to fuel the entire body through a network of arteries, arterioles, and capillaries. The cycle repeats itself as venules and veins return oxygen-depleted blood back to the superior and inferior vena cava and finally to the heart.[10] **Figure 9.1** illustrates the pathway of blood flow through the heart.

Each cardiac cycle has a period of **systole** and **diastole**. Systole refers to active pumping of blood out of the heart by the ventricles. Diastole is when the ventricles are relaxed and blood flows from the atria to refill the ventricles. There are several equations used to measure the proper function of the cardiovascular system. **Stroke volume** is the amount of blood pumped per heartbeat. It can be calculated

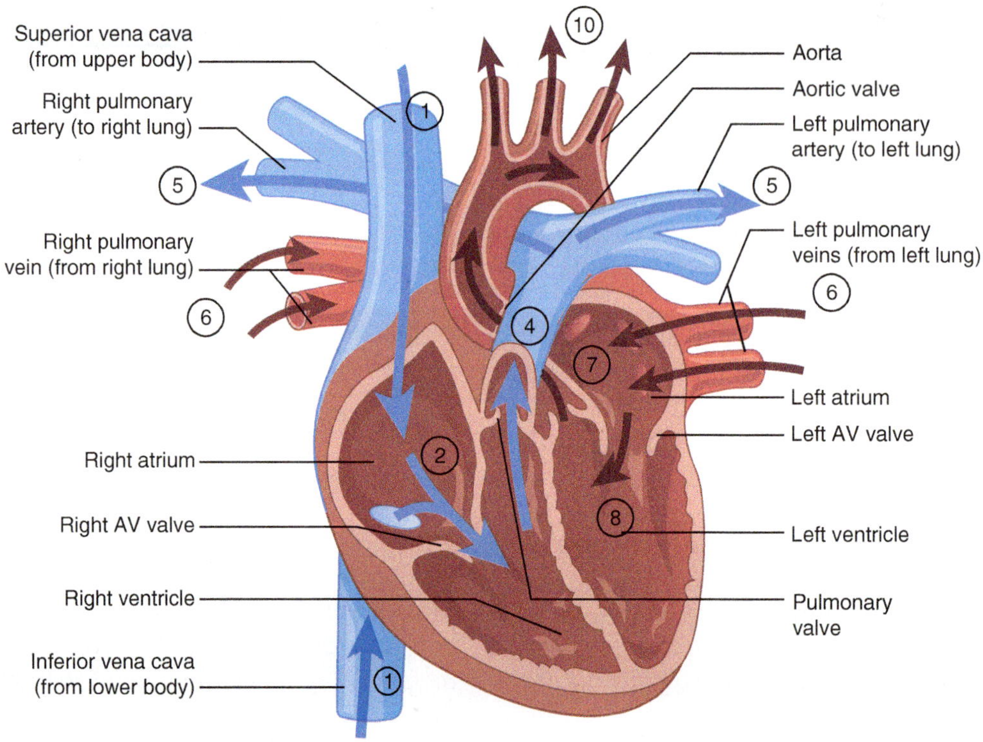

Figure 9.1 Pathway of Blood Flow Through the Heart

as the blood volume in the ventricle at the end of diastole (end-diastolic volume) minus the blood volume in the ventricle at the end of systole (end-systolic volume). **Cardiac output** is a measure of blood pumped per minute that is calculated by multiplying the stroke volume by the heart rate. **Ejection fraction (EF)** is typically used to measure heart function or contractility in patients with HF (**Box 9.1**). It represents the amount of blood being pumped out of the ventricle each time it contracts. EF is the percentage of blood in the ventricle at the end of diastole that is pumped out during systole; the equation is stroke volume (amount of blood pumped out) divided by end-diastolic volume (amount of blood left in the chamber). A normal EF is between 55% and 80%. **Mean arterial pressure (MAP)** is defined as the average pressure that pushes blood through the arteries during a cardiac cycle. MAP is a product of cardiac output and **total peripheral resistance** (resistance of blood flow in systemic circulation). MAP can also be approximated as diastolic pressure plus one-third of the difference between systolic and diastolic pressures.[9] These measurements make it possible to closely monitor the effects of diseases of the cardiovascular system.

For the heart to effectively pump blood throughout the body, electrical activity (action potential) exists within a network of intercalated discs between **myocytes** (heart cells). Electrical activity is started at the sinoatrial (SA) node, which causes the left and right atrium to contract by means of depolarization. The electrical impulse travels to the atrioventricular (AV) node, atrioventricular bundle (bundle of His), right and left bundle branches, and finally to **Purkinje fibers** that spread throughout the right and left ventricles. An **electrocardiogram** (EKG or ECG) can be used to measure the heart's electrical activity by placing electrodes on the body surface that can detect the activity in the extracellular fluid.[9] **Figure 9.2** illustrates the cardiac conduction system, and **Figure 9.3** displays the stages of an electrocardiogram measuring the heart's electrical activity.

CVD describes a collection of conditions in which the proper function of the heart and circulatory system is interrupted. One modifiable pathway that is a culprit

Box 9.1 Equations Measuring Cardiac Function

Stroke volume (SV) = End Diastolic Volume (EDV) − End Systolic Volume (ESV)

Cardiac Output = SV × Heart Rate (HR) in beats per minute (bpm)

Ejection Fraction = SV/EDV

CASE STUDY INTRODUCTION

Carl is a 55-year-old male referred for medical nutrition therapy (MNT) after being diagnosed with dyslipidemia. At his initial visit to the nutrition clinic, he discloses that he works over 60 hours/week as an accountant and relies on fast food choices for meals during the day. His spouse prepares family meals for dinner, and he does not want to complain or change their cooking habits. He admits that he does not exercise but tries to play outside with his daughters on the weekends.

Anthropometric Data:

Weight: 95 kg
Height: 178 cm
BMI: 30 kg/m^2
Waist circumference: 107 cm

Biochemical Data:

Total cholesterol (TC) 299 (Desirable: <200 mg/dL)
Low-density lipoprotein cholesterol (LDL-C) 179 (Desirable: <100 mg/dL)
High-density lipoprotein cholesterol (HDL-C) 28 (Desirable: ≥40 mg/dL)
Triglycerides 155 (Desirable: <150 mg/dL)
Non-high-density lipoprotein cholesterol (non-HDL-C) 271 mg/dL (Desirable: <139 mg/dL)

Clinical Data:

Past Medical History: HTN, dyslipidemia (newly diagnosed)
Medications: metoprolol
Vital Signs: Blood pressure 160/73 mm Hg, Temperature 98.6°F, Heart rate 70 beats/min
Nutrition-Focused Physical Exam: Appears well nourished, android body type

Dietary Data:

24-Hour Diet Recall
Breakfast (6 am): 2 cups of coffee (cream and sugar added)
Lunch (12 pm): Large steak and cheese sandwich, snack-sized chips, 12 ounces of soda
Snack (3 pm): 2 cookies, or a donut, or a fruit cup
Snack (6 pm): Peanut butter and jelly sandwich or bologna (2 slices) and cheese (1 slice) with a little mayonnaise on white bread
Dinner (8 pm): Large serving of spaghetti and meatballs (3 large homemade ricotta meatballs), homemade marinara sauce, 2 dinner rolls with butter, garden side salad (lettuce, cucumber, tomato) with ranch dressing, 8 ounces of water, sometimes wine (6-ounce glass)
Snack (10 pm): Ice cream with fruit (large bowl)
Physical Activity: Plays outside with daughter on weekends, otherwise sedentary

Questions

1. What risk factors does Carl have for CVD at this point?
2. How would you interpret Carl's biochemical data?
3. After assessing Carl's diet recall and evaluating Carl's eating pattern and food/beverage choices, write two Problem/Etiology/Signs and Symptoms (PES) statements for Carl identifying Carl's active nutrition issues.
4. Identify the nutrition interventions you would like to initiate for Carl to address the problems identified in your PES statements.
5. What indices are included in your monitoring and evaluation plan? Why?

for the disruption of cardiovascular function is atherosclerosis. Atherosclerosis describes an active inflammatory process leading to the buildup of plaque that narrows and thickens artery walls and restricts normal blood flow.[1,4] The type of heart disease associated with atherosclerosis is ASCVD. ASCVD is mainly defined as coronary heart disease (CHD) or coronary artery disease (CAD), cerebrovascular disease, and peripheral artery disease (PAD), depending on the location of the blocked arteries from plaques in the heart, brain, or extremities resulting in reduced blood flow. The inflammation associated with atherosclerosis assaults the inner endothelial lining of the arteries. As the endothelium becomes weakened from continued exposure to stressors (high serum cholesterol levels, high serum blood glucose levels, cigarette toxins, or hemodynamic

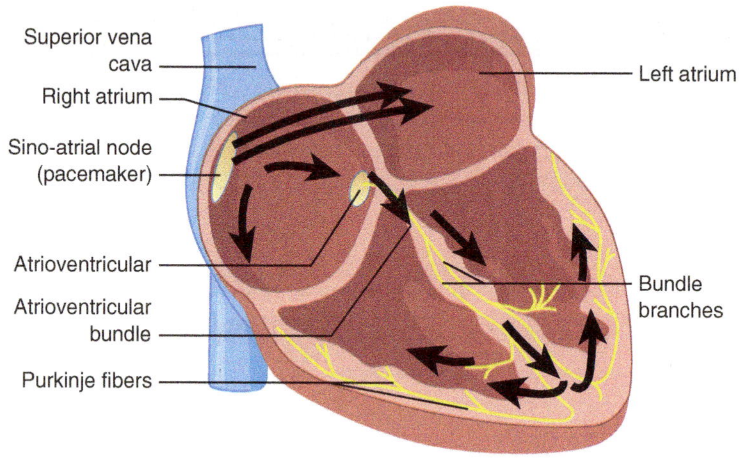

Figure 9.2 Cardiac Conduction System

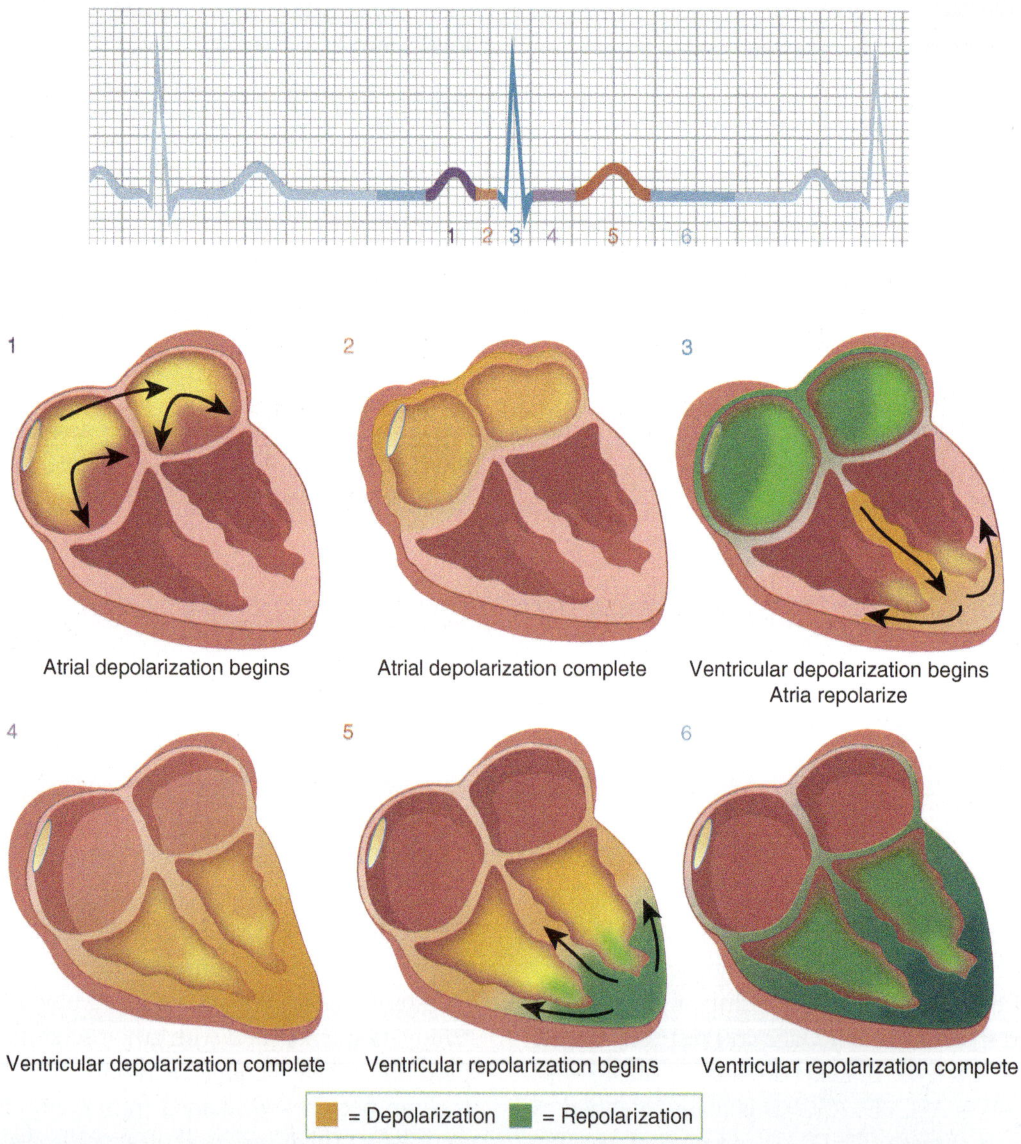

Figure 9.3 Electrocardiogram and Electrical Activity of the Myocardium

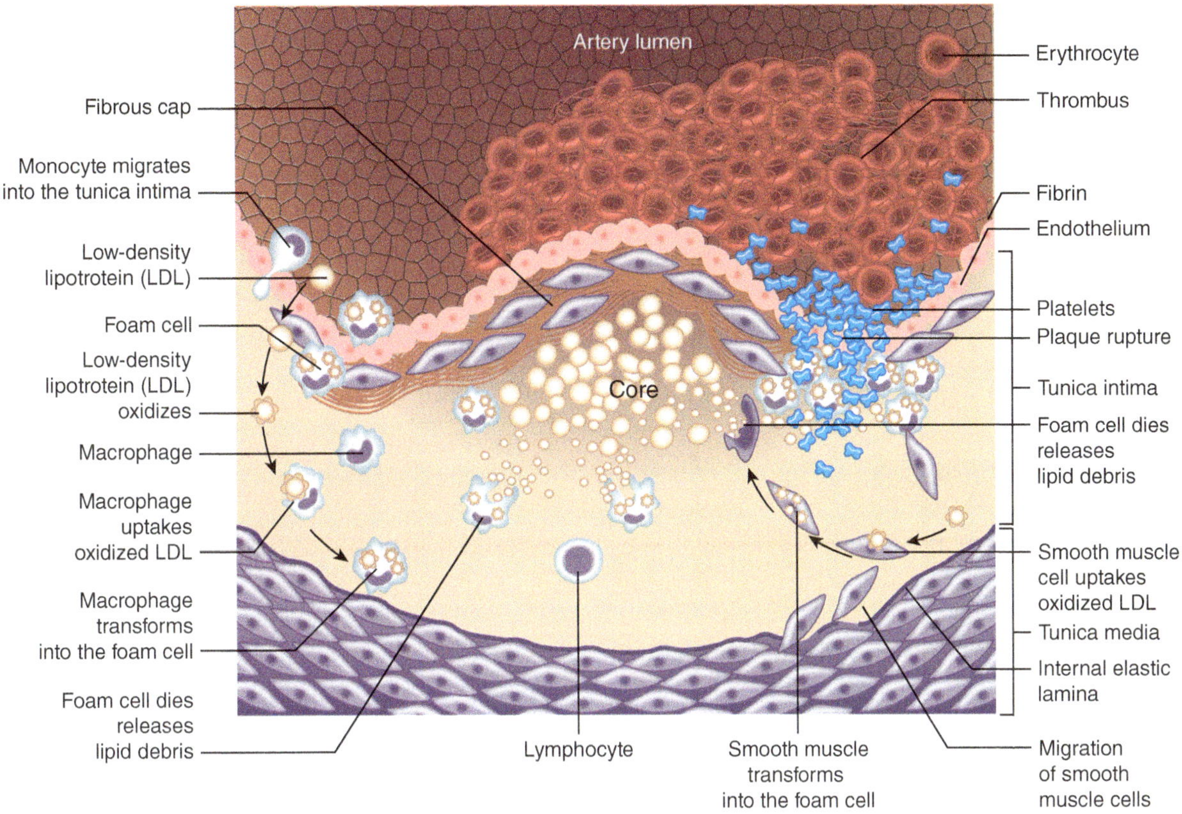

Figure 9.4 Factors Associated with Vulnerable Plaque Formation

disturbance), it is more likely to host high levels of low-density lipoprotein cholesterol (LDL-C). High levels of LDL-C embedded in the endothelial cells undergo enzymatic alterations, become oxidized, and can cause cell death within the endothelium. This triggers an inflammatory cascade, activating release of lymphocytes and monocytes. The monocytes become macrophages and engulf the oxidized LDL-C to form **foam cells** and the lipid core of atherosclerotic plaque. A fibrous cap covers the core. If the fibrous cap is thin and the lipid core is thick, the plaque is said to be vulnerable. **Vulnerable plaque** is a thin cap fibroatheroma and it is the most at risk of rupture.[11] **Figure 9.4** illustrates cholesterol and plaque formation. Plaques can become calcified, narrowing the artery and causing stenosis.[9] If a vulnerable plaque ruptures, the outcome is **thrombosis**, the formation of a blood clot that interferes with normal blood flow. A blood clot that breaks free and travels to another area of the body is referred to as an **embolism**.[11] The final location of the blockage determines the CVD event.

CORE CONCEPT 2

Exposure to stressors such as high serum cholesterol, hyperglycemia and toxins, weakens the endothelial lining, triggering an inflammatory cascade that results in oxidized LDL-C and formation of foam cells.

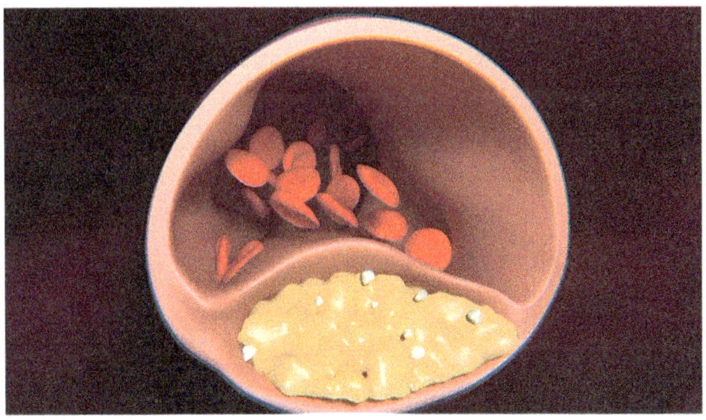

Reproduced from U.S. Centers for Disease Control and Prevention. LDL and HDL Cholesterol and Triglycerides. CDC. Published May 15, 2024. Accessed January 12, 2026. https://www.cdc.gov/cholesterol/about/ldl-and-hdl-cholesterol-and-triglycerides.html

Cardiovascular Disease Clinical Course

Risk Factor Assessment and ASCVD Prevention

The single most important means to prevent ASCVD and HF is to promote a healthy lifestyle throughout the lifespan. The American Heart Association and American College of Cardiology (AHA/ACC) and multi-council guideline in 2019 on the Primary Prevention of CVD recommends adults ages 20–39 years assess traditional ASCVD risk factors (smoking, overweight or obesity, HTN, diabetes mellitus [DM], high cholesterol, and a family history of heart disease) at least every 4–6 years. Asymptomatic adults ages 40–75 years are recommended to routinely assess traditional CVD risk factors using a 10-year ASCVD risk estimator available for download and use at the ACC website to assess ASCVD risk for primary prevention and before the initiation of pharmacological treatments.[4] The calculator uses the following ASCVD risk factors: male sex, older age, race, dyslipidemia, history of DM, on HTN treatment, smoking status, on a statin, and on aspirin therapy.[12] Additional CVD risk factors include overweight and obesity, physical inactivity, and suboptimal diet.[4,5] Many of these risk factors are modifiable and can be prevented or improved with early intervention; refer to **Table 9.1**. The 10-year risk for ASCVD is calculated and categorized as low risk (<5%), borderline risk (5–7.4%), intermediate risk (7.5–19.9%), and high risk (≥20%).[12] For adults over 75 years, open discussion between a clinician and the patient about possible ASCVD preventative therapies that are age appropriate should be conducted.[4] The Academy of Nutrition and Dietetics (AND) recommends that medical nutrition therapy (MNT) is provided by a registered dietitian (RD) for the following CVD risk factors: overweight/obesity, disorders of lipid metabolism, DM, and/or HTN.[13,14] This chapter will provide a review of the nutrition management of disorders of lipid metabolism and HTN for the prevention and management of CVD. This text has additional chapters dedicated to MNT for weight management (Chapter 7 *Weight and Health*) and DM (Chapter 8 *Nutrition in Diabetes Mellitus*).

Table 9.1 Modifiable Versus Nonmodifiable Risk Factors for CVD[4]

Modifiable Risk Factors	Nonmodifiable Risk Factors
■ Diet ■ Dyslipidemia (on a statin) ■ Elevated blood pressure (on HTN treatment) ■ Obesity/overweight ■ Aspirin use ■ Physical inactivity ■ Smoking/secondhand smoke	■ Male sex ■ Older age ■ Race

Disorders of Lipid Metabolism

Lipid molecules include cholesterol, triglycerides (TG), and phospholipids. Cholesterol is a necessary part of cell membranes, steroid hormones, and bile acids, and it is composed of four carbon rings and a carbon ring tail.[15] Triglycerides are essential for the transport of fat. They are structurally made up of a three-carbon glycerol backbone and three fatty acid chains. Both cholesterol and TGs travel as part of the core of **lipoproteins** (refer to **Figure 9.5**).

> **CORE CONCEPT 3**
>
> Many atherosclerotic cardiovascular disease risk factors are modifiable and can be prevented or improved with early intervention; these include dyslipidemia, diabetes mellitus, hypertension, obesity/overweight, physical inactivity, diet, and tobacco use/secondhand smoke. Nonmodifiable risk factors include male sex, older age, and race.

Phospholipids are essential components of cell membranes, and they consist of a glycerol molecule and two fatty acid chains. Phospholipids and free cholesterol join with protein molecules (**apolipoproteins**) to make up the outer layer of lipoproteins.[16] Lipoproteins are responsible for the transport and delivery of fatty acids; there are several types classified by density.[15] Triglyceride-rich lipoproteins are the least dense; examples include chylomicrons, chylomicron remnants, intermediate-density lipoprotein (IDL), and very-low-density lipoproteins (VLDL). VLDL is produced in the liver and transports fatty acids and LDL-C.[15,16] VLDL eventually breaks down into IDL. IDL can be accepted by receptors in liver cells or broken down to LDL-C, a type of higher density lipoproteins. LDL-C can then be accepted by LDL-C receptors in mainly liver cells and numerous tissues. Besides LDL-C, higher density lipoproteins include HDL-C and **lipoprotein(a)**, abbreviated Lp(a). Normal lipoprotein transport moves TGs from the intestine to the liver and then on to storage sites such as fat tissue and utilization sites, mainly muscle[16].

LDL-C, containing mainly one atherogenic **apolipoprotein B100** (apoB100 or apoB), is the dominant cholesterol in high concentration causing atherosclerosis.[17] Elevated levels of circulating LDL-C create a favorable environment for oxidation and atherosclerosis. Serum LDL-C can become elevated due to weight gain, diet choices, inactivity, and defects of the receptors on liver and peripheral cells that usually bind LDL-C.[15]

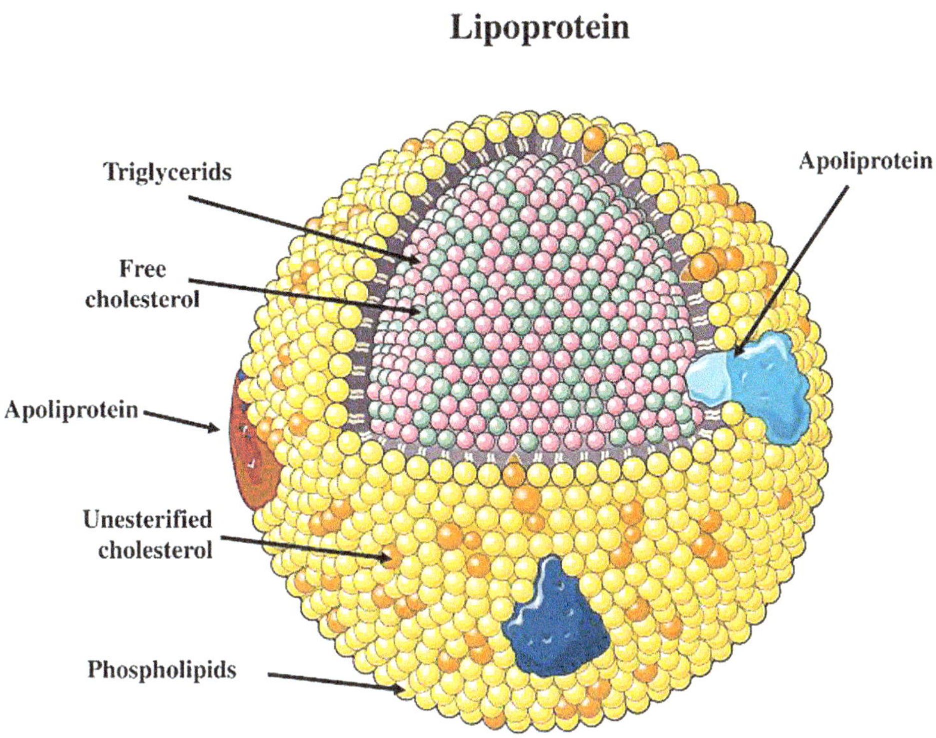

Figure 9.5 The Structure of Lipoproteins

Lp(a) is a heterogeneous liver-derived lipoprotein having similar size and structure as LDL-C (both contain one apoB) (**Figure 9.6**).[17] It is also atherogenic as well as prothrombotic, possibly contributing to blood clots due to the apolipoprotein (a) tail's property.[18,19] In fact, all lipoproteins containing apoB are atherogenic, including chylomicron remnants, IDL, VLDL, LDL-C, and Lp(a).[5,17] HDL-C, which does not contain apoB, seems non-atherogenic. Elevated levels of HDL-C are protective against CAD. HDL-C facilitates reverse transport of cholesterol from the bloodstream to the liver for conversion to bile acids and elimination, and thus prevents LDL-C oxidation and atherosclerosis.[15,16] Non-HDL-C comprises all atherogenic apoB-containing lipoproteins, calculated as the total cholesterol level minus the anti-atherogenic HDL-C level, and is considered as more problematic than LDL-C alone.[5]

Dyslipidemia refers to alterations in the normal transport of lipids and lipoproteins that contribute to atherosclerosis and CVD risk. Dyslipidemia is diagnosed when a blood test detects abnormal levels of circulating lipids. It may include any combination of elevated total cholesterol (>200 mg/dL), LDL-C (≥100 mg/dL), TG (>150 mg/dL), and/or reduced HDL-C (<40 mg/dL for men, and <50 mg/dL for women).[16,20,21] **Hypertriglyceridemia** refers to elevated fasting serum TG levels (>150 mg/dL). It can occur within dyslipidemia, or it can be an independent lipid metabolism disorder.[20,21] Hypertriglyceridemia involves elevated TGs and increases the risk of ASCVD.[21] Moreover, hypertriglyceridemia is frequently linked to DM and metabolic syndrome. This is because insulin resistance is a frequent contributor to high serum TG levels. The amount of free fatty acids increases as serum glucose levels rise, and the liver uses them to synthesize TGs. The liver then packs these TGs into VLDL and releases them into the bloodstream and thus serum TGs levels rise.[20,21] Hypertriglyceridemia is also associated with liver steatosis and metabolic dysfunction–associated steatohepatitis due to insulin resistance. Severe hypertriglyceridemia (TG >500 mg/dL) increases the risk of acute pancreatitis due to the accumulation of free fatty acid breakdown triggering inflammation.[21,22] The average total cholesterol for Americans aged ≥20 years is about 187 mg/dL. Nearly 25 million adults or about 10% of adults aged 20 years and over in the United States have a total serum cholesterol value ≥240 mg/dL. The average LDL-C for Americans aged ≥20 years is about 110 mg/dL. Over 63 million adults aged 20 years or 25.5% of adults have an elevated LDL-C >130 mg/dL.[3]

Due to the dominant atherogenicity, long-standing evidence from lipid-lowering trials, and relatively affordable cost, LDL-C remains as the primary therapeutic target for ASCVD risk prevention and reduction.[5,17]

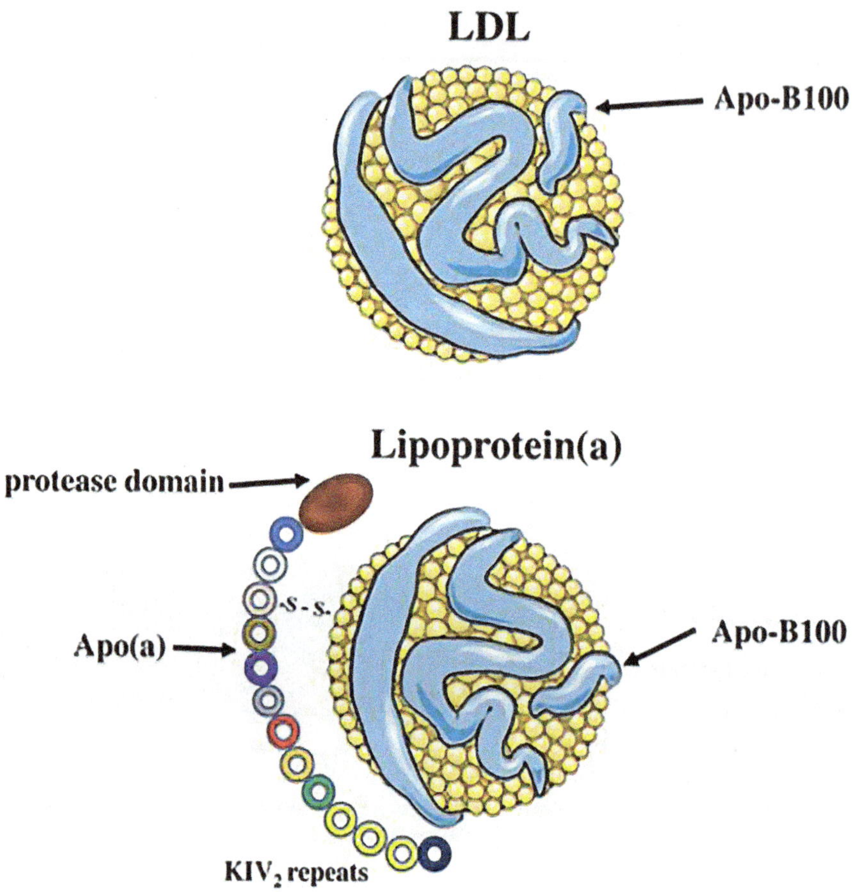

Figure 9.6 Structures of LDL-C and Lp(a)

Reproduced from Lampsas S, Xenou M, Oikonomou E, et al. Lipoprotein(a) in atherosclerotic diseases: from pathophysiology to diagnosis and treatment. Molecules. 2023;28(3):969. doi:10.3390/molecules28030969. https://creativecommons.org/licenses/by/3.0/

The goal of LDL for a general healthy population is <100 mg/dL. As for patients with very high ASCVD risk factors, the goal of LDL is lowered to <70 mg/dL.[5,17,23–26] Recommended standard lipid lab tests to diagnosis dyslipidemia and/or hypertriglyceridemia include total cholesterol, LDL-C, HDL-C, and TGs.[5,27] If TGs are ≥400 mg/dL, the LDL-C level could be underestimated, so that calculating the non-HDL-C, or obtaining a lab of direct LDL-C measurement is better to assess actual LDL-C level and ASCVD risk.[5,20,22] Advanced lipid lab tests may be considered for patients under specific circumstances including Lp(a) and apoB.[5] The 2018 ACC/AHA and multi-society Guideline on the Management of Blood Cholesterol suggests routinely screening lipid profile every 4–6 years for the general population 40 years and older is a key component of primary CVD prevention. Screening for younger adults 20–39 years of age for the same frequency is reasonable.[5] Testing for elevated apoB and Lp(a) is not used in routine lipid profile-level testing but in advanced testing as secondary targets for refined treatment of genetic disorders of lipid metabolism and/or assessment of risk in patients with borderline/intermediate ASCVD risk groups.[5,28–30] ApoB testing gives the actual number of atherogenic lipoprotein particles instead of their lipid content and more accurately represents ASCVD risk. When cholesterol is within optimal target levels, an ApoB test can be a better predictor to determine if pure hypertriglyceridemia is the atherogenic condition. The optimal ApoB is <90 mg/dL.[5,24,25,28] Lp(a) is usually used as an independent genetic risk factor to predict and diagnose ASCVD risk when patients have family a history of premature CAD and/or familial hypercholesterolemia.[5,28] However, as evidence has evolved, testing Lp(a) has become more prominent in most guidelines around the world. ACC has an update in 2023 as expert analysis stating testing for Lp(a) once in a lifetime is recommended for most individuals with increased ASCVD risk, because an individual's Lp(a) level is 80–90% inherited, and its level remains stable, typically after age of 5 through an individual's lifetime regardless of lifestyle or sex, except in certain acute inflammatory states.[28,29,31] Lp(a) level exhibits racial differences in that Black people have significant higher Lp(a) levels than White or Asian people, about 1.6- to 2-fold higher.[31] The optimal Lp(a) is <30 mg/dL.[24,29,30] **Table 9.2** illustrates how lipid lab values are interpreted.[17,23–25,29]

CASE STUDY REVISITED

Six weeks after his initial visit, Carl returns to returns for an appointment with the RD at the lipid clinic. His data are as follows:

Anthropometric Data:

Weight: 100 kg
Height: 178 cm
BMI: 30 kg/m^2
Waist circumference: 109 cm

Biochemical Data:

Total cholesterol (TC) 280 (Desirable: <200 mg/dL)
Low-density lipoprotein cholesterol (LDL-C) 167 (Desirable: <100 mg/dL)
High-density lipoprotein cholesterol (HDL-C) 25 (Desirable: ≥40 mg/dL)
Triglycerides 180 (Desirable: <150 mg/dL)
Non-high-density lipoprotein cholesterol (non-HDL-C): 255 mg/dL (Desirable: <139 mg/dL)

Clinical Data:

Medications: furosemide (recently added), metoprolol
Vital Signs: Blood pressure 150/68 mm Hg, Temperature 98.6°F, Heart rate 89 beats/min
Nutrition-Focused Physical Exam: Well-nourished, android body type

Dietary Data:

24-Hour Diet Recall
Breakfast (6 am): 2 cups of coffee (2% milk and sugar added), 2 cups sweetened whole grain cereal with 2% milk
Lunch (12 pm): Large turkey and cheese sub, snack-sized potato chips, 12 ounces of soda, oatmeal cookie
Snack (3 pm): Apple slices with 4 tbsp peanut butter, cheese, and crackers
Dinner (8 pm): 6–9 ounces grilled salmon, 3 cups pasta primavera (olive oil and about 1 cup vegetables), 2 slices of garlic bread, large salad (lettuce, tomato, cucumber, olives, chickpeas, feta cheese, low-fat ranch dressing), 8 ounces of water
Snack (10 pm): 1½ cups low-fat frozen yogurt (sometimes the entire pint), fruit
Physical Activity: Remains sedentary

Questions

1. How does Carl's diet compare to his last visit?
2. Identify changes that Carl has made and how they relate to his anthropometric and laboratory data.
3. Assess Carl's PES statements from his initial visit. Identify if each statement remains an active issue or if the PES statement has been resolved. If the PES statement remains an active issue, has improvement in the issue been noted? If the issue has been resolved, write a new PES statement.

Table 9.2 Interpreting Lipid Laboratory Values

Total Cholesterol Level	Category
<200 mg/dL	Desirable
200–239 mg/dL	Borderline high
≥240 mg/dL	High
LDL Cholesterol Level	**Category**
<70 mg/dL	For patients with very high ASCVD risk* as secondary prevention
<100 mg/dL	Optimal
100–129 mg/dL	Near optimal/above optimal
130–159 mg/dL	Borderline high

(continues)

Table 9.2 Interpreting Lipid Laboratory Values *(continued)*

160–189 mg/dL	High
≥190 mg/dL	Very high
HDL Cholesterol Level	**Category**
<40 mg/dL for males <50 mg/dL for females	A major risk factor for CVD
40–59 mg/dL	Normal
≥60 mg/dL	Protective against CVD
Non-HDL Cholesterol Level	**Category**
<100 mg/dL	For patients with very high ASCVD risk* as secondary prevention
<120 mg/dL for <19 years of age <130 mg/dL for >20 years of age	Desirable
130–159 mg/dL	Above desirable
160–189 mg/dL	Borderline high
190–219 mg/dL	High
>220 mg/dL	Very high
Triglycerides	**Category**
<150 mg/dL	Normal
150–199 mg/dL	Borderline high
200–499 mg/dL	High
≥500 mg/dL	Very high
Advanced Lipid Testing	
ApoB	**Category**
<90 mg/dL	Optimal
90–119 mg/dL	Moderately high
>120 mg/dL	High
Lp(a)	**Category**
<30 mg/dL	Optimal
30–50 mg/dL	Moderately high
>50 mg/dL	High

*Very high ASCVD risk refers to an individual with 2 or more major ASCVD events (recent Acute Coronary Syndrome <12 months, a history of MI, history of ischemic stroke or symptomatic PAD; or 1 major ASCVD event and 2 or more high risk factors such as older age ≥65 years; FH; previous bypass surgery or percutaneous intervention; DM; HTN; CKD; smoking; and LDL-C ≥100 mg/dL despite maximal statin therapy and ezetimibe; or a history of HF.[26]

Data from Jacobson TA, Ito MK, Maki KC, et al. National Lipid Association recommendations for patient-centered management of dyslipidemia: part 1—full report. J Clin Lipidol. 2015;9(2):129-169. doi:10.1016/j.jacl.2015.02.003; Martin SS, Blaha MJ, Elshazly MB, et al. Comparison of a novel method vs the Friedewald equation for estimating low-density lipoprotein cholesterol levels from the standard lipid profile. *JAMA*. 2013;310(19):2061-2068. doi:10.1001/jama.2013.28053224; Jellinger PS, Handelsman Y, Rosenblit PD, et al. American Association of Clinical Endocrinologists and American College of Endocrinology guidelines for management of dyslipidemia and prevention of cardiovascular disease. *Endocr Pract*. 2017;23(Suppl 2):1-87. doi:10.4158/ep171764.Appgl25; Academy of Nutrition and Dietetics. Nutrition Care Manual. Cardiovascular disease: general guidance—nutritional indicators. Accessed July 13, 2024. https://www.nutritioncaremanual.org/topic.cfm?ncm_category_id=1&lv1=272984&lv2=35987&lv3=255518&ncm_toc_id=267296&ncm_heading=Nutrition%20Care; Alebna PL, Mehta A. An update on lipoprotein(a): the latest on testing, treatment, and guideline recommendations. *J Am Coll Cardiol*. 2023;September 13.

Nonmodifiable risk factors for dyslipidemia include genetics and increasing age.[5,13] One genetic disorder, **familial hypercholesterolemia (FH)**, is caused by defective LDL-C receptors leading to LDL-C levels greater than the 95th percentile for age and sex.[15,32] FH is diagnosed with a combination of LDL-C levels, family history of premature CAD, and **xanthomas** (subcutaneous yellow patches caused by deposits of excess lipid).[32] FH, if left untreated, can result in significant increased risk of CAD; 50% of men and 30% of women with untreated FH will have a coronary event before reaching 50 years of age for men and 60 years of age for women. Identifying and treating FH early can reduce CVD risk by approximately 80%.[32,33] Modifiable risk factors for dyslipidemia include tobacco smoking/secondhand smoke, diet choices (high saturated fat/trans fat, excess energy, inadequate fiber intake, and added sugar intake), overweight/obesity, physical inactivity, HTN, and DM.[4,5] Nonmodifiable risk factors for hypertriglyceridemia include genetic defects in reduced or absent lipoprotein lipase, which increases risk for pancreatitis. Modifiable risk factors for hypertriglyceridemia are similar to dyslipidemia, but some marked characteristics in diet choices include excess simple sugar intake, low-fat and high-refined carbohydrate diet, and excess alcohol consumption.[21] MNT for disorders of lipid metabolism addresses these modifiable risk factors.

CORE CONCEPT 4

Dyslipidemia refers to alterations in the normal transport of lipids and lipoproteins that contribute to major ASCVD risk. Modifiable risk factors for dyslipidemia include tobacco use/secondhand smoke, diet choices of high saturated fat/trans fat intake, excess energy, inadequate fiber intake, added sugar intake, overweight/obesity, physical inactivity, hypertension, and diabetes mellitus.

CORE CONCEPT 5

Hypertriglyceridemia refers to elevated fasting serum TG levels (>150 mg/dL) occurring within dyslipidemia or as an independent lipid metabolism disorder. Modifiable risk factors for hypertriglyceridemia are similar to dyslipidemia but have some marked characteristics in dietary choices including excess simple sugar intake, a low-fat and high-refined carbohydrate diet, and excess alcohol consumption.

Nutritional Management in Disorders of Lipid Metabolism

According to the 2018 AHA/ACC and multi-society Guideline on the Management of Blood Cholesterol and the 2019 ACC/AHA Guideline on the Primary Prevention of CVD suggested for cholesterol management and CVD prevention, much attention should be given to intensive lifestyle changes for reducing lifetime ASCVD risk in all ages, including tobacco cessation/avoidance of secondhand smoke, weight loss, diet modification, and physical activity.[4,5] Unfortunately, many Americans are falling short of dietary goals. Reported in the 2020–2025 Dietary Guidelines for Americans (DGAs), the National Health and Nutrition Examination Survey (NHANES) data show the average intake of fruit and vegetables, dairy, whole grains, seafoods, and plant-based protein (beans, peas, and lentils) were well underconsumed by most adults, while refined grains, added sugar, saturated fat, and sodium were overconsumed. About 60–65% of adults exceeded the limit for added sugar. More than 70% of adults exceed the recommendations for saturated fat. Nearly all men and about 80% of women consume too much sodium daily.[34] RDs are essential in making ASCVD prevention a reality by providing the knowledge and facilitating the behavior change necessary to make lasting lifestyle changes. Working with an RD providing MNT sessions over 6–12 weeks can lead to a decreased intake of energy (232–710 kcal/day), total fat (5–8%), and saturated fat (2–4%). These changes can result in a decrease in TC (7–21%), LDL-C (7–22%), and TG (11–31%). A greater improvement in cholesterol levels is demonstrated as more time is spent at MNT visits with an RD.[35]

PRACTICE POINT

Individuals with disorders of lipid metabolism should be referred to an RD for MNT as part of CVD prevention/comprehensive medical treatment.

Nutrition Assessment in Cardiovascular Disease

A nutrition assessment involves the collection of information related to the following categories: food/nutrition intake and related history; anthropometric measurements; biochemical data, medical tests, and procedures; nutrition-focused physical findings;

and client history. In the patient with dyslipidemia, it is important to acquire a complete recall of food/beverage intake and to identify choices high in saturated and trans fat, sodium, and added sugar. During the recall, additional information is collected regarding medication and herbal supplement use, food allergies/intolerances, knowledge/beliefs/attitudes toward nutrition and diet change, eating behaviors, frequency of eating out, access to food, and physical activity.[27] Anthropometric data includes height, weight, usual body weight (UBW), weight history, body mass index (BMI), waist circumference (WC), and waist-to-hip ratio (WHR). WC and WHR are essential to collect because BMI does not accurately predict CVD in adults older than 65 years of age. Elevated BMI, WC, and WHR increase the risk of CVD. In this population, biochemical data includes a standard lipid profile of TC, HDL-C, LDL-C, non-HDL-C, TG, blood pressure, and fasting glucose. Additional labs may include 25-OH vitamin D, hemoglobin A1c (HbA1c) in patients with known DM, thyroid function tests, liver function tests, a coagulation profile of prothrombin time and international normalized ratio (to assess arterial thrombosis risk), and other blood chemistries such as blood urea nitrogen, creatinine, sodium, and other electrolytes. Sometimes, Lp(a), ApoB, C-reactive protein (CRP), and insulin sensitivity measures are performed. The physical exam should include observation of fat distribution, muscle wasting, fluid retention, shortness of breath, presence of xanthomas, xanthelasma (refer to **Figure 9.7**), corneal arcus, palmar discolorations, and/or odor of cigarette smoke or alcohol. Finally, client history involves a review of age, sex, race/ethnicity, nutrition-related medical, family, and social history.[27,35] **Table 9.3** summarizes the information collected during the nutrition assessment for patients with disorders of lipid metabolism, HTN, and patients at risk for HF.[27,35,89,133]

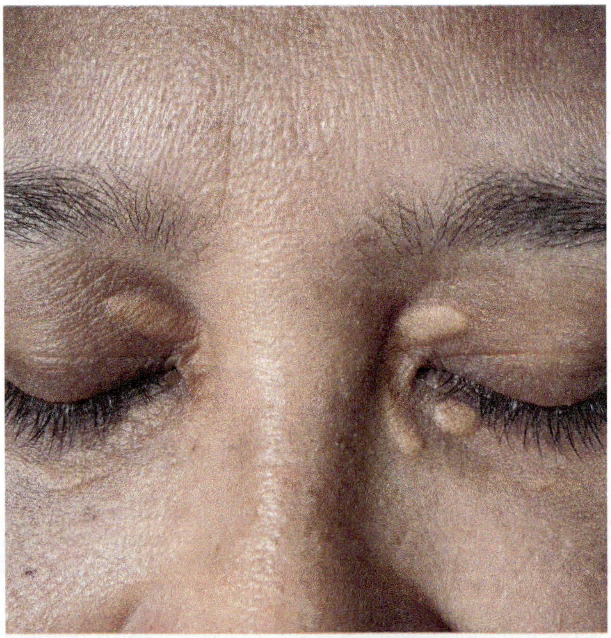

Figure 9.7 Xanthelasma—Yellow Deposits on the Eyelids

Medications in Disorders of Lipid Metabolism

Nutrition assessment involves a review of a patient's medication regimen. Statins are the preferred medication of choice for primary prevention and treatment of disorders of lipid metabolism by AHA/ACC and multi-society guidelines, and many patients are treated with statins alone.[4,5] Choices of alternative medication or add-on therapies for hypercholesterolemia include ezetimibe, bempedonic acid, and bile acid–binding resins. New agents of proprotein convertase subtilisin/kexin type 9 (PCSK9) inhibitors and a siRNA agent may be considered in combination with diet and a maximally tolerated statin therapy in adults with FH or for secondary prevention in patients with very high risk of new ASCVD events. Fibrates and omega-3 fatty acids may be used alone or in combination with statins for hypertriglyceridemia treatment.[5,36,37] Niacin was previously recommended for patients with hypercholesterolemia and hypertriglyceridemia is now not commonly recommended.

Statins interfere with the enzyme HMG-CoA reductase, which is the rate-limiting step in cholesterol synthesis. Low cholesterol production causes the liver to up-regulate hepatic LDL receptors, which remove cholesterol from the plasma. Statins also decrease CRP and have anti-inflammatory effects, thus stabilizing atherosclerotic plaque. They reduce LDL-C by 18–55%, TG by 7–30%, and increase HDL-C by 5%–15%.[16,36,37] Myalgia, or muscle pain, is a side effect of statins. Reducing the statin dose to a tolerated level or stopping statins may be indicated. Possible dietary supplementation with vitamin D if vitamin D deficiency is present and/or CoQ10 daily for possible myalgia symptom relief, but current evidence is limited and with mixed results.[38,39]

Ezetimibe, a cholesterol absorption inhibitor, is used as the most common non-statin agent. It inhibits cholesterol absorption at the small intestinal level, so that decreased cholesterol absorption from the gastrointestinal (GI) track reduces delivery of cholesterol to the liver eventually leading to decreased hepatic cholesterol storage and increased blood clearance of cholesterol. It reduces LDL-C by 18%, TG by 8%, and increases HDL-C by 1%.[5,16,36,37]

Table 9.3 Nutrition Assessment for Dyslipidemia and/or Hypertension

Nutrition Assessment Category	Data Collected
Food/nutrition intake and related history	■ Usual recall of food/beverage intake, including alcohol and smoking status ■ Food choices high in saturated fat, trans fat, sodium, and added sugar ■ Frequency of eating out/convenience foods ■ Medication and dietary supplement regimen ■ Knowledge/beliefs/attitudes toward nutrition; readiness to change ■ Nutrition education history ■ Food allergies/intolerances ■ Symptoms of nausea, vomiting, diarrhea, constipation ■ Eating behaviors ■ Access to food, ability to feed self, food environment including who food shops/cooks ■ Past and current physical activity
Anthropometric measurements	■ Height, weight ■ Weight history, UBW ■ BMI ■ WC ■ WHR
Biochemical data, medical tests, and procedures	■ TC ■ HDL-C ■ LDL-C ■ Non-HDL-C ■ Triglyceride ■ ApoB ■ Blood pressure ■ Lipoprotein(a) ■ Fasting glucose, HbA1c ■ Sodium and other electrolytes ■ BUN, creatinine ■ Liver function tests ■ 25-OH vitamin D ■ Thyroid function tests ■ C-reactive protein (CRP) ■ Glomerular filtration rate (GFR) ■ Prothrombin time (PT), international normalized ratio (INR)
Nutrition-focused physical findings	■ Fat distribution pattern ■ Fluid retention, shortness of breath ■ Xanthomas, xanthelasma, corneal arcus, palmar discoloration ■ Odor of cigarette smoke or alcohol
Client history	■ Age, sex, race/ethnicity ■ Medical history ■ Family history ■ Social history

Bempedoic acid, an ACL (adenosine triphosphate citrate lyase) inhibitor works by inhibiting APT citrate lyase, an enzyme upstream to HMG-CoA reductase in the cholesterol synthesis pathway in the liver and thus lowering LDL-C. It decreases LDL-C by 15–36%.[16,36,37]

Bile acid sequestrants are bile acid-binding resins that block the reabsorption of bile acids in the intestine, allowing removal of a large portion of bile acids, thus the liver subsequently produces more bile from cholesterol. An increase in cholesterol catabolism to bile acids leads to an increase in hepatic LDL-C receptors activity, which reduces cholesterol levels. They reduce LDL-C by 15–30%, may increase TG, and increase HDL-C by 3–5%. A side effect of this mechanism is the potential for decreased absorption of fat, fat-soluble vitamins, calcium, iron, zinc, magnesium, beta-carotene, and folate.[16,36,37]

PCSK9 inhibitors prevent LDL-C receptor degradation so that the number of LDL-C surface receptors increases, which can lead to a reduction in plasma cholesterol levels. Inclisiran, a siRNA agent, inhibits mRNA codes for PCSK9, and thus prevents LDL-C receptor breakdown and increases LDL-C uptake by more than 50% via hepatocytes. PCSK9 inhibitors and the siRNA agent are powerful LDL-C-lowering agents and generally well tolerated, but long-term safety remains unclear. Ezetimibe, PCSK9 inhibitors, and inclisiran are limited to patients on maximally tolerated statin therapy (with or without ezetimibe) with persistently elevated LDL-C (≥70 mg/dL) and with ASCVD, at high risk to very-high risk for ASCVD, and/or with FH.[5,36,37]

Fibrates and omega-3 fatty acids can be used in severe hypertriglyceridemia (TG ≥500 mg/dL). Fibrates enhance lipoprotein lipase activity to break down VLDL-C by increasing TG removal and thus can reduce LDL-C by 5–20%, reducing TGs by 20–50%, and increasing HDL-C by 10–20%. Fibrates should be used cautiously for those with kidney impairment as they may exacerbate renal insufficiency. Fibrates are contraindicated in patients with active liver disease or unexplained persistent liver function abnormalities. Addition of fibrates, specifically from gemfibrozil to statins, may raise risk of myalgia.[36,37]

Omega-3 fatty acids, derived from fish oil containing eicosapentaenoic acid (EPA) alone, or EPA and docosahexaenoic acid (DHA), also increase lipoprotein lipase activity and can decrease TGs by 30–40%. It is used as an adjunct to diet for the treatment of adults with severe hypertriglyceridemia, and it is used as an adjunct for adults with established CVD on maximally tolerated statin therapy with elevated TG ≥150 mg/dL. It is reasonable to be used in secondary prevention of CAD with hypertriglyceridemia, FH, and adverse outcomes in patients with HF.[5,36,40]

Niacin is currently not commonly used as a primary medication treatment for dyslipidemia. It is a class of water-soluble vitamin B-complex (vitamin B3) that might decrease cholesterol and TGs, because niacinamide, formed from niacin conversion, is needed for lipid metabolism, tissue respiration, and glycogenolysis. It has no effect on cholesterol synthesis.[37] However, niacin used in patients intolerant to statins in older studies had no evidence of benefit in dyslipidemia treatment for current-day patients, and it can increase all-cause mortality with no CVD advantage when used with statins.[41,42]

The 2018 AHA/ACC and multi-society blood cholesterol guideline recommends moderate-intensity statin therapy (daily dose lowers LDL-C by 30–50%) or high-intensity statin therapy (daily dose lowers LDL-C by 50%) for the following four groups: individuals with clinical ASCVD, severe hypercholesterolemia with LDL-C ≥190 mg/dL, ages 40–75 years with DM and LDL-C ≥70 mg/dL, and 40–75 years of age adults without DM and with LDL-C ≥70 mg/dL and a 7.5% or over for estimated 10-year ASCVD risk. The guideline focuses on the maximum of statin therapy rather than providing specific LDL-C and HDL-C targets.[5] Correcting disorders of lipid metabolism with statins can result in a 21% decrease in the rate of CAD progressing to HF. **Table 9.4** illustrates the nutrition implications of medications used for the treatment of elevated blood cholesterol.[5,16,36,43] The AHA/ACC and multi-society guideline does not include the use of plant stanols, sterol esters, stanols, red yeast Chinese rice supplements, or other herbs and dietary supplements for the treatment of disorders of lipid metabolism.[5] However, the 2022 ACC Expert Consensus Decision Pathway states that plant stanols and sterols and soluble fibers may be considered as dietary adjuncts for lowering LDL-C for patients with dyslipidemia.[44] If a patient reports the use of alternative therapies, the RD should ensure that the patient's physician and pharmacist are aware of these therapies and that the risks versus the potential benefits are addressed.

PRACTICE POINT

The gold standard for estimating energy needs in individuals with disorders of lipid metabolism is indirect calorimetry. When this method is not possible, predictive equations can be used.

Energy Needs in Disorders of Lipid Metabolism

Nutrition assessment includes a calculation of energy needs. The gold standard for estimating energy needs for individuals with dyslipidemia is indirect calorimetry. When this method is not possible, predictive equations (Mifflin–St Jeor, Harris–Benedict) can be used.[45]

Nutrition Intervention in Cardiovascular Disease

MNT for disorders of lipid metabolism focuses on the achievement of a healthy body weight and optimal lipid values with a combination of increased physical activity and a therapeutic dietary pattern that emphasizes a variety of fruits and vegetables, whole grains, lean protein, low-fat dairy, and heart-healthy fats, and limits intakes of sweets, sugar sweetened beverages, red meat, and alcohol in moderation. To achieve optimal lipid management, adults with or without CVD

Table 9.4 Cholesterol Medications and Nutrition Implications

Medication	Potential Side Effect	Nutrition Intervention
Statins (atorvastatin, rosuvastatin, simvastatin)	■ Nausea, abdominal pain, constipation, diarrhea, indigestion, gas ■ Medication metabolism is affected by grapefruit juice	■ Monitor gastrointestinal symptoms and provide diet recommendations for symptom relief; consider small, frequent meals ■ Encourage avoidance of grapefruit juice with lovastatin and simvastatin; avoidance of large quantities (≥50 mL to 1.2 L/day of grapefruit juice with atorvastatin)
	■ Myalgia[38,39]	■ Possible dietary supplementation with vitamin D if vitamin D deficiency presents and/or CoQ10 daily for possible symptom relief, current evidence is limited and with mixed results
ACL inhibitor (bempedoic acid)	■ Abdominal pain or discomfort	■ Monitor gastrointestinal symptoms and provide diet recommendations for symptom relief; consider small, frequent meals
Bile acid absorption inhibitors (cholestyramine; colestipol; colesevelam)	■ Anorexia, weight change, tongue irritation, nausea, vomiting, abdominal pain, constipation, diarrhea, indigestion, gas ■ May decrease absorption of fat-soluble vitamins (A, D, E, K), calcium, iron, zinc, magnesium, beta-carotene, and folate	■ Monitor weight and gastrointestinal symptoms and provide diet recommendations for symptom relief; consider small, frequent meals ■ Monitor levels of fat-soluble vitamins, calcium, iron, zinc, magnesium, and folate and replete as needed ■ Educate on food sources of nutrients that may need to be consumed in larger quantities and separate from medication to prevent deficiencies
Cholesterol absorption inhibitors (ezetimibe)	■ Diarrhea	■ Monitor for diarrhea and provide diet recommendations for symptom relief
Fibrates (fenofibrate; gemfibrozil)	■ Taste changes, nausea, vomiting, abdominal pain, constipation, diarrhea, indigestion, gas	■ Monitor gastrointestinal symptoms and provide diet recommendations for symptom relief; consider small, frequent meals
PCSK9 Inhibitors (alirocumab and evolocumab) and siRNA agent (inclisiran)	■ Neurocognitive effects of confusion, dementia, memory impairment	■ Monitor neurocognitive symptoms and weight and provide diet recommendations; modified consistency diets may be helpful for adults with difficulty chewing or swallowing
Omega-3 fatty acids derived from fish oils (icosapent ethyl [EPA only]; omega-3 acid ethyl esters [EPA and DHA])	■ Eructation (burping), indigestion, altered taste, constipation, gout	■ Monitor and provide diet recommendations for symptom relief; take the medications with food

Data from Grundy SM, Stone NJ, Bailey AL, et al. 2018 AHA/ACC/AACVPR/AAPA/ABC/ACPM/ADA/AGS/APhA/ASPC/NLA/PCNA guideline on the management of blood cholesterol: a report of the American College of Cardiology/American Heart Association Task Force on Clinical Practice Guidelines. *Circulation*. 2019;139(25):e1082-e1143. doi:10.1161/CIR.0000000000000625.; Mann DL, Zipes DP, Libby P, Bonow RO, Braunwald E, eds. *Braunwald's Heart Disease: A Textbook of Cardiovascular Medicine*. 10th ed. Philadelphia, PA: Elsevier Saunders; 2015.; Sisson E, Ingram J, Babalola R, Alhomoud I. Quick Guide to Medications. 12th ed. Chicago, IL: American Association of Diabetes Educators; 2022.; Pronsky ZM, ed. *Food Medication Interactions*. 18th ed. 2015.

should consider reducing dietary saturated fat intake, as it will likely reduce total cholesterol and atherogenic LDL-C, and possible CVD events.[5,46–48] The AND's Evidence Analysis Library (EAL) Saturated Fat Guideline 2021–2023 and the Nutrition Care Manual (NCM) General Guidance for Disorders of Lipids Metabolism 2017 recommend appropriate individualized dietary patterns by an RD, such as Dietary Approaches to Stop Hypertension (DASH), healthy U.S.-style, Mediterranean-style, and vegetarian/vegan diets with a goal of reducing saturated fat intake by reducing the total amount of saturated fat rather than reducing specific sources of saturated fat, and replacing saturated fat intake with polyunsaturated fat.[27,45] These goals confer with the CVD prevention clinical practice guidelines from the 2021 AHA Dietary Guidance to Improve Cardiovascular Health Scientific Statement, and the 2013 AHA/ACC/National Heart, Lung, and Blood Institute (NHLBI) Guideline on Lifestyle Management to Reduce Cardiovascular Risk. The AHA recommends a diet pattern with minimally processed foods that emphasizes vegetables, fruits, whole grains, healthy sources of protein (low-fat and fat-free dairy products, poultry, fish and seafood, legumes, nuts, and lean cuts of meat or poultry) and non-tropical vegetable oils, and limits intake of ultra-processed foods, sweets, sugar-sweetened beverages, red meats, and alcohol.[13,49]

The Mediterranean Diet

The Mediterranean diet can be moderate in calories and low in sodium, added sugar, and saturated fat that emphasizes mostly plant-based foods including minimally processed vegetables, fruits, whole grains, legumes, nuts, and seeds as excellent sources of fiber, unsaturated fat, lean protein, vitamins, minerals, and other nutrients. Although low in saturated fat, this diet is relatively rich in polyunsaturated fat. The recommended fat sources are olives and olive oil (especially extra virgin olive oil), avocado, nuts and seeds, seafood that is rich in omega-3 polyunsaturated fatty acids (PUFAs), while limiting red meats, high-fat dairy, and processed meats. Alcohol in moderation with meals/dinner is also a part of the Mediterranean diet and red wine is preferred; however, people who do not drink are not encouraged to start.[50–52] **Table 9.5** presents components of the Mediterranean diet.[34,52]

Table 9.5 The Mediterranean Diet

Food Group	Servings per Day					
	1600 Calories	2000 Calories	2600 Calories	Serving Sizes	Examples and Notes	Significance of Each Food Group to the Mediterranean Eating Plan
Grains	5	6	9	1 slice bread 1 oz dry cereal† ½ cup cooked rice, pasta, or cereal	Amaranth, barley, brown rice, buckwheat, corn teff, millet, oatmeal, quinoa, rye sorghum, whole wheat bread and rolls, whole wheat pasta	Major sources of energy and fiber; focus on whole grains
Vegetables	2	2 ½	3 ½	1 cup raw leafy vegetable ½ cup cut-up raw or cooked vegetable ½ cup vegetable juice	Broccoli, carrots, collards, corns green beans, green peas, potatoes, kale, lima beans, spinach, squash, sweet potatoes, tomatoes	Rich sources of potassium, magnesium, and fiber; focus on a variety of vegetables with different colors and low sodium
Fruits	2	2 ½	2 ½	1 medium fruit ¼ cup dried fruit ½ cup fresh, frozen, or canned fruit ½ cup fruit juice	Apples, apricots, bananas, dates, grapes, mangoes, melons, oranges, peaches, pineapples, raisins, strawberries, tangerines	Important sources of potassium, magnesium, and fiber; focus on a variety of whole fruits, canned fruits without sugar, dried fruits; limit fruit juice

Food Group	Servings per Day					
	1600 Calories	2000 Calories	2600 Calories	Serving Sizes	Examples and Notes	Significance of Each Food Group to the Mediterranean Eating Plan
Fat-free or low-fat milk and milk products, and dairy alternatives	2	2	2 ½	1 cup milk or yogurt 1½ oz cheese	Fat-free (skim) or low-fat (1%) milk or low added sugar yogurt, cheeses, fortified low added sugar soymilk or soy yogurt	Major sources of calcium and protein
Lean protein foods	5 ½	6 ½	7 ½	1 oz cooked fish, shrimp, clams, scallops, fatty fish of tuna, salmon, herring, sardines; 1 egg; 1 oz cooked lean red meat or lean poultry	Select seafood a few times per week, especially fatty fish: salmon, mackerel, anchovies, sardines, and herring; some eggs. Select only lean meats and poultry; trim away visible fat; broil, roast, or poach; remove skin from poultry	Rich sources of protein, omega-3-rich PUFA from fatty fish, and magnesium
Nuts, seeds, and legumes and plant protein-based meat alternatives	4 per week	5 per week	5 per week	⅓ cup or 1½ oz nuts 2 tbsp peanut butter 2 tbsp or ½ oz seeds ½ cup cooked legumes (dry beans and peas)	Select unsalted nuts and seeds. Almonds, hazelnuts, mixed nuts, peanuts, and peanut butter, walnuts, sunflower seeds, kidney beans, lentils, split peas, reduced-sodium veggie burgers/sausages	Rich sources of energy, magnesium protein, and fiber
Fats and oils[§]	~5	6	7.5	1 tsp soft margarine, 1 tsp vegetable oil, 1 tbsp low-fat mayonnaise, 2 tbsp low-fat, low-sodium salad dressing	Olives, avocado, unsaturated vegetable oils such as extra virgin olive oil, peanut oil, vegetable oil–based margarines and spreads	Major source of energy and PUFA. The Mediterranean diet has an average 30–35% of calories as fat and oils, including fat in or added to foods mainly from extra virgin olive oil, nuts and seeds, and seafoods
Limit calories for other use	120 kcal/day	240 kcal/day	300 kcal/day		Snacks and desserts contain sugar and/or saturated fat (ice cream, donuts, etc.); salt and seasoning blends contain salt, fried foods	Limits added sugar, refined starches, saturated fat, or sodium

[†] Serving sizes vary between ½ cup and 1¼ cups, depending on cereal type. Check the product's Nutrition Facts label.

[§] Fat content changes serving amounts for fats and oils. For example, 1 tbsp of regular salad dressing equals one serving; 1 tbsp of a low-fat dressing equals one-half serving; 1 tbsp of a fat-free dressing equals zero servings.

Abbreviations: oz, ounce; tbsp, tablespoon; tsp, teaspoon.

Data from U.S. Department of Agriculture and U.S. Department of Health and Human Services. *Dietary Guidelines for Americans 2020–2025*: Healthy Mediterranean-Style Dietary Pattern for Ages 2 and Older, With Daily or Weekly Amounts from Food Groups, Subgroups, and Components. Accessed January 12, 2026. https://www.dietaryguidelines.gov/sites/default/files/2020-12/Dietary_Guidelines_for_Americans_2020-2025.pdf (Table A3-5, p. 149); Academy of Nutrition and Dietetics. *Nutrition Care Manual*. Healthful Mediterranean nutrition therapy. 2022. Accessed January 12, 2026

The Spanish PREvencion con DIeta MEDiterranea (PREDIMED) multicenter randomized controlled trial is the largest study to evaluate the Mediterranean diet and its long-term effects on primary prevention of CVD without calorie restriction. Over 7,400 participants with high CVD risk were randomly enrolled in either a Mediterranean diet supplemented with extra virgin olive oil, a Mediterranean diet supplemented with mixed nuts, or a controlled diet aimed to reduce all dietary fat. The trial was stopped early at 4.8 years instead of the planned 6 years, as it showed significant relative risk reduction of CVD incidence of MI, stroke, or CVD death by approximately 30% in the Mediterranean diet groups compared to low-fat diet controls. Although, a few years later, the original results of PREDIMED trial were retracted and then republished due to deviations of study protocols related to the randomization process, the main finding of a Mediterranean diet and its risk reduction of major CVD incidence compared to a low-fat diet remained similar.[53–55] The EAL suggests that in the general population, the Mediterranean diet may be more effective to reduce TGs and LDL-C compared to other therapeutic diets. It may decrease blood pressure compared to a standard diet, but it may not be superior to other therapeutic diets. No studies were identified to evaluate blood sugar control or weight changes in the Mediterranean diet compared to other diets. For adults with CVD, there is no significant effect on blood lipids nor blood pressure for having a Mediterranean diet pattern compared to other therapeutic diets. In addition, no studies were identified to evaluate the Mediterranean diet's effect on blood sugar control nor weight in adults with CVD. The Mediterranean diet may reduce weight, LDL-C, and systolic blood pressure in individuals with overweight and obesity, and it may improve dyslipidemia and blood sugar control in patients with type 2 DM.[51] Thus, the Mediterranean diet may be more beneficial as a primary CVD prevention diet for patients with high CVD risk due to other comorbidities such as overweight and obesity or type 2 DM. For patients with CVD, choosing an individualized therapeutic diet that best suits them is reasonable.

In addition to recommended dietary patterns, AND and the NCM provide recommendations for macronutrient intake for individuals with disorders of lipid metabolism. They recommend 20–35% of calories from fat (<7% calories from saturated fat) and to achieve a target of 5–6% of energy from saturated fat, 15–20% of calories from protein, and 45–60% of calories from carbohydrate, with an emphasis on high-fiber choices.[27,35,47,56–58] Diet recommendations require consideration of estimated energy needs, personal and cultural food preferences, and medical history, social history, and psychological history. An RD is critical in individualizing these general guidelines and ensuring long-term diet compliance for best outcomes. Along with nutrition education, an RD can facilitate behavior change by using motivational interviewing, assessing patient's readiness for behavior change, addressing barriers to change, and allowing the patient to establish personal diet goals that are specific, measurable, achievable, realistic, and timely.

Reduction of Saturated/Trans Fat Intake

For patients with disorders of lipid metabolism, the EAL and NCM recommend <7% daily calories from saturated fat, with a goal of 5–6% of daily calories, while AHA/ACC recommends a slightly lower intake of 5–6% of daily calories from saturated fat. Of note, it is difficult for an individual to achieve a saturated fat intake <10% of total energy if one's intake of total fat is about 30–35% of total energy.[5,27,35,45,47,56,58] The current national average consumption is 11–12% of calories from saturated fat (239 calories/day), according to 2020–2025 DGA, with top three leading sources from other foods (20%), sandwiches (19%), and desserts and sweet snacks (11%).[34] Calories from trans fat is suggested to be as low as possible.[57–59] A diet low in saturated fat and trans fat that reduces LDL-C and non-HDL-C by 3–7% is considered an effective intervention.[57]

An RD can assist in education related to dietary intake of fat and facilitate lasting behavior change. Nutrition intervention involves the identification of food sources of the different types of fat. Saturated fat is a fully hydrogenated fatty acid that is solid at room temperature, originating mainly from animal sources, including high-fat meats, especially red meat, fried meat, full-fat dairy (whole milk, cream, cheese, yogurt), butter, lard, and beef tallow. Saturated fat also exists in some plant sources including tropical vegetable oils such as palm and palm kernel oil, coconut oil, and cocoa butter in food products.[58] Trans fat is a partially hydrogenated oil, which increases LDL-C levels and has been most strongly associated with adverse cardiovascular outcomes.[48] Trans fat sources include some fried and processed foods, stick margarine, traditional vegetable shortening, baked goods, processed sweets, and any food containing the ingredient "partially hydrogenated oil."[56] As of June 2018, the major source of artificial trans fat in the food market, partially hydrogenated oil, is no longer

Generally Recognized as Safe (GRAS) by the Food and Drug Administration (FDA) and is no longer added to foods.[34] Trans fat is also naturally found in small amounts in meat and dairy products due to the fermentation process in animals' rumens.[34,59] The nutrition facts label is mandated by the FDA to list quantity of both saturated fat and trans fat. Besides education on identifying food sources of saturated fat and trans fat, MNT also includes education related to interpreting nutrition facts labels to choose foods with zero grams of trans fat and less than 3 grams of saturated fat per serving.

Replacement of Saturated/Trans Fat with Other Unsaturated Fat or High-Fiber Carbohydrates

Besides reducing the amount of saturated fat intake, calories from saturated and trans fat should be replaced with PUFAs, mainly omega-3-rich PUFA, followed by monounsaturated fatty acids (MUFAs), and finally high-fiber carbohydrates for the largest benefit to lower blood lipids.[13,15,45,46,60] The World Health Organization and the Food and Agricultural Organization of United Nations have set the acceptable macronutrient distribution range (AMDR) for PUFAs up to 11% of total energy. AND suggests increasing PUFA intake by focusing on increasing omega-3-rich PUFA, aiming for at least 0.5–2% of total energy per day. Since there is no established AMDR for MUFA, the currently recommended MUFA consumption levels are calculated from total fat intake, subtracting the amount of saturated fat and recommended PUFA. AND suggests a moderate MUFA intake of 15–20% of energy intake, while keeping total fat within 20–35% of total energy.[56] These recommendations are justified by a systematic review of evidence from clinical trials. Randomized controlled trials (RCTs) have illustrated that a modified diet can result in a decrease of LDL-C by 11–13 mg/dL or 11% when a diet consisting of 5–6% saturated fat, 26–27% total fat, 15–18% protein, and 55–59% carbohydrate is compared to a diet consisting of 14–15% saturated fat, 34–38% total fat, 13–15% protein, and 48–51% carbohydrate.[13,15] Additional RCTs have demonstrated that a 1% decrease in calories from saturated fat correlates with a 1.2–1.8 mg/dL decrease in LDL-C. The largest decrease in LDL-C is seen when saturated fat is replaced with PUFAs. Replacing saturated fat with PUFAs also lowers TGs by about 0.4 mg/dL and HDL-C by about 0.2 mg/dL. Replacing saturated fat with PUFAs can lower CVD risk by about 10% if 5% total energy is substituted.[56] When MUFAs are used to replace saturated fat, TGs can increase by about 0.2 mg/dL and HDL-C can be lowered by about 1.2 mg/dL. If saturated fat is replaced with carbohydrate, TGs can increase by 1.9 mg/dL and HDL-C can be lowered by about 0.4 mg/dL. If 1% of calories from trans fat are replaced with MUFA or PUFA, LDL-C can be lowered by 1.5 and 2.0 mg/dL, respectively. Additionally, TGs can be lowered by about 1.2 and 1.3 mg/dL, and HDL-C can be increased by 0.4 and 0.5 mg/dL, respectively.[13] A meta-analysis of prospective cohort studies concluded that as little as a 2% increase in calories from trans fat correlates with a 23% increased risk of CHD.[61] Although previous guidelines have also encouraged a reduction in dietary cholesterol intake, the AHA/ACC review of current evidence concluded that there are insufficient findings to suggest that decreasing dietary cholesterol decreases LDL-C.[13] Currently consuming dietary cholesterol in moderation (<200 mg dietary cholesterol/day) and choosing a heart-healthy dietary pattern that is naturally low in dietary cholesterol is suggested.[57,58]

For patients to make diet changes, tasty and easy alternatives need to be provided. An RD can work with patients to develop a meal plan that emphasizes heart-healthy PUFAs and MUFAs.[46,56] Examples include fatty fish containing omega-3-rich PUFAs, olive and canola oil, nuts, seeds, and avocados. Instead of instructing patients to eliminate foods high in saturated and trans fat, ideas can be provided for substitutions; for example, replacing butter with olive oil, grilling salmon burgers instead of traditional burgers, and replacing sour cream with low-fat Greek yogurt. **Table 9.6** provides suggestions for adding unsaturated fats to the diet.[46,58] **Table 9.7** illustrates ways to decrease saturated fat intake.

Dietary and Supplementation of Omega-3 Fatty Acids

Omega-3 fatty acids and their derivatives of EPA and DHA, types of polyunsaturated fat, have been demonstrated to maintain cell membrane fluidity, reduce blood viscosity, clotting tendency, and promote the formation of anti-inflammatory mediators. Omega-3 fatty acids may modestly decrease atherosclerosis, blood pressure, left ventricular mass, and heart rate with an increase in stroke volume.[45,48,62-66] Two or more servings per week of

Table 9.6 Guidelines for Increasing Unsaturated Fat Intake

Easy Ways to Choose More Unsaturated Fats Each Day
■ Add slices (3 tbsp) of avocado to a sandwich ■ Order grilled or baked salmon when eating out ■ Make tuna salad using light tuna and light mayonnaise ■ Snack on trail mix made with 2–3 tbsp of nuts (almonds, walnuts, peanuts), 2 tbsp dried fruit, and ½ cup whole grain cereal ■ Spread an apple half with 1–2 tbsp of peanut butter, or have a handful of almonds with a piece of fruit for a quick snack ■ Add 2 tbsp of crushed walnuts or almond slivers to yogurt or cereal ■ Try 1 tbsp olive oil and vinegar as a topping on sandwiches and salads ■ Sprinkle 2 tbsp of sunflower or pumpkin seeds onto salads or cooked veggies ■ Add 1 tbsp of flaxseed to oatmeal or hot cereal ■ Try 1–2 tbsp of almond butter on wheat crackers as a snack

Table 9.7 Guidelines for Decreasing Saturated Fat Intake

Low Saturated Fat *Choose MORE Often*	High Saturated Fat *Choose LESS Often*
■ Low-fat or skim milk	■ Whole milk, cream, half & half
■ Low-fat yogurt, low-fat Greek yogurt	■ Whole milk yogurt
■ Cheese made with Low-fat or skim milk	■ Whole milk cheese
■ Low-fat sour cream	■ Sour cream
■ Lean animal meats (loin, leg, round, extra lean hamburger, venison)	■ High-fat animal meats (ribs, T-bone steak, regular hamburger meat, bacon, sausage, pepperoni, salami, hot dogs)
■ Light meat poultry without skin	■ Dark meat poultry with skin
■ Grilled, baked, broiled, steamed, braised, boiled, roasted foods	■ Fried foods
■ Olive, canola oil	■ Palm, palm kernel oil
■ Heart-healthy spread	■ Stick butter

fatty fish is associated with 30–45% reduced risk of death from cardiac events in the general population.[35] The EAL recommendation for dietary omega-3 fatty acid intake for ASCVD prevention is two 4-ounce servings of fatty fish weekly, which provides a daily dose of 250–500 mg of EPA and DHA. In patients with ASCVD, the recommendation increases to two or more 4-ounce servings of fatty fish per week.[35,64,67,68] It is important to note that there is a risk of exposure to mercury, polychlorinated biphenyls, and other contaminants from some types of seafood. The AHA states that if fish is consumed within the guidelines set by the FDA and Environmental Protection Agency (EPA), the benefits of eating fish outweigh the risks for middle-aged and older men and postmenopausal women. High-risk populations (pregnant women, children) are advised to avoid fish high in mercury and choose up to 12 ounces per week of fish lower in mercury. There are online resources available from the AHA, FDA, and EPA to classify fish that are high in omega-3 fatty acids and low in mercury, such as salmon, haddock, and sardines.[69]

Supplementation of omega-3 fatty acids primarily from fish oil has provided mixed results,[48] but a dose of 1 gram/day EPA + DHA from fish or fish-oil supplements has been shown to decrease risk of death from cardiac events in patients with CVD.[68] Supplementing with 2 grams/day EPA + DHA may be beneficial for patients with HF to improve quality of life and reduce signs and symptoms of HF if taken for one year. However, omega-3 fatty acids may increase the effects of blood thinning agents such as warfarin, aspirin, clopidogrel, and vitamin E. The appropriateness of the dosage and duration of omega-3 fatty acids for patients with HF is unclear.[70] A dose of supplemental 2–4 grams/day EPA+DHA may be beneficial to reduce serum TG levels.[67] If unable to meet recommendations from dietary sources and no contraindications exist, supplementation of 850 mg/day EPA+DHA may be warranted (1 gram fish oil supplement provides 200–800 mg EPA+DHA).[67,68] Fish oil supplementation is contraindicated in patients with angina or chest pain, and implantable cardioverter defibrillators (ICDs). Studies have presented increased cardiac mortality and sudden death rates in patients with angina taking 3 grams/day fish oil supplementation as well as an increased incidence of arrhythmia in patients with ICDs taking 1.8 grams/day fish oil supplementation.[67,71,72] The potential adverse effects of fish oil supplementation are a reason to recommend food sources before supplements.

Fiber

The NCM fiber recommendations are 21–25 grams for women, and 25–38 grams daily for men, including 7–13 grams of soluble fiber.[47] According to the 2020–2025 DGA, more than 90% of women and 97% of men in the general population do not meet recommended intakes for dietary fiber.[34] Meeting fiber goals, in addition to other guidelines discussed previously, can further reduce total cholesterol by 2–3% and LDL-C by up to 7%.[35] A meta-analysis of 10 prospective cohort studies found that an increase of 10 grams/day of fiber was associated with a 12% decrease in cardiac events and a 30% decrease in cardiac deaths.[62] A study including 68 men and women found that an intake of 30 grams/day fiber with 13 grams/day soluble fiber resulted in decreased total cholesterol and LDL/HDL ratio.[41] A study of 36 men who were overweight and whose increased fiber intake to 30 grams/day illustrated a 17% decrease in small LDL-C, 6.2% decrease in LDL-C, and 5% decrease in LDL/HDL ratio.[41] When providing MNT for disorders of lipid metabolism, an RD can identify and encourage consumption of fiber-rich foods such as whole grains, fruits, vegetables, nuts and seeds, and beans and advise patients to drink plenty of water or fluid daily (about 9 to 12 cups of fluid if no contraindication) to help with GI symptoms when increasing fiber intake.[73]

Nuts and Seeds

Nuts and seeds can be recommended as a source of unsaturated fat that may help to improve disorders of lipid metabolism when used to replace saturated and trans fats and consumed in small portions, as they have greater caloric density. Nuts and seeds can also be a source of omega-3 fatty acids for patients consuming a vegetarian/vegan diet. The EAL states that there is fair evidence to suggest that the consumption of 5 ounces of nuts per week is associated with reduced risk of MI based on results from the Nurses' Health Study.[13] Nuts and seeds high in omega-3 fatty acids include walnuts and walnut oil, ground flaxseed and flax oil, pumpkin seeds, and chia seeds.[35,67]

Plant Stanols and Sterols

Plant stanols and sterols (about 2–3 grams/day) have been considered for individuals with disorders of lipid metabolism by the NCM because they compete with cholesterol for absorption in the small intestine. Intake levels that may result in reduced TGs and LDL-C are 0.8–3 grams/day. The average intake from natural sources of plant stanols and sterols from nuts, vegetable oils, fruits, and vegetables is only 0.2 grams/day. Fortified spreads contain 0.5–1.7 grams/tbsp.[47,62,74] Phytosterolemia (also known as "sitosterolemia") is a rare autosomal recessively inherited lipid metabolic disorder of elevated serum and tissue sterol levels due to increased intestinal absorption and decreased biliary excretion of plant sterols. Individuals with this condition should avoid foods fortified with stanols and sterols. Taking a dose beyond 3 grams/day does not provide additional CVD protective benefit.[47]

Added Sugar

Added sugar can contribute to weight gain, which is a risk factor for dyslipidemia and hypertriglyceridemia. The 2020–2025 DGAs suggest about 60% of men and 65% of women consume more than 10% of daily calories as added sugar, which is the recommended limit.[34] Average daily intake of added sugar is approximately 330 kcal for men and 250 kcal for women. Top sources of added sugar are in the forms of sugar-sweetened beverages (40%) including sweetened coffee and/or tea; desserts and sweet snacks, candies, and sweetened breakfast cereals (30%); and other foods (30%).[34] The AHA recommends reducing added sugar to no more than 6% of total calories per day, which is about 100 calories/day (6 teaspoons of sugar) for women and 150 calories/day (9 teaspoons of sugar) for men.[75] MNT for disorders of lipid metabolism includes the identification and reduction of sugars and syrups that are added to foods during processing, preparation, or at the table, and using alternatives such as whole fruits.

Physical Activity

As a part of MNT for disorders of lipid metabolism, the EAL recommends at least 2 days/week of resistance exercise and moderate intensity physical activity for at least 30 minutes on most days of the week.[35,47] The 2018 AHA/ACC and multi-society blood cholesterol guidelines recommend that aerobic physical activity of three to four times per week for an average of 40 minutes at moderate-to-vigorous intensity can reduce LDL-C by 3–6 mg/dL.[3,5] However, only slightly over 24% of American adults are meeting the aerobic physical activity guidelines and participating in strength training ≥2 days/week.[3]

PRACTICE POINT

Physical activity on most days of the week is recommended as part of MNT for CVD prevention and comprehensive medical treatment.

Vitamin and Mineral Supplements

The EAL states that vitamin E, vitamin C, and/or beta-carotene supplements should not be recommended as there is no evidence of CVD benefit and there is the potential for harm.[35] The Journal of the American College of Cardiology reports that folic acid and vitamin B complex have moderate quality for stroke prevention; no CVD preventive effect was found for multivitamins, vitamin D, calcium, and vitamin C. An increased risk for all-cause mortality of 10% was found for niacin combined with a statin.[41,42]

Medium Chain Triglyceride Supplements

Medium-chain triglyceride (MCT) oil supplements are a primary supplement containing increased saturated fat content that is marketed for weight loss. MCT oil contains mainly medium-chain fatty acids that are metabolized differently than long-chain fatty acids including saturated fat, PUFA, and MUFA. MCT is absorbed directly through the portal system instead of undergoing beta-oxidation through the lymphatic system like long-chain fatty acids, so it is less likely to reform TGs and be stored as fat in adipose tissue. MCT oil is only approved for medical use in patients with fat malabsorption who cannot metabolize long-chain fatty acids properly. Additionally, natural MCT oil contains high saturated fat, mainly from coconut oil, palm oil, and milk fat and current research lacks evidence on the effects of MCT oil on LDL-C and total cholesterol levels. Safety and toxicity dosages are also not established,[56,76] so MCT oil is not recommended for patients with CVD.

Alcohol

In moderation, alcohol consumption may be a part of a healthy dietary pattern. The EAL guidelines define moderation as one drink per day for women and two drinks per day for men.[47,58] Individuals who do not currently consume alcohol should not be encouraged to start.[47,58] Alcohol should be limited or eliminated for patients with hypertriglyceridemia.[77]

Smoking Cessation

Smoking cessation and avoidance of secondhand smoke is an important element of CVD prevention and treatment.[5] During MNT, an RD can refer a patient to the appropriate smoking cessation programs, and/or direct the patient to have further smoking cessation discussion and treatment with their primary care physician.

Nutrition Interventions for Hypertriglyceridemia

For patients with hypertriglyceridemia, nutrition intervention is similar to disorders of lipid metabolism as addressed above for management of blood lipids targeting LDL-C and non-HDL-C lowering. In addition, the NCM suggests avoiding high fat and carbohydrate (especially refined carbohydrate) intake, reducing serum glucose to <100 mg/dL for those with elevated glucose, and maintaining a healthy weight. For patients with severe hypertriglyceridemia, the NCM recommends a very low-fat diet pattern of <15% of energy from fat and elimination of alcohol to prevent pancreatitis.[21,77]

PRACTICE POINT

As part of MNT for disorders of lipid metabolism, recommendations for lowering LDL-C and non-HDL-C include a reduction of calories from saturated and trans fat, and an individualized dietary pattern that emphasizes vegetables, fruits, whole grains, low-fat dairy, lean protein, preferably plant protein, and unsaturated fat. As part of MNT for hypertriglyceridemia, lowering blood glucose is also important if fasting blood glucose and/or HbA1c are above normal range.

Nutrition Monitoring and Evaluation in Cardiovascular Disease

The monitoring and evaluation portion of MNT for disorders of lipid metabolism involves a review of the nutrition assessment categories: food/nutrition intake and related history; anthropometric measurements; biochemical data, medical tests, and procedures; nutrition-focused physical findings; and client history.[27] Refer to Table 9.3 for data to monitor patient progress toward established goals and outcomes.

Hypertension Clinical Course

Hypertension (HTN) is chronic elevated arterial BP. It is the leading risk factor for CVD, and suboptimal BP control is the most common attributor. About 1.28 billion adults aged 30–79 years old have HTN worldwide.[78] The prevalence of HTN in the United States is over 45% of all adults ≥20 years old, which is equivalent to 122.4 million adults.[3] The prevalence of high BP is higher in men than women (50.4% in men vs. 43.0% in women), increasing with advancing age (28.5% in men 20–44 years of age vs. 76.5% in men 75 and above years of age), and is higher in Black people than in White people, Hispanic people, and Asians (57.5% and 58.4% vs. 48.9% and 42.6% vs. 50.3% and 35.3% vs. 50.2% and 37.6%, respectively, in men and women).[3] HTN is associated with increased risk for CVD events of CAD, coronary revascularization, stroke, or HF by 25%, and it attributes to 34% incidents of end stage kidney disease.[3] HTN causes over 124,000 deaths in the United States annually.[3] HTN is estimated to cost over $50 billion per year for healthcare cost.[3] **Primary (essential) HTN** refers to high BP that is not the result of another disease; it originates from both genetic and environmental factors. Primary HTN accounts for ≥90% of HTN cases.[79,80] HTN has been referred to as a silent killer because there are usually no symptoms associated with high BP. Data show that 38% of adults in the United States are not aware that they have HTN.[3] The outcomes can be severe, including stroke, MI, HF, PAD, kidney failure, and death. HTN causes vascular stress, which creates an environment for atherosclerosis and thrombosis.[79] Chronic elevated BP results in myocyte hypertrophy, myocardial scarring, and loss of myocardial contractile tissue in the incidence of MI. These conditions promote the development of HF by an average of slightly over 14 years.[80] HTN is present in >80% of patients in HF. The incidence of HF increases to 1.6 times in those with systolic BP in the 120–139 mm Hg range, to 2.2 times in those with systolic BP of 140–150 mm Hg, and to 2.6 times in those with systolic blood BP ≥160 mm Hg.[3]

HTN is a condition in which the force of blood pushing against arterial walls is increased. **Systolic blood pressure** is the force caused when the heart is actively pumping blood. **Diastolic blood pressure** is the force when the heart is at rest. A BP reading lists systolic over diastolic BP. Normal BP is defined as BP less than 120/80 mm Hg.[9] The 2017 ACC/AHA and multi-society Guideline for the Prevention, Detection, Evaluation, and Management of High Blood Pressure in Adults has an updated categorization for BP ranges, and the definition of hypertension is tightened to 130/80 mm Hg and higher.[81] Previously, the hypertension threshold was at 140/90 mm Hg from the Seventh Report of the Joint National Committee on Prevention, Detection, Evaluation, and Treatment of High Blood Pressure (JNC 7 report) published in 2003.[82] This update is based on observational studies for the association between both systolic and diastolic BP and CVD risk, RCTs of lifestyle changes for BP reduction, and RCTs of antihypertensive

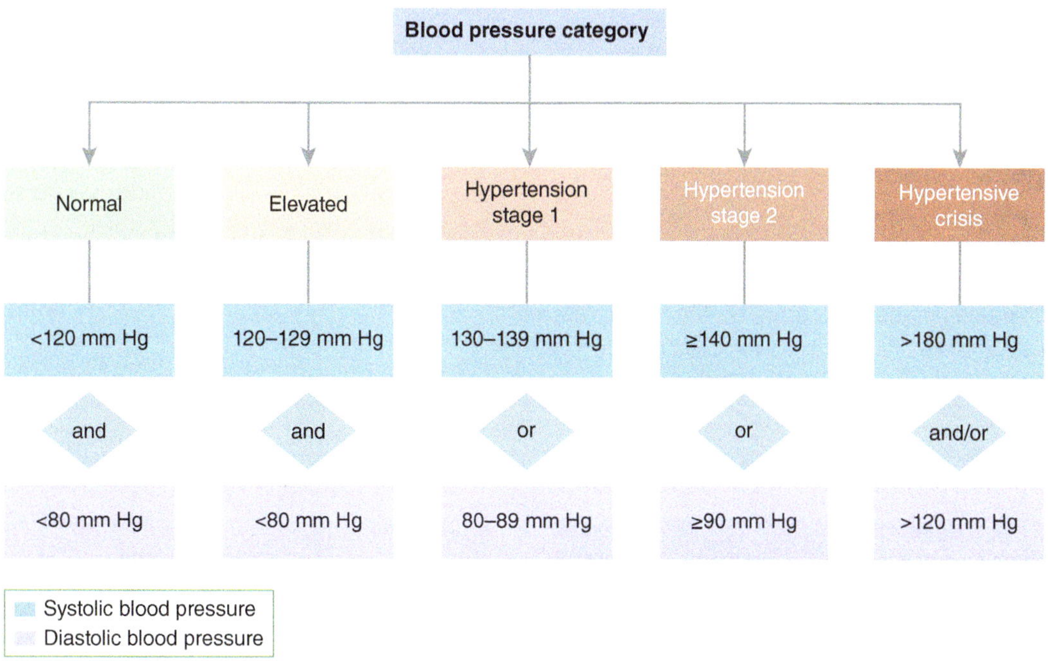

Figure 9.8 Categories of Blood Pressure in Adults

CASE STUDY REVISITED

One year later, Carl is now 56 years old. He returns for another follow-up visit with his RD. He reports a lot of stress at work and an inability to maintain his nutrition goals as previously established. Over the past year he had bouts of chest pain and angina. A cardiac catheterization was performed, showing 90% occlusion in his left anterior descending coronary artery. An angioplasty was performed at the time of the exam. In addition to his other medications, his doctor added atorvastatin. Carl believes that dietary modification is no longer necessary because he is now on these medications.

Questions

1. How would you explain to Carl the importance of lifestyle change in combination with pharmacotherapy for dyslipidemia and HTN?
2. Describe how MNT can be tailored for Carl to address both dyslipidemia and HTN.
3. Write 1 PES statement for Carl identifying Carl's active nutrition issue(s).

An elevated body mass index categorized as overweight or obese increases cardiovascular morbidity and mortality risk.

medication treatment for CVD prevention. Refer to **Figure 9.8** for detailed categories of BP in adults. HTN should be diagnosed by the average of at least two careful readings obtained on at least two occasions as >130/80 mm Hg or at a single occasion as ≥180/110 mm Hg. BP should be properly measured after a 5-minute rest, in a seated position with feet on the floor uncrossed, and arm supported at heart level.[81]

Conditions that may promote elevated BP include sympathetic nervous system hyperactivity, abnormal cardiovascular or kidney development, renin–angiotensin system activity, defect in natriuresis (which usually brings blood pressure back to normal after high salt intake), and increased intracellular sodium and calcium. Obesity may lead to HTN by causing increased intravascular volume, elevated cardiac output, and activation of the renin–angiotensin system.[23,79] Risk factors for HTN include relatively fixed risk factors of family history of HTN, male sex, increased age, low socioeconomic/educational status, obstructive sleep apnea, chronic CKD, and psychosocial stress; and modifiable risk factors of overweight/obesity, dyslipidemia, DM, suboptimal diet including high salt intake, excessive alcohol intake, physical inactivity, smoking, and secondhand smoking.[4,81]

Nutritional Management in Hypertension

Studies have indicated that counseling patients to reduce sodium intake by about 1150 mg/day results in lowering BP by 3–4 mm Hg systolic and 1–2 mm Hg diastolic.[13] Both ACC/AHA and NCM/EAL suggest that a healthful diet with sodium reduction, possible potassium supplementation preferably through diet if no contraindication, limiting alcohol intake, weight control, and regular exercise with appropriate intensity are fundamental lifestyle approaches to prevent HTN in individuals at high risk for developing BP-related CVD, improve BP control, and reduce the need for antihypertensive medication in individuals with HTN. The NCM also suggests limiting unhealthy fat intake as part of lifestyle interventions of HTN.[81,83–86] MNT for HTN involves educating patients on reduced-sodium intake and the DASH (Dietary Approaches to Stop Hypertension) dietary pattern, and motivational interviewing to facilitate behavior change. A patient's readiness to change and personal motivators drive MNT sessions. The EAL indicates a strong body of evidence showing that MNT for HTN provided every other week for at least three sessions in the first 3 months can achieve reductions in systolic BP up to 10 mm Hg and in diastolic BP up to 6 mm Hg.[84–85]

CORE CONCEPT 6

Nutrition intervention for hypertension includes sodium restriction which lowers blood pressure in a dose-response manner.

PRACTICE POINT

Individuals with HTN should be referred to an RD for MNT as part of CVD prevention and nonpharmacological management.

Nutrition Assessment in Hypertension

The nutrition assessment categories for individuals with HTN are the same as those described for dyslipidemia.[25,83] Table 9.3 identifies data collected during the assessment of patients with disorders of lipid metabolism, dyslipidemia, HTN, and patients at risk for HF.

Medications in Hypertension

According to the 2017 ACC/AHA and multi-society HTN guideline, adults with an estimated 10-year ASCVD risk <10%, and an elevated BP or stage 1 HTN should be managed with lifestyle modification and have a repeat BP measured within 3–6 months after initiating behavior change. Adults with an estimated 10-year ASCVD risk ≥10% and stage 1 or 2 HTN should be managed with a combination of lifestyle modifications and antihypertensive medication therapy, and after initiating both therapies, have a repeat BP measured 1 month later. For adults with a normal BP, repeating a BP measurement annually is reasonable. Patients with HTN crisis should be monitored closely and assessed for organ damage. The goal of HTN management is to reach an average BP of <130/80 mm Hg for most patients.[81]

A detailed assessment of the patient's medication regimen is useful to address the many food/nutrient–medication interactions associated with antihypertensive medications. The 2017 ACC/AHA and multi-society HTN guideline maintained the same suggestions for initiating antihypertensive medication as the 2014 Evidence-Based Guideline for the Management of High Blood Pressure in Adults from the Eighth Joint National Committee. It recommends the use of a thiazide-type diuretic, calcium channel blocker (CCB), angiotensin-converting enzyme inhibitor (ACEI), or angiotensin receptor blocker (ARB) as initial antihypertensive treatment. In the general Black population without HF or CKD, initial therapy should be with a thiazide-type diuretic or CCB.[36,81,87] Secondary agents can be added including loop diuretics, potassium-sparing diuretics, aldosterone antagonist diuretics, beta blockers, direct renin inhibitors, alpha-1 blockers, central alpha-agonist and other centrally acting drugs, and direct vasodilators. When initiating antihypertensive medication therapy, many patients are started on one agent, but for patients with stage 2 HTN, two drugs from different classes may be initiated. Many patients that start on one agent will eventually need two or more medications from different classes for optimal BP control.[81] **Table 9.8** provides

Table 9.8 Antihypertensive Medication Classes and Nutrition Implications

Medication	Potential Side Effect	Nutrition Intervention
Primary Agents		
Thiazide-type diuretics ▪ Decrease excess fluid volume ▪ e.g., hydochlorothiazide	▪ K+, Mg+ depletion ▪ Elevated blood glucose (BG) ▪ Elevated lipids	▪ Monitor and replete K+ and Mg+; educate on food sources of each ▪ Maintain BG within normal limits; educate on BG control ▪ Monitor lipids; provide MNT for dyslipidemia
Calcium channel blockers (CCBs) ▪ Block calcium channels in the heart to decrease heart rate and contractility or block peripheral calcium channels to cause vasodilation ▪ e.g., diltiazem, verapamil, amlodipine, nifedipine	▪ Metabolism is affected by grapefruit juice	▪ Encourage limited grapefruit juice consumption
Angiotensin-converting enzyme inhibitors (ACEIs) ▪ Block conversion of angiotensin I to angiotensin II to decrease vasoconstriction ▪ e.g., lisinopril, fosinopril	▪ Hyperkalemia ▪ Nausea, vomiting, abdominal pain	▪ Educate on <2000 mg/day K+; provide a list of foods containing K+; monitor serum K+ ▪ Educate on small frequent meals as tolerated; monitor adequacy of oral intake

(continues)

Table 9.8 Antihypertensive Medication Classes and Nutrition Implications (continued)

Medication	Potential Side Effect	Nutrition Intervention
Angiotensin receptor blockers (ARBs) ■ Block angiotensin II receptors to decrease vasoconstriction ■ e.g., valsartan, losartan	■ Hyperkalemia ■ Zinc deficiency	■ Educate on <2000 mg/day K+; provide list of foods containing K+; monitor serum K+ ■ Monitor and replete zinc; educate on food sources of zinc
Secondary Agents		
Loop diuretics ■ Decrease excess fluid volume ■ e.g., furosemide	■ K+, Mg++, Ca++ depletion ■ Elevated BG ■ Anorexia, nausea, vomiting	■ Monitor and replete K+, Mg++, Ca++; educate on food sources of each ■ Maintain BG within normal limits; educate on BG control ■ Educate on small frequent meals as tolerated; monitor adequacy of oral intake
Potassium-sparing diuretics ■ Decrease excess fluid volume ■ e.g., spironolactone	■ Hyperkalemia	■ Educate on <2000 mg/day K+; provide list of foods containing K+; monitor serum K+
Beta-blockers ■ Decrease heart rate and cardiac output ■ e.g., metoprolol, carvedilol, atenolol	■ Hyperkalemia	■ Educate on <2000 mg/day K+; provide a list of foods containing K+; monitor serum K+

Data from Sisson E, Ingram J, Babalola R, Alhomoud I. Quick Guide to Medications. 12th ed. Chicago, IL: American Association of Diabetes Educators; 2022.; Pronsky ZM, Ayoob K, eds. Food Medication Interactions. 18th ed. 2015.; Dunn SP, Bleske B, Dorsch M, Macaulay T, Van Tassell B, Vardeny O. Nutrition and heart failure: impact of drug therapies and management strategies. *Nutr Clin Pract.* 2009;24(1):60-75.; Charney P. *Academy of Nutrition and Dietetics Pocket Guide to Nutrition Assessment.* 4th ed. Chicago, IL: Academy of Nutrition & Dietetics; 2022.

an overview of common antihypertensive medications and their nutrition implications.[36,43,63,88]

Energy Needs in Hypertension

Similar to disorders of lipid metabolism, MNT for HTN involves assessing energy needs using indirect calorimetry or predictive equations (Mifflin–St Jeor, Harris–Benedict).[83]

Nutrition Intervention in Hypertension

The dietary pattern recommended by the 2017 ACC/AHA and multi-society guideline for HTN in adults for BP lowering is a combination of the DASH diet, reduced-sodium intake, with possible potassium supplementation preferably through diet, if no contradiction of CKD or on potassium sparing medications, and limited alcohol consumption.[81] The DASH diet is also recommended by the NCM as an essential part of MNT for HTN, and by the 2020–2025 DGA as an optimal dietary pattern for healthy Americans.[34,86] Individually, both the DASH diet and reduced-sodium intake have the potential to lower BP; the benefit is maximized with a combination of both the DASH diet with a low sodium intake of <1500 mg sodium/day.[13,49,86,89]

DASH Diet and Sodium Reduction

The DASH diet developed by NHLBI in the 1990s emphasizes whole grains, fruits, vegetables, low-fat dairy, nuts, fish, lean meats, and unsaturated fats. It is naturally high in calcium, fiber, potassium, and magnesium, and low in total fat, saturated fat, cholesterol, and sodium (<2300 mg/day). **Table 9.9** illustrates the components of the DASH diet.[90-92] An RCT of 412 individuals found that when comparing a high-sodium (8700 mg sodium/day) control diet to a low-sodium DASH diet (2900 mg sodium/day), the reduction in systolic BP was 7.1 mm Hg in those without HTN and 11.5 mm Hg in those with HTN.[91] Another RCT of 144 patients with overweight or obesity with high BP achieved the following reductions in BP: 16.1/9.9 mm Hg with the DASH diet and weight management; 11.2/7.5 mm Hg with the DASH diet alone; and 3.4/3.8 mm Hg with a control diet. The DASH diet plus weight management group also benefited from reduced left ventricular mass, which is a factor that may increase HF, cardiac arrest, or stroke risk.[93]

Table 9.9 The Dietary Approaches to Stop Hypertension (DASH) Diet

	Servings per Day					
	1600 Calories	**2000 Calories**	**2600 Calories**	**Serving Sizes**	**Examples and Notes**	**Significance of Each Food Group to the DASH Eating Plan**
Grains*	6	6–8	10–11	1 slice bread 1 oz dry cereal[†] ½ cup cooked rice, pasta, or cereal	Whole wheat bread and rolls, whole wheat pasta, English muffin, pita bread, bagel, cereals, grits, oatmeal, brown rice, unsalted pretzels and popcorn	Major sources of energy and fiber
Vegetables	3–4	4–5	5–6	1 cup raw leafy vegetable ½ cup cut-up raw or cooked vegetable ½ cup vegetable juice	Broccoli, carrots, collards, green beans, green peas, kale, lima beans, potatoes, spinach, squash, sweet potatoes, tomatoes	Rich sources of potassium, magnesium, and fiber
Fruits	4	4–5	5–6	1 medium fruit ¼ cup dried fruit ½ cup fresh, frozen, or canned fruit ½ cup fruit juice	Apples, apricots, bananas, dates, grapes, oranges, mangoes, melons, peaches, pineapples, raisins, strawberries, tangerines	Important sources of potassium, magnesium, and fiber
Fat-free or low-fat milk and milk products	2–3	2–3	3	1 cup milk or yogurt 1½ oz cheese	Fat-free (skim) or low-fat (1%) milk or buttermilk; fat-free, low-fat, or reduced-fat cheese; fat-free or low-fat regular or frozen yogurt	Major sources of calcium and protein
Lean meats, poultry, and fish	3–6	6 or less	6	1 oz cooked meats, poultry, or fish 1 egg	Select only lean meats; trim away visible fat; broil, roast, or poach; remove skin from poultry	Rich sources of protein and magnesium
Nuts, seeds, and legumes	3 per week	4–5 per week	1 daily	⅓ cup or 1½ oz nuts 2 tbsp peanut butter 2 tbsp or ½ oz seeds ½ cup cooked legumes (dry beans and peas)	Almonds, hazelnuts, mixed nuts, peanuts, walnuts, sunflower seeds, peanut butter, kidney beans, lentils, split peas	Rich sources of energy, magnesium, protein, and fiber
Fats and oils[§]	2	2–3	3	1 tsp soft margarine 1 tsp vegetable oil 1 tbsp mayonnaise 2 tbsp salad dressing	Soft margarine, vegetable oil (such as canola, corn, olive, or safflower), low-fat mayonnaise, light salad dressing	The DASH study had 27% of calories as fat, including fat in or added to foods
Sweets and added sugars	0	5 or less per week	<2 daily	1 tbsp sugar 1 tbsp jelly or jam ½ cup sorbet, gelatin 1 cup lemonade	Fruit-flavored gelatin, fruit punch, hard candy, jelly, maple syrup, sorbet and ices, sugar	Sweets should be low in fat

*Whole grains are recommended for most grain servings as a good source of fiber and nutrients.

† Serving sizes vary between ½ cup and 1¼ cups, depending on cereal type. Check the product's Nutrition Facts label.

§ Fat content changes serving amounts for fats and oils. For example, 1 tbsp of regular salad dressing equals one serving; 1 tbsp of a low-fat dressing equals one-half serving; 1 tbsp of a fat-free dressing equals zero servings.

Abbreviations: oz, ounce; tbsp, tablespoon; tsp, teaspoon.

Modified from National Heart, Lung, and Blood Institute. *Your Guide to Lowering Your Blood Pressure with DASH*. Accessed January 12, 2026. https://www.nhlbi.nih.gov/files/docs/public/heart/new_dash.pdf. (Table, p. 3)

High sodium intake is associated with elevated BP and negative effects on the blood vessels, heart, and kidneys.[94] The EAL states that lowering sodium intake to 1500–2000 mg/day in adults with HTN achieved a reduction up to 12 mm Hg of systolic BP and up to 6 mm Hg of diastolic BP.[84] The evidence compiled by the AHA/ACC illustrates that in adults with a baseline BP of 120 to 150/80 to 95 mm Hg, reducing sodium intake to 2400 or 1500 mg/day (from 3300 mg/day) decreases BP by 2/1 and 7/3 mm Hg, respectively.[13] This reduction in BP is demonstrated in both sexes as well as in Black and non-Black adults. A meta-analysis of 167 trials concluded that in patients with HTN, a reduced-sodium diet decreased systolic BP by about 5, 6, and 10 mm Hg in White, Black, and Asian participants, respectively.[95] Another meta-analysis of 28 RCTs found that modestly reducing sodium intake resulted in reducing systolic BP by about 5 mm Hg in patients with HTN and by about 2 mm Hg in individuals without HTN.[96] An RCT of 20 individuals with untreated HTN showed that BP fell from 163/100 to 147/91 mm Hg when sodium intake was decreased from 11,200 to 2900 mg/day.[97] There is a clear relationship between the reduction of dietary sodium intake and improvements in BP, and therefore modification of CVD risk factors.

High sodium intake has also been found to be associated with left ventricular hypertrophy, which is a risk factor for CVD outcomes.[98] Three studies have illustrated that reducing sodium intake decreases left ventricular mass; the sodium reductions ranged from 2000 to 5000 mg/day and the study durations from 6 weeks to 4 years. Two of the studies combined reduced-sodium intake with additional diet and lifestyle changes.[99–101]

In addition to illustrating that decreased sodium intake modifies risk factors for CVD, studies have also indicated a direct relationship between sodium intake and CVD. A meta-analysis of 13 prospective cohort studies found that an increase in sodium intake of 5000 mg/day was associated with a 23% increase in the risk of stroke and a 14% increase in the risk of CVD.[102] In a meta-analysis of seven RCTs, individual trials showed a trend toward reduced-sodium intake and decreased CVD and stroke events; when data were pooled, the result was a statistically significant 20% reduction in CVD and stroke events.[103] This confers with data from a long-term follow-up of phase I and phase II of the Trials of Hypertension Prevention. An analysis of 3126 participants from both trials found that a sodium reduction led to a significant 25% decrease in CVD and stroke events.[104] A challenge has come from observational studies that have suggested a relationship between sodium reduction and increased risk of CVD and stroke in 2011.[105,106] The AHA has reviewed the evidence and has published a statement that the findings were based on secondary analyses from studies not originally intended to suggest a relationship between sodium intake and CVD/stroke. Suggested reasons for careful consideration of the results include measurement error, residual confounding, and reverse causality.[94] The current AHA/ACC guidelines continue to recommend reduced-sodium intake for the prevention and management of CVD.[4,13,49,81]

The ACC/AHA recommendation is optimally a sodium intake of <1500 mg/day, but aim for at least 1000 mg sodium/day reduction from current amount for most adults.[81] The 2020–2025 DGAs recommend <2300 mg/day sodium intake for all healthy adults and individuals with HTN, DM, and/or CKD.[34] The NCM 2018's MNT for HTN guideline has been updated to recommend lowering consumption of sodium to no more than 1500–2300 mg/day for patients with HTN.[86] Current estimations of national sodium intake for people over 1 year of age in the United States is 3393 mg/day.[34] Most sodium consumed in the United States comes from salt added during commercial food processing and preparation and foods prepared at restaurants.[34] Significant sodium consumption in the United States can also be attributed to processed foods such as breads, grains, cereals, soups, sauces, and cured meats.[49,107] The 2020–2025 DGA indicates top food sources of sodium are coming from sandwiches (21%), other sources (19%), and within rice, pasta, and other grain-based mixed dishes (8%).[34] Advice to follow a sodium restriction can be overwhelming given the plethora of high-sodium food choices in grocery stores and restaurants.

MNT provided by an RD is critical for individuals with HTN. Nutrition intervention can provide the necessary education and support needed for a successful diet change. The DASH diet is complex, and an RD can facilitate adjusting to this dietary pattern by creating individualized dietary plans that meet cultural considerations, food preferences, and additional nutrient needs unique to each patient. The education piece of MNT for HTN incorporates information regarding daily sodium goals, food sources of sodium, low- and high-sodium choices, low-sodium cooking strategies, strategies to choose low-sodium meals or cooking methods when eating away from home, and development of an individualized diet pattern that meets the DASH diet guidelines. An RD can address barriers to change, such a busy lifestyle, by providing ideas and recipes to illustrate that cooking fresh, healthy foods can be a fast and easy alternative to relying on high-sodium convenience foods. Another common barrier is the misconception that a low-sodium diet is a bland diet. This can be overcome by showing ways to preserve the flavor and appeal of food with a variety of herbs and spices when cooking. Commercial non-salt seasoning blends are widely available. Important goals are to replace salt with other herbs and spices and using vinegar, citrus, and spicy aroma vegetables such as garlic, onion, jalapeño, and ginger since just 1 tsp of added salt contains 2300 mg of sodium; to read food labels to choose foods with less than 140–300 mg of sodium per serving; to order foods with less salt/soy sauce/cooked without sodium at restaurants; and choose fewer sandwiches with high sodium condiments, cheese, or cold cuts. Refer to **Table 9.10** for a list of food choices that can be suggested to replace high-sodium foods. Over several MNT sessions, an RD can provide education and motivation for behavior change essential for the nutrition management of HTN.

PRACTICE POINT

MNT for HTN involves educating patients on the DASH diet, reduced-sodium intake with possible potassium supplementation preferably through diet, if no contraindications, weight loss if applicable, physical activity, and limited alcohol consumption.

Table 9.10 Substitutions for High-Sodium Food Choices

Low Sodium *Choose MORE Often*	High Sodium *Choose LESS Often*
▪ Fresh meat, poultry, fish	▪ Breaded and processed meats, poultry, fish
▪ Low-sodium deli meat, rinsed tuna	▪ Deli meat, canned tuna
▪ Swiss cheese, mozzarella cheese	▪ Hard cheese, cottage cheese
▪ Low-sodium bread and rolls	▪ Salted bread and rolls
▪ Rice, pasta	▪ Commercial pasta or rice mixes
▪ Fresh or frozen fruits and veggies	▪ Canned goods, pickled veggies
▪ Low-sodium soup	▪ Soup and bouillon
▪ Vinegar, low-sodium dressing	▪ Salad dressing, soy sauce

Other Effective Nonpharmacological Therapies for Blood Pressure Reduction

Potassium

In addition to sodium reduction, the ACC/AHA and multi-society guideline suggests increasing dietary potassium intake, if no contradictions of CKD or potassium sparing medication use.[81] Increased dietary potassium intake reduces sodium reabsorption at the proximal and distal nephron of the kidneys and promotes sodium excretion. The ACC/AHA and multi-society guideline recommends aiming for 3500–5000 mg potassium daily to benefit BP reduction of 4/5 mm Hg for patients with HTN, and 2 mm Hg for people without HTN.[81] Eating a diet high in potassium is especially beneficial for patients who cannot reduce dietary sodium intake.[81,108,109] The EAL indicates that increasing dietary potassium consumption up to 2000 mg/day increases the likelihood of diastolic BP control.[84] Potassium-rich foods include most leafy greens, tomato and tomato products, citrus fruits, bananas, bran cereals, legumes, nuts and seeds, and dairy and dairy alternatives.[110] The DASH diet is naturally rich in potassium. The EAL states that if adults with HTN cannot meet the Dietary Reference Intake (DRI) for potassium (3400 mg/day for men, 2600 mg/day for women) and have no risk nor harm contradictions, potassium supplementation up to about 3700 mg/day may be recommended to reduce systolic BP by 3–13 mm Hg and diastolic BP up to 8 mm Hg.[84]

Alcohol

Excessive alcohol intake is a risk factor for HTN. A reduction in alcohol intake may reduce systolic BP by 2–4 mm Hg. Individuals with HTN should be instructed to only consume alcohol in moderation (one drink per day for women and two drinks per day for men). Abstinence from alcohol for heavy drinkers reduces systolic BP up to 28 mm Hg and diastolic BP up to 18 mm Hg. Individuals who do not drink should not start drinking alcohol.[49,89]

Physical Activity

Increasing physical activity with a structured program is another effective behavior modification for BP reduction. Both the EAL and the AHA/ACC recommend physical activity 3–4 times per week for an average of 40 minutes at moderate-to-vigorous intensity. This level of physical activity can reduce systolic BP by 2–5 mm Hg and diastolic BP by 1–4 mm Hg.[81,83] The 2017 ACC/AHA and multi-society guideline for HTN recommends resistance training of 90–150 minutes/week alone, results in BP reduction of 2–4 mm Hg.[81] It also recommends isometric resistance training or handgrips, for 2 minutes of four repetitions, three sessions per week for 8–10 weeks leading to BP reduction of 4–5 mm Hg.[81,111,112]

Smoking Cessation

Smoking cessation and avoidance of secondhand smoke is an important element of CVD prevention and treatment.[4,81] During MNT, an RD can refer a patient to the appropriate smoking cessation programs, and/or direct the patient to have further smoking cessation discussion with their primary care physician.

Vitamin D

The EAL suggests adequate intake of vitamin D to meet the DRI (600–800 IU/day).[113] Data is inconclusive on vitamin D status or intake for BP control in patients with HTN.[84]

Calcium

The EAL suggests adequate intake of dietary calcium to meet the DRI (1000–1200 mg/day). [113] For patients with HTN, at least 800 mg/day of dietary calcium intake reduced systolic BP up to 4 mm Hg and diastolic BP up to 2 mm Hg.[84] If patients with HTN cannot meet the DRI for dietary calcium, supplementation of 1000–1500 mg calcium daily is recommended. Calcium supplementation at this level reduced systolic BP up to 3 mm Hg and diastolic BP up to 2.5 mm Hg.[84]

Magnesium

The EAL suggests adequate intake of dietary magnesium to meet the DRI (310–320 mg/day for women, 400–420 mg/day for men).[114] Data is unclear on the relationship between dietary magnesium and BP in patients with HTN. If patients with HTN cannot meet the DRI for magnesium through diet, supplementation of 240–1000 mg magnesium daily is reasonable. Magnesium supplementation at this level reduced systolic BP by 1–5.6 mm Hg and diastolic BP by 1–2.8 mm Hg.[84]

Salt Substitutes

Salt substitutes, now a popular salt alternative, can reduce or replace the mineral sodium in regular edible salt (sodium chloride), with other substances, such as potassium. The benefits of salt substitutes are to reduce sodium intake while supplementing potassium intake but not compromising the salty taste. A recent meta-analysis including 23 studies of 32,073 participants showed a significant lowering of systolic BP by 4.8 mm Hg, and diastolic BP by 1.48 mm Hg and reduced all-cause mortality by 12% in both those with and without HTN, when using lower sodium salt substitutes instead of regular salt.[115] The chief concern of supplementing potassium is risk of hyperkalemia, or high serum potassium, which may weaken muscles and damage the heart. This meta-analysis found no significant adverse effects of hyperkalemia in the studies, although the potassium chloride salt substitute increased serum potassium level by 0.1 mmol/L.[115] Using potassium chloride salt could help with BP management. However, there is no information from AND on using salt substitutes, and there are limited guidelines on recommendations of salt substitutes by different institutes. The ACC/AHA suggests that patients with CKD who have hyperkalemia or end-stage kidney disease (ESKD) not on dialysis, patients on potassium-sparing diuretics, patients prescribed potassium supplements, or patients that have another contraindication should not use salt substitutes.[81,116] There is limited evidence to support the use of salt substitutes in the general population without HTN due to the concerns of possibilities of individuals having undiagnosed advanced CKD misusing such potassium-enriched substitutes.

Monosodium Glutamate (MSG)

Monosodium glutamate (MSG), the salt form of glutamate acid, is widely used in Asian-themed cooking as a flavor enhancer. The flavor from MSG is called "umami," or savoriness, and is the fifth basic taste along with sweet, sour, bitter, and spicy. It is naturally present in some foods such as tomatoes, mushrooms, seaweed, and cheese, and can be produced through fermentation of starch, sugar beets, sugar cane, and molasses. The synthetic form can be used as an additive in some restaurant meals, soups, canned vegetables, and deli meat. The FDA recognizes MSG as GRAS, and it requires MSG to be listed on the nutrition facts panel. Some MSG-sensitive individuals may have adverse reactions such as headache or nausea after ingesting foods containing MSG. Currently the FDA suggests that consuming foods with 3 grams or more of MSG might introduce these transient mild symptoms. It is unlikely that food would contain this amount of MSG level since a typical serving of food contains 0.5 grams of MSG. The EAL states that in healthy adults there is inconsistent results related to MSG reactions, and ingestion of MSG for adults with asthma did not worsen symptoms.[118] MSG contains less sodium than sodium chloride (about one-third of sodium compared to table salt). AND and the EAL currently do not have guidelines on MSG intake and there is no guideline from AHA/ACC on MSG intake. Use MSG in moderation for patients with HTN and/or CVD.

Nutrition Monitoring and Evaluation in Hypertension

Like disorders of lipid metabolism, the monitoring and evaluation portion of MNT for HTN involves a review of the nutrition assessment categories described in Table 9.3. Specific goals and outcomes can be monitored and evaluated at each follow-up visit. Examples for the patient with HTN include BMI, WC, diet recall, sodium intake, and BP (ACC/AHA guidelines recommend a BP goal of <130/80 mm Hg).[81]

Overweight/Obesity and Cardiovascular Disease Clinical Course

Overweight (BMI ≥25–29.9 kg/m^2) and obesity (BMI >30 kg/m^2) are risk factors for disorders of lipid metabolism, HTN, DM, CAD, stroke, and HF. An elevated BMI increases risk of morbidity and mortality from cardiovascular events.[119,120] Lower BMI thresholds for Asian adults is recommended. Overweight in the Asian population is defined as BMI ≥23 to <27.5 kg/m^2, while obesity is defined as a BMI ≥27.5 kg/m^2.[3] WC is also an important measure because it distinguishes between android (apple-shaped) body type and gynoid (pear-shaped) body type. Android obesity, associated with an increased risk of CVD, is a WC of >35 inches in women and >40 inches in men. WC cutoffs for Asians are adjusted to a WC of >31 inches in Asian women and >35 inches in Asian men.[3]

The AHA/ACC guideline indicates that a weight loss of 3–5% can lead to clinically significant reduction in some CVD risk factors.[120] A 3 kg, or 6.6 lb, weight loss has been associated with a 15 mg/dL decrease in TGs; a 5–8 kg, or 11–17.6 lb, weight loss can lead to a 5 mg/dL decrease in LDL-C and a 2–3 mg/dL increase in HDL-C.[120] Weight management also contributes to BP reduction. A 5% weight loss correlates with a 3/2 mm Hg reduction in BP.[120] The ACC/AHA suggests that individuals who are overweight aim to lose at least 1 kg or 2.2 lb, which may reduce BP by 1 mm Hg.[81] Following the DASH diet, which is low in saturated fat and refined carbohydrates, may also be beneficial for weight loss if patients are overweight/obese. Refer to Chapter 7, *Weight and Health*, for more information on the nutritional management of obesity.

CORE CONCEPT 7

An elevated body mass index categorized as overweight or obese increases cardiovascular morbidity and mortality risk.

PRACTICE POINT

A weight loss of 3–5% can lead to clinically significant reduction in some CVD risk factors.

Diabetes Mellitus and Cardiovascular Disease Clinical Course

Type 2 DM in patients increases CVD risk by 2- to 3-fold, with women showing an increased higher risk than men (2.5-fold vs. 1.7-fold increased risk, respectively).[121] Both DM and CVD have overlapping risk factors of HTN, overweight/obesity, dyslipidemia, hyperglycemia, suboptimal dietary intake, and physical inactivity. CVD prevention should consider regulation of blood sugar as a key target for intervention. Currently fewer than 20% of adults in the United States with DM are at target for the three important measurements of HbA1c, BP, and LDL-C.[3,121,122]

Current studies indicate pharmacotherapies of glucose-lowering agents, such as glucagon-like peptide-1 receptor agonists (GLP-1 RAs) and sodium-glucose cotransporter 2 inhibitors (SGLT2i), can lead to reductions in major adverse cardiac events of CVD mortality, nonfatal MI, HF, and all-cause mortality by not only regulating blood sugar, but also regulating BP.[121] These glucose-lowering agents are also commonly prescribed to patients with CVD.

CORE CONCEPT 8

Type 2 diabetes mellitus (DM) increases risk for cardiovascular disease development by 2- to 3-fold, as both conditions have many overlapping risk factors of overweight/obesity, dyslipidemia, hyperglycemia, hypertension, suboptimal dietary choices, and physical inactivity.

CASE STUDY REVISITED

Acute Hospital Admission Note

Several years later, Carl is now 60 years old and experiences an episode of increasing chest pain and dyspnea accompanied by nausea, vomiting, and feeling "unwell." He presents to the Emergency Department where an ECG is done indicating ST-elevation myocardial infarction. This is confirmed by elevated troponin levels. Upon hospital admission, a cardiac catheterization reveals 100% occlusion in his left and right coronary arteries. His EF = 35%. Carl undergoes a coronary artery bypass graft surgery and is recovering well.

Carl's spouse passed away and his daughter is now away at college. He lives alone, although his siblings live nearby.

Anthropometric Data:

Weight: 110 kg
Height: 178 cm
BMI: 34.7 kg/m^2

Biochemical Data:

Sodium 134 (135–145 mEq/L)
Potassium 3.5 (3.6–5.0 mEq/L)
Chloride 99 (98–110 mEq/L)
Carbon dioxide 23 (20–30 mEq/L)
Blood urea nitrogen 20 (6–24 mg/dL)
Creatinine 0.8 (0.4–1.3 mg/dL)
Glucose 130 (70–139 mg/dL)
Calcium 8.9 (8.5–10.5 mg/dL)
Phosphorus 4.5 (2.7–4.5 mg/dL)
Magnesium 1.7 (1.3–2.1 mg/dL)
Albumin 4.0 (3.5–5.0 g/dL)
Prealbumin 26 (17–36 g/dL)

Clinical Data:

Past Medical History: HTN, dyslipidemia, CAD, s/p angioplasty, obesity, depressive disorder

Medications: atorvastatin, furosemide, gemfibrozil, metoprolol, warfarin

Vital Signs: Blood pressure 159/80 mm Hg, Temperature 99.9°F, Heart rate 90 beats/min

Nutrition-Focused Physical Exam: No evidence of muscle wasting, mild lower extremity edema, android body type, some shortness of breath noted

Dietary Data:

24-Hour Diet Recall

Since his spouse passed away, Carl has relied primarily on convenience foods. Appetite remains good.

Breakfast (9 am): 1 cup coffee with 2% milk and sugar, 2 cups unsweetened whole grain cereal with 1 cup 2% milk, banana

Lunch (12 pm): Canned tomato soup and cheese sandwich, or cheese and crackers, or tuna sandwich with mayo

Snack (3 pm): Chocolate pudding or granola bar

Dinner (6 pm): Frozen pizza; or macaroni and cheese with canned peas; or spaghetti with canned tomato sauce, frozen broccoli, and frozen garlic bread

Physical Activity: Sedentary prior to admission

Diet Prescription: 2000 mg sodium, heart-healthy diet

Questions

1. Assess the sodium content of Carl's diet prior to admission.
2. Write two PES statements for Carl identifying Carl's active nutrition issues.
3. Identify the nutrition interventions you would like to initiate for Carl to address the problems identified in your PES statements.
4. What indices are included in your monitoring and evaluation plan? Why?
5. Outline the components of the nutrition education that should be provided to Carl after his CABG surgery.

RDs can help patients with DM work on behavior change targeting increasing physical activity and improving diet thereby reducing blood glucose, dyslipidemia, BP, and weight. The EAL indicates that studies show that MNT provided by an RD has fair evidence in aiding adults with type 2 DM in reduction of total cholesterol by 8–28 mg/dL, LDL-C by 8–22 mg/dL, TGs by 15–153 mg/dL, likely increase of HDL-C by

2.4–6 mg/dL, and likely reduction of systolic BP and diastolic BP by 3.2–9 mm Hg/2.5–5.3 mm Hg.[13,123] Refer to Chapter 8, *Nutrition in Diabetes Mellitus*, for more information on nutritional therapy for DM.

Cardiovascular Disease Outcomes

The CVD outcomes of HTN and atherosclerosis can result in further outcomes of CAD, angina pectoris, MI, stroke, PAD, and HF. **Coronary artery disease (CAD)** is the leading cause of CVD death in the United States, at 40.3%.[3] CAD refers to atherosclerosis affecting the arteries that supply blood to the heart. CAD is also referred to as coronary heart disease (CHD) and **ischemic heart disease**. **Angina pectoris**, or stable chest pain, is a symptom of CAD, but individuals may be asymptomatic until a coronary event. When a blockage occurs in one or several of the coronary arteries that supply blood to the heart, the result can be a **myocardial infarction (MI)**, often referred to as a heart attack. MIs can be fatal. Nonfatal MI increases the risk of developing HF by decreasing functional heart myocytes, scaring heart tissue, causing left ventricular remodeling, and breaking down myocardium (heart muscle).[2] An MI occurs every 40 seconds. Each year, 805,000 Americans experience an MI.[3] **Ischemic cardiomyopathy** is a type of HF in which the left ventricle is enlarged because of decreased blood supply to the heart muscle due to CAD and MI. If atherosclerosis leads to an embolism in the cerebral arteries that supply the brain, the result can be an ischemic **stroke**.[2] Stroke causes 1 in every 21 deaths in the United States, where it is the second cause of CVD death at 17.5%.[3] Atherosclerosis can also narrow the arteries that deliver blood to the legs, arms, stomach, or kidneys in the case of **peripheral artery disease (PAD)**. The early stages of PAD in the extremities can cause cramping, pain, and discomfort. Untreated PAD can result in gangrene and limb amputation.[2,124]

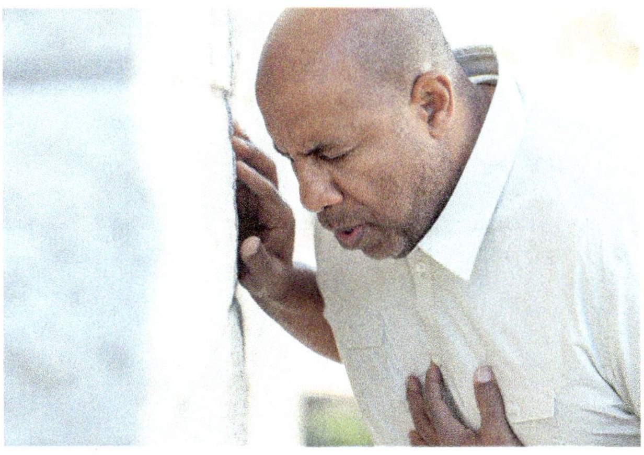

Advanced Coronary Artery Disease Diagnosis and Surgical Treatment

CAD can be diagnosed using computed tomography (CT) scans, magnetic resonance imaging (MRI), cardiac catheterization, and angiography. **Cardiac catheterization** is a common yet invasive procedure where a catheter is inserted into a large blood vessel leading to the heart. Measures of BP and flow can be used to assess heart function and parameters such as ejection fraction. Cardiac catheterizations commonly include an **angiogram**, where a contrast dye that can be observed on x-ray is injected through the catheter. The flow of contrast dye can be followed to determine stenosis or narrowing of specific arteries. When significant stenosis is found, **percutaneous coronary intervention (PCI)**, also called **percutaneous transluminal coronary angioplasty (PTCA)**, is performed by expanding a balloon-tipped catheter at the site and placing a stent.[9] Figures 9.9A and B illustrate cardiac catheterization and PCI.

If PCI is not possible, a surgical option is **coronary artery bypass graft (CABG)**, in which the stenosis is bypassed with the placement of an artificial or saphenous vein graft.[9] Patients should receive a nutrition assessment prior to and post cardiac surgery. A BMI >30 kg/m² is associated with an increased rate of postoperative deep sternal wound and saphenous vein harvest site infections.[125,126] Malnutrition is a risk factor for morbidity and mortality in patients post cardiac surgery.[127] A study of 5,168 patients found that BMI <20 kg/m² was associated with increased mortality after cardiopulmonary bypass.[126] Nutrition support may be warranted for patients with malnutrition before and/or after cardiac surgery. Nutrition support for the cardiac population is discussed later in this chapter.

During CABG surgery, **cardiopulmonary bypass** is used to perform the work of the heart and lungs temporarily. Associated risks include ischemic damage to the bowel and bacterial translocation.[125] For this reason, it is important to monitor postoperative GI function before advancing a patient's diet. After CABG surgery, a patient is instructed to consume a low-sodium, high-protein diet to aid in wound healing. The long-term MNT for a patient post CABG is to start or continue to follow an individualized heart-healthy diet as discussed previously. A comprehensive secondary prevention for CVD, such as after experiencing a nonfatal MI, or status post a CABG surgery, is for qualified patients to participate in a cardiac rehabilitation (CR) program to improve functional capacity, learn about a heart-healthy diet, manage stress, quit smoking if applicable, and improve overall quality of life. CR is discussed later in this chapter.

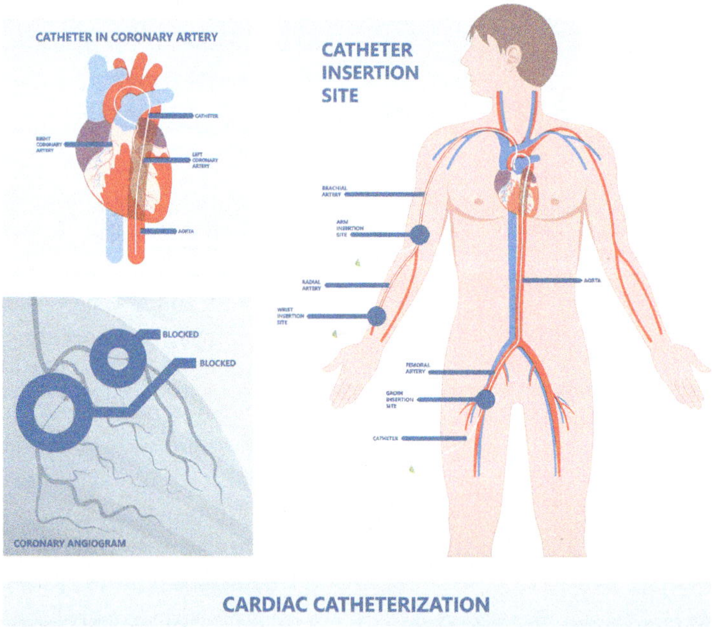

A

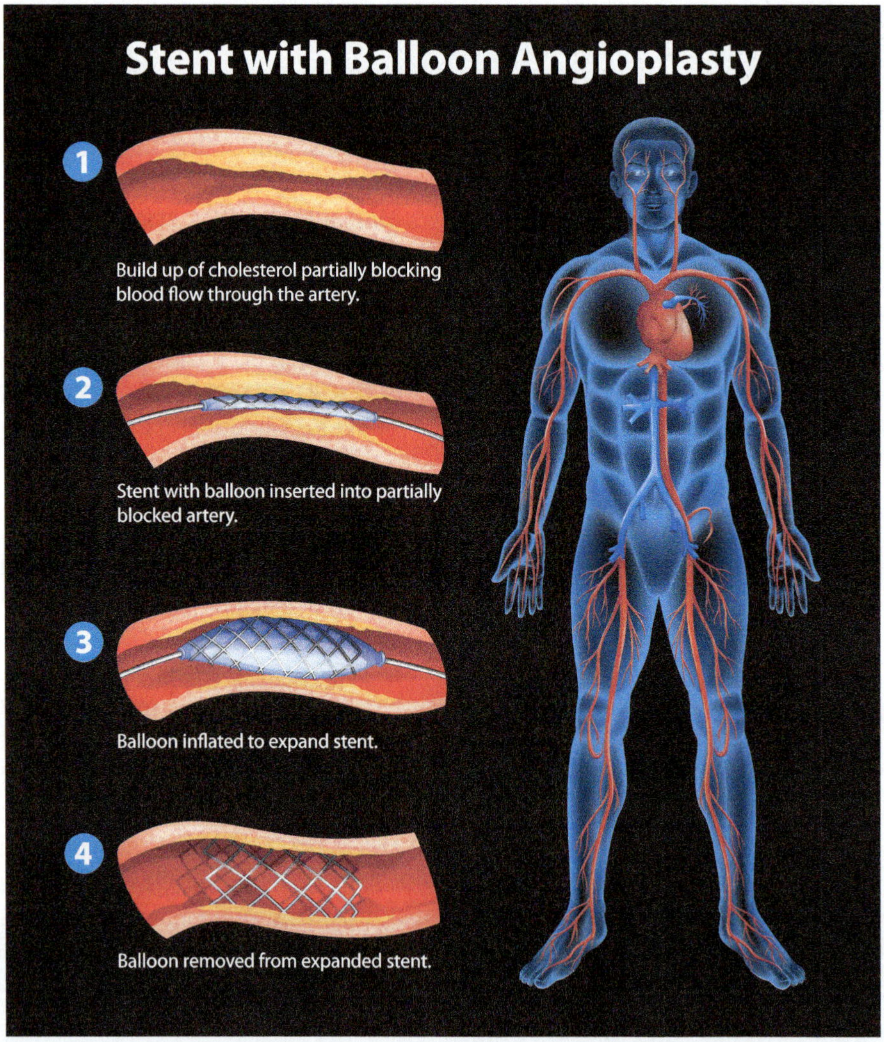

B

Figure 9.9 **A.** Cardiac Catheterization with Angiogram. **B.** Stent Angioplasty

A: © Af Pepermpron/Shutterstock; B: © Af BlueRingMedia/Shutterstock

CASE STUDY REVISITED

Four years later, Carl's CVD has progressed to heart failure. He presents to the hospital with shortness of breath, fatigue, decreased exercise tolerance, and recent weight loss and is diagnosed with acute decompensated heart failure. He reports that he no longer has an interest in food and he has been instructed by his RD to follow a low-sodium diet. He recalls that he used to be a "big guy," but now the weight is melting off.

Anthropometric Data:

Weight: 65 kg
Height: 178 cm
BMI: 20.4 kg/m^2
Estimated dry weight: 63 kg

Weight history
70 kg (6 months ago); 75 kg (12 months ago); 95 kg (15 years ago)

Biochemical Data:

Sodium 134 (136–145 mEq/L)
Potassium 3.2 (3.4–5.0 mEq/L)
Chloride 99 (96–106 mEq/L)
Carbon dioxide 23 (22–31 mEq/L)
Blood urea nitrogen 17 (8–20 mg/dL)
Creatinine 0.7 (0.7–1.3 mg/dL)
Glucose 110 (70–139 mg/dL)

Calcium 9.0 (8.5–10.5 mg/dL)
Phosphorus 4.0 (2.5–4.5 mg/dL)
Magnesium 1.5 (1.5–2.7 mg/dL)
Albumin 3.5 (3.5–5.5 g/dL)
Prealbumin 8 (16–30 g/dL)
B-type natriuretic peptide (BNP) 1,800 pg/mL (<300 pg/mL)

Clinical Data:

Past Medical History: HTN, dyslipidemia, CAD, s/p angioplasty, MI, CABG, obesity, depressive disorder, advanced HF

Medications: atorvastatin, furosemide, gemfibrozil, metoprolol, multivitamin/mineral supplement, warfarin

Nutrition-Focused Physical Exam: Bilateral temporal muscle wasting, lower extremity edema

Dietary Data:

24-Hour Dietary Recall

Breakfast (9 am): 1 cup of coffee (cream and sugar added), toast with butter

Lunch (12 pm): Usually skips lunch

Snack (3 pm): Crackers and peanut butter, 8 ounces of milk

Dinner (6 pm): Frozen dinner (meat or chicken with rice and vegetable), usually eats about 50%

Physical Activity: Sedentary

Questions

1. What additional nutrition assessment data can be collected as part of subjective global assessment (SGA)? Why is SGA useful in Carl's current situation?
2. How would you describe Carl's nutritional status and nutritional risk factors?
3. How would you estimate Carl's current protein and energy needs?
4. Write two PES statements for Carl identifying Carl's current active nutrition issues.
5. Identify the nutrition interventions you would like to initiate for Carl to address the problems identified in your PES statements.
6. What indices are included in your monitoring and evaluation plan? Why?

Heart Failure Clinical Course

Chronic and progressive HF is often the final stage of CVD and related conditions. The prevalence of HF is increasing over time with the aging population and the increasing rate of CVD. It is estimated that 56.2 million people have HF globally. Approximately 6.7 million adults have HF in the United States, equating to 2.3% of the population, and the number of individuals with HF is predicted to increase by 46% to more than 8 million from the year 2012 to 2030. A greater burden is observed in the Black community than in the White population, Hispanic people, or Asians (3.8% and 3.3% vs. 2.9% and 1.6% vs. 1.8% and 1.6% vs. 1.4% and 0.5%, respectively, in men and women), and slightly greater incidence is demonstrated in women than men (505,000 incidents vs. 495,000 incidents, respectively). The total cost of HF care in the United States is more than $30 billion annually. HF has led to over 85,000 deaths annually in the United States, where over 50% of HF deaths are due to CVD causes. HF can be caused by damage to heart tissue. CAD, HTN, cigarette smoking, obesity, and DM are common causes attributed to HF (20% vs. 20% vs. 14% vs. 12% vs. 12%, respectively).[3]

Heart failure (HF) refers to the heart's inability to provide the body with adequate oxygenated blood due to symptomatic structural or functional impairment of ventricular filling or ejection of blood. Right-sided HF is when the heart cannot pump adequate blood to the lungs to be oxygenated. Left-sided HF is when the heart is unable to pump adequate oxygenated blood to the entire body. HF can also be distinguished as systolic and diastolic. Systolic HF refers to ventricular hypertrophy that leads to decreased pumping during systole. The result is HF with a reduced ejection fraction labeled as HFrEF, defined as left ventricular ejection fraction (LVEF) ≤40%. HF can also exist with a preserved EF, labeled as HFpEF, classified as LVEF ≥50%. HFpEF represents most of the HF population and its prevalence is increasing; HFpEF is usually related to diastolic HF. Diastolic HF is classified as a thickening of the ventricle cavity as opposed to an enlargement of the whole ventricle. The reduced cavity size results in decreased filling capacity during diastole. Patients with LVEF between 41% and 49% are classified as HF with mildly reduced EF, labeled as HFmrEF. While there are many ways to differentiate HF, it is also possible for many types of HF to occur at the same time.[9,128,129]

HF can result in fatigue, dyspnea, fluid retention, lack of appetite, nausea, malnutrition, and death. In the case of HF, cardiac output and arterial pressure are decreased. The inability to increase cardiac output leads to symptoms of fatigue and decreased exercise tolerance. Fluid accumulation occurs to compensate for decreased arterial pressure and can result in edema and **dyspnea** (shortness of breath). **Acute decompensated heart failure (ADHF)** is a rapid onset of HF symptoms that requires immediate treatment.[9]

Common HF risks include MI, HTN, and valvular heart disease. Other risks include familial cardiomyopathy, older age, male sex, exposure to cardiotoxic agents for cancer and other treatments, HTN, type 2 DM, obesity, dyslipidemia, CKD, dietary factors, sedentary lifestyle, sleep-disordered breathing, and smoking.[128] Maintaining a healthy weight, BP, blood glucose, healthy eating, exercising regularly, and not smoking have been associated with a lower lifetime risk of developing HF. BP is a key risk factor for HF as over 80% of patients with HF also have HTN. The treatment goal of BP for patients with CVD risk ≥10% is <130/80 mm Hg.[128] Many of the modifiable risk factors associated with HF are the same for CVD. For this reason, the 2022 AHA/ACC/Heart Failure Society of America (HFSA) Guideline for the Management of HF recommends using similar preventative measures for both CVD and HF.[4,128] The focus is on starting prevention at the earliest stage of HF to prevent or alleviate HF symptoms and improve quality of life.

HF has been classified by both the ACC/AHA and the New York Heart Association (NYHA). The ACC/AHA stages focus on HF disease development and progression, while the NYHA classes are based on symptoms and functional capacity for patients in symptomatic (Stage C) and advanced HF (Stage D).[128] **Table 9.11** presents these classification systems.[128] The NYHA classification is widely used in clinical practice as a subjective assessment to determine treatments for patients and can change over treatment time. It is an independent predictor of mortality.[128]

Early treatment of HF involves pharmacotherapy along with placement of an ICD and/or cardiac resynchronization therapy (CRT) when appropriate. The gold standard treatment of advanced HF is heart transplantation.[128] An option for patients awaiting heart transplantation and those who suffer acute cardiogenic shock is the implantation of a ventricular assist device (VAD). A VAD can also be used as destination therapy in patients with HF who are not eligible for heart transplantation. The most common type of VAD is a **left ventricular assist device (LVAD)**; this is a surgically implanted mechanical pump that supports the heart function by pumping blood from the left ventricle to the aorta to circulate oxygen-rich blood throughout the body. **Figure 9.10** displays an LVAD. Other VADs include right ventricular assist devices (RVADs) and bi-ventricular assist devices (BIVADs). Advances in VAD technology have made the devices smaller, more reliable, and longer lasting. VADs can be used for both temporary treatment and destination therapy at various stages of HF. In the case of heart transplantation, the VAD is removed and replaced with a donor organ.[129–131]

Table 9.11 Heart Failure Classification

New York Heart Association (NYHA) Functional Classification	
Class	**Patient Symptoms**
Class I (Normal)	No limitation of physical activity. Ordinary physical activity does not cause symptoms of HF.
Class II (Mild)	Slight limitation of physical activity. Ordinary physical activity results in symptoms of HF.
Class III (Moderate)	Marked limitation of physical activity. Comfortable at rest, but less than ordinary activity causes symptoms of HF.
Class IV (Severe)	Unable to carry out any physical activity without symptoms of HF, or symptoms of HF at rest.
ACC/AHA Classification	
Stage	***Description***
A: At Risk for HF	At high risk for HF but without structural heart disease or symptoms of HF.
B: Pre-HF	Structural heart disease, evidence for increased filling pressures, or patients with risk factors and increased biomarker of B-type peptides or cardiac troponin, but without signs or symptoms of HF.
C: Symptomatic HF	Structural heart disease with prior or current symptoms of HF.
D: Advanced HF	Marked HF symptoms that interfere with daily life requiring specialized interventions.

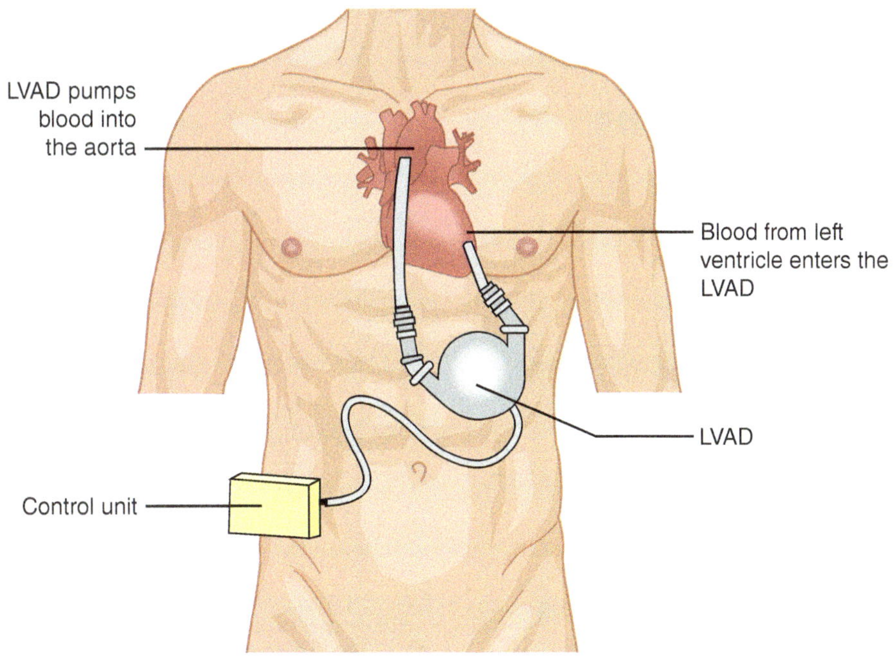

Figure 9.10 Left Ventricular Assist Device (LVAD)

Refer to Chapter 16, *Nutrition in Solid Organ Transplantation*, for more information on MNT for heart transplantation.

CORE CONCEPT 9

Heart failure (HF) refers to the heart's inability to provide the body with adequate oxygenated blood due to symptomatic structural or functional impairment of ventricular filling or ejection of blood. HF can result in fatigue, dyspnea, fluid retention, lack of appetite, nausea, malnutrition, and death.

PRACTICE POINT

MNT for HF can result in improvements in dietary patterns, edema, fatigue, and quality of life.

Nutritional Management in Heart Failure

The EAL recommends that all patients with HF be referred to an RD for MNT. An initial visit (at least 45 minutes) and one to three follow-ups (at least 30 minutes each) may result in improvements in dietary pattern, quality of life, edema, and fatigue, especially in patients with HF classified as NYHA Class IV and/or AHA Stage D advanced HF.[70,132,133]

Nutrition Assessment in Heart Failure

The nutrition assessment of the patient with HF includes the following: food/nutrition intake and related history; anthropometric measurements; biochemical data, medical tests, and procedures; nutrition-focused physical findings; and client history. Table 9.3 describes data collected for each category for patients at risk of HF. For patients with HF, focus on the following biochemical data: chem-10 lab panel (sodium, potassium, chloride, bicarbonate, blood urea nitrogen, creatinine, blood glucose, calcium, magnesium, and phosphorus), HbA1c, standard lipid panel, hemoglobin, hematocrit, serum iron, albumin, prealbumin, total protein, B-type natriuretic peptide (BNP, a biomarker of HF), and C reactive protein (CRP). Albumin and prealbumin should be measured and monitored because they correlate with disease outcome in several studies. However, albumin and prealbumin are influenced by several factors not related to nutrition status and should not be used as independent nutrition markers. Additional anthropometric measurements in this patient population include estimated dry weight (EDW) and ideal body weight (IBW).[132]

A useful assessment tool for the HF population is the **subjective global assessment (SGA)**. SGA evaluates weight change, dietary intake, GI symptoms, functional impairment, muscle wasting, and fat loss.[88,134,135] **Table 9.12** illustrates the components of the SGA. The SGA helps to classify patients with HF as well-nourished, mild-to-moderately malnourished, and severely malnourished.[88,134,135]

PRACTICE POINT

A useful assessment tool for the HF population is the subjective global assessment (SGA). The SGA evaluates weight change, dietary intake, GI symptoms, functional impairment, muscle wasting, and fat loss.

Table 9.12 Subjective Global Assessment

Components of Subjective Global Assessment	
Weight change	▪ Weight change over 2 weeks, 6 months, and 1 year ▪ Intentional versus unintentional weight change ▪ Actual weight and clothing size changes
Dietary intake	▪ Changes over time ▪ Restrictions
Gastrointestinal symptoms	▪ Nausea, vomiting, diarrhea ▪ Anorexia, dysphagia
Functional impairment	▪ Hand grip strength
Muscle wasting and subcutaneous fat loss	▪ Muscle stores: bicep, tricep, quadricep, deltoid, temple ▪ Fat stores: tricep, chest, eyes, perioral, interosseous, palmar
Edema (including ascites)	▪ Hands, sacral, lower extremities

Data from Charney P. *Academy of Nutrition and Dietetics Pocket Guide to Nutrition Assessment*. 4th ed. Chicago, IL: Academy of Nutrition & Dietetics; 2022.; Detsky AS, McLaughlin JR, Baker JP, et al. What is subjective global assessment of nutritional status? *JPEN J Parenter Enteral Nutr*. 1987;11(1):8-13. doi:10.1177/014860718701100108; Academy of Nutrition and Dietetics. Nutrition Care Manual. McCann A. Nutrition-Focused Physical Findings: Subjective Global Assessment. Accessed July 20, 2024. https://www.nutritioncaremanual.org

Medications in Heart Failure

Patients with HF are often prescribed multiple medications with nutrition-related implications. Table 9.8 lists classes of medications that may be taken by patients with HF, mainly ACEIs or ARB, beta blockers, mineralocorticoid receptor antagonists (MRA), and diuretics for HTN management, fluid control, LV dysfunction, and congestive symptoms; statins can also be taken to prevent symptomatic HF and adverse CVD events. The 2022 AHA/ACC/HFSA HF guideline also adds SGLT2i for patients with type 2 DM and either established or at high risk for CVD, and/or for patients with symptomatic chronic HFrEF as the choice of medication to prevent or reduce hospitalizations for HF and cardiovascular mortality.[128] Additional classes of medications are presented in **Table 9.13**. Possible drug–nutrient interactions are assessed to prevent and address potential adverse reactions.[43,63]

Energy Needs in Heart Failure

Indirect calorimetry is the ideal way to assess energy needs in patients with HF. When this method is not available, appropriate energy needs calculations such as the Mifflin–St Jeor or Harris–Benedict can be used. A stress factor should be added to account for increased resting energy expenditure in patients with HF. The NCM suggests calculating daily protein needs as 1.12 g/kg/day in well-nourished patients with HF and 1.37 g/kg/day in nutritionally depleted patients with HF.[70,132,133] Actual protein delivery may need to be modified in the case of patients with acute kidney injury, depending on the treatment method. Fluid restriction in patients with HF may be needed to improve clinical symptoms and quality of life.[132]

Obesity in Heart Failure

Obesity increases the risk of HF that for every 1-unit BMI increase, the incidence of HF increases by 5% in men and 7% in women.[136] The prevalence of overweight is about 29–40%, and obesity is about 30–49% in the HF population.[137] Factors that contribute to weight gain in patients with HF include decreased exercise tolerance, excessive calorie intake, volume overload, and medications.[74,138] Obesity can be identified in the HF population with the anthropometric measurements of BMI (based on EDW), WC, and WHR. The outcomes associated with overweight/obesity include infection and poor wound healing, as well as increased incidence of comorbidities such as dyslipidemia, HTN, and insulin resistance.[74,138] While elevated BMI has associated risks, it has also been found to be linked to a decreased mortality rate in the HF population. The protective effect of elevated BMI in patients with HF has been termed the **"obesity paradox."**[139] The reason for the protective effect of obesity in HF is not well understood. One suggested reason is that HF may be found earlier in patients with an elevated BMI as compared to those with a lower BMI; low BMI may be indicative of disease progression. Another possible explanation is that a greater metabolic reserve allows individuals with obesity to handle metabolic stress better than those with a lower BMI. Increased adipose tissue in

Table 9.13 Drug–Nutrient Interactions

Medication Class	Potential Side Effect	Nutrition Intervention
Anticoagulants (warfarin) Prevent blood clots	▪ Interact with vitamin K ▪ Interact with additional herbs and supplements	▪ Educate on consistent intake of foods high in vitamin K; provide a list of foods containing vitamin K ▪ Encourage patients to talk with their physician before taking vitamin E, fish oil, or herbal supplements
Inotropes (digoxin) Stimulate the heart to contract	▪ Hypo- or hyperkalemia ▪ Decreased Ca+, Mg+ ▪ Interactions with herbal supplements ▪ Anorexia, weight loss, nausea, vomiting, diarrhea ▪ Arrhythmias when combined with Ca+/Vitamin D supplementation	▪ Monitor K+; replete or restrict as indicated; educate on food sources ▪ Monitor Ca++ and Mg++; replete as indicated; educate on food sources ▪ Avoid St. John's wort; caution with aloe, foxglove, hawthorn ▪ Educate on small frequent meals as tolerated; monitor adequacy of oral intake ▪ Use caution with Ca++/vitamin D supplementation; educate on food sources as an alternative

patients with obesity may play a role in neutralizing the effects of **tumor necrosis factor-alpha**, which typically contributes to muscle wasting in patients with HF.[139]

Now as more studies have emerged, the paradoxical relationship is specifically evident in patients with HF who are overweight or have class 1 obesity (BMI of 30 to <35 kg/m^2). A large meta-analysis including 89 studies and over 1.3 million patients supported this finding, but it also demonstrated that the "obesity paradox" protective effect is diminished after 5 years of follow-up.[140] Additionally for patients who are underweight, higher risk for mortality is demonstrated in both short-term within 6 months and long-term over 6 months. For patients with more severe obesity (BMI ≥35 kg/m^2), a higher mortality risk in the long-term is demonstrated. This study concluded a J-shape relationship between BMI and mortality rate.[140] Thus, for patients with HF with a BMI <18.5 kg/m^2, appropriate weight gain is suggested, and for patients with HF with a BMI ≥35 kg/m^2, achieving intentional weight loss of at least ≥5–10% to improve symptoms and cardiac function may be reasonable.[137] The difficulty with using BMI to classify patients with HF in these studies is that it is not possible to identify whether protective factors are related to increased lean body mass or increased fat tissue. Cardiorespiratory fitness, the functional capacity and cardiovascular health developed by exercise, is now suggested to may be the best predictor of outcomes of HF.[141,142] The role of the RD is to weigh the risks and benefits of each patient's BMI when performing nutrition assessments.

PRACTICE POINT

While elevated BMI has associated risks, it has also been found to be linked to a decreased mortality rate in the HF population. The protective effect of elevated BMI in patients with HF has been termed the "obesity paradox." A possible J-shape relationship exists between BMI and mortality in patients with HF with the lowest mortality rate exhibited in patients with HF who are overweight or with class 1 obesity.

Cardiac Cachexia

Hippocrates (460–370 BCE) described cardiac cachexia as follows: "The flesh is consumed and becomes water...the shoulders, clavicles, chest and thighs melt away. This illness is fatal."[143] **Cardiac cachexia** is an uncontrollable loss of weight that includes muscle, fat, and eventually bone loss. This condition affects an estimated 5–15% of patients with HF and is associated with a 20–40% mortality rate annually.[63,138,144–146] Cardiac cachexia is a clinical indicator of advanced HF. An observational prospective analysis of 208 patients previously hospitalized due to HF found that malnutrition was an independent risk factor for mortality. The findings were mortality rates of 56%, 23.5%, and 11.3% after 12 months in the malnourished, at risk of malnutrition, and adequate nutrition status groups, respectively. After 32 months, the mortality rates increased to 80.8%, 42.4%, and 26.6% in each group, respectively. Associations were found among malnutrition and cognitive impairment, low prealbumin levels, and low BMI.[147] Similar results were found in a retrospective analysis of 154 patients with HF; the mortality rates were 26.5% in the malnourished group, 42% in the at risk of malnutrition group, and 6.7% in the well-nourished group.[131]

Contributing factors to cardiac cachexia include metabolic malfunction, decreased calorie intake (due to anorexia, early satiety, volume overload, nausea, depressive disorder, medications, taste changes, and increased cytokine levels), loss of lean body mass (from decreased intake, tissue hypoxia, aging, decreased exercise, inflammation, and medications), malabsorption (due to intestinal edema and decreased GI perfusion), and increased losses (from diarrhea and diuresis).[63,138,144,148] Cardiac cachexia does not have a standard definition. A nutrition assessment should look for the criteria of more than 5–7.5% unintentional weight loss over 6–12 months and a BMI <20 kg/m^2 (in patients younger than 65 years) or a BMI <22 kg/m^2 (in patients older than 65 years). In addition, patients with cardiac cachexia will have at least three of the following: albumin <3.5 grams/L, decreased total protein levels, anemia, elevated TG, elevated blood glucose, elevated lactic acid, decreased muscle strength, fatigue, anorexia, decreased lean body mass, and ongoing inflammation (elevated norepinephrine, epinephrine, cortisol, and tumor necrosis factor-alpha).[145,146,148,149]

Cardiac cachexia is thought to involve the function of the immune, metabolic, and neurohormonal systems within the body. An inflammatory response caused from hypoxia, decreased heart function, and increased GI permeability from bowel edema results in an elevation of tumor necrosis factor-alpha. Tumor necrosis factor-alpha stimulates catabolic processes that result in muscle breakdown, anorexia, and decreased exercise tolerance. The muscle breakdown exacerbates further inflammatory response.[145] Patients with cardiac cachexia have been found to have increased levels of the stress hormones norepinephrine, epinephrine, and cortisol.[150] This explanation of the mechanism of cardiac cachexia progression helps to explain why the condition is not reversible with nutrition intervention. Adequate nutrition will not reverse cardiac cachexia, but it does have the potential to diminish the negative outcomes of the condition.[145] Cardiac cachexia should be addressed as early as possible to mitigate the outcomes of increased rate of infection, poor wound healing, decubitus ulcers, bacterial overgrowth, malabsorption, loss of lean body mass, and overall morbidity and mortality.[63,138]

CORE CONCEPT 10

Cardiac cachexia is an uncontrollable loss of weight that includes muscle, fat, and eventually bone loss. It is associated with a 20–40% mortality rate annually. The condition is not reversible with nutrition intervention, but adequate nutrition may diminish negative outcomes.

Nutrition Intervention in Heart Failure

The overall goal of MNT in the patient with HF is to achieve optimal nutrition status to manage current HF, slow disease progression, and prepare the best surgical outcomes if/when left ventricular access device and/or heart transplant is indicated. An RD will ensure adequate daily calorie and protein intake and compliance with diet recommendations. In the case that a patient with HF is unable to meet nutrition needs with oral intake, nutrition support may be warranted.

Individualized Sodium Modification and Fluid Restriction

Sodium restriction is often used as a common nutrition intervention for patients with symptomatic HF. Currently, the AHA recommends a sodium restriction to <2300 mg/day for achieving general cardiovascular health, with optimal aim of ≤1500 mg sodium/day for most adults.[151] The 2020–2025 DGAs recommend <2300 mg/day sodium intake for all adults and individuals with HTN, DM, and/or CKD.[34] However, the 2022 AHA/ACC/HFSA HF guideline points out that the evidence for such sodium restriction recommendation is graded low as there is no trial to support this sodium restriction level in the HF population.[128] In small RCTs, aggressive sodium restriction to 800 mg/day for patients in ADHF during hospitalization did not lower weight, congestion, diuretic use, readmission rate, or all-cause mortality.[152,153] A pilot RCT indicated a sodium restriction to 1500 mg reduced urinary sodium and improved quality of life; however, it did not improve clinical outcomes.[154] Another pilot RCT had a sodium restriction of 1500 mg/day vs. 2300 mg/day showed improvement in BNP levels and quality of life in the lowered sodium intake group.[155] A third pilot RCT providing home delivery meals of 1500 mg sodium/day presented improvement in clinical outcomes and reduction in the readmission rate, but results were nonsignificant.[156] RCTs also showed that even with prepared meals or home visits, reducing sodium intake through diet is difficult for patients with HF to achieve.[157] The MNT for HF in the NCM 2023 suggests a sodium-modified diet for AHA Stage C HF by avoiding excessive sodium intake for symptom alleviation. It agrees with the 2022 HF guideline by using a sodium restriction diet with caution as it is often related to reduced energy and micronutrient intake.[132] The 2022 AHA/ACC/HFSA HF guideline and EAL's HF Guideline 2017 suggest a sodium intake of 2000–3000 mg/day for the HF population as this improves NYHA functional class and leg edema in patients with HFrEF. Previously, the EAL suggested a sodium restricted diet of sodium <2000 mg/day.[128,133,158]

Both the NCM and EAL suggest individualizing fluid intake/restriction based on measurement of fluid intake and output.[132,133] Fluid restriction is usually prescribed to patients with hyponatremia in acute HF with a modest improvement in hyponatremia (serum sodium <130 mg/dL). The AHA/ACC/HFSA 2022 HF guideline states that for patients with advanced HF and hyponatremia, it is unclear if fluid restriction reduces congestive symptoms.[128] However, it states that for patients with HFrEF, not in advanced HF, fluid and sodium restriction improve NYHA functional classification and leg edema.[128] The EAL previously suggested a fluid restriction of 1.4–1.9 L/day, now suggests 1–2 L fluid per day for patients with HF (NYHA Classes I–IV/AHA Stages B, C, D).[133] The EAL indicates that in patients with HF (NYHA Classes I-IV/AHA Stages B and C), those who had 2800 mg sodium intake per day had a significantly lowered readmission rate, length of stay, and mortality rate than those who had 1800mg sodium intake per day when restricting fluid to 1 L/day. However, those consuming 2800 mg sodium/day had significantly higher mortality rate than those consuming only 1900 mg sodium/day when fluid was liberalized to 2–2.4 L/day. The EAL reports for patients with advanced HF (NYHA Class IV/AHA Stage D), frequent high sodium consumption and fluid intake was associated with congestion and increased risk of death or deterioration. For patients with advanced HF, fluid intake over 2 L/day is associated with hyponatremia.[70] Thus, currently, an individualized sodium-modified diet with sodium intake of 2000–3000 mg/day and possible fluid restriction of 1–2 L/day (those who have a higher sodium intake should consume a lower fluid intake) seems reasonable for most patients with HF (NYHA Classes I-IV/ AHA Stages B, C, D). For patients with AHA Stage A HF, consider using nutrition interventions addressed in disorders of lipid metabolism and HTN sections to prevent development of symptomatic HF.

The role of the RD is to educate patients and encourage compliance with a well-balanced, individualized sodium-modified/fluid restricted diet. The education piece includes identifying low versus high sodium foods, suggesting replacements for the saltshaker (herbs, spices, citrus, etc.), encouraging patients to cook fresh foods instead of processed foods, reviewing nutrition labels to identify sodium content, and developing an individualized meal plan. Regarding fluid, the RD can explain the reason for the restriction, illustrate fluid goals in terms that make sense to patients (2 L equals 8 cups), identify foods that count as fluids (all foods that are liquid at room temperature such as soup, ice cream, popsicles, and ice chips), and educate patients on fluid measurement by utilizing fluid intake logs and familiarity with measurements of cups, glasses, and bowls. In addition to providing nutritional information, the importance of decreasing sodium and fluid intake can be explained with motivators that matter to each patient (increased quality of life, fewer sick days, more time with family). Self-monitoring of weight should also be discussed with patients with HF as unexpected weight gain in a short period of time could be a sign of fluid retention. Patients with HF should weigh themselves daily and may keep a weight log. They should contact healthcare providers if a weight gain of 1.4 kg or 3 lb or more in 1–2 days, and/or 2.3 kg or 5 lb or more in a week is noted. The RD may also provide education on signs and symptoms of fluid retention such as increased swelling in extremities, shortness of breath, orthopnea, and difficulty breathing when lying flat.[132,159] An RD can provide positive reasons for behavior change, highlight ways to preserve the taste of food, discuss strategies for overcoming cravings and thirst, and give tips on enjoying social events, showing cultural sensitivity, and gaining support from family and friends. The overall goal is to assist patients in adhering to sodium modification and possible fluid restriction to achieve increased quality of life, decreased HF symptoms, and decreased hospitalizations.

Heart-Healthy Eating Patterns

The reason for emphasizing heart-healthy eating patterns in the HF population is to decrease the risk of cardiac events and prevent/manage the comorbidities of HTN, CAD, and DM. The "Disorders of Lipid Metabolism" section of this chapter has a review of common heart-healthy eating patterns. An RD can help combine recommendations for multiple conditions. An example is **Table 9.14**, which illustrates a sample heart-healthy meal plan with approximately 2000 mg/day of sodium and less than 2 L/day of fluid.

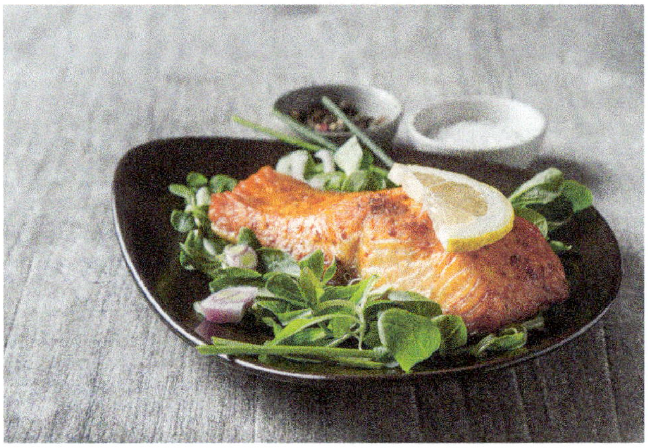

Blood Glucose Management

Patients with HF benefit from blood glucose management to decrease complications. An increase of HbA1c of 1% correlates with an 8–16% increase in the risk of hospitalization for HF and death.[63] HbA1c >8% may be a contraindication for cardiac surgery.[132] Chapter 8 *Nutrition in Diabetes Mellitus* provides a detailed description of DM and MNT for blood glucose control.

Nutrient Deficiencies

MNT for HF includes addressing possible nutrient deficiencies. Reasons for nutrient deficiencies in the HF population include overall decreased dietary intake and losses due to diuretics.[160] One goal of MNT is to ensure adequate micronutrient intake to reduce adverse events. **Table 9.15** describes possible nutrient deficiencies and treatment.[43,63,149,160–163]

Table 9.14 Heart Healthy, <2000 mg/day Sodium, <1.5 L/Day Fluid

Breakfast 1 cup oatmeal, 1 tsp cinnamon 1–2 tbsp almond slivers 1 banana or 1 cup blueberries 1 cup low fat milk	**Snack** 6 oz Greek yogurt (0% fat) ½ cup strawberries 1 cup water
Lunch 2 slices whole grain bread 3 oz roast turkey, lettuce, tomatoes 2 tsp low-fat mayo 1½ cup veggie sticks 1 orange, 1 cup seltzer water	**Snack** 1 mozzarella string cheese 6 whole grain crackers 1 cup lemon water
Dinner 4 oz grilled salmon with lemon zest 1–2 cups spinach salad (2 tsp vinegar, 1 tbsp olive oil, 2 tbsp cranberries, 2 tbsp walnuts) 1 cup brown rice	**Snack** Baked apple slices with cinnamon 1–2 tbsp natural peanut butter 1 cup water

Dietary Supplements

An estimated one in every three patients with HF uses complementary and/or alternative medicines. It is the role of the medical team, including the RD, to assist patients in evaluating nutrition supplement claims.[133,164] Precautions should be taken to avoid possible supplement–medication interactions. Evaluating dietary supplement regimens can help to prevent adverse reactions in patients with HF.

Coenzyme Q

It has been theorized that coenzyme Q may improve systolic heart function, but there is limited evidence to support this claim. Coenzyme Q should not be taken with gemfibrozil, tricyclic antidepressants, statins, beta blockers, or warfarin due to interactions. Adverse reactions associated with coenzyme Q are transient nausea, maculopapular rash, epigastric pain, dizziness, photophobia, and irritability. Current research is unclear of supporting the use of coenzyme Q in patients with HF.[70,164]

Hawthorn

In a meta-analysis of eight RCTs, hawthorn was found to improve maximal workload, pressure-heart rate

Table 9.15 Possible Nutrient Deficiencies in the Heart Failure Population

Zinc Deficiency[43,63]	
Risk factors for deficiency	ACE inhibitors, angiotension II receptor blockers, thiazide diuretics, diarrhea, alcohol use disorder
Symptoms	Dysgeusia, poor wound healing, dry skin, poor appetite, weakness, facial rash (butterfly shape)
Treatment	220 mg/day zinc sulfate
Food sources	Wheat germ, liver, turkey, beef, pork, beans, cashews, soy nuts, sunflower seeds
Thiamine Deficiency[43,63,149,161]	
Risk factors for deficiency	Alcohol use disorder, loop diuretic use, malnutrition, older age, HF, vomiting/diarrhea, malabsorption, gastric bypass, frequent hospitalization
Symptoms	Cardiovascular, GI, and nervous system impairment *Wet Beriberi:* sodium retention, peripheral vasodilation, biventricular HF
Treatment	100–200 mg/day thiamine for 4 weeks; 100 mg/day IV or IM for 5 days if symptomatic deficiency
Food sources	Enriched grains, organ meats, wheat germ, pork, peas, peanuts, sunflower seeds, rice bran, soybeans, soy milk, tofu, brewer's yeast, beans
Vitamin D Deficiency[63,162,163]	
Risk factors for deficiency	Poor oral intake, malabsorption, decreased sun exposure, steroid administration
Symptoms	Osteopenia, secondary hyperparathyroidism, cardiomyopathy, alteration of renin-angiotensin axis, may affect vascular endothelium (inflammation, thrombosis, cell proliferation), altered Ca++ channel fluxes
Treatment	50,000 IU ergocalciferol once weekly for 6–8 weeks
Food sources	Fatty fish, egg yolk, liver, fortified dairy products

Clinical Roundtable

Topic: Nutritional Management of Poor Intake with Advanced Heart Failure

Background: Advanced heart failure symptoms often lead to decreased appetite and inadequate food/beverage intake. Given the risk of malnutrition in this population, interventions aimed at adequate energy and protein intake are common. Increasing nutritional intake in patients with multiple dietary restrictions prescribed for heart failure can be a challenge for the RD.

Roundtable Discussion

1. What would you recommend to address this issue?
2. Would you prescribe nutrition supplement drinks when a patient is on a fluid restriction?
3. Would you suggest using appetite stimulants?
4. Which medication(s) would you recommend?
5. How will you illustrate the benefits versus the potential risks?
6. How would you monitor for measurable outcomes based on your recommendations?

products, and symptoms of fatigue and dyspnea with doses ranging from 160 to 1800 mg/day.[165] The risks associated with hawthorn in the HF population include interactions with beta-blockers, calcium channel blockers, digoxin, and nitrates. Adverse reactions include dizziness and vertigo. Currently there is limited evidence to support the use of hawthorn in patients with HF.[164,165]

B-Complex Vitamins

While B-complex vitamins have been demonstrated to decrease homocysteine levels, studies have failed to show any significant reduction in cardiovascular morbidity or mortality. In addition, there has been evidence to support the risk of restenosis in patients with a history of MI or recent stent who were taking either 0.8–1.2 mg/day folic acid or 0.06–0.4 mg/day B12 supplementation in combination with other vitamins.[165] Currently, routine supplementation of B vitamins is not recommended for patients with HF. Exceptions include the case of micronutrient deficiencies, alcohol-related cardiomyopathy, and macrocytic anemia.[63,70]

Antioxidants

A review of RCTs does not support the use of vitamin E, vitamin C, or beta-carotene supplements in patients with HF. Food sources of antioxidants should be encouraged rather than supplementation.[63]

Vitamin E

The risks of vitamin E supplementation in patients with HF outweigh the benefits. Observational studies suggest a decreased risk of CAD associated with vitamin E, but RCTs fail to support the theory. An increased incidence of HF was found to be associated with 400 IU/day vitamin E supplementation in the HOPE trial. This trial included 9541 adults with a 7-year follow-up. High doses of vitamin E supplementation (>400 IU/day) may be associated with mortality. For these reasons, vitamin E supplementation is not recommended for the HF population.[63,166]

Vitamin D

Vitamin D supplementation of 2000 IU daily for 6 weeks did not cause adverse effects in patients with HF. However, current research is unclear on the dosage and duration of vitamin D supplementation for patients with HF due to drug interactions between vitamin D and common medications. Vitamin D supplements are not recommended for patients with HF unless vitamin D deficiency is present.[70]

Iron

Currently, there is no evidence to report a benefit for iron supplementation in patients with HF on quality measures of readmission rates, length of stay, mortality, quality of life, or kidney function. Iron supplementation is not suggested for patients with HF.[70]

Nutrition Intervention in the Case of Cardiac Cachexia

MNT for cardiac cachexia will not reverse the condition but can aid in the prevention of further loss of muscle, fat, and bone mass.[63] The RD can assist patients with cardiac cachexia in meeting their estimated energy, protein, and nutrient needs. A calorie count can be helpful to monitor oral intake. Decreased intake and early satiety can be addressed with small/frequent meals, nutrition supplement drinks/snacks, and an appetite-stimulating medication, such as megestrol acetate. Studies have demonstrated that a dose of 160 mg/day of megestrol acetate may improve appetite within 1 week, but potential weight gain requires a higher dose (480–800 mg/day) for a longer duration. Side effects include edema, elevated blood glucose, adrenal suppression, elevated liver enzymes, and increased risk of deep vein thrombosis.[144] Oral nutrition supplements for patients with cardiac cachexia may be indicated. If a patient is unable to meet at least 70% of calorie and protein needs with oral intake, nutrition support is warranted.

Nutrition Monitoring and Evaluation in Heart Failure

The monitoring and evaluation portion of MNT for HF involves a review of all data collected during the nutrition assessment. Patient progress toward desired goals and outcomes should be documented. Monitoring and evaluation of the patient with HF may include the following: weight change, hand grip strength, muscle and fat stores, edema, adequacy of protein/energy intake, compliance with sodium modification/fluid restriction, activity tolerance, medication/dietary supplement regimen, symptoms related to food intake, chem-10 lab panel, HbA1c, standard lipid panel, hemoglobin, hematocrit, serum iron, albumin, prealbumin, total protein, BNP, CRP, and nutrition quality of life.[132]

PRACTICE POINT

The overall goal of MNT in the patient with HF is to achieve optimal nutrition status to manage current HF, slow disease progression, and prepare for the best surgical outcomes if/when left ventricular assist device and/or heart transplantation is indicated.

Nutrition Support in Cardiovascular Disease

Nutrition support is initiated at times when the patient with CVD is otherwise unable to meet calorie, protein, fat, fluid, and nutrient needs with oral intake. Nutrition support may be warranted in the case of malnutrition, cardiac cachexia, or intubation due to ADHF and/or cardiogenic shock. **Cardiogenic shock** is a severe, life-threatening condition of systemic hypoperfusion. This can be an outcome of MI or advanced HF in addition to multiple other causes.[167] Damage to the heart muscle leads to decreased cardiac output and MAP. Shock results in pulmonary congestion, systemic inflammation, and acidosis. Treatment may include mechanical ventilation, fluid resuscitation, vasopressors, and **intra-aortic balloon pump (IABP)** support. **Vasopressors** increase BP and MAP by constricting blood vessels. Examples include norepinephrine, dopamine, and dobutamine. An IABP provides short-term mechanical support to increase cardiac output. A balloon is placed in the aorta via the femoral artery without the need for invasive surgery. In the case of MI, treatment may continue with PCI or CABG. In the case of HF, treatment may continue with the placement of a VAD.[167] Special consideration should be made when providing nutrition support to this patient population. Cardiogenic shock decreases blood supply to the gut, therefore increasing gut permeability and bacterial translocation. In addition, the following factors increase risk of bowel ischemia: vasopressors, IABP, mechanical ventilation, decreased cardiac output, CKD, and a history of MI, PAD, or stroke.[125]

Enteral nutrition (EN) is the recommended route of feeding for patients with cardiac conditions when normal GI function exists.[168–172] This guideline is supported by the Critical Care Guidelines from the American Society of Parenteral and Enteral Nutrition (ASPEN) and the Society of Critical Care Medicine (SCCM), the European Society for Clinical Nutrition and Metabolism (ESPEN), along with the Academy of Nutrition and Dietetics' EAL. EN decreases the rate of infection and complications when compared to parenteral nutrition (PN). When provided appropriately, EN can improve preoperative left ventricular end-diastolic volume and immune defense. In the postoperative patient population, EN can decrease infection rate, preserve kidney function, prevent mucosal atrophy, preserve GI microbiota balance, improve gut perfusion, and decrease length of hospital stay.[169,170,173] A trial that provided EN to nine patients with cardiac conditions on the first postoperative day found the following results: increased cardiac index and splanchnic blood flow, decreased MAP by 10%, stable heart rate, and tolerance of EN. These patients received 130% of measured energy expenditure while medically managed with dobutamine and norepinephrine to maintain MAP of 70 mm Hg.[174] An additional study illustrated that EN was tolerated in patients post cardiothoracic surgery medically managed with dopamine and norepinephrine when EN was started within 2–3 days of surgery, and advanced slowly over 4–6 days.[175]

When estimating calorie and protein needs in patients with cardiac conditions, the gold standard is to use indirect calorimetry.[169,170] If indirect calorimetry is not available, use predictive equations to estimate

CASE STUDY REVISITED

Carl's condition has worsened during his hospital admission. He is now requiring mechanical ventilation as a result of pulmonary edema. The team is planning for LVAD surgery while he awaits a heart transplant.

Questions

1. What additional information is needed to determine if Carl should be started on nutrition support? If indicated, what nutrition support recommendations should be provided to the medical/surgical team?
2. Assess Carl's PES statements from his initial visit. Identify if each statement remains an active issue or if the PES statement has been resolved. If the PES statement remains an active issue, has improvement in the issue been noted? If the issue has been resolved, write a new PES statement.
3. Identify the nutrition interventions you would like to initiate for Carl to address the problems identified in your PES statements.
4. What indices are included in your monitoring and evaluation plan? Why?

energy needs, specifically the Penn State equation or the modified Penn State equation in patients older than 60 years with a BMI >30 kg/m^2 for patients on mechanically ventilation.[170] Protein needs for patients with cardiac conditions requiring nutrition support can be estimated as 1.5–2 g/kg/day UBW for patients with BMI <30 kg/m^2 and 1.5–2 g/kg/day using IBW in patients with a BMI >30 kg/m^2.[125]

ASPEN/SCCM, ESPEN, and the EAL recommend starting EN within 24–48 hours of intensive care unit (ICU) admission following fluid resuscitation.[168-171] EN should only be initiated when a patient is hemodynamically stable, vasopressor dose is decreased, MAP is 60–70 mm Hg, and intra-abdominal pressure is >20 mm Hg. A feeding tube can be placed in the stomach as the standard approach or sometimes in the small bowel in the cases of high aspiration risk, supine position, heavy sedation, and high gastric residual volumes.[125,168,171,172] A fluid-restricted formula is usually required in this population due to the presence of edema. Additional protein modulars may be used to meet elevated protein requirements to achieve positive nitrogen balance. Additional immune modulators such as selenium and fish oil may be considered to reduce inflammatory response for patients with complex and prolonged surgical procedures.[127] The ASPEN/SCCM recommendation is to initiate continuous EN at 10–20 mL/hour and advance to reach the goal rate within 48–72 hours as tolerated. EN may be advanced slowly if patients are at risk of or showing signs of refeeding syndrome (metabolic or electrolyte alternations due to reintroduction of nutrition for malnourished patients) in 3–4 days.[125,127,171,172] Patients on EN are monitored for the following: MAP, vasopressor doses, ventilatory requirements, aspiration, abdominal pain/distention, nasogastric tube output, absence of stool/flatus/bowel sounds, ileus, diarrhea, dilated and thickened bowel loops, and metabolic acidosis. Some of these symptoms can be resolved with troubleshooting. In the case of high gastric residual volume, the EN route should be into the small bowel (postpyloric feeding) and prokinetic agents may be provided, if needed.[168,170,172] Diarrhea can be addressed with a isotonic, fiber-free formula; other causes of diarrhea should always be explored (sorbitol-containing medications, antibiotics, *Clostridium difficile*, and large volumes of fluid to the small intestine).[168] In the case of sudden worsening of hemodynamic status or GI function, gastric aspiration volume >500 mL/6 hours, EN should be held.[170] EN protocols can establish standards for initiating and advancing EN, monitoring for tolerance, troubleshooting common side effects, and holding EN. Having an EN protocol in place reduces ICU and hospital length of stay and number of days of ventilation.[176] Refer to Chapter 6, *Nutrition in Critical Illness,* for more information on nutrition management of patients in the ICU.

PN can be supplemental to EN or replace EN. PN is indicated in the case of mesenteric ischemia, GI dysfunction, or intolerance of adequate energy from EN. PN should not be started until all reasonable strategies to improve EN tolerance have been exhausted.[168–170] ASPEN suggests not starting PN until 7 days postoperatively in well-nourished patients, while an earlier start can be considered in malnourished patients.[168,169] However, ESPEN suggests initiating supplement PN between day 4 and day 7 of ICU stay.[170] Once initiated, the risk of infection can be decreased with intensive insulin therapy for blood glucose

CASE STUDY REVISITED

Carl receives an LVAD and remains hospitalized while he awaits his heart transplant. After 1 month, Carl undergoes a heart transplant and recovers well and discharges home. After 6 months post-transplant, Carl is trying to improve his lifestyle to optimize his cardiac health by exercising through walking a few times a week but is limited by fatigue. He is also working to improve his eating habits by trying to cook with less sodium but forgets what other nutrition advice he received several years ago. He eats a lot of premade products for convenience to save time and energy. He has some life stressors including that he is fully responsible for the household chores as he lives alone now and has not yet returned to work since his surgery.

Questions

1. What are your recommendations for Carl to help his cardiac condition and improve his nutrition quality of life?
2. Carl's CVD progression has been followed from his initial dyslipidemia diagnosis to the complications of advanced HF and heart transplant course. What can be learned from his case in its entirety? At what other time periods may Carl have been referred to a CR program to delay/reverse disease progression?

Clinical Controversy

The New Dietary Guidelines: Implications for Medical Nutrition Therapy

The US Department of Agriculture and US Department of Health and Human Services recently released the 2025 Dietary Guidelines for Americans (DGA). 1 These Dietary Guidelines are updated every 5 years and serve as the cornerstone of nutrition program and policy planning, which in turn can influence school lunch programs, SNAP benefits and nutrition education to the public. Central to the new guidelines is a theme to "Eat Real Foods", prioritizing nutrient dense, whole foods with limits to ultra processed foods, added sugars and refined carbohydrates. Protein and vegetables serve as the foundation for achieving healthy eating patterns as represented by the new Dietary Food Pyramid which appears as an upside-down version of the previous 2020 DGA edition.

Many of these suggestions are evidence-based and are supported by nutrition professionals. Research has demonstrated the negative association between increased consumption of ultra processed foods and risk of cardiac disease and mortality. 2 Similarly, current advice to lower sodium intake is consistent with previous recommendations as there is a well-known dose response relationship between sodium intake and blood pressure as well as cardiovascular events. 3 However, other aspects of the guidelines are controversial. For example, the DGAs define healthy fats as any that are in their whole, natural state. This includes both plant and animal-based fats. Use of butter and beef tallow as appropriate alternatives to plant-based fats such as olive and canola oil are allowed despite their higher saturated fat content. Furthermore, directives to consume a high protein diet that includes red meat along with full fat dairy, while still limiting saturated fat intake to less than 10% of total calories can be a challenge and are not supported by research. Experts fear that some of this messaging may lead to unnecessary high protein and saturated fat intakes, along with avoidance of whole grains, which can be helpful for prevention and progression of heart disease and associated conditions. This controversy has direct implications for Medical Nutrition Therapy in patients with heart disease.

Questions

1. What are the challenges around diet education on the new guidelines? Consider advice on reducing ultra-processed foods and replacing them with fresh produce.
2. Do you agree with the revised food pyramid? Why or why not?

References

1. U.S. Department of Agriculture and U.S. Department of Health and Human Services. *Dietary Guidelines for Americans*, 2025-2030. 10th Edition. January 2026. Available at DietaryGuidelines.gov.
2. Lane M M, Gamage E, Du S, Ashtree D N, McGuinness A J, Gauci S et al. Ultra-processed food exposure and adverse health outcomes: umbrella review of epidemiological meta-analyses *BMJ* 2024; 384 :e077310 doi:10.1136/bmj-2023-077310
3. Filippini T, Malavolti M, Whelton PK, Naska A, Orsini N, Vinceti M. Blood Pressure Effects of Sodium Reduction: Dose-Response Meta-Analysis of Experimental Studies. Circulation. 2021 Apr 20;143(16):1542-1567. doi: 10.1161/CIRCULATIONAHA.120.050371. Epub 2021 Feb 15. PMID: 33586450; PMCID: PMC8055199

PRACTICE POINT

Nutrition support can be initiated at times when the patient with CVD is otherwise unable to meet calorie, protein, fluid, and nutrient needs with oral intake. Nutrition support may be warranted in the case of malnutrition, cardiac cachexia, or intubation due to acute decompensated heart failure and/or cardiogenic shock.

management and protocols for preventing central line bacteremia. In the cardiac population, care should be taken to minimize PN volume and ensure that TGs remain <400 mg/dL.[125,176]

Once a patient is no longer requiring mechanical ventilation and GI function is confirmed, an oral diet can be advanced as tolerated. Intake can be monitored with calorie counts, and nutrition support may be discontinued when the patient is able to meet at least 70% of energy and protein needs with oral intake.

Cardiac Rehabilitation as Secondary Prevention

Cardiac rehabilitation services (CR) are an evidence-based, team-based, physician-supervised multimodal behavioral and medical rehabilitative program that aims to improve cardiovascular health as a secondary prevention method for those with established CVD and/or at increased risk for developing CVD. The benefits of CR are increasing the functional capacity of patients after their cardiovascular events/surgeries, reducing risks for future CVD events, alleviating and/or decreasing anginal pain, reducing disability, improving quality of life, and reducing total and cardiac morbidity and mortality rates.[177,178] Although unclear for the mechanism for reduction of cardiovascular mortality in patients receiving CR, assumptions include improved myocardial revascularization, mitigated fatal dysrhythmias, improved cardiac risk factor measures, improved cardiac fitness, and increased patient surveillance.[178] A meta-analysis has indicated that CR significantly decreases recurrent MI and mortality rates.[177] One observational study found that patients post CABG participating in a CR program, a 10-year absolute risk reduction in all-cause mortality of more than 12% was demonstrated.[177] Patients who participated in CR had a 20–30% reduction in readmission in the year after experiencing a cardiac event.[177] The AHA/ACC states all patients with chronic coronary disease and appropriate indications should be referred to a CR program for outcome improvement.[179]

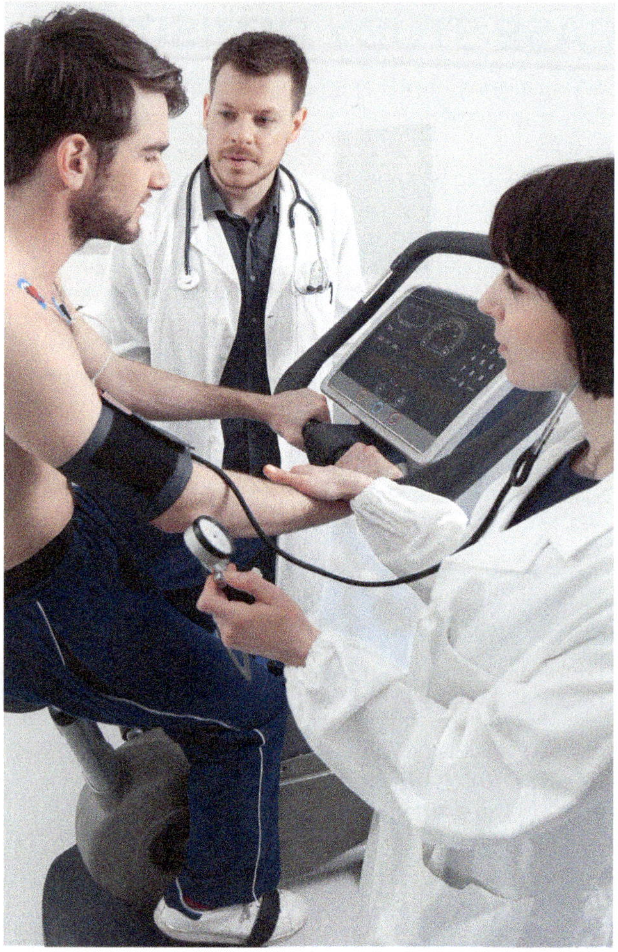

CR is usually classified in three phases. Phase I refers to a brief period of inpatient rehabilitation during hospitalization related to CVD events/medical procedures with patient education on treatment options for current symptoms, risk factors discussion, and lifestyle and dietary modification suggestions. Phase I of CR is now less formalized due to short durations of hospital stay. Phase II refers to a physician-supervised outpatient (at the outpatient department of a hospital or a clinic) usually with a heart rhythm–monitored exercise program postdischarge. This cardiac rehabilitative exercise program usually consists of 36 sessions. This is when the most intensive lifestyle modification therapies are delivered, and an RD can play a vital role. Most of the time, a CR program is commonly referred to as phase II of a CR program. This section of text is mainly dedicated to phase II CR. Phase III refers to a continuation of unmonitored exercise with a comprehensive wellness plan that helps patients continue making heart-healthy lifestyle choices.[179,180]

The phase II CR program usually consists of these core components: physician-prescribed aerobic exercise training, cardiac lifestyle risk factor modification (nutritional counseling on a heart-healthy diet, weight management, BP management, lipid management, DM management, tobacco cessation, and physical activity counseling), psychosocial assessment, and outcomes assessment.[179,181,182] This range of measures targets modifiable ASCVD risk factors. The phase II CR program is a team effort that requires a group of medical specialists including physicians, registered nurses, and exercise physiologists, with the addition of RDs, possibly psychiatrists, and social workers to deliver such a medically supervised rehabilitative exercise with patient education.

Medicare and most commercial insurances provide coverage for both phase I and phase II CR service. Phase III of CR is generally not specifically addressed by Medicare coverage. Criteria for a patient to be qualified for a referral to a phase II CR program includes at least one of the following conditions: an acute MI (within the preceding 12 months), a CABG surgery, current stable angina pectoris, heart valve repair or replacement, PCI or coronary stenting, a heart or heart–lung transplant, and chronic HF with LVEF ≤35% and NYHA Class II to IV symptoms despite being on optimal HF therapy for at least 6 weeks.[181-184]

Currently there are two types of phase II CR services: the traditional cardiac rehabilitation (TCR) and the intensive cardiac rehabilitation (ICR). TCR, which has been approved by the Centers for Medicare and Medicaid (CMS) since 1982, is typically 36 supervised aerobic exercise session programs that each last for 30–60 minutes delivered three times a week during a 12-week period including some form of education. ICR services are furnished in a more rigorous manner by increasing the frequency and number of specific interventions to improve CVD outcomes in decreasing LDL-C, TGs, BMI, systolic and diastolic BP, and the need for cholesterol, BP, and DM medications. The length for an ICR program is doubled to 72 sessions: typically, 36 supervised 30–60 minutes exercise sessions plus 36 formal and structural heart health education sessions delivered in conjunction, three times a week during a 12-week period. Nationally CMS-approved ICR programs currently include Dr. Ornish's Program for Reversing Heart Disease, the Pritikin Program, and the Benson-Henry Institute Cardiac Wellness Program, which are all multicomponent intervention programs including supervised exercise, nutrition counseling, and behavioral education each with a different focus.[185] Among Medicare beneficiaries, ICR is associated with a 12% lower mortality than TCR, but no difference has been found in nonfatal cardiac events or hospitalizations due to CVD between ICR and TCR. Additionally, higher attendance to either ICR or TCR is associated with lower mortality.[186]

Despite the frequent recommendations for a CR program for patients with CVD, CR has been underutilized. Approximately 80% of patients post MI, 60% of patients after a PCI or coronary angioplasty, and 10.5% of patients with HF were referred to CR. Approximately 35% of patients with a history of acute MI received subsequent CR.[187] Besides a referral gap, there is also an enrollment gap. Among patients referred, only about 50% enrolled and participated in CR. Moreover, CR completion rate (≥36 sessions) is <30%. Ethnic people of color, those ≥65 years old, women, those with less than a college education, caregiver responsibilities, multiple comorbidities, limited program access, and/or insufficient health insurance coverage are less likely to utilize CR.[177,188] It is estimated that if CR completion rates improved to 70% or more, approximately 25,000 deaths and 180,000 hospitalizations would be prevented annually.[189,190] Lack of physician endorsement of CR, especially from a cardiologist or a cardiac surgeon, greatly reduces patient enrollment rate. Additionally, the limited availability of CR services nationwide, especially in rural areas, limits CR referrals. Moreover, the high cost of maintaining the program with relatively low reimbursement rates could be a disincentive.[191] To improve participation and completion of CR, novel models to deliver CR as home-based, remote, and virtual services are being developed, tested, and implemented. CMS approved Telehealth CR during COVID-19 as a temporary addition due to the COVID-19 Public Health Emergency (PHE).[190]

RDs play an important role in CR to educate, guide, and support patients with CVD for a healthier lifestyle. An RD can deliver MNT for CVD and/or HF via individual counseling and/or group-class

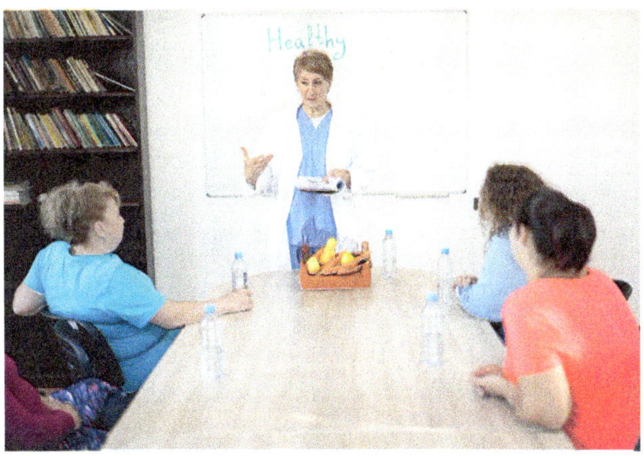

settings with follow-ups when patients come to their CR sessions. An RD will also need to be familiar with MNT for common CVD comorbidities, such as overweight/obesity, HTN, dyslipidemia, DM, and CKD. An RD may additionally receive training in ECG interpretation, BP monitoring, blood glucose monitoring, exercise stress testing, external counter pulsation therapy to alleviate anginal pain of patients, patient functional capacity assessment during exercise therapy, and cardiopulmonary resuscitation (CPR), a life-saving technique used in emergency situations when an individual is in cardiac or cardiopulmonary arrest. A pilot study showed that expanding the role of an RD above the standard scope of nutrition practice is a cost-effective method to provide nutrition intervention in a CR setting.[192] However, a systematic review suggests that currently there is lack of guidance of standard nutrition practice in the CR setting.[193] More research for high-quality nutrition interventions that optimize and maintain nutrition improvements in patients with CVD attending CR is needed.

CORE CONCEPT 11

Cardiac rehabilitation as a secondary prevention includes physician-prescribed aerobic exercise training, cardiac lifestyle risk factor modification including nutrition counseling on a heart-healthy diet, weight and diabetes management, tobacco cessation, psychosocial support and outcomes assessment.

Chapter Summary

Cardiovascular disease (CVD) is a group of disorders of the heart and blood vessels. Atherosclerotic cardiovascular disease (ASCVD), the heart blood vessel disease that is mainly atherosclerotic in origin, is the major underlying cause of CVD, and remains the leading cause of morbidity and mortality globally. Atherosclerosis is the buildup of cholesterol deposits, or plaques, in the heart's blood vessels resulting in thickening and hardening of the arterial wall. ASCVD is mainly defined as coronary heart disease (CHD) or coronary artery disease (CAD), cerebrovascular disease, and peripheral artery disease (PAD) depending on the location of the plaque. Atherosclerotic plaques can erode or rupture, causing thrombosis and a closure of the blood vessel, resulting in myocardial infarction (MI) or heart attack, stroke, extremity ischemia, and death. Heart failure (HF) is the final stage of CVD and its related conditions. CVD is currently the number one cause of death worldwide. Prevention and early management are critical to improving outcomes. Medical nutrition therapy (MNT) is an integral part of the prevention and management of CVD and related conditions.

Key Terms

cardiovascular disease (CVD), atherosclerotic cardiovascular disease (ASCVD), atherosclerosis, myocardium, systole, diastole, stroke volume, cardiac output, ejection fraction (EF), mean arterial pressure (MAP), total peripheral resistance, myocytes, Purkinje fibers, electrocardiogram, foam cells, vulnerable plaque, thrombosis, embolism, lipoproteins, apolipoproteins, lipoprotein(a), apolipoprotein B100, dyslipidemia, hypertriglyceridemia, familial hypercholesterolemia (FH), xanthomas, hypertension (HTN), primary (essential) HTN, systolic blood pressure, diastolic blood pressure, coronary artery disease (CAD), ischemic heart disease, angina pectoris, myocardial infarction (MI), ischemic cardiomyopathy, stroke, peripheral artery disease (PAD), cardiac catheterization, angiogram, percutaneous coronary intervention (PCI), percutaneous transluminal coronary angioplasty (PTCA), coronary artery bypass graft (CABG), cardiopulmonary bypass, heart failure (HF), dyspnea, acute decompensated heart failure (ADHF), left ventricular assist device (LVAD), subjective global assessment (SGA), obesity paradox, cardiac cachexia, tumor necrosis factor-alpha, cardiogenic shock, vasopressors, intra-aortic balloon pump (IABP), cardiac rehabilitation

Acknowledgments

The author acknowledges Alexis Madej for contributions to the previous version of this chapter.

References

1. Frąk W, Wojtasińska A, Lisińska W, Młynarska E, Franczyk B, Rysz J. Pathophysiology of cardiovascular diseases: new insights into molecular mechanisms of atherosclerosis, arterial hypertension, and coronary artery disease. *Biomedicines*. 2022;10(8). doi:10.3390/biomedicines10081938
2. Kusumoto F. Cardiovascular Disorders: Heart disease. In: Hammer G, McPhee S, eds. *Pathophysiology of Disease: An Introduction to Clinical Medicine*. 7th ed. McGraw-Hill Education; 2013.
3. Martin SS, Aday AW, Almarzooq ZI, et al. 2024 Heart disease and stroke statistics: a report of US and global data from the American Heart Association. *Circulation*. 2024;149(8):e347–e913. doi:10.1161/CIR.0000000000001209
4. Arnett DK, Blumenthal RS, Albert MA, et al. 2019 ACC/AHA Guideline on the Primary Prevention of Cardiovascular Disease: A Report of the American College of Cardiology/American Heart Association Task Force on Clinical Practice Guidelines. *Circulation*. 2019;140(11):e596–e646. doi:10.1161/CIR.0000000000000678
5. Grundy SM, Stone NJ, Bailey AL, et al. 2018 AHA/ACC/AACVPR/AAPA/ABC/ACPM/ADA/AGS/APhA/ASPC/NLA/PCNA Guideline on the Management of Blood Cholesterol :A Report of the American College of Cardiology/American Heart Association Task Force on Clinical Practice Guidelines. *Circulation*. 2019;139(25):e1082–e1143. doi:10.1161/CIR.0000000000000625
6. U.S. Centers for Disease Control and Prevention. About Heart Disease. Updated May 15, 2024. Accessed July 13, 2024. https://www.cdc.gov/heart-disease/about/index.html
7. U.S. Centers for Disease Control and Prevention. Heart Disease Facts. Updated May 15, 2024. Accessed July 13, 2024. https://www.cdc.gov/heart-disease/data-research/facts-stats/index.html
8. World Health Organization. Cardiovascular Disease (CVDs). Updated June 11, 2021. Accessed July 13, 2024. https://www.who.int/news-room/fact-sheets/detail/cardiovascular-diseases-(cvds)
9. Harris DM. The Peripheral Vascular System. *Mohrman and Heller's Cardiovascular Physiology*. 10th Ed. McGraw-Hill; 2023.
10. Gray H, Lewis WH. *Anatomy of the Human Body*. 20th ed .Bartleby.com; 2000.
11. Stefanadis C, Antoniou CK, Tsiachris D, Pietri P. Coronary atherosclerotic vulnerable plaque: current perspectives. *J Am Heart Assoc*. 2017;6(3). doi:10.1161/jaha.117.005543
12. American College of Cardiology. ASCVD Risk Estimator Plus. Accessed July 29, 2024. https://tools.acc.org/ascvd-risk-estimator-plus/#!/calculate/estimate
13. Eckel RH, Jakicic JM, Ard JD, et al. 2013 AHA/ACC Guideline on Lifestyle Management to Reduce Cardiovascular Risk. *Circulation*. 2014;129(25_suppl_2):S76–S99. doi:10.1161/01.cir.0000437740.48606.d1
14. Dietetics AoNa. Evidence Analysis Library. Accessed July 29, 2023. https://www.andeal.org/
15. Sacks FM, Lichtenstein AH, Wu JHY, et al. Dietary fats and cardiovascular disease: a presidential advisory from the American Heart Association. *Circulation*. 2017;136(3):e1–e23. doi:10.1161/CIR.0000000000000510
16. Mann DL ZD, Libby P, Bonow RO, Braunwald E, eds. *Braunwald's Heart Disease: A Textbook of Cardiovascular Medicine*. Elsevier Saunders; 2015.
17. Jacobson TA, Ito MK, Maki KC, et al. National lipid association recommendations for patient-centered management of dyslipidemia: part 1—full report. *J Clin Lipidol*. 2015;9(2):129–169. doi:10.1016/j.jacl.2015.02.003
18. DynaMedex. *Lipoprotein(a) and Cardiovascular Disease*. EBSCO Information Services; 2024.
19. Maranhão RC, Carvalho PO, Strunz CC, Pileggi F. Lipoprotein (a): structure, pathophysiology and clinical implications. *Arq Bras Cardiol*. Jul 2014;103(1):76–84. doi:10.5935/abc.20140101
20. Karanchi H MV, Wyne K. *Hypertriglyceridemia*. StatPearls; 2024.
21. Academy of Nutrition and Dietetics, Nutrition Care Manual. Hypertriglyceridemia. Accessed July 13, 2024. https://www.nutritioncaremanual.org/topic.cfm?ncm_category_id=1&lv1=272984&lv2=35987&lv3=8477&ncm_toc_id=8477&ncm_heading=Nutrition%20Care
22. Yang AL, McNabb-Baltar J. Hypertriglyceridemia and acute pancreatitis. *Pancreatology*. 2020/07/01/ 2020;20(5):795–800. doi:10.1016/j.pan.2020.06.005
23. Martin SS, Blaha MJ, Elshazly MB, et al. Comparison of a novel method vs the Friedewald equation for estimating low-density lipoprotein cholesterol levels from the standard lipid profile. *JAMA*. 2013;310(19):2061–2068. doi:10.1001/jama.2013.280532
24. Jellinger PS, Handelsman Y, Rosenblit PD, et al. American Association of Clinical Endocrinologists and American College of Endocrinology Guidelines for Management of Dyslipidemia and Prevention of Cardiovascular Disease. *Endocr Pract*. 2017;23(Suppl 2):1–87. doi:10.4158/ep171764.Appgl
25. Academy of Nutrition and Dietetics, Nutrition Care Manual. Cardiovascular Disease: General Guidance-Nutritional Indicators. Accessed July 13, 2024. https://www.nutritioncaremanual.org/topic.cfm?ncm_category_id=1&lv1=272984&lv2=35987&lv3=255518&ncm_toc_id=267296&ncm_heading=Nutrition%20Care
26. Wong ND. Identifying the very-high-risk atherosclerotic cardiovascular disease patient. *J Am Coll Cardiol*. 2019;74(20):2508–2510. doi:10.1016/j.jacc.2019.09.023
27. Academy of Nutrition and Dietetics, Nutrition Care Manual. General Guidance for Disorders of Lipid Metabolism. Accessed July 13, 2024. https://www.nutritioncaremanual.org/topic.cfm?ncm_category_id=1&lv1=272984&lv2=35987&lv3=255518&ncm_toc_id=273664&ncm_heading=Nutrition%20Care
28. Wu H, Luan Ja, Forgetta V, et al. Utility of genetically predicted Lp(a) (lipoprotein [a]) and ApoB levels for cardiovascular risk assessment. *Circ Genom Precis Med*. 2021;14(5):e003312 .doi:10.1161/CIRCGEN.121.003312
29. Alebna PL, Mehta A. An update on lipoprotein(a): the latest on testing, treatment, and guideline recommendations .Expert analysis. *J Am Coll Cardiol*. September 13, 2023.
30. Wilson DP, Jacobson TA, Jones PH, et al. Use of lipoprotein(a) in clinical practice: a biomarker whose time has come. A scientific statement from the National Lipid Association. *J Clin Lipidol*. 2019;13(3):374–392. doi:10.1016/j.jacl.2019.04.010
31. Enkhmaa B, Anuurad E, Berglund L. Lipoprotein (a): impact by ethnicity and environmental and medical conditions. *J Lipid Res*. 2016;57(7):1111–1125. doi:10.1194/jlr.R051904
32. Civeira F. Guidelines for the diagnosis and management of heterozygous familial hypercholesterolemia. *Atherosclerosis*. 2004;173(1):55–68. doi:10.1016/j.atherosclerosis.2003.11.010

33. U.S. Centers for Disease Control and Prevention. About Familial Hypercholesterolemia. Updated May 15, 2024. Accessed July 13, 2024. https://www.cdc.gov/heart-disease-family-history/about/about-familial-hypercholesterolemia.html
34. U.S. Department of Agriculture and U.S. Department of Health and Human Services. *Dietary Guidelines for Americans, 2020–2025*. 9th ed. 2020.
35. Academy of Nutrition and Dietetics, Evidence Analysis Library. Disorders of Lipid Metabolism- Major Recommendations. Accessed October 4, 2017. http://www.andeal.org/topic.cfm?menu=5300&cat=4530.
36. Sisson E, Ingram J, Babalola R, Alhomoud I. *Quick Guide to Medications*. 12th ed. American Association of Diabetes Educators; 2022.
37. DynaMedex. *Management of Dislypidemias*. EBSCO Information Services; 2024.
38. Kennedy C, Köller Y, Surkova E. Effect of Coenzyme Q10 on statin-associated myalgia and adherence to statin therapy: a systematic review and meta-analysis. *Atherosclerosis*. 2020;299:1–8. doi:10.1016/j.atherosclerosis.2020.03.006
39. DynaMedex. *Statin-Associated Muscle Symptoms*. EBSCO Information Services.
40. DynaMedex. *Omega-3-acid Ethyl Esters, In: Merative Micromedex DRUGDEX (electronic version)*. Merative Healthcare Solutions/EBSCO Information Services.
41. Jenkins DJ, Kendall CW, Vuksan V, et al. Soluble fiber intake at a dose approved by the US Food and Drug Administration for a claim of health benefits: serum lipid risk factors for cardiovascular disease assessed in a randomized controlled crossover trial. *Am J Clin Nutr*. 2002;75(5):834–839. doi:10.1093/ajcn/75.5.834
42. Jenkins DJA, Spence JD, Giovannucci EL, et al. Supplemental vitamins and minerals for cardiovascular disease prevention and treatment: JACC Focus Seminar. *J Am Coll Cardiol*. 2021;77(4):423–436. doi:10.1016/j.jacc.2020.09.619
43. Pronsky ZM ED, Ayoob K. *Food-Medication Interactions*. 18th ed. Food Medication Interactions; 2015.
44. Lloyd-Jones DM, Morris PB, Ballantyne CM, et al. 2022 ACC Expert consensus decision pathway on the role of nonstatin therapies for LDL-cholesterol lowering in the management of atherosclerotic cardiovascular disease risk. *J Am Coll Cardiol*. 2022;80(14):1366–1418. doi:10.1016/j.jacc.2022.07.006
45. Academy of Nutrition and Dietetics, Evidence Analysis Library. Saturated Fat (DLM-SF) Guideline - Executive Summary of Recommendations. Accessed July 29, 2024. https://www.andeal.org/topic.cfm?menu=5300&cat=6215
46. Academy of Nutrition and Dietetics, Evidence Analysis Library. Saturated Fat (DLM-SF) Systematic Review. Accessed July 29, 2024. https://www.andeal.org/topic.cfm?menu=5300&cat=5890
47. Academy of Nutrition and Dietetics, Nutrition Care Manual. Summary of Nutrition Interventions for Cardiovascular Disease. Accessed July 30, 2024. https://www.nutritioncaremanual.org/topic.cfm?ncm_category_id=1&lv1=272984&lv2=255501&lv3=272406&ncm_toc_id=272406&ncm_heading=Nutrition%20Care
48. Yu E, Malik VS, Hu FB. Cardiovascular disease prevention by diet modification: JACC Health Promotion Series. *J Am Coll Cardiol*. 2018;72(8):914–926. doi:10.1016/j.jacc.2018.02.085
49. Lichtenstein AH, Appel LJ, Vadiveloo M, et al. 2021 Dietary guidance to improve cardiovascular health: a scientific statement from the American Heart Association. *Circulation*. 2021;144(23):e472–e487. doi:10.1161/CIR.0000000000001031
50. Tosti V, Bertozzi B, Fontana L. Health benefits of the Mediterranean diet: metabolic and molecular mechanisms. *J Gerontol A Biol Sci Med Sci*. 2018;73(3):318–326. doi:10.1093/gerona/glx227
51. Academy of Nutrition and Dietetics, Evidence Analysis Library. Mediterranean Diet and Cardiovascular Risk Factors (MDCRF) Umbrella Review. Accessed July 13, 2024. https://www.andeal.org/topic.cfm?menu=6083&cat=6186
52. Academy of Nutrition and Dietetics, Nutrition Care Manual. General, Healthful Mediterranean Nutrition Therapy. Accessed July 30, 2024. https://www.nutritioncaremanual.org/client_ed.cfm?ncm_client_ed_id=408
53. Estruch R, Ros E, Salas-Salvadó J, et al. Primary prevention of cardiovascular disease with a Mediterranean diet. *NEJM*. 2013;368(14):1279–1290. doi:10.1056/NEJMoa1200303
54. Estruch R, Ros E, Salas-Salvadó J, et al. Primary Prevention of cardiovascular disease with a Mediterranean diet supplemented with extra-virgin olive oil or nuts. *NEJM*. 2018;378(25):e34. doi:10.1056/NEJMoa1800389
55. Kargin D, Tomaino L, Serra-Majem L. Experimental outcomes of the Mediterranean diet: lessons learned from the predimed randomized controlled trial. *Nutrients*. 2019;11(12). doi:10.3390/nu11122991
56. Vannice G, Rasmussen H. Position of the Academy of Nutrition and Dietetics: Dietary fatty acids for healthy adults. *J Acad Nutr Diet*. 2014;114(1):136–153. doi:10.1016/j.jand.2013.11.001
57. Academy of Nutrition and Dietetics, Nutrition Care Manual. Cardiovascular Disease: General Guidance. Accessed July 13, 2024. https://www.nutritioncaremanual.org/topic.cfm?ncm_category_id=1&lv1=272984&lv2=255501&lv3=271996&ncm_toc_id=271996&ncm_heading=Nutrition%20Care
58. Academy of Nutrition and Dietetics, Nutrition Care Manual. LDL Cholesterol-Lowering Nutrition Therapy. Accessed July 30, 2024. https://www.nutritioncaremanual.org/client_ed.cfm?ncm_client_ed_id=466
59. Eckel RH, Borra S, Lichtenstein AH, Yin-Piazza SY. Understanding the complexity of trans fatty acid reduction in the American diet: American Heart Association Trans Fat Conference 2006: report of the Trans Fat Conference Planning Group. *Circulation*. 2007;115(16):2231–2246. doi:10.1161/circulationaha.106.181947
60. Johnson SA, Kirkpatrick CF, Miller NH, Carson JAS, Handu D, Moloney L. Saturated fat intake and the prevention and management of cardiovascular disease in adults: an Academy of Nutrition and Dietetics evidence-based nutrition practice guideline. *J Acad Nutr Diet*. Dec 2023;123(12):1808–1830. doi:10.1016/j.jand.2023.07.017
61. Mozaffarian D, Katan MB, Ascherio A, Stampfer MJ, Willett WC. Trans fatty acids and cardiovascular disease. *NEJM*. 2006;354(15):1601–1613. doi:10.1056/NEJMra054035
62. Van Horn L, McCoin M, Kris-Etherton PM, et al. The evidence for dietary prevention and treatment of cardiovascular disease. *J Am Diet Assoc*. 2008;108(2):287–331. doi:10.1016/j.jada.2007.10.050
63. Dunn SP, Bleske B, Dorsch M, Macaulay T, Van Tassell B, Vardeny O. Nutrition and heart failure: impact of drug therapies and management strategies. *Nutr Clin Pract*. 2009;24(1):60–75. doi:10.1177/0884533608329299
64. Mozaffarian D, Gottdiener JS, Siscovick DS. Intake of tuna or other broiled or baked fish versus fried fish and

cardiac structure, function, and hemodynamics. *Am J Cardiol*. 2006;97(2):216–222. doi:10.1016/j.amjcard.2005.08.025
65. Bucher HC, Hengstler P, Schindler C, Meier G. N-3 polyunsaturated fatty acids in coronary heart disease: a meta-analysis of randomized controlled trials. *Am J Med*. Mar 2002;112(4):298–304. doi:10.1016/s0002-9343(01)01114-7
66. Mozaffarian D. Fish and n-3 fatty acids for the prevention of fatal coronary heart disease and sudden cardiac death. *Am J Clin Nutr*. Jun 2008;87(6):1991s–1996s. doi:10.1093/ajcn/87.6.1991S
67. Academy of Nutrition and Dietetics, Nutrition Care Manual. Heart-Healthy Fats: Omega-3 Fatty Acids. Accessed July 30, 2024. https://www.nutritioncaremanual.org/client_ed.cfm?ncm_client_ed_id=102
68. Wang C, Harris WS, Chung M, et al. n-3 Fatty acids from fish or fish-oil supplements, but not alpha-linolenic acid, benefit cardiovascular disease outcomes in primary- and secondary-prevention studies: a systematic review. *Am J Clin Nutr*. 2006;84(1):5–17. doi:10.1093/ajcn/84.1.5
69. U.S. Food & Drug Administration. Advice about Eating Fish. Updated March 5, 2024. Accessed July 13, 2024. https://www.fda.gov/food/consumers/advice-about-eating-fish
70. Academy of Nutrition and Dietetics, Evidence Analysis Library. Heart Failure (HF) Systematic Review. Accessed July 13, 2024. https://www.andeal.org/topic.cfm?menu=5289&cat=5361
71. Burr ML, Ashfield-Watt PA, Dunstan FD, et al. Lack of benefit of dietary advice to men with angina: results of a controlled trial. *Eur J Clin Nutr*. Feb 2003;57(2):193–200. doi:10.1038/sj.ejcn.1601539
72. Raitt MH, Connor WE, Morris C, et al. Fish oil supplementation and risk of ventricular tachycardia and ventricular fibrillation in patients with implantable defibrillators: a randomized controlled trial. *JAMA*. Jun 15 2005;293(23):2884–2891. doi:10.1001/jama.293.23.2884
73. Academy of Nutrition and Dietetics, Nutrition Care Manual. Heart-Healthy Fiber Tips. Accessed July 30, 2024. https://www.nutritioncaremanual.org/client_ed.cfm?ncm_client_ed_id=101
74. Retelny VS, Neuendorf A, Roth JL. Nutrition protocols for the prevention of cardiovascular disease. *Nutr Clin Pract*. 2008;23(5):468–476. doi:10.1177/0884533608323425
75. Johnson RK, Appel LJ, Brands M, et al. Dietary sugars intake and cardiovascular health. *Circulation*. 2009;120(11):1011–1020. doi:10.1161/CIRCULATIONAHA.109.192627
76. Jadhav HB, Annapure US. Triglycerides of medium-chain fatty acids: a concise review. *J Food Sci Technol*. 2023;60(8):2143–2152. doi:10.1007/s13197-022-05499-w
77. Academy of Nutrition and Dietetics, Nutrition Care Manual. High Triglycerides Nutrition Therapy. Accessed July 30, 2024. https://www.nutritioncaremanual.org/client_ed.cfm?ncm_client_ed_id=109
78. World Health Organization. Hypertension. Updated March 16, 2023. Accessed July 20, 2024. https://www.who.int/news-room/fact-sheets/detail/hypertension
79. Sutters M. Overview: Systemic Hypertension. In: Papadakis MA, McPhee SJ, Rabow MW, McQuaid KR, eds. *Current Medical Diagnosis & Treatment 2023*. McGraw-Hill Education; 2023.
80. Tackling G, Borhade M. *Hypertensive Heart Disease*. StatPearls; 2024.
81. Reboussin DM, Allen NB, Griswold ME, et al. Systematic review for the 2017 ACC/AHA/AAPA/ABC/ACPM/AGS/APhA/ASH/ASPC/NMA/PCNA Guideline for the Prevention, Detection, Evaluation, and Management of High Blood Pressure in Adults: A Report of the American College of Cardiology/American Heart Association Task Force on Clinical Practice Guidelines. *Hypertension*. 2018;71(6):e116–e135. doi:10.1161/HYP.0000000000000067
82. Whelton P, Carey R, Aronow W, et al. 2017 ACC/AHA/AAPA/ABC/ACPM/AGS/APhA/ASH/ASPC/NMA/PCNA Guideline for the Prevention, Detection, Evaluation, and Management of High Blood Pressure in Adults: A Report of the American College of Cardiology/American Heart Association Task Force on Clinical Practice Guidelines. *JACC*. 2018;71(19):e127–e248. doi:10.1016/j.jacc.2017.11.006
83. Academy of Nutrition and Dietetics, Nutrition Care Manual. Hypertension. Accessed July 20, 2024. https://www.nutritioncaremanual.org/topic.cfm?ncm_category_id=1&lv1=272984&lv2=8480&ncm_toc_id=8480&ncm_heading=Nutrition%20Care
84. Academy of Nutrition and Dietetics, Evidence Analysis Library. Hypertension Systematic Review. Accessed July 13, 2024. https://www.andeal.org/topic.cfm?menu=5285&cat=5132
85. Academy of Nutrition and Dietetics, Evidence Analysis Library. Pre-Hypertension and Hypertension Systematic Review. Accessed July 13, 2024. https://www.andeal.org/topic.cfm?menu=5285&cat=6243
86. Academy of Nutrition and Dietetics, Nutrition Care Manual. Hypertension Nutrition Therapy. Accessed July 20, 2024. https://www.nutritioncaremanual.org/client_ed.cfm?ncm_client_ed_id=99
87. James PA, Oparil S, Carter BL, et al. 2014 evidence-based guideline for the management of high blood pressure in adults: report from the panel members appointed to the Eighth Joint National Committee (JNC 8). *JAMA*. 2014;311(5):507–520. doi:10.1001/jama.2013.284427
88. Charney P. *Academy of Nutrition and Dietetics Pocket Guide to Nutrition Assessment*. 4th ed. Academy of Nutrition & Dietetics; 2022.
89. Academy of Nutrition and Dietetics, Nutrition Care Manual Hypertension Guideline- Major Recommendations. Accessed July 13, 2024. https://www.andeal.org/topic.cfm?menu=5285&cat=5592
90. U.S. Department of Health and Human Services, National Institutes of Health, National Heart, Lung, and Blood Institute. Your guide to lowering blood pressure with DASH - DASH eating plan. 2006. Accessed July 30, 2024. https://www.nhlbi.nih.gov/files/docs/public/heart/new_dash.pdf
91. Sacks FM, Svetkey LP, Vollmer WM, et al. Effects on blood pressure of reduced dietary sodium and the Dietary Approaches to Stop Hypertension (DASH) diet. DASH-Sodium Collaborative Research Group. *NEJM*. 2001;344(1):3–10. doi:10.1056/nejm200101043440101
92. National Heart, Lung, and Blood Institute. The Science Behind the DASH Eating Plan. Updated December 29, 2021. Accessed July 20, 2024. https://www.nhlbi.nih.gov/education/dash/research
93. Blumenthal JA, Babyak MA, Hinderliter A, et al. Effects of the DASH diet alone and in combination with exercise and weight loss on blood pressure and cardiovascular biomarkers in men and women with high blood pressure: the ENCORE study. *Arch Intern Med*. 2010;170(2):126–135. doi:10.1001/archinternmed.2009.470
94. Whelton PK, Appel LJ, Sacco RL, et al. Sodium, blood pressure, and cardiovascular disease. *Circulation*. 2012;126(24):2880–2889. doi:10.1161/CIR.0b013e318279acbf
95. Graudal NA, Hubeck-Graudal T, Jürgens G. Effects of low-sodium diet vs. high-sodium diet on blood pressure, renin, aldosterone, catecholamines, cholesterol, and triglyceride (Cochrane Review). *Am J Hypertens*. 2012;25(1):1–15. doi:10.1038/ajh.2011.210

96. He FJ, MacGregor GA. Effect of modest salt reduction on blood pressure: a meta-analysis of randomized trials. Implications for public health. *J Hum Hypertens*. 2002;16(11):761–770. doi:10.1038/sj.jhh.1001459
97. MacGregor GA, Markandu ND, Sagnella GA, Singer DR, Cappuccio FP. Double-blind study of three sodium intakes and long-term effects of sodium restriction in essential hypertension. *Lancet*. 1989;2(8674):1244–1247. doi:10.1016/s0140-6736(89)91852-7
98. He FJ, Burnier M, Macgregor GA. Nutrition in cardiovascular disease: salt in hypertension and heart failure. *Eur Heart J*. 2011;32(24):3073–3080. doi:10.1093/eurheartj/ehr194
99. Ferrara LA, de Simone G, Pasanisi F, Mancini M, Mancini M. Left ventricular mass reduction during salt depletion in arterial hypertension. *Hypertension*. 1984;6(5):755–759. doi:10.1161/01.HYP.6.5.755
100. Liebson PR, Grandits GA, Dianzumba S, et al. Comparison of five antihypertensive monotherapies and placebo for change in left ventricular mass in patients receiving nutritional-hygienic therapy in the Treatment of Mild Hypertension Study (TOMHS). *Circulation*. 1995;91(3):698–706. doi:10.1161/01.cir.91.3.698
101. Jula AM, Karanko HM. Effects on left ventricular hypertrophy of long-term nonpharmacological treatment with sodium restriction in mild-to-moderate essential hypertension. *Circulation*. 1994;89(3):1023–1031. doi:10.1161/01.cir.89.3.1023
102. Strazzullo P, D'Elia L, Kandala NB, Cappuccio FP. Salt intake, stroke, and cardiovascular disease: meta-analysis of prospective studies. *BMJ*. 2009;339:b4567. doi:10.1136/bmj.b4567
103. Taylor RS, Ashton KE, Moxham T, Hooper L, Ebrahim S. Reduced dietary salt for the prevention of cardiovascular disease: a meta-analysis of randomized controlled trials (Cochrane review). *Am J Hypertens*. 2011;24(8):843–853. doi:10.1038/ajh.2011.115
104. Cook NR, Cutler JA, Obarzanek E, et al. Long term effects of dietary sodium reduction on cardiovascular disease outcomes: observational follow-up of the trials of hypertension prevention (TOHP). *BMJ*. 2007;334(7599):885–888. doi:10.1136/bmj.39147.604896.55
105. Ekinci EI, Clarke S, Thomas MC, et al. Dietary salt intake and mortality in patients with type 2 diabetes. *Diabetes Care*. 2011;34(3):703–709. doi:10.2337/dc10-1723
106. Stolarz-Skrzypek K, Kuznetsova T, Thijs L, et al. Fatal and nonfatal outcomes, incidence of hypertension, and blood pressure changes in relation to urinary sodium excretion. *JAMA*. 2011;305(17):1777–1785. doi:10.1001/jama.2011.574
107. Academy of Nutrition and Dietetics, Nutrition Care Manual. Low-Sodium Nutrition Therapy. Accessed July 30, 2024.
108. Whelton PK, He J, Cutler JA, et al. Effects of oral potassium on blood pressure. Meta-analysis of randomized controlled clinical trials. *JAMA*. May 28 1997;277(20):1624–1632. doi:10.1001/jama.1997.03540440058033
109. National Academies of Sciences, Engineering, and Medicine; Health and Medicine Division; Food and Nutrition Board; Committee to Review the Dietary Reference Intakes for Sodium and Potassium. 4, Potassium: Dietary Reference Intakes for Adequacy. In: Oria M, Harrison M, Stallings V, eds. *Dietary Reference Intakes for Sodium and Potassium*. National Library of Medicine National Center for Biotechnology Information; 2019.
110. Academy of Nutrition and Dietetics, Nutrition Care Manual. Potassium Content of Foods. Accessed July 20, 2024. https://www.nutritioncaremanual.org/client_ed.cfm?ncm_client_ed_id=153
111. Carlson DJ, Dieberg G, Hess NC, Millar PJ, Smart NA. Isometric exercise training for blood pressure management: a systematic review and meta-analysis. *Mayo Clin Proc*. 2014;89(3):327–334. doi:10.1016/j.mayocp.2013.10.030
112. Inder JD, Carlson DJ, Dieberg G, McFarlane JR, Hess NC, Smart NA. Isometric exercise training for blood pressure management: a systematic review and meta-analysis to optimize benefit. *Hypertens Res*. Feb 2016;39(2):88–94. doi:10.1038/hr.2015.111
113. Institute of Medicine (US) Committee to Review Dietary Reference Intakes for Vitamin D and Calcium. 5, Dietary Reference Intakes for Adequacy. In: Ross AC TC, Yaktine AL, et al., ed. *Dietary Reference Intakes for Calcium and Vitamin D*. National Academies Press, U.S.; 2011.
114. Institute of Medicine (US) Standing Committee on the Scientific Evaluation of Dietary Reference Intakes. 6 Magnesium. *Dietary Reference Intakes for Calcium, Phosphorus, Magnesium, Vitamin D, and Fluoride*. National Academies Press, U.S.; 1997.
115. Tsai YC, Tsao YP, Huang CJ, et al. Effectiveness of salt substitute on cardiovascular outcomes: a systematic review and meta-analysis. *J Clin Hypertens (Greenwich)*. 2022;24(9):1147–1160. doi:10.1111/jch.14562
116. Xu X, Zeng L, Jha V, et al. Potassium-enriched salt substitutes: a review of recommendations in clinical management guidelines. *Hypertension*. 2024;81(3):400–414. doi:10.1161/HYPERTENSIONAHA.123.21343
117. U.S. Food & Drug Administration. Questions and Answers on Monosodium glutamate (MSG). Updated January 4, 2018. Accessed July 20, 2024. https://www.fda.gov/food/food-additives-petitions/questions-and-answers-monosodium-glutamate-msg
118. Academy of Nutrition and Dietetics, Evidence Analysis Library. Umami (UM) and Sodium Intake Scoping Review. Accessed July 20, 2024. https://www.andeal.org/topic.cfm?menu=5280
119. Kenchaiah S, Evans JC, Levy D, et al. Obesity and the risk of heart failure. *NEJM*. 2002;347(5):305–313. doi:10.1056/NEJMoa020245
120. Jensen MD, Ryan DH, Apovian CM, et al. 2013 AHA/ACC/TOS Guideline for the management of overweight and obesity in adults. *Circulation*. 2014;129(25_suppl_2):S102–S138. doi:10.1161/01.cir.0000437739.71477.ee
121. Schwarz PEH, Timpel P, Harst L, et al. Blood sugar regulation for cardiovascular health promotion and disease prevention: JACC Health Promotion Series. *J Am Coll Cardiol*. 2018;72(15):1829–1844. doi:10.1016/j.jacc.2018.07.081
122. American Diabetes Association Professional Practice Committee. 10. Cardiovascular Disease and Risk Management: Standards of Care in Diabetes—2024. *Diabetes Care*. 2023;47(Supplement_1):S179–S218. doi:10.2337/dc24-S010
123. Academy of Nutrition and Dietetics, Evidence Analysis Library. Diabetes (DM) Type 1 and 2 Systematic Review. Accessed July 30, 2024. https://www.andeal.org/topic.cfm?menu=5305&pcat=5491&cat=5161
124. American Heart Association. Answers by heart. Cardiovascular conditions. What is peripheral vascular disease? 2021. Accessed July 30, 2024. https://www.heart.org/-/media/Files/Health-Topics/Answers-by-Heart/What-is-Peripheral-Artery-Disease.pdf

125. Cresci G, Hummell AC, Raheem SA, Cole D. Nutrition intervention in the critically ill cardiothoracic patient. *Nutr Clin Pract.* 2012;27(3):323–334. doi:10.1177/0884533612444135
126. Engelman DT, Adams DH, Byrne JG, et al. Impact of body mass index and albumin on morbidity and mortality after cardiac surgery. *J Thorac Cardiovasc Surg.* 1999;118(5):866–873. doi:10.1016/s0022-5223(99)70056-5
127. Stoppe C, Goetzenich A, Whitman G, et al. Role of nutrition support in adult cardiac surgery: a consensus statement from an International Multidisciplinary Expert Group on Nutrition in Cardiac Surgery. *Crit Care.* Jun 5 2017;21(1):131. doi:10.1186/s13054-017-1690-5
128. Heidenreich PA, Bozkurt B, Aguilar D, et al. 2022 AHA/ACC/HFSA Guideline for the Management of Heart Failure: a report of the American College of Cardiology/American Heart Association Joint Committee on Clinical Practice Guidelines. *Circulation.* 2022;145(18):e895–e1032. doi:10.1161/CIR.0000000000001063
129. Fuster V, Harrington RA, Narula J, Eapen ZJ. *Hurst's The Heart.* 14th ed. McGraw-Hill Education; 2017.
130. National Heart, Lung, and Blood Institute. Heart Failure Treatment. Updated March 24, 2022. Accessed July 13, 2024. https://www.nhlbi.nih.gov/health/heart-failure/treatment
131. Aggarwal A, Kumar A, Gregory MP, et al. Nutrition assessment in advanced heart failure patients evaluated for ventricular assist devices or cardiac transplantation. *Nutr Clin Pract.* 2013;28(1):112–119. doi:10.1177/0884533612457948
132. Academy of Nutrition and Dietetics, Nutrition Care Manual. Heart Failure. Accessed July 20, 2024. https://www.nutritioncaremanual.org/topic.cfm?ncm_category_id=1&lv1=272984&lv2=275292&lv3=275293&ncm_toc_id=275293&ncm_heading=Nutrition%20Care
133. Academy of Nutrition and Dietetics, Evidence Analysis Library. Heart Failure (HF) Guideline- Major Recommendations. Accessed July 13, 2024. https://www.andeal.org/topic.cfm?menu=5289&cat=5579
134. Detsky AS, McLaughlin JR, Baker JP, et al. What is subjective global assessment of nutritional status? *JPEN.* 1987;11(1): 8–13. doi:10.1177/014860718701100108
135. Academy of Nutrition and Dietetics, Nutrition Care Manual, McCann. Nutrition-Focused Physical Findings: Subjective Global Assessment. Accessed July 20, 2024. https://www.nutritioncaremanual.org/topic.cfm?ncm_toc_id=267679
136. Powell-Wiley TM, Poirier P, Burke LE, et al. Obesity and cardiovascular disease: a scientific statement from the American Heart Association. *Circulation.* 2021;143(21):e984–e1010. doi:10.1161/CIR.0000000000000973
137. Elagizi A, Carbone S, Lavie CJ, Mehra MR, Ventura HO. Implications of obesity across the heart failure continuum. *Prog Cardiovasc Dis.* Sep–Oct 2020;63(5):561–569. doi:10.1016/j.pcad.2020.09.005
138. Lennie TA. Nutrition self-care in heart failure: state of the science. *J Cardiovasc Nurs.* 2008;23(3):197–204. doi:10.1097/01.Jcn.0000317426.14092.60
139. Oreopoulos A, Padwal R, Kalantar-Zadeh K, Fonarow GC, Norris CM, McAlister FA. Body mass index and mortality in heart failure: a meta-analysis. *Am Heart J.* Jul 2008;156(1):13–22. doi:10.1016/j.ahj.2008.02.014
140. Wang ZJ, Zhou YJ, Galper BZ, Gao F, Yeh RW, Mauri L. Association of body mass index with mortality and cardiovascular events for patients with coronary artery disease: a systematic review and meta-analysis. *BMJ Heart.* 2015;101(20):8. doi:10.1136/heartjnl-2014-307119
141. Lavie CJ, Ventura HO. The obesity paradox in heart failure. *JACC: Heart Failure.* 2015;3(11):927–930. doi:10.1016/j.jchf.2015.07.009
142. Oktay AA, Lavie CJ, Ventura HO. Obesity and the obesity paradox in heart failure. In: Vasan RS, Sawyer DB, eds. *Encyclopedia of Cardiovascular Research and Medicine.* Elsevier; 2018:546–564.
143. Katz AM, Katz PB. Diseases of the heart in the works of Hippocrates. Br Heart J. 1962;24(3):257-264. doi:10.1136/hrt.24.3.257
144. Gottschlich M. *The A.S.P.E.N. Nutrition Support Core Curriculum: A Case-Based Approach: The Adult Patient.* A.S.P.E.N; 2007.
145. Carlson H, Cahlin C. Managing the effects of cardiac cachexia. *J Hospice Palliative Nurs.* 2014;16:6. doi:10.1097/NJH.0000000000000039
146. Krysztofiak H, Wleklik M, Migaj J, et al. Cardiac cachexia: a well-known but challenging complication of heart failure. *Clin Interv Aging.* 2020;15:2041–2051. doi:10.2147/cia.S273967
147. Bonilla-Palomas JL, Gámez-López AL, Anguita-Sánchez MP, et al. Influencia de la desnutrición en la mortalidad a largo plazo de pacientes hospitalizados por insuficiencia cardiaca [Impact of malnutrition on long-term mortality in hospitalized patients with heart failure]. *Rev Esp Cardiol.* 2011;64(9):752–758. doi:10.1016/j.recesp.2011.03.009
148. Anker SD, Coats AJ. Cardiac cachexia: a syndrome with impaired survival and immune and neuroendocrine activation. *Chest.* 1999;115(3):836–847. doi:10.1378/chest.115.3.836
149. Sandek A, Doehner W, Anker SD, von Haehling S. Nutrition in heart failure: an update. *Curr Opin Clin Nutr Metab Care.* 2009;12(4):384–391. doi:10.1097/MCO.0b013e32832cdb0f
150. Anker SD, Chua TP, Ponikowski P, et al. Hormonal changes and catabolic/anabolic imbalance in chronic heart failure and their importance for cardiac cachexia. *Circulation.* 1997;96(2):526–534. doi:10.1161/01.cir.96.2.526
151. American Heart Association. How much sodium should I eat per day? Updated Jan 5. Accessed July 30, 2024. https://www.heart.org/en/healthy-living/healthy-eating/eat-smart/sodium/how-much-sodium-should-i-eat-per-day
152. Aliti GB, Rabelo ER, Clausell N, Rohde LE, Biolo A, Beck-da-Silva L. Aggressive fluid and sodium restriction in acute decompensated heart failure: a randomized clinical trial. *JAMA Intern Med.* 2013;173(12):1058–1064. doi:10.1001/jamainternmed.2013.552
153. Machado d'Almeida KS, Rabelo-Silva ER, Souza GC, et al. Aggressive fluid and sodium restriction in decompensated heart failure with preserved ejection fraction: results from a randomized clinical trial. *Nutrition.* 2018;54:111–117. doi:10.1016/j.nut.2018.02.007
154. Kalogeropoulos A, Papadimitriou L, Georgiopoulou VV, Dunbar SB, Skopicki H, Butler J. Low- Versus moderate-sodium diet in patients with recent hospitalization for heart failure: The PROHIBIT (Prevent Adverse Outcomes in Heart Failure by Limiting Sodium) Pilot Study. *Circ Heart Fail.* 2020;13(1):e006389. doi:10.1161/circheartfailure.119.006389
155. Colin-Ramirez E, McAlister FA, Zheng Y, Sharma S, Ezekowitz JA. Changes in dietary intake and nutritional status associated with a significant reduction in sodium intake in patients with heart failure. A sub-analysis of the SODIUM-HF pilot study. *Clin Nutr ESPEN.* 2016;11:e26–e32. doi:10.1016/j.clnesp.2015.11.002

156. Hummel SL, Karmally W, Gillespie BW, et al. Home-delivered meals postdischarge from heart failure hospitalization. *Circ Heart Fail.* 2018;11(8):e004886. doi:10.1161/circheartfailure.117.004886
157. Welsh D, Lennie TA, Marcinek R, et al. Low-sodium diet self-management intervention in heart failure: pilot study results. *Eur J Cardiovasc Nurs.* 2013;12(1):87–95.doi:10.1177/1474515111435604
158. Philipson H, Ekman I, Forslund HB, Swedberg K, Schaufelberger M. Salt and fluid restriction is effective in patients with chronic heart failure. *Eur J Heart Fail.* 2013;15(11):1304–1310. doi:10.1093/eurjhf/hft097
159. Academy of Nutrition and Dietetics, Nutrition Care Manual. Fluid-Restricted Nutrition Therapy. Accessed July 20, 2024. https://www.nutritioncaremanual.org/client_ed.cfm?ncm_client_ed_id=413
160. Azizi-Namini P, Ahmed M, Yan AT, Keith M. The role of B vitamins in the management of heart failure. *Nutr Clin Pract.* 2012;27(3):363–374. doi:10.1177/0884533612444539
161. Wooley JA. Characteristics of thiamin and its relevance to the management of heart failure. *Nutr Clin Pract.* 2008;23(5):487–493. doi:10.1177/0884533608323430
162. U.S. Department of Health and Human Services and National Institutes of Health Office of Dietary Supplements. Dietary Supplement Fact Sheet: Vitamin D. Updated November 8, 2022. Accessed July 30, 2024. https://ods.od.nih.gov/factsheets/VitaminD-Consumer/
163. Fiscella K, Franks P. Vitamin D, race, and cardiovascular mortality: findings from a national US sample. *Ann Fam Med.* 2010;8(1):11–18. doi:10.1370/afm.1035
164. Escott-Stump S. *Nutrition & Diagnosis-Related Care.* 9th ed. Lippincott Williams & Wilkins; 2021.
165. Academy of Nutrition and Dietetics Evidence Analysis Library. Heart Failure Major Recommendations (Previous Version). http://www.andeal.org/topic.cfm?menu=5289. Accessed August 15, 2014.
166. Yusuf S, Dagenais G, Pogue J, Bosch J, Sleight P. Vitamin E supplementation and cardiovascular events in high-risk patients. *NEJM.* 2000;342(3):154–160. doi:10.1056/nejm200001203420302
167. Ingbar DH, Thiele H. Cardiogenic shock and pulmonary edema. In: Loscalzo J, Fauci A, Kasper D, Hauser S, Longo D, Jameson JL, eds. *Harrison's Principles of Internal Medicine.* 21st ed. McGraw-Hill Education; 2022.
168. McClave SA, Taylor BE, Martindale RG, et al. Guidelines for the Provision and Assessment of Nutrition Support Therapy in the Adult Critically Ill Patient: Society of Critical Care Medicine (SCCM) and American Society for Parenteral and Enteral Nutrition (A.S.P.E.N.). *JPEN.* 2016;40(2):159–211. doi:10.1177/0148607115621863
169. ASPEN Nutrition. ASPEN International Nutrition Guidelines for Adult Perioperative Cardiac Patients: Protocol. Clinical Guidelines. *JPEN.* March 20 2024. Accessed December26,2024.https://www.nutritioncare.org/uploadedFiles/Documents/Guidelines_and_Clinical_Resources/Protocol%20ASPEN%20International%20Nutrition%20Guidelines%20for%20Adult%20Perioperative%20Cardiac%20Patients%203.20.24.pdf.
170. Singer P, Blaser AR, Berger MM, et al. ESPEN practical and partially revised guideline: Clinical nutrition in the intensive care unit. *Clin Nutr.* 2023;42(9):1671–1689. doi:10.1016/j.clnu.2023.07.011
171. Academy of Nutrition and Dietetics, Nutrition Care Manual. Enteral Nutrition. Accessed July 20, 2023. https://www.nutritioncaremanual.org/topic.cfm?ncm_category_id=1&lv1=255693&lv2=275367&lv3=275373&ncm_toc_id=275373&ncm_heading=Nutrition%20Care
172. Academy of Nutrition and Dietetics, Evidence Analysis Library. Critical Illness (CI) Guideline: Major Recommendations. Accessed July 30, 2024. https://www.andeal.org/topic.cfm?menu=5302&cat=4801
173. Academy of Nutrition and Dietetics, Evidence Analysis Library. Critical Illness (CI) Systematic Review. Accessed July 30, 2024. https://www.andeal.org/topic.cfm?menu=5302&cat=4063
174. Revelly JP, Tappy L, Berger MM, Gersbach P, Cayeux C, Chioléro R. Early metabolic and splanchnic responses to enteral nutrition in postoperative cardiac surgery patients with circulatory compromise. *Intensive Care Med.* 2001;27(3):540–547. doi:10.1007/s001340100855
175. Berger MM, Revelly JP, Cayeux MC, Chiolero RL. Enteral nutrition in critically ill patients with severe hemodynamic failure after cardiopulmonary bypass. *Clin Nutr.* 2005;24(1):124–132. doi:10.1016/j.clnu.2004.08.005
176. Widlicka A. Enteral nutrition in the cardiothoracic intensive care unit: challenges and considerations. *Nutr Clin Pract.* 2008;23(5):510–520. doi:10.1177/0884533608323422
177. Thomas RJ, Balady G, Banka G, et al. 2018 ACC/AHA Clinical Performance and Quality Measures for Cardiac Rehabilitation. *J Am Coll Cardiol.* 2018;71(16):1814–1837.doi:10.1016/j.jacc.2018.01.004
178. Heran BS, Chen JM, Ebrahim S, et al. Exercise-based cardiac rehabilitation for coronary heart disease. *Cochrane Database Syst Rev.* 2011;(7):Cd001800. doi:10.1002/14651858.CD001800.pub2
179. Virani SS, Newby LK, Arnold SV, et al. 2023 AHA/ACC/ACCP/ASPC/NLA/PCNA Guideline for the Management of Patients with Chronic Coronary Disease: a report of the American Heart Association/American College of Cardiology Joint Committee on Clinical Practice Guidelines. *Circulation.* 2023;148(9):e9–e119. doi:10.1161/CIR.0000000000001168
180. McMahon SR, Ades PA, Thompson PD. The role of cardiac rehabilitation in patients with heart disease. *Trends Cardiovasc Med.* 2017;27(6):420–425. doi:10.1016/j.tcm.2017.02.005
181. U.S. Centers for Medicare & Medicaid Services, Medicare Learning Network. Conditions of Coverage for Outpatient Cardiac Rehabilitation Programs. 2022. Accessed July 20, 2024. https://www.hhs.gov/guidance/sites/default/files/hhs-guidance-documents/MLN7561577__002___LCBfinal_.pdf
182. Brown TM, Pack QR, Aberegg E, et al. Core Components of Cardiac Rehabilitation Programs: 2024 Update: A Scientific Statement From the American Heart Association and the American Association of Cardiovascular and Pulmonary Rehabilitation. *Circulation.* 2024;150(18):e328–e347. doi:10.1161/CIR.0000000000001289
183. U.S. Centers for Medicare & Medicaid Services. Cardiac Rehabilitation Programs. Accessed July 20, 2024. https://www.cms.gov/medicare-coverage-database/view/ncd.aspx?ncdid=36&ncdver=1&doctype=all&year=2023&sortBy=title&bc=14
184. U.S. Centers for Medicare & Medicaid Services. Decision Memorandum for Coverage of Cardiac Rehabilitation

(CR)Programs for Chronic Heart Failure (HF). Accessed July 20, 2024. https://www.cms.gov/medicare-coverage-database/view/ncacal-decision-memo.aspx?proposed=N&NCAId=270

185. U.S. Centers for Medicare & Medicaid Services. Intensive Cardiac Rehabilitation (ICR) Programs. Updated September 6, 2023. Accessed July 20, 2024. https://www.cms.gov/medicare/coverage/approved-facilities-trials-registries/cardiac-rehab-programs

186. Husaini M, Deych E, Waken RJ, et al. Intensive versus traditional cardiac rehabilitation: mortality and cardiovascular outcomes in a 2016–2020 retrospective Medicare cohort. *Circ Cardiovasc Quality Outcomes*. 2023;16(12):e010131. doi:10.1161/CIRCOUTCOMES.123.010131

187. Fang J, Ayala C, Luncheon C, Ritchey M, Loustalot F. Use of outpatient cardiac rehabilitation among heart attack survivors — 20 states and the District of Columbia, 2013 and four states, 2015. Report. *MMWR*. 2017;66(33):5. doi:http://dx.doi.org/10.15585/mmwr.mm6633a1

188. Peacock JM, Styles E, Johnson S, et al. Surveillance of the initiation of, participation in, and completion of cardiac rehabilitation in Minnesota, 2017–2018. *Prev Chronic Dis*. 2023;20(220324). doi:10.5888/pcd20.220324

189. Ritchey MD, Maresh S, McNeely J, et al. Tracking cardiac rehabilitation participation and completion among Medicare beneficiaries to inform the efforts of a national initiative. *Circ Cardiovasc Quality Outcomes*. 2020;13(1):e005902. doi:10.1161/CIRCOUTCOMES.119.005902

190. Oehler A, Battel L, Poornima IG. Cardiac Rehabilitation and Health Care Disparities in the Post-COVID-19 Era. Expert Analysis. *Am Coll Cardol*. September 25, 2023; Accessed December 26, 2024. https://www.acc.org/Latest-in-Cardiology/Articles/2023/09/25/14/05/Cardiac-Rehabilitation-and-Health-Care-Disparities-in-the-Post-COVID-19-Era.

191. American Association of Cardiovascular and Pulmonary Rehabilitation. *Cardiac Rehabilitation Summary for Payers*. Accessed July 20, 2024. https://www.aacvpr.org/Portals/0/Docs/Practice/CR%20summary%20for%20payers_FINAL_5-15-19.pdf

192. Albert DL, Lounsbury P. Expanding the role of a clinical dietitian in cardiac rehabilitation: a pilot study. Poster Session. *J Acad Nutr Diet*. 2007;107(8). doi:10.1016/j.jada.2007.05.285

193. Kocanda L, Schumacher TL, Plotnikoff RC, et al. Effectiveness and reporting of nutrition interventions in cardiac rehabilitation programmes: a systematic review. *Eur J Cardiovasc Nurs*. 2022;22(1):1–12. doi:10.1093/eurjcn/zvac033

CHAPTER 10

Nutritional Management of Gastrointestinal Maldigestion

Rachel Wilkinson-Bartlett

CHAPTER OUTLINE

CORE CONCEPTS

1. Any disease state that impairs normal digestion or absorption requires medical nutrition therapy at all stages of treatment to improve quality of life and prevent any secondary nutritional deficiencies.
2. The digestive system relies on the cooperation of a complex network of gastrointestinal and accessory organs to accomplish its functions in digestion and absorption.
3. Although digestion must first occur to allow for proper absorption, the two processes are entirely distinct in purpose and function.
4. While maldigestion and malabsorption are distinguishable in a pathophysiological sense, the two disorders often occur together clinically.
5. Gastric surgery indicates a number of concerning nutritional implications that may occur during the postoperative period. Nutrition interventions should be tailored to each individual depending on the symptoms and clinical manifestations that arise.
6. Acute pancreatitis and chronic pancreatitis differ substantially in their respective nutritional requirements. For both disease states, it is crucial to provide sufficient energy to meet increased needs, adapt care plans in regard to individual symptoms, and intervene with nutrition support when necessary.
7. Any changes to the integrity of the GI anatomy will alter function and impact how the body digests and ultimately absorbs nutrients.
8. Gastroesophageal reflux disease is a common condition with various possible medical, surgical, and nutritional treatments. It is important for RDs to be well versed in the most up-to-date treatment options for these patients, individualizing interventions to target the cause of reflux.

LEARNING OBJECTIVES

1. Describe the key mechanisms of digestion.
2. Define and differentiate between maldigestion and malabsorption.
3. Identify factors that cause maldigestion.
4. Discuss the different types of gastric surgery for maldigestion.
5. Define pancreatitis (acute and chronic) and explain the differences in pathophysiology.
6. Formulate appropriate medical nutrition therapy for acute and chronic pancreatitis.
7. Describe gastroesophageal reflux disease and identify various treatment options (medical, surgical, and nutritional/lifestyle).

Introduction

There is no bodily system more readily involved in maintaining nutritional status than the gastrointestinal (GI) tract and its accessory organs. Together, these structures form a digestive system with one true purpose—to extract nutrients from food that is consumed (digestion) and relay them to the body in a usable form (absorption).[1] Normal digestion and absorption occur at numerous points along the tract, encompassing all of the structures from mouth to anus, and require integration of the nervous, endocrine, and circulatory systems.[2] Given this complexity, there are countless areas where the system can fail. Thus, a wide range of diagnoses may account for an individual's poor nutritional status through impairment of digestion, absorption, or both.

Pathology of the digestive system hovers near the top of the list of most commonly treated healthcare complaints in the United States, accounting for nearly 50 million ambulatory visits and more than 20 million hospitalizations annually.[3] For all disease states affecting digestion and absorption, nutrition therapy is a crucial component of both prevention and treatment.[4] Given the complexity of GI disorders and treatment, this chapter will cover the nutritional management of maldigestion, while Chapter 11 will detail nutritional management of gastrointestinal malabsorption.

CORE CONCEPT 1

Any disease state that impairs normal digestion or absorption requires medical nutrition therapy at all stages of treatment to improve quality of life and prevent any secondary nutritional deficiencies.

Note: The digestive system is an immensely complex system, and there are many disorders that arise when the system fails. This chapter addresses those that most directly influence nutritional status by impairing normal digestion. There are several other conditions involving the digestive system that most often occur secondary to disease states. As these may not have direct impact on the body's utilization of foods, they are covered in other chapters.

Functional Anatomy of the Digestive System

The body's digestive system is a powerhouse. At the most basic level, this system maintains an individual's nourishment through four inter-reliant processes: ingestion, digestion, absorption, and excretion.[2] Efficiency in completing these processes relies on interaction and cooperation within a network of GI and accessory organs (**Figure 10.1**).[5]

The GI tract (also referred to as the "alimentary canal" or the "gut") is a long, muscular tube with openings at the mouth and the anus. This continuation of the external environment can be divided into two main categories: the upper digestive tract, which includes the oral cavity, esophagus, and the stomach; and the lower digestive tract, comprising the small and large intestines. A third category supports digestion and absorption by providing the secretions necessary for these processes to occur. This group, which consists of the salivary glands, the liver, the gallbladder, and the pancreas, is collectively referred to as the "accessory organs"; each connects to the GI system at a specific point along the tract via ducts that allow for transfer of the secretions.[1,2,5] For example, pancreatic juices empty into the proximal portion of the small intestine (the **duodenum**) through the sphincter of Oddi. This relationship is critical, as digestive enzymes contained in the solution are required by half of all ingested carbohydrates and protein and almost all ingested lipids.[2]

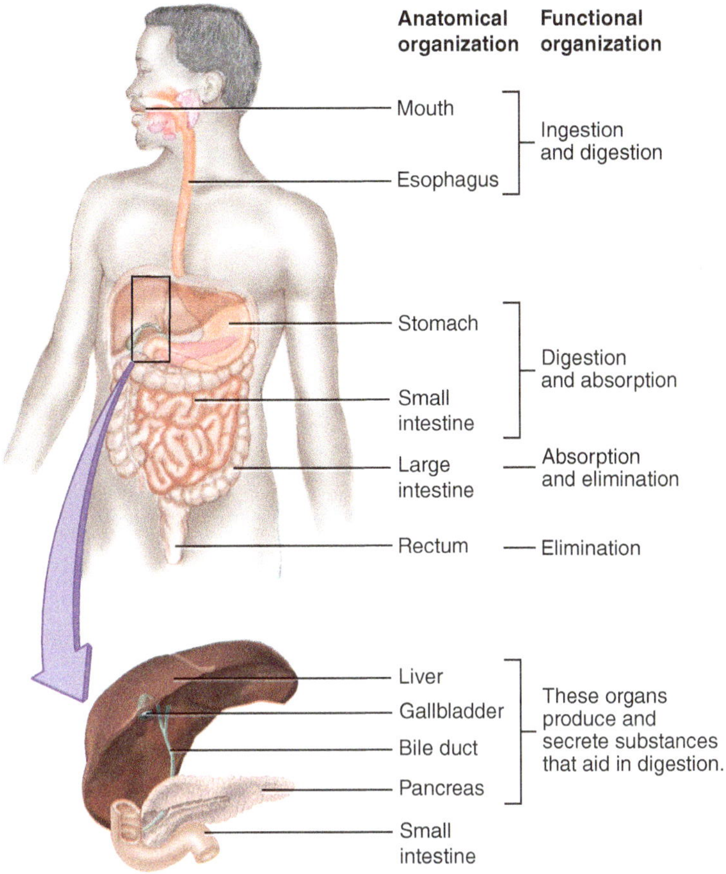

Figure 10.1 Anatomic and Functional Organization of the GI Tract

CASE STUDY INTRODUCTION

Janice is a 56-year-old female who is admitted to the outpatient clinic following a gastric surgery 6 weeks ago for gastric cancer. Since her surgery, Janice has experienced some gastrointestinal tolerance. By report, she has frequent watery stools that occur soon after eating. Her information is below.

Anthropometric Data:

Adm Weight: 75 kg
Height: 165 cm
BMI: 27.5 kg/m^2

Weight History
90 kg 6 months ago (UBW)
80 kg 6 weeks ago

Biochemical Data:

Sodium 140 (136–145 mEq/L)
Potassium 3.1 (3.5–5.0 mEq/L)
Chloride 100 (96–106 mEq/L)
Carbon dioxide 19 (22–31 mEq/L)
Blood urea nitrogen 22 (8–20 mg/dL)
Creatinine 0.8 (0.7–1.3 mg/dL)
Glucose 120 (70–139 mg/dL)
Serum osmolality 290 (275–295 mOsm/kg)
25-OH vitamin D12 (20–100 ng/mL)
Vitamin B12 and iron labs are pending.

Magnesium 1.2 (1.5–2.7 mg/dL)
Calcium 8.0 (8.5–10.5 mg/dL)
Phosphorus 2.4 (2.5–4.5 mg/dL)
Albumin 2.6 (3.5–5.5 g/dL)
Hemoglobin 11.1 (14–18 g/dL)
Hematocrit 36.4 (40–50%)
Mean corpuscular volume 89 (80–100 fL)
Red cell distribution width 58 (39–46 fL)

Clinical Data:

Past Medical History: Gastric cancer s/p resection, hypertension, prediabetes, gastroesophageal reflux disease (GERD), hyperlipidemia

Medications: chlorothiazide, cobalamin, metformin, omeprazole, pravastatin

Vital Signs: Blood pressure 140/69 mm Hg, Temperature 98.6°F, Heart rate 120 beats/min

Nutrition-Focused Physical Exam: Patient appears alert. Mild muscle wasting evident in clavicular region. Oral exam reveals good dentition and slightly enlarged, smooth, glossy tongue. Skin is pale, nails appear brittle.

Dietary Data:

Dietary History: Janice has a fair appetite. Since leaving the hospital, her diet transitioned to a regular diet. She follows 6 small meals throughout the day. She has 6 or more stools per day. Her diarrhea occurs approximately 30 minutes after eating each meal. These episodes are often accompanied by dizziness and perspiration. She does not note any odor or fatty substance in her stool.

24-Hour Diet Recall:

Breakfast (7:30 am): Two scrambled eggs, one cup of cereal with low fat milk, 6 oz coffee, cream and 2 sugars

Midmorning snack (10 am): 1 cup tea with milk and sugar, ½ jelly donut

Lunch (12:30 pm): 1/2 tuna salad sandwich on white bread, 4 oz grape or apple juice, 1 cup chocolate pudding

Midday snack (3 pm): 4 oz chocolate milk, 1 small blueberry muffin

Dinner (7 pm): 3 oz baked fish, 1/2 cup mashed potatoes, 1/2 cooked carrots, 1 cup canned peaches

Evening snack (9 pm): Peanut butter and jelly on white bread

Questions

1. What are Janice's nutritional risk factors?
2. Describe the possible physiologic symptoms that may occur given Janice's surgery.
3. Write two Nutrition Diagnosis statements for Janice identifying the Problem/Etiology/Signs and Symptoms (PES) of Janice's active nutrition issues.
4. Identify the nutrition interventions you would like to initiate for Janice to address the problems identified in your PES statements.
5. What biochemical indices should be included in your monitoring and evaluation plan? Why?

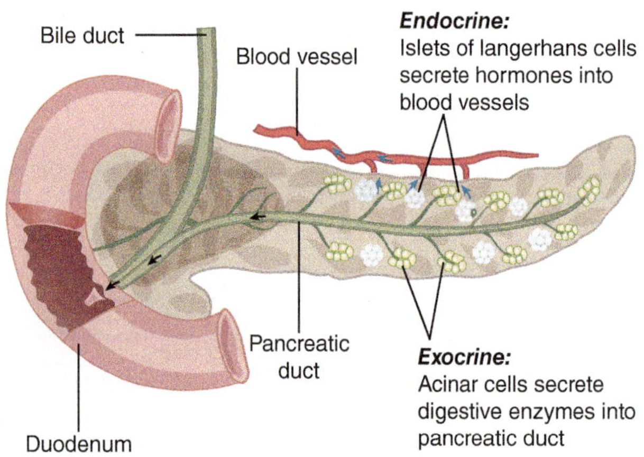

Figure 10.2 The Pancreas Performs Both Endocrine and Exocrine Functions

The pancreas is vital to the digestive system. This complex organ has both exocrine and endocrine functions (illustrated in **Figure 10.2**). The endocrine cells, made up of the islets of Langerhans, release hormones into the bloodstream.[6] These hormones include insulin and glucagon. The exocrine pancreas makes up most of the organ. These cells, called "acinar cells," produce enzymes that assist with digestion, including protease, pancreatic lipase, and amylase.[6]

A number of anatomical characteristics separate the digestive system from other organ structures and allow for completion of its unique functions. First, four distinct layers comprise the wall of the GI tract throughout the entirety of the tract: (1) mucosa, (2) submucosa, (3) muscularis externa, and (4) serosa (**Figure 10.3**). Each layer has a specific responsibility when moving ingested food particles through the digestion and absorption processes, including the secretion of enzymes and control of muscle movement and blood flow. Second, the enlarged surface area of the small intestine, created by the folds of Kerckring, the villi, and the microvilli's **brush border** (an array of microvilli on the membrane of epithelial cells), maximizes the capacity for absorption (**Figure 10.4**). Third, the contraction of both smooth (involuntary) and striated (voluntary) muscles allows for passage of food

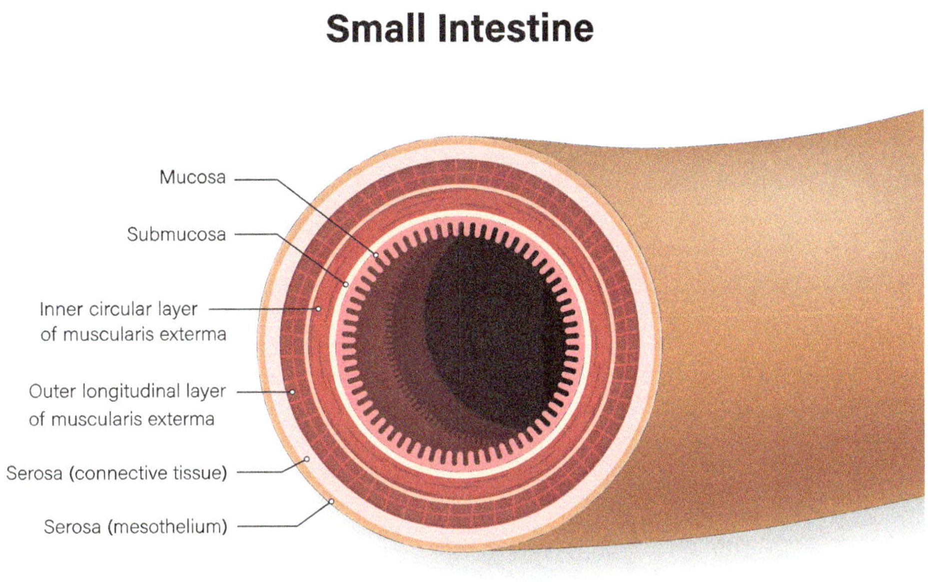

Figure 10.3 Four Layers Comprise the GI Tract Wall Throughout the Entirety of the Tract

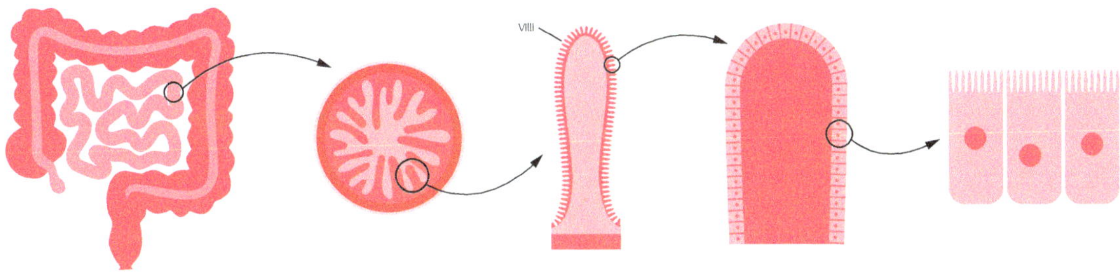

Figure 10.4 Intestinal Folding

particles (via **peristalsis**, the involuntary contraction and constriction of smooth muscle in wavelike patterns to propel a food bolus down the esophagus and upper GI tract), as well as for the opening and closing of sphincters, down the tract. Neural involvement in GI function, which regulates both muscle movement and secretions, is made possible by the enteric nervous system and its strategic positioning within the wall of the GI tract.[2,7] Each characteristic is fundamentally necessary for completing the normal processes of digestion and absorption.

CORE CONCEPT 2

The digestive system relies on the cooperation of a complex network of gastrointestinal and accessory organs to accomplish its functions in digestion and absorption.

Overview of Digestion and Absorption

The pathways through which the body obtains usable nutrients are unavoidably intertwined; absorption cannot occur without digestion as a precursor. Although the two processes are coordinated in action, they are distinctly separate. **Digestion** can be defined as the mechanical or enzymatic breakdown of food to its constituents. The term **absorption** describes the movement of these digested particles from the external environment and into the cells of the GI tract to be utilized by the body.[2] Understanding the mechanisms of normal nutrient digestion and absorption will yield greater understanding of the nutritional implications that arise when these processes are impaired.

CORE CONCEPT 3

Although digestion must first occur to allow for proper absorption, the two processes are entirely distinct in purpose and function.

Impaired digestive processes decrease the body's ability to maintain its nutritional status. Just as digestion and absorption are two separate processes, maldigestion and malabsorption are physiologically distinct. The term **maldigestion** is used in cases when the breakdown of macronutrients is impaired.[8] Theoretically, it is the failure of the enzymatic processes of digestion. Maldigestion often denotes the inability of the digestive system to access or utilize digestive enzymes, as would occur in gastric surgery or pancreatitis.[9] **Malabsorption** occurs as a result of defective mucosal uptake or transport of inadequately digested nutrients.[8,9] There is a range of diagnoses linked to the presence of malabsorption, and addressing each would extend beyond the scope of this chapter. The majority of associated disorders involve pathophysiology of the small intestine,[10] where the greatest amount of absorption occurs,[2] but are also present in diseases of the pancreas, liver, biliary tract, and stomach.[10] Both maldigestion and malabsorption occur from damage to the normal anatomy of one or more of the many components of the digestive system.

Differentiating between maldigestion and malabsorption is important in a pathophysiologic sense. Understanding the mechanisms behind the progression of disease, and whether the symptoms are occurring from issues with digestion or absorption, is helpful in determining the best course of treatment. **Table 10.1** provides a list of signs and symptoms of both maldigestion and malabsorption. The distinction is not always useful clinically: maldigestion and malabsorption present with similar clinical markers. Because digestive and absorptive processes are so intimately connected, the term **malassimilation** may be used to describe cases where both maldigestion and malabsorption occur.[9] Although maldigestion and malabsorption are two separate conditions, they often occur in tandem in a clinical context.

CORE CONCEPT 4

While maldigestion and malabsorption are distinguishable in a pathophysiologic sense, the two disorders often occur together clinically.

Table 10.1 Common Signs and Symptoms of Maldigestion and Malabsorption

Gastrointestinal	Nutrient Deficiency
Diarrhea	Glossitis
Steatorrhea	Cheilosis
Flatulence	Stomatitis
Bloating, distention	Signs of bleeding
Abdominal pain	Easy bruising
Emesis	Bone pain
Edema	Weakness, fatigue
Ascites	Muscle weakness
Blood in stool	Weight loss, cachexia

Data from Malik Z. Overview of Malabsorption. *Merck Manual Professional Edition*. Merck & Co., Inc; reviewed/revised March 2025. Accessed January 12, 2026. https://www.merckmanuals.com/professional/gastrointestinal-disorders/malabsorption-syndromes/overview-of-malabsorption

Key Mechanisms of Digestion

The breakdown of food into absorbable nutrients begins in the oral cavity and progresses through the remaining GI structures in sequence:

1. The swallowing mechanism passes digesta into the esophagus as a **bolus** (a ball of food).
2. The bolus moves through the stomach, where it mixes with gastric juices to become **chyme**.
3. Chyme passes into the small intestine, where the majority of digestive processes occur.
4. Any remaining undigested matter moves into the large intestine (colon).

Digestive processes take place in both the lumen of the GI tract and on the brush border. At each location, digestive enzymes act on the carbohydrates, protein, and lipids contained in food, reducing the digesta into forms the body is capable of utilizing. The various necessary enzymes are secreted by the mouth, stomach, pancreas, and small intestine. Ultimately, carbohydrates are reduced to the monosaccharides glucose, fructose, and galactose; lipids to glycerol, free fatty acids, and monoglycerides; and proteins, which are first broken down into polypeptides, and then to individual amino acids.[1,2,7]

Medical Nutrition Therapy for Disorders of Digestion

Gastric Surgery

A typical gastric surgery involves a resection of the stomach as indicated for treatment of trauma or disease to the upper GI tract and the reconstructive procedure that follows. The most common diseases requiring gastrectomy include peptic ulcer disease (PUD) and gastric cancer.[11,12] Although surgical treatment of PUD has declined, it is still used in patients with intractable disease not responding to medical management. Gastric resection was historically the primary approach used to treat patients with PUD. High recurrence rates of PUD helped identify the role of the vagus nerve in gastric acid secretion. Hence, a vagotomy is a surgical procedure for PUD that is still used today.[13,14] A **selective vagotomy** eliminates innervation from the vagus nerve to parietal cells of the proximal stomach, decreasing the secretion of gastric acid and reducing cellular response to gastrin. In a **total (truncal) vagotomy**, parietal cell innervation is severed and the portion of the vagus nerve that controls gastric emptying is eliminated. To correct for complications related to decreased gastric emptying, total vagotomy procedures are completed with a **pyloroplasty,** which enlarges the pyloric sphincter.[11] The decision to use the option of gastric resection depends on the extent of the damaged stomach that would require removal.

Pyloroplasty and gastric resection procedures are always followed by subsequent reconstruction, generally through a gastroduodenostomy (Billroth I), a gastrojejunostomy (Billroth II), or a Roux-en-Y. **Figure 10.5** depicts Billroth I and Billroth II, while **Figure 10.6** details a Roux-en-Y procedure. A Billroth I procedure involves partial **gastrectomy** or pyloroplasty with a reconstruction consisting of an **anastomosis** of the proximal end of the duodenum to the distal end of the stomach.[11] Billroth II procedures create a similar anastomosis, but instead connect the proximal end of the jejunum to the distal end of the stomach following a partial gastrectomy. A "blind loop" of the duodenum

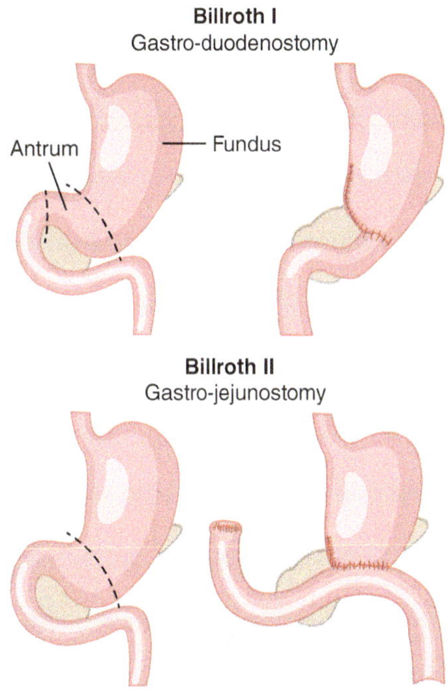

Figure 10.5 Pyloroplasty and Gastric Resection Procedures Are Always Followed by Subsequent Reconstruction, Generally Through a Gastroduodenostomy (Billroth I) and a Gastrojejunostomy (Billroth II)

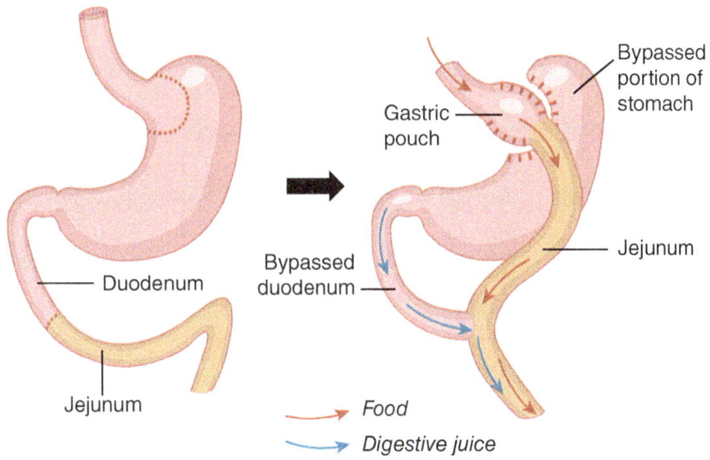

Figure 10.6 The Roux-en-Y Creates a Small Gastric Pouch by Removing the Top Part of the Stomach from Its Remaining Portion. The Jejunum Is Anastomosed to This Newly Created Gastric Pouch

is created in order to facilitate continued flow of bile salts and pancreatic enzymes.[13] The Roux-en-Y (gastric bypass) yields similar results to the Billroth II, but creates a small pouch following the gastric resection with anastomosis of the jejunum to the upper portion of the stomach.[12] Other types of anastomoses can be done depending on the disease or condition. The Billroth I, Billroth II, and Roux-en-Y are the three most common surgical procedures for treating gastric cancers. These surgical procedures may include various types of reconstruction or anastomosis depending on patient circumstances, and to reduce commons symptoms of gastritis and bile reflux.[15]

Despite the etiology, many of the same surgical techniques, particularly the Roux-en-Y, are used to treat GI disorders as well as obesity.[16,17] Thus, a patient who has had bariatric surgery is at risk for similar nutritional complications and should follow a comparable medical nutrition therapy plan as an individual who underwent a nonelective gastric surgery.

Medical Nutrition Therapy

When portions of the stomach are resected or rerouted during gastric surgery, normal digestive mechanisms may be altered or lost altogether. Changes to the stomach that affect holding capacity, gastric emptying, and enzyme secretion are responsible for the most common nutrition-related postoperative complications. Those with significant nutritional implications include gastric stasis, fat maldigestion, select nutrient deficiencies, and dumping syndrome.[18] Symptoms may be prevented, reduced, or eliminated through appropriate nutrition interventions.

Gastric Stasis. The occurrence of **gastric stasis** is a concern for all patients during the postoperative period but is most common in surgical procedures that include a total vagotomy. Gastric stasis, or **gastroparesis**, is the delayed gastric emptying that occurs when vagus innervation, and thus control, are eliminated. Patients typically present with nausea and vomiting, anorexia, bloating, and/or early satiety—all of which severely limit oral intake. In addition, those who present with gastric stasis are at an increased risk for developing small intestine bacterial overgrowth, which will be discussed later in the chapter.[18]

The management of gastric stasis typically involves the use of prokinetic and antiemetic medications combined with careful nutrition interventions. Dietary modifications are made based on the individual and their symptoms. Consuming small, frequent meals throughout the day will help to decrease bloating, early satiety, and the severity of nausea and vomiting. Many patients may experience exacerbated symptoms when consuming solid foods but have no difficulty with liquid intake. For this subgroup, it may be necessary to increase calories from liquids or pureed foods. In many cases, an oral nutritional supplement (ONS) may be recommended. If symptoms persist, patients will likely benefit from the adoption of a low-fat, low-fiber diet since foods of this nature tend to have faster gastric emptying rates than their high-fat, high-fiber counterparts. However, liquid fats do not pose a problem and should not be excluded; most are well tolerated and serve as a source of extra calories. In addition, patients should avoid the intake of alcohol and carbonated beverages, which are known to slow gastric emptying. Light exercise postprandially may help to speed up gastric emptying rates and facilitate proper digestion.[18]

PRACTICE POINT

Patients who present with gastric stasis should consume small, frequent meals and will likely require increased calories in liquid forms. Although solid fats are not often well tolerated, liquid fats can help provide necessary energy.

Fat Maldigestion. In a functioning digestive system, chief cells of the stomach secrete gastric lipase to initiate lipid digestion. Following gastric resection and/or reconstruction, there is a marked decrease in gastric secretions and the necessary digestive enzymes. When lipids cannot be digested properly and are not subsequently absorbed, patients present with symptoms of fat malabsorption. This manifests primarily as greasy, foul-smelling diarrhea known as **steatorrhea**, which indicates undigested fat excretion in the stool. Patients may also report cramping and abdominal pain.

For many patients, it will be necessary to initiate a low-fat diet. This recommendation is often paired with the inclusion of a **medium-chain triglyceride (MCT)** oil supplement. MCTs are indicated for patients with fat maldigestion and malabsorption because they do not follow the conventional channels for lipid digestion; instead, MCTs are absorbed directly into portal circulation and immediately transported to the liver for oxidation.[19] It is generally suggested to increase intake of MCT oil slowly, as large amounts can cause GI symptoms such as abdominal discomfort, cramping, nausea, vomiting, diarrhea, and bloating.[19] Additionally, it is important to note that MCT oil is not particularly palatable, so it may be best to mix with fat-free beverages or low-fat foods such as applesauce or oatmeal.

Regardless, the amount of caloric intake from dietary lipids should be no higher than 30% for all individuals experiencing steatorrhea. The use of exogenous lipase may be initiated to aid in digestive processes. For cases of prolonged fat maldigestion, it is of the utmost importance to monitor the status of the fat-soluble vitamins A, D, E, and K and replete deficiencies as necessary.

PRACTICE POINT

Although fat intake should provide no more than 30% of caloric intake for patients with fat malabsorption, it remains an important source of energy. MCT oil supplements may be indicated for patients with severe or chronic fat malabsorption.

Nutrient Deficiencies. For many patients, the changes to digestive processes that occur following gastric surgery lead to maldigestion and malabsorption, and thus deficiency, of a number of micronutrients. Most often, patients present clinically with iron, folate, and/or vitamin B12 deficiency, but other common nutrient deficiencies include calcium, copper, thiamine, zinc, and vitamins D and C.[20] Note that micronutrient deficiencies develop slowly and may not manifest until years after the gastric procedure. Continued monitoring of the nutrients of concern is necessary.

It is common for patients to develop iron deficiency anemia, pernicious anemia, or macrocytic anemia postoperatively; anemias arise due to inadequate intake or malabsorption of iron, vitamin B12, and/or folate. Although clinicians monitor all symptoms of deficiency-related anemias, members of the medical team are highly attuned to those associated with vitamin B12 and iron because the mechanisms for occurrence are so well understood.[20]

Vitamin B12 becomes an issue when secretion of **intrinsic factor**, which typically occurs via the parietal cells of the stomach, is diminished following gastric surgery. Intrinsic factor is necessary for absorption of the vitamin.[2,18] Iron deficiency, the most common postoperative deficiency, may be attributed to one or two factors. First, gastric surgeries (specifically, gastrectomies) can lead to rapid transit of food particles through the duodenum, decreasing absorption time. Second, gastric acid that is secreted by the stomach is a key player in the conversion of ferric ions to ferrous ions—the form of iron most easily absorbed.[18] Some patients report a new intolerance and thus avoidance of red meat following surgery, one of the primary sources of heme iron. Regardless of the cause, all deficiencies are treated through supplementation, whether orally or via injection or intravenous infusion.[18,20]

Vitamin D deficiency can occur when the duodenum, its primary site of absorption, is bypassed. Because vitamin D is a fat-soluble vitamin, it can also become deficient with fat malabsorption as previously described. Calcium deficiency is common with gastric surgery and can be exacerbated by lack of vitamin D. Along with calcium, trace minerals zinc, copper, and selenium can become deficient due to malabsorption and bypass of the duodenum, where they are primarily absorbed as well.[20] **Table 10.2** presents common micronutrient deficiencies following gastric surgery.

Dumping Syndrome. **Dumping syndrome (DS)** is not only the most common complication of gastric surgery—it is the most intrusive. DS describes a range of symptoms that occur when stomach contents are released too quickly and in too large of a volume into the small intestine. This creates a hyperosmolar overload, which the body overcompensates for by drawing excess fluid into the intestine. DS is subdivided into two forms: early and late; classification depends on the length of time following ingestion of a meal that symptoms arise. It is likely the result of a combination of factors, including changes in gastric emptying, changes to innervation of the stomach, and changes in the function of the pyloric sphincter.[21]

Early DS, which accounts for more than 75% of cases, manifests 10–30 minutes postprandially as a combination of GI and vasomotor symptoms. The typical GI symptoms—abdominal pain, bloating, nausea, vomiting, and explosive diarrhea—occur as a direct result of the hyperosmolar content and influx of fluid into the intestine. Electrolyte imbalances can occur due to GI losses with diarrhea. Vasomotor symptoms include headache, flushing, fatigue, dizziness, perspiration, palpitations, and hypotension, and are likely the consequence of hormone fluctuations. The expression of these symptoms will vary based on the individual.[18,22]

The remaining 25% of cases are classified as late DS (patients rarely experience symptoms common to both categories). Late dumping manifests anywhere from 1 to 3 hours after a meal with systemic, vascular symptoms. It is thought to be the result of reactive hypoglycemia: the rapid delivery of carbohydrates to the small intestine is followed by rapid absorption of glucose into circulation, which the body counters with an exaggerated release of insulin. Associated

Table 10.2 Micronutrient Deficiency, Etiology and Clinical Manifestations Following Gastric Surgery

Vitamins	Etiology	Clinical Manifestations
Vitamin B12	Lack of gastric acidity and production of intrinsic factor due to resection of parietal cells	Macrocytic anemia, neurological complications, numbness, poor coordination, swollen red tongue, bleeding gums
Fat-Soluble Vitamins A, D, E, K	Fat maldigestion, improper mixing with bile acid	Bone loss, impaired blood clotting, immune impairment, night blindness, hyperkeratosis
Folate	Duodenal bypassing, vitamin B12 deficiency	Macrocytic anemia, fatigue, shortness of breath, memory loss, pregnancy risk for neural tube defects
Vitamin C	Poor diet postsurgery	Scurvy, bleeding gums, bruising
Thiamine	Jejunal bypassing, vomiting	Beriberi: nerve and muscle abnormalities, heart failure Wernicke–Korsakoff syndrome: irritability fatigue, anorexia, numbness, weakness
Trace Elements		
Iron	Lack of gastric acidity to solubilize and stabilize ferric ion for absorption, duodenal bypassing	Anemia, pale skin, dizziness, heart palpitations, shortness of breath, cold extremities
Calcium	Fat malabsorption, duodenal bypassing	Osteoporosis, muscle spasms, weak nails, tooth decay
Zinc	Duodenal bypassing	Poor healing, dermatitis, hair loss
Copper	Duodenal bypassing	Fatigue, pallor, joint pain, numbness
Selenium	Duodenal bypassing	Cardiomyopathy, muscle weakness, fatigue, hair loss

Data from Gasmi A, Bjørklund G, Mujawdiya PK, et al. Micronutrient deficiencies in patients after bariatric surgery. *Eur J Nutr*. 2022;61:55-67. doi:10.1007/s00394-021-02619-8

symptoms include perspiration, weakness, confusion, and shakiness.[18,21,22]

The majority of patients with DS respond to a course of treatment that includes nutrition therapy. Pharmacologic agents like acarbose and octreotide can be used to correct hypoglycemia, delay gastric emptying, decrease postprandial vasodilation, and increase the absorption of water in the intestine. Regardless, dietary modifications are unavoidable. Patients will work to identify foods that trigger episodes of dumping. Generally, foods that exacerbate symptoms and should be avoided are those containing lactose or the simple sugars sucrose, fructose, or sugar alcohols (xylitol, mannitol, and sorbitol). Carbohydrate intake should instead consist primarily of complex carbohydrate choices. A high fiber diet that includes protein and fat at each meal in increased amounts will counterbalance the caloric deficit created by the decreased intake of refined carbohydrates. It is crucial that patients continue to meet daily energy needs to avoid unintentional weight loss.[14,21,22]

Distributing daily intake into small, frequent meals, along with slow and thorough chewing, will help to prevent large amounts of undigested food from reaching the small intestine too quickly. Fluid intake should be limited, if not completely restricted, during mealtimes. Patients should wait at least 30 minutes after finishing a meal to drink liquids.[14,22] It may be helpful for patients to lie in the supine position postprandially to delay gastric emptying and minimize vasomotor symptoms. For those who experience severe hypoglycemic episodes, supplementation of dietary fiber has been proven effective to delay glucose absorption and prolong transit time.[21,22]

CORE CONCEPT 5

Gastric surgery indicates a number of concerning nutritional implications that may occur during the postoperative period. Nutrition interventions should be tailored to each individual depending on the symptoms and clinical manifestations that arise.

Nutrition Assessment. All patients recovering from gastric surgery are at nutritional risk. Throughout the postoperative period, individuals are monitored for the physical manifestations and biochemical indicators of the nutritional complications, including unexplained weight loss, inadequate intake, food intolerances, or other parameters consistent with malnutrition.[23] Weight loss following a gastric procedure is well documented, and unintended weight loss is of nutritional concern for nonelective procedures. Postprandial fullness is the main culprit, but weight loss may also result from inadequate intake due to DS symptoms or malabsorption.[18]

A complete nutrition assessment should address the patient's dietary history, anthropometric values, and other physical indicators of nutritional status, biochemical indices, and clinical parameters. Evaluation of dietary habits that typically exacerbate symptoms, including consumption of simple carbohydrates, caffeine, dairy foods, and/or fluids with meals, is critical. Symptoms that would interfere with normal eating patterns, such as nausea, vomiting, constipation, and diarrhea, may be addressed through nutrition interventions. Biochemical assessments should consider values associated with anemia (complete blood count, iron studies, vitamin B12, folate), fluid and electrolyte status, additional micronutrients of concern (copper, vitamin A, vitamin D, and thiamine), and transport proteins (albumin, prealbumin).[23]

Nutrition Intervention. Enhanced recovery after surgery (ERAS) is a concept that is used to improve recovery after surgery, reduce risk of complications, and shorten hospital stays. It involves an interprofessional, multimodal approach that essentially follows the patient through their operative phases of care. Strategies include patient education, guidelines for pre- and postoperative nutrition therapy, and early mobilization after surgery. Advances in this program have led to ERAS protocols and evidence-based guidelines for many different surgical subsets including hip and knee replacement, cardiac surgery, cardiac, liver, and pancreatic disease, a wide range of oncology conditions, and bariatric surgery.[24]

A major goal of ERAS is to reduce metabolic stress during the perioperative phase of care (preparation for surgery, surgery, and after surgery) in order to improve surgical outcomes. Presurgical interventions focus on nutrition, physical activity, and stress reduction. Nutritional assessment is recommended prior to surgery. Patients should be provided with nutrition support if they are malnourished, unlikely to eat perioperatively for 5 days, or if they have a history of poor oral intake. Use of an ONS and/or enteral nutrition (EN) is the optimal mode of therapy.

One key element in the ERAS program for patients undergoing surgery is to reduce perioperative fasting. Traditional protocols that include prolonged periods of fasting are no longer recommended. Allowing solids until 6 hours prior to surgery and clear liquids up to 2 hours prior to surgery has not been associated with added surgical risk of aspiration or regurgitation and reduces stress upon the patient. Use of carbohydrate clear liquid solutions is also recommended and has been associated with increased patient comfort without complications. Caution should be taken in patients with gastroparesis or severe diabetes.

Another key component of the ERAS protocol is early oral nutrition following surgery. In most cases, oral intake, particularly clear liquids, can be provided within a few hours postsurgery. This relies heavily on the individual patient and procedure. Other postsurgical interventions include reduction of factors that may interfere with GI tolerance, minimized time on postoperative paralytics, and early mobilization to facilitate protein synthesis and muscle function. **Table 10.3** displays the basic elements of the ERAS protocol for gastric surgery.[25,26]

It is easier to prevent the occurrence of nutritional complications than to correct it. For example, vitamin B12 supplementation is initiated for all patients following gastric surgery, before the manifestations of pernicious anemia arise.[18] As gastric procedures modify the anatomy of the digestive tract, all patients, regardless of the presence of the associated complications, will require dietary modifications in addition to supplementation. An individual's postoperative status, including prior medical history, will have a significant impact on their current nutritional requirements.[23] Thus, nutrition interventions should be individualized and will require adjustments based on the development of new or alleviation of existing symptoms.[18] A nutrition intervention should first ensure that the patient continues to maintain daily energy needs. Adequate caloric and protein intakes are necessary to promote optimal postoperative healing. This is accomplished through small, frequent meals that exclude foods known to exacerbate symptoms. Refer to **Table 10.4** for a list of common foods to be limited or avoided altogether. If progression to solid food is delayed, it may be necessary to recommend appropriate nutrition support.[18,24] Studies have demonstrated that, if warranted, postoperative early EN is safe and well tolerated.[27]

Nutrition education should also be provided to help minimize the symptoms of micronutrient deficiency, early and late DS, and maldigestion or malabsorption. Nutrition counseling ensures adequate

Table 10.3 ERAS Guidelines for Patients Undergoing Gastric Surgery

Surgery Type	Preoperative	Intraoperative	Postoperative
Bariatric Surgery	Preoperative information Patient education Carbohydrate loading Reduced fasting times Prehabilitation/exercise Cessation of smoking and alcohol consumption	Fluid management Prophylactic management of nausea/vomiting Anesthesia protocols Airway management Nasogastric tube Abdominal drainage	Pain management Early ambulation Early nutrition
Surgery for Gastric Cancer	Preoperative nutrition Malnutrition screening Nutrition support	Minimally invasive surgery (laparoscopy, robotic surgery, hybrid procedures) Nasogastric/nasojejunal decompression Early mobilization	Early postoperative diet ■ Oral liquids on day one ■ Nutrition support if unable to meet 60% of estimated energy needs Limit abdominal drainage Early mobilization

Data from Desiderio J, Trastulli S, D'Andrea V, Parisi A. Enhanced recovery after surgery for gastric cancer (ERAS-GC): optimizing patient outcome. *Transl Gastroenterol Hepatol*. 2020;5:11. doi:10.21037/tgh.2019.10.04; Huh YJ, Kim DJ. Enhanced recovery after surgery in bariatric surgery. *J Metab Bariatr Surg*. 2021;10(2):47-54. doi:10.17476/jmbs.2021.10.2.47

Table 10.4 Foods to Limit or Avoid Following Gastric Surgery

Food Group	Foods to Limit or Avoid
Dairy Products	■ Chocolate milk or other dairy products made with added sugar • It may be necessary to choose lactose-free products or soy milk.
Protein Foods	■ Fried meat, poultry, or fish ■ Deli meats ■ Sausage, hot dogs, bacon ■ Tough or chewy meats ■ Dried beans and peas ■ Nuts and chunky nut butters
Vegetables	■ All raw vegetables (excluding lettuce) ■ Any cooked vegetables served with skins or seeds ■ Beets ■ Gas-producing vegetables, including broccoli, Brussels sprouts, cabbage, and cauliflower ■ Collards, mustard, and turnip greens ■ Corn ■ Potato skins
Fruits	■ All raw fruits except banana and melons ■ Dried fruits, including prunes and raisins ■ Any fruit juice ■ Canned fruit in sugar or syrup
Beverages	■ Any caffeinated or carbonated beverage ■ Alcohol-containing beverages ■ Beverages made with sugar, corn syrup, or honey ■ Fruit juices and other fruit drinks • Do not drink milk or other beverages with meals or snacks. After consuming solid foods, wait a minimum of 30 minutes before having a beverage.
Other	■ Sugar ■ Honey, syrup ■ Sorbitol, xylitol

Data from Academy of Nutrition and Dietetics. Gastric surgery nutrition therapy. *Nutrition Care Manual*. Academy of Nutrition and Dietetics; 2015.

calorie and protein intake, prevents weight loss, and improves quality of life for many of these patients.[28]

Nutrition Monitoring and Evaluation. Monitoring and evaluation of patient response to therapy should include assessment of weight and weight history, GI tolerance related to specific foods, and stool frequency and patterns. Biochemical indices for monitoring anemia, fat-soluble vitamins, and any nutrients of concern based on surgical history and dietary intake. Fluid and electrolyte status should be assessed to screen for dehydration and hypoglycemia.

Pancreatitis

Pancreatitis, in both its acute and chronic forms, is an inflammatory disorder of the pancreas. Both disease states require different approaches to nutritional management.[29] The pancreas plays a dual role in endocrine and exocrine activities. As part of its endocrine function, the pancreas secretes digestive enzymes including amylase, lipase, protease. The pancreas also has a primary role in endocrine function by secreting insulin and glucagon (**Figure 10.7**). Although acute pancreatitis has less impact on digestive functions than chronic pancreatitis, pancreatic exocrine functions are more impacted by disease progression in chronic pancreatitis. All patients with acute pancreatitis require nutrition intervention, while many may require nutritional support. Chronic pancreatitis, on the other hand, has a direct impact on the digestive and absorptive abilities of the GI system, negatively affecting the patient's nutritional status. Any abnormality

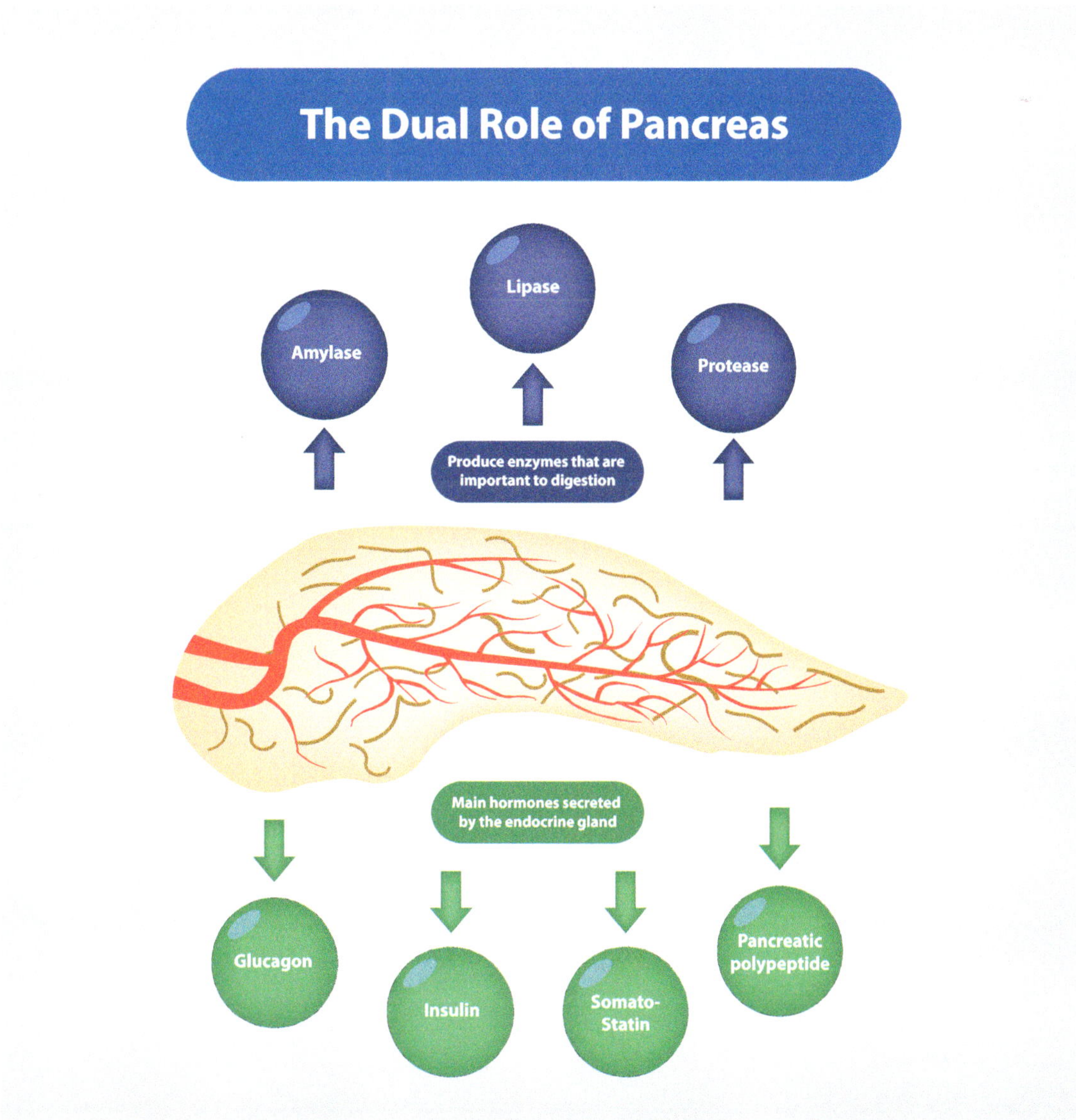

Figure 10.7 Normal Secretory Function of the Pancreas

Table 10.5 Common Etiologies for Acute Pancreatitis*

Etiology	Susceptibility Factor
Lifestyle Factors	■ Alcohol use disorder (>2 alcohol containing drinks per day [average]) ■ Obesity (BMI >30) ■ Heavy smoking history ■ Illegal drug use
Duct Obstruction	■ Gallstones or biliary sludge ■ Post-endoscopic cholangiopancreatography (ERCP) ■ Tumors ■ Anatomical abnormalities ■ Parasites
Metabolic Abnormalities	■ Hyperlipidemia ■ Hypercalcemia ■ Acidosis
Medications (*partial list*)	■ Acetaminophen ■ Azathioprine ■ Erythromycin ■ Estrogen ■ Hydrochlorothiazide ■ Nonsteroidal anti-inflammatory drugs ■ Tetracycline
Genetic Factors	■ Cystic fibrosis gene (*CFTR*) ■ Trypsinogen gene (*PRSS1*) ■ Pancreatic secretory trypsin inhibitor gene (*SPINK1*)
Infectious	■ Viral infection ■ Bacterial infection
Trauma	■ Blunt or penetrating ■ Surgical

*A number of cases (20%) are idiopathic.[29]

Data from Papachristou G, Singh V, Whitcomb DC. Acute pancreatitis. In: *Textbook of Clinical Gastroenterology and Hepatology*. Wiley-Blackwell; 2012:518-524. doi:10.1002/9781118321386.ch69. Accessed January 22, 2025.

involving the exocrine functions of the pancreas will have considerable nutritional implications.

Acute Pancreatitis

Acute pancreatitis (AP) is an extremely common disorder of the digestive system, most often the result of a biliary tract obstruction or alcohol use disorder. Refer to **Table 10.5** for a more comprehensive list of common etiologies.

Regardless of the initial cause, all cases of AP manifest as inflammation of the pancreas, as indicated in **Figure 10.8**. This figure depicts a gallstone blockage, which is a common, but not the only cause of acute pancreatitis. Although the exact mechanism of pancreatic injury in AP is not fully understood, the

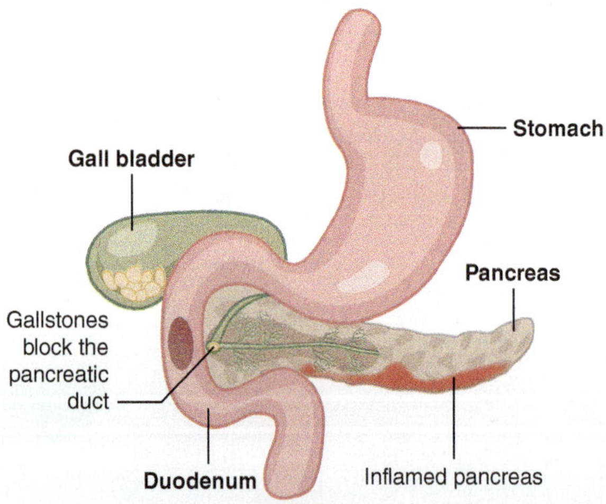

Figure 10.8 Acute Pancreatitis Is Represented Here as the Result of Gallstones Blocking the Pancreatic Duct

Table 10.6 Revised Atlanta Classification System with Clinical Implications

	Revised Atlanta Classification (2012)	Implications
Mild	■ No organ failure ■ No systemic inflammation or local complications	■ Typically does not require abdominal imaging ■ Frequently discharged within 3–7 days of onset of illness
Moderate	■ Transient organ failure (defined as organ failure lasting <48 hours) ■ Local systemic complications without persistent organ failure (>48 hours)	■ Organ failure includes respiratory, cardiovascular, and renal failure ■ Local complications include interstitial pancreatitis and necrotizing pancreatitis ■ May require a longer hospital stay ■ Typically associated with a higher mortality rate
Severe	■ Persistent organ failure (>48 hours)	■ Persistent organ failure may affect single or multiple organs ■ Patients with persistent organ failure usually present with one or more local complications ■ Associated with increased risk of death (mortality reported to be as great as 50%)

Data from Banks PA, Bollen TL, Dervenis C, et al. Classification of acute pancreatitis—2012: revision of the Atlanta classification and definitions by international consensus. *Gut*. 2013;62(1):102-111.

most common theory involves irregular activation of pancreatic digestive enzymes. Premature stimulation of trypsin within the pancreas results in autodigestion of the pancreatic cells, triggering an immune response. The enzymes released by the destroyed cells eventually move into circulation, to be later detected by elevated serum amylase and lipase levels. Patients typically present with nausea, vomiting, steatorrhea, and abdominal pain that may radiate to the back.[29–32]

A clinical diagnosis is made upon admission based on the presence of at least two of the following three criteria:

1. Sudden onset of abdominal pain characteristic of AP
2. Serum amylase and/or lipase levels three (or more) times the upper limit of normal values
3. Findings characteristic of AP on abdominal imaging studies (contrast-enhanced computed tomography, magnetic resonance imaging, or transabdominal ultrasound)

Additionally, although most AP cases resolve without causing significant harm, it is not uncommon for immune system involvement to extend beyond the pancreas and trigger a systemic inflammatory response. The 15% of patients who develop multiorgan involvement and/or pancreatic necrosis within the first 72 hours of diagnosis have prolonged hospital stays, as well as significant increases in morbidity and mortality.[29,30]

Classification. Once AP is determined as the definitive diagnosis, a scoring system is then used to classify the severity of the disease state. Of the many classification tools available, most consider both the level of systemic inflammation and the level of extrapancreatic organ dysfunction. Although there are a number of useful systems, including Ranson's Criteria, Acute Physiology and Chronic Health Evaluation (APACHE II), and the Bedside Index for Severity of Acute Pancreatitis (BISAP), the newly revised Atlanta classification is the most applicable system in the clinical setting. Under this method, clinical severity is stratified into three categories: mild, moderate, and severe. The revised Atlanta clarification is described in more detail in **Table 10.6**.[30,33]

If the patient improves rapidly without organ failure or systemic complications, the disease falls into the mild AP category. If local or systemic complications arise, but cannot be classified as persistent (lasting more than 48 hours), the disease is defined as moderate AP. Finally, if persistent organ failure affecting single or multiple organ(s) occurs, the disease is regarded as severe AP and is associated with high morbidity and mortality rates.[29,33] Classification guides provide guidance for determining the best course of treatment. When the Atlanta system is used, the mild, moderate, and severe classifications help determine the necessary extent of dietary intervention. Most notably, these levels provide the most reliable indication of patients who will require nutrition support.[29,30]

Treatment. The primary treatment for AP involves early, aggressive fluid resuscitation and pain treatment immediately upon admission. Resuscitation with lactated Ringer's solution rather than normal saline solution has been associated with decreased severity of AP, likely related to a reduction in C-reactive protein

(CRP) levels.[34] The treatment plan will also provide management of respiratory and kidney function, treatment of infection, and, when warranted, nutrition support.[29,31,33] For a patient with AP, it is critical to prevent stimulation of the pancreas and thus reduce the release of its digestive secretions. Pancreatic rest is accomplished through the implementation of **NPO** (*nil per os*, or nothing by mouth) status; without food entering the digestive tract, there is no trigger prompting pancreatic stimulation.[31]

Pancreatitis represents a highly catabolic state in body.[30] For the majority of patients, this is not terribly concerning, as mild AP will have little impact on metabolism or nutritional status.[30] In addition, oral intake is typically restored within 3–5 days of hospitalization, when the symptoms of nausea, vomiting, and abdominal pain resolve.[29,30] Past studies have suggested feeding should begin first with clear liquids and progress to foods as tolerated.[30,32] However, the 2016 American Society for Parenteral and Enteral Nutrition (ASPEN) guidelines recommend patients with mild disease advance to a normal diet rather than a clear liquid diet initially, as this has been demonstrated to decrease hospital length of stay.[35] There is strong consensus that the diet should be advanced as soon as tolerated without waiting for normalization of serum lipase concentration.[36]

Patients classified with severe AP have elevated nutrition needs as a result of increased energy expenditure and high protein catabolism rates.[35] Energy requirements are similar to that during critical illness in adults. ASPEN guidelines recommend a calorie range of 12–25 kcal/kg with protein ranging between 1.2 and 2 grams/kg depending on severity of illness.[35] The European Society for Clinical Nutrition and Metabolism (ESPEN) recommends 20–25 kcal/kg/day, with a protein target of 1.3 grams/kg/day. A lower target for protein is suggested in the event of acute kidney injury, which often accompanies AP[37] Both recommend nutrition support early in the course of the disease.[35,37]

Nutrition Support. Nutrition support is indicated for all patients with severe necrotizing pancreatitis (pancreatitis associated with necrosis or pancreatic tissue death) and in more moderate cases if oral nutrition is not possible due to pain or other symptoms after more than 5 days.[36] EN is preferred over parenteral nutrition (PN) because it is associated with reduced infectious and systemic complications and hospital length of stay, and is less expensive.[36,38,42,43] Strong evidence suggests that the risks of multiorgan failure and mortality are significantly less for patients provided EN when compared to those receiving PN.[38]

There are no specific contraindications for EN use in acute pancreatitis. Position statements from both societies confirm that tube feeding can be executed successfully even when severe AP is accompanied by complications such as pseudocysts, ascites, and/or **fistulas**, which are abnormal passages or connections between two body parts.[35,36] Most patients tolerate standard polymeric intact protein enteral formulas, although a peptide-based MCT oil–containing formula may be indicated if significant maldigestion is present.[35–38]

The recommendation for route of EN is slightly controversial. Some clinicians feel that nasojejunal (NJ) tube placement is superior to nasogastric (NG) tube placement because it provides greater pancreatic rest.[30] However, substantial evidence indicates that NG feeding—which is simpler, less expensive, and easier to implement—is equally as effective as NJ feeding for patients with severe AP.[38–42] Per ESPEN consensus, NJ feeding would only be preferred in the case of digestive intolerance.[36] Regardless of the route implemented, the timing of EN support is also considered important. When started within the first 48 hours of admission, EN improves GI function, reduces inflammation, decreases hospital length of stay, and reduces the risk of multiorgan involvement and infection.[41] Based on the abundance of evidence, early EN is currently recommended in this population.[36,38,42,43]

In some cases, EN may need to be supplemented with or replaced by PN. Although associated with greater complications,[42] this route is indicated for patients unable to tolerate the EN route or when complications to the digestive tract render EN administration impossible.[36,43] When using PN, it is suggested that the energy goal be reduced by 70% to prevent overfeeding, particularly in the early stage of care. In addition, parenteral glutamine, if available, at a dose of 0.20 grams/kg/day is suggested, given its potential benefits on surgical outcome.[36]

Oral feeding can be attempted once symptoms normalize if it does not result in pain or further complications. This typically begins with initiation of liquids, then a low-fat solid diet, progressing to a more normalized intake as tolerated. EN or PN feedings may be gradually weaned as oral intake improves over time.[36,43]

PRACTICE POINT

Enteral nutrition is the recommended method of nutrition support for patients with severe acute pancreatitis and should be started within 48 hours of admission. The nasogastric route is acceptable unless digestive intolerance is noted.

⚠ Clinical Controversy

Nasogastric Versus Nasojejunal Tube Feeding in Acute Pancreatitis

Enteral nutrition during acute pancreatitis is the optimal mode of feeding in patients with AP and may even alter the course of an inflammatory state if provided early. However, the type of tube feeding placement remains controversial. A recent meta-analysis by Dutta et al. found no difference in efficacy between nasogastric and nasojejunal feedings in patients with respect to mortality, infection rate, and tolerance of feedings. This is significant since nasogastric feeding tubes are often easily placed, enabling early initiation of feedings which is also favorable in this population. In contrast with this recommendation are the findings of O'Keefe et al. where nasogastric feedings were associated with a higher rate of feeding failure (55%), which improved with nasojejunal feeding. Because nutrition support is so important in acute pancreatitis, determining the optimal route of administration is important.

Question

1. Read the referenced articles. Compare study design and findings. What would your recommendation be regarding EN route of administration for patients with acute pancreatitis?

References

1. Dutta- AK, Goel A, Kirubakaran R, Chacko A, Tharyan P. Nasogastric versus nasojejunal tube feeding for severe acute pancreatitis. *Cochrane Database Syst Rev*. 2020;3(3):CD010582. doi:10.1002/14651858.CD010582.pub2
2. O'Keefe S, Graham T, Coté GA, Whitcomb DC, Evans A, Soni D. Early enteral feeding in severe acute pancreatitis: a randomized clinical trial between gastric vs distal jejunal feeding. *Tech Innov Gastrointest Endosc*. 2023;25(4):337-346. doi:10.1016/j.tige.2023.06.002

Chronic Pancreatitis

The hallmark of **chronic pancreatitis (CP)** is progressive, long-standing inflammation of the pancreas leading to fibrosis and gradual loss of both exocrine and endocrine functions. CP presents as one of two recognized forms—small-duct or large-duct—and can take several years to develop. The disease is complex and pathogenesis is controversial. The most common cause, responsible for upwards of 80% of cases, is excessive alcohol consumption. However, there are several other contributing factors. For many patients, CP occurs as the result of a mixture of environmental factors (alcohol use disorder, tobacco use, suboptimal nutrition, and/or occupational chemical exposure) and genetic predisposition. In addition, CP may accompany a hereditary condition or autoimmune disease. Approximately 20% of cases are classified as idiopathic.[36,44–46]

For all patients with CP, the continuous inflammation causes irreversible damage. Fibrous tissue replaces the normal parenchyma of the pancreas and results in the loss of islets and acinar cells. The resulting loss of function can manifest as diabetes mellitus (type 3c) and/or as decline in pancreatic exocrine function in varying degrees, respectively. These changes to pancreatic structure wreak havoc on the normal digestion and absorption of nutrients. In addition, almost all patients with CP report significant upper abdominal pain that may radiate to the back. Refer to **Table 10.7** for the most common clinical presentations of CP.[36,44–47]

Table 10.7 Clinical Features of Chronic Pancreatitis

Abdominal Pain	▪ In upper abdomen, may radiate to the back ▪ Exacerbated by eating and/or drinking (especially alcohol) ▪ **Type A Pain:** recurrent episodic pain ▪ **Type B Pain:** continuous pain
Pancreatic Exocrine Insufficiency (PEI)	▪ Maldigestion ▪ Steatorrhea ▪ Weight loss
Diabetes Mellitus (DM)	▪ Type 3c DM ▪ Endocrine hormone deficiencies • Insufficient glucagon and insulin
Rare Complications	▪ Pseudocysts ▪ Splenic vein thrombosis ▪ Nausea and vomiting ▪ Jaundice ▪ Pale, clay-colored stools

Data from Afghani E, Sinha A, Singh VK. An overview of the diagnosis and management of nutrition in chronic pancreatitis. *Nutr Clin Pract*. 2014;29(3):295-311.; Berberat PO, Ceyhan GO, Dambrauskas Z, Büchler MW, Friess H. Chronic pancreatitis. In: *Textbook of Clinical Gastroenterology and Hepatology*. Wiley-Blackwell; 2012:525-532.

Nutrition Intervention. All treatment of CP begins with conservative, noninvasive measures for pain control and nutrition management to correct the consequences of exocrine insufficiency. This will include counseling against any exacerbating factors. Patients should receive thorough education on abstinence from alcohol, smoking cessation, and limiting excessive dietary fat. More extreme measures, including endoscopic treatment or surgical intervention, are only considered when conventional therapy fails to control pain or other complications.[48] The therapy required by each of the primary complications will be discussed in detail in the following sections.

Abdominal Pain. Almost all patients with CP experience debilitating abdominal pain. It serves as the primary reason many seek initial medical care, but it is also the most difficult to correct. This type of pain typically worsens postprandially, especially following the consumption of a high-fat meal. Both recurrent and continuous abdominal pain are associated with decreased appetite, weight loss, and eventual malnutrition.[47–49]

Although abdominal pain may be corrected surgically, the first line of treatment is always non-narcotic analgesics and/or nonsteroidal anti-inflammatory agents for pain relief. For those with severe pain that does not subside after initial intervention, narcotic analgesics are prescribed; most will require this route for pain management. Because medical therapy is largely ineffective, many patients ultimately require endoscopic or surgical treatment. Surgical procedures indicated by intractable abdominal pain involve drainage and/or resection and will be discussed later in the chapter.[40,41] Interestingly, there is strong evidence that exogenous enzyme supplementation for pancreatic insufficiency can be used to treat pain in patients with CP. The mechanism by which enzyme therapy alleviates pain is thought to occur through a reduction in pancreatic secretions and thus ductal pressure.[44,50]

Pancreatic Exocrine Insufficiency. The primary nutritional concern for patients with CP is maldigestion due to deficiency of pancreatic enzymes. **Pancreatic exocrine insufficiency (PEI)**, formally defined as a reduction in pancreatic enzyme activity below the threshold necessary for normal digestion, is directly related to destruction of acinar cell mass and the associated decrease in levels of the enzymes lipase, amylase, and trypsin.[39,44]

The most common and reliable indication of exocrine insufficiency is bulky, foul-smelling stools indicative of excess excretion of fat. As pancreatic lipase is responsible for 90% of all lipid digestion, PEI is primarily associated with maldigestion of fat leading to steatorrhea. Decreased secretion of amylase impacts carbohydrate metabolism and may lead to starch excretion in the feces (**amylorrhea**), abdominal distention, and/or flatulence. In addition, the loss of pancreatic trypsin leads to maldigestion of protein, which can manifest as edema, ascites, and/or **azotorrhea** (excess nitrogen in the urine or feces). Because the body has additional mechanisms for carbohydrate and protein breakdown that do not require pancreatic enzymes, fat maldigestion remains the primary concern. Any maldigestion and subsequent malabsorption can cause unintentional weight loss, micronutrient deficiencies, and malnutrition. Early diagnosis of PEI is crucial to prevent or reduce these complications. Criteria for diagnosing PEI include a fecal fat test following a high fat diet of 100 grams. This method requires a 3-day stool sample collection and relies on patient adherence. Alternatively, fecal elastase can be measured in stools; a method that is widespread and inexpensive. Elastase levels below 200 micrograms/gram are considered abnormal. Low levels of elastase (<50 mcg/gram) are diagnostic of steatorrhea.[40,41,51]

Most patients can be managed by dietary interventions to reduce steatorrhea and supplement calories. This generally includes maintenance of adequate intake, with the highest level of fat that will not result in steatorrhea or abdominal pain. Most importantly, all patients with PEI will benefit from supplementation with exogenous **pancreatic enzyme replacement therapy (PERT)**. Nutrition therapy will focus on alleviating PEI-related symptoms, limiting both weight loss and micronutrient deficiencies, and, above all, preventing malnutrition.[39,40,44,45,50]

Pancreatic Enzyme Replacement Therapy. The best way to improve the nutritional status of a patient with PEI is by initiating PERT immediately upon diagnosis. Supplementation with exogenous pancreatic enzymes is associated with alleviation of symptoms (steatorrhea and abdominal pain) and improvement in body weight; in addition, because the enzymes are safe, well tolerated, and easy to administer, PERT has become the gold standard of treatment for the maldigestion associated with CP.[29,40,43,45,51]

Pancreatic enzymes with each oral feeding distributed throughout the meal ensure adequate digestion and absorption. Consuming 4–5 meals per day along and taking acid-reducing agents will also help the efficacy of enzymes. Dietary fat restriction should be avoided to augment caloric intake and fat-soluble vitamin availability.[51] **Pancreatic enzyme preparations (PEP)**, called "pancrelipase" or "pancreatin," contain a mixture of the digestive enzymes amylase, lipase, and protease. The enteric-coated tablets are taken orally and designed to withstand the

Table 10.8 Pancreatic Enzyme Preparations (PEP) Approved for Use

- Creon
  - Enteric
  - Delayed-release capsule
- Zenpep
  - Enteric
  - Delayed-release capsule
- Pancreaze
  - Enteric
  - Delayed-release capsule
- Ultresa
  - Enteric
  - Delayed-release capsule
- Pertzye
  - Enteric
  - Delayed-release capsule
- Viokace
  - Nonenteric
  - Tablet

Generic, pancrelipase.

Data from Afghani E, Sinha A, Singh VK. An overview of the diagnosis and management of nutrition in chronic pancreatitis. *Nutr Clin Pract*. 2014;29(3):295–311; Muniraj T, Aslanian HR, Farrell J, Jamidar PA. Chronic pancreatitis, a comprehensive review. part II: Diagnosis, complications, and management. *Dis Mon*. 2015;61(1):5–37.

acidic environment of the stomach to prevent denaturation of the enzymes before reaching the duodenum.[46] Refer to **Table 10.8** for a more detailed list of brand name medications for PEP.

Administration should be individualized per patient and per meal, according to body weight, severity of exocrine insufficiency, and fat composition of food. Initial dosage usually includes 20,000 units of lipase, but most patients require between 25,000 and 75,000 units per meal; generally, approximately 2,000 units of lipase are needed per gram of fat.[39,43] While correct dosing allows for optimal digestion in the GI tract lumen, timing of administration is equally as important. Enzymes must be taken to facilitate interaction with both nutrients and the intestinal lumen at the same time. There is evidence that the optimal timing of PEP dosing in relation to food consumption with pancreatitis is during and after a meal, and not prior.[44,51,52]

When administered in the correct dose and with correct timing, PERT will aid in the digestion of fats, protein, and carbohydrates; increase absorption of micronutrients; alleviate steatorrhea; and help to maintain normal nutritional status for patients with PEI.[46]

PRACTICE POINT

Every patient with PEI should be treated with pancreatic enzyme replacement therapy (PERT). A dose ranging from 20,000 to 75,000 USP units of lipase per meal and about half of that amount (~20,000 USP units) per snack should be initiated. The most important parameters for monitoring success are body weight and improvement in GI symptoms.

Nutrient Deficiency and Malnutrition. Patients with CP, especially those also diagnosed with PEI, are at increased risk for nutrient deficiency and malnutrition as a result of maldigestion, malabsorption, and poor oral intake. Because the etiology for most cases of CP is alcohol use disorder, many patients enter the disease state with an already-impaired nutritional status.[48] The development and severity of malnutrition is two-fold. First, maldigestion and malabsorption force the body to deplete its energy and nutrient stores. Second, there is increased metabolic activity as a result of the disease process; patients with CP have resting energy expenditure 30–50% above normal.[44,47]

Thorough nutritional screening will identify all patients at risk for nutrient deficiencies and malnutrition. The major cause—maldigestion of macronutrients—is corrected in large part by the initiation of PERT. However, nutrition interventions must ensure sufficient intake to meet the increased caloric needs of the patient. Typically, a diet providing at least 35 kcal/kg of body weight/day through small, frequent meals will meet the energy demands of CP. Most patients will not require a fat restriction due to supplementation with PERT; however, if fat intake is not fully tolerated, MCTs can be added to the diet without exacerbation because they do not require lipase for digestion.[30,47,50]

Nutrition Support. Most patients with CP can be treated adequately with typical oral food intake and PERT. Some patients may require additional calories and protein through an ONS between meals. PERT therapy should be coordinated with ONS as well. Patients who are malnourished or who have difficulty meeting their needs orally may require tube feeding to overcome calorie deficits. Enteral nutrition therapy should be individualized in these patients. Both bolus and continuous feeding can be used. Generally, a standard polymeric feeding is well tolerated, although some patients may require elemental feedings if GI intolerance is present. Patients receiving pancreatic enzymes are generally prescribed a low fiber formula as fiber can interact with pancreatic enzyme function.

Timing of pancreatic enzymes for tube fed patients can also be a challenge. A lipase cartridge system can be used to coordinate pancreatic enzymes with tube feeding delivery.[53] This is described in more detail in Chapter 21, *Nutrition in Cystic Fibrosis*. Only a small number of patients will need nutrition support through PN.[27]

Nutrition Monitoring and Evaluation. Nutrition therapy for patients with CP must always include monitoring for and repletion of any micronutrient deficiencies. Nutrients of concern are primarily the fat-soluble vitamins A, D, E, and K; deficiency of these vitamins correlates directly with severity of steatorrhea but may also be the result of suboptimal intake. Increased losses and malabsorption may also contribute to deficiencies of vitamin B12, calcium, zinc, magnesium, copper, folate, and/or thiamine.[30,47,50] Additionally, it is important to note that those with CP are at high risk of developing either osteoporosis or osteopenia, with an estimated incidence of two out of three people. A dual-energy x-ray absorptiometry (DXA) should be used to identify osteopathy.[37]

PRACTICE POINT

It is critical to provide adequate protein (1.2–1.5 grams protein/kg/day) and energy intake (35 kcal/kg/day) to meet the increased demands of CP and prevent the development of malnutrition.

CORE CONCEPT 6

Acute pancreatitis and chronic pancreatitis differ substantially in their respective nutritional requirements. For both disease states, it is crucial to provide sufficient energy to meet increased needs, adapt care plans in regard to individual symptoms, and intervene with nutrition support when necessary.

Pancreatic Surgery

Pancreatic procedures that alter the GI anatomy are massively complex and associated with a number of surgical complications and debilitating nutritional implications postoperatively. Surgery of this nature is indicated in one of two cases: to treat pancreatic malignancies or when pain management in CP cannot be controlled through noninvasive treatment.[53] Refer to **Table 10.9** for common CP complications that require surgical intervention.

Table 10.9 Indications for Surgical Intervention in Chronic Pancreatitis

Chronic Abdominal Pain	■ Pain does not resolve with conservative medical treatment ■ Prolonged medication use results in narcotic dependency
Obstruction	■ Common bile duct and/or pancreatic duct obstruction ■ Duodenal obstruction ■ Portal and/or splenic vein obstruction
Malignancies	■ Mass lesion in pancreatic head ■ Suspected pancreatic cancer
Pancreatic Complications	■ Ductal rupture ■ Persistent or symptomatic pseudocyst ■ Pancreatic fistula unresponsive to other therapy ■ Pancreatic ascites unresponsive to medical therapy

Data from Afghani E, Sinha A, Singh VK. An overview of the diagnosis and management of nutrition in chronic pancreatitis. *Nutr Clin Pract.* 2014;29(3):295-311.; Berberat PO, Ceyhan GO, Dambrauskas Z, Büchler MW, Friess H. Chronic pancreatitis. In: *Textbook of Clinical Gastroenterology and Hepatology*. Wiley-Blackwell; 2012:525-532. doi:10.1002/9781118321386.ch70. Accessed January 22, 2025.; Berry AJ. Pancreatic surgery: indications, complications, and implications for nutrition intervention. *Nutr Clin Pract.* 2013;28(3):330-357.

There are two primary categories of procedures used for patients with pancreatitis: those that involve decompression (or drainage) and those that involve resection. A growing area of surgical intervention combines the two mechanisms. Refer to **Table 10.10** for the most frequently used techniques. Regardless of the method, the goal for surgical intervention is first, to eliminate pain and second, to preserve as much of the pancreatic anatomy as possible.[53]

Nutrition Implications. Disruption to the anatomy of the digestive system has a substantial impact on normal digestive and absorptive processes.[54] Many of the associated complications will appear similar to those found in patients in the postoperative period for gastric surgery. Here, it will be helpful to consider the instrumental role of pancreatic exocrine and endocrine functions for utilization of nutrients, as well as the implications of involving the small intestine in reconstructive procedures, when studying the nutritional implications of pancreatic surgery. For example, note that many patients with CP also experience PEI preoperatively. The disruption to pancreatic structure

Table 10.10 Common Methods for Pancreatic Procedures

Drainage Procedures	■ **Pancreaticojejunostomy** • Puestow procedure • Partington–Rochelle procedure ■ Reduce intra-pancreatic pressure by draining the main pancreatic duct ■ Prevent the loss of pancreatic function by preserving pancreatic tissue
Procedures Involving Resection	■ **Pancreaticoduodenectomy** (**Figure 10.9**) • Classic Whipple procedure • Pylorus-preserving procedure • Left pancreatic resection ■ Indications: contracted duct, inflamed pancreatic mass, suspicious of pancreatic carcinoma
Procedures Combining Resection *and* Drainage	■ **Pancreatic head resection** • Duodenum-preserving: Beger operation • Local: Frey operation • Central: Büchler–Farkas operation ■ Extremely effective for pain management (90% long-term success rate for relief) ■ Allows for good preservation of pancreatic function

Data from Berberat PO, Ceyhan GO, Dambrauskas Z, Büchler MW, Friess H. Chronic pancreatitis. In: *Textbook of Clinical Gastroenterology and Hepatology*. Wiley-Blackwell; 2012:525-532. doi:10.1002/9781118321386.ch70. Accessed January 22, 2025.; Berry AJ. Pancreatic surgery: indications, complications, and implications for nutrition intervention. *Nutr Clin Pract*. 2013;28(3):330-357.

that occurs during surgery does little to remedy the insufficiency; instead, existing conditions will often worsen and a number of new cases will arise.[49] Upwards of 80% of individuals will experience some degree of PEI following pancreatic resection and all will require PERT to achieve normal fat digestion and absorption.[55–57] If unrecognized and untreated, patients are at risk for unintentional weight loss and nutrient deficiencies.[54] In addition, compromising the structural integrity of the pancreas will affect endocrine functions; 20–50% of patients develop diabetes from decreased insulin production following surgery and will require thorough education on the management of blood glucose.[58]

The leading cause of postoperative complications for patients post pancreatic surgery is delayed gastric emptying (DGE). The exact pathophysiology of DGE is largely unknown, and there are several hypothesized causes. DGE can have a severe impact on a patient's nutritional status, and can delay initiation of oral feedings and prolong the hospital stay.[55] Symptoms of concern include nausea, vomiting, bloating, early satiety, and abdominal pain.[58] The medical nutrition therapy for these patients is nearly identical to those who experience DGE following gastric resection: maintain intake to meet energy needs through small, frequent meals high in protein and low in solid fats and fiber.[59]

Nutrition Intervention. General operative nutrition guidelines recommend small, frequent meals that include protein and limit fat to less than 30% of total caloric intake. In addition, eating slowly and

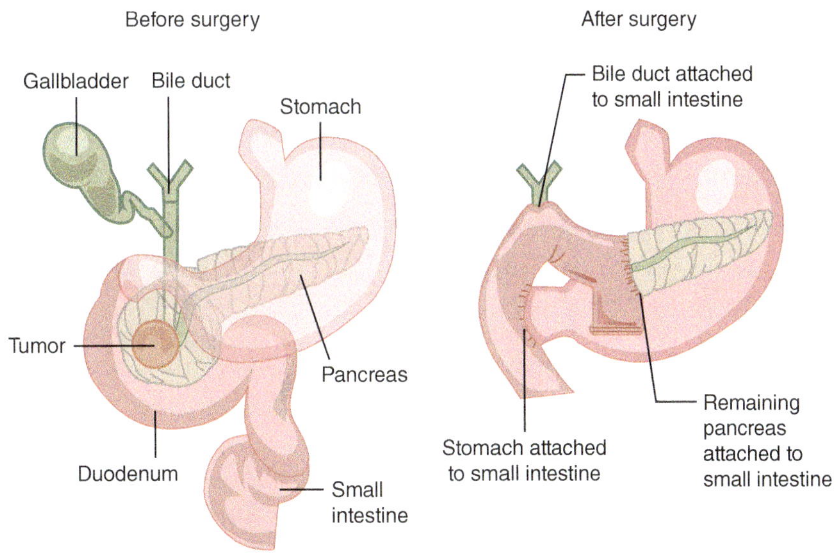

Figure 10.9 Pancreaticoduodenectomy Using the Classic Whipple Procedure

CASE STUDY REVISITED

Janice presents for a regularly scheduled follow-up appointment with her surgeon 12 weeks later. Her diarrhea has resolved, and she is tolerating a regular diet. However, she is still having acid reflux. What additional advice might you recommend?

Anthropometric Data:

Current weight: 78 kg
Height: 165 cm
BMI: 28.7 kg/m^2

Clinical Data:

Medications: calcium citrate plus vitamin D, chlorothiazide, lansoprazole, multivitamin with minerals, pravastatin, vitamin B12 (sublingual), vitamin D

Vital Signs: Blood pressure 120/76 mm Hg, Temperature 98.6°F

Nutrition-Focused Physical Exam: Patient appears well. Good skin tone. Hair and nails are less brittle. Oral exam appears normal. Patient demonstrating a frequent dry cough during exam.

Dietary Data:

Dietary History: Janice trying her best to follow a "healthy diet." She has returned to work and notes that her schedule is busy. She often eats "on the run" at work and relies on take out as well.

24-Hour Diet Recall:

Breakfast: Two slices whole wheat toast, 1 avocado, 2 fried eggs

Lunch: Fried chicken sandwich, lettuce and tomato, diet soda (at work)

Dinner: Usually take out, stir fry noodles with spicy meat sauce, glass of wine (6 oz)

Evening snack: Brownie with milk

Questions

1. What foods do you inform her may be causing her symptoms?
2. Assess Janice's previous PES statements. Identify if each statement remains an active issue or if the PES statement has been resolved. If the PES statement remains an active issue, has improvement in the issue been noted? If the issue has been resolved, write a new PES statement.
3. What strategies might she incorporate to reduce her acid reflux symptoms?
4. How might this differ from previous recommendations?

chewing food thoroughly will help to facilitate proper digestive progress in the GI tract. Simple sugars and sugar alcohols should be avoided in both foods and drinks. Fluid intake should be limited at mealtimes; the majority should occur 30–40 minutes postprandially. Finally, early identification and management of malnutrition improves quality of life for patients postoperatively; often, interventions include nutrition support in the form of EN and/or PN.[55]

CORE CONCEPT 7

Any changes to the integrity of the GI anatomy will alter function and impact how the body digests and ultimately absorbs nutrients.

Nutrition Monitoring and Evaluation. Monitoring weight and indicators of malnutrition is important following pancreatic surgery. Gastrointestinal symptoms and response to PEI therapy should be evaluated.

Gastroesophageal Reflux Disease

Gastroesophageal reflux disease (GERD) is a common digestive disorder, with estimated prevalence between 10% and 20% in the Western Hemisphere.[60] Normally, the lower esophageal sphincter opens when food passes from the esophagus to the stomach, and then immediately closes to prevent any food or stomach acid from moving back into the esophagus. **Figure 10.10** displays a relaxed or weakened lower

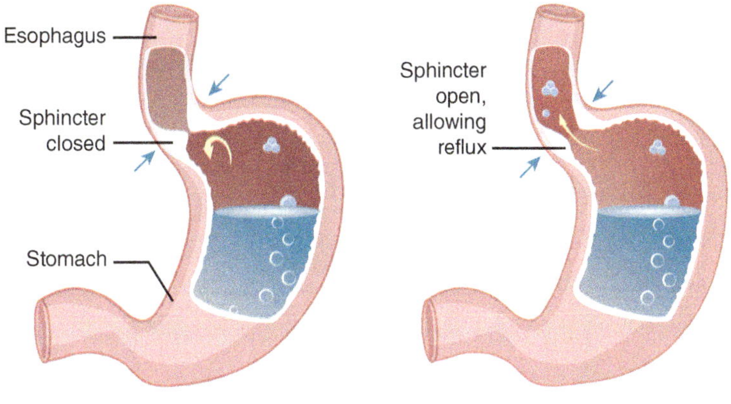

Figure 10.10 Gastroesophageal Reflux Disease is Characterized by an Open Esophageal Sphincter, Allowing Reflux into the Esophagus

esophageal sphincter, which is now open and allowing reflux to occur.

Typically, symptoms of GERD include heartburn and regurgitation of stomach acid. Other symptoms may include abdominal pain, bad breath, epigastric pressure, cough, sore throat, dental erosions, wheezing, or difficulty swallowing.[60,61] Diagnosis may be made based on history and symptoms, although further testing may be necessary to rule out further complications. Over time, untreated GERD can lead to erosive esophagitis, pulmonary disease, esophageal adenocarcinoma, Barrett's esophagus, and peptic stricture.[60] Treatment can include medication, surgery, and/or nutrition and lifestyle modifications.

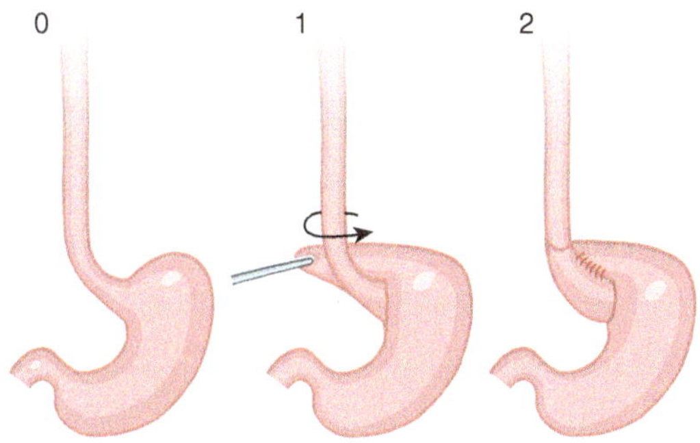

Figure 10.11 The Nissen Fundoplication Surgery Wraps the Stomach Around the Lower Esophagus to Improve the Integrity of the Lower Esophageal Sphincter to Reduce Reflux

Medical and Surgical Treatment. Medical treatment of GERD typically involves the use of acid-suppressing medications, such as proton-pump inhibitors (PPIs). This medication is taken 30–60 minutes prior to eating a meal to reduce the production of acid in the stomach.[60] If the patient's symptoms do not improve with medical therapy, surgical options may be considered.

Surgical intervention can be beneficial for patients who do not have symptom improvement with medication, do not wish to take medication daily, have additional complications such as hiatal hernia or severe obesity, or show symptoms of continued erosion despite treatment. A **Nissen fundoplication** is a procedure where the top portion of the stomach is wrapped around the lower esophagus to improve the integrity of the lower esophageal sphincter and reduce reflux.[62] **Figure 10.11** illustrates how the sphincter is now reinforced and tightened. For patients with obesity, gastric bypass may be recommended as a treatment for GERD, as Nissen fundoplication has been shown to be less beneficial in these patients.[60] The Roux-en-Y gastric bypass has been demonstrated to be most favorable in reduction of GERD symptoms as well as other obesity-related comorbidities.

Nutrition Assessment and Intervention. When a patient reports reflux, it is helpful to get a detailed dietary recall to assess any potential trigger foods in the diet. Foods that may cause increased reflux include high fat foods, chocolate, alcohol, mint, spicy foods, caffeine, and acidic foods.[56] Consuming smaller, more frequent meals as opposed to larger meals may reduce reflux as well.[61,63] **Figure 10.12** presents several causes and risk factors for GERD.

Accurate anthropometric measurements are also helpful in assessing whether the reflux may be related to obesity, as increasing BMI is associated with increasing GERD symptoms. In fact, weight loss of up to 10% has been demonstrated to be effective in reducing chronic medication use and improving the effects of the patient's current PPI.[64,65]

Other than weight loss and avoidance of trigger foods, there are a few other strategies that can help

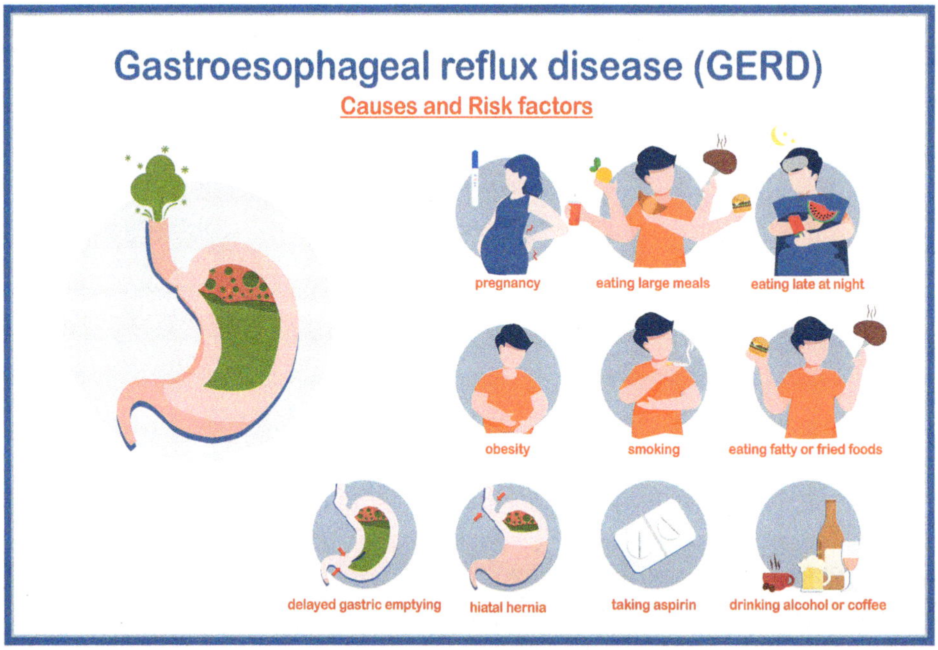

Figure 10.12 Nutritional and Lifestyle Factors Associated with GERD

patients improve symptoms. Quitting smoking and wearing loose-fitting clothing may be beneficial. Notably, waiting at least 3 hours after eating to lie down and elevating the head of the bed have been demonstrated to decrease reflux.[61] Patients may need instruction on meal timing and meal planning to improve satiety and avoid late night meals and snacks.

CORE CONCEPT 8

GERD is a common condition with various possible medical, surgical, and nutritional treatments. It is important for RDs to be well versed in the most up-to-date treatment options for these patients, individualizing interventions to target the cause of reflux.

Clinical Roundtable

Topic: Nutrition and Lifestyle Interventions for Gastroesophageal Reflux Disease (GERD)

Background: Frequent GERD symptoms are becoming more common and afflict up to 20% of North Americans. GERD is one of the most common gastrointestinal disorders, negatively impacting productivity and healthcare costs. Dietary modifications commonly proposed include avoidance of certain foods such as fat, chocolate, alcohol, mint, citrus, tomato, coffee, and tea. The timing and size of meals is also considered to be an important factor. Lifestyle changes include weight reduction and cessation of smoking. Pharmacological interventions with acid-reducing medications (antacids) are common, contributing to the financial burden of the disease. In addition, the long-term consequences of GERD on quality of life and health, including the risk of esophageal adenocarcinoma, support the need for better management of this disorder. Unfortunately, individuals with moderate to severe symptoms of GERD commonly follow some (avoiding citrus and tomato products, and certain types of alcohol), but not all dietary modifications. This suggests that progress can be made in lifestyle management techniques. At the same time, lack of adherence to recommended dietary changes is concerning. Furthermore, the combination of weight reduction and smoking cessation may be challenging for many patients. What would be your approach to nonpharmacological management of GERD?

References

1. Shaqran TM, Ismaeel MM, Alnuaman AA, et al. Epidemiology, causes, and management of gastroesophageal reflux disease: a systematic review. *Cureus*. 2023;15(10):e47420. doi:10.7759/cureus.47420

Chapter Summary

Proper digestion is crucial to obtaining adequate levels of nutrients from the foods we eat. Problems with digestion can occur at any point in the GI tract, leading to a wide variety of conditions. RDs have the opportunity to take the lead in treatment of these patients, providing the support they need to maintain their weight and overall nutritional status while dealing with complex diseases. Chapter 11 will continue the discussion of the GI tract, focusing on disorders of absorption.

Key Terms

duodenum, brush border, peristalsis, digestion, absorption, maldigestion, malabsorption, malassimilation, bolus, chyme, selective vagotomy, total (truncal) vagotomy, pyloroplasty, gastrectomy, anastomosis, gastric stasis, gastroparesis, steatorrhea, medium-chain triglyceride (MCT), intrinsic factor, dumping syndrome (DS), Pancreatitis, acute pancreatitis (AP), NPO, fistula, chronic pancreatitis (CP), pancreatic exocrine insufficiency (PEI), pancreatic enzyme preparations (PEP), amylorrhea, azotorrhea, pancreatic enzyme replacement therapy (PERT), gastroesophageal reflux disease (GERD), Nissen fundoplication

Acknowledgments

The author acknowledges V. Paige Murphy for contributions to the previous version of this chapter.

References

1. Joneja JMV. *Digestion, Diet, and Disease: Irritable Bowel Syndrome and Gastrointestinal Function.* Rutgers University Press; 2004.
2. Gropper SS, Smith JL. The digestive system: mechanism for nourishing the body. In: *Advanced Nutrition and Human Metabolism.* 6th ed. Wadsworth Cengage Learning; 2013:33–62.
3. Digestive Diseases Statistics for the United States. U.S. Department of Health and Human Services, National Institute of Diabetes and Digestive and Kidney Diseases. Updated 2014. Accessed December 3, 2024. https://www.niddk.nih.gov/health-information/health-statistics/digestive-diseases
4. Montgomery SC, Williams CM, Maxwell IV PJ. Nutritional support of patient with inflammatory bowel disease. *Surg Clin North Am.* 2015;95(6):1271–1279.
5. Barrett KE. Functional anatomy of the GI tract and organs draining into it. In: *Gastrointestinal Physiology.* 2nd ed. McGraw-Hill; 2014.
6. The Pancreas. Johns Hopkins University. Accessed January 22, 2025. https://www.hopkinsmedicine.org/health/conditions-and-diseases/the-pancreas.
7. Towers E, Tischler M. *Gastrointestinal Physiology: A Clinical Approach.* Springer International Publishing; 2014.
8. Rogers AI, Madanick RD. Maldigestion and malabsorption. In: Hawkey CJ, Bosch J, Richter JE, Garcia-Tsao G, Chan FKL, eds. *Textbook of Clinical Gastroenterology and Hepatology.* Wiley-Blackwell; 2012:279–287.
9. WGO practice guideline: Malabsorption. 2015. World Gastroenterology Organization (WGO). Accessed December 29, 2024. http://www.worldgastroenterology.org/guidelines/global-guidelines
10. Högenauer C, Hammer HF. Maldigestion and malabsorption. In: Feldman M, Friedman LS, Brandt LJ, eds. *Sleisenger and Fordtran's Gastrointestinal and Liver Disease.* 10th ed. Elsevier, Saunders; 2016:1788–1823.
11. Yeldiz A. Truncal vagotomy, gastrojejunostomy and braun anastomosis technique in the surgical treatment of intractable peptic ulcer. *Haydarpasa Numune Med J.* 2021;61(1):105–109.
12. Wang Y, Xu Y, Meng FJ, Cai XL, Yu WM, Zhang MZ. Comparison between Billroth II and Billroth II + Braun anastomosis in gastrectomy for gastric cancer. *J Surg Res.* 2024;303:670–678. doi:10.1016/j.jss.2024.09.044.17
13. Olufajo OA, Wilson A, Yehayes B, Zeineddin A, Cornwell EE, Williams M. Trends in the surgical management and outcomes of complicated peptic ulcer disease. *The American Surgeon*™. 2020;86(7):856–864. doi:10.1177/0003134820939929
14. Adkisson C, Weithorn D. Minimally invasive treatment of ulcer disease: laparoscopic Graham patch, laparoscopic vagotomy and antrectomy. In: Chen H, Lindeman B., eds. *Illustrative Handbook of General Surgery.* Springer; 2024. doi:10.1007/978-3-031-63878-7_19
15. Li XG, Song QY, Wu D, et al. Does the addition of Braun anastomosis to Billroth II reconstruction on laparoscopic-assisted distal gastrectomy benefit patients? *World J Gastrointest Oncol.* 2022;14(6):1141–1147. doi:10.4251/wjgo.v14.i6.1141
16. Chacon D, Bernardino T, Geraghty F, et al. Bariatric surgery with Roux-en-Y gastric bypass or sleeve gastrectomy for treatment of obesity and comorbidities: current evidence and practice. *Cureus.* 2022;14(6):e25762. doi:10.7759/cureus.25762
17. The American Society for Metabolic and Bariatric Surgery. Bariatric Procedures. Updated May 2021; Accessed December 3, 2024. https://asmbs.org/patients/bariatric-surgery-procedures
18. Rogers C. Postgastrectomy nutrition. *Nutri Clin Pract.* 2011; 26:126–136. doi:10.1177/0884533611400070
19. Shah ND. The use of medium-chain triglycerides in gastrointestinal disorders. *Pract Gastroenterol.* 2017;160:20–28.
20. Gasmi A, Bjørklund G, Mujawdiya PK, et al. Micronutrients deficiencies in patients after bariatric surgery. *Eur J Nutr.* 2022;61:55–67 . doi:10.1007/s00394-021-02619-820
21. Scarpellini E, Arts J, Karamanolis G, et al. International consensus on the diagnosis and management of dumping syndrome. *Nat Rev Endocrinol.* 2020;16:448–466. doi:10.1038/s41574-020-0357-5

22. D'hoedt A, Vanuytsel T. Dumping syndrome after bariatric surgery: prevalence, pathophysiology and role in weight reduction – a systematic review. *Acta Gastro-Enterologica Belgica*. 2023;86;(3):417–427.
23. Academy of Nutrition and Dietetics. *Nutrition Care Manual*. Gastric surgery. https://www.nutritioncaremanual.org/topic.cfm?ncm_category_id=1&lv1=5522&lv2=19309&ncm_toc_id=19309&ncm_heading=Nutrition%20Care Accessed January 4, 2025.
24. ERAS® Society. Guidelines. Accessed December 5, 2024. https://erassociety.org/guidelines/
25. Desiderio J, Trastulli S, D'Andrea V, Parisi A. Enhanced recovery after surgery for gastric cancer (ERAS-GC): optimizing patient outcome. *Transl Gastroenterol Hepatol*. 2020;5:11. doi:10.21037/tgh.2019.10.04
26. Huh YJ, Kim DJ. Enhanced recovery after surgery in bariatric surgery. *J Metab Bariatr Surg*. 2021;10(2):47–54. doi:10.17476/jmbs.2021.10.2.47
27. Kubota T, Shoda K, Konishi H, Okamoto K, Otsuji E. Nutrition update in gastric cancer surgery. *Ann Gastroenterol Surg*. 2020;4:360–368. doi:10.1002/ags3.12351
28. Yan H, He F, Wei J, et al. Effects of individualized dietary counseling on nutritional status and quality of life in postdischarge patients after surgery for gastric cancer: a randomized clinical trial. *Front Oncol*. 2023;13:1058187. doi:10.3389/fonc.2023.1058187
29. Lankisch PG, Apte M, Banks PA. Acute pancreatitis. *Lancet*. 2015;386(9988):85–96.
30. Papachristou G, Singh V, Whitcomb DC. Acute pancreatitis. In: Hawkey CJ, Bosch J, Richter JE, Garcia-Tsao G, Chan FKL, eds. *Textbook of Clinical Gastroenterology and Hepatology*. Wiley-Blackwell; 2012:518–524.
31. Academy of Nutrition and Dietetics. Pancreatitis. In: *Nutrition Care Manual*. 2022. https://www.nutritioncaremanual.org/topic.cfm?ncm_category_id=1&lv1=5522&lv2=275088&ncm_toc_id=275088&ncm_heading=Nutrition%20Care.Accessed January 4, 2025.
32. Petrov MS, McIlroy K, Grayson L, Phillips ARJ, Windsor JA. Early nasogastric tube feeding versus nil per os in mild to moderate acute pancreatitis: a randomized controlled trial. *Clin Nutr*. 2013;32(5):697–703.
33. Banks PA, Bollen TL, Dervenis C, et al. Classification of acute pancreatitis—2012: revision of the Atlanta classification and definitions by international consensus. *Gut*. 2013;62(1): 102–111.
34. Kayhan S, Selcan Akyol B, Ergul M, Baysan C. The effect of type of fluid on disease severity in acute pancreatitis treatment. *Eur Rev Med Pharmacol Sci*. 2021;25(23):7460–7467.
35. McClave S, Taylor B, Martindale R, et al. Guidelines for the Provision and Assessment of Nutrition Support Therapy in the Adult Critically Ill Patient: Society of Critical Care Medicine (SCCM) and American Society for Parenteral and Enteral Nutrition (ASPEN). *JPEN*. 2016;40(2):185–186.
36. Arvanitakis M, et al. ESPEN guideline on clinical nutrition in acute and chronic pancreatitis. *Clin Nutr*. 2020;39:612–631.
37. Singer P, Blaser AR, Berger MM, et al. ESPEN guideline on clinical nutrition in the intensive care unit. *Clin Nutr*. 2019;38(1):48–79.
38. Sun J-K, Lv C, Gao L, Mao W, Li W, Ke L. Nutrition therapy in critically ill patients with severe acute pancreatitis. *Nutr Clin Pract*. 2024; 39:271–280. doi:10.1002/ncp.11135
39. Olah A, Romics Jr. L. Enteral nutrition in acute pancreatitis: A review of the current evidence. *World J Gastroenterol*. 2014;20(43):16123–16131.
40. Dutta AK, Goel A, Kirubakaran R, Chacko A, Tharyan P. Nasogastric versus nasojejunal tube feeding for severe acute pancreatitis. *Cochrane Database Systemat Rev*. 2020;3:CD010582. doi:10.1002/14651858.CD010582.pub2
41. Carlin-Ronquillo A, Benites-Goñi H, Diaz-Arocutipa C, et al. Nasogastric versus nasojejunal tube feeding for severe acute pancreatitis: a systematic review of randomized controlled trials. *Rev Gastroenterol Peru*. 2023;43(3):207–216. doi:10.47892/rgp.2023.433.1542
42. Qi D, Yu B, Huang J, Peng M. Meta-analysis of early enteral nutrition provided within 24 hours of admission on clinical outcomes in acute Pancreatitis. *JPEN*. 2018;42: 1139–1147. doi:10.1002/jpen.1139
43. Crockett SD, Wani S, Gardner TB, et al. American Gastroenterological Association Institute guideline on initial management of acute pancreatitis. *Gastroenterol*. 2018;154(4):1096–1101.
44. Afghani E, Sinha A, Singh VK. An overview of the diagnosis and management of nutrition in chronic pancreatitis. *Nutr Clin Pract*. 2014;29(3):295–311.
45. Berberat PO, Ceyhan GO, Dambrauskas Z, Büchler MW, Friess H. Chronic pancreatitis. In: Hawkey CJ, Bosch J, Richter JE, Garcia-Tsao G, Chan FKL, eds. *Textbook of Clinical Gastroenterology and Hepatology*. Wiley-Blackwell; 2012:525–532.
46. Braganza JM, Lee SH, McCloy RF, McMahon MJ. Chronic pancreatitis. *Lancet*. 2011;377(9772):1184–1197.
47. Rasmussen HH, Irgun O, Olesen SS, Drewes AM, Holst M. Nutrition in chronic pancreatitis. *World J Gastroenterol*. 2013;19(42):7267–7275.
48. Muniraj T, Aslanian HR, Farrell J, Jamidar PA. Chronic pancreatitis, a comprehensive review. Part II: Diagnosis, complications, and management. *Dis Mon*. 2015;61(1):5–37.
49. Muniraj T, Aslanian HR, Farrell J, Jamidar PA. Chronic pancreatitis, a comprehensive review and update. part I: Epidemiology, etiology, risk factors, genetics, pathophysiology, and clinical features. *Dis Mon*. 2014;60(12):530–550.
50. Sikkens ECM, Cahen DL, Kuipers EJ, Bruno MJ. Pancreatic enzyme replacement therapy in chronic pancreatitis. *Best Pract Res Clin Gastroenterol*. 2010;24(3):337–347.
51. Vege SS, Chari ST. Chronic pancreatitis *N Engl J Med*. 2022;386:869–878 doi:10.1056/NEJMcp1809396
52. Berry AJ. Pancreatic enzyme replacement during pancreatic insufficiency. *Nutr Clin Pract*. 2014;29(3):312–321.
53. O'Brien SJ, Omer E. Chronic pancreatitis and nutrition therapy. *Nutr Clin Pract*. 2019;34:S13–S26. doi;10.1002/ncp.10379
54. Berry AJ. Pancreatic surgery: Indications, complications, and implications for nutrition intervention. *Nutr Clin Pract*. 2013;28(3):330–357.
55. Gianotti L, Besselink MG, Sandini M, et al. Nutritional support and therapy in pancreatic surgery: a position paper of the International Study Group on Pancreatic Surgery (ISGPS). *Surgery*. 2018;164(5):1035–1048. doi:10.1016/j.surg.2018.05.040
56. Domínguez-Muñoz JE. Pancreatic enzyme replacement therapy: exocrine pancreatic insufficiency after gastrointestinal surgery. *HPB*. 2009;11(Suppl. 3):3–6.
57. Friess H, Michalski CW. Diagnosing exocrine pancreatic insufficiency after surgery: when and which patients to treat. *HPB*. 2009;11(Suppl. 3):7–10.
58. Marcason W. What is the Whipple procedure and what is the appropriate nutrition therapy for it? *J Acad Nutr Diet*. 2015;115(1):168.
59. Parrish CR. Nutritional considerations in the patient with gastroparesis. *Gastroenterol Clin North Am*. 2015;44(1):83–95.

60. Badillo R, Francis D. Diagnosis and treatment of gastroesophageal reflux disease. *World J Gastrointest Pharmacol Ther*. 2014;5(3):105–112.
61. Johnson A. *Gastroesophageal reflux*. Academy of Nutrition and Dietetics. Published November 22, 2021. Reviewed September 26, 2023. Accessed January 6, 2025. https://www.eatright.org/health/health-conditions/digestive-and-gastrointestinal/gastroesophageal-reflux
62. GERD Surgery. Mayo Clinic. Updated 2017. Accessed December 8, 2024. https://www.mayoclinic.org/diseases-conditions/gerd/multimedia/gerd-surgery/img-20006950
63. Newberry C, Lynch K. The role of diet in the development and management of gastroesophageal reflux disease: why we feel the burn. *J Thorac Dis*. 2019 Aug;11(Suppl 12):S1594–S1601. doi:10.21037/jtd.2019.06.42
64. de Bortoli N, Guidi G, Martinucci I, et al. Voluntary and controlled weight loss can reduce symptoms and proton pump inhibitor use and dosage in patients with gastroesophageal reflux disease: a comparative study. *Dis Esophagus*. 2014;29(2):197–204.
65. Ness-Jensen E, Hveem K, El-Serag H, et al. Lifestyle intervention in gastroesophageal reflux disease. *Clin Gastroenterol Hepatol*. 2016;14(2):175–182.

CHAPTER 11

Nutritional Management of Gastrointestinal Malabsorption

Rachel Wilkinson-Bartlett

CHAPTER OUTLINE

Core Concepts
Introduction
Celiac Disease (CD)
Irritable Bowel Syndrome (IBS)
Non-Celiac Gluten/Wheat Sensitivity
Inflammatory Bowel Disease (IBD)
Increased Intestinal Permeability
Helicobacter pylori
Small Intestinal Bacterial Overgrowth (SIBO)
Bowel Surgery and Short Bowel Syndrome (SBS)
Monitoring and Evaluation

CORE CONCEPTS

1. Celiac disease, once diagnosed, can be managed with careful adherence to the gluten-free diet. This requires extensive patient education and monitoring. Until patients reach an asymptomatic state, and the damage is allowed to heal, there are a number of deficiencies and/or intolerances that may occur.
2. Diet plays an important role in the management of irritable bowel syndrome. It is important not to overly restrict the diet as a means to improve gastrointestinal symptoms, as this can lead to disordered eating, nutrient deficiencies, and malnutrition.
3. Patients with non-celiac gluten/wheat sensitivity (NCGS/NCWS) may also benefit from a gluten-free diet. Although there is no current best practice guideline for medical nutrition therapy for NCGS/NCWS, RDs can help patients create an individualized diet that minimizes the symptoms.
4. Inflammatory bowel disease is associated with a wide range of nutritional implications that center on malnutrition. Adequate intake, whether in the form of nutritional support or oral intake, is required.
5. Careful assessment of the patient's nutritional status and gastrointestinal symptoms will direct nutritional intervention in increased intestinal permeability also known as "leaky gut syndrome," such as limiting alcohol and practicing stress management. Clinicians should be wary of "easy fix" fad diets that patients may be following.

6. Deficiencies in iron, vitamin C, vitamin A, alpha-tocopherol, vitamin B12, folic acid, nickel, and selenium are possible in patients with *Helicobacter pylori*. Patients with this infection should be monitored closely for both nutrient deficiency and unintentional weight loss.
7. Small intestinal bacterial overgrowth is often associated and occurs concurrently with a number of other disorders related to maldigestion and malabsorption. Nutrition therapy plays a critical role in the treatment of this patient population.
8. In surgical resections of the gastrointestinal tract, the amount of bowel removed, remaining functional bowel, and the location from which the resection is made are key determinants as to whether digestive and absorptive processes can be maintained postoperatively and if prolonged nutrition intervention is necessary.

LEARNING OBJECTIVES

1. Describe the key mechanism of absorption.
2. Identify factors that cause malabsorption.
3. Define the abnormalities leading to celiac disease and their manifestations.
4. Describe medical nutrition therapy for individuals with celiac disease.
5. Explain potential medical nutrition therapy approaches for patients with irritable bowel syndrome.
6. Distinguish key differences between ulcerative colitis and Crohn's disease.
7. Discuss nutritional implications during and following medical treatment for inflammatory bowel disease.
8. Discuss the RD's role in treatment of patients with *Helicobacter pylori* infection.
9. Identify risk of malnutrition and specific deficiencies associated with short bowel syndrome.
10. Recognize the phases of intestinal adaptation to short bowel syndrome and discuss associated medical nutrition therapy.

Introduction

The gastrointestinal (GI) tract functions to both digest and absorb nutrients. This chapter will focus on absorption, which moves digested particles of food from outside the cells into the cells of the GI tract for further utilization. Malabsorption can occur as a result of two things: (1) inadequately digested nutrients are transported or (2) mucosal uptake of nutrients is flawed. Medical nutrition therapy is a key part of treatment for patients with malabsorptive conditions, and registered dietitians (RDs) have a recognized and important role in implementing these strategies.

Key Mechanisms of Absorption

Once food particles have been broken down into their simplest constituents via digestion, these nutrients cross the barrier between the lumen of the GI tract and the internal environment of the body. This is the process of absorption.[1]

Although select components of the digesta are absorbed within the stomach (water, alcohol, and select minerals), most absorption occurs in the small intestine. Refer to **Figures 11.1** and **11.2** for a visual representation of absorption sites. Absorptive processes for most micro- and macronutrients begin in the duodenum and continue throughout the middle and distal portions of the small intestine—the **jejunum** and the **ileum**, respectively.[2] Finger-like projections (the villi) of the GI tract wall contain intestinal absorptive cells called **enterocytes**. The mechanism by which nutrients are absorbed into enterocytes depends on a number of factors: (1) the solubility of the nutrient, (2) the concentration or electrical gradient, and (3) the size of the molecule to be absorbed.[2] The majority of food components pass into circulation after binding to transport proteins, crossing the epithelium through the process of diffusion.[1] Other absorption methods include facilitated diffusion and active transport; occasionally, nutrients enter through pinocytosis, endocytosis, or a paracellular route.[2]

The remaining digesta empties from the ileum into the cecum of the large intestine. From there, the matter continues through the ascending, transverse, descending, and sigmoid sections, where colonic epithelial cells work to primarily absorb water, sodium, and chloride. When this process is complete, any unabsorbed materials have been dehydrated to form feces and pass through the distal end of the tract, the anus. Normal defecated material will contain *only* sloughed GI cells, inorganic matter, water, and insignificant amounts of unabsorbed nutrients, constituents of digestive juices, fiber, and bacteria.[1,2]

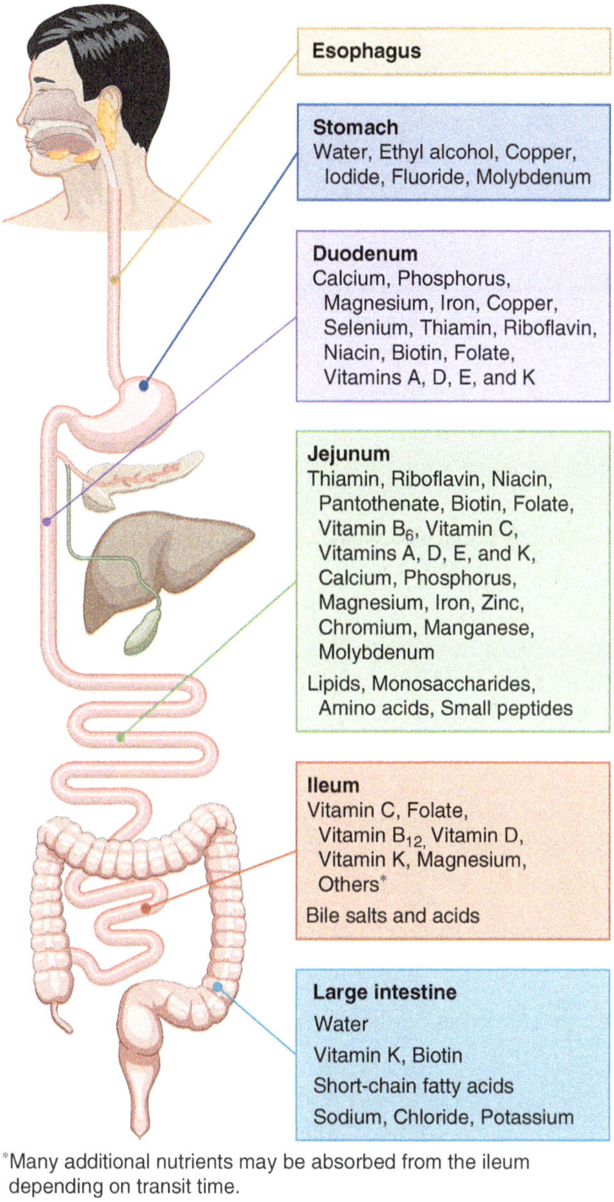

Figure 11.1 Absorptive Sites Within the GI Tract

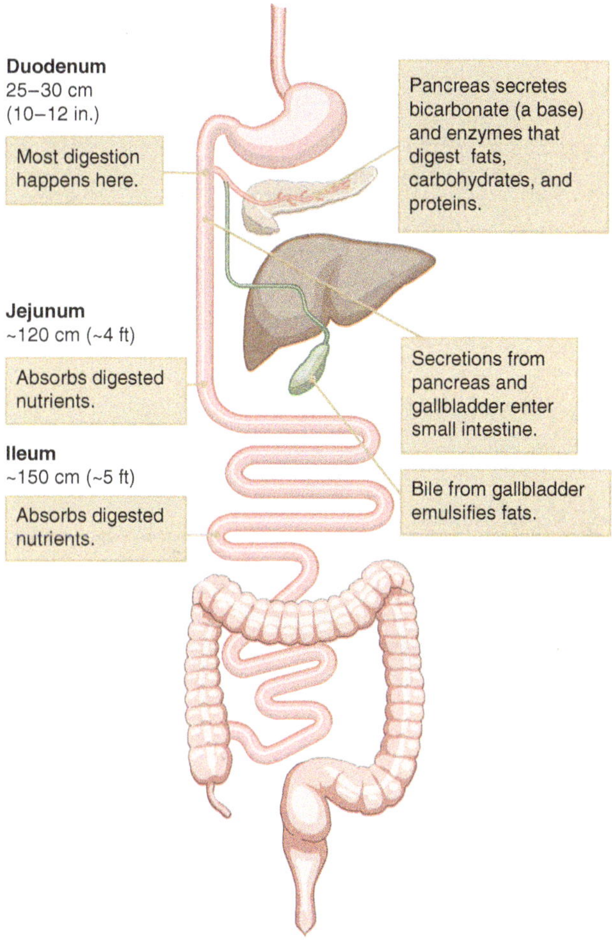

Figure 11.2 The Small Intestine The duodenum is mainly responsible for digesting food; the jejunum and ileum primarily deal with absorption of food. The duodenum secretes mucus, enzymes, and hormones along with other digestive juices from assisting organs to aid digestion. All along the intestinal walls, nutrients are absorbed into blood and lymph. Undigested materials are passed on to the large intestine

Medical Nutrition Therapy for Disorders of Absorption

Malnutrition is common in patients with GI disorders. Depending on the disease state, both macronutrient and micronutrient deficiencies can exist, often concurrently. Nutritional assessment in patients with GI disease should be comprehensive, deriving from anthropometric, biochemical, clinical, and dietary information. Weight history and muscle wasting can identify protein-calorie malnutrition. Diet history should be thorough, exploring omission of food groups due to intolerance or adherence to special diets. A food diary spanning over several days can help identify symptoms associated with consumption of foods. Patients should be asked about nausea, vomiting, abdominal pain, and diarrhea. A description of stool patterns with respect to timing of meals, as well as stool characteristics, can be helpful in identifying causes as well as potential nutrient deficiencies. A nutrition-focused physical exam can detect muscle and fat loss as well as micronutrient deficiencies. While risk of micronutrient deficiency can vary according to disease, anemia and bone disease are common in many GI disorders. Biochemical analysis of iron, vitamin B12, folate, calcium, and vitamin D can be used to corroborate intake information and physical exam findings. In those conditions where micronutrient deficiencies are predictable, preemptive supplementation and routine screening for anemia and bone demineralization are recommended.[3,4]

CASE STUDY INTRODUCTION

Daniel is a 24-year-old male who was referred to the gastroenterology outpatient clinic by his primary care physician. The patient presents with complaints of significant diarrhea for the past 3 weeks. Daniel contacted his physician when the episode did not respond to over-the-counter antidiarrheal medications. The following clinical information was taken during his initial appointment.

Anthropometric Data:

Current Weight: 62.8 kg
Height: 175 cm
BMI: 20.5 kg/m^2

Weight history
UBW: 70 kg (6 months ago)

Biochemical Data:

Labs are pending.

Clinical Data:

Past Medical History: None
Medications: Antidiarrheal caplets (over the counter)
Vital Signs: Blood pressure 127/83 mm Hg, Temperature 99.5°F
Nutrition-Focused Physical Exam: Patient appears pale and fatigued. Abdominal exam reveals some distention, and patient reports pain when mild abdominal pressure applied. Skin is dry, intact, and warm to touch; no wounds noted. Oral exam reveals dry mucosa and tongue. No lesions observed. Good dentition noted.

Dietary Data:

Diet History: Typically follows a diet with no restrictions. Patient reports that he occasionally experiences loose stools, particularly after eating fatty foods. More recently, he has followed a "bland diet" based on what he has read online.
24-Hour Diet Recall:
Breakfast (6:30 am): 1 slice of toast with jelly, coffee with cream.
Lunch (12:30 pm): 1 bowl of elbow macaroni (about 1 and 1/2 cups cooked); butter (1 tbsp), parmesan cheese (1 tbsp).
Dinner (6:30 pm): Baked chicken, 1 cup of white rice, 1/2 cup carrots, water.

Questions

1. What are Daniel's nutritional risk factors?
2. Describe the possible pathophysiologic etiology associated with Daniel's symptoms.
3. Write two Nutrition Diagnosis statements for Daniel identifying the Problem/Etiology/Signs and Symptoms (PES) of Daniel's active nutrition issues.
4. Identify the nutrition interventions you would like to initiate for Daniel to address the problems identified in your PES statements.
5. What should be included in your monitoring and evaluation plan? Why?

Celiac Disease (CD)

Perhaps the most well-understood autoimmune disorder, **celiac disease (CD)** is characterized by inflammatory injury to the intestinal mucosa following gluten ingestion. An inappropriate immune response is triggered by specific sequences of amino acids found in the **prolamin** fractions of wheat, barley, and rye. CD pathogenesis can only occur in individuals with an incredibly specific genetic profile that includes human leukocyte antigen (HLA)-DQ2 or DQ8 alleles.[4]

Damage to the mucosal surface appears in a "patchy," sporadic pattern, most evident in the proximal portion of the small intestine. Structural changes to the normal villous structure flatten the epithelial wall, decreasing the surface area and thus capacity for absorption, as presented in **Figure 11.3**. As a result, undiagnosed or untreated CD is associated with significant malabsorption of both macro- and micronutrients.[4]

Diagnostic procedures begin with an initial assessment of serologic values. The highly sensitive and specific immunoglobulin A-transglutaminase assay is the most readily used approach when CD is suspected. In some cases, genetic testing for HLA-DQ2 or DQ8 alleles can be helpful to confirm diagnosis. Other important measures include tissue transglutaminase, endomysial antibody, and/or deamidated antigliadin

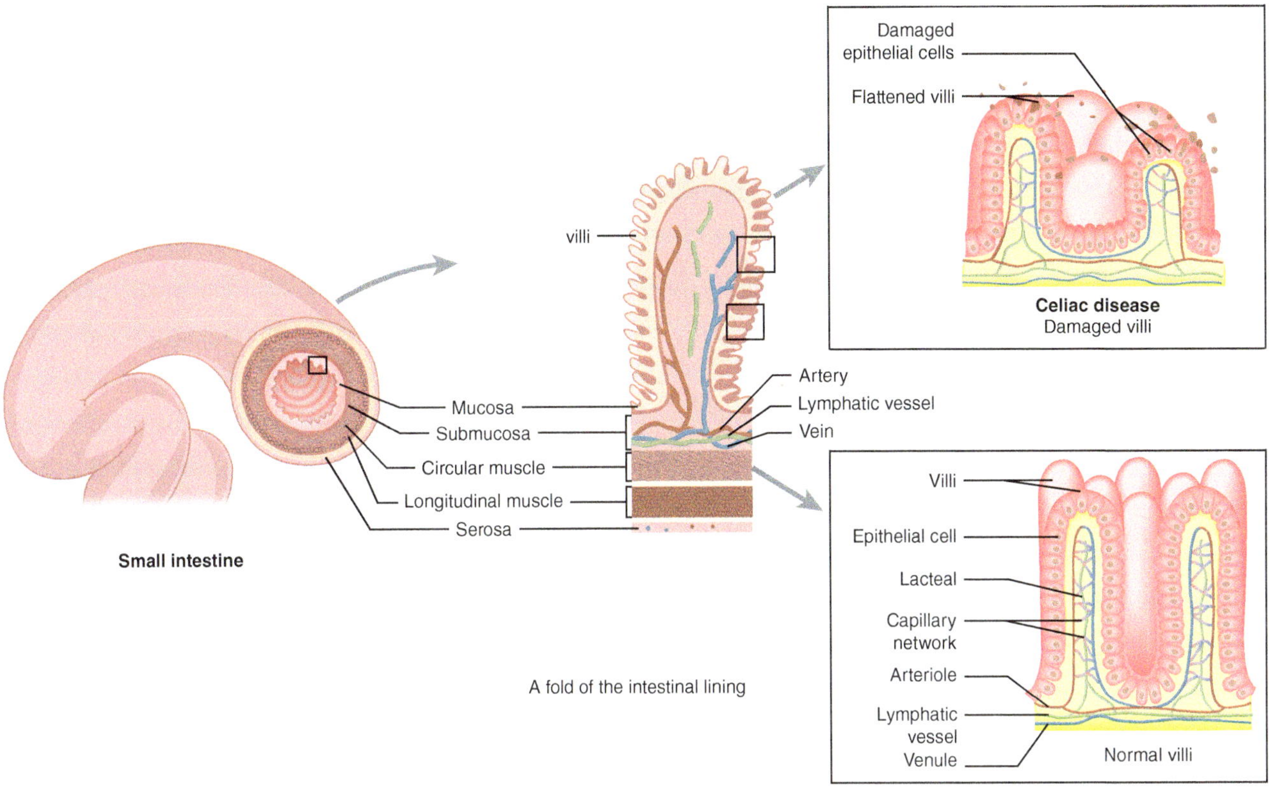

Figure 11.3 Structural Changes to the Normal Villous Structure Flatten the Epithelial Wall, Decreasing the Surface Area and Thus Capacity for Absorption

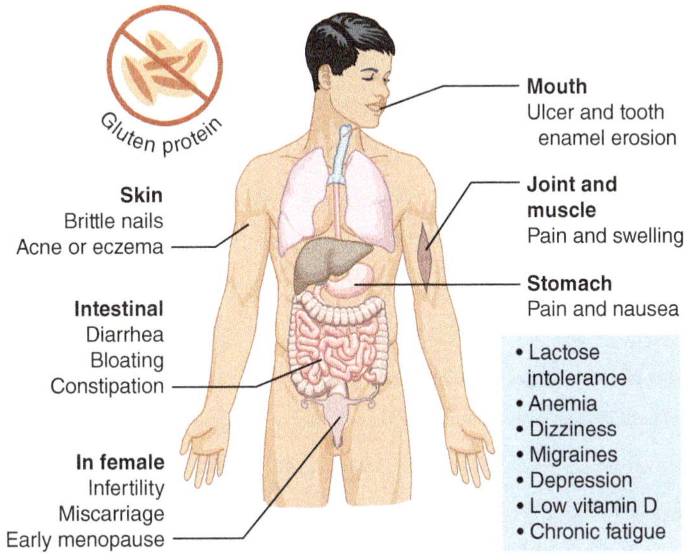

Figure 11.4 Manifestations of Celiac Disease by Location in the Body

peptide. All individuals with positive values will have the diagnosis confirmed by a duodenal biopsy. During the procedure, several specimens are taken due to the intermittent nature of the disease. CD diagnoses are supported by clinical improvement after a gluten-free diet is implemented.[4]

Clinical Manifestations

The clinical manifestations of CD exist on a wide spectrum of both GI and extraintestinal manifestations. Refer to **Figure 11.4** for a list of manifestations by location in the body. Symptoms present in children and adults at similar rates, the severity of which varies greatly among individuals and on the degree of affected intestine, as described in **Table 11.1**. Although there is a classic profile for CD, marked by chronic diarrhea, weight loss, and fatigue, the vast majority of patients present with atypical symptoms, and some report no GI symptoms whatsoever.[3,4]

As a result of the broad range of presentations, one of the biggest clinical barriers for patients with CD is misdiagnosis. For more than 50% of new patients, CD is initially undiagnosed or misdiagnosed. Most often, patients will report multiple, mild symptoms common to a number of other GI disorders. Without appropriate serologic testing and/or biopsy procedures, a false conclusion is easy to make. The most common misdiagnosis for patients with CD is irritable bowel syndrome.[4]

It is important to note other long-term health concerns associated with CD. White males with CD have a significantly higher risk of developing coronary artery disease (CAD) compared to those without CD.[5] Additionally, patients with both CD and CAD have a higher prevalence of hyperlipidemia, iron deficiency anemia, and type 2 diabetes compared to those with CAD only.[5] It is plausible that the underlying systemic inflammation found in CD may contribute to this association.[6] Following a strict gluten-free diet helps decrease this inflammation, although it is unclear whether that will in turn decrease the risk of CAD. This is an area where future research is warranted.

Table 11.1 Clinical Manifestations of Celiac Disease

Classical Presentation	▪ Chronic diarrhea ▪ Iron deficiency anemia ▪ Weight loss ▪ Abdominal pain ▪ Malaise and fatigue ▪ Irritability ▪ Depression ▪ Abdominal distention ▪ Anorexia
Gastrointestinal	▪ Flatulence ▪ Dyspepsia ▪ Bloating ▪ Vomiting ▪ Constipation ▪ Steatorrhea ▪ Recurrent or severe aphthous stomatitis ▪ Symptomatic lactose intolerance
Extraintestinal	▪ Ataxia ▪ Peripheral neuropathy ▪ Muscle weakness ▪ Sensory loss ▪ Macrocytic anemia (folate deficiency) ▪ Elevated prothrombin time (vitamin K deficiency) ▪ Hypocalcemia ▪ Vitamin D deficiency ▪ Osteopenic bone disease ▪ Arthralgia ▪ Dental enamel defects ▪ Male and female infertility, miscarriage ▪ Malignancies
Superficial	▪ Short stature ▪ Clubbing ▪ Edema ▪ Dermatitis herpetiformis
Pediatric-Specific	▪ Impaired growth ▪ Weight faltering (previously failure to thrive) ▪ Delayed puberty ▪ Hypotonia ▪ Behavioral problems, such as poor academic performance

Data from Leffler DA, Cárdenas A, Kelly CP. Celiac disease. In: *Textbook of Clinical Gastroenterology and Hepatology*. Wiley-Blackwell; 2012:288-298. doi:10.1002/9781118321386.ch40. Accessed January 22, 2025.; Academy of Nutrition and Dietetics. Celiac disease. Nutrition Care Manual. Accessed January 22, 2025.

Nutrition Intervention

The only effective treatment for patients with CD is a lifelong commitment to avoidance of dietary gluten. A strict gluten-free diet (GFD) allows the intestinal mucosa to heal and prevents any future symptoms or complications from occurring. Because as little as 50 mg of gluten/day can cause continued enteropathy, patients with CD require extensive education on foods containing the offensive prolamins of wheat, barley, and rye (gliadin, hordein, and secalin, respectively). Refer to **Table 11.2** for a list of safe and unsafe food sources for individuals following a GFD. In addition, counseling should include information on label reading and cross-contamination. First, gluten is present in many of the ingredients widely used in processed foods. There are several nonfood items, including supplements, medications, and makeup such as mascara and lipstick, which can be sources of gluten. Second, the potential for cross-contamination in processing, storage, and transport both in industry

Table 11.2 Safe and Unsafe Foods and Ingredients for the Gluten-Free Diet

Contain Gluten (Unsafe)	Processed Foods That May contain Gluten (Unsafe)	Gluten-Free Foods (Safe)
■ Wheat • All varieties, including einkorn, emmer, spelt, and kamut • Wheat starch, wheat bran, wheat germ, cracked wheat, hydrolyzed wheat protein ■ Barley ■ Rye ■ Triticale (crossbreed of wheat and rye) ■ Brewer's yeast ■ Dextrin ■ Malt ■ Modified food starch ■ Starch ■ Most flour varieties • Bromated flour, durum flour, enriched flour, farina, graham flour, phosphated flour, self-rising flour, semolina, white/wheat flour	■ Bouillon cubes ■ Brown rice syrup ■ Candy ■ Chewing gum ■ Communion wafers ■ French fries ■ Gravy varieties ■ Imitation fish ■ Matzo, matzo meal ■ Potato chips ■ Prepared sauces ■ Processed meats ■ Rice mixes ■ Seasoned tortilla chips ■ Soups ■ Soy sauce ■ Vegetables in sauce	■ Amaranth ■ Arrowroot ■ Buckwheat ■ Cassava (manioc) ■ Corn ■ Finger millet (ragi) ■ Flax ■ Legumes ■ Lentils ■ Mesquite ■ Millet ■ Montina ■ Nuts ■ Oats* ■ Potatoes ■ Quinoa ■ Rice ■ Sago ■ Seeds ■ Sorghum ■ Soy ■ Tapioca ■ Teff (or tef) ■ Wild rice ■ Yucca

*Oats are often contaminated by wheat or barley because of growing and processing practices. It is generally recommended that newly diagnosed patients abstain from consuming oats, while all patients with CD should purchase oats designated as gluten-free.

Data from Academy of Nutrition and Dietetics. Celiac Disease. Nutrition Care Manual. Academy of Nutrition and Dietetics. Accessed January 22, 2025.; Kaukinen K, Makharia GK, Gibson PR, Murray JA. Practical insights into gluten-free diets. *Nat Rev Gastroenterol Hepatol*. 2015;12(10):580-591.; National Institute of Diabetes and Digestive and Kidney Diseases. Celiac disease. U.S. Department of Health and Human Services. Updated October 2020. Accessed January 22, 2025. https://www.niddk.nih.gov/health-information/health-topics/digestive-diseases/celiac-disease/Pages/facts.aspx#examples

and at home is significant. Complete elimination of gluten from the diet is difficult and requires diligence to maintain.[4,7,8]

Due to the varying degrees of damage that can occur to the small intestine, patients with new diagnoses of CD may present with varying degrees of malabsorption. Many patients present with micronutrient deficiencies—most often as iron, vitamin B12, and/or folate, zinc, calcium, and vitamin D, which are responsible for the anemias and/or bone disorders many patients experience. Nutrient deficiencies of this kind occur because the proximal portion of the intestine, where CD causes the most significant damage, is the primary location for absorption. In addition to the GFD, all patients with clinical evidence of malabsorption should be supplemented to replete any deficiencies. Many eating patterns within the GFD are also associated with deficiency, depending on the level of patient reliance on processed, low-nutrient-density foods, or avoidance of food groups. As most prepacked gluten-free foods are made with refined flour, these products are not enriched with the B vitamins and iron, nor do they provide enough fiber. Patients should be educated on meal planning tips that are both in accordance with the GFD and allow for adequate nutrient intake.[4,9,10]

Many patients with CD also develop secondary lactose intolerance. For many, the reduced levels of the enzyme lactase are temporary and will regenerate as the GFD allows the intestine to heal. For these individuals, it is beneficial to follow a lactose-free diet until their symptoms have resolved. Given 3–6 months of treatment (and thus mucosal repair), dairy products can be reintroduced if tolerated. Vitamin D and calcium levels should be carefully monitored.[4,9]

CORE CONCEPT 1

Celiac disease, once diagnosed, can be managed with careful adherence to the gluten-free diet. This requires extensive patient education and monitoring. Until patients reach an asymptomatic state and the damage is allowed to heal, there are several deficiencies and/or intolerances that may occur.

PRACTICE POINT

The gluten-free diet is the only treatment for patients with celiac disease. With careful adherence, most individuals will notice symptomatic improvement within only 48 hours and full clinical remission after 3–6 months.

PRACTICE POINT

It is important to assess micronutrient deficiencies common to patients with celiac disease, which include iron, vitamin B12, folate, zinc, calcium, and vitamin D.

Irritable Bowel Syndrome (IBS)

As the most frequently diagnosed digestive disorder, yet one of the most complex and controversial, **irritable bowel syndrome (IBS)** presents an interesting challenge for the clinical team. IBS is a functional GI disorder characterized by recurrent abdominal pain and altered bowel habits, the pathophysiology of which is only partially understood. There is little consensus on the true pathogenesis of the disease and even less agreement on the best treatment approach to address the wide range of symptoms. It is necessary to acknowledge that the science surrounding IBS continues to evolve.[11,12]

In addition, although there are dietary components to both the manifestations and treatment of the disease, IBS does not fit neatly into a discussion on digestion and absorption. However, nutrition therapy is at the center of current research. Given both the increasingly high prevalence and debate surrounding the syndrome, this chapter would be incomplete without a discussion of IBS.

Fundamentals of IBS

Common etiology indicates that IBS has peak incidence in the 20-year and 30-year age groups; occurs predominantly in females; and is preceded by anxiety, depression, and/or a severe adverse life event in more than half of patients. However, there is no single, agreed-upon cause. Instead, the symptoms of IBS are thought to result from both central brain and peripheral GI abnormalities. Current evidence supports four main contributing factors:

1. Abnormal GI motility
2. **Visceral hypersensitivity** (the experience of pain within the internal organs)
3. Altered brain–gut communication
4. Psychosocial factors: depression, anxiety, and/or **somatization** (complaint of recurrent medical symptoms of unknown cause)

The relationship among irregular GI motility, sensation, and the brain is dependent on the enteric nervous system and its regulation of the GI system. IBS may also be influenced by genetic predisposition, chronic low-grade inflammation, and/or dietary intolerances.[11,13,14]

Bowel habits vary between constipation and diarrhea within the IBS classification, often within the same patient. Thus, an IBS diagnosis is further specific as one of the following classifications:

1. IBS-C: Constipation Predominant
2. IBS-D: Diarrhea Predominant
3. IBS-M: Mixed, Constipation and Diarrhea
4. IBS-U: Unspecific

Individuals may alternate between the classifications over time. However, given the varying classifications and an abundance of additional GI and non-GI symptoms, the presentation of IBS is often confusing and contradictory. Clinicians use the Rome III Diagnostic Criteria to eliminate differential diagnoses and confirm the presence of IBS. Diagnosis relies heavily upon the clinical manifestations of IBS.[11,15] Diagnostic criteria includes recurrent abdominal pain or discomfort (at least 3 days/month in the last 3 months) as well as two or more of the following three factors: (1) abdominal pain/discomfort improves with defecation, (2) change in frequency of stool is associated with the onset of abdominal pain/discomfort, or (3) change in appearance of stool is associated with the onset of abdominal pain/discomfort.[15]

Clinical Presentation

As indicated by the varying classifications of IBS, there is irregularity in terms of bowel habits, frequency, and consistency for this population. Patients will present with constipation, diarrhea, or both, most often accompanied by lower abdominal pain and uncomfortable distention. Other common GI-related symptoms include incomplete fecal evacuation, straining or difficulty with bowel movements, mucus in the stool, excessive flatulence, urgency, and/or incontinence.[11,14,16]

Episodic abdominal pain is one of the most common physical manifestations found in IBS and is often the reason individuals seek initial medical consultation. For many, the pain is described as severe and debilitating but cannot be pinpointed to a specific location. Instead, patients describe bilateral pain in the general abdominal area that often radiates to the back and/or perianal region. Exacerbation of pain is often associated with eating, accompanied by increased urgency of bowel movements following a meal. Pain of this nature may be relieved by defecation, but this is not consistent throughout the IBS population.[14] Many researchers feel that this exhausting pain can be attributed to the initial presentation of visceral hypersensitivity. Theoretically, patients would experience an enhanced sensitivity to colonic distention in the GI tract, resulting in a reduced threshold for pain.[17]

There is a wide range of non-GI, psychological symptoms noticed in patients with IBS. Extraintestinal manifestations are not often associated with other GI disorders, so their presence may help to influence the initial IBS diagnosis. As previously mentioned, anxiety, depression, and somatization are common concurrent conditions. Other non-GI symptoms include medically unexplained headaches, fatigue, lethargy, palpitations, sleep disturbances, and neck, chest, and/or back pain.[11,14]

PRACTICE POINT

Due to the strong influence of psychological factors on IBS presentation, there is an unfortunate stigma surrounding the disorder. Many patients are made to feel that the symptoms they experience are the result of hypochondriasis. However, both the GI and non-GI symptoms experienced by patients with IBS are real and can be debilitating.

Nutrition Intervention

Unfortunately, because of the varying manifestations of IBS, current interventions are not uniformly successful. There are a few treatments that can be used to minimize symptoms. The most common approach is a combination of pharmacologic, psychosocial, and nutritional therapies. Medication use may include antidiarrheal agents, antispasmodics, antidepressants, and/or selective serotonin reuptake inhibitors, among others, all of which work to control abdominal pain, bloating, or consistency of the stool. The efficacy of pharmacologic intervention is inconsistent, and many patients with IBS rely on complementary therapies. For example, some individuals will find relief with cognitive behavior therapy or GI-directed hypnotherapy.[11,12,16] Most patients (approximately 70%), however, believe that intolerance to specific foods and/or the overall act of eating is responsible for their symptoms. Diet modifications are extremely prevalent in this population, and nutrition interventions continue to be of interest.[18]

It is understandable why there is no one specific dietary intervention used in cases of IBS. The varying components of effective nutrition therapy are based on the patient's presenting symptoms, identification of food intolerances, and/or potential allergies, and adjustment for energy and nutrient needs. The symptoms of IBS often lead to changes in oral intake, which can subsequently result in nutrient deficiencies, dehydration, and unintentional weight loss.[11] Many different dietary approaches have been utilized in both clinical and academic settings; however, the low FODMAP diet is perhaps the most well-researched and consistently recommended.

Based on the subjective association between intake and exacerbation of GI symptoms, patients identify many food items as important triggers. For example, IBS is historically associated with lactose intolerance. Patients may also present with aversions to gluten, caffeine, alcohol, and/or high-fat foods. As a result, nutrition therapy must involve the identification of foods not tolerated. The diet may then be adjusted to allow for a trial elimination of these foods. It is important to closely monitor the patient's presenting symptoms; ongoing elimination diets that are presented to have little impact on symptoms are unnecessary and may ultimately impact nutrition status. There is warranted concern regarding nutritionally inadequate diets in this population.[11,13,14]

Other, more general, nutrition recommendations include normalizing eating patterns and consuming 5–6 small meals each day to ensure adequacy of all nutrients. Increasing fiber through whole grains, fresh fruits and vegetables, seeds, and nuts may be beneficial for some patients, but will worsen symptoms in others. If an increase in dietary fiber is favorable, increase fluids accordingly. A low-fat diet is often better tolerated in this population. IBS symptoms may be worsened by high fat intake, as this stimulates both bile and pancreatic secretions, which can lead to changes in both frequency and consistency of stool.[11] Patients may also benefit from omitting foods that increase gas and flatulence (e.g., beans, cabbage, and onions). Depending on the adequacy of oral intake, it may be necessary to implement a general multivitamin or other micronutrient supplementation in accordance with any identified deficiencies.[11,13,19,20] Another intervention that has attracted considerable attention for the potential in decreasing IBS symptoms includes the introduction of probiotics to the diet.[11]

CORE CONCEPT 2

Diet plays an important role in the management of irritable bowel syndrome. It is important not to overly restrict the diet as a means to improve gastrointestinal symptoms, as this can lead to disordered eating, nutrient deficiencies, and malnutrition.

Low FODMAP Diet

The acronym FODMAP represents **F**ermentable **O**ligo-, **D**i-, and **M**onosaccharides **a**nd **P**olyols—carbohydrates grouped together based on the length of their chains.[20] Researchers at Monash University in Melbourne, Australia, theorized that ingestion of any one of the FODMAP constituents would worsen the symptoms of digestive disorders, including IBS, and the **low FODMAP diet** was born (refer to **Figure 11.5**). Short-chain carbohydrates (FODMAPs) are poorly absorbed by the small intestine and thus pass into the colon, where they can trigger GI symptoms through two separate mechanisms. First, the highly osmotic nature of FODMAPs draws excess fluid into the lumen of the intestine. Second, colonic bacteria rapidly ferment any unabsorbed FODMAPs, inducing gas production. Both occurrences cause luminal distention, contributing to the excess bloating, flatulence, cramping, and diarrhea observed in IBS.[13,20–22]

Oligosaccharides are carbohydrates of 3–10 linked monosaccharide units found in foods such as fructans and galactans. They pose an issue for patients with IBS because the human body does not produce the enzymes necessary for their digestion. The specific **disaccharide** (two monosaccharides linked) of concern is lactose, which is only considered a FODMAP if there are insufficient levels of lactase. Free fructose is a simple sugar (**monosaccharide**); as one of the simplest constituents of carbohydrates, fructose requires no digestion. However, fructose becomes a FODMAP when the amount ingested exceeds that of glucose. In a functioning GI tract, absorption of fructose would follow an alternative mechanism and there would be little to no issue. However, in individuals with IBS, this route is often impaired, resulting in fructose malabsorption. Finally, **polyols** are sugar alcohols. The absorption of polyols (or sugar alcohols) across the

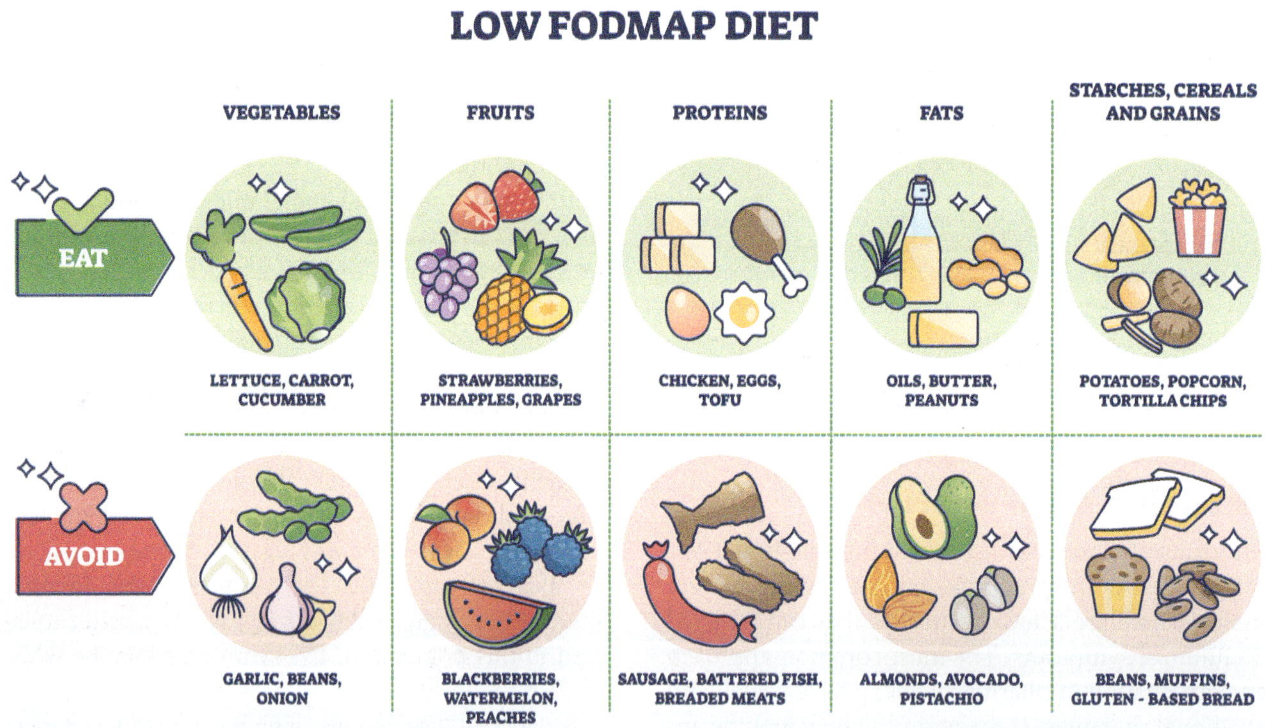
LOW FODMAP DIET
VEGETABLES
FRUITS
PROTEINS
FATS
STARCHES, CEREALS AND GRAINS
EAT
LETTUCE, CARROT, CUCUMBER
STRAWBERRIES, PINEAPPLES, GRAPES
CHICKEN, EGGS, TOFU
OILS, BUTTER, PEANUTS
POTATOES, POPCORN, TORTILLA CHIPS
AVOID
GARLIC, BEANS, ONION
BLACKBERRIES, WATERMELON, PEACHES
SAUSAGE, BATTERED FISH, BREADED MEATS
ALMONDS, AVOCADO, PISTACHIO
BEANS, MUFFINS, GLUTEN - BASED BREAD

Figure 11.5 Low FODMAP Diet

Table 11.3 FODMAP Components with High FODMAP Foods to Avoid

Oligosaccharides	Disaccharides	Monosaccharides	Polyols
Fructans, Galactans	**Lactose**	**Fructose**	**Sorbitol, Mannitol, Maltitol, Xylitol, Erythritol, Polydextrose, Isomalt**
▪ Apples ▪ Artichokes ▪ Asparagus ▪ Barley ▪ Beets ▪ Brussels sprouts ▪ Broccoli ▪ Cabbage ▪ Chickpeas ▪ Fennel ▪ Garlic ▪ Leeks ▪ Legumes ▪ Lentils ▪ Okra ▪ Onions ▪ Peaches ▪ Peas ▪ Persimmon ▪ Pistachios ▪ Rye ▪ Shallots ▪ Watermelon ▪ Wheat	▪ Dairy foods • Cheese (soft and fresh) • Custard • Ice cream • Milk (cow, goat, and sheep; regular and low-fat) • Yogurt	▪ Apples ▪ Artichokes ▪ Asparagus ▪ Canned fruits in natural juice ▪ Cherries ▪ Honey ▪ High-fructose corn syrup ▪ Mangoes ▪ Peaches ▪ Pears ▪ Sugar snap peas ▪ Watermelon ▪ *Large total fructose dose*: concentrated fruit sources, large servings of fruit, dried fruit, fruit juice	▪ Apples ▪ Apricots ▪ Artificial sweeteners ▪ Avocado ▪ Cauliflower ▪ Cherries ▪ Mushrooms ▪ Nectarines ▪ Peaches ▪ Pears ▪ Plums ▪ Prunes ▪ Snow peas ▪ Watermelon

Data from Marcason W. What is the FODMAP diet? J Acad Nutr Diet. 2012;112(10):1696.; Monash University. Low FODMAP diet for irritable bowel syndrome. Accessed January 25, 2025. https://www.monashfodmap.com/ibs-central/i-have-ibs/starting-the-low-fodmap-diet/; Mansueto P, Seidita A, D'Alcamo A, Carroccio A. Role of FODMAPs in patients with irritable bowel syndrome. Nutr Clin Pract. 2015;30(5):665-682.

intestinal barrier is slow; moreover, the GI tract is capable of absorbing only approximately one-third of what is consumed.[23] Refer to **Table 11.3** for the foods highest in each of the FODMAP constituents.

The rationale supported by many studies is that avoidance of foods high in FODMAPs will reduce fermentation and distention in the GI tract and thus a number of the associated symptoms. Evidence from several trials supports the reduction of symptoms, including abdominal pain and bloating, in patients with IBS who closely adhere to the low FODMAP diet.[24–26]

The research does not present the low FODMAP diet as a cure but instead supports its use as the first line of treatment for improving quality of life. Researchers and clinicians express some concern with the safety of long-term FODMAP restriction, primarily in regard to the nutritional inadequacies associated with any form of elimination diet. It would not be recommended to trial a strict low FODMAP diet for patients with eating disorders or disordered eating, those with malnutrition or at risk for malnutrition, those who are food insecure, or those with uncontrolled psychiatric disorders, as this could lead to over-restriction and further concern of nutrient deficiencies.[24] In addition to nutritional inadequacies, another concern with the low FODMAP diet is short-term changes in GI microbiota, including reduction in the beneficial *Bifidobacteria*.[25]

The low FODMAP diet restriction phase should last 4–6 weeks, followed by a reintroduction phase, and ultimately, an individualized plan to follow long-term.[24] Clinicians recommend a gradual stepwise reintroduction of small amounts of individual FODMAP foods to assess tolerance. The goal is to determine appropriate tolerance amounts so that some FODMAP foods can be consumed in the diet long term. While challenging a high FODMAP food, it is best to wait until symptoms are under control to minimize the influence of other high FODMAP foods not being challenged at that time. Essentially, each food should be

Table 11.4 Example Food and Symptom Log for the FODMAP Reintroduction Phase

Test: Fructose			
Day 1	Symptom(s) Present	Timing/Onset of Symptom(s)	Severity of Symptom(s)
1 teaspoon honey			
Day 2	Symptom(s) Present	Timing/Onset of Symptom(s)	Severity of Symptom(s)
2 teaspoons honey			
Day 3	Symptom(s) Present	Timing/Onset of Symptom(s)	Severity of Symptom(s)
1 tablespoon honey			
Day 4–7 Washout			

Repeat for each high FODMAP food group. Stop each challenge when/if symptoms arise. Recommend to follow closely with RD during reintroduction phase.
Data from Monash University. Practical Tips for FODMAP Reintroduction. *FODMAP Blog*. Published 2019. Accessed August 7, 2024. https://www.monashfodmap.com/blog/practical-tips-fodmap-reintroduction/

tested separately to better assess tolerance.[26] A food and symptom diary is a helpful tool to use during this time to track symptoms during reintroduction. Once the reintroduction phase is completed, the RD should work with the patient to construct a plan that is as liberal as possible while avoiding or limiting foods that cause symptoms. **Table 11.4** provides a sample reintroduction schedule for high FODMAP food groups. The current evidence for the low FODMAP diet presents markedly more strengths than weaknesses, with the majority of studies supporting its role in symptom relief for patients with IBS.[11,13,14,20,23,27]

Probiotics

Probiotics are live microorganisms often sold as dietary supplements or as components of foods (e.g., yogurt) that are intended to have health benefits through interaction with the body's normal flora. Research on general probiotic use is still evolving, and there is mixed evidence that specific strains may be useful in alleviating the symptoms associated with IBS.[28,29]

The relationship between a functioning human GI tract and the complex community of bacteria it houses is mutually beneficial. A number of studies suggest that imbalances or abnormalities in this normal flora may influence the severity of the GI-related symptoms common to IBS.[29,30] Theoretically, this indicates the potential for probiotic supplementation as a corrective treatment. There are numerous proposed ways through which probiotics may positively influence IBS pathophysiology:

- Stimulation of goblet cells to produce mucus that enhances GI barrier function, normalizes bowel movements, and reduces visceral hypersensitivity
- Improvement of GI motility and/or acceleration of transit time
- Protection against pathogenic bacteria
- Modulation of the GI inflammatory response and colonic fermentation
- Stabilization of intestinal permeability and the colonic microbiota

There is still much to be understood in terms of how probiotics affect GI function, and the exact pathophysiological mechanism(s) that probiotics impact has yet to be determined. Although studies are inconsistent, some research has indicated improvement in abdominal distention, pain and/or discomfort, flatulence, and altered bowel movements.[16,30–36] The exact species or strains that are the most beneficial for this population remain unclear.[31,32] Although the most widely used species of probiotics are *Lactobacillus* and *Bifidobacterium*, there are a number of individual strains that have been presented to impact different components of IBS.

In addition to the disagreement regarding the best probiotic strain, there is no set dosage for use in IBS. In light of current evidence, probiotics may be used to supplement other forms of primary treatment; they are not meant to serve as the only method for symptom relief. Given the current state of research, it may be best to take a natural approach regarding probiotic intake, recommending probiotic-rich foods such as yogurt, kombucha, miso, kefir, pickles, and sauerkraut.[11] When making a patient recommendation, refer to the most current clinical evidence and reevaluate after a minimum of 4 weeks of consistent use.[11,20,31,36]

PRACTICE POINT

Research surrounding diet interventions for IBS continues to evolve. Implementing any elimination diet should occur on a trial basis, with careful monitoring of how each may affect the patient's symptoms. Always consult the most current evidence before making any recommendations.

Non-Celiac Gluten/Wheat Sensitivity

The GFD is not only popular among those with celiac disease, but also with patients who have **non-celiac gluten/wheat sensitivity (NCGS/NCWS)**. This condition is both controversial and not well defined in the literature.[37,38] Evidence has not been able to pinpoint how gluten might cause GI symptoms without inflammation of the GI tract. It is also possible that gluten is not the main culprit, but rather fructans, which are abundant in wheat, or amylase-trypsin inhibitors (ATIs), both of which may be present with gluten. ATIs are water-soluble cereal proteins used as a natural defense by plants.[39] It was previously believed that NCGS/NCWS did not appear to cause intestinal damage, making malabsorption less likely; however, this perspective has been challenged. Research has demonstrated that systemic immune activation is triggered in those with NCGS/NCWS by noting increase in serum levels of SCD14 (a protein made by macrophages) and lipopolysaccharide-binding protein (LBP) (an acute phase reactant), antibody reactivity to microbial antigens, as well as improvement in immune activation markers such as FABP2 when following a strict GFD.[40] There is additionally some speculation that NCGS/NCWS is closely related to IBS, as both the GFD and low FODMAP diet have provided symptom relief in recent trials.[37]

It is important for the care team to first eliminate celiac disease as the cause of symptoms, as that will determine whether strict avoidance of gluten is necessary.[38] Once this disease is ruled out, the RD can assist in helping the patient reduce symptoms with dietary intervention.

The goal of nutrition intervention for patients with NCGS/NCWS at this time is symptom relief. Some patients may benefit from strict elimination of gluten, while others may be able to tolerate some level of this protein.[38] Further research is certainly needed in this area, particularly given newer research showing potential systemic inflammation with ingestion of wheat and/or gluten.[40] The low FODMAP diet can also be trialed in this population with the help of an experienced RD.[37] Frequent reassessment of nutritional status and GI symptoms will help direct interventions.

CORE CONCEPT 3

Patients with non-celiac gluten/wheat sensitivity (NCGS/NCWS) may also benefit from a gluten-free diet. Although there is no current best practice guideline for medical nutrition therapy for NCGS/NCWS, RDs can help patients create an individualized diet that minimizes their symptoms.

CASE STUDY REVISITED

At the gastroenterology clinic, the medical team begins a diagnostic workup to identify the source of Daniel's excessive diarrhea and unintentional weight loss. The team probes for his medical history, which reveals no previous gastrointestinal disorder or surgery. However, Daniel reports that over the years he has had bouts of diarrhea in the past that would not really bother him. In addition, Daniel confirms that over the past 6 months, his diarrhea has become more frequent; his stools occasionally show signs of oil in the feces that would indicate steatorrhea. There is no presence of blood in the stool. Daniel also reveals that his diarrhea is accompanied by considerable abdominal pain that is not always relieved by defecation. In addition, his bowel movements are preceded by extreme urgency.

When questioned on his personal history, Daniel does not report any alarming psychosocial abnormalities. He reports experiencing fatigue and moderate stress at his job, but no symptoms of anxiety or depression. Daniel claims no history of substance abuse. He does have a 4-year history of tobacco use and consumes alcohol on occasion.

Questions

1. Think back to the case presentation. Do you agree with your original description of Daniel's illness?
2. There are many sources of malabsorption that are indicated by excessive diarrhea and weight loss. What distinguishing features of Daniel's symptoms are important? Are there any specific questions you would ask, biochemical lab values you would consider, or other procedures you would require to confirm a diagnosis?

This heavily debated condition presents a unique opportunity for RDs to become involved in research to find the best diet for these patients.

Inflammatory Bowel Disease (IBD)

Among the many complex disorders covered within this chapter, **inflammatory bowel disease (IBD)** is perhaps one of the most intricate and involved. Much of the etiology behind this group of disorders remains unclear, making it difficult for researchers and practitioners to target specific treatments or therapies. In terms of nutrition, the existing evidence base (which is often unclear, conflicting, or weak) is a source of significant confusion. It is abundantly clear that diet plays a pivotal role in the disease process for these patients, both as a potential component of the pathogenesis and in the subsequent treatment.[41] This patient population often presents with strong, predetermined beliefs about the impact of diet on the IBD clinical course and in exacerbating or alleviating symptoms.[42] When considered in the context of the documented toll that the natural progression of IBD takes on nutritional status, these reasons indicate the importance of the RD in prevention and management.

IBD encompasses a group of chronic, relapsing-remitting immune disorders that originate in the GI tract. The two major forms of IBD, **ulcerative colitis (UC)** and **Crohn's disease**, represent intrinsically distinct conditions that share several overlapping features. The pathomechanisms behind IBD are largely undefined, although a single cause-and-effect relationship is improbable. As with many inflammatory disorders, IBD is thought to arise from an interaction among genetic factors, environmental influences, and other endogenous modifiers that lead to the disruption of the intestinal mucosa. An uncontrolled immune-mediated response leads to the release of inflammatory cytokines and overproduction of immune factors causing intestinal barrier disruption. One of the most pronounced alterations in the immune response is the hyperactivity of T helper cells, which maintain an active disease state.[43,44] Dysbiosis or changes in GI microbiota appear to be related to the onset of disease.[45,46] Within this context, diet has been proposed as a potential modulator in the disease process.[47] The leading hypothesis is that there is an aberrant immune response to GI microbiota in a genetically susceptible host, triggering cycles of inflammation and healing.[43–47]

Distinguishing Features of Ulcerative Colitis and Crohn's Disease

Although similar in many aspects of clinical presentation, UC and Crohn's disease are fundamentally different disorders. The most prominent distinction is the location of the inflammatory process; UC is characterized by inflammation that is limited to the mucosal layer of the colon, while Crohn's disease triggers transmural inflammation that can affect any organ of the GI tract from mouth to anus. Refer to **Table 11.5** for the most commonly involved sites. **Figure 11.6** demonstrates these key differences between Crohn's disease and UC. As a result, each disorder has a notably different impact on its respective patient population, meaning discernable disease

Table 11.5 Common Locations of GI Involvement for Crohn's Disease Patients

Location of Affected Tract	Percentage of Presenting Patients
Small bowel (typically distal ileum, or ileitis)	80%; 30% have ileitis exclusively
Ileum and colon (ileocolitis)	50%
Colon	20%
Perianal disease	30%
Mouth	5–15%
Gastroduodenal	5–15%
Esophagus	>5%
Proximal small bowel	>5%

Data from Peppercorn MA, Kane SV. Clinical manifestations, diagnosis, and prognosis of Crohn disease in adults. UpToDate. Updated August 20, 2023. Accessed January 22, 2025.

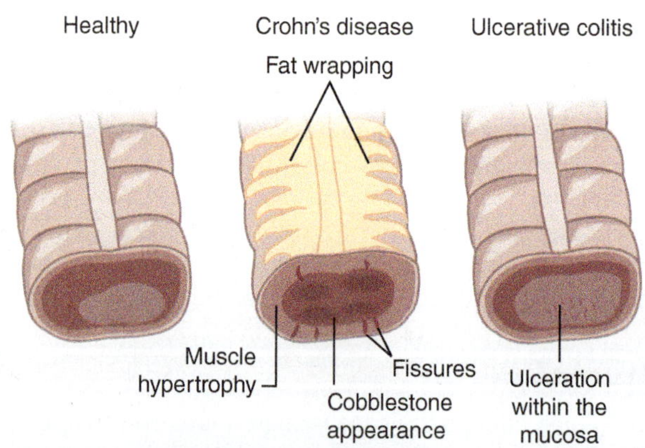

Figure 11.6 Key Differences Between Crohn's disease and Ulcerative Colitis

Clinical Roundtable

Topic: Diet as an Etiological Factor in Inflammatory Bowel Disease (IBD)

Background: The increase in worldwide incidence of IBD, especially in recently industrialized nations, has led to an interesting discussion on the role of diet as an environmental factor in the largely unidentified etiology of the disease. Why? The sharp rise in the incidence trend has paralleled the social and economic advances that are accompanied by a shift toward a more Western lifestyle; this includes, of course, dietary changes.[50-53]

The surge in new cases in accordance with increased consumption of more refined and processed foods (the so-called "Western diet") suggests a strong role of diet in the pathogenesis of IBD. There are several proposed mechanisms that may explain why dietary factors have such a significant impact:

- Direct effect of dietary antigens on inflammatory processes
- Diet-induced alterations of gene expression that affect the transcription factors involved in regulation of intestinal inflammation
- Changes to the composition or homeostasis of GI microbiome
- Shifts in GI permeability secondary to diet composition

Researchers now agree that dietary factors play an underestimated role in the pathogenesis and course of IBD. The question arises about which foods may be involved? Components of the Western diet, which is high in fat and protein but low in fruits and vegetables, have taken much of the blame.[50,51] The dietary components that can be considered risk factors for IBD development are as follows:

- **Cow's milk:** Data suggest a likely relationship between hypersensitivity to cow's milk at an early age and subsequent development of IBD, particularly ulcerative colitis (UC).
- **Refined carbohydrates:** As one of the first dietary factors to be implicated, high intakes of sugar and refined carbohydrates are associated with increased risk of both UC and Crohn's disease. In addition, a high intake of overall carbohydrates has been linked to increased risk for onset of Crohn's disease.
- **Dietary fat:** Both the type and the amount of fat are linked to increased risk of UC and Crohn's disease—this includes high dietary intakes of total fat and high ratios of omega-6 to omega-3 fatty acids, particularly a high intake of linoleic acid, which is metabolized to arachidonic acid and has proinflammatory properties.
- **Animal proteins:** Increased consumption of high-fat meats has been suspected as a risk factor for both Crohn's disease and UC.
- **Fast food:** Studies have identified an increased relative risk of IBD when individuals consume fast food at least twice per week.
- **Preservatives:** A number of additives used for the preservation of foods, like dietary sulfur, have been linked with increased numbers of UC cases.

Roundtable Discussion

The identification of food components that impact IBD development has significant implications for necessary shifts in dietary patterns and is an important consideration for those already diagnosed (whether in remission or periods of relapse). How might this be incorporated into your education and care plan for a patient with IBD? How will you evaluate the efficacy of avoiding these dietary components?

courses and chief complaints. These differences impact all other components of the disease process, including nutritional implications and treatment options. For example, the cardinal symptom of UC, identified in over 90% of patients at presentation, is chronic, bloody diarrhea. However, because of the variability in disease location that occurs with Crohn's, the presenting symptoms are less consistent than those noticed in UC. In general, nonspecific symptoms like fatigue, prolonged diarrhea (not typically accompanied by blood), abdominal pain, weight loss, and fever are the hallmarks of Crohn's disease. Carefully examine **Table 11.6** for a comprehensive comparison of UC and Crohn's disease.[44,48,49]

CASE STUDY REVISITED

Daniel is diagnosed with Crohn's disease as the explicit source of malabsorption.

Questions

1. What typical features differentiate Crohn's disease from ulcerative colitis?
2. How will this change the nutrition therapy you choose to initiate?

Table 11.6 Clinical Distinction Between Ulcerative Colitis and Crohn's Disease

	Ulcerative Colitis (UC)	Crohn's Disease
Disease Distribution	▪ Inflammatory process limited to the mucosal layer of the colon ▪ Commonly involves the rectum, may extend proximally (but only within the large intestine) ▪ Inflammation is continuous and circumferential	▪ Inflammatory process occurs transmurally from mouth to anus ▪ Patchy, asymmetrical involvement ▪ Unlike UC, often extends into perianal disease (anal fissures and/or anorectal abscess) but with rectal sparing
Clinical Presentation	*Onset of symptoms is gradual and intermittent:* ▪ Diarrhea, typically bloody ▪ Frequent bowel movements, small in volume secondary to rectal inflammation ▪ Colicky abdominal pain ▪ Urgency associated with defecation ▪ **Tenesmus** (cramping, rectal pain) ▪ Incontinence ▪ Patients with primarily distal disease may present with constipation accompanied by blood and/or mucus discharge	*Symptoms may exist for years before diagnosis:* ▪ Cramp-like abdominal pain ▪ Prolonged diarrhea without bleeding, may fluctuate over time ▪ Transmural inflammation is linked with sinus tracts that can lead to: • Fistula formation (common, unlike in UC); symptoms depend on the site of the fistula • *Phlegmon* formation • *Abscess* formation ▪ *Perianal disease*: • Perianal pain, drainage from large skin tags, anal fissures, perirectal abscesses, and anorectal fistulas ▪ Other potential GI involvement: • Oral: aphthous ulcers, pain • Esophageal: odynophagia, dysphagia • Gastroduodenal: upper abdominal pain • Gallstones may form secondary to reduced bile acid
Systemic Symptoms	▪ Fever ▪ Chronic fatigue ▪ Unintended weight loss ▪ Dyspnea or palpitations • Secondary to anemia	▪ Chronic fatigue ▪ Unintended weight loss ▪ Fever (occurs less frequently)
Physical Examination	▪ Evidence of blood in rectum ▪ Mild to moderate UC: • Otherwise normal ▪ Moderate to severe UC: • Abdominal tenderness to palpitation • Hypotension • Tachycardia • Pallor ▪ For those with prolonged diarrhea: • Evidence of muscle wasting • Loss of subcutaneous fat • Peripheral edema resulting from weight loss and malnutrition	▪ May be normal or show nonspecific signs (pallor, weight loss) ▪ *More specific signs:* • Perianal lesions • Perianal skin tags • Sinus tracts • Abdominal tenderness

Diagnosis	■ Presence of diarrhea for >4 weeks with hematochezia and urgency ■ Evidence of active inflammation on endoscopy and chronic changes on biopsy ■ Exclusion of other causes of colitis by • History (i.e., infectious, recent travel, nonsteroidal anti-inflammatory drug [NSAID]/medication exposure) • Laboratory studies (i.e., stool studies for toxins to rule out infection, fecal calprotectin, serologic testing for sexually transmitted diseases) • Endoscopy (colon and ileum) and biopsy	■ Established with endoscopic findings or imaging studies in a patient with a compatible clinical history ■ Colonoscopy is the most appropriate initial test for those with predominant diarrhea, while imaging studies are used for patients with abdominal pain ■ Exclude differential diagnoses
Endoscopic Findings	■ Punctate (i.e., studded) ulceration appears, may become confluent, and leaves islands of inflammatory tissue ■ Erythematous appearance (i.e., redness): loss of vascular markings due to engorgement of the mucosa ■ Mucosa also appears granular, hyperemic, and friable (bleeds easily) ■ **Pseudopolyps** ("inflammatory polyps") and mucosal bridging may develop ■ Over time, shortening of the colon and a reduction in diameter occur as a result of thickening/contracture of mucosal layer ■ Additional findings may include: • Petechiae (small red and/or purple spots) • Exudate (fluid secretions) • Edema • Erosions	■ Ileocolonic involvement: • Focal ulcerations adjacent to areas of normal appearing mucosa • Polypoid mucosal changes give "cobblestone" appearance ■ Skip areas of involvement • Segments of normal-appearing bowel interrupted by large areas of disease • Different from the continuous involvement noticed in UC ■ Transmural nature of inflammation results in fibrotic strictures and fistulas ■ Pseudopolyps (as noticed in UC) are often present
Histologic Features (via Biopsy)	■ Crypt cell abnormalities • Crypt branching • Shortening and disarray • Crypt atrophy • Crypt abscesses: collections of neutrophils that migrate across crypt epithelium into the lumen ■ Epithelial cell abnormalities • Goblet cell mucin depletion • Paneth cell metaplasia ■ Inflammatory features • Increased lamina propria cellularity • Basal plasmacytosis • Basal lymphoid aggregates • Lamina propria eosinophils	■ Focal ulcerations ■ Abnormal mucosal architecture ■ Increased cellularity of the lamina propria with infiltration of neutrophils ■ **Granulomas** (seldom found in UC) • "Histological hallmark" • A collection of monocytes and/or macrophages and other inflammatory cells with or without giant cells • Reported in as many as 70% of patients with Crohn's disease

(continues)

Table 11.6 Clinical Distinction Between Ulcerative Colitis and Crohn's Disease *(continued)*

	Ulcerative Colitis (UC)	Crohn's Disease
Extraintestinal Manifestations	▪ **Musculoskeletal** • Peripheral arthritis • Spondyloarthropathy, which may progress to ankylosing spondylitis • Osteoporosis, osteopenia, and osteonecrosis ▪ **Ocular** • Uveitis, iritis, or episcleritis ▪ **Dermatological** • Erythema nodosum and/or pyoderma gangrenosum ▪ **Hepatobiliary** • Sclerosing cholangitis • Fatty liver • Autoimmune liver disease ▪ **Hematopoietic** • Venous and arterial thromboembolism • Anemia	
Acute and Chronic Complications	▪ Severe bleeding and/or massive hemorrhage ▪ Fulminant colitis • >10 stools per day • Continuous bleeding • Abdominal pain • Distention • Acute, severe toxic symptoms: fever and anorexia • High risk of developing toxic megacolon ▪ Toxic megacolon: colonic diameter >6 cm or cecal diameter >9 cm and the presence of systemic toxicity ▪ Perforation • Typically, the result of toxic megacolon • May occur during the first episode of UC due to the lack of scarring from prior episodes of colitis ▪ Strictures: narrowing of the colon, may cause symptoms of obstruction ▪ Dysplasia and colorectal cancer: increased risk related to severity and duration of disease	▪ **Fibrostenosis** (narrowing), which may result in small bowel obstruction ▪ Short bowel syndrome (SBS), if multiple surgeries are necessary secondary to reoccurrence ▪ Dysplasia and colorectal cancer: increased risk related to severity and duration of disease ▪ Fistulae formation between the lumen of the GI tract and mesentery and/or another organ or the abdominal wall or skin ▪ Abscess formation ▪ Bleeding • While diarrhea is characteristically non-bloody, rapid bleeding is an uncommon but life-threatening complication ▪ Malnutrition ▪ Bone disease • Osteopenic bone disease and osteoporosis

Data from Shanahan F. Ulcerative colitis. In: McDonald JWD, Burroughs AK, Feagan BG, eds. *Textbook of Clinical Gastroenterology and Hepatology*. Hoboken, NJ: Wiley-Blackwell; 2012:355-371.; Rubin DT, Ananthakrishnan AN, Siegel CA, Sauer BG, Long MD. ACG clinical guideline: ulcerative colitis in adults. *Am J Gastroenterol*. 2019;114(3):384-413. doi:10.14309/ajg.0000000000000152; Lichtenstein GR, Loftus EV Jr, Isaacs KL, Regueiro MD, Gerson LB, Sands BE. ACG clinical guideline: management of Crohn's disease in adults. *Am J Gastroenterol*. 2018;113(4):481-517.

Both UC and Crohn's disease occur as intermittent exacerbations of symptoms followed by periods of remission; the length of time spent in either of the phases is extremely individual and cannot be predicted.

The severity of symptoms will range from mild to severe; this can change on a person-to-person basis or over time within the same disease course. Although objective measures for disease activity exist (indices like Truelove and Witt's for use in UC and the Crohn's Disease Activity Index), most clinicians do not utilize any formal activity index in daily practice and instead focus on GI and extraintestinal manifestations. Disease severity has important implications for predicting clinical outcomes. Patients with UC typically experience long periods of completely asymptomatic remission; two-thirds of patients will have at least one relapse in the 10 years following diagnosis, with a small percentage experiencing continued symptoms with no complete remission.[48] According to guidelines published by the American College of Gastroenterology, only 20–30% of patients with Crohn's disease will be without symptoms. For most patients, symptoms of Crohn's disease are intermittent; only a minority have continuously active symptomatic disease.[44,49]

Medical Management of IBD

With no specific, curative treatments identified, the management of IBD involves pharmacologic and nutritional measures. The overarching goal of treatment is to induce and maintain remission, with secondary, but significant objectives that include correction of nutritional status, prevention of complications, and facilitation of mucosal healing. While the accomplishment of each goal contributes to improved quality of life, a more concrete outcome is the avoidance of surgical intervention. This, however, is often inevitable. Furthermore, in Crohn's disease, patients have a 50% risk of recurrence of symptoms following surgery.[44,49]

Induction of Remission. The bulk of IBD's medical management emphasizes anti-inflammatory and/or immunosuppressive pharmacotherapy. Due to the relapsing nature of the disease, patients with IBD will require treatment that is highly individualized to fit the needs of the initial presentation or current flare-up. Pharmacologic therapy to induce remission includes a carefully monitored combination of systemic aminosalicylates, corticosteroids, immunosuppressive agents, antibiotic treatment, and other biological therapies like anti-tumor necrosis factor (anti-TNF) drugs, integrin blockers, and interleukin blockers.[49] These agents may also be effective for maintenance of remission—refer to **Table 11.7**. However, many of these medications are potentially toxic and can cause incredibly damaging side effects. For example, corticosteroids, which present a wide range of negative repercussions when used long term, are prescribed at high dosages when necessary to induce remission in moderate-to-severe disease courses. Once remission has been reached and maintained, the goal then becomes to taper steroids and avoid future use.[44,49]

Enteral nutrition (EN) has been identified as a strategy to both induce and maintain remission in patients with Crohn's disease, although not for those with UC. Some studies have demonstrated remission rates equal to or beyond that of corticosteroid use.[50] This will be discussed in further detail in a subsequent section.

Maintenance of Remission. Once remission is achieved, the long-term goals are to maintain an asymptomatic state for as long as possible and, similarly, to minimize the frequency and/or severity of relapses. Most patients with IBD can be successfully maintained—meaning a return to a normal function and high quality of life—with aminosalicylates and an occasional course of corticosteroid treatment. There is a potential role for nutritional support in the maintenance of remission to be discussed later.[44,49,50]

Surgical Intervention. Although surgical intervention (in the form of bowel resection and/or reconstruction) is often considered the last resort for patients with IBD, it should not be delayed if there is clear clinical decline despite aggressive pharmacologic therapy or failure of pharmacologic therapy altogether. In addition, acute complications, such as **toxic megacolon** in UC or evidence of dysplasia indicating colorectal cancer, are well-defined indications for surgery. Modest approximations suggest that one-fifth of all patients with IBD will require intestinal resection based on intractable symptoms, bowel obstruction, or perforation.[44,49,50] Surgical intervention involving bowel resection causes significant changes to the integrity of the GI tract, which introduces new challenges to an already complicated nutritional status. Refer to the section of this chapter entitled "Bowel Surgery and Short Bowel Syndrome (SBS)" for more information on this topic.

Medical Nutrition Therapy

An IBD diagnosis is accompanied by various nutritional challenges. At the most basic level, the common

Table 11.7 Pharmacologic Agents for Induction or Maintenance of Remission in Inflammatory Bowel Disease

	Ulcerative Colitis	Crohn's Disease
Aminosalicylates	**For Mild to Moderate:** cornerstone treatment of active disease and for maintenance of remission	**For Mild to Moderate:** effective in induction of remission and maintenance of remission
Corticosteroids	**For Moderate to Severe:** prescribed at high dosage to bring condition under control, then tapered	**For Severe Active Disease:** effective in induction of remission
Immuno-suppressants	**Cyclosporine, for Severe:** used because of its rapid action, but must be closely supervised; not to be used as a routine oral therapy or long term	**Azathioprine, for Maintenance of Remission:** maintenance therapy presented effective in clinical trials compared to placebo **Methotrexate, for Maintenance of Remission:** used as second-line for patients unresponsive to azathioprine (may also be used for improving symptoms in active disease)
Antibiotics (metronidazole, ciprofloxacin)		**For Mild to Moderate:** used for antibacterial action despite no identification of a causative microorganism
Anti-TNF-α (infliximab, adalimumab, golimumab, certolizumab)	**For Severe:** safer (but more expensive) alternative to cyclosporine; effective rescue therapy for induction of remission	**For Severe Active Disease:** effective in induction of remission, useful for retreatment after relapse
Integrin blockers (vedolizumab, natalizumab)	**Vedolizumab, for Moderate to Severe:** used when conventional therapy or TNF-alpha antagonists were not tolerated or effective; prevents white blood cells from entering the GI tract and causing inflammation	**Vedolizumab, for Moderate to Severe:** used when conventional therapy or TNF-alpha antagonists were not tolerated or effective; prevents white blood cells from entering the GI tract and causing inflammation **Natalizumab, for Moderate to Severe:** used when unresponsive to other types of therapy; prevents white blood cells from entering the GI tract and causing inflammation
Interleukin blockers (ustekinumab)	**For Moderate to Severe:** decreases inflammation in the GI tract by targeting interleukin-12 and interleukin-23	**For Moderate to Severe:** decreases inflammation in the GI tract by targeting interleukin-12 and interleukin-23

Data from Shanahan F. Ulcerative colitis. In: *Textbook of Clinical Gastroenterology and Hepatology*. Wiley-Blackwell; 2012:355–371. doi:10.1002/9781118321386.ch49; Vermeire S, Van Assche G, Rutgeerts P. Crohn's disease. In: *Textbook of Clinical Gastroenterology and Hepatology*. Wiley-Blackwell; 2012:372–393. doi:10.1002/9781118321386.ch50; Biologics and Inflammatory Bowel Disease (IBD). UChicago Medicine. Accessed August 8, 2024. https://www.uchicagomedicine.org/conditions-services/inflammatory-bowel-disease/treatment/biologics-and-inflammatory-bowel-disease-ibd-crohns-colitis

sequelae of the inflammatory process (uncontrolled pain, nausea, fever, and/or diarrhea) are associated with a number of consequences that negatively affect nutritional status: loss of appetite, decreased dietary intake, malabsorption, and/or altered nutrient metabolism.[47,51–53] Because the inflammatory process of Crohn's disease can occur at any point along the GI tract, with specific involvement of the small intestine (where the majority of absorption occurs), nutritional implications are generally more drastic for this patient population when compared to those with UC.[52] The disruption of GI tract function and the associated symptoms of pain, nausea, and diarrhea contribute to significant reductions in dietary intake and impaired nutrient utilization. Important challenges related to these changes include malabsorption, unintended weight loss, malnutrition, micronutrient deficiencies, and impaired bone health.[51]

Malabsorption

The specific type of malabsorption (bile acid or bile salt malabsorption) that results from the inflammatory processes of IBD is noticed primarily in patients with Crohn's disease that have involvement of the small intestine. In a healthy GI tract, most bile acids will be absorbed by receptors in the distal ileum after they are used for the digestion and absorption of dietary lipids. Bile salt malabsorption will occur when more than 50 cm of terminal ileum is diseased. Unabsorbed bile salts travel into the colon and draw increased fluid into the lumen, resulting in secretory diarrhea. More importantly, however, if more than 100 cm of the terminal ileum is affected, the amount of bile salts lost from malabsorption will deplete all stores and outweigh the body's ability to compensate, triggering a dangerous cascade of fat maldigestion/malabsorption, steatorrhea, weight loss, and ultimately malnutrition.[50–52]

Weight Loss and Reduced Muscle Mass

Although unintended weight loss and reductions in muscle mass are becoming increasingly less common due to advances in nutrition therapy, these implications remain important indicators of nutritional status for this patient population. General weight loss, observed in up to 70% of patients with IBD, is largely related to malabsorption, decreased oral intake, or a combination of the two. It is most pronounced in those with acute exacerbations of or widespread Crohn's disease.[50,53,54] In addition, some degree of lean body mass (LBM) depletion is estimated to occur in more than half of individuals with IBD, with significant muscle wasting observed in one-fifth of patients with prolonged symptomatic periods. Reductions in muscle mass are directly related to disease activity, as the inflammatory process amplifies protein catabolism; reductions may also be due, in part, to corticosteroid treatment and/or decreased physical activity. Regardless, loss of LBM beyond 10% is associated with increased morbidity for this patient population.[55,56]

Malnutrition

Although malnutrition is most readily identified in those with Crohn's disease affecting the small intestine, its effects are widespread and can impact any individual within this patient population, even during periods of remission. Malnutrition, recognized as protein-energy malnutrition (PEM), is one of the most influential factors on poor clinical outcomes associated with the disease process. As it depends largely on disease activity, PEM is reported in 20–85% of patients.[50] Malnutrition (accompanied by weight loss) is the third most common clinical feature identified in Crohn's disease, preceded only by diarrhea and abdominal pain. **Figure 11.7** presents the typical factors

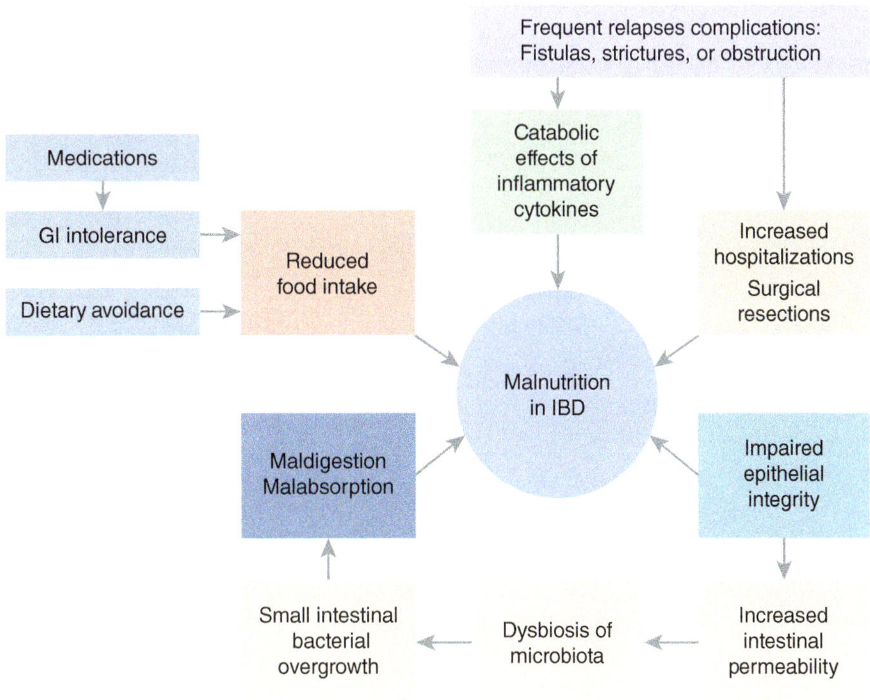

Figure 11.7 Causes of Malnutrition in Inflammatory Bowel Disease

Data from Hou JK, Lee D, Lewis J. Diet and inflammatory bowel disease: review of patient-targeted recommendations. *Clin Gastroenterol Hepatol*. 2014;12(10):1592-1600.; Yamamoto T, Nakahigashi M, Saniabadi AR. Diet and inflammatory bowel disease: epidemiology and treatment. *Aliment Pharmacol Ther*. 2009;30(2):99-112.; Forbes A, Goldesgeyme E, Paulon E. Nutrition in inflammatory bowel disease. *JPEN J Parenter Enteral Nutr*. 2011;35(5):571-580.; DeLegge MH. Nutrition and dietary interventions in adults with inflammatory bowel disease. In: UpToDate, Post TW, ed. UpToDate. Wolters Kluwer; Updated December 17, 2015. Accessed November 30, 2017. https://www.uptodate.com/contents/nutrition-and-dietary-interventions-in-adults-with-inflammatory-bowel-disease; Vagianos K, Bector S, McConnell J, Bernstein CN. Nutrition assessment of patients with inflammatory bowel disease. *JPEN J Parenter Enteral Nutr*. 2007;31(4):311-319.

Table 11.8 Common Nutrient Deficiencies in Inflammatory Bowel Disease and Suggested Dosing

Deficiency	Risk Factor for Deficiency	Recommended Dosing
Iron	Blood loss (UC) Small intestinal bacterial overgrowth	100 mg/day oral (divided in doses) Vitamin C (to improve absorption) For severe anemia, parenteral iron should be considered
Calcium	Vitamin D deficiency Bile acid/fat malabsorption (CD) Corticosteroid use (UC and CD)	■ 9–18 years: 1300 mg/day ■ 19–51years: 1000 mg/day ■ 51–70 years 1000 mg/day (males) 1200 mg/day (females) ■ 71+ yrs: 1300 mg/day
Vitamin D	Bile acid/fat malabsorption (CD) Small intestinal bacterial overgrowth Corticosteroid use (UC and CD)	1500–2000 IU/day-maintenance 3000–6000 IU/day-higher dose if on glucocorticoids, malabsorption
Vitamin B12	Gastric or ileal resection (CD) Terminal ileal involvement (CD)	1000 mcg/day oral
Folate	Small intestinal bacterial overgrowth Restrictive diets Sulfasalazine, methotrexate	1 mg/day
Magnesium	Chronic dsiarrhea	150 mg elemental 4 times daily
Zinc	Chronic diarrhea Fistulizing disease (CD)	50 mg elemental zinc (monitor for copper deficiency due to antagonism)

Data from Crohn's & Colitis Foundation. Nutrition resources for health care professionals: common nutrient deficiencies in IBD. Developed January 2017. Accessed December 2024. https://www.crohnscolitisfoundation.org/sites/default/files/legacy/science-and-professionals/nutrition-resource-/micronutrient-deficiency-fact.pdf

that contribute to malnutrition, related to both the pathology and treatment of IBD.[3,53,54,57]

Micronutrient Deficiencies

In the context of reduced intake, chronic diarrhea, malabsorption, and GI blood loss, a variety of micronutrient deficiencies are common to IBD. Evidence suggests that even patients who appear well nourished according to anthropometric measures, even during periods of remission, can mask baseline vitamin and mineral deficiencies. Deficiencies may result as manifestations of disease activity or location:

1. **Disease activity:** Iron deficiency anemia, which occurs secondary to chronic GI blood loss, is present in up to 80% of patients with UC
2. **Disease location**: Patients with Crohn's disease centralized in the terminal ileum will be more likely to experience vitamin B12 deficiency due to the loss of absorption site and/or fat-soluble vitamin deficiency (fat malabsorption attributed to bile acid deficiency).

Beyond the pathophysiology of IBD, some pharmacological treatments can contribute to further complications by either causing or exacerbating deficiencies. **Table 11.8** lists the most identified nutrient deficiencies.[3,53,54,57]

Bone Disease

Due to the high prevalence of malnutrition and micronutrient deficiencies, osteoporosis and/or osteomalacia are common problems for the patient with IBD; nearly 50% of patients are affected by some degree of bone disease. First, the most plausible explanation for reductions in bone mineral density is malabsorption of calcium and vitamin D. Second, long-term use of glucocorticoid therapy is associated with significant bone loss; in fact, it is the most common cause of secondary osteoporosis. Third, self-imposed restrictions of dairy products are widespread; inadequate calcium intake is reported in more than one-third of patients, accompanied by inadequate vitamin D intakes and low serum vitamin D concentrations. This represents a critical area for nutrition intervention.[54]

Nutrition Intervention

The focus of dietary intervention is to maximize or correct nutritional status, maintain adequate macro- and micronutrient intake levels, and assist in identifying and avoiding foods that may exacerbate symptoms. Preserving nutritional status is critical for the prevention of long-term health consequences, minimizing the potential for relapse and improving surgical outcomes. Planned periods of nutritional optimization and use of Enhanced Recovery After Surgery (ERAS) protocols can help maintain or correct nutritional status for patients planned for bowel surgery. The role of diet in the management of IBD, particularly as a therapeutic approach to inducing remission, continues to evolve.[51–58] Refer to Chapter 10, *Nutritional Management of Gastrointestinal Maldigestion*, for a description of ERAS protocol for GI surgery.

Nutrition Support

In the context of IBD management, nutrition support can be divided into three basic categories with fundamentally different objectives: enteral nutrition for correcting malnutrition, enteral nutrition as a tool to modify the underlying disease process (to induce or maintain remission), and recourse parenteral nutrition when enteral support is contraindicated.[50]

Enteral Nutrition–Role in Correcting Malnutrition. EN support is indicated to improve or correct the nutritional status of patients who present with signs of malnutrition. Current European Society of Clinical Nutrition and Metabolism (ESPEN) guidelines recommend that EN be provided as supportive therapy if oral intake is insufficient.[59] Patients who have lost >5% of normal body weight, those with a body mass index (BMI) of <18.5 kg/m^2, or those with continuing weight loss despite pharmacologic intervention, are considered candidates for EN support.[59] Because poor nutritional status is a risk factor for patients requiring surgical intervention, a period of nutritional optimization is sometimes needed. Preoperative nutrition optimization for 6–10 weeks has been associated with improved nutritional status, decreased inflammation, and better surgical outcomes.[41,52,58–62] When planning EN support, energy targets should consider current nutritional status, active versus remission state, surgical plans, and other stressors that may elevate energy expenditure. For protein, 1 gram/kg protein/day during remission and 1.2–1.5 grams/kg/day during active stages of Crohn's disease is recommended.[52,59]

PRACTICE POINT

EN is recommended for patients who have lost >5% of normal body weight, have a BMI of <18.5 kg/m^2, or are continuing to lose weight despite pharmacologic intervention.

PRACTICE POINT

Nutritional optimization for 6–10 weeks prior to surgery can improve nutritional status in patients at risk.

Role in Inducing or Maintaining Remission. Several studies have presented the therapeutic efficacy of EN during active Crohn's Disease.[47,50,51,53,55,56,59] EN downregulates proinflammatory cytokines to actively reduce intestinal inflammation. As evidence of this, normalization of numerous inflammatory markers (C-reactive protein, interleukins) begins almost immediately after initiation of feedings.[50,55,56] One of the biggest differences between remission maintained by pharmacologic treatment and remission achieved via EN is the added benefit of mucosal healing. EN-induced remission is associated with higher rates of mucosal healing (one of the treatment goals of IBD), as compared to corticosteroids.[53,58] The presence of luminal nutrients stimulates the production of hormones and growth factors within the GI tract that facilitate mucosal healing.[63] EN may also play a role in shifting the biodiversity of the microbiome, helping to rid of pathogenic bacteria, thereby reducing antigen exposure.[45,53,58,64]

Exclusive enteral nutrition (EEN) refers to the use of complete nutritional formulas as the sole source of dietary intake over a time spanning anywhere from 6 to 10 weeks. This approach eliminates all food from the diet, thereby decreasing the risk of exposure to factors within the normal diet that may be inflammatory. EEN is the first line of therapy in pediatric patients with active Crohn's disease where it has been presented to effectively induce remission while supporting growth and mucosal healing. In this population, EEN has been presented to be equally or more effective than corticosteroids, with fewer side effects, making it particularly desirable in children.[53,58,64]

Unlike the pediatric population, studies in adult patients with Crohn's disease have presented EEN to be less effective than corticosteroids to date. This may be due to barriers such as decreased palatability of diet and poor adherence in the adult population. Another concern is that once EEN ends, and a typical diet is resumed, remission reoccurs.[65] For these reasons, EEN is not currently recommended by ESPEN or the American College of Gastroenterology for inducing remission in the adult population.[49,59,64] However, a partial enteral nutrition (PEN) combined with a Crohn's disease elimination diet has been presented to be as effective as EEN for inducing remission in adult patients with mild-to-moderate active Crohn's disease.[59]

EEN can also be used for those with enterocutaneous fistulas, active inflammatory strictures, stenosis, or preoperatively as described above.[61–63,66,67] Provision of EEN by feeding tube ending distal to fistulas or stenosis can be used.[59] The recommended duration of EEN may change pending the reason for use; for example, 6–8 weeks to induce remission, 4–12 weeks as a bridge while awaiting maintenance therapy to reach therapeutic range, 4 or more weeks for preoperative support, and 6–12 weeks for management of abdominal fistula or abscess.[66] There is no difference in therapeutic efficacy among elemental, semi-elemental, and polymeric formulas for the induction or maintenance of remission in Crohn's disease. Consider that polymeric feeds are generally less hyperosmolar and are easier to flavor if consumed orally. It is important to note that the use of nutrition support as a means of inducing or maintaining remission applies only to those with Crohn's disease. There is no evidence that EN is an effective therapy for active UC. Nutrition support is only indicated for patients with UC for the purpose of correcting malnutrition.[59]

PRACTICE POINT

The use of nutrition support as a means of inducing or maintaining remission applies only to those with Crohn's disease.

Parenteral Nutrition. The use of parenteral (PN) support is—as it is for many chronically ill patients—controversial for the IBD population. PN should only be used when EN is contraindicated or attempts at enteral feeding have failed. Special circumstances that call for the use of PN include cases of severe malnutrition, high-output fistulas, obstruction, toxic megacolon, or during the preoperative period. Traditionally, PN was used to induce bowel rest in patients with debilitating and/or long-standing flare-ups, but this practice is no longer recommended. Research and clinical outcomes have illustrated that the use of PN during a period of bowel rest is not effective for either UC or Crohn's disease. Instead, PN should serve as a short-term solution until nutritional status is corrected and/or until conversion to EN becomes appropriate.[41,50,59] Intravenous fluids are indicated to maintain hydration status in those with high-output stomas unable to keep up with demand orally.[68]

PRACTICE POINT

Indications for PN include those with intractable vomiting, severe diarrhea, anastomotic leak, severe shock, intestinal ischemia, intestinal fistula with high output, severe stenotic disease, short bowel syndrome, or a perforated GI tract.

There are several shortcomings to PN use in the clinical setting. First, PN is associated with significant risks for the patient (including central venous line sepsis) and much higher medical costs. Second, PN does not have the same therapeutic effects on the intestinal lumen that are noticed when EN is employed as a remission induction or maintenance treatment; PN is not indicated as a therapy for UC and Crohn's disease. Although PN may be necessary to correct nutritional deficiency, it is important to consider the risks of using PN for an extended period. Careful monitoring is required.[4,45,50,52,69]

PRACTICE POINT

If indicated, PN should be introduced cautiously and progressively with close monitoring, as in all other high-risk contexts; many patients who require PN for malnutrition may have had prolonged malnutrition and may be at high risk for refeeding syndrome.

Micronutrient Supplementation

Given the high prevalence of micronutrient deficiencies noted in both UC and Crohn's Disease, a daily multivitamin supplement should be instituted immediately following diagnosis. Keep in mind that these deficiencies are observed at all degrees of disease severity, even in patients who show no sign of malnutrition according to anthropometric measures, particularly given the prevalence of food avoidance and frequent disordered eating in this population.[57–59,68] Supplementation beyond the daily multivitamin may also be necessary depending on the course of the disease. Additional supplements often used in this population include iron, calcium, vitamin D, vitamin B12, and folate. Any supplement recommendation should be accompanied by careful consideration of the type, brand, and dosage. Many ingredients in vitamin and mineral supplements can cause additional GI symptoms in those with IBD (lactose, sugar alcohol, artificial coloring, etc.). The biggest challenge is iron supplementation, which is necessary based on the incredibly high incidence of deficiency. Approximately 25% of patients will react poorly to an oral iron supplement, which manifests as worsening symptoms or disease activity.[56,57] To maintain adequate 25-hydroxy vitamin D levels, those with IBD require at least 2000 IU cholecalciferol daily, with higher doses recommended during active disease, or with malabsorption.[65] For mild IBD activity with mild-to-moderate anemia (Hgb 10–12 grams/dL for women or Hgb 10–13 grams/dL in men), iron supplementation can be attempted by the oral route. Intravenous supplementation should be used in adults with moderate-to-severe anemia or for those who do not tolerate oral iron.[51] Refer back to Table 11.8 for the recommended dosing for key nutrients of concern in IBD.

PRACTICE POINT

All patients with IBD must be monitored for appropriate iron, calcium, vitamin D, vitamin B12, and folate intake due to the high prevalence of these nutrient deficiencies.

PRACTICE POINT

Those taking sulfasalazine or methotrexate should supplement with 1–2 mg folic acid daily, as taking these medications can lead to lower folate stores in the body.

Individualized Diets

Counseling this population on oral intake, both during times of remission and active flare-ups of the disease, can be problematic. There is no single recommendation that can be made for a specific diet. Instead, patients will require special tailoring to develop a plan that ensures sufficient intake in terms of both energy and nutrients and identifies any trigger foods. In addition, this plan must take the disease course, the type of pharmacology used, and past surgical history into consideration.[69–71]

It is common for patients to self-restrict and/or avoid certain foods or food groups in an attempt to alleviate ongoing symptoms or prevent triggering active disease. Trigger foods will be identified as exacerbations of symptoms or the disease course. Removing foods from the diet and assessing for the presence of symptoms during that time can be helpful.

PRACTICE POINT

Exclusion diets are safest and most effective when the patient is concurrently receiving supplemental or total EN, as this ensures that diet quality will be maintained as foods are removed.

While trigger foods are largely individual, the most commonly recognized are dairy products and fiber-containing foods. Other problematic foods include processed meat, soft drinks, citrus fruits, and alcohol-containing beverages. Any food identified as a trigger should be avoided, particularly during a flare-up. Nevertheless, this is difficult to generalize; what prompts a symptom in one patient may be well tolerated in another. As a result of the tendency to avoid certain foods, these patients are at a high risk for insufficient dietary intake. An important component of nutrition therapy will be to help patients identify these foods and compose a plan that limits these foods without sacrificing diet quality. Overall, a well-balanced diet with as minimal restrictions as possible is encouraged.[4,41,50,59,72]

Defined Diets

An area of expanding IBD research centers around **defined diets**, which are dietary regimens based on an underlying theory or ideology of how food interacts with the body. Although the evidence is still highly controversial and lacks rigorous scientific backing, the use of such diets has grown in the patient population due to the lay literature and online searching. It is important to be aware of the several defined diets that have been publicized as successful antidotes to intestinal inflammation. These diets include a low FODMAP diet, a special carbohydrate diet, pre- and probiotics, and an omega-3 fatty acid diet. At a practical level, these diets are difficult to follow, may cause unnecessary financial burden, and are associated with a high deficiency risk due to their restrictive nature. In addition, they have not been proven beneficial.[47,49,59,70,73]

The Crohn's Disease Exclusion Diet (CDED) is one of the few defined diets that in combination with PEN has consistently proven beneficial during active Crohn's disease in adults. This diet encourages fruit and vegetable intake as a means of promoting release of short-chain fatty acids from the microbiome. The diet includes a mandatory intake of 5 foods: eggs, chicken, potato, apple, and banana. Food additives, gluten, dairy, and red meat are excluded. Studies show that use of the CDED with PEN providing 50% of energy intake can improve disease activity and decrease inflammation.[59,70,73] **Table 11.9** presents diet interventions that are commonly used in IBD.

The Bottom Line

This population is often receptive to nutrition counseling and may actively seek professional guidance.

Table 11.9 Diet Interventions Considered for Use in Inflammatory Bowel Disease

Diet	Description
Exclusive Enteral Nutrition (EEN) [64–66]	Provision of nutritionally complete formula improves dysbiosis Avoids all other sources of food to decrease inflammation
Partial Enteral Nutrition (PEN) and Crohn's Disease Exclusion Diet (CDED)[58,59]	Provision of 50% of calories as enteral nutrition Rest of calories come from foods allowed (fruits, vegetables, grains, oat, rice)
The Low FODMAP Diet[46,58]	Restriction of short-chain carbohydrates that are poorly absorbed in the small intestine to reduce GI symptoms that are also common to IBD
The Specific Carbohydrate Diet (SCD)[46,58]	Strict elimination of all complex carbohydrates (disaccharides and polysaccharides) on the basis that bacterial fermentation of maldigested carbohydrates contributes to intestinal inflammation and/or bacterial and yeast overgrowth Monosaccharides are the only permitted carbohydrates
High-Fiber Diet[46, 53]	Fiber has a beneficial effect on GI bacteria, producing short-chain fatty acids that can stimulate water and sodium absorption in the colon and promote mucosal healing May not be appropriate for patients with strictures
Mediterranean Diet[58,59]	Fruits and vegetables, whole grains, legumes, seafood, nuts olive oil Avoids red meat, processed foods, sweets

Patients with both UC and Crohn's disease will have a strong interest in any dietary modifications that can be made as part of the management plan. However, data indicate that while up to 90% of patients consider dietary guidance an important factor, only 20% feel they receive adequate information. It is of the utmost importance that careful time and consideration is spent with each patient, developing a plan that all parties involved feel meets the needs of the individual.

CORE CONCEPT 4

IBD is associated with a wide range of nutritional implications that center on malnutrition. Adequate intake, whether in the form of nutritional support or oral intake, is required.

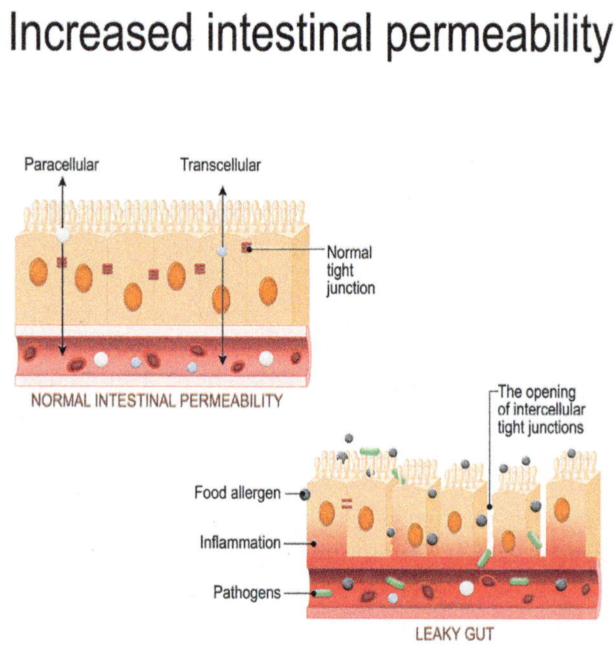

Figure 11.8 Intestinal Permeability

Increased Intestinal Permeability

Increased **intestinal permeability (IP)**, sometimes referred to as "leaky gut syndrome," is a highly debated condition in nutrition and gastroenterology. A quick internet search of **"leaky gut"** will lead to a plethora of fad diets promising relief, but research on this syndrome has only just begun. In medical nutrition therapy, IP is explained by the opening of tight junctions that enable pathogens and other substances to pass into the system circulation (**Figure 11.8**). This can be due to endogenous factors, such as stress and intestinal inflammation, as well as exogenous factors such as food antigens, and substances such as alcohol, creating an inflammatory environment.[74,75] While the cells lining the small intestine allow for transport of molecules into the bloodstream, exactly how inflammation is related to larger molecules and microorganisms progressing through this barrier is unknown. Some research has presented that this increased permeability may be related to IBD, as the dysfunctional structure and integrity of the GI tract can lead to increased inflammation and therefore worse IBD outcomes.[74] The protein zonulin functions to open spaces between intestinal cells and allow substances to pass, while keeping out harmful bacteria and toxins. Interestingly, this protein is unregulated in both celiac disease and type 1 diabetes.[75] Whether this is a cause or an effect of IP remains to be discovered.

Other contributing factors to IP include nonsteroidal anti-inflammatory drug (NSAID) use, excessive alcohol intake, radiation, chemotherapy, bacterial infections, and increased stress.[75]

Medical Diagnosis

A lactulose–mannitol challenge may be used as a test to determine presence of IP. A patient would come into the clinic and consume a solution that includes both sugars, then supply urine over the course of 6 hours. The aim of the test is to assess the ratio of lactulose to mannitol recovered in the urine, with a normal result being less than 0.03%. A higher rate may indicate increased permeability of these sugars from the small intestine into the bloodstream, leading to a potential diagnosis of IP. The issue with this test is that many factors can influence the test, such as patient size, duration of urine collection, and geographical location.[75]

The 51-chromium-labeled ethylenediaminetetraacetic acid (51-Cr-EDTA) permeability test has a similar aim as the lactulose–mannitol challenge. In this test, a patient ingests radio labeled EDTA, and urine is again collected over time to assess whether the chemical is recovered in the urine. Similar issues arise with the accuracy of this test, suggesting its use may or may not be clinically relevant.[75]

Larazotide acetate is a medication currently being considered for treatment in patients who have celiac disease and symptoms suggestive of leaky gut despite strict adherence to the gluten-free diet. This medication serves as a tight-junction regulator.[73] Clinical trials are currently underway, making this an exciting area of preliminary research.

Zonulin may be a good surrogate marker to show that the intestinal barrier function is impaired, thus allowing for IP. Serum zonulin levels have correlated with lactulose–mannitol challenge results in several studies.[75]

Nutrition Intervention

Nutrition intervention recommendations for IP are in the initial stages. Several studies have presented that dietary patterns can directly influence GI microbiota. It is suggested that the microorganisms present in our GI tract may have an influence on modulating inflammation as well as regulating tight junction function. Diets high in fat, sugar, animal proteins, and alcohol may negatively impact the GI microbiota and increase intestinal permeability, whereas diets high in fiber, fruits, and vegetables have the opposite effect. The MaPLE randomized controlled trial demonstrated that a dietary pattern rich in polyphenols may be beneficial in reducing the risk of IP, potentially due to their antioxidant, anti-inflammatory, and immunomodulatory activity both in the GI tract and systemically throughout the body. This study recommended a diet with 700 mg total polyphenols daily (including berries, blood orange, pomegranate juice, green tea, Renetta apple, dark chocolate) for 8 weeks, and showed reduced intestinal permeability by reduced zonulin levels.[75]

Some practical suggestions may include the following:

1. Provide instruction and support for patients with celiac disease to ensure they follow the GFD strictly
2. Utilize MyPlate to promote an overall healthy diet
3. Recommend increased intake of overall fiber intake, vegetables, and fruits
4. Recommend decreased intake of added sugar and saturated/trans fats
5. Choose leaner animal protein options if incorporated in the diet
6. Promote stress management techniques
7. Review alcohol intake
8. Recommend patient discuss NSAID usage with their physician if this is a regularly taken medication

As more is discovered in research about IP etiology and treatment, RDs will have the ability to provide more up-to-date recommendations to help these patients reduce symptoms.

CORE CONCEPT 5

Careful assessment of the patient's nutritional status and GI symptoms will direct nutritional intervention in IP such as limiting alcohol and practicing stress management. Clinicians should be wary of "easy fix" fad diets that patients may be following.

Helicobacter pylori

Helicobacter pylori (*H. pylori*) is a bacterial infection that colonizes the stomach by moving through the mucosal lining, attaching to gastric epithelial cells, and releasing cytotoxins to allow for generation of more bacteria.[76,77] This infection can lead to a host of medical conditions, from general gastritis to peptic or duodenal ulcer, mucosal-associated lymphoid tissue lymphoma, and gastric cancer. In fact, *H. pylori* infection is implicated in 75% of gastric cancer cases worldwide.[76] **Figure 11.9** presents the bacteria penetrating the mucosal lining and leading to an ulcer. Transmission of these bacteria is due to interhuman contact and is strongly associated with low socioeconomic status.

Medical Treatment

Medical therapy for elimination of *H. pylori* infection is a 7-day combination therapy of four drugs: a proton-pump inhibitor (PPI) and three antibiotics (clarithromycin, amoxicillin, and metronidazole). The use of multiple types of antibiotic medications reflects the discovery of antibiotic resistance with certain strains of *H. pylori*. The eradication of *H. pylori* is important for the prevention of secondary diseases as well as the standard therapy for treating peptic ulcer disease.[78]

Besides the use of PPI and antibiotics, probiotics have received some support for an additional benefit in the treatment of *H. pylori* and peptic ulcer disease.[79] The mechanism behind this theory is that probiotics are able to attach to the gastric epithelial cells and provide immune system support. In patients with diarrhea, probiotic use was able to decrease this symptom. Additional studies must assess the most beneficial probiotic strain, frequency, dose, and length of treatment.

In animal studies, there has been some evidence that those fed a diet rich in whole-grains, vegetables, beans, nuts, seeds, and mushrooms produced a favorable microbiome, which is theorized to be due to the prebiotic and anti-inflammatory nature of these foods.[80] After *H. pylori* infection, there is a documented decrease in the diversity of GI bacteria.[81] Future research should explore this interplay between the microbiome, *H. pylori* infection, and diet patterns.

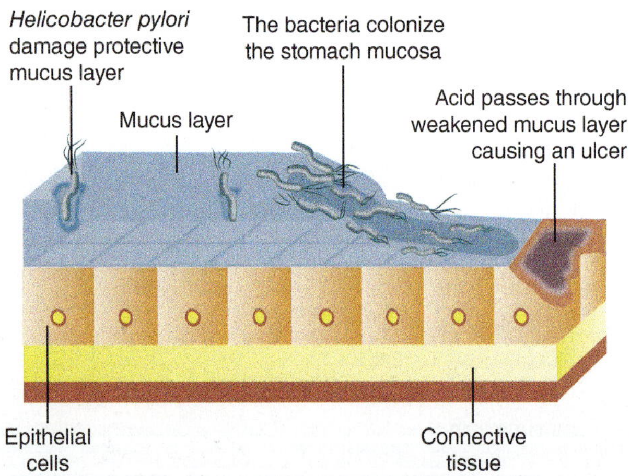

Figure 11.9 Bacterial Penetration of the Mucosal Lining Leads to Peptic Ulcer

Nutrition Intervention

Attention to micronutrient status is important since *H. pylori* has been known to cause deficiencies in iron, vitamin C, vitamin A, alpha-tocopherol, vitamin B12, folic acid, zinc, nickel, and selenium.[76,77] The infection has been speculated to affect insulin resistance, obesity, and lipid profiles.[77] Perhaps most importantly, *H. pylori* has been linked to malnutrition, particularly in children of developing nations. It is imperative that the RD assesses whether a patient has any signs of nutrient deficiency or unintentional weight loss.

Eradication of *H. pylori* using PPI and antibiotic combination therapy usually corrects micronutrient deficiencies because the bacteria are no longer sequestering these nutrients for their own proliferation. It is still important to monitor these micronutrient levels and provide supplementation as necessary. Limited research has suggested that avoidance of high levels of zinc, nickel, and iron may assist in quicker elimination of the bacteria as *H. pylori* requires these minerals to grow[76]; however, this must be weighed against the detrimental effects of becoming deficient in these nutrients.

In the case of unintentional weight loss, nutritional advice should be provided to help the patient safely regain weight and improve overall nutritional status through a general healthy diet.

CORE CONCEPT 6

Deficiencies in iron, vitamin C, vitamin A, alpha-tocopherol, vitamin B12, folic acid, nickel, and selenium are possible in patients with *H. pylori*. Patients with this infection should be monitored closely for both nutrient deficiency and unintentional weight loss.

Small Intestinal Bacterial Overgrowth (SIBO)

The human GI tract is home to more than 10 times more bacteria than the body has cells. This normal flora is part of a mutually beneficial relationship shared with the digestive tract, helping to maintain normal GI and immune functions. Most bacteria are contained in the colon, with smaller amounts found in the small intestine, where abnormal amounts would interfere with the digestion and absorption of food. If a disproportionate number of bacteria (typically of the colonic nature) invade the small intestine, the overgrowth competes with the body for ingested nutrients and can impair the individual's nutritional status. This condition is referred to as **small intestinal bacterial overgrowth (SIBO)**.[82–89]

SIBO occurs secondary to several clinical conditions, such as those listed in **Table 11.10**. It is typical in cases of diminished gastric acid secretion or disordered GI motility; however, SIBO is also linked to other non-intestinal disease states including autoimmune, endocrine, cardiovascular, and renal, as well as obesity.[82–84] Most bacteria that enter the digestive tract via ingestion are eliminated within the acidic environment of the stomach. Any that survive long enough to pass into the small intestine are

Table 11.10 Clinical Conditions Associated with Small Intestinal Bowel Overgrowth

Disturbances in Small Intestinal Transit and/or Motility	▪ Autonomic visceral neuropathy ▪ Blind loops of the small intestine ▪ Changes with aging ▪ Chronic intestinal pseudo-obstruction ▪ Disordered migrating motor complex ▪ Intestinal stricture ▪ Surgical alteration of normal small intestinal anatomy
Disturbances in Gastric Acid Secretion	▪ Achlorhydria ▪ Acid suppression via medication ▪ Chronic atrophic gastritis ▪ Gastric resection
Associated Diagnoses	▪ Acute and chronic pancreatitis ▪ Celiac disease ▪ Chronic radiation enteropathy ▪ Diabetes mellitus ▪ Diverticulosis/diverticulitis ▪ End-stage renal disease ▪ End-stage liver disease ▪ Fibromyalgia ▪ Gastroesophageal reflux disease ▪ Hypothyroidism ▪ Immunodeficiency syndrome(s) ▪ Inflammatory bowel disease (primarily Crohn's disease) ▪ Irritable bowel syndrome ▪ Recurrent antibiotic use ▪ Short bowel syndrome

Data from Roszkowska P, Klimczak E, Ostrycharz E, Rączka A, Wojciechowska-Koszko I, Dybus A, Cheng YH, Yu YH, Mazgaj S, Hukowska-Szematowicz B. Small intestinal bacterial overgrowth (SIBO) and twelve groups of related diseases—current state of knowledge. *Biomedicines*. 2024;12(5):1030. doi:10.3390/biomedicines12051030 subsequently cleared; normal motility is thus a major defense system against bacterial colonization of the small intestine, due in part to the action of the **migrating motor complex (MMC)**. The MMC, or "intestinal housekeeper," produces a cleansing wave every 90–120 minutes during times of fasting. This wave sweeps the contents of the small intestine toward the colon, effectively removing any unwanted bacteria from the area. As such, one of the most common underlying causes of SIBO is impairment of the MMC—reduced frequency or complete loss of MMC movements occurs in an estimated 70% of patients with SIBO.[89]

SIBO is formally defined when >100,000 colony-forming units of bacteria per milliliter of intestinal juice are found in the proximal small intestine.[87] Although the bacterial strains are typically nonpathogenic in nature, such dramatic changes in the normal flora have a massive impact on nutritional status. The clinical manifestations that occur are primarily the result of malabsorption, caused by both bacterial competition for ingested nutrients and damage to the small intestinal epithelium. Patients can experience bloating, abdominal pain, and diarrhea among other symptoms.[85–89]

Diagnosis

Typically, bacterial abnormalities are identified using direct culture from the jejunum, considered to be the gold standard for diagnosis. As the intestinal bacterial flora is often out of reach of instrumentation, this method is not appropriate when assessing for SIBO. Traditionally, the SIBO diagnosis is made using a hydrogen breath test. During the test, patients are given a predetermined amount of lactulose or glucose, and all gases exhaled are measured over the course of several hours. Theoretically, any small intestinal bacteria will feed off the sugar; this bacterial fermentation produces methane and/or hydrogen gas, depending on the type of bacteria present. The gases are subsequently expelled by the lungs. Because the human body is unable to produce methane or hydrogen gas, their presence in the breath is indicative of SIBO; the test is positive if the patient produces a minimum of 20 ppm hydrogen and/or methane within the first 2 hours following administration. The hydrogen breath tests can be confounded by intestinal transit times and are criticized for a lack of specificity and high rates of false positives. This continues to be debated in the clinical arena.[85–87]

Consequences of Overgrowth on Absorption

Some degree of nutrient malabsorption is virtually guaranteed with the SIBO diagnosis. While there are several reasons why it occurs, malabsorption is primarily attributed to competition for nutrients and/or damage to absorptive surfaces.[88–90]

One of the most common complications of SIBO is fat malabsorption. As part of the normal absorptive process, digested lipids (monoglycerides and fatty acids) combine with phospholipids and bile acid to form **micelles**. Micelles transport the otherwise poorly absorbed substrates to the surface of the enterocyte, where they are taken up by the body. In the presence of SIBO, intraluminal bacteria cause the deconjugation of bile acid; if the concentration of conjugated bile acids drops below the threshold necessary for micellar formation, as is often the case, absorption of fats is impaired. It is thus extremely common for patients to present with chronic steatorrhea. Improper micellar formation and/or fat malabsorption will often lead to deficiencies of the fat-soluble vitamins.[90]

Bacterial activity in the GI lumen has been presented to indirectly damage the absorptive mucosa; when this occurs, carbohydrate and protein absorption may also be affected. Mucosal injury and decreased brush border enzyme activity primarily interfere with carbohydrate uptake; in this case, bacterial flora ferment the carbohydrate substrates before they are made available to the host. Although severe protein malnutrition is extremely rare in SIBO patients, GI bacteria similarly compete with the host for protein substrates. Overall absorptive dysfunction and mucosal injury, along with decreased levels of the enterokinases necessary for pancreatic protease activation, contribute to decreased amino acid and peptide uptake.[91]

Finally, SIBO's effect can extend beyond macronutrient malabsorption, inhibiting uptake of several micronutrients. As mentioned, fat malabsorption is linked with deficiencies of the fat-soluble vitamins (primarily vitamins A, D, and E; because vitamin K is synthesized by the bacterial microflora, deficiency is rarely noticed). In addition, bacteria within the intestinal lumen readily utilize vitamin B12 before it can be absorbed. Deficiencies of thiamine and nicotinamide, although less common, have also been reported for similar reasons. In contrast, folate levels are often elevated in this population; the GI bacteria synthesize the vitamin, which is subsequently absorbed by the body.[83,86–91]

Clinical Presentation

Symptoms will vary depending on both the type of bacteria colonizing the small intestine and the nature of any underlying intestinal abnormality that preceded SIBO. There are a number of clinical features common to most SIBO cases: excess intestinal gas, abdominal distention and bloating, diarrhea, and pain or discomfort. Refer to **Table 11.11** for a more comprehensive patient profile.[83,91]

The classical manifestations of SIBO are largely the result of bacterial interaction with ingested food; within this context, symptoms may be exacerbated postprandially or may occur secondary to malabsorption. For example, bacteria that prefer to metabolize carbohydrates will produce excess gas and cause significant intestinal distention, while those that metabolize bile salts and therefore inhibit fat absorption will contribute to chronic steatorrhea. When these symptoms reduce or alter normal food intake, as is often the case, the disease state is further complicated. Most patients identify postprandial bloating and/or nausea as the culprits behind decreased oral intake. Correcting nutritional status remains a priority.[89–92]

Table 11.11 Clinical Characteristics of Small Intestinal Bowel Overgrowth

Gastrointestinal Symptoms	■ Abdominal discomfort, pain, and/or cramping ■ Belching ■ Constipation ■ Diarrhea and/or steatorrhea ■ Distention (especially postprandial bloating) ■ Early satiety ■ Flatulence ■ Lactose intolerance ■ Nausea ■ Weight loss
Extraintestinal Symptoms	■ Anemia ■ Depression ■ Eczema ■ Fatigue ■ Headaches or loss of concentration ■ Impaired night vision ■ Joint pain ■ Neuropathy ■ Osteomalacia
Biochemical Abnormalities	■ Micronutrient deficiencies • Vitamin A • Vitamin B12 • Vitamin D • Vitamin E • Iron ■ Hypoproteinemia, hypoalbuminemia

Data from Roszkowska P, Klimczak E, Ostrycharz E, Rączka A, Wojciechowska-Koszko I, Dybus A, Cheng YH, Yu YH, Mazgaj S, Hukowska-Szematowicz B. Small intestinal bacterial overgrowth (SIBO) and twelve groups of related diseases—current state of knowledge. *Biomedicines*. 2024;12(5):1030. doi:10.3390/biomedicines12051030

Medical Treatment

There are three primary components to the treatment of SIBO:

1. Correct (or treat) the underlying cause.
2. Eliminate bacterial overgrowth via antibiotic therapy.
3. Address any nutritional implications, including deficiencies.

Regardless of the pathogenesis behind the diminished acid production and/or motility impairment that ultimately resulted in SIBO, any excess bacteria colonizing the small intestine must be eradicated. Therefore, antibiotic therapy forms the cornerstone of treatment. In some cases where antibiotic use is contraindicated (allergies and/or limited response), patients are fed with an **elemental formula**. Elemental formulas provide nutrients in predigested forms and are thought to be absorbed within the first few feet of the small intestine. Research presents that, because the nutrients are absorbed before reaching the bacteria, which are subsequently starved, elemental diets provide a safe and effective alternative to treating the overgrowth. Most patients are prescribed Rifaximin because of its efficacy within the digestive tract: 99.6% will remain in the GI tract without being absorbed. SIBO has a high recurrence rate (nearly 50%) within 9 months following antibiotic treatment if the underlying cause is also not addressed.[92–94]

Nutrition Intervention

Nutrition interventions are critical to successful management of SIBO. While there are a number of overarching goals to be met through nutrition therapy, including symptom management, correction of nutritional deficiencies, and recurrence prevention, all interventions should be individualized to meet the patient's specific needs.[89,91–95]

Although symptoms associated with malabsorption may begin to improve shortly after treatment begins, it is important for patients to initially avoid foods that contribute to intestinal fermentation. The damage caused by SIBO results in decreased secretion of the brush border enzymes lactase, sucrase, and maltase; because the epithelium takes time to repair and regenerate, the reduction in these enzymes may continue after the overgrowth has been treated. Undigested and unabsorbed lactose, sucrose, and maltose become substrates for bacterial fermentation; thus, restricting intake of sugars and starches can help prevent prolonged bloating and abnormal bowel movements while the intestine heals. Patients with IBS who also have SIBO are often prescribed a low FODMAP diet. However, it remains inconclusive whether a low FODMAP diet is useful in reducing the symptoms associated with SIBO alone.[95] At this time, diet therapy should focus on helping the patient develop a symptom management plan that is customized per individual tolerances.[53]

There are a number of other dietary modifications that can be made to reduce specific symptoms. For example, for patients with persistent steatorrhea, a decrease in or restriction of fat intake may be beneficial at the beginning of treatment.[86] Others who present with enduring and/or uncomfortable flatus may find relief from eliminating nonabsorbable sugar alcohols (sorbitol, aspartame, and saccharine) from the diet. Choosing more omega-3 fatty acids as opposed to omega-6 fatty acids may assist in lowering inflammation.[82] Aerophagia—the involuntary swallowing of air—occurs in all individuals via normal activities such as chewing gum or drinking beverages through a straw. This, however, may be irritating to the SIBO patient population and can be avoided to help reduce abdominal distention.[89]

PRACTICE POINT

Encourage patients to maintain a log that will track intake and symptoms. This provides for identification of foods or food groups that continue to exacerbate the symptoms of malabsorption, which can be avoided at the beginning of treatment through a careful elimination diet and reintroduced once symptoms resolve.

It may be difficult to correct nutrient deficiencies when digestive symptoms persist, as this indicates that a certain degree of the brush border of the intestinal tract remains damaged. In patients with documented steatorrhea, the use of MCTs can help to facilitate absorption of fatty acids. As symptoms subside, however, all nutrient deficiencies should be identified and corrected. Again, SIBO typically interferes with fat-soluble vitamins (A, D, and E), vitamin B12, and iron; however, other deficiencies are not uncommon.[82,86,89]

PRACTICE POINT

When recommending supplementation of micronutrients, be sure to select brands without fillers or other ingredients such as gluten and/or sugars that may continue intestinal fermentation and/or irritation.

Finally, nutrition therapy can play a role in promoting the actions of the MMC. This will be critical in preventing the recurrence of bacterial overgrowth. Because the MMC is deactivated when eating, the most important consideration will be meal spacing. Individuals prone to SIBO should be encouraged to distribute meals evenly throughout the day, typically every 3–5 hours, and to avoid or limit between-meal snacking; both modifications will allow sufficient time for the cleansing wave to remove waste from the small intestine.[82,85]

The goal of nutritional intervention for this population is the same as that for all disease states: the optimization of nutritional status. In severe cases of SIBO, individuals may present with weight loss and/or malnutrition. For these patients, nutritional supplements should be provided, and careful monitoring of weight and markers of nutritional status is necessary. Although uncommon, PN may be indicated to provide nutrition to the severely malnourished patient; however, this is associated with a number of secondary complications and should only be used when all other options for nutrient repletion have been exhausted.[84,86] The bottom line remains: the RD plays an integral role in helping patients with SIBO to alleviate symptoms, optimize digestion, and improve nutritional status.[82]

PRACTICE POINT

When evaluating clients with undiagnosed GI complaints, SIBO should always be on the RD's radar. The most important concerns when working with this population include maintaining adequate nutritional intake through a customized dietary approach, correcting nutrient deficiencies, and maximizing digestion.

CORE CONCEPT 7

Small intestinal bacterial overgrowth is often associated with and occurs concurrently with a number of other disorders related to maldigestion and malabsorption. Nutrition therapy plays a critical role in the treatment of this patient population.

Clinical Controversy

Topic: Do probiotics have a place at the table for small intestinal bacterial overgrowth (SIBO) treatment?

Although antibiotic use currently serves as the first line of treatment for eliminating inappropriate bacterial overgrowth of the small intestine, it is not a guaranteed solution. The most common concerns with antibiotic treatment in the context of SIBO involve poor patient tolerance and diminished efficacy with long-term use. More importantly, there is a large potential for rebound colonization after treatment is complete. Interest in the use of probiotics as a potential treatment for SIBO and as a means for preventing recurrence has grown. However, the evidence is largely preliminary and is, in many cases, controversial.[82–90]

The biggest barrier to probiotic use in this population is the limited availability of high-quality trials specific to patients with SIBO. As clinicians in an evidence-based practice, this is certainly cause for apprehension for many RDs. There is sufficient evidence demonstrating the benefit of probiotic use to the disordered GI tract at large. There are several identified mechanisms for how these benefits occur:

1. Competition with pathogens for adherence to the intestinal epithelium and mucosa
2. Production of bacteriocins (produced by bacteria to kill or inhibit bacterial strains closely related to produced bacteria)
3. Inhibition of bacterial translocation
4. Enhancement of mucosal barrier function
5. Downregulation of inflammatory processes
6. Modulation of GI motor and sensory responses and signaling between luminal bacteria, the intestinal epithelium, and the immune system

The results from preliminary and pilot trials are encouraging. Most studies have focused on bacterial strains from the genus *Lactobacillus*, which have been proven effective for other GI-related conditions.[82,83]

Studies are difficult to compare due to the vast differences in study populations, probiotic species used, and clinical outcomes. These limitations, when combined with the small sample sizes of each study, hamper the generalization of the results.[85–90]

The beneficial effects of prebiotics need to be confirmed with double-blind, randomized, placebo-controlled trials of notably larger sample sizes. Before the recommendation for probiotic use in this patient population can be solidified, these trials must demonstrate the following:

1. The most favorable bacterial strain and/or combination of strains
2. Appropriate dosage and dose effects
3. The therapeutic role of probiotics as initial therapy or in maintenance/suppression
4. Clinical relevance

Because antibiotic therapy cannot correct the underlying microflora imbalances in SIBO, recurrences of overgrowth and the accompanying symptoms following this treatment method are common. Probiotics appear to be viable alternatives or adjuncts to conventional treatment of SIBO by helping to rebalance the GI flora and improving overall function of the GI tract. Current evidence presents support for the reduction of symptoms and overall reduction of inappropriate bacterial overgrowth, but the use of probiotics within this population necessitates further research.[82,83,85]

Read the two articles below. Critique their study design and findings. How do they compare? What is the clinical relevance of their findings? What are your recommendations based on the findings of these papers?

References

1. Wagner NRF, Lopes MCP, Fernandes R, et al. Effects of probiotic use on gastrointestinal symptoms in the late postoperative period of bariatric surgery: a cross-over, randomized, triple-blind, placebo-controlled study. *Obes Surg*. 2024;34(4):1306–1315. doi:10.1007/s11695-024-07117-4
2. Redondo-Cuevas L, Belloch L, Martín-Carbonell V, et al. Do herbal supplements and probiotics complement antibiotics and diet in the management of SIBO? A randomized clinical trial. *Nutrients*. 2024;16(7):1083. doi: 10.3390/nu16071083

Bowel Surgery and Short Bowel Syndrome (SBS)

As with any disease state, surgical interventions for disorders of the small and large intestines are used only when more conventional methods of care fail. If extensive damage to the bowel occurs as the result of chronic disease or obstruction, function in that area is understandably lost and that section requires removal.[96] For example, it is common for a patient with Crohn's disease to require surgery related to uncontrolled inflammation or for complications secondary to the disease progression. In any case, surgical management typically involves resection to remove the damaged bowel and a reconstruction to allow digestive processes to occur with as much normalcy as possible. The extent of resection and procedure of choice depends on the preemptive diagnosis and degree of damage. The nutritional implications and necessary interventions also depend on the area and amount of the bowel that is removed.[96] Different sections of the small and large intestines have different responsibilities in terms of digestion and absorption. Any changes to the integrity of the GI tract will have significant consequences on nutritional status postoperatively.

Bowel Resection

There are a number of diagnoses involving the GI tract that, when all other treatment approaches have been exhausted, warrant surgical intervention. These conditions often involve intestinal inflammation, obstruction, or acute injury. The magnitude of the refractory disease and the extent of damage determine the amount of bowel to be resected. As portions of the small and/or large intestine are removed, the segments that remain may be reattached to one another, forming an **anastomosis**. When necessary, an artificial opening referred to as a **stoma** is created to form a new path for fecal excretion; this type of procedure, called an **ostomy**, will be discussed in more detail later in the chapter. **Figure 11.10** depicts a stoma formed from part of the colon brought through the abdominal wall. The goal is to leave as much functional bowel as possible and to facilitate relatively normal digestive processes.[96,97]

Although all patients are at high risk for malabsorption and subsequent malnutrition following bowel resection, the needs of each individual will vary greatly. The postoperative nutritional implications and thus the care plan to be implemented primarily depend on the location and amount of remaining bowel. However, clinical manifestations

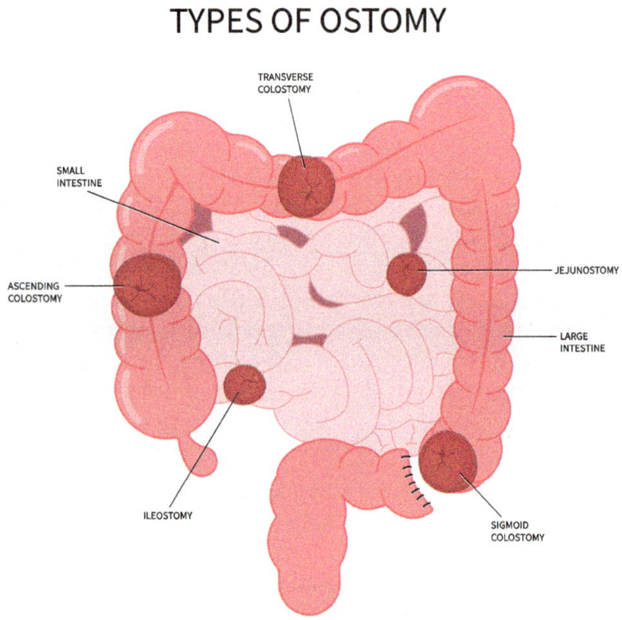

Figure 11.10 Types of Ostomies Created in Bowel Surgery

CASE STUDY REVISITED

Despite the efforts of the medical team, Daniel's Crohn's disease remains poorly controlled. He has a number of relapses that deplete his nutritional status quickly. Two years after his diagnosis, Daniel underwent a Type II surgery with a jejuno-ileal anastomosis. Although his colon is in continuity, he has lost his entire ileum. He remained in the hospital for 3 weeks during his acute phase and received a combination of IV fluids and parenteral and enteral nutrition with some oral intake. He comes to see the RD 1 week after discharge. He remains on EN and PN but reports that his oral intake is improving. His appetite is good, and he has even gained some weight back.

Anthropometric Data:

Current Weight: 65 kg
Height: 175 cm
BMI: 21.2 kg/m^2

Weight history
UBW: 70 kg (2.5 years ago)
Pre-surgery weight: 59 kg (6 weeks ago)
Weight upon discharge from hospital: 63 kg

Biochemical Data:

Sodium 138 (136–145 mEq/L)
Potassium 4.1 (3.5–5.0 mEq/L)
Chloride 100 (96–106 mEq/L)
Carbon dioxide 24 (22–31 mEq/L)
Blood urea nitrogen 18 (8–20 mg/dL)
Creatinine 0.8 (0.7–1.3 mg/dL)
Glucose 135 (70–139 mg/dL)
Serum osmolality 280 (275–295 mOsm/kg)
25-OH vitamin D 18 (20–40 ng/mL)
Magnesium 1.2 (1.5–2.7 mg/dL)
Calcium 8.0 (8.5–10.5 mg/dL)
Phosphorus 3.8 (2.5–4.5 mg/dL)
Albumin 3.0 (3.5–5.5 grams/dL)
Hemoglobin 11.1 (14–18 grams/dL)
Hematocrit 36.4 (40–50%)
Mean corpuscular volume 120 (80–100 fL)

Clinical Data:

Past Medical History: Crohn's disease, short bowel syndrome
Medications: Bile acid sequestrant, glucagon-like peptide-2 analog, glutamine, H_2 blockers, loperamide, MVI
Vital Signs: Blood pressure 130/68 mm Hg, Temperature 96.5°F
Nutrition-focused Physical Exam: Patient appears pale but alert and energetic. Abdominal feels soft and non-tender. Skin is dry, intact, and warm to touch, no bruising noted. Oral exam reveals smooth pink, magenta tongue, and good dentition.

Dietary Data:

Diet History: Patient reports some intolerance to fatty foods, however much improved.
24-Hour Diet Recall:
Breakfast (6:30 am): Hard-boiled egg (2), avocado toast (2 slices white bread, ½ avocado), coffee with cream
Mid-morning snack: Oral nutrition supplement, cheese and crackers
Lunch (12:30 pm): Sandwich (turkey, tuna, or ham), mayo, white bread, lettuce, tomato, soda
Dinner (6:30 pm): Baked or fried fish, 1 baked potato with butter, sour cream, salt, iceberg lettuce with oil and vinegar
Evening snack: Milk and cereal, or ice cream, or oral nutrition supplement

Questions

1. What are your dietary recommendations for Daniel during the adaptation phase?
2. List the potential nutritional implications given his surgery? What labs might you request?
3. Assess Daniel's original PES statements. Identify if each statement remains an active issue or if the PES statement has been resolved. If the PES statement remains an active issue, has improvement in the issue been noted? If the issue has been resolved, write a new PES statement.

are not only related to the length of the remaining bowel. The most obvious consideration is the difference in function at each segment of the GI tract, with careful attention to which area may have been lost. It is also critical to recognize that some portions of the intestine are more capable of adapting and compensating for loss of absorptive capacity than others. Lastly, having the presence of the ileocecal valve and a functional colon in continuity with the small bowel is beneficial. When the colon is not present, severe electrolyte imbalances and dehydration can occur, and often malnutrition ensues.[98] Accordingly, the three factors that most affect nutritional status in this patient population are as follows:

1. The sections of the small and/or large intestine that remain
2. The functional capacity of the remaining intestine
3. The presence of the ileocecal valve

Absorption Affected by Resection Site

The tasks of the small and large intestines differ. Each portion is designed specifically to facilitate the absorption of nutrients, fluid, and electrolytes.

Considering the area of resection can help the clinician predict the nutritional challenges a patient will face postoperatively before any complications occur.[98]

Duodenal Resection. The most proximal portion of the small intestine, the duodenum (approximately 25–30 cm in length), is a digestive dynamo. Not only is it the preferred site of absorption for many micronutrients, but it is also the location at which the pancreatic enzymes and bile salts enter the GI tract. Loss of the duodenum would be catastrophic to normal digestion and absorption. Fortunately, it is rarely resected or involved in bowel reconstructive procedures.[99]

Jejunal Resection. More than 90% of nutrient absorption occurs within the first 100–150 cm of the small intestine. This area encompasses the duodenum and the proximal portion of the jejunum, meaning that the jejunum (approximately 200–300 cm in length in its entirety) has a similarly critical role in facilitating absorptive processes. In addition, jejunal enterohormones (cholecystokinin, secretin, gastric inhibitory peptide, and vasoactive inhibitory peptide) are key to normal digestion and absorption. When segments of the jejunum are removed, the resulting reduction in surface area and decreased transit time indicates significant potential for impaired nutrient absorption.[99]

The ileum can adapt both structurally and functionally to perform the lost functions of the jejunum. Jejunal resections are thus typically well tolerated when enough of the ileum remains to compensate. Documented patient outcomes are notably better for jejunal resections when compared to ileal resections.[99,100]

Ileal Resection. The ileum (approximately 300–400 cm in length) has an absorptive capacity nearly double that of the jejunum with a much slower intrinsic motility. Here, an intestinal feedback mechanism known as the **ileal brake** is triggered when undigested nutrients enter the ileum. Ileal brake activation delays gastric emptying and slows transit time in the proximal portions of the small intestine, allowing extended contact time between nutrients and the mucosa. This mechanism, which facilitates greater nutrient absorption, is one of the key factors allowing the ileum to compensate for any decreased absorption in the jejunum.[99–102] In addition, the ileum is the only location for absorption of bile salts and the vitamin B12–intrinsic factor complex.[98–99]

Significant resections of the ileum, especially from the terminal portion, are problematic. If more than 100 cm of terminal ileum are lost, hepatic synthesis of bile salts cannot compensate for intestinal losses and the bile salt pool is not maintained. Without bile salts, undigested fat is excreted in feces, causing severe steatorrhea and potential fat-soluble vitamin deficiency. If more than 60 cm of terminal ileum is lost, absorption of vitamin B12 is readily impaired. Most patients will require supplementation of both vitamin B12 and the fat-soluble vitamins. Loss of the distal ileum and thus the function of the ileal break leads to rapid gastric emptying and small intestine transit time, closely mimicking what is noticed in dumping syndrome. In cases of complete ileal resection, most patients will rely on long-term PN for sustenance and survival.[96,98,99,102,103]

The Ileocecal Valve. The **ileocecal (IC) valve** separates the ileum of the small intestine from the cecum of the large intestine. The importance of the IC valve is twofold. First, it plays a pivotal role in preventing the reflux of colonic contents into the ileum. Second, the IC valve maintains slow control over the passage of digesta from the ileum into the colon, increasing nutrient/mucosa contact time in the small intestine.[99] When this crucial area is removed as part of the surgical resection, there is considerable loss of absorptive function. More importantly, however, loss of the IC valve places the patient at considerable risk for developing SIBO within whatever small intestine remains. The presence or absence of the IC valve is an essential consideration when determining nutritional implications postoperatively.[98,102]

Colonic Involvement. Although little nutrient absorption occurs past the small intestine, the large intestine (approximately 160 cm in length) is the central site for fluid and electrolyte reabsorption. Whereas a normal colon recovers between 1 and 1.5 L of electrolyte-rich fluid daily, this capacity can increase by three- to fivefold if necessary for compensation. Regardless, preservation of the colon is imperative for the maintenance of hydration status. Of equal importance, the colon can help to compensate for decreased jejunal carbohydrate absorption if necessary; maintaining half (or more) of the colon is equivalent to maintaining 50 cm of functional small intestine. Outcomes are significantly better in patients able to retain colonic function.[98,100]

CORE CONCEPT 8

In surgical resections of the GI tract, the amount of bowel removed, remaining functional bowel, and the location from which the resection is made are key determinants as to whether digestive and absorptive processes can be maintained postoperatively and if prolonged nutrition intervention is necessary.

Bowel Reconstruction

If intestinal damage extends into the bowel, warranting removal of the colon and/or rectum, it will be necessary to surgically create a new pathway for fecal excretion. This type of procedure, referred to as an "ostomy," removes colonic involvement from the digestive pathway altogether. Instead, a piece of the intestine is brought through an incision in the abdominal wall; this segment, called the "stoma," connects to a plastic pouch **appliance**. Once the ostomy is in place, bowel movements naturally empty through the stoma and into the appliance. On an individual basis, ostomies provide either a temporary or a permanent solution.[104]

Ostomy procedures are further categorized based on the portion of the intestine that serves as the stoma. The two most readily utilized techniques are the **ileostomy**, which may involve removal of the colon and the rectum and connects the distal end of the ileum as the stoma, and the **colostomy**, which utilizes a portion of the colon as the stoma after removal of the rectum. In extreme cases of widespread damage, when ileal surface area or function is lost, a **jejunostomy** may be used to connect the distal jejunum as the stoma. For all patients, however, the extent of nutritional implications will relate more to the initial amount and type of bowel resection than to the presence of an ostomy itself. As previously addressed, a bowel resection will alter intestinal motility, absorptive capacity, and production of waste. While placement of the stoma will not exacerbate the nutritional consequences of the resection, its location does play a role in determining the type of fecal matter produced.[97,104,105]

Jejunostomy

Patients who have received an end jejunostomy require the most intensive nutritional interventions because they lack both the ileum and the colon in continuity. The remaining jejunum is incapable of compensating for the loss of ileal and colonic function. Therefore, these patients are subject to significant malabsorption of macro- and micronutrients, as well as high-volume fluid and electrolyte losses.[98,106]

Ileostomy

An ileostomy placement indicates resection of the terminal ileum and colon, and therefore loss of the important IC valve. Absence of the IC valve results in increased motility throughout the proximal small intestine, shortening the length of contact time between nutrients and absorptive mucosa. If transit time is sufficiently altered, absorption of both macro- and micronutrients will be impaired. The nutrient of most concern is vitamin B12, which requires receptors located in the distal end of the ileum to be absorbed. Finally, and perhaps most importantly, patients with ileostomies struggle to maintain proper hydration status without a continuous colon to reabsorb water and electrolytes.[97,98]

Without the opportunity to pass through the colon, where fluid is reabsorbed and stool is shaped, ileostomy output manifests as watery, less-formed waste. In the initial weeks following surgery, output averages at 1200 mL/day, but may settle to 600 mL/day as the body adjusts.[97]

Colostomy

A colostomy is further specified as one of three types based on the portion of the colon that is used as the stoma. In an ascending colostomy, the least common of the three, the stoma is created using the ascending colon and exits via the right abdominal wall. This indicates that all but the first segment of the colon has been resected. Output from an ascending colostomy will be much more watery when compared to the remaining two procedures. The second variation, a descending colostomy, utilizes either the descending or the sigmoid colon to create the stoma, which will then exit through the left lower abdomen. **Figure 11.11** provides a visual image of a descending colostomy. Output is generally semi-formed or fully formed because it has passed through ascending and transverse sections of the colon. This is the most common of the colostomy procedures. Finally, a transverse colostomy can be created using one or two stomas from any portion of the transverse colon. If there are two openings, the procedure is referred to as a "double-barrel colostomy," with one to pass semi-formed stool and the other to pass mucus.[105]

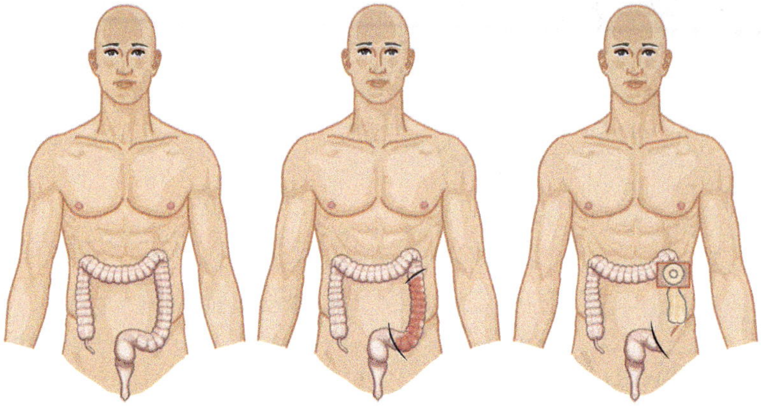

Figure 11.11 A Colostomy Is Placed Depending on the Disease-Affected Portion of the Colon. There Are Three Major Types of Colostomy, Ascending, Descending, and Transverse; Presented Here Is a Descending Colostomy

Nutritional Implications of Bowel Resection and Bypass: Common Guidelines

Any patient is at high risk for nutritional implications postoperatively. This patient population is especially vulnerable, considering the following:

1. The significant changes to the GI anatomy that will possibly affect the processes of digestion and absorption
2. The strong potential for malnutrition from the preceding disease state that likely existed prior to surgery

The location at which the resection was made and the ability for the remaining bowel to compensate for intestinal losses are extremely important. Many patients, particularly those who have undergone multiple surgeries or who have received extensive bowel resection, will develop short bowel syndrome. This common condition will be discussed in its entirety in the following section and will guide much of the nutrition intervention patients will require. There is a set of general guidelines that apply to all members of this patient population in the immediate postoperative period.[96,99,107]

Nutrition Intervention: Postoperative Diet Progression

The traditional approach following bowel surgery involves progression from a clear liquid diet to a more normalized meal plan, but many patients with extensive resection will require nutrition support in the form of EN and/or PN as the healing process begins. Focus should remain on encouraging oral intake, providing fluid and electrolytes, and stimulation to the GI tract with minimal digestion. Eventually, the patient will be advanced to a low-fiber diet that provides adequate energy, protein, fluid, and electrolytes. Smaller, more frequent meals are often better tolerated. As oral intake increases, adequate fluid intake is encouraged.[96,97,105]

Nutrition therapy will primarily focus on ensuring adequate absorption to optimize nutritional status postoperatively and promote healing. In addition, there are a number of diet modifications that can help in the alleviation of symptoms; for example, patients are encouraged to avoid gas- and/or odor-producing foods and foods that may exacerbate diarrhea. Limiting concentrated sugars and concentrated carbohydrates can reduce the likelihood of diarrhea. Other nutrition-related goals include avoiding alcohol and caffeine, as well as foods that may be harder to digest such as nuts, seeds, skins, and peels, decreasing the risk of obstruction, and maintaining hydration status through proper fluid and electrolyte balance. As always, diet recommendations will be highly individualized. Patients should be considered at risk for developing malnutrition until able to consume a normalized diet without symptoms (which may include cramping, nausea, vomiting, excessive flatulence, or diarrhea).[97,105]

Nutrition support in the form of EN or PN or both is necessitated when patients are unable to meet energy needs orally or when postoperative complications, such as obstructions, fistulas, or anastomotic leaks, arise. Cases of malnutrition are common. Be cognizant of indications that the patient requires supplemental or complete support, including evidence of malabsorption, fluid and electrolyte imbalance, weight loss, decreased muscle mass, and/or micronutrient deficiencies. PN use is not unusual in this population.[96,98]

Nutritional Implications of Bowel Resection and Bypass: Short Bowel Syndrome (SBS)

Short bowel syndrome (SBS) broadly encompasses any malabsorption related to decreased absorptive surface area and/or loss of functional capacity in the small intestine. For the vast majority of cases, SBS occurs in the aftermath of surgical resection or bypass. Etiologic factors include extensive surgery for Crohn's disease, mesenteric infarction, and cancer. The degree of severity will depend on the length of resection, as well as the quality and location of the remaining bowel. The presence or absence of a continuous colon (in other words, whether or not the patient received an ostomy) will also be influential in SBS development. Because of chronic fluid, nutrient, and electrolyte malabsorption, patients will rely on bowel adaptation and a combination of pharmacologic and nutritional therapies for survival.[98,103]

It is important to note that because of the extreme heterogeneity in this patient population, it is difficult to develop uniform scientific trials. Large, prospective, randomized studies do not exist. Therefore, all recommendations for patients with SBS are based on best practice from small clinical trials and the guidance of experienced clinicians.[98]

Pathophysiology

In a typical adult, the length of the small intestine varies between 300 and 800 cm, approximately half of which can be removed without significant issue. However, when extensive bowel resection is necessary, patients may be left with 100 cm or less of functioning small intestine. While there is no fixed bowel length necessary for SBS diagnosis, resections of this nature—with loss of two-thirds or more of the small intestine—loosely define the disorder. Within the context of bowel length, there are two clinical distinctions of SBS. The first contains patients with approximately 100–120 cm of remaining bowel without continuity of the colon (those with a small bowel ostomy). The second encompasses those with continuity of the colon with 50 cm or less of remaining small bowel; for this group, the presence of the IC valve and functioning colon significantly improve absorptive capacity. These categorizations can be further divided based on which specific segments of the small intestine remain. Resection of the duodenum and terminal ileum will be more detrimental to patients than resection of the jejunum. Regardless, in the presence of any degree of SBS, severe malabsorption is inevitable. Both groups heavily rely on the ability of the remaining bowel to compensate for the lost absorptive surface and function; this process is known as "intestinal adaptation."[98,99,102,103,108]

Phases of Recovery in Short Bowel Syndrome

There are three phases of postoperative rehabilitation for bowel resection: the acute phase, the adaptation phase, and the maintenance phase. The acute phase begins immediately following surgery and generally lasts up to 4 weeks. During this time, there are large enteric losses, which can lead to metabolic imbalances. Close monitoring of total output and provision of intravenous fluid and electrolytes are required. Once the patient is stabilized hemodynamically, PN can be instituted. As the patient stabilizes, they will enter the most crucial period of recovery: the adaptation phase. This phase, which lasts 1–2 years,[98,109] is marked by both structural and functional changes in the remaining bowel to allow for compensation of lost surface area. Structural changes include the lengthening of the bowel, while functional changes include mechanisms to decrease intestinal transit to allow more time for nutrient absorption. The list of potential adaptations includes the following:

1. Villous hypertrophy: Significant increases in villi height and crypt depth (structural)
2. Slight increase in the length and diameter of the residual bowel (structural)
3. Alterations in motility, enzyme activity, and hormonal responses (functional)

While the exact mechanism of these changes remains unknown, the sum effect of the adaptation period is a sizeable increase in the remaining bowel's absorptive capacity. The RD plays a critical role: the adaptations occur only if nutrients are presented to the intestinal lumen. This importance cannot be overstated; a gradual increase in nutrient exposure through oral intake is the most powerful stimulus to intestinal adaptation. The time that the patient spends in the adaptation phase must be maximized to its full potential. Once an individual enters the maintenance phase, it is unlikely that any other structural or functional changes will occur to the GI tract (**Figure 11.12**).[98,99,102,103]

PRACTICE POINT

Transition patients to a complex oral diet as early as possible in the postoperative recovery period to stimulate the necessary adaptive changes within the remaining intestinal tract.

SBS manifestations are most aptly controlled through pharmacologic treatment and medical nutrition therapy. The overarching goal is the prevention of malnutrition and chronic dehydration through adequate absorption of nutrients and fluids. A number of medications, listed in **Table 11.12**, will help to slow

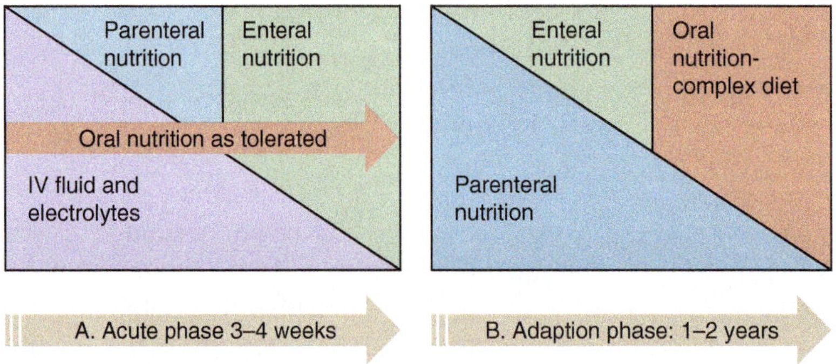

Figure 11.12 Primary Mode of Nutrition Therapy During the Acute and Adaptive Phase of Recovery from Short Bowel Surgery

Data from Wędrychowicz A, Zając A, Tomasik P. Advances in nutritional therapy in inflammatory bowel diseases: review. *World J Gastroenterol.* 2016;22(3):1045-1066.; Yamamoto T, Nakahigashi M, Saniabadi AR. Diet and inflammatory bowel disease: epidemiology and treatment. *Aliment Pharmacol Ther.* 2009;30(2):99-112.; Teitelbaum JE. Nutrient deficiencies in inflammatory bowel disease. UpToDate. Updated February 22, 2017. Accessed November 30, 2017. https://www.uptodate.com/contents/nutrient-deficiencies-in-inflammatory-bowel-disease.

Table 11.12 Pharmacological Treatment Options for Short Bowel Syndrome

Drug Category	Action
Antimotility/Antidiarrheal Agents *Common examples:* loperamide, diphenoxylate, atropine, codeine, deodorized tincture of opium (DTO), clonidine	Used to slow peristalsis and improve absorption of fluid, electrolytes, and nutrients
Antisecretory Agents Histamine H_2 antagonists (H_2 blockers) *Common examples:* famotidine, ranitidine, cimetidine Proton pump inhibitors (PPIs) *Common examples:* omeprazole, lansoprazole, pantoprazole Somatostatin analogues *Common examples:* octreotide	Used to decrease gastric acid secretion, diarrheal losses, and risk for peptic ulcer disease
Gastrointestinal Support *Antibiotic therapy, pancreatic enzyme replacement therapy, bile acid sequestrants, lactase*	Used to treat bacterial overgrowth, assist with carbohydrate and fat absorption
Anabolic Agents Oral solution Glutamine Growth Hormone Teduglutide (a glucagon-like peptide-2 analog)	Drugs used to provide anabolic support the GI tract and decrease reliance and volume of PN needed.
Parenteral Infusion Therapy *May vary from saline infusions to full PN support*	Needed to maintain fluid and electrolyte balance postoperatively as bowel function normalizes

Data from Massironi S, Cavalcoli F, Rausa E, Invernizzi P, Braga M, Vecchi M. Understanding short bowel syndrome: current status and future perspectives. *Dig Liver Dis.* 2020;52(3):253–261.

intestinal transit, while others will minimize the gastric acid hypersecretion that is common to this patient population; management of both will improve absorption rates. This section will focus on the dietary modifications that, when made based on personal tolerance and procedure type, will ensure that the energy and fluid needs of the patient are met while minimizing any nutrition-related symptoms that arise.[98,102,103]

Nutrition support may be required either temporarily in the postoperative period or on a more long-term basis depending on the specific needs of the patient. An SBS diagnosis does not necessarily indicate **intestinal failure**, which is clinically defined when an individual is unable to maintain nutritional autonomy and thus requires long-term PN.[108]

Medical Nutrition Therapy

For patients in the postoperative adaptation phase, the most prudent nutritional goal is stimulation through maximized use of remaining GI tracts with provision of adequate energy, fluid, and electrolytes. It is common for patients to be fed via PN and supplemented with additional IV fluids in the period immediately following surgery. At this point, PN serves as the primary source of nutrition and hydration until the bowel begins to adapt. Ultimately, the intention is to wean all patients from nutrition support. Nutritional autonomy can be accomplished in many cases, especially for those with a colon in continuity and/or a minimum of 100 cm of functional small bowel remaining. Even if maximal adaptation of the bowel is achieved, the vast majority of patients will experience malabsorption of at least 30% of nutrients ingested.[98,99,109,110]

PRACTICE POINT

Encourage patients to consume nutrient-dense foods that are higher in calories than necessary to meet energy needs. Aim for 45–60 kcal/kg/day. Patients may need to ingest 200–400% over needs to offset the malabsorption experienced in this condition.

PRACTICE POINT

Weaning from PN can be initiated when the patient tolerates oral nutrition without excessive stool or ostomy output. Continue to monitor output as the weaning process progresses, in addition to weight status to include either weight maintenance or appropriate weight gain. If necessary, oral intake can be supplemented with enteral feedings.

Table 11.13 Diet Composition for Short Bowel Syndrome, With and Without Colon Continuity

	Small Bowel Ostomies *(no colon in continuity)*	Intact Colon *(colon in continuity)*
Meal Frequency and Distribution	4–6 small meals per day	3 meals + 2 snacks per day
Carbohydrates	40–50% total caloric intake	50–60% total caloric intake
Protein	20–30% total caloric intake	20–30% total caloric intake
Fat	30–40% total caloric intake	20–30% total caloric intake
Oxalate Restriction	Not generally required	Restriction necessary

Data from Matarese LE, O'Keefe SJ, Kandil HM, Bond G, Costa G, Abu-Elmagd K. Short bowel syndrome: clinical guidelines for nutrition management. *Nutr Clin Pract*. 2005;20:493–502.; Wall EA. An overview of short bowel syndrome management: adherence, adaptation, and practical recommendations. *J Acad Nutr Diet*. 2013;113(9):1200-1208.; Fessler TA. A dietary challenge: maximizing bowel adaptation in short bowel syndrome. Today's Dietitian. 2007;9(1):40.

The secondary nutritional goal for patients with SBS is management of symptoms related to both the postoperative recovery period and to malabsorption. This patient population is extremely heterogeneous; dietary modifications vary depending on differences in GI anatomy and functional capacity of the remaining mucosa. Depending on these factors, patients may present with nausea, vomiting, obstruction, diarrhea, and/or dehydration. Each symptom has its own dietary modification. For example, chronic diarrhea is exacerbated by a diet high in concentrated simple sugars, which should be avoided because of their increased hyperosmotic load.[96,102,105]

Diet Composition

In terms of specific macronutrients, diet composition will vary depending on the location and length of remaining bowel. Currently, there are two specific sets of recommendations that were developed based on whether the patient has the colon in continuity. A summarization of the two sets is provided in **Table 11.13**.[102,103,109] There are also recommendations to be made for each individual macronutrient. The most important factor when developing an individualized diet prescription is including complex and varied macronutrients that will stimulate the digestive tract.[99]

Both carbohydrate type and amount are incredibly important for this patient population. Complex carbohydrates, which are generally well tolerated, should comprise approximately 50% of the dietary intake, with an increased goal (closer to 60%) for patients with a colon in continuity. Fiber, in both the soluble and insoluble forms, is a crucial dietary inclusion. Soluble fiber plays a role in slowing gastric emptying and intestinal transit time, contributing to greater nutrient–mucosa exposure and thus increased absorption rates. Moreover, it is essential in promoting intestinal adaptation as the bowel adjusts postoperatively.[103] Although insoluble fiber also slows intestinal transit time, it is generally more useful in bulking the stool for patients with watery fecal or ostomy output. The rationale for emphasizing carbohydrates—especially fiber—for those with an intact colon is a concept called **salvage absorption**: the normal flora will ferment any unabsorbed carbohydrates that enter the colon to short-chain fatty acids, which are subsequently absorbed and utilized. This can serve as a significant source of energy for patients with SBS; salvage absorption can add up to 500 calories daily. One final consideration in the context of carbohydrates is lactose intake, which is often avoided in this population because of concern regarding lactose intolerance. However, most patients will tolerate lactose in the diet, making restriction unnecessary.[102,103,107]

Most patients with SBS have little difficulty tolerating protein intake, meaning that normal consumption can be encouraged. The general guideline for patients with and without a colon in continuity is protein as 20% of daily energy intake. There is no evidence in the literature to support the benefit of one protein source over another, but high biological value sources will provide more absorbable and better utilized protein and overall calories when compared to plant sources.[102]

The level of optimal fat intake in the postoperative diet is heavily debated. Fat provides substantial energy and essential fatty acids. Patients with ostomies, or no colon in continuity, benefit from moderately high amounts of fat (30–40% of daily calories) in the diet; consumption at this level helps to increase the potential that energy is absorbed. Levels should be lower for those with an intact colon (approximately 20–30% of caloric intake) to maximize absorption and minimize output.[102,103] The controversy is that for many patients, especially those with an intact colon, fat malabsorption and steatorrhea can be severe. One of the long-term complications of chronic fat malabsorption is **oxalate nephrolithiasis**, or kidney stones. Normally, oxalate from food will bind to calcium, leaving little that can be absorbed by the colon. However, if unabsorbed fatty acids enter the colon, they will bind to calcium in the lumen instead, meaning that oxalate ions are free to be absorbed. Eventually, free oxalate ions circulate through the kidney for excretion; increased levels tend to cause stones, reported in nearly 60% of those with an intact colon. For this reason, these patients are recommended to consume lower levels of fat (to decrease the risk of fat malabsorption) than their counterparts without a colon in continuity (who are not at increased risk for this complication) and to avoid foods high in oxalate, such as those listed in **Table 11.14**. As always, make recommendations based on individual needs and tolerance.[99,102,103]

Table 11.14 High-Oxalate Foods and Beverages to Limit with Short Bowel Syndrome and Intact Colon

Beverages	Black tea, chocolate-containing beverages (chocolate milk, hot chocolate, cocoa, Ovaltine), cola, draft (dark) beers, instant coffee, juice made from high-oxalate fruits, soy beverages
Fruits	Apricots, blackberries, blueberries, cherries, concord grapes, currants, elderberries, figs, gooseberries, kiwi, lemons, limes, oranges, pear, plums, rhubarb, strawberries, tangerines
Nuts and Seeds	Almonds, cashews, peanuts, pecans, all variations of nut butters, sesame seeds, soy nuts, tahini
Starches	Amaranth, buckwheat, cereal (bran or other high fiber), fruit cake, grits, pretzels, taro, wheat bran, wheat germ, whole wheat bread, whole wheat flour
Vegetables	Artichoke, asparagus, beans (baked, green, dried, kidney, wax), beets, beet greens, carrots, celery, chicory, chives, collards, dandelion greens, eggplant, endive, escarole, kale, leeks, okra, olives, peppers (chili and green), potatoes, red cabbage, rutabaga, spinach, summer squash, sweet potato, Swiss chard, tomatoes, zucchini
Miscellaneous	Black pepper (>1 tsp), chocolate, marmalade, parsley, soy products

Data from Parrish CR. The clinician's guide to short bowel syndrome. *Pract Gastroenterol.* 2005;XXIX(9):67–106.; UPMC Nutrition Services. Low oxalate diet. University of Pittsburgh Medical Center Web site. Updated 2016. Accessed December 24, 2024. http://www.upmc.com/patients-visitors/education/nutrition/Pages/low-oxalate-diet.aspx

Fluid and Electrolyte Needs

Fluid and electrolyte management can be one of the most difficult components of nutrition care for this patient population because of the massive increase in losses. The trend presented throughout this section continues here: needs differ on an individual basis depending on the remaining GI anatomy.[110] Many patients with extensive resection will have a **net secretory response** to both dietary and fluid intake; these patients will excrete more water and sodium than can be ingested, resulting in increased dehydration and electrolyte depletion.[99,108] Those with small bowel ostomies or with limited remaining colon length are at especially high risk and will have much higher fluid requirements than those with a colon in continuity.[98,102,108]

Intravenous fluid support will be necessary in the period immediately following surgery. The volume of urine produced should guide the total amount of IV and oral fluid delivered. An additional consideration for determining requirements is the composition of stool output or ostomy effluent; account for any increased losses by increasing the fluid provided. Initial fluid and electrolyte needs will be greater until the bowel is given appropriate time to adapt. The goal for ostomy output following surgery is approximately 1–1.5 L/day; this may decrease to approximately 600 mL/day for patients with an ileostomy and to 200–600 mL/day for those with a colostomy.[97,98,105,110]

PRACTICE POINT

A guideline for determining IV fluid support postoperatively in SBS is that patients with >1.5 L stool output and <800 mL urine output in 24 hours will have difficulty maintaining hydration and electrolyte balance without IV infusion therapy. Set a goal for the patient to produce at least 1200 mL of urine daily.

Generally, oral fluid intake should always exceed losses (whether via stool or stoma output) to prevent dehydration. Patients at an increased risk for dehydration may require **oral rehydration solutions (ORS)**—dilute glucose–water mixtures containing electrolytes. Commercially available ORS drinks contain a specific ratio of water, glucose, and sodium to utilize the glucose–sodium active transport mechanism at the intestinal brush border. Because of this pathway, ORS can be absorbed even in the presence of significant diarrhea; ORS solutions are thus an effective way to maintain hydration status.[98,99,102,110]

PRACTICE POINT

ORS that contains 70–90 mEq of Na and 20 grams of glucose/L has been presented to result in positive sodium and fluid balance. To maximize the benefit of ORS, patients should replace both hypertonic (juices, soft drinks) and hypotonic (plain water) beverages with ORS as much as possible.

PRACTICE POINT

ORS beverages, although incredibly useful, are typically not considered palatable by patients. Begin with a goal of 1 L/day and increase the volume to meet needs (usually 2–3 L/day) if the patient demonstrates ability and/or willingness to sip throughout the day.

Additional Micronutrient Considerations

All patients will require a daily multivitamin with minerals postoperatively, preferably in a chewable or liquid form to facilitate maximum nutrient absorption. Any additional supplemental needs will vary on an individual basis. Deficiencies secondary to malabsorption are not unusual.[102,103]

There are two specific nutrients (or groups of nutrients) that require careful attention. First, vitamin B12 becomes a concern for this population when >60 cm of terminal ileum has been removed; as previously discussed, this is the location of vitamin B12–intrinsic factor complex absorption. Patients with ileal resections require routine monitoring of serum vitamin B12 and methylmalonic acid (a marker of vitamin B12 status), often needing injections to prevent or correct deficits.[102,103,108] Second, the divalent cations—calcium, magnesium, and zinc—are deficiency risks in the setting of decreased absorption and increased excretion.[102,103]

PRACTICE POINT

Use caution when supplementing magnesium, as certain forms are poorly absorbed and act as a cathartic. The safest forms of magnesium include the slow-releasing magnesium lactate or magnesium gluconate, which do not increase output or cause other GI symptoms as much as other forms of magnesium (especially magnesium oxide).

PRACTICE POINT

Calcium supplementation at 1000–1500 mg/day can help to reduce the risk of oxalate nephrolithiasis by binding to dietary oxalate.

Finally, be aware that osteoporosis, anemia, and fat-soluble vitamin deficiencies are also common for patients with SBS on a long-term basis. Persistent monitoring of the associated nutrients can help to prevent these secondary conditions.[99]

Oral Diet Modifications

For patients able to consume an oral diet, there are some small, but effective, modifications that will help to minimize symptoms:

1. Take small bites when eating and chew thoroughly before swallowing to help facilitate full digestion by the altered GI tract.
2. Consume small, frequent meals, distributed evenly throughout the day.
3. Drink liquids separately from meals; sip slowly throughout the day.
4. Avoid simple or concentrated sugars, which may exacerbate osmotic diarrhea, in both food and beverages.
5. Avoid practices and/or products that increase bloating through swallowed air, such as chewing gum, drinking through a straw, carbonated beverages, smoking, chewing tobacco, or eating meals too quickly.
6. Avoid foods that can cause increased gas formation and/or odor: alcohol, asparagus, beans, broccoli, Brussels sprouts, cabbage, cauliflower, eggs, fish.
7. Increase consumption of foods that decrease odor, like buttermilk, cranberry juice, kefir, parsley, yogurt.
8. Increase consumption of foods that help to thicken stool, including applesauce, bananas/banana flakes, cheese, pasta, pectin, potatoes, rice.
9. Consuming the largest meal of the day mid-afternoon, versus in the evening, can help to decrease output overnight (for those who find this is an issue).
10. Liberalize added salt, especially for patients with small bowel ostomies.

Adding these simple adjustments to the normal pattern of eating can help increase patient comfort with oral feedings and will be advantageous to optimizing digestion and absorption.[97–99,105]

Intestinal Failure

After the initial postoperative period (when PN support is necessary for all patients with SBS as the lone source of energy, fluid, and electrolytes) approximately 50% of patients may gradually decrease dependence on PN/IV support with progression to the oral diet already discussed. Unfortunately, many cannot be fully weaned and will thus require long-term PN/IV support. This group is made up of those unable to absorb more than one-third of oral intake (when attempted) and/or those whose extensive resections left little functional bowel length remaining. **Table 11.15** presents the characteristics of the three major types of surgery leading to SBS and characteristics that may lead to chronic intestinal failure. It can be noticed that in Type I, where the intestine ends with the jejunum (thus a loss of ileum and colon), the risk for PN is high. Conversely, when the ileal cecal valve and colon

Table 11.15 Main Surgical Procedures Involved in Short Bowel Syndrome and Their Characteristics

Type of Surgery	Type I End Jejunostomy	Type II Jejuno-colonic Anastomosis	Type III Jejuno-ileal Anastomosis
Description	Complete resection of ileum and colon. Jejunum remains and represents end of GI tract	Complete resection of the ileum, partial resection of the colon	Jejunal resection, >10 cm of terminal ileum remains along with colon
Presence of ileocecal valve	No	No	Yes
Preservation of colon	No	Partial	Complete
Clinical manifestations	Dehydration	Weight loss, malnutrition	Major malnutrition rare
Risk for need for PN Support	High	Moderate-supplemental PN may be needed	None-PN rarely required

Data from Massironi S, Cavalcoli F, Rausa E, Invernizzi P, Braga M, Vecchi M. Understanding short bowel syndrome: current status and future perspectives. *Dig Liver Dis*. 2020;52(3):253-261.; Aksan A, Farrag K, Blumenstein I, Schröder O, Dignass AU, Stein J. Chronic intestinal failure and short bowel syndrome in Crohn's disease. *World J Gastroenterol*. 2021;27(24):3440-3465. doi:10.3748/wjg.v27.i24.3440 are preserved, the need for PN is unlikely. Regardless, if full PN/IV support is required throughout the duration of the adaptation period, the likelihood of permanent intestinal failure (and thus long-term nutrition support) is 95%. The initiation of home PN/IV support as cycled infusions will maintain quality of life—and create a sort of normalcy—for these individuals[98,100,102,103,109]

PRACTICE POINT

Support provided on a long-term basis at home will vary greatly from the short-term PN provided in the postoperative hospital setting in terms of delivery. Mimic the anticipated home PN regimen prior to discharge from the hospital to assess tolerance and make any necessary corrections.

Monitoring and Evaluation

SBS is a complex and highly individualized condition. Successful management requires coordination of medical, nutritional, and pharmaceutical therapies with the goal of providing the energy, nutrients, and fluid required for survival. Frequent follow-ups are required for close monitoring of the nutritional status of the patient. The dietary prescription will likely change as the adaptation period progresses and beyond, when necessary, to treat nutrient deficiencies and/or potential complications common to this population.

Monitoring of nutritional status and response to diet intervention in malabsorptive disorders should be individualized according to the specific malabsorptive condition, past medical history, symptoms experienced by the patient, and planned interventions. Assessment of dietary intake using food records, which includes a log of symptoms such as pain, anorexia, nausea, vomiting, and diarrhea, should be obtained. All patients should have routine weight checks at least every 6 months. A nutrition-focused physical exam should evaluate muscle and subcutaneous fat stores, presence of edema, and signs of protein-calorie malnutrition. Serial measures of muscle and fat mass using skinfold thickness and circumference measures can also be used to assess changes in body composition. Evaluation of hair, skin, nails, and mouth can be used to screen for micronutrient status. In patients at risk for vitamin D deficiency due to malabsorption or medications, parathyroid hormone, total calcium, and 25-OH vitamin D values should be measured every 6 months, with yearly measures of bone mineral density. Blood tests for anemia (iron, vitamin B12, and folate), electrolytes, calcium, phosphorus, and magnesium should be considered. Patients with fat malabsorption or steatorrhea should have levels of all fat-soluble vitamins as well as trace minerals assessed.[3,110,111]

Chapter Summary

A functioning GI tract is necessary to maintain nutritional status and overall health. Any procedure or disease that damages the integrity of one or more of the many components of this system will have immense implications for the patient. The RD plays a critical role in providing highly individualized nutrition interventions that address both adequate intake and the etiology of the specific disease. As the evidence continues to grow and new interventions are presented in the literature and the lay press, it is important to remain cognizant and informed within this progressive field.

Key Terms

jejunum, ileum, enterocytes, celiac disease (CD), prolamin, irritable bowel syndrome (IBS), somatization, visceral hypersensitivity, low FODMAP diet, oligosaccharide, disaccharide, monosaccharide, polyols, probiotics, non-celiac gluten/wheat sensitivity (NCGS/NCWS), inflammatory bowel disease (IBD), Crohn's disease, ulcerative colitis (UC), toxic megacolon, defined diets, intestinal permeability (IP), leaky gut, *Helicobacter pylori*, small intestinal bacterial overgrowth (SIBO), migrating motor complex (MMC), micelles, elemental formula, anastomosis, stoma, ostomy, ileocecal (IC) valve, ileal brake, appliance, colostomy, ileostomy, jejunostomy, short bowel syndrome (SBS), intestinal failure, salvage absorption, oxalate nephrolithiasis, net secretory response, oral rehydration solutions (ORS)

Acknowledgments

The author acknowledges V. Paige Murphy for contributions to the previous version of this chapter.

References

1. Joneja JMV. *Digestion, Diet, and Disease: Irritable Bowel Syndrome and Gastrointestinal Function*. Rutgers University Press; 2004.
2. Gropper SS, Smith JL. The digestive system: mechanism for nourishing the body. In: Gropper SS, Smith JL, eds. *Advanced Nutrition and Human Metabolism*. 6th ed. Wadsworth Cengage Learning; 2013:33–62.
3. Jeejeebhoy KN, Duerksen DR. Malnutrition in gastrointestinal disorders: detection and nutritional assessment. *Gastroenterol Clin North Am*. 2018;47(1):1–22. doi:10.1016/j.gtc.2017.09.002
4. Pinto-Sanchez MI, Blom JJ, Gibson PR, Armstrong D. Nutrition assessment and management in celiac disease. *Gastroenterol*. 2024;167:116–131.
5. Haider B, Naylor P, Das A, Haider S, Ehrinpreis M. Celiac disease patients with coronary artery disease: a nationwide population-based study. *Cureus*. 2022;14(6):e26151.
6. Wang Y, Chen B, Ciaccio EJ, et al. Celiac disease and the risk of cardiovascular diseases. *Int J Mol Sci*. 2023;24(12):9974.
7. See JA, Kaukinen K, Makharia GK, Gibson PR, Murray JA. Practical insights into gluten free diets. *Nat Rev Gastroenterol Hepatol*. 2015;12(10):580–591.
8. National Institute of Diabetes and Digestive and Kidney Disorders. Celiac disease. U.S. Department of Health and Human Services, Health Information. Published June 2015. Reviewed October 2020. Accessed December 15, 2024. http://www.niddk.nih.gov/health-information/health-topics/digestive-diseases/celiac-disease/Pages/facts.aspx#examples
9. Lebovits J, Lee AR. Micronutrient considerations for celiac disease. *Pract Gastroenterol*. 2023;27:26–42.
10. Mędza A, Szlagatys-Sidorkiewicz A. Nutritional status and metabolism in celiac disease: narrative review. *J Clin Med*. 2023;12(15):5107. doi:10.3390/jcm12155107
11. Academy of Nutrition and Dietetics. *Nutrition Care Manual*. Irritable bowel syndrome (IBS). https://www.nutritioncaremanual.org/topic.cfm?ncm_category_id=1&lv1=5522&lv2=275334&lv3=275345&ncm_toc_id=275345&ncm_heading=Nutrition%20Care. Accessed August 7, 2024.
12. Wald A, Rakel D. Behavioral and complementary approaches for treatment of irritable bowel syndrome. *Nutr Clin Pract*. 2008;23(3):284–292.
13. Böhn L, Störsrud S, Liljebo T, et al. Diet low in FODMAPs reduces symptoms of irritable bowel syndrome as well as traditional dietary advice: a randomized control trial. *Gastroenterol*. 2015;149(6):1399–1407.
14. Spiller R. Irritable bowel syndrome. In: Hawkey CJ, Bosch J, Richter JE, Garcia-Tsao G, Chan FKL, eds. *Textbook of Clinical Gastroenterology and Hepatology*. Wiley-Blackwell; 2012:472–481.
15. Rome Foundation. Rome IV diagnostic criteria for irritable bowel syndrome. Updated 2021. Accessed April 9, 2026 https://theromefoundation.org/wp-content/uploads/RomeCritieraLaunch.pdf
16. Goodoory VC, Khasawneh M, Black CJ, Quigley EMM, Moayyedi P, Ford AC. Efficacy of probiotics in irritable bowel syndrome: systematic review and meta-analysis. *Gastroenterol*. 2023;165(5):1206–1218. doi:10.1053/j.gastro.2023.07.018
17. Zhou Q, Verne GN. New insights into visceral hypersensitivity—clinical implications in IBS. *Nat Rev Gastroenterol Hepatol*. 2011;8(6):349–355.
18. Lacy BE. The science, evidence, and practice of dietary interventions in irritable bowel syndrome. *Clin Gastroenterol Hepatol*. 2015;13(11):1899–1906.
19. Academy of Nutrition and Dietetics. *Nutrition Care Manual*. Irritable bowel syndrome (2023). https://www.nutritioncaremanual.org/topic.cfm?ncm_category_id=1&lv1=5522&lv2=275334&lv3=275335&ncm_toc_id=275335&ncm_heading=Nutrition%20Care Accessed January 4, 2025.
20. Marcason W. What is the FODMAP diet? *J Acad Nutr Diet*. 2012;112(10):1696.
21. Monash University. FODMAPs and Irritable Bowel Syndrome. Published 2019. Accessed January 4, 2025. https://www.monashfodmap.com/about-fodmap-and-ibs/
22. Gibson PR, Varney J, Malakar S, Muir JG. Food components and irritable bowel syndrome. *Gastroenterol*. 2015;148(6):1158–1174.
23. Mansueto P, Seidita A, D'Alcamo A, Carroccio A. Role of FODMAPs in patients with irritable bowel syndrome. *Nutr Clin Pract*. 2015;30(5):665–682.
24. Chey W, Hashash J, Manning L, Chang L. AGA clinical practice update on the role of diet in irritable bowel syndrome: expert review. *J Gastroenterol*. 2022;162(6):1737–1745.
25. Black C, Staudacher H, Ford A. Efficacy of a low FODMAP diet in irritable bowel syndrome: systematic review and network meta-analysis. *Gut*. 2022;71(11):1117–1126.
26. Monash University. *FODMAP Blog*. Practical Tips for FODMAP Reintroduction. https://www.monashfodmap.com/blog/practical-tips-fodmap-reintroduction/. Published 2019. Accessed August 7, 2024.
27. Halmos EP, Power VA, Shepherd SJ, Gibson PR, Muir JG. A diet low in FODMAPs reduces symptoms of irritable bowel syndrome. *Gastroenterol*. 2014;146(1):67–75.
28. Probiotics: In depth. National Institutes of Health (NIH): National Center for Complementary and Integrative Health (NCCIH). https://nccih.nih.gov/health/probiotics/introduction.htm. Last updated August 2019. Accessed December 29, 2024.
29. Clauson ER, Crawford P. What you must know before you recommend a probiotic. *J Fam Pract*. 2015;64(3):151–155.
30. Spiller R. Review article: Probiotics and prebiotics in irritable bowel syndrome. *Aliment Pharmacol Ther*. 2008;28(4):385–396.
31. Santos AR, Whorwell PJ. Irritable bowel syndrome: The problem and the problem of treating it - is there a role for probiotics? *Proc Nutr Soc*. 2014;73(4):470–476.
32. Ford AC, Quigley EMM, Lacy BE, et al. Efficacy of prebiotics, probiotics, and synbiotics in irritable bowel syndrome and chronic idiopathic constipation: systematic review and meta-analysis. *Am J Gastroenterol*. 2014;109(10):1546–1562.
33. Tiequn B, Guanqun C, Shuo Z. Therapeutic effects of lactobacillus in treating irritable bowel syndrome: a meta-analysis. *Intern Med*. 2015;54(3):243–249.
34. Mullin GE. Probiotics and digestive disease. *Nutr Clin Pract*. 2012;27(2):300–302.

35. Quigley EMM. Prebiotics and probiotics: their role in the management of gastrointestinal disorders in adults. *Nutr Clin Pract*. 2012;27(2):195–200.
36. Moran C, Shanahan F. Editorial: Probiotics and IBS - where are we now? *Aliment Pharmacol Ther.* 2014;40(3):318.
37. Leung J, Crowe SE. Food allergy and food intolerance. In: Buckman A, ed. *Nutrition Care of the Patient with Gastrointestinal Disease*. Taylor & Francis Group. 2015:63–88.
38. Gibson PR, Skodje GI, Lundin KE. Non-coeliac gluten sensitivity. *J Gastroenterol Hepatol*. 2017;32(1):86–89.
39. Call L, Haider E, D'Amico S, et al. Synthesis and accumulation of amylase-trypsin inhibitors and changes in carbohydrate profile during grain development of bread wheat (*Triticum aestivum* L). *BMC Plant Biol.* 2021;21(113).
40. Cárdenas-Torres FI, Cabrera-Chávez F, Figueroa-Salcido OG, Ontiveros N. Non-celiac gluten sensitivity: an update. *Medicina*. 2021;57(6):526.
41. Lin A, Micic D. Nutrition considerations in inflammatory bowel disease. *Nutr Clin Pract*. 2021;36(2):298–311. doi:10.1002/ncp.10628
42. Hou JK, Lee D, Lewis J. Diet and inflammatory bowel disease: review of patient-targeted recommendations. *Clin Gastroenterol Hepatol*. 2014;12(10):1592–1600.
43. Petagna L, Antonelli A, Ganini C, et al. Pathophysiology of Crohn's disease inflammation and recurrence. *Biology Direct*. 2020;15(1):23–33.
44. Shanahan F. Ulcerative colitis. In: Hawkey CJ, Bosch J, Richter JE, Garcia-Tsao G, Chan FKL, eds. *Textbook of Clinical Gastroenterology and Hepatology.* Wiley-Blackwell; 2012:355–371.
45. Shan Y, Lee M, Chang EB. The gut microbiome and inflammatory bowel diseases. *Ann Rev Med*. 2022;73:455–468.
46. Aldars-García L, Chaparro M, Gisbert JP. Systematic review: The gut microbiome and its potential clinical application in inflammatory bowel disease. *Microorganisms*. 2021; 9(5):977. doi:10.3390/microorganisms9050977
47. Wark G, Samocha-Bonet, D, Ghaly S, Danta M. The role of diet in the pathogenesis and management of inflammatory bowel disease: a review. *Nutrients*. 2020;13(1):135.
48. Rubin D, Ananthakrishnan A, Siegel C, Sauer B, Long M. ACG clinical guideline: ulcerative colitis in adults. *Am J Gastroenterol*. 2019;114(3):384–413. doi:10.14309/ajg.0000000000000152
49. Lichtenstein G, Loftus E, Isaacs K, Regueiro M, Gerson L, Sands B. ACG Clinical Guideline: Management of Crohn's Disease in Adults. *Am J Gastroenterol*. 2018;113(4):481–517.
50. Forbes A, Goldesgeyme E, Paulon E. Nutrition in inflammatory bowel disease. *JPEN*. 2011;35(5):571–580.
51. Kikut J, Konecka N, Ziętek M, Ziętek M, Kulpa D, Szczukoet Ml. Diet supporting therapy for inflammatory bowel diseases. *Eur J Nutr*.2021;60:2275–2291. doi:10.1007/s00394-021-02489-0
52. Durchschein F, Petrisch W, Hammer HF. Diet therapy for inflammatory bowel diseases: the established and the new. *World J Gastroenterol*. 2016;22(7):2179–2194.
53. Balestrieri P, Ribolsi M, Guarino MPL, Emerenziani S, Altomare A, Cicala M. Nutritional aspects in inflammatory bowel diseases. *Nutrients*. 2020;12(2):372. doi:10.3390/nu12020372
54. Jabłońska B, Mrowiec S. Nutritional status and its detection in patients with inflammatory bowel diseases. *Nutrients*. 2023;15(8):1991. doi:10.3390/nu15081991
55. Wędrychowicz A, Zajac A, Tomasik P. Advances in nutritional therapy in inflammatory bowel diseases: review. *World J Gastroenterol*. 2016;22(3):1045–1066.
56. Yamamoto T, Nakahigashi M, Saniabadi AR. Review article: diet and inflammatory bowel disease - epidemiology and treatment. *Aliment Pharmacol Ther*. 2009;30(2):99–112.
57. Crohn's and Colitis Foundation: Nutrition Resources for Health Care Professionals. Common Nutrient Deficiencies in IBD. Developed January 2017. Accessed December 2024. https://www.crohnscolitisfoundation.org/sites/default/files/legacy/science-and-professionals/nutrition-resource-/micronutrient-deficiency-fact.pdf
58. Reznikov EA, Suskind DL. Current nutritional therapies in inflammatory bowel disease: improving clinical remission rates and sustainability of long-term dietary therapies. *Nutrients*. 2023;15(3):668. doi:10.3390/nu15030668
59. Bischoff SC, Bager P, Escher J, et al. ESPEN guideline on clinical nutrition in inflammatory bowel disease. *Clin Nutr*. 2023;42(3):352–379.
60. Brennan GT, Ha I, Hogan C, et al. Does preoperative enteral or parenteral nutrition reduce postoperative complications in Crohn's disease patients: a meta-analysis. *Eur J Gastroenterol Hepatol*. 2018;30(9):997–1002.
61. Wang H, Zuo L, Zhao J, et al. Impact of preoperative exclusive enteral nutrition on postoperative complications and recurrence after bowel resection in patients with active Crohn's disease. *World J Surg*. 2016;40(8):1993–2000.
62. Guo Z, Guo D, Gong J, et al. Preoperative nutritional therapy reduces the risk of anastomotic leakage in patients with Crohn's disease requiring resections. *Gastroenterol Res Pract*. 2016;5017856.
63. Heerasing N, Thompson B, Hendy P, et al. Exclusive enteral nutrition provides an effective bridge to safer interval elective surgery for adults with Crohn's disease. *Aliment Pharmacol Ther.* 2017;45(5):660–669.
64. Diederen K, Li JV, Donachie GE, et al. Exclusive enteral nutrition mediates gut microbial and metabolic changes that are associated with remission in children with Crohn's disease. *Sci Rep*. 2020;10(1):18879.
65. de Sire R, Nardone OM, Testa T, Calabrese G, Caiazzo A, Castiglione F. Exclusive enteral nutrition in adult Crohn's disease: an overview of clinical practice and perceived barriers. *Clin Exp Gastroenterol*. 2021;14:493–501. doi:10.2147/CEG.S267172
66. Academy of Nutrition and Dietetics. *Nutrition Care Manual*. Inflammatory Bowel Disease: Crohn's Disease, Ulcerative Colitis (2022). Accessed August 8, 2024. https://www.nutritioncaremanual.org/topic.cfm?ncm_category_id=1&lv1=5522&lv2=275071&lv3=275082&ncm_toc_id=275082&ncm_heading=Nutrition%20Care
67. Day A, Wood J, Melton S, Bryant R. Exclusive enteral nutrition: an optimal care pathway for use in adult patients with active Crohn's disease. *Gastroenterol Hepatol*. 2020;4(2):260–266.
68. Bischoff SC, Escher J, Hébuterne X, et al. ESPEN practical guideline: clinical nutrition in inflammatory bowel disease. *Clin Nutr.* 2020;39(3):632–653.
69. Richman E, Rhodes JM. Review article: evidence-based dietary advice for patients with inflammatory bowel disease. *Aliment Pharmacol Ther*. 2013;38(10):1156–1171.
70. Prince A, Whelan K, Moosa A, Lomer MCE, Reidlinger DP. Nutritional problems in inflammatory bowel disease: the patient perspective. *J Crohns Colitis*. 2011;5(5):443–450.
71. Gkikas K, Svolos V, Hansen R, Russell RK, Gerasimidis K. Take-home messages from 20 years of progress in dietary

therapy of inflammatory bowel disease. *Ann Nutr Metab.* 2023;79(6):476–484. doi:10.1159/000535007

72. Ruemmele FM. Role of diet in inflammatory bowel disease. *Ann Nutr Metab.* 2016;68(Suppl 1):33–41.
73. Yanai H, Levine A, Hirsch A, et al. The Crohn's disease exclusion diet for induction and maintenance of remission in adults with mild-to-moderate Crohn's disease (CDED-AD): an open-label, pilot, randomized trial. *Lancet Gastroenterol Hepatol.* 2022;7:49–59.
74. Michielan A, D'Inca R. Intestinal permeability in inflammatory bowel disease: pathogenesis, clinical evaluation, and therapy of leaky gut. *Mediators Inflam.* 2015;2015:628157. doi:10.1155/2015/628157
75. Del Bo C, Bernardi S, Cherubini A, et al. A polyphenol-rich dietary pattern improves intestinal permeability, evaluated as serum zolulin levels, in older subjects: the MaPLE randomised controlled trial. *Clin Nutr.* 2021;40(5):3006–3018.
76. Haley PK, Gaddy JA. Nutrition and *Helicobacter pylori*: host diet and nutritional immunity influence bacterial virulence and disease outcome. *Gastroenterol Res Pract.* 2016;2016: 3019362. doi:10.1155/2016/3019362
77. Franceschi F, Tortora A, Di Renzo T, et al. Role of *Helicobacter pylori* infection on nutrition and metabolism. *World J Gastroenterol.* 2014;20(36):12809–12817.
78. Hsu PI, Wu DC, Chen WC, et al. Randomized controlled trial comparing 7-day triple, 10-day sequential, and 7-day concomitant therapies for *Helicobacter pylori* infection. *Antimicrob Agents Chemother.* 2014;58(10):5936–5942.
79. Boltin D. Probiotics in *Helicobacter pylori*-induced peptic ulcer disease. *Best Pract Res Clin Gastroenterol.* 2016;30(1):99–109.
80. Rueda-Robles A, Rubio-Tomás T, Plaza-Diaz J, Álvarez-Mercado AI. Impact of dietary patterns on *H. pylori* infection and the modulation of microbiota to counteract its effect. a narrative review. *Pathogens.* 2021;10(7):875.
81. Ozbey G, Sproston E, Hanafiah A. *Helicobacter pylori* infection and gastric microbiota. *Euroasian J Hepatogastroenterol.* 2020;10(1):36–41.
82. Roszkowska P, Klimczak E, Ostrycharz E, et al. Small intestinal bacterial overgrowth (SIBO) and twelve groups of related diseases—current state of knowledge. *Biomedicines.* 2024;12(5):1030.
83. Sroka N, Rydzewska-Rosołowska A, Kakareko K, Rosołowski M, Głowińska I, Hryszko T. Show me what you have inside—the complex interplay between SIBO and multiple medical conditions—a systematic review. *Nutrients.* 2023;15(1):90. doi:10.3390/nu15010090
84. Losurdo G, D'Abramo FS, Indellicati G, Lillo C, Ierardi E, Di Leo A. The influence of small intestinal bacterial overgrowth in digestive and extra-intestinal disorders. *Int J Mol Sci.* 2020;21(10):3531. doi:10.3390/ijms21103531
85. Quigley EMM, Murray JA, Pimentel M. AGA clinical practice update on small intestinal bacterial overgrowth: expert review. *Gastroenterol.* 2020;159(4):1526–1532. doi:10.1053/j.gastro.2020.06.090
86. Rezaie A, Buresi M, Lembo A, et al. Hydrogen and methane-based breath testing in gastrointestinal disorders: the North American consensus. *Am J Gastroenterol.* 2017;112(5):775–784.
87. Kashyap P, Moayyedi P, Quigley EMM, Simren M, Vanner S. Critical appraisal of the SIBO hypothesis and breath testing: a clinical practice update endorsed by the European Society of Neurogastroenterology and Motility (ESNM) and the American Neurogastroenterology and Motility Society (ANMS). *Neurogastroenterol Motil.* 2024;36:e14817. doi:10.1111/nmo.14817
88. Bushyhead D, Quivley EMM. Small intestinal bacterial overgrowth—pathophysiology and its implications for definition and management. *Gastroenterol.* 2022;163(3):593–607.
89. Knez E, Kadac-Czapska K, Grembecka M. The importance of food quality, gut motility, and microbiome in SIBO development and treatment. *Nutrition.* 2024;124:112464. doi:10.1016/j.nut.2024.112464
90. Montoro-Huguet MA, Belloc B, Domínguez-Cajal M. Small and large intestine: malabsorption of nutrients. *Nutrients.* 2021;13(4):1254. doi:10.3390/nu1304125490
91. Adike A, DiBaise JK. Small intestinal bacterial overgrowth: nutritional implications, diagnosis, and management. *Gastroenterol Clin N Am.* 2018;47(1):193–208. doi:10.1016/j.gtc.2017.09.008
92. Shanab AA, Quera RM, Quigley EMM. Small intestinal bacterial overgrowth. In: Hawkey CJ, Bosch J, Richter JE, Garcia-Tsao G, Chan FKL, eds. *Textbook of Clinical Gastroenterology and Hepatology.* Wiley-Blackwell; 2012:305–310.
93. Rezaie A, Pimental M, Rao SS. How to test and treat small intestinal bacterial overgrowth: an evidence-based approach. *Curr Gastroenterol Rep.* 2016;18(2):8–19.
94. Bohm M, Siwiec RM, Wo JM. Diagnosis and management of small intestinal bacterial overgrowth. *Nutr Clin Pract.* 2013;28(3):289–299.
95. Ginnebaugh B, Chey WD, Saad R. Small intestinal bacterial overgrowth. *Gastroenterol Clin.* 2020;49(3):571–587.
96. Academy of Nutrition and Dietetics. *Nutrition Care Manual.* Bowel resection. https://www.nutritioncaremanual.org/topic.cfm?ncm_category_id=1&lv1=5522&lv2=144839&lv3=267421&ncm_toc_id=267421&ncm_heading=Nutrition%20Care Accessed January 4, 2025.
97. Academy of Nutrition and Dietetics. *Nutrition Care Manual.* Ileostomy. Accessed January 4, 2025. https://www.nutritioncaremanual.org/topic.cfm?ncm_category_id=1&lv1=5522&lv2=19729&lv3=268565&ncm_toc_id=268565&ncm_heading=Nutrition%20Care
98. Massironi S, Cavalcoli F, Rausa E, Invernizzi P, Braga M, Vecchi M. Understanding short bowel syndrome: Current status and future perspectives. *Digest Liver Dis.* 2020; 52(3):253–261.
99. Weimann A, Braga M, Carli F, et al. ESPEN practical guideline: clinical nutrition in surgery. *Clin Nutr.* 2021;40(7):4745–4761. doi:10.1016/j.clnu.2021.03.031
100. Jeppesen PB. Spectrum of short bowel syndrome in adults: intestinal insufficiency to intestinal failure. *JPEN.* 2014;38(suppl 1):8S–13S.
101. van Avesaat M, Troost FJ, Ripken D, Hendriks HF, Masclee AAM. Ileal brake activation: macronutrient-specific effects on eating behavior? *Int J Obes.* 2015;39(2):235–243.
102. Cuerda C, Pironi L, Arends J, et al. ESPEN practical guideline: clinical nutrition in chronic intestinal failure. *Clin Nutr.* 2021;40(9):5196–5220. doi:10.1016/j.clnu.2021.07.002
103. Wall EA. An overview of short bowel syndrome management: adherence, adaptation, and practical recommendations. *J Acad Nutr Diet.* 2013;113(9):1200–1208.
104. Ostomy Expanded Information. American Society of Colon and Rectal Surgeons. Accessed January 4, 2025. https://fascrs.org/patients/diseases-and-conditions/a-z/ostomy-expanded-version.
105. Academy of Nutrition and Dietetics. *Nutrition Care Manual.* Colostomy. https://www.nutritioncaremanual.org/topic.cfm?ncm_category_id=1&lv1=5522&lv2=19799&ncm_toc_id=19799&ncm_heading=Nutrition%20Care Accessed January 4, 2025.

106. Tappenden KA. Pathophysiology of short bowel syndrome: considerations of resected and residual anatomy. *JPEN*. 2014;38(suppl 1):14S–22S.
107. Rocha R, de J Santos G, Santana G. Influence of nutritional status in the postoperative period of patients with inflammatory bowel disease. *World J Gastrointest Pharmacol Ther*. 2021;12(5):90–99. doi:10.4292/wjgpt.v12.i5.90
108. Jackson CS, Buchman AL. Short bowel syndrome. In: Hawkey CJ, Bosch J, Richter JE, Garcia-Tsao G, Chan FKL, eds. *Textbook of Clinical Gastroenterology and Hepatology*. Wiley-Blackwell; 2012:299–304.
109. Aksan A, Farrag K, Blumenstein I, Schröder O, Dignass AU, Stein J. Chronic intestinal failure and short bowel syndrome in Crohn's disease. *World J Gastroenterol*. 2021;27(24): 3440–3465. doi:10.3748/wjg.v27.i24.3440
110. Montoro-Huguet MA, Belloc B, Domínguez-Cajal M. Small and large intestine: malabsorption of nutrients. *Nutrients*. 2021;13:1254. doi:10.3390/nu13041254
111. UPMC Nutrition Services. Low oxalate diet. University of Pittsburgh Medical Center. Updated 2016. Accessed December 27, 2024. https://share.upmc.com/2016/01/help-prevent-kidney-stones-with-a-low-oxalate-diet/

CHAPTER 12

Nutrition in Kidney Disease

Yijie (Claire) Cheng
Haewook Han
Judith Kirk

CHAPTER OUTLINE

CORE CONCEPTS

1. The prevalence of chronic kidney disease is increasing due to the rising rates of risk factors such as diabetes and hypertension, as well as an aging population.
2. Medical nutrition therapy is a necessary component of chronic kidney disease management and can improve outcomes by preventing malnutrition and slowing disease progression.
3. For patients with acute kidney injury, temporary protein restriction may be needed depending on clinical status. For patients with nephrotic syndrome, it is important to avoid overconsumption of protein unless determined necessary by clinical status. Both types of kidney disease may or may not progress to needing renal replacement therapy.
4. Prevention is a key component in the management of chronic kidney disease and involves treatment of underlying conditions, such as diabetes and hypertension.
5. Malnutrition risk increases as the glomerular filtration rate decreases and may complicate the management of chronic kidney disease due to protein, fluid, and/or micronutrient restrictions.

6. Protein is a necessary macronutrient in the diet of patients with chronic kidney disease, and despite controversy regarding the possibility that protein restriction improves outcomes, these patients must be able to eat a balanced, palatable diet that provides adequate energy and protein to prevent loss of lean body mass.
7. Patients receiving renal replacement therapy can tolerate higher protein, fluid, and electrolyte levels than patients with chronic kidney disease alone, so recommendations should be individualized to each patient.

LEARNING OBJECTIVES

1. Describe the functions of the kidneys.
2. Identify the prevalence and differentiate the different stages of kidney disease.
3. Explain the importance of medical nutrition therapy on the progression of kidney disease.
4. Assess the nutritional needs of individuals in all stages of chronic kidney disease (CKD).
5. Outline the nutritional management of polycystic kidney disease.
6. Identify the different types of kidney stones and the corresponding nutritional interventions.

Introduction and Epidemiology

Globally, over 800 million people have chronic kidney disease (CKD), and it is one of the leading causes of death.[1] CKD contributes to disability, decreased quality of life, and increased healthcare costs.[2] In the United States, there are approximately 35.5 million adults (14% of the population) with CKD, and about 90% of patients are not aware that they have CKD due to absence of symptoms.[3] The prevalence of CKD is slightly higher in females (14%) than males (12%).[3] There are different stages of CKD, and kidney failure is called **end-stage kidney disease (ESKD)**, which requires **renal replacement therapy (RRT)**, such as dialysis and kidney transplantation, to survive. In 2020, over 130,000 people started RRT, and currently there are approximately 800,000 individuals in the United States living with ESKD, 69% of whom receive dialysis and 31% are post kidney transplant.[3] The most common causes of CKD are diabetes, hypertension, glomerulonephritis, other causes, including cystic kidney disease, as well as unknown causes. In this chapter, the causes of CKD and nutritional management to help stabilize kidney function to prevent ESKD will be discussed.

CORE CONCEPT 1

The prevalence of chronic kidney disease is increasing due to the rising rates of risk factors such as diabetes and hypertension, as well as an aging population.

Physiology and Functions of Kidneys

The kidneys are located on both sides of the vertebrae. The usual size of the kidneys is approximately 11–12 cm long (fist size) and 150 grams. The kidneys are divided into two main regions: the cortex and the medulla (**Figure 12.1**), which contain the functional units of the kidney, the **nephrons**. On average, each kidney contains about 1 million nephrons but the number can vary among individuals.[4] The nephron consists of two parts: the **glomerulus**, where blood is filtered, and the **tubule**, where reabsorption and secretion occur. Kidneys regulate fluid volume, acid–base balance, control blood pressure with water and solutes, and excrete metabolic waste products.

Filtration

Filtration of the blood is a passive process that relies on blood pressure created by adequate cardiac output, which is the amount of blood pumped by the heart per minute, and the diameter of the renal artery, both of which determine the amount of blood flowing into the nephrons.[4] Initially, blood flows into the renal corpuscle of the nephron through the afferent arteriole and enters the glomerular space. The glomerulus allows fluid and waste to pass into the **Bowman's capsule** while preventing red blood cells and large macromolecules such as protein from getting through (these return to the bloodstream through the efferent arteriole). The resulting **ultrafiltrate** (filtrate made once waste is filtered from the blood), proceeds to the second step of the filtration process by entering the renal tubules to be further modified.

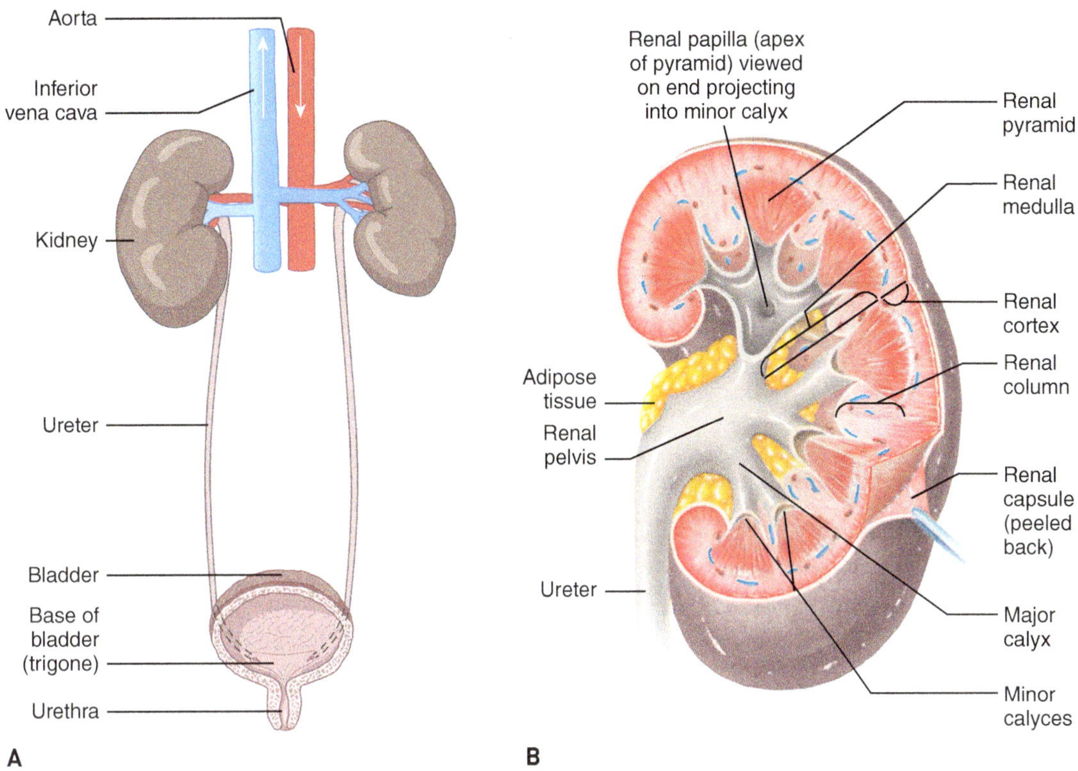

Figure 12.1 Anatomy of the Urinary System and Kidney

Reabsorption

The tubules, which include the proximal convoluted tubule, the loop of Henle, and finally, the distal convoluted tubule, and the collecting duct reabsorb the ultrafiltrate. Each section of the tubule has a different permeability, secreting and absorbing various components of the ultrafiltrate (**Table 12.1**). For example, the proximal convoluted tubule is responsible for reabsorbing nutrients (glucose, amino acids, sodium, bicarbonate, potassium, chloride, calcium, and phosphate), while the descending loop of Henle reabsorbs water.

Urine is produced and funneled into the collecting duct and renal pelvis, which narrows into a single ureter per kidney. The **ureters** bring urine to the bladder, which can then be released from the body.[4] Through this process, the nephrons filter 1600 L of blood per day, producing approximately 180 L of ultrafiltrate, resulting in approximately 1–2 L of urine output daily depending on fluid intake. The structure of the kidney and urinary system is illustrated in Figure 12.1, and the structure of the nephron is illustrated in **Figure 12.2**.[5]

While the etiology of a renal insult can be multifactorial in nature, kidney disease is characterized by an acute or progressive loss of functioning nephrons, which unfolds in a pattern of systemic hypertension, proteinuria, and a gradual decline in **glomerular filtration rate (GFR)**, the amount of plasma filtered through the glomeruli within a given period.[6] Initially, the kidneys can compensate for the loss of nephrons and maintain overall GFR. Because the same amount of blood must flow through the kidney despite now having fewer nephrons capable of filtering the blood, the kidneys activate the renin–angiotensin system to increase afferent arteriole vasodilation and concurrently constrict the efferent arteriole vessel.[7] As a result, each remaining functional nephron takes on more pressure from the systemic circulation, a process known as **adaptive hyperfiltration**.[7] A sustained increase in blood volume and subsequent pressure leads to scarring (glomerulosclerosis) due to thickening of the walls and narrowing of the lumen of glomerular arterioles (arteriolosclerosis). In CKD, this syndrome of glomerular hypertrophy, glomerular hypertension with resulting macrophage infiltration and accumulation of extracellular matrix components, eventually leads to loss of nephron function, causing ESKD.[8] Disease progression is associated with uncontrolled diabetes, poorly controlled blood pressure, and high levels of protein in the urine, which contribute to continually decreasing GFR. A graphic representation of this process can be found in **Figure 12.3**.

Table 12.1 Flow of Fluid Through the Nephron in a Normal and Compromised Kidney Function

Nephron Component	Normal Function	Compromised Function
Glomerulus	Produces filtrate from blood	Filtration is slow and incomplete Waste products unable to be eliminated Proteins are lost through the pores of the glomerulus and are excreted in the urine
Proximal Convoluted Tubule	Reabsorbs two-thirds of filtrate Reabsorption site of glucose and amino acids Reabsorbs a major fraction of sodium, bicarbonate, calcium, phosphorus, and potassium through active transport	Impaired reabsorption of filtrate Glucosuria, aminoaciduria, renal tubular acidosis, bicarbonate, metabolic acidosis Sodium and potassium wasting Hypophosphatemia, vitamin D deficiency
Loop of Henle	**Descending limb** Creates a concentration gradient Reabsorbs water but impermeable to sodium, with the purpose of concentrating urine **Ascending limb** Reabsorbs electrolytes but is impermeable to water	Dilute urine Distal renal tubular acidosis
Distal Convoluted Tubule	Concentrates urine when the body needs to conserve water, as it is permeable to water only in the presence of antidiuretic hormone (ADH)	ADH is persistently present dueto decreased blood flow throughthe kidneys Kidneys conserve water to raise blood volume, leading to fluid retention
Collecting Duct	Permeability regulated by ADH and aldosterone Urine is formed and travels through the ureter to the bladder	Insufficient removal of waste products from the blood enter the urine Azotemia results

Data from Skorecki K, Chertow GM, Marsden PA, Taal MW, Yu ASL, eds. *Brenner and Rector's The Kidney*. 10th ed. Philadelphia, PA: Elsevier; 2015.

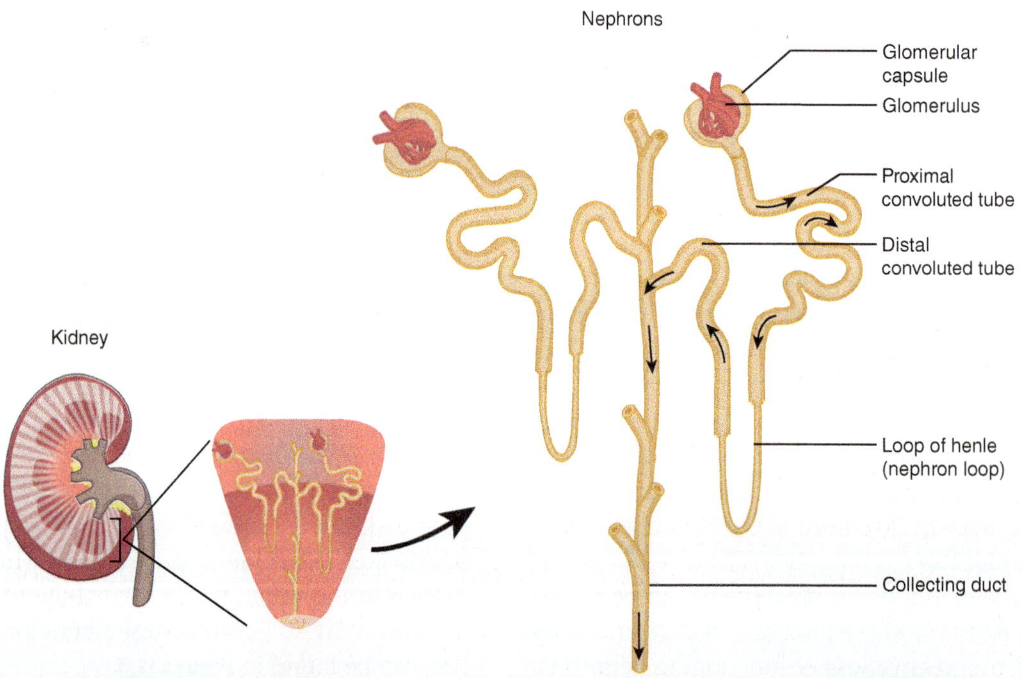

Figure 12.2 Physiology of a Nephron

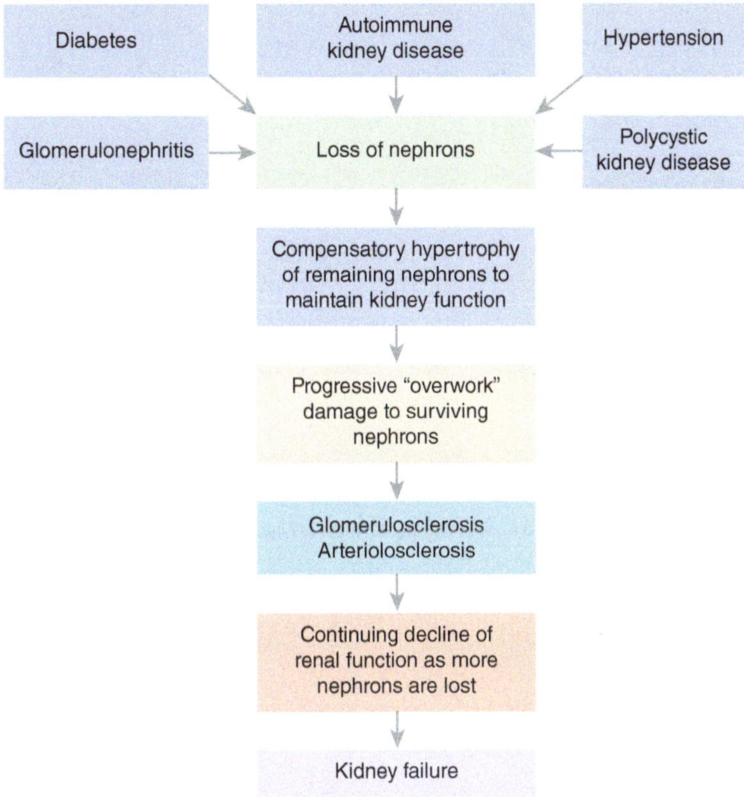

Figure 12.3 Progression of Chronic Kidney Disease

CASE STUDY INTRODUCTION

Dean is a 33-year-old Black male who presents to the hospital with 3 days of acute cough, worsening dyspnea with minimal exertion, orthopnea, and paroxysmal nocturnal dyspnea (shortness of breath that worsens at night). Upon inquiry, he reports experiencing weakness and some shortness of breath in the past 3 months, which he attributed to having a newborn daughter at home and studying for the bar exam. His symptoms progressively worsened and eventually led to this admission. He also reports foamy, dark-colored urine and increased frequency of nocturnal urination. He lives with his wife and newborn daughter. Dean states that his grandmother died of kidney disease at age 65.

Anthropometric Data:

Height: 175 cm
Weight: 85 kg
BMI: 28 kg/m^2

Weight History
Usual body weight: 83 kg 3 months ago

Biochemical Data:

Sodium 137 (136–145 mEq/L)
Potassium 4.5 (3.5–5.0 mEq/L)
Chloride 104 (96–106 mEq/L)
Carbon dioxide 29 (22–31 mEq/L)
Blood urea nitrogen 82 (8–20 mg/dL)
Creatinine 2.1 (0.7–1.3 mg/dL)
Glucose 98 (70–139 mg/dL)

Calcium 8.9 (8.5–10.5 mg/dL)
Phosphorus 3.8 (2.5–4.5 mg/dL)
Magnesium 1.9 (1.5–2.7 mg/dL)
Albumin 3.5 (3.5–5.5 g/dL)
Hemoglobin 15.7 (14–18 g/dL)
Hematocrit 42% (40%–50%)

Clinical Data:

Past Medical History: No significant past medical history
Medications: No medications

Vital Signs: Blood pressure: 178/96 mm Hg, Temperature 98.6°F, Heart rate 120 beats/min
Nutrition-Focused Physical Exam: Dean appears well nourished and physically fit, with +1 edema on his bilateral lower extremities. Skin appears dry; no wounds noted. Oral exam unremarkable with intact dentition, normal tongue.

Dietary Data:

24-Hour Diet Recall:
Breakfast (5:30 am): 16 oz coffee with cream, bran muffin, banana, 6 oz orange juice
Lunch (12 pm): Cobb salad with 1 cup kale, 1 cup iceberg lettuce, 1 egg, 2 tablespoons bacon bits, ½ avocado, ¼ cup ranch dressing, 12 oz diet cola
Snack (4 pm): 20 oz blended sweetened coffee drink, blueberry scone
At home appetizer with wife (7 pm): cheese with crackers, two glasses wine
Dinner (8:30 pm): 8 oz baked chicken, 2 cups rosemary roasted potatoes, 1 cup zucchini sautéed in butter
Evening snack (11 pm): 8 oz skim milk and 2 oatmeal cookies
Diet Prescription: No added salt diet (3–4 grams Na) diet

Questions

1. What are Dean's CKD risk factors?
2. What physiologic complications of CKD does Dean exhibit?
3. How would you interpret Dean's labs?

Regulation of Blood Pressure

The kidneys can regulate blood pressure in two ways. If blood pressure is elevated or decreased, the kidneys can adjust the amount of urine formed to eliminate or conserve body fluid, a mechanism hormonally regulated through arginine vasopressin, also known as **antidiuretic hormone (ADH)**. The release of ADH is influenced by the osmolarity or solute concentration of extracellular fluid (ECF). Decreased ECF osmolarity inhibits ADH secretion, so the kidneys excrete more urine. Conversely, increased ECF osmolarity stimulates ADH secretion, so the kidneys reabsorb more fluid and excrete less urine, which can help to maintain appropriate blood pressure. The kidneys are also the main site of action of the renin–angiotensin–aldosterone system (RAAS). When there is a decrease in blood pressure, perfusion can be compromised, leading to reduced blood flow to body tissues, as well as the kidneys. **Figure 12.4** outlines the steps in RAAS activation.

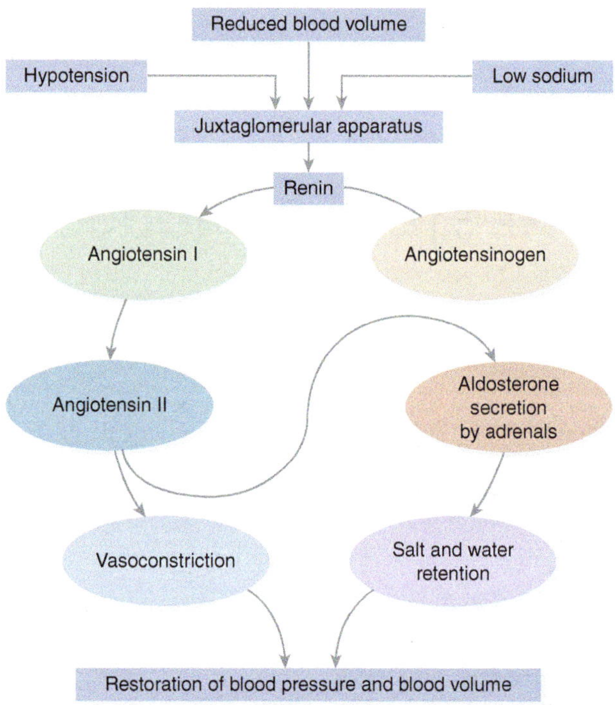

Figure 12.4 The Role of the Kidney in the Regulation of Blood Pressure and Blood Volume

Maintenance of Body Fluid Composition and Acid-Base Balance

Kidneys regulate both intracellular and extracellular fluid by retention or excretion of electrolytes.The concentration of water, sodium, potassium, calcium, phosphate, and hydrogen is tightly regulated to maintain normal cellular function.

One of the key roles of the kidneys is to maintain fluid and electrolyte balance by controlling the secretion and reabsorption of blood components, regulating ECF volume and osmolarity. The kidneys can concentrate urine up to 1200 milliosmoles (mOsm) and can dilute urine to as little as 50 mOsm, depending on the volume of excess fluid present and the amount of solute that must be released. The kidneys can excrete up to 12 L or as little as 500 mL of urine daily. This function of kidneys is critical for blood pressure regulation.

The kidneys also play a role in blood pH regulation. Acids and bases are metabolically produced, and a narrow parameter of pH must be maintained for appropriate organ system function. Primarily through the renal tubules, the kidneys maintain pH balance by excreting or reabsorbing acid or bicarbonate or producing new bicarbonate. For example, the kidney reabsorbs bicarbonate in the tubules and releases hydrogen ions in the urine when pH decreases below normal levels.

Excretion of Waste Products and Foreign Substances

Another function of the kidney is to filter and eliminate waste products and toxins from the blood. Normal metabolism produces byproducts that must be removed from the body. At least 500 mL of urine output is necessary to rid the body of the average 600 mOsm of solute that is generated daily through normal metabolism.[9] The solute load includes **nitrogenous waste**, such as urea, creatinine, and ammonia, which are end products of protein metabolism. The kidneys also excrete foreign substances, including a wide range of pharmacologic and exogenous toxic compounds in the urine.

Production of Hormones

The kidney produces and/or releases hormones, including those that control the production of red blood cells, activate vitamin D, and regulate blood pressure, as described above. The kidney secretes **erythropoietin (EPO)**, a glycoprotein hormone that promotes maturation of progenitor erythroid cells into mature red blood cells in the bone marrow. Interstitial fibroblasts produce erythropoietin in response to the hypoxia inducible factor, which regulates responses to low oxygen levels.

The kidney also activates 25-hydroxyvitamin D to 1,25-dihydroxyvitamin D3, also known as "calcitriol," the active form of vitamin D. The final hydroxylation of vitamin D to its active form is achieved by the proximal tubule cells in response to parathyroid hormone. The kidney further participates in bone homeostasis by regulating blood levels of calcium and phosphorus through parathyroid hormone regulation.

When the kidneys do not function properly, the effects are far reaching. Kidney failure leads to the inability of the kidney to perform its normal homeostatic control mechanisms, as well as its excretory and endocrine functions. This can lead to a buildup of waste products, fluid overload, electrolyte abnormalities, acid–base disturbances, anemia, and bone and mineral disorders, among other conditions.

Measurement of Kidney Function

Glomerular Filtration Rate (GFR)

GFR is the product of the average filtration rate of each single nephron (the filtering unit of the kidneys) multiplied by the number of nephrons in both kidneys. Normal GFR levels vary considerably according to age, sex, body size, physical activity, diet, pharmacologic therapy, and physiologic states such as pregnancy, and it declines with age. For GFR to be standardized for differences in kidney size (kidney size is proportional to body size), GFR is typically indexed for body surface area, which is computed from height and weight, and then expressed per 1.73 m^2 surface area, which was the mean body surface area of young females and males at the time indexing was first proposed. Typical average GFR values are approximately 120 and 130 mL/min/1.73 m^2 for young females and males, respectively.[10]

Reductions in GFR can be due to a decline in the nephron number or a decline in the average single-nephron GFR resulting from physiologic or hemodynamic alterations. GFR cannot be measured directly in humans; however, GFR can be calculated from serum creatinine levels, cystatin C levels, or both (**estimated GFR [eGFR]**).

Calculation of Estimated Glomerular Filtration Rate (eGFR)

GFR is the best measure of kidney function and is used to stage the degree of kidney failure, so its calculation plays a critical role in diagnosing kidney disease. There are several methods to calculate eGFR developed over the past few decades.[10] eGFR is based on various parameters and can be calculated by several equations. Some are based on creatinine (eGFRcr). These include the Cockcroft–Gault formula, the Modification of Diet in Renal Disease study (MDRD) equation, and the 2009 and 2021 Chronic Kidney Disease Epidemiology (CKD-EPI) equations. Some are based on cystatin C (eGFRcys). These include the Chronic Kidney Disease in Children (CKiD U25) Cystatin C equation and the 2012 Chronic Kidney Disease Epidemiology (CKD-EPI) Cystatin C equation. Others use both creatinine and cystatin C (eGFRcr-cy). These

CASE STUDY REVISITED

Dean is diagnosed with CKD due to IgA nephropathy. His age is 33 years, his creatinine is now 3.4 mg/dL, and his serum cystatin C is 2.0 mg/L (0.8–1.2 mg/L). He received appropriate treatment upon admission and was discharged with instruction to follow up regularly with an outpatient nephrologist.

Based on the CKD-EPI Creatinine equation, Dean's eGFR is 26 mL/min/1.73 m^2.

Based on the CKD-EPI Cystatin C equation, Dean's eGFR is 35 mL/min/1.73 m^2.

Questions

1. Compare the results. How do you account for the differences in eGFR?
2. What stage is Dean's CKD?
3. Write two Problem/Etiology/Signs and Symptoms (PES) statements for Dean identifying Dean's active issues.
4. Identify the interventions you would like to initiate for Dean to address the problems identified in your PES statements.What do you suggest based on his diet recall?
5. What biochemical indices should be included in your monitoring and evaluation plan? Why?
6. Why is it important for Dean to have regular follow-up appointments with an outpatient nephrologist?

are the 2012 and 2021 Chronic Kidney Disease Epidemiology (CKD-EPI) Creatinine-Cystatin C equations. **Table 12.2** provides a summary of the different eGFR calculation equations modified from the reference.[10]

CKD-EPI Creatinine–Cystatin C, 2021: Preferred Method

GFR estimates based on cystatin C alone are not more accurate than creatinine-based estimating equations overall, but it may be more accurate in selected clinical settings. It is the combination of the two markers that generally results in the most accurate estimate in populations with and without CKD. The CKD-EPI 2012 cystatin C and creatinine–cystatin C equations were developed with cystatin C that was measured with assays traceable to the international reference standard in a large database of subjects with diverse characteristics. Kidney Disease: Improving Global Outcomes (KDIGO) guidelines recommend use of the 2012 CKD-EPI equation if cystatin C is measured.[11] The 2021 CKD-EPI creatinine–cystatin C[12] was developed without inclusion of race as a factor in its calculation which could delay a CKD diagnosis, particularly in the Black population. This race-free equation serves to address concerns about possible racial bias and seeks to eliminate structural racism in health care. Its use is recommended by the American Society of Nephrology (ASN) and National Kidney Foundation (NKF).[12]

Stages of CKD

There are 5 progressive stages of CKD (stages 1–5) based on eGFR calculation. Stage 5D typically refers to a patient in stage 5 who is undergoing dialysis. According to the KDIGO guidelines, CKD stages with proteinuria are classified based on the eGFR alongside the level of albuminuria (proteinuria), categorized as A1 (normal), A2 (moderately increased), and A3 (severely increased), with stage 1 CKD indicating kidney damage with a normal eGFR (>90 mL/min/1.73m²) and detectable proteinuria, progressing through stages with decreasing eGFR and potentially increasing levels of proteinuria in the urine (**Figure 12.5**).[11]

Types of Kidney Disease

There are several types of kidney disease. If kidney failure occurs suddenly, it is called **acute kidney injury (AKI),** and most patients with AKI can recover kidney function with medical treatment of its cause. If eGFR is decreased for more than 3 months, it is **chronic kidney disease (CKD)** and patients with CKD do not regain kidney function.[13]

There are underlying causes of CKD progression, and the goal of medical treatment and medical nutrition therapy (MNT) is to control existing causes to preserve current kidney function. Kidney disease may be hereditary or non-hereditary, and may be caused by immunological reactions, tissue ischemia, exogenic toxic agents like medications, drugs, inflammatory infiltrates, direct trauma, and chronic conditions such as hypertension and diabetes.[14] Renal blood flow is estimated to be 400 mL/100 gram tissue per minute, which is higher compared to many other well-perfused organs such as the heart, liver, and brain. In addition, glomerular filtration is dependent on

Table 12.2 Various Methods to Estimate Glomerular Filtration Rate

Creatinine-Based Equation	
Cockcroft–Gault Formula	C_{cr} (mL/min) = (140 − age) × weight/72 × Scr × 0.85 [if female]
Modification of Diet in Renal Disease (MDRD) Study Equation	GFR (mL/min/1.73 m^2) = 175 × S Cr $^{-1.154}$ × age$^{-0.203}$ × 0.742 [if female] × 1.210 [if Black]
2009 Chronic Kidney Disease Epidemiology (CKD-EPI) Equation	GFR (mL/min/1.73 m^2) = 141 × min (Scr/κ, 1)α × max(Scr/κ, 1) $^{-1.209}$ × 0.993^{Age} × 1.018 [if female] × 1.157 [if Black] where κ is 0.7 for females and 0.9 for males, α is −0.329 for females and −0.411 for males, min indicates the minimum of Scr/κ or 1, and max indicates the maximum of Scr/κ or 1
2021 Chronic Kidney Disease Epidemiology (CKD-EPI) Equation	GFR (mL/min/1.73 m^2) = 142 × min (Scr/κ,1) ^{α} × max(Scr/κ,1)$^{-1.200}$ × 0.9938 ^{age} × 1.012 [if female] where κ is 0.7 for females and 0.9 for males, α is −0.241 for females and −0.302 for males, min indicates the minimum of Scr/κ or 1, max indicates the maximum of Scr/κ or 1
Cystatin C-Based Equations	
Chronic Kidney Disease in Children (CKiD U25) Cystatin C Equation (Pediatric and Young Adults to Age 25)	GFR = K × 1/Scys where K for males 1–14 y, 87.2 × 1.011$^{(age - 15)}$; 15–17 y, 87.2 × 0.960$^{(age - 15)}$; 18–25 y, 77.1; and K for females: 1–11 y, 79.9 × 1.004$^{(age - 12)}$; 12–17 y, 79.9 × 0.974$^{(age - 12)}$; 18–25 y, 68.3
2012 Chronic Kidney Disease Epidemiology (CKD-EPI) Cystatin C Equation	133 × min (Scys/0.8, 1) $^{-0.499}$ × max (Scys/0.8, 1)$^{-1.328}$ × 0.996^{Age} × 0.932 [if female] where Scys is serum cystatin C, min indicates the minimum of Scr/κ or 1, and max indicates the maximum of Scr/κ or 1
Creatinine–Cystatin C-Based Equations	
2012 Chronic Kidney Disease Epidemiology (CKD-EPI) Creatinine–Cystatin C Equation	135 × min(Scr/κ, 1)α × max (Scr/κ, 1)$^{-0.601}$ × min (Scys/0.8, 1)$^{-0.375}$ × max (Scys/0.8, 1)$^{-0.711}$ × 0.995^{Age} × 0.969 [if female] × 1.08 [if black] where Scr is serum creatinine, Scys is serum cystatin C, κ is 0.7 for females and 0.9 for males, α is −0.248 for females and −0.207 for males, min indicates the minimum of Scr/κ or 1, and max indicates the maximum of Scr/κ or 1
2021 Chronic Kidney Disease Epidemiology (CKD-EPI) Creatinine–Cystatin C Equation	GFR (mL/min/1.73 m^2) = 135 × min (Scr/k,1)^{α} × max (Scr/κ,1)$^{-0.544}$ × min (Scys/0.8,1)$^{-0.323}$ × max (Scys/0.8,1)$^{-0.778}$ × 0.9961^{age} × 0.963 [if female] where κ is 0.7 for females and 0.9 for males, α is −0.219 for females and −0.144 for males, min indicates the minimum of Scr/κ or 1, max indicates the maximum of Scr/κ or 1

Data from Inker LA, Levey AS. Assessment of kidney function in acute and chronic settings. In: Gilbert SJ, Weiner DE, Bomback AS, Perazella MA, Rifkin DE, eds. *National Kidney Foundation's Primer on Kidney Diseases*. 8th ed. Elsevier; 2023:26-32.

intraglomerular pressure. These factors make glomerular capillaries vulnerable to hemodynamic insults and circulatory substances.[14]

Other forms of kidney disease include IgA nephropathy, pyelonephritis, nephrotic syndrome, polycystic kidney disease (PKD), and kidney stones.[15] In this chapter, AKI, CKD, ESKD, nephrotic syndrome, PKD, and kidney stones will be discussed in detail.

Nutrition Assessment in Kidney Disease

Introduction

Nutrition assessment is important for all patients with CKD to provide appropriate dietary interventions to prevent protein energy wasting (PEW) and help slow

Chronic Kidney Disease (CKD) Stages and urine albumin creatinine ratio		Urine Albumin Creatinine Ratio (UACR) Albuminuria [urine albumin (mg)/creatinine (g)]		
CKD stage	eGFR (mL/min/1.73 m^2)	A1 (< 30 mg/g) Normal to mildly elevated	A2 (30–300 mg/g) Moderate	A3 (>300 mg/g) Severe
G1	≥ 90	Low	Mild	Moderate
G2	60–89	Low	Mild	Moderate
G3a	45–59	Mild	Moderate	High
G3b	30–44	Moderate	High	High
G4	15–29	High	High	Very high
G5	<15	Very high	Very high	Very high

Figure 12.5 Prediction of Progression of CKD Risk Based upon Urine Albumin Creatinine Ratio

GFR and albuminuria grid to reflect the risk of progression by intensity of coloring (green, yellow, orange, red, and deep red). The numbers of the boxes are a guide to the frequency monitoring (number of times per year).

Data from Chapter 2: Definition, identification, and prediction of CKD progression. *Kidney Int Suppl* (2011). 2013;3(1):63–72. doi:10.1038/kisup.2012.65

the progression of CKD in its early stages. In general, nutrition assessment includes anthropometric, biochemical, clinical, and dietary assessment, and subjective global assessment (SGA) or nutrition-focused physical examination (NFPE). Appetite assessment along with dialysis kinetic adequacy evaluation is unique for patients undergoing hemodialysis. The Kidney Disease Outcome Quality Initiative (KDOQI) guidelines provide standards for each nutrition goal for patients with kidney disease.[16]

CORE CONCEPT 2

Medical nutrition therapy is a necessary component of chronic kidney disease management and can improve outcomes by preventing malnutrition and slowing disease progression.

Anthropometric Assessment

Anthropometric measurement is used to assess body composition including weight, height, frame size, body mass index (BMI), skinfolds, and muscle circumferences. Bioelectrical impedance analysis (BIA) and dual energy x-ray absorptiometry (DXA) can be used for body composition, although this occurs more commonly in the research setting. Refer to Chapter 1, *Nutrition Assessment,* for additional information related to anthropometric measurement collection and interpretation.

Body Weight

Body weight is usually measured during clinic visits for patients with CKD. Weight and weight history are important to assess fluid balance and determine the presence of malnutrition. There are several types of body weight, including ideal body weight (IBW) and **standard body weight (SBW)**, which is based on the National Health and Nutrition Evaluation Survey (NHANES III) data.[17] Percentage of IBW or SBW is the patient's actual body weight expressed as a percentage of a defined "normal" body weight for Americans of a similar frame size, sex, height, and age.[18,19]

$$\%SBW = (\text{actual weight}/SBW) \times 100$$

Table 12.3 provides an interpretation of percentage of SBW as it relates to nutritional status in the CKD population.

SBW may also be used to estimate the **adjusted edema-free body weight (aBWef)** in patients undergoing dialysis with edema who are either obese or underweight.[18,19] This adjusted weight is important to use when determining energy and calorie intake goals for patients with edema, as failure to do so may result in over- or underestimation of needs, which could further complicate the disease process. The formula for calculating aBWef is as follows[18,19]:

$$aBWef = BWef + ([SBW - BWef] \times 0.25)$$

Comparison of actual weight to usual body weight (UBW or %UBW) can also be used to determine whether a patient has lost or gained weight, especially over a

Table 12.3 Interpretation of Percentage of Standard Body Weight (SBW)

SBW	<70%	<90%	90–110%	115–130%	130–150%	>150%
Nutritional Status	Severely malnourished	Mild to moderately malnourished	Well nourished; recommended target for maintenance dialysis patients	Mildly obese	Moderately obese	Severely obese

Data from National Kidney Foundation. K/DOQI clinical practice guidelines for chronic kidney disease: evaluation, classification, and stratification. *Am J Kidney Dis*. 2002;39(2 suppl 1):S1-S266. https://www2.kidney.org/professionals/kdoqi/guidelines_nutrition/nut_appx07a.html.

certain period of time. It can be used for patients new to dialysis to determine whether weight loss is due to fluid removal versus muscle and/or fat loss. Low %UBW can be an indicator of decreased nutritional status.

Height

Height is the best method to determine stature. To measure height, the registered dietitian (RD) or other clinician should follow a standardized process to obtain an accurate and consistent measurement. If a patient is not able to stand, there are height surrogates that can be used to estimate height, including arm span, half arm span, and/or knee height measurements.[20–22]

Body mass index (BMI)

The World Health Organization provides BMI categories used for standardized assessment, with overweight defined as >25 kg/m^2 and obesity as >30 kg/m^2.[23] This categorization can be applied to patients with CKD.

Determination of Frame Size

Frame size can be used to provide a more accurate determination of desirable or ideal weight. Weight range varies by frame size; therefore, it can help identify a patient's weight status, which can then optimize their nutrition plan. Frame size can be determined using elbow breadth.[21]

Biochemical Assessment

Biochemical tests commonly measured in CKD include:

Electrolytes: sodium, potassium, chloride, carbon dioxide

Measures of kidney function: blood urea nitrogen, serum creatinine, cystatin C, eGFR

Proteins: albumin, prealbumin, C-reactive protein

Lipid profile: total cholesterol, low-density lipoprotein (LDL) cholesterol, high-density lipoprotein (HDL) cholesterol, and triglycerides

Hematological parameters: hemoglobin, iron, ferritin, transferrin, and percentage saturation of transferrin

Bone mineral disorder markers: corrected calcium, phosphorus, parathyroid hormone (PTH), vitamin D

Refer to Chapter 2, *Biochemical Assessment*, for additional information related to biochemical measures and interpretation.

Electrolytes

Sodium

Sodium is the major extracellular cation that plays an important role in maintaining fluid homeostasis. Blood sodium level is not a reflection of dietary intake. Hyponatremia in CKD can be seen with uncontrolled diabetes, excess diuretic administration with water consumption, and the syndrome of inappropriate diuretic hormone (SIADH). Elevated blood sodium usually occurs with dehydration.

Potassium

Potassium is a major intracellular cation, and it can be either elevated or decreased in CKD. Blood potassium levels can be elevated by medications (RAAS blockade, potassium-sparing diuretics), hydration status (dehydration), metabolic acidosis, uncontrolled diabetes, lab error (hemolysis), and high dietary potassium intake.

Chloride/Carbon Dioxide

Chloride and carbon dioxide are indicators of acid–base balance, which is controlled by the kidneys.

Elevated chloride and low carbon dioxide levels are often seen with metabolic acidosis in CKD.

Kidney Function

Blood Urea Nitrogen (BUN)

BUN is a measure of urea, which is a metabolic by-product of protein metabolism, as well as exogenous protein intake. Although many factors can lead to an increased BUN level (dehydration, gastrointestinal or GI bleeding, catabolism), a high BUN may be a reflection of an altered excretion rate that occurs in CKD.

Serum Creatinine

Creatinine is a breakdown product of muscle and can be affected by dietary meat intake. Since creatinine is cleared by the kidney, an elevated creatinine level may signify altered kidney function. It is most frequently used for the eGFR calculation.

Cystatin C

Cystatin C is a protein produced in the body and filtered by the kidneys. Unlike BUN and creatinine, cystatin C is not affected by diet. Cystatin C is an important marker of kidney function and can improve the accuracy of kidney disease diagnosis when evaluated in conjunction with creatinine.

eGFR

There are several formulas used to calculate eGFR, as discussed earlier, with the most accurate equation using both creatinine and cystatin C.[10]

Proteins

Albumin

Albumin is a visceral protein and may be a good indication of nutritional status in a patient without acute illness. A major disadvantage of albumin is its long half-life (14–21 days), which decreases its sensitivity to short-term nutritional changes. Albumin is also a predictor of hospitalization and mortality in patients with CKD.[19] Decreased serum albumin can be an indication of malnutrition, liver disease, or acute inflammation.[24] Low albumin levels are a hallmark of nephrotic syndrome, to be covered later in this chapter.

Prealbumin

Prealbumin, also known as "transthyretin," is another negative acute phase visceral protein but has a shorter half-life (2–3 days), which makes it more responsive to short-term dietary changes. Prealbumin levels can be falsely elevated in CKD due to decreased catabolism by the kidneys.

C-Reactive Protein (CRP)

CRP is a positive acute phase protein and is an indication of inflammation. When the CRP level is high, it is likely that negative acute phase proteins, such as albumin and prealbumin, would be low for reasons such as fever, infection, and acute illness. An elevated CRP level would indicate that albumin and prealbumin should not be interpreted as nutritional markers in an inflammatory state.

Lipid Profile

Total cholesterol, LDL-cholesterol, HDL-cholesterol, and triglycerides are usually measured. A low total cholesterol is usually correlated with poor nutritional status, and other lipid levels are related to cardiovascular disease. In nephrotic syndrome or advanced CKD, lipid levels may be elevated.[25,26]

Hematological Parameters

Anemia is common in patients with CKD, especially in advanced stages of CKD, due to low production of erythropoietin (EPO), which promotes production of red blood cells. In CKD, an acceptable hemoglobin level is slightly lower than the typical reference range because of lower production of EPO. Iron should be repleted in patients with CKD for heme synthesis. A ferritin level can be checked since it may reflect the storage form of iron. As a positive acute phase protein, ferritin levels may be confounded (increased) by inflammation. To monitor for adequate iron status in patients with CKD, transferrin saturation (TSAT) is calculated. This will determine whether the patient needs iron supplementation, which can be provided as either oral or intravenous (IV) iron.[27]

Bone Mineral Disorder (CKD-BMD) Markers

CKD-BMD is a complicated disorder involving calcium, phosphorus, parathyroid hormone (PTH), and vitamin D metabolism. These blood levels are checked in patients with CKD routinely to prevent CKD-BMD. **Figure 12.6** provides an overview of normal calcium and phosphorus homeostasis.[28]

Calcium

Calcium is stored mainly in the bones and has many important physiological functions in the body. Eighty

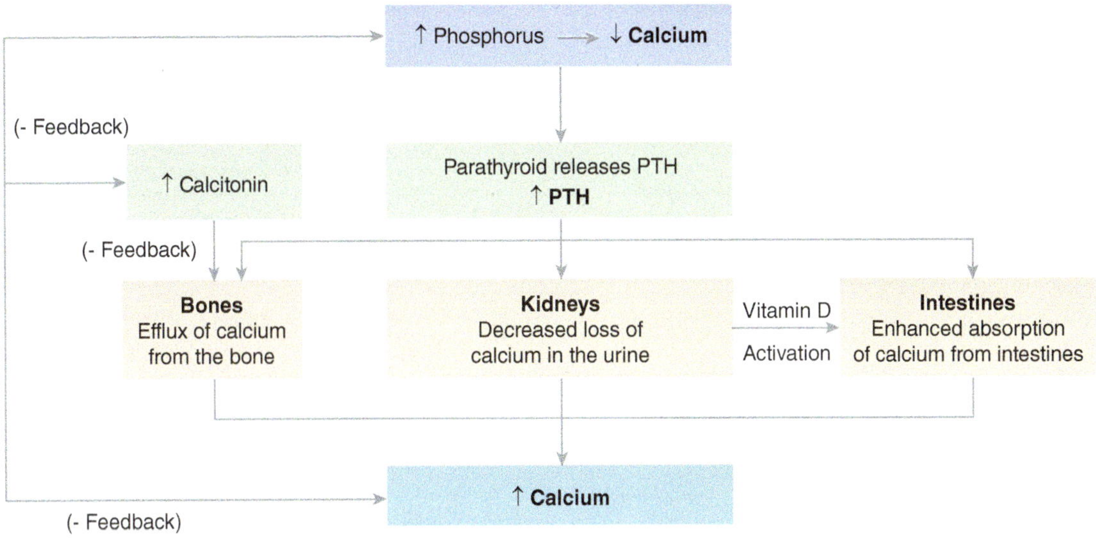

Figure 12.6 Mechanism Involved in Calcium and Phosphorus Homeostasis in Normal Physiology

Data from Kraft MD. Phosphorus and calcium: a review for the adult nutrition support clinician. *Nutr Clin Pract.* 2015;30(1):21-33. doi:10.1177/0884533614565251

percent of calcium is bound to albumin in the blood. When the patient has malnutrition or inflammation, corrected calcium should be calculated to prevent extra unnecessary supplementation, which is not desirable for patients with CKD.[19,29]

Phosphorus

Most phosphorus is present in the bone as a calcium–phosphate complex. Elevation of blood phosphorus is often seen in advanced stages of CKD due to decreased excretion via the kidneys. A low phosphorus level can be an indicator of malnutrition as a reflection of poor intake in patients with CKD. **Phosphate binders** can be used for control of phosphorus levels in the blood in advanced CKD.[29]

Parathyroid hormone (PTH)

PTH level is measured in the blood and is affected by blood calcium levels and active vitamin D (1,25 $(OH)_2$ D_3). An acceptable PTH level range is higher than normal with CKD progression. With low blood calcium levels, PTH is secreted and can cause bone to release calcium into blood, potentially compromising bone health.[19,29]

Vitamin D

Vitamin D is important for calcium homeostasis, and active vitamin D increases GI calcium absorption. Circulating vitamin D $(OH)D_3$ is measured in the blood, and maintaining a normal range is important for patients with CKD.[19,29] **Table 12.4** provides a summary of labs commonly checked with CKD.[19]

Dietary Assessment

Collection of a diet history can determine whether patients are consuming adequate food and nutrients to achieve or maintain an appropriate nutritional status. There are three commonly used food intake records.[29]

24-Hour Food Recall

RDs can collect patient's dietary intake over the previous 24 hours. Although it may not represent usual intake, it is useful to assess a patient's energy and protein consumption.[19]

3-Day Food Record

The 3-day food record is the most useful dietary intake record, especially for patients undergoing hemodialysis (HD). This food record can represent a dialysis day, a non-dialysis day, and one weekend day during which patients typically have different food consumption patterns. For this reason, it is a preferred method of evaluating protein and calorie consumption for patients on HD.[19]

Food Frequency Questionnaire

The food frequency questionnaire has been developed to establish how frequently patients eat specific foods/food groups within a specified time period (daily, weekly, or monthly, for example). However, it is not

Table 12.4 Biochemical Indices of CKD Range

Test	Reference Range	CKD Range
Creatinine	0.7–1.3 mg/dL	2–15 mg/dL (varies by stages)
Albumin	3.5–5.5 g/dL	WNL >4 g/dL
Prealbumin	16–30 mg/dL	>30 mg/dL
Parathyroid hormone	10–65 pg/mL	<110 stage 4, <200 Stage 5 2–9X normal ESKD
Vitamin D	20–100 ng/mL	WNL
Calcium	8.5–10.5 mg/dL	8.5–10.0 mg/dL
Phosphorus	2.5–4.5 mg/dL	3.0–5.5 mg/dL
Potassium	3.5–5.0 mEq/L Range varies by institutes	3.5–5.5 mEq/L 3.5–6.0 mEq/L**
Sodium	136–145 mEq/L	WNL
Hemoglobin	12–16 g/dL Females 14–18 g/dL Males	11–12 grams/dL or 10–12 grams/dL
Transferrin saturation	15–50% Females 20–50% Males	>20%
Iron	50–160 ug/dL Females 60–175 ug/dL Males	WNL
Ferritin	10–150 ng/mL Females 12–300 ng/mL Males	CKD>100 ng/mL HD >200 ng/mL
Blood urea nitrogen	8–20 mg/dL	60–80 mg/dL Varies by stage
Cholesterol	<200 mg	WNL <150 mg: nutrition evaluation
Alkaline phosphatase	30–120 U/L	WNL
C-reactive protein (CRP)	≤/0.8 mg/dL	WNL
Adequacy of dialysis ▪ Hemodialysis ▪ Peritoneal dialysis		Kt/V >1.2 (minimal) Kt/V >1.7

**Acceptable for dialysis
WNL, within normal limits/same as reference range.

Data from Ikizler TA, Burrowes JD, Byham-Gray LD, et al. KDOQI clinical practice guideline for nutrition in CKD: 2020 update. *Am J Kidney Dis*. 2020;76(3 suppl 1):S1-S107.

commonly used for patients with CKD or ESKD to evaluate overall dietary intake.

Nutrition-Focused Physical Exam (NFPE)

The NFPE is a total body, head-to-toe assessment. The NFPE can identify signs of malnutrition, including nutrient deficiencies and possible toxicity of both macro- and micronutrients including protein, vitamin A, iron, vitamin C, zinc, essential fatty acids, and B vitamins. The NFPE also includes evaluation of muscle and fat stores in the body, which are affected by nutritional status. Fluid retention and handgrip strength can be evaluated with NFPE, especially for patients with ESKD.

Specific Nutritional Assessment for Patients on Dialysis

Appetite and Diet Assessment Tool (ADAT)

Appetite assessment is a nutrition-specific tool that is usually used among patients on HD to evaluate prevalence of anorexia.[30] A poor score on the ADAT is associated with poor nutritional status, which can lead to hospitalization and increase risk of death.[30]

Subjective Global Assessment-Malnutrition-Inflammation Score (SGA-MIS)

Subjective global assessment (SGA) is usually used to assess a patient's nutritional status and diagnose malnutrition. It can be completed by any clinician using their own judgment as the assessment is not objective. The SGA is useful for all patients, especially those who are followed on a regular basis, which includes patients with CKD. The SGA allows clinicians to monitor physical changes as a reflection of overall nutritional status.[31–33]

The SGA-MIS is a combined assessment tool used to evaluate a patient's nutritional status by incorporating elements from the standard SGA and lab markers of inflammation such as albumin and transferrin to diagnose inflammation-related malnutrition and clinical outcomes.[34]

Handgrip Strength

Handgrip strength is measured by a handheld dynamometer. It is a reliable measurement of upper extremity strength, which can provide information about protein-energy and functional status and can help to identify malnutrition.[19]

Dialysis Adequacy

Dialysis adequacy is the measure of how thoroughly a patient's blood is being dialyzed. The measurement is called **urea kinetic modeling (UKM)**, and it is measured monthly based on the dialysis dose. Kt/V is the fractional clearance of urea as a function of its distribution volume.[19] **K** represents the delivered dialyzer urea clearance measured in L/min plus residual kidney clearance (except for patients without urine output), **t** is the treatment time (in minutes), and **V** is the patient's volume (in mL) of distribution of urea.[18,19]

The goal of adequacy varies depending on treatment modality—hemodialysis versus peritoneal dialysis. If adequacy is not achieved to the goal, the dialysis treatment should be adjusted. Kt/V also provides the benefit of nutrition assessment of **normalized protein nitrogen appearance (nPNA)**. This is the validated amount of daily protein consumed and it is useful to predict morbidity and mortality of patients on dialysis.[35]

PRACTICE POINT

There are various types of nutritional assessment tools to assess patients with kidney disease. The RD should understand each method and choose the correct tools for the different types of patients with kidney disease.

PRACTICE POINT

Nutrition assessment in ESKD should include urea kinetic modeling, subjective global assessment, and calculation of the malnutrition inflammation score to identify malnutrition, protein energy wasting, and inflammation, which affects morbidity and mortality in ESKD.

Kidney Disease Outcomes Quality Initiatives (KDOQI)

The **Kidney Disease Outcome Quality Initiative (KDOQI)** is a group of comprehensive, evidence-based clinical practice guidelines in nephrology.[19] They were first developed by the National Kidney Foundation (NKF) in 1995 and published in 1997. These guidelines have now become broadly accepted to guide quality care for patients with kidney disease in the United States and worldwide.[36] The KDOQI guidelines can be accessed through the *American Journal of Kidney Disease*, covering the following topics: hemodialysis and peritoneal dialysis adequacy; vascular access and anemia in chronic kidney failure; nutrition in CKD (children and adults); the evaluation, classification, and stratification of CKD; bone metabolism and disease in CKD (children and adults); clinical practice recommendations for dyslipidemia, anemia, diabetes, and cardiovascular diseases in CKD; and practice for functioning recipients of a kidney transplant.[19] In 2003, **Kidney Disease: Improving Global Outcomes (KDIGO)** was established when a group of nephrology experts aimed to improve the care and outcomes of people with kidney disease worldwide.[29]

KDOQI and KDIGO are two different entities, although their guidelines overlap in many topics.

The first KDOQI guidelines for nutrition were published in 2000, focusing on the nutrition management of CKD. Over the years, the guidelines were regularly updated with accumulation of new evidence and adoption of an increasingly rigorous development process. The most recent version—KDOQI Clinical Practice Guideline for Nutrition in CKD: 2020 Update[19]—was developed through a joint effort with the Academy of Nutrition and Dietetics and covers six primary topics: (1) nutrition assessment, (2) medical nutrition therapy, (3) dietary protein and energy intake, (4) nutrition supplementation, (5) micronutrients, and (6) electrolytes. The guideline development followed the 5-step systematic review process from the Academy Evidence Analysis Center.[37] Identified publications were screened by a preselected expert panel based on preestablished inclusion and exclusion criteria. The final included publications were then reviewed for data extraction, evidence-grading, and summarization into recommendations. Detailed rationales are also provided under each recommendation in these guidelines.[19] Key takeaways and recommendations of the 2020 KDOQI nutrition guidelines are summarized in **Table 12.5**.

Table 12.5 Summary of KDOQI Nutrition Recommendations for CKD

Nutrient	CKD Stages	Recommendation	Comments
Energy	1–5D metabolically stable	25–35 kcal/kg/day	Adjust energy needs based on age, sex, physical activity, body composition, concurrent illness, or presence of inflammation
Protein	3–5 without diabetes	0.55–0.60 gram/kg/day	Dietary and keto acid/amino acid analogs combined
	3–5 with diabetes	0.6–0.8 gram/kg/day	Higher protein goal to optimize glycemic control
	5D on HD/PD, without diabetes	1.0–1.2 grams/kg/day	
	5D on HD/PD, with diabetes	1.0–1.2 grams/kg/day	Higher dietary protein may need to be considered if poor glycemic control
EFA	3–5	~2.0 grams/day LC n-3 PUFA	To lower serum triglyceride level
	5D on HD/PD	1.3-4.0 grams/day LC n-3 PUFA	To improve lipid profile
Vitamin C	1–5D, who are at risk of deficiency	Male: >90 mg/day Female: >75 mg/day	
Calcium	3–4 not on vitamin D analogs	800–1000 mg/day	Including dietary, supplement, and calcium-based binders
	5D	Personalize	Adjust based on vitamin D analogs
Phosphorus	3–5D	Personalize to avoid hyperphosphatemia	Consider bioavailability of phosphorus, additives > animal > vegetable
Potassium	3–5D	Personalize to avoid hyperkalemia	
Sodium	3–5D	<2.3 grams/day	
Vitamin K	Not to routinely supplement if patient is on anticoagulation therapy		
Vitamin A, E	Not to routinely supplement due to risk of toxicity. If supplementation is warranted, care should be taken to avoid excessive doses.		

MHD, maintenance hemodialysis.

LC n-3 PUFA, long-chain omega-3 polyunsaturated fatty acids.

EFA, essential fatty acids.

Data from Ikizler TA, Burrowes JD, Byham-Gray LD, et al. KDOQI clinical practice guideline for nutrition in CKD: 2020 update. *Am J Kidney Dis*. 2020;76(3 suppl 1):S1-S107.

Acute Kidney Injury

Acute kidney injury (AKI), also known as "acute renal failure," is a sudden decline in kidney function characterized by a rapid reduction in GFR and urine volume.[13] AKI leads to water, sodium, and metabolic product retention due to decreased urinary excretion capacity. Therefore, patients often present with increased serum levels of creatinine (Cr), blood urea nitrogen (BUN), potassium, phosphorus, and, in some cases, magnesium. AKI can develop in previously healthy kidneys, or on top of already existing CKD. AKI is clinically reversible once the underlying causes are appropriately addressed. A small portion of patients may need temporary RRT during the recovery process. However, if the underlying insult persists, repeated AKI and nonreversible renal function damage may occur. As of 2022, the rate of newly diagnosed AKI in the United States reached 242 per 1000 patient-year (compared to 80 per 1000 patient-year in 2007).[38] AKI may last for days or weeks, or longer if it progresses to CKD. The recovery rate data is limited but a reported 62% of patients with AKI completely or partially recovered their kidney function.[13]

Etiology

The causes of AKI are complex, as any condition that results in a clinically significant reduction in intravascular volume or pressure or kidney damage may lead to AKI.[39] These conditions include, but are not limited to, cancer, sepsis, shock, GI diseases, liver diseases, cardiac insufficiency, trauma, and post-renal transplant. The etiologies of AKI are divided into three categories: prerenal causes, postrenal causes, and intrinsic or tubulointerstitial causes.

CASE STUDY REVISITED

Three months later, Dean presents to the hospital again, with worsening shortness of breath, drowsiness, nausea, and significant loss of appetite and reduced urine output for 3 days. His wife reports that Dean has not followed up with an outpatient nephrologist since last discharged. He tries his best to follow the diet prescription at home (low sodium and modified protein). However, due to the stress of taking the bar exam, Dean would get fast-food takeout once or twice a week. He stopped studying 3 days ago, when he had acute worsening of the above symptoms. His eGFR based on his serum creatinine is 15 mL/min/1.73 m^2 at the time of presentation. After 2 days of inpatient treatment, where he received continuous renal replacement therapy, Dean feels significantly better and his eGFR gradually improved to 33 mL/min/1.73 m^2.

Anthropometric Data (on Admission):

Weight: 89 kg

Usual Body Weight: 85 kg

Biochemical Data (on Admission):

Sodium 129 (136–145 mEq/L)
Potassium 5.8 (3.5–5.0 mEq/L)
Chloride 100 (96–106 mEq/L)
Carbon dioxide 27 (22–31 mEq/L)
Blood urea nitrogen 96 (8–20 mg/dL)
Creatinine 4.9 (0.7–1.3 mg/dL)
Glucose 69 (70–139 mg/dL)
Calcium 6.7 (8.5–10.5 mg/dL)
Phosphorus 6.3 (2.7–4.5 mg/dL)
eGFR (based on creatinine) 15 mL/min/1.73 m^2

Dietary Data (on Admission):

24-Hour Dietary Recall

Breakfast: Skipped due to loss of appetite
Lunch: Couple bites of chicken nuggets from McDonald's
Snack: 8 oz orange juice
Dinner: A dinner roll with butter.
(Low dietary intake in the past 3 days per wife)

Questions

1. Why did Dean's eGFR drop significantly but then recover after treatment? What is this condition called?
2. Would you change your diet prescription while Dean is receiving treatment and recovering to his baseline?
3. What is your nutritional concern if Dean's condition did not improve as expected?

Prerenal AKI is a result of inadequate kidney perfusion, leading to reduced oxygen and nutrient delivery to nephrons and ultimately compromising GFR.[40] Kidney hypoperfusion can be caused by (1) hypovolemia from excessive fluid loss due to severe burns, hemorrhage, persistent vomiting or diarrhea, increased ostomy or drain output, over-diuresis, and significantly reduced oral intake; (2) hypotension due to cardiogenic shock, heart failure, massive pulmonary embolism, sepsis, anaphylaxis; (3) renal vasoconstriction due to iodinated contrast used in imaging, hepatorenal syndrome, nonsteroidal anti-inflammatory drugs (NSAIDs); and (4) glomerular efferent arteriolar vasodilation caused by angiotensin-converting enzyme (ACE) inhibitors and angiotensin receptor blockers.[16,39] Prerenal AKI usually improves with volume repletion and can recover if addressed promptly.

Postrenal AKI is caused by obstructions that impede urine outflow, which may cause urine backflow and exert an adverse force on renal filtration. Common causes of obstruction include cancers (prostate, gynecological, bladder, etc.), nephrolithiasis (kidney stones), blood clots, and strictures. Patients can recover from postrenal AKI with early intervention to resolve the underlying obstruction.

Intrinsic AKI is caused by conditions affecting the glomerulus or tubule. For example, prolonged kidney ischemia may result in acute tubular necrosis (ATN) leading to intrinsic AKI. ATN is the most common cause of intrinsic AKI. Some medications or autoimmune conditions may cause acute interstitial nephritis (AIN), which can also result in intrinsic AKI. Other common contributors include glomerulonephritis and intratubular obstruction. Intrinsic AKI does not improve with volume repletion. It may recover over time, but depending on the degree of kidney function impairment, full recovery may not always be possible. **Table 12.6** outlines the causes of AKI,[39] and **Table 12.7** provides an overview of medications associated with AKI.[41]

Table 12.6 Causes of Acute Kidney Injury

Category	Etiology	Common Causes*
Prerenal	Reduced renal perfusion	Severe burns, hemorrhage, persistent vomiting or diarrhea, increased ostomy output, over diuresis, hypotension, renal vasoconstriction, etc.
Postrenal	Obstructions that impede urine outflow	Prostate, gynecological, bladder cancer, nephrolithiasis (kidney stone), blood clots, structures, etc.
Intrinsic	Glomerulus or tubule damage	Ischemia, autoimmune conditions, glomerulonephritis, some medications, etc.

*Please note that this is not a complete list of causes.

Data from Goyal A, Daneshpajouhnejad P, Hashmi MF, Bashir K. Acute *kidney injury*. StatPearls. 2024.

Table 12.7 Medications Associated with Acute Kidney Injury

Angiotensin-converting enzyme inhibitors	Vancomycin	Radiocontrast agents
Angiotensin receptor blockers	Colistin/polymyxins	Bisphosphonates
Antacids (PPI, histamine-2 blockers)	Amphotericin B products	Immunotherapies
Sodium-glucose cotransporter-2 inhibitors (SGLT2 inhibitors)	Antiviral agents (cidofovir, tenofovir, adefovir)	Antiangiogenesis drugs
Calcineurin inhibitors	Analgesics (foscarnet, acetaminophen overdose, NSAIDs)	Anticonvulsants
Aminoglycosides	Chemotherapeutic agents	Lithium

Please note that this is not a complete list of medications.
NSAIDs, nonsteroidal anti-inflammatory drugs; PPI, proton pump inhibitor.

Data from Perazella MA, Rosner MH. Drug-induced acute kidney injury. *Clin J Am Soc Nephrol*. 2022;17(8):1220-1233.

Table 12.8 Acute Kidney Injury Stating Criteria

Stage	Urine Output	Serum Creatinine (SCr)
1	Amount: <0.5 mL/kg/hour Duration: for 6–12 hours	>0.3 mg/dL increase or 1.5–1.9 times baseline
2	Amount: <0.5 mL/kg/hour Duration: for >12 hours	2.0–2.9 times baseline
3	Amount: <0.3 mL/kg/hour Duration: for >24 hours OR No urine output for >12 hours	3.0 times baseline or increase in SCr to >4.0 mg/dL

eGFR, estimated glomerular filtration rate.

Data from Khwaja A. KDIGO clinical practice guidelines for acute kidney injury. Nephron *Clin Pract*. 2012;120(4):c179-c184. doi:10.1159/000339789.

Diagnosis

There are multiple diagnostic tools for AKI, such as RIFLE (Risk, Injury, Failure, Loss, and End-stage), AKIN (Acute Kidney Injury Network), and KDIGO.[16] KDIGO is the most used among all three. It combines criteria from RIFLE and AKIN. Based on the KDIGO criteria, the presence of any of the following is sufficient to make an AKI diagnosis: (1) a serum creatinine increase by 0.3 mg/dL or more within 48 hours, (2) a serum creatinine increase to 1.5 times or more compared to a baseline level in the prior 7 days, and (3) urine volume reduction to less than 0.5 mL/kg/hour for at least 6 hours. KDIGO has also developed an AKI staging system to facilitate early detection and early intervention (**Table 12.8**).[42]

Medical Treatment

AKI treatment is similar to CKD and ESKD treatment in some ways. The length of AKI treatment is shorter unless it progresses to CKD or ESKD. Close monitoring of kidney function and urine output is essential during AKI treatment.[39] To distinguish prerenal AKI and ATN, a fluid challenge may be implemented if a patient's clinical condition allows, as prerenal AKI usually improves with fluid repletion, although ATN does not. In the hospital setting, the nephrology team should be consulted, if indicated. As it is important to avoid further renal insult, nephrotoxic medications should be avoided, and the medical team should review the patient's current medication list to renally adjust dosage, if indicated. Diuretics may be needed to treat volume overload. However, a careful balance is required to avoid overdiuresis because this can adversely contribute to AKI. Patients may have elevated serum potassium and/or phosphorus levels. In these cases, dietary restrictions of high potassium and high phosphorus foods may be necessary, with or without potassium or phosphorus binders. In acute hyperkalemia that predisposes patients to cardiac arrhythmia, insulin, IV dextrose, and calcium gluconate can be used to drive intracellular potassium shift and stabilize the cardiac membrane. Sometimes, RRT is needed until kidney function recovers. The medical team should also focus on treating the underlying cause of AKI. This may require vasoactive medications or surgery depending on the etiology of AKI.

Nutrition Intervention

Patients with AKI have acutely reduced kidney function, which may lead to uremia, metabolic acidosis, electrolytes imbalance, and fluid retention.[43] These are all relevant to nutrition care and should be considered when formulating a nutrition intervention plan. Currently, MNT for AKI is dependent on expert consensus from KDIGO[42] and the American Society of Parenteral and Enteral Nutrition (ASPEN),[44] with appropriate clinical judgment when necessary.

CORE CONCEPT 3

For patients with acute kidney injury, temporary protein restriction may be needed depending on clinical status. For patients with nephrotic syndrome, it is important to avoid overconsumption of protein unless determined necessary by clinical status. Both types of kidney disease may or may not progress to needing RRT.

Energy

The estimated energy needs of patients with AKI should be based on underlying clinical conditions. ASPEN recommends indirect calorimetry, when possible.[44] This is considered to be the gold standard for energy estimation. If indirect calorimetry is not feasible, energy requirements should be individualized by utilizing current existing clinical guidelines and clinical judgment. The KDIGO Clinical Practice Guidelines for Acute Kidney Injury[42] recommend a total intake of 20–30 kcal/kg/day for patients at all stages of AKI. In cases of severe catabolic state such as trauma, sepsis, severe burn, metastatic and cachexic cancer, severe malabsorption, and continuous renal replacement therapy (CRRT) in the intensive care unit (ICU), a higher calorie goal may be required. An early study has suggested that patients who are critically ill with sepsis and AKI had 30% increased energy needs compared to controls with normal kidney function and free of sepsis.[45] It is also essential to avoid overfeeding in this population, as it may adversely contribute to volume status, electrolyte imbalance, and uremia in patients with AKI.

PRACTICE POINT

Indirect calorimetry is the gold standard for determining energy requirements in patients with AKI to avoid overfeeding.

Protein

The protein requirement of patients with AKI largely depends on the underlying disease and how AKI is being treated at the time of assessment. In CKD, a lower protein goal is usually recommended for patients with impaired kidney function who are not on dialysis to reduce uremia and to preserve kidney function. For example, KDOQI guidelines[42] recommend 0.55–0.60 gram/kg/day protein for patients with stage 3–5 CKD who are without diabetes and not on dialysis. However, in AKI, it is important to consider that AKI could be short-lived, and temporary reduction in protein provision may not be clinically meaningful. KDIGO guidelines recommend a usual protein provision of 0.8–1.0 gram/kg/day for non-catabolic patients with AKI who are not on dialysis.[42] Protein restriction with a purpose to prevent or delay the initiation of dialysis in AKI is not recommended.[43] For patients with AKI who are on dialysis, 1.0–1.5 grams/kg/day protein is recommended. For those who are in a hypermetabolic state on CRRT, up to 2.5 grams/kg/day is recommended.[43] CRRT aims to achieve solute and fluid removal over 24-hour period.[46] It is required for patients with AKI/ESKD who are hemodynamically unstable in the ICU and cannot tolerate traditional intermittent dialysis. CRRT is known to cause protein and amino acid loss through ultrafiltration and filter membrane, about 10.4 grams/day median loss.[47] An early study found 2.5 grams/kg/day parenteral protein provision in patients receiving CRRT helped to achieve a slightly negative or positive nitrogen balance in a catabolic state while still allowed reasonable azotemic control.[48] In addition to protein intake, KDIGO also recommends carbohydrate intake of 3–5 grams/kg/day (maximum 7 grams/kg/day) and fat intake of 0.8–1.0 gram/kg/day in the AKI population to better meet calorie needs.[42]

PRACTICE POINT

In AKI, it is important to balance increased energy and protein needs with compromised protein metabolism.

Fluid and Sodium

Fluid overload is a common comorbidity in patients with oliguria and anuria due to AKI. It is associated with increased mortality in this population and should be minimized in the clinical setting.[49] Fluid requirements of patients with AKI should be determined after considering multiple factors[16]: remaining kidney function and urine output, serum sodium levels, fluid status, presence of edema and third spacing, whether the patient is on RRT, and if any other fluid losses are present. As the clinical course changes, fluid requirements should be adjusted accordingly to best meet the patient's needs. The goal is to provide adequate fluid to replace losses (due to ostomy output, nausea, vomiting, drains, insensible losses, for example) to prevent further renal insult and to minimize fluid overload. Patients with the aforementioned fluid losses and those who are regularly receiving RRT may need more fluid input than those who are not in those conditions. Fluid input may come from oral intake and/or IV administration. Although IV fluid contributes more significantly to volume status,[19] oral fluid restriction may still be necessary. It is often difficult to determine a daily fluid allowance for these patients due to clinical complexity. Clinicians may start with a 1–1.5 L daily fluid restriction and adjust as needed based on the patient's clinical course. Dietary sodium restriction is recommended for patients with CKD; however, there is limited data to support a similar recommendation for patients with AKI.

Potassium and Phosphorus

Hyperkalemia and hyperphosphatemia are two common electrolyte disturbances in patients with AKI due to reduced kidney excretion of these electrolytes. Hyperkalemia and hyperphosphatemia may occur alone or together. Patients with AKI usually have one or multiple underlying diseases. In cases of trauma, tissue damage, and tumor lysis syndrome, potassium and phosphorus will be released from damaged cells and cause elevated serum levels.[16,43] Metabolic acidosis, potassium-sparing diuretics, and potassium-containing medications can contribute to hyperkalemia. As previously mentioned, acute hyperkalemia can be managed by insulin and IV dextrose to promote an intracellular shift. Phosphorus is rich in processed food in the form of nonorganic phosphate additives. Phosphorus is also naturally rich in animal protein foods. Dietary potassium and phosphorus restriction may be needed to help maintain normal serum levels. It is important to note that not every patient requires strict potassium and/or phosphorus restriction; restriction should be individualized. If restriction is needed, start by cutting foods highest in potassium and phosphorus until serum levels normalize. Potassium and phosphorus binders can also be used if dietary restriction alone does not achieve the desired result. As AKI gradually improves, dietary restrictions should be lifted when appropriate.

Monitoring and Evaluation

Patients with AKI should be monitored to assess for improvement in kidney function. This would include ongoing assessment of urine output and fluid balance to assess for volume depletion or edema. It is also important to monitor electrolyte levels, particularly sodium, potassium, chloride, carbon dioxide, serum creatinine, BUN, phosphorus, and magnesium levels. Trending weight is another metric to monitor; however, fluid shifts and fluid overload may make body weight as well as nutrition-focused physical examination findings difficult to interpret. Assessment of oral intake and/or nutritional support adequacy is critical to ensure appropriate energy and protein provision.

CASE STUDY REVISITED

Dean's CKD continues to worsen. Another 6 months later, his eGFR is 20 mL/min/1.73 m^2. He is admitted to the hospital and nutrition is again consulted. Dean reports he has worsening edema in his legs and arms and continues to experience dyspnea at night and with minimal exertion. Due to his significant fatigue, he has put his studies on hold.

Anthropometric Data:

Weight: 88 kg

Usual body weight: 85 kg

Biochemical Data:

Sodium 127 (136–145 mEq/L)
Potassium 6.3 (3.5–5.0 mEq/L)
Chloride 117 (96–106 mEq/L)
Carbon dioxide 16 (22–31 mEq/L)
Blood urea nitrogen 95 (8–20 mg/dL)

Creatinine 4.2 (0.7–1.3 mg/dL)
Glucose 90 (70–139 mg/dL)
Calcium 6.4 (8.5–10.5 mg/dL)
Phosphorus 6.7 (2.5–4.5 mg/dL)
eGFR (based on creatinine) 15 mL/min/1.73 m^2
UACR 90 mg/g (<30 mg/g)

Dietary Data:

Diet Prescription: 2 grams sodium, 2 grams potassium diet

Questions

1. What stage is Dean's CKD now?
2. What are the nutrition priorities for Dean?
3. How are his labs a reflection of his physical presentation and anthropometric and clinical data?
4. How would you interpret Dean's weight trend in comparison to his first visit a year ago?
5. Assess Dean's PES statement(s) from the previous RD encounter. Identify if each statement remains an active issue or if the PES statement has been resolved. If the PES statement remains an active issue, is it being addressed and/or has improvement in the issue been noted? If the issue has been resolved, write a new PES statement.
6. Identify the interventions you would like to initiate for Dean to address the problems identified in your PES statements.

Chronic Kidney Disease

According to the 2024 KDIGO clinical practice guidelines[50] for the evaluation and management of chronic kidney disease, CKD is defined as abnormalities of the kidney lasting longer than 3 months, either structural or functional, with implications for health. CKD affects >10% of the population worldwide, amounting to >800 million individuals.[1] CKD can be classified into five stages. People with early stages of CKD are often asymptomatic until more advanced stages are reached. Symptoms may include foamy urine (a sign of proteinuria), urinating more or less than usual (reflecting glomerular hypertension as a temporary compensation, and decline in kidney function, respectively), fatigue, nausea, loss of appetite, shortness of breath, swelling of lower extremities, and unintentional weight loss.[51] CKD involves complex, comorbid conditions, including malnutrition, cardiovascular disease, hypertension, dyslipidemia, and bone and mineral metabolism disorders. The consequence of CKD progression is ESKD, which requires lifelong RRT or kidney transplantation. Therefore, early detection, education, and intervention are key to preventing the progression of CKD. Refer to Chapter 16, *Nutrition in Solid Organ Transplantation,* for additional information related to nutritional management in kidney transplantation.

Classification and Diagnosis of CKD

CKD can be classified based on cause, eGFR category, and albuminuria category. With eGFR, it is classified into five stages[50]: G1 normal or high (eGFR ≥90 mL/min/1.73 m^2), G2 mildly decreased (eGFR 60–89 mL/min/1.73 m^2), G3a mildly to moderately decreased (eGFR 45–59 mL/min/1.73 m^2), G3b moderately to severely decreased (eGFR 30–44 mL/min/1.73 m^2), G4 severely decreased (eGFR 15–29 mL/min/1.73 m^2), and G5 kidney failure (eGFR ≤15 mL/min/1.73 m^2). With the level of albuminuria, it can be classified into three categories: A1 normal to mildly increased (<30 mg/gram), A2 moderately increased (30–300 mg/gram), A3 severely increased (>300 mg/gram). **Table 12.9** shows the KDIGO diagnosis of CKD by GFR and albuminuria categories. CKD is diagnosed by the presence of kidney damage marker or decline in eGFR <60 mL/min/1.73 m^2.[50]

Causes of CKD

CKD has various causes and may be multifactorial. Common causes of CKD are summarized in **Figure 12.7**.[52] Diabetes and hypertension are the two leading causes of CKD, accounting for 41% and 18% of the cases, respectively, followed by glomerulonephritis, and other causes including cystic diseases (especially **polycystic kidney disease**, which will be discussed later in this chapter). Some common other causes are family history of CKD, age 60 years or older, ethnic groups (Black people, Hispano people, Asians, Pacific Islanders, and Indigenous Americans have higher risk compared to White people), obesity, autoimmune diseases, urinary tract and systemic infection, overuse of pain medications, exposure to renal toxic medications or chemicals, direct kidney injury, and loss of a kidney.[16]

Diabetes

Diabetes has three devastating manifestations: retinopathy, nephropathy, and neuropathy. In diabetic nephropathy, chronic hyperglycemia induces slow

Table 12.9 Stages of CKD on eGFR and Criteria of Albuminuria

Stage of CKD			Albuminuria Categories	
Stage	eGFR (mL/min/1.73 m^2)		Description	Range (mg/g albumin)
G1	>90	Normal or high	A1 Normal to mildly increased	<30 mg/gram <3 mg/mmol
G2	60–89	Mildly decreased		
G3a	45–59	Mildly to moderately decreased	A2 Moderately increased	30–300 mg/gram 3–30 mg/mmol
G3b	30–44	Moderately to severely decreased		
G4	15–29	Severely decreased	A3 Severely increased	>300 mg/gram >30 mg/mmol
G5	<15	Kidney failure		

Data from Kidney Disease: Improving Global Outcomes CKDWG. KDIGO 2024 clinical practice guideline for the evaluation and management of chronic kidney disease. *Kidney Int*. 2024;105(4S):S117-S314.

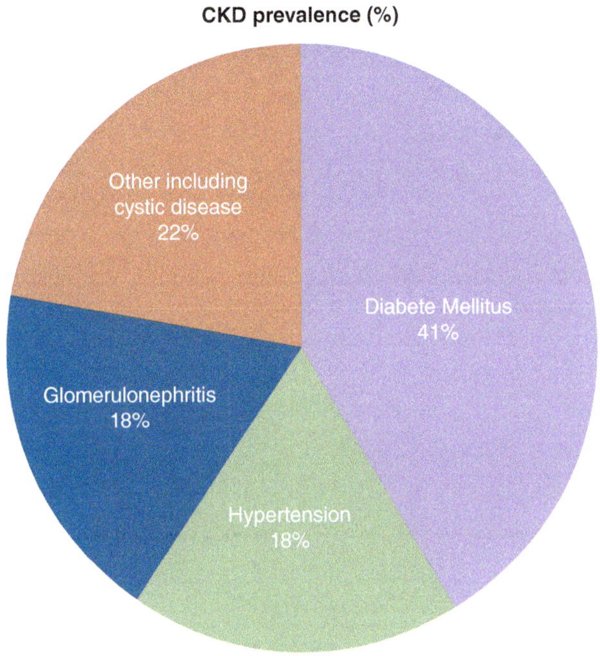

Figure 12.7 Causes of CKD

Data from Xie Y, Bowe B, Mokdad AH, et al. Analysis of the Global Burden of Disease study highlights the global, regional, and national trends of chronic kidney disease epidemiology from 1990 to 2016. *Kidney Int.* 2018;94(3):567-581.

but progressive damage to the renal microvasculature (damage to blood vessels). If not controlled, this can ultimately compromise renal filtration and cause CKD.[53] CKD caused by diabetes can be referred to as diabetic kidney disease (DKD). The goal of DKD management mainly focuses on glycemic control to slow down the microvascular damage, usually through dietary modifications and glucose-lowering medications. According to 2020 KDIGO Diabetes Management in CKD Guidelines,[54] physical activity, nutrition therapy, and weight loss are recommended before starting antihyperglycemic medications. If lifestyle modifications do not produce the desired results, metformin is used as the first-line therapy. Metformin can only be used when eGFR is higher than 30 mL/min/1.73 m^2 because it is renally excreted. Sodium-glucose co-transporter-2 inhibitors (SGLT-2) and glucagon-like peptide-1 (GLP-1) receptor agonists are two new classes of medications approved to treat diabetes. SGLT-2 inhibitors lower blood glucose by reducing renal glucose reabsorption. They also help to lower blood pressure, reduce cardiovascular events, and can induce modest weight loss. Clinical trials have demonstrated renal-protective effects of SGLT-2 inhibitors as they can help to slow CKD progression and reduce albuminuria.[55] When metformin and SGLT-2 inhibitors are not sufficient to achieve glycemic control, additional agents can be added. GLP-1 receptor agonists are preferred due to their effect on reducing cardiovascular events, the potential to prevent severe albuminuria, and slow eGFR decline.[54] The 2024 KDIGO guidelines for CKD[50] recommend a glycemic control goal of hemoglobin A1c between 6.5% and 8.0% in patients with CKD and diabetes not on dialysis.

Hypertension

Hypertension and CKD are two intertwined conditions. On one hand, hypertension causes blood vessel damage and reduces the number of functioning nephrons, leading to CKD. On the other hand, CKD causes sodium retention, volume expansion, and upregulation of RAAS and can lead to worsening hypertension.[56] RAAS is an important hormonal system that regulates blood pressure and fluid status of human body. Upregulation of RAAS leads to vasoconstriction and sodium reabsorption, which in turn leads to increased serum osmolarity and expanded vascular volume contributing to hypertension. RAAS inhibitors (RAASi) are a class of medications that include an ACE inhibitor (ACEi) and angiotensin II receptor blocker (ARB). These medications are widely used to treat hypertension. The 2021 KDIGO guidelines for blood pressure management in CKD[57] recommend the use of RAASi therapy in patients with hypertension, CKD, and moderately to severely increased albuminuria, with or without diabetes, as evidence is strong that the therapy helps to control blood pressure in this population as well as lower proteinuria. A goal of blood pressure <120 mmHg is recommended by KDIGO, if tolerated.

Other Causes

Glomerulonephritis (GN) means inflammation of the kidney, specifically the glomerulus. It is a diverse group of disorders and often immune-mediated.[58] Patients who have GN may notice urine that is dark (due to blood in the urine) and frothy (due to a large amount of protein in the urine).[59] Mild GN may be asymptomatic and can be fully treated. If not treated, GN can result in long-term kidney damage and CKD development. Autoimmune diseases, PKD, frequent urinary tract infections, obesity, and long-term use of NSAIDS are risk factors for GN. PKD will be discussed later in this chapter.

CORE CONCEPT 4

Prevention is a key component in the management of chronic kidney disease and involves treatment of underlying conditions, such as diabetes and hypertension.

Nutrition Intervention

Nutrition recommendations for CKD should follow the 2020 KDOQI nutrition guidelines, which are summarized in **Table 12.10**.[19] To quickly recap, energy prescription should be around 25–35 kcal/kg/day, with the low end being appropriate for patients with CKD not on dialysis who have relatively low metabolic demand (for example, older age, inactivity, without acute health issues, or other chronic complications). The high end would be more appropriate for patients with CKD who are either on dialysis, or in acute distress or have chronic complications that increases metabolic demands, or both. Energy requirements should always be further individualized based on patient's clinical status. A protein recommendation of 0.55–0.6 gram/kg/day is appropriate for CKD stage 3–5 patients without diabetes, and 0.6–0.8 gram/kg/day for those who with diabetes to optimize glycemic control. For patients who are on dialysis, 1.0–1.2 grams/kg/day is recommended due to increased protein loss. Again, protein needs should also be further individualized to best meet each patient's needs. The KDOQI 2020 guidelines no longer recommend specific phosphorus and potassium restrictions. It is suggested that these micronutrients be individualized based on serum levels. Sodium recommendation remains <2.3 grams/day. In addition to the recommendations made by the guidelines, RDs should also consider a balanced plate—as these calculations may not always yield a balanced proportion of each macronutrient. For example, in some patients, protein may be restricted due to CKD and carbohydrate may be limited due to diabetes. If the patient has a high metabolic demand, fat should be significantly increased to help meet energy requirements. This may or may not be desirable depending on the patient's clinical status and food preferences. A reasonable compromise on the protein or carbohydrate restrictions could be made if it is deemed appropriate by the multidisciplinary team. Refer to **Figure 12.8** for a renal-appropriate balanced plate.

It has been suggested that a vegetarian diet is suitable for patients with CKD. According to the NKF, a vegetarian diet is safe and beneficial for patients with CKD with careful planning as it may help to prevent infection, build muscle, maintain a healthy weight, and slow CKD progression.[60] A 2023 systematic review[61] found inconsistent results—with some studies reporting an increased eGFR in patients with CKD assigned to follow a vegetarian diet and others reporting no difference. RDs should use clinical judgment when

Table 12.10 Nutrition Recommendations for Stages 3–5 CKD (Not on Dialysis)

Nutrient	Recommendation
Protein without diabetes with diabetes	 0.55–0.60 gram/kg/day; 0.28–0.43 gram/kg/day with ketoacid/amino acid analogs 0.60–0.80 grams/kg/day
Energy	25–35 kcal/kg/day
Sodium for blood pressure for proteinuria and dry weight	 <100 mmol/day (or 2.3 grams/day) <100 mmol/day (or 2.3 grams/day) and pharmacologic intervention Reduced sodium intake as an adjunctive lifestyle modification strategy to achieve better volume control and desirable body weight (BW)
Potassium	Adjust dietary potassium intake to maintain serum levels within normal range In patients with hyper- or hypokalemia, dietary or supplemental intake should be based on the patient's individual needs and clinical judgment
Calcium	800–1000 mg/day. Including dietary, supplement, and calcium-based binders
Phosphorus	Adjust dietary phosphorus intake to maintain serum levels within normal range Consider the bioavailability of the phosphorus sources
Micronutrients	Not routinely supplemented unless insufficiency

Data from Ikizler TA, Burrowes JD, Byham-Gray LD, et al. KDOQI clinical practice guideline for nutrition in CKD: 2020 update. *Am J Kidney Dis*. 2020;76(3 suppl 1):S1-S107.

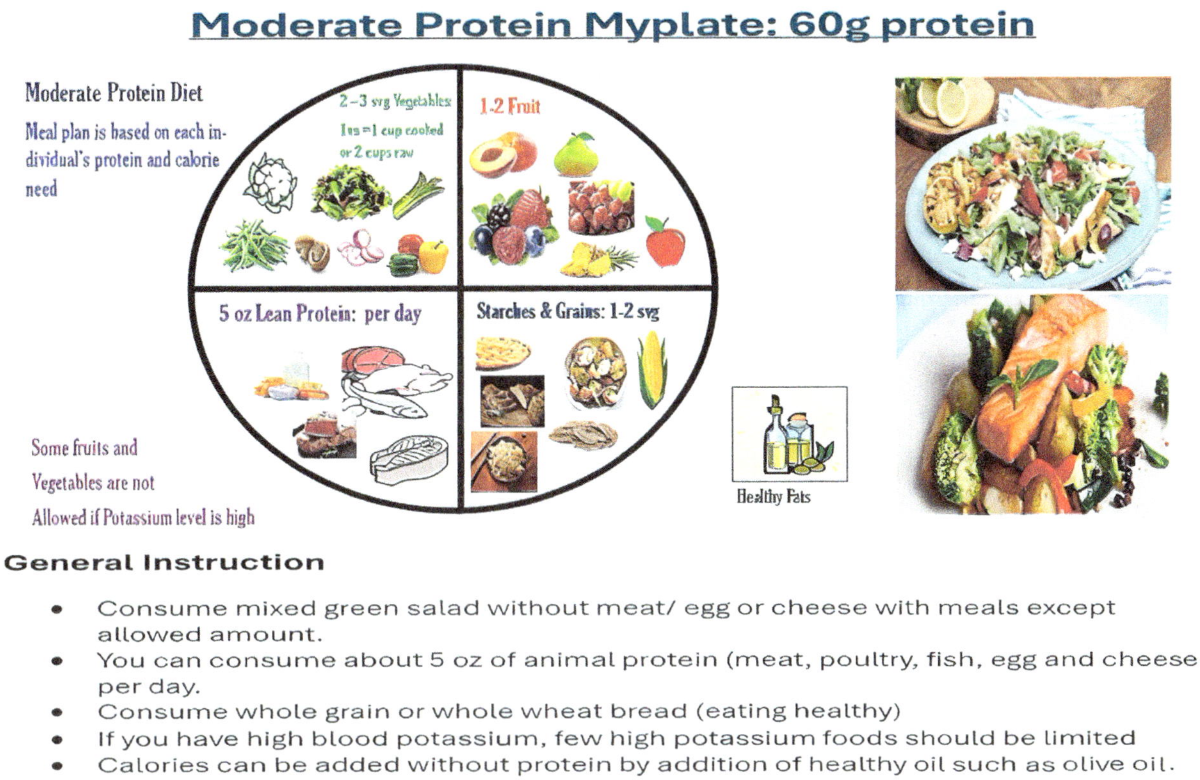

Figure 12.8 60-Gram Moderate Protein Meal Plan

Permission from Haewook Han PhD, RD, LDN, FNKF

considering vegetarian diets in patients with CKD. When the patient is otherwise healthy and not at risk for malnutrition, switching from an animal protein–based diet to a more plant-based diet may insert health benefits if serum potassium levels are within normal limits. For patients who are malnourished or at risk for developing malnutrition, a vegetarian diet (which is naturally more restrictive) may increase a patient's risk of developing deficiencies. Patients with CKD who follow a vegetarian diet should be regularly followed by RDs for careful dietary planning.

CORE CONCEPT 5

Malnutrition risk increases as the glomerular filtration rate decreases and may complicate the management of chronic kidney disease due to protein, fluid, and/or micronutrient restrictions.

CORE CONCEPT 6

Protein is a necessary macronutrient in the diet of patients with chronic kidney disease, and despite controversy regarding the possibility that protein restriction improves outcomes, patients must be able to eat a balanced, palatable diet that provides adequate energy and protein to prevent loss of lean body mass.

Monitoring and Evaluation

Patients with CKD should be monitored for signs of fluid overload including weight trends, particularly changes to edema-free body weight, and nutrition-focused physical findings of edema. Electrolyte levels, particularly sodium, potassium, chloride, and carbon dioxide, as well as serum creatinine, BUN, phosphorus, and magnesium levels should also be checked regularly. Iron studies (hemoglobin, iron, ferritin, TSAT), lipid panel (total cholesterol, HDL-cholesterol, LDL cholesterol, triglycerides), and bone mineral disorder markers (corrected calcium, PTH, and vitamin D) can be intermittently evaluated. Assessment of oral intake is critical to ensure appropriate energy, protein, and fluid provision. As CKD progresses, uremia and metabolic acidosis can cause nausea, which can lead to decreased appetite and intake. Additionally, the restrictive nature of the diet can be a barrier to optimal intake. Ensuring patient comprehension of their individualized diet recommendations is key to appropriate diet selections.

End-Stage Kidney Disease/Kidney Failure

End-stage kidney disease (ESKD), **end-stage renal disease (ESRD)**, and kidney failure are three terms used interchangeably in the medical field. They all refer to the condition in which kidneys have stopped working and are not able to remove waste products and extra water from the body. The 2020 KDIGO nomenclature for kidney function and disease report[62] suggests that clinicians use "kidney failure" rather than "end-stage" to describe such a condition. The 2024 KDIGO guidelines[50] define kidney failure as GFR <15 mL/min/1.73 m^2. In adults with CKD, the probability of progression to kidney failure within 5 years was 14.5% for stage G3a, 16.5% for stage G3b, and 20.4% for stage G4.[63] Once this stage is reached, an individual can no longer survive without RRT, such as dialysis. Dialysis is defined as a mean to remove waste metabolites and extra water from body by the process of diffusion and ultrafiltration.[64] Dialysis can be classified into hemodialysis (HD) and peritoneal dialysis (PD).

Although these treatments are available, patients have the right to refuse RRT as a step toward ending their life in the setting of this debilitating, irreversible disease. If patients do not feel that their quality of life justifies undergoing this time-consuming and expensive treatment, they may decide to forego or withdraw the therapy and initiate the dying process. Many patients with stage 5 and 5D CKD may also have other diseases that may further diminish their quality of life. This decision involves the RD because MNT may no longer be appropriate for the patient; they may wish to receive comfort measures including a liberal, unrestricted diet in their end-of-life care.

Dialysis Access

Hemodialysis requires vascular access. Temporary access sites include central venous catheters inserted in the internal jugular or subclavian vein (in rare cases, the femoral vein). Permanent access includes the arteriovenous fistula (AV fistula) and arteriovenous graft (AV graft). AV fistula is the most durable access for HD and it is associated with the lowest rates of complications.[65] It is created surgically by creating an anastomosis between an artery and a vein, usually the radiocephalic area. Arterial blood has a high flow rate, whereas venous blood has lower pressure. Allowing a high-flow artery to connect with a low-pressure vein results in dilation and wall-thickening of the vein. This process is called "arterialization." Once the arterialization matures, it can be used for cannulation and HD. An AV graft is created by surgically placing a tunneled polytetrafluoroethylene graft to connect an artery and vein. An AV graft is more prone to infection and therefore is usually not considered unless other options have been exhausted. **Figure 12.9** presents the structure of an AV fistula and AV graft. Unlike access for HD, PD access is a silicone tube implanted on the abdominal wall.[66]

Hemodialysis

In **hemodialysis (HD)**, a dialysis machine delivers blood from the patient to the dialyzer, cleanses the blood using a prescribed bath (dialysate), and returns the blood to the patient. Blood and dialysate (containing sodium bicarbonate, sodium chloride, acid concentrate, and deionized water) flow across a semipermeable dialysis membrane in a countercurrent manner to effectively remove small solutes by diffusion, such as urea and creatinine.[64,67] Excess water is removed by ultrafiltration carried out by the dialysis machine. The amount of solute and water removal is related to the ultrafiltration rate and length of dialysis. Refer to **Figure 12.10** for demonstrations of HD.

Types of Hemodialysis

Conventional/In-Center Hemodialysis

Conventional HD is usually carried out in dialysis centers, and it is currently the most widespread HD modality.[68] It usually includes three treatments per week on nonconsecutive days, each lasting about 4 hours. Patients are assigned to Monday/Wednesday/Friday (MWF) sessions, or Tuesday/Thursday/Saturday (TTS) sessions. In-center HD has many advantages[68]: patients are assisted by medical staff during dialysis hours, they can be followed up by a nephrologist or RD in the center, and they are accompanied by people who are in similar health conditions, etc. Disadvantages are also obvious: patients are tied to a 3 times/week schedule, which limits work, exercise, and travel; older adults may need rides to travel between their home and the dialysis center; risk of missing dialysis sessions when rides are unavailable (e.g., extreme weather that makes travel unsafe or impossible); finally, patients are more exposed to a healthcare milieu, which can increase their risk

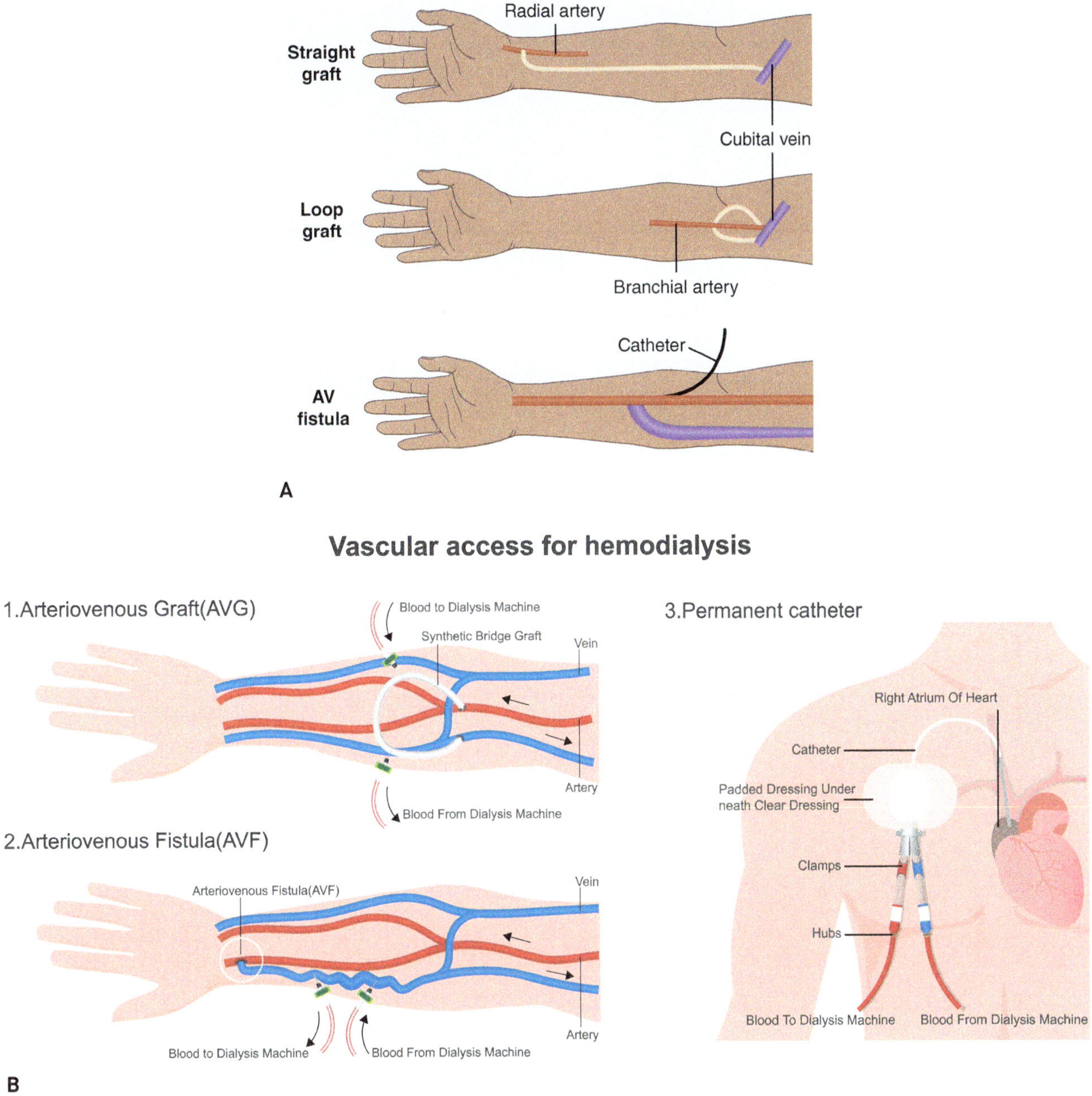

Figure 12.9 **A.** Arteriovenous Fistula vs. Arteriovenous Graft. **B.** Vascular Access for Hemodialysis

CASE STUDY REVISITED

Two years later, Dean is in Stage 5 CKD and has decided to initiate in-center hemodialysis.

Anthropometric Data:

Weight: 80 kg

Usual Body Weight: 85 kg

Biochemical Data:

Sodium 131 (136–145 mEq/L)
Potassium 5.6 (3.5–5.0 mEq/L)
Chloride 113 (96–106 mEq/L)
Carbon dioxide 17 (22–31 mEq/L)
Blood urea nitrogen 78 (8–20 mg/dL)

Creatinine 2.5 (0.7–1.3 mg/dL)
Glucose 79 (70–139 mg/dL)
Calcium 9.5 (8.5–10.5 mg/dL)
Phosphorus 4.9 (2.5–4.5 mg/dL)
Hemoglobin 10.7 (14–18 g/dL)
Hematocrit 22% (40%–50%)

Clinical Data:

Medications: Includes calcium acetate 3 with meals and 1 with snacks
Nutrition-Focused Physical Exam: Dean appears tired with some notable edema in his upper and lower extremities.
Urine output: 1 L daily

Dietary Data:

24-Hour Diet Recall:
Breakfast (8 am): 1 cup corn flakes with 4 oz low-fat milk, 8 oz coffee with nondairy creamer
Lunch (12 pm): 1½ cups pasta with olive oil, green beans, 1 oz baked chicken, 12 oz ginger ale
Dinner (7 pm): 2 oz baked fish, 2 cups white rice, 6 spears fresh asparagus, 12 oz water
Diet prescription: 2 grams sodium, 2 grams potassium, low-phosphorus diet

Questions

1. How would you assess Dean's weight loss?
2. How would you assess Dean's labs?
3. Assess Dean's PES statement(s) from the previous RD encounter. Identify if each statement remains an active issue or if the PES statement has been resolved. If the PES statement remains an active issue, is it being addressed and/or has improvement in the issue been noted? If the issue has been resolved, write a new PES statement.
4. Identify the interventions you would like to initiate for Dean to address the problems identified in your PES statements. What specific diet changes do you suggest for Dean as he initiates hemodialysis?

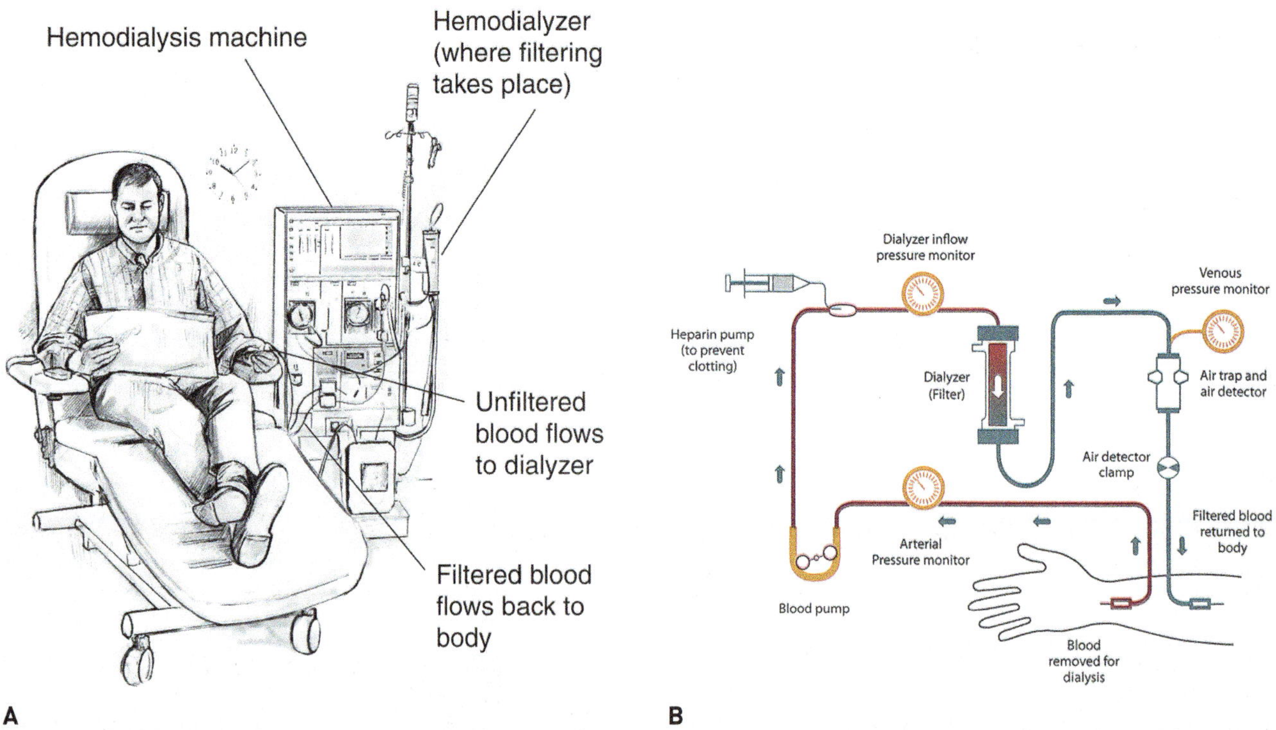

Figure 12.10 **A.** Hemodialysis Procedure **B.** Passage of Blood through a Dialyzer

A: Reproduced from National Institute of Diabetes and Digestive and Kidney Diseases, National Institutes of Health. https://www.niddk.nih.gov/news/media-library/17866; **B:** Reproduced from National Institute of Diabetes and Digestive and Kidney Diseases, National Institutes of Health. Hemodialysis. https://www.niddk.nih.gov/health-information/kidney-disease/kidney-failure/hemodialysis

of being exposed to pathogens, especially during the pandemic.[68] A study found that U.S. patients on home HD had 30–50% lower odds of getting COVID-19 and 30–60% lower odds of being hospitalized for COVID-19, compared to patients who received in-center HD.[69]

Satellite Hemodialysis

Patients on dialysis who are medically stable, but do not have a suitable home or dialysis partner to carry out home HD, can choose satellite HD. A satellite HD facility provides maintenance HD but without the highly specialized medical care as those provided in a specialized dialysis center.[68] The services available at a satellite HD facility may vary across different countries. Some sites may have a nephrologist, but some may not. Some sites may be called "self-care" HD centers where patients perform their own dialysis treatment with little professional assistance.

Home Hemodialysis

Home HD usually delivers a higher dialysis dose (could be customized to 5–7 times/week), and is associated with higher quality of life and lower societal burden.[68] Home HD may improve outcomes for a longer and better survival. However, it is important to keep in mind that only the most motivated, adherent, and medically stable patients will be selected as candidates for home HD. This population may naturally have better outcomes than those who are medically unstable, not motivated, and nonadherent. Home HD requires a high level of patient and caregiver participation. Barriers to home HD include medical instability, patient's fear of adverse events, psychosocial issues, caregiver burden, and government agency (lack of funding for home HD therapy).

Continuous Renal Replacement Therapy (CRRT)

Continuous renal replacement therapy (CRRT) is continuous hemodialysis over 24 hours. It removes solute and excess water at a much slower pace compared to regular HD (which removes solute and water over 4 hours). CRRT is usually for patients who are critically ill, hemodynamically unstable, and unable to tolerate regular HD since CRRT avoids rapid fluid shifts. CRRT requires close medical and nutrition monitoring as this population has elevated metabolic demands and protein losses during CRRT.[70]

Peritoneal Dialysis

In **peritoneal dialysis (PD)**, the peritoneum, a smooth tissue that lines the abdominopelvic cavity and surrounds the abdominal organs, is used as a natural semipermeable membrane.[66] PD dialysate is hyperosmotic as it contains dextrose, usually 1.5%, 2.5%, or 4.5%. Hyperosmolar dialysate that contains dextrose is infused into the abdominal cavity and is allowed to dwell for hours or overnight. During this process, dialysate is in close contact with the peritoneum and capillaries, allowing solutes and water to diffuse into dialysate. As water enters dialysate, its osmolarity gradually decreases and dialysate will eventually lose its osmotic gradient against blood in capillaries. For this reason, the dialysate needs to be changed regularly.

Patients on PD can be classified into "high transporters" or "low transporters."[66] High transporters reach creatinine and urea equilibrium quickly, and also absorb dextrose quickly, which results in a rapid loss of osmotic gradient. High transporters can benefit from short dwell time and more frequent dialysate exchange. On the other hand, low transporters reach creatinine and urea equilibrium slowly and the osmotic gradient can last longer. Low transporters can benefit from longer dwell time and less frequent dialysate exchange. The amount of dextrose absorption during PD may vary with dextrose concentration, dwell time, and individual's membrane characteristic.[71]

PD has multiple advantages[68]: better survival, more mobility and flexibility, and continuous treatment allows better solute and water removal allowing patients to follow a less restricted diet. PD helps to preserve residual kidney function, functions as a bridge to kidney transplant, and does not require vascular access. Figure 12.11 shows a patient receiving PD.

Types of Peritoneal Dialysis

Continuous Ambulatory Peritoneal Dialysis (CAPD)

With **continuous ambulatory peritoneal dialysis (CAPD)**, the abdominal cavity is always filled with dialysate. Patients usually receive a prescription of 2–2.5 L dialysate per bag with 3–5 exchanges daily. The exchange needs to be completed manually by draining the old dialysate via gravity and infusing fresh dialysate to allow another 3–5 hours of dwell time.

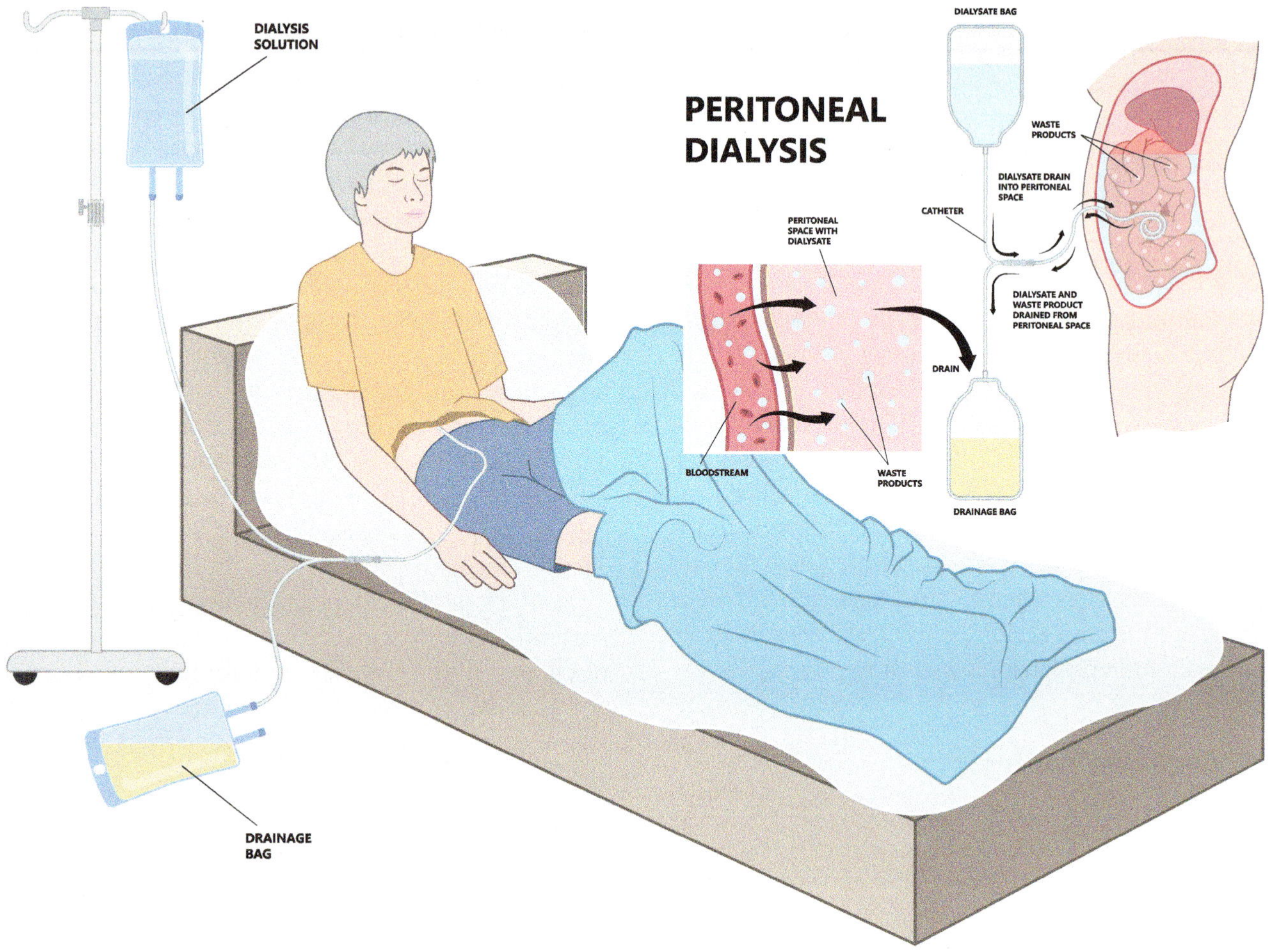

Figure 12.11 Peritoneal Dialysis

Automated Peritoneal Dialysis (APD)

In APD, dialysate exchanges are completely or partially carried out by machine. There are two forms of APD. The first one is **continuous cycling peritoneal dialysis (CCPD)**. CCPD is usually conducted overnight during sleep, using a machine to perform the dialysate exchanges. During the day, dialysate is maintained in the abdominal cavity and the patient may or may not need to perform manual exchanges based upon a physician's prescription. Another type is nocturnal intermittent peritoneal dialysis (NIPD). This method is like CCPD, except that the patient will not have dialysate dwelling during the day.

Nutrition Intervention

Protein calorie wasting is common among patients receiving dialysis. Nutritional goals should improve overall nutritional status and prevent poor outcomes associated with dialysis, such as hospitalization and increased morbidity and mortality. **Figure 12.12** shows the consequences of how poor nutrition can affect patients on dialysis.

Energy and Protein

Please refer to **Table 12.11** for the 2020 KDOQI nutrition recommendations for the dialysis population. To recap, the 2020 KDOQI guidelines recommend 25–35 kcal/kg/day energy with 1.0–1.2 grams/kg/day protein.[19] Energy and protein needs should be individually adjusted to best meet patients' clinical status. It is important to keep in mind that patients on PD may absorb a considerable amount of dextrose from dialysate (around 300 kcal/day), although this may vary with varying dialysis prescriptions.[71] Protein requirements of patients on CRRT may be as high as 2.0–2.5 grams/kg/day.[70]

Sodium and Fluid

Sodium and fluid recommendations also require individualization. These should be based on factors

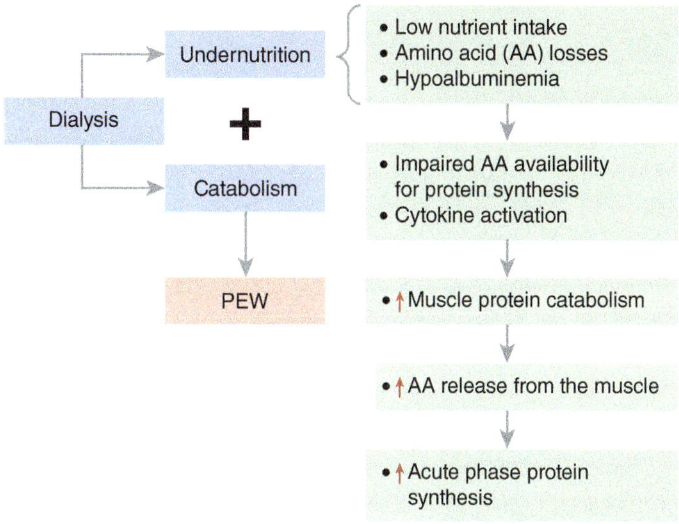

Figure 12.12 How Dialysis and Poor Nutrient Intake Leads to Protein Energy Wasting (PEW)

Data from Ikizler TA, Cano NJ, Franch H, et al. Prevention and treatment of protein energy wasting in chronic kidney disease patients: a consensus statement by the International Society of Renal Nutrition and Metabolism. *Kidney Int.* 2013;84(6):1096-1107.; Carrero JJ, Stenvinkel P, Cuppari L, et al. Etiology of the protein-energy wasting syndrome in chronic kidney disease: a consensus statement from the International Society of Renal Nutrition and Metabolism (ISRNM). *J Ren Nutr.* 2013;23(2):77-90.

Table 12.11 KDOQI Nutrition Recommendation for ESKD

Nutrient	Recommendation for HD	Recommendation for PD
Protein	1.0–1.2 grams/kg/day	
Energy	25–35 kcal/kg	
Fluid	1–1.5 L/day	1.3 L based on urine output
Sodium	<100 mmol/day (less than 2.3 grams/day)	
Potassium	Adjust dietary potassium intake to maintain serum levels within normal range In patients with hyper- or hypokalemia, dietary or supplemental intake should be based on the patient's individual needs and clinical judgment	
Calcium	Avoid excessive calcium loads and avoid calcium-based binders	
Phosphorus	Adjust dietary phosphorus intake to maintain serum levels within normal range Consider the bioavailability of the phosphorus sources	
Micronutrients	Water-soluble vitamins: usually supplemented Fat-soluble vitamins: avoid supplements except vitamin D if insufficient Other micronutrients: not usually supplemented	

Data from Ikizler TA, Burrowes JD, Byham-Gray LD, et al. KDOQI clinical practice guideline for nutrition in CKD: 2020 update. *Am J Kidney Dis.* 2020;76(3 suppl 1):S1-S107.

including a patient's fluid status, urine output, blood pressure, interdialytic weight gains (IDWG), and residual kidney function. For both patients on HD or PD, a sodium intake of <2.3 grams/day is still the ideal recommendation.[16] For patients on HD who can produce >1 L urine/day, a 2 L fluid/day recommendation is reasonable. For patients on HD who produce <1 L urine/day, fluid should be restricted to 1–1.5 L/day. For patients with oliguria on HD, a fluid allowance should be 750 mL daily plus the amount of urine output over 24 hours. For example, if a patient with oliguria on HD urinates 600 mL/day, the recommended fluid restriction would be 1350 mL/day. For patients on PD, daily fluid intake should be adequate to maintain a daily fluid balance and avoid hypertonic exchanges.

Clinical Roundtable

Topic: Balancing Protein Restriction with Malnutrition in CKD

Background: Protein is an essential part of the diet and is needed to maintain lean body mass. It is even more important to prevent malnutrition during chronic illness because malnutrition can contribute to poor outcomes. Consuming a diet high in animal protein can increase the release of glucagon, insulin-like growth factor, and kinins, and can increase reabsorption of sodium in the proximal tubule, all of which have been shown to increase GFR.[1] An increase in GFR in kidney disease is not preferable, because this can put higher stress on the damaged kidneys and exacerbate the damage to cause an ultimate decline in kidney function. Some studies have shown that limiting dietary protein slows the progression of CKD and delays the need for RRT,[1-4] and others have found that protein restriction may increase mortality risk.[5] Others have come up inconclusive, or have found that plant-based protein intake does not have as severe an effect on kidney function as animal protein sources.[6,7] In the absence of conclusive evidence as to whether or not protein restriction in CKD improves survival or increases malnutrition-related mortality, clinicians must analyze the available research and use their clinical judgment when following professional guidelines from sources such as KDIGO and KDOQI.

Roundtable Discussion: Consider the risks and benefits associated with dietary protein restriction during CKD.

1. Do you think protein should be restricted in all patients with CKD?
2. Are there any situations in which dietary protein restriction would benefit a patient?
3. How would you educate your patient on a protein restriction of 0.8 gram/kg/day, and what are some techniques you could suggest to increase the palatability and caloric density of a protein-restricted meal plan?

References

1. Chapman AB, Rahbari-Oskoui FF, Cook J, Rizk DV. 39 - Polycystic and other cystic kidney diseases. In: Gilbert SJ, Weiner DE, Bomback AS, Perazella MA, Rifkin DE, eds. *National Kidney Foundation's Primer on Kidney Diseases*. 8th ed. Elsevier; 2023:375–386.
2. Dell KM. The spectrum of polycystic kidney disease in children. *Adv Chronic Kidney Dis*. 2011;18(5): 339–347. doi:10.1053/j.ackd.2011.05.001
3. Sans-Atxer L, Joly D. Tolvaptan in the treatment of autosomal dominant polycystic kidney disease: patient selection and special considerations. *Int J Nephrol Renovasc Dis*. 2018;11:41–51. doi:10.2147/ijnrd.S125942
4. Chebib FT, Nowak KL, Chonchol MB, et al. Polycystic kidney disease diet: what is known and what is safe. *Clin J Am Soc Nephrol*. 2024;19(5): 664–682. doi:10.2215/CJN.0000000000000326
5. Torres JA, Kruger SL, Broderick C, et al. Ketosis ameliorates renal cyst growth in polycystic kidney disease. *Cell Metab*. 2019;30(6):1007–1023 e5. doi:10.1016/j.cmet.2019.09.012
6. Torres JA, Rezaei M, Broderick C, et al. Crystal deposition triggers tubule dilation that accelerates cystogenesis in polycystic kidney disease. *J Clin Invest*. 2019;129(10):4506–4522. doi:10.1172/JCI128503
7. Cukoski S, Lindemann CH, Arjune S, et al. Feasibility and impact of ketogenic dietary interventions in polycystic kidney disease: KETO-ADPKD-a randomized controlled trial. *Cell Rep Med*. 2023;4(11):101283. doi:10.1016/j.xcrm.2023.101283

Potassium, Phosphorus, and Calcium

The 2020 KDOQI guidelines no longer recommend specific potassium and phosphorus restrictions. Serum levels should be monitored and maintained in the goal range. But for patients with persistent hyperkalemia or hyperphosphatemia, diet counseling to avoid higher potassium/phosphorus sources is recommended. Potassium and phosphorus binder medications are also an option. Potassium is better controlled with PD than HD, and patients on PD may be encouraged to add potassium sources to their diet if their levels are trending down. Calcium should also be maintained within the goal range. Total calcium intake should be around 800–1000 mg/day, including dietary sources, supplements, and calcium-containing binders.[16]

Water-soluble vitamins (thiamine, riboflavin, folic acid, vitamin B6, vitamin B12, niacin, biotin, pantothenic acid, vitamin C) should be supplemented as needed. A dialysis-specific vitamin that contains a mixture of water-soluble vitamins is recommended daily.

CORE CONCEPT 7

Patients receiving renal replacement therapy can tolerate higher protein, fluid, and electrolyte levels than patients with chronic kidney disease alone, so recommendations should be individualized to each patient.

Dialysis Adequacy

Kinetic modeling is used to evaluate the effectiveness of HD treatment. Kinetic modeling involves complex mathematical processes using computerized systems, but the basic equation used is Kt/V, where **K** stands for dialyzer clearance in milliliters/minute, **t** stands for the amount of time spent on treatment, and **v** stands for the patient's total body water volume.[72] A Kt/v of 1.2 or better is recommended. Another method of determining dialysis efficacy is the calculation of the **urea reduction ratio (URR)**. This calculation indicates the reduction in the amount of urea as a result of the treatment. A goal of at least 65% clearance is recommended. Kt/V and URR are more useful when used to determine the weekly average after all dialysis treatments because the results can vary greatly depending on the patient and the day of treatment. An abnormally low Kt/V should not be a cause for concern if the patient's weekly average Kt/V meets the goal of 1.2.[72]

In PD, the peritoneal equilibration test (PET) is done by collecting a blood sample and samples of used dialysate solutions.[73] PET measures how much dextrose was absorbed and how much urea and creatinine entered the dialysate during a 4-hour dwell. From these data, Kt/V can be calculated.

PRACTICE POINT

Patients receiving renal replacement therapy should have recommendations individualized to each patient. This includes the patient's treatment, diet, and cultural and social considerations.

PRACTICE POINT

Nutrition intervention needs to be ongoing and collaborative with the interdisciplinary team to assist patients in attaining and maintaining a higher quality of life.

Monitoring and Evaluation

Monitoring oral intake is important in the dialysis population. There are several factors that can negatively impact food intake, including uremia, which can lead to nausea and vomiting, especially for those new to dialysis; fatigue, which is a common side effect of HD and anemia; early satiety due to the dialysate dwelling in the peritoneum in PD; constipation due to reduced fluid intake and possibly reduced activity; possible taste changes; and confusion related to the complexity of the diet. Psychosocial impacts of the dialysis regimen, which can also affect appetite and intake, include depression due to lower quality of life, and loneliness and possible reduced income due to the frequency of dialysis therapy interfering with the ability to work. Since protein guidelines are more liberalized once a patient with CKD starts dialysis, ensuring a patient is not overly restricting their protein intake is key. Evaluation of intake on both HD and non-HD days is important to assess overall (average) energy and protein provision, especially as patients may eat significantly less on HD days due to fatigue. Biochemical assessment is critical with regular evaluation of electrolytes including sodium, potassium, chloride, bicarbonate, and creatinine, BUN, phosphorus, and magnesium. It is important to note that the increased levels are common in patients with CKD on dialysis. Low or normal biochemical values may be an indicator of poor intake. Intermittent assessment of iron studies, lipid panels, bone mineral disorder makers, and proteins such as albumin, prealbumin, and CRP are important components of care. Checking glucose and hemoglobin A1c levels is vital for those with DKD and may be helpful for those on PD due to the passive glucose absorption of the dialysate. The nutrition-focused physical exam should be monitoring for signs of protein energy wasting, including muscle or fat wasting, as well as edema. Patients with CKD on dialysis should be monitored for changes in post-dialysis weights to track trends since fluid fluctuations are common. Finally, assessment of dialysis adequacy is vital through kinetic modeling, urea reduction ratio, and peritoneal equilibrium testing.

Nephrotic Syndrome

Nephrotic syndrome is a clinical condition characterized by massive protein loss via urine (proteinuria, or >3.5 grams/day), which results in hypoalbuminemia (<30 g/L) and other complications including, but not limited to, hyperlipidemia, hypercoagulability, edema, volume overload, hypocalcemia, and bone abnormalities.[74] Nephrotic syndrome affects people of all ages but is more common in children (1.15–16.9 per 100,000 children),[75] especially males before adolescence. In adults, it affects both sexes equally.

The nephron is the functional unit of the kidney consisting of the glomerulus, which contains capillaries optimized for filtration. Nephrotic syndrome occurs when the glomerulus structures (basement membrane, endothelial surface, or podocytes) are damaged, leading to the loss of large protein molecules.[74] This could result in multiple complications,

⚠ Clinical Controversy

Intradialytic Parenteral Nutrition

Due to the high risk of malnutrition associated with long-term HD, it is imperative to find a method of nutrient administration to replace those nutrients lost during HD that has been clinically proven to improve outcomes. **Intradialytic parenteral nutrition (IDPN)** has been proposed as a way to prevent the development of malnutrition during long-term HD in patients with CKD, with an advantage being ease-of-use. The infusion can occur simultaneously with HD because it is possible to use the same venous access for both therapies. Studies such as that by Marsen et al. demonstrated that IDPN improves the nutritional status of patients with CKD on long-term HD. However, other studies such as a systematic review by Anderson et al. found that IDPN did not improve clinically relevant outcomes and does not recommend broad usage of IDPN.

Questions

1. Based upon this research, discuss how you would proceed with a patient on long-term HD showing signs of malnutrition in whom enteral nutrition is contraindicated.
2. How would you balance the risks associated with PN with the patient's need for adequate nutrition?

References

1. Marsen TA, Beer J, Mann H, German. IDPN-Trial group. Intradialytic parenteral nutrition in maintenance hemodialysis patients suffering from protein-energy wasting. Results of a multicenter, open, prospective, randomized trial. *Clin Nutr.* 2017;36:107–117.
2. Anderson J, Peterson K, Bourne D, Boundy E. Effectiveness of intradialytic parenteral nutrition in treating protein-energy wasting in hemodialysis: a rapid systematic review. *J Ren Nutr.* 2019;29(5):361–369.

including hypoalbuminemia, hypercoagulability, dyslipidemia, infection, and bone mineral density disease.

Multiple Complications of Nephrotic Syndrome

Hypoalbuminemia

Albumin is the most abundant protein in the blood. The loss of albumin through urine can cause hypoalbuminemia and lead to reduced plasma oncotic pressure. This drives water into interstitial spaces and can lead to peripheral edema.

Hypercoagulability

Anticoagulant proteins are also lost through urine, manifesting as hypercoagulability and can predispose patients to arterial and venous thrombosis.[76]

Dyslipidemia

Lipid metabolism is altered in nephrotic syndrome.[77] Due to the loss of protein through urine, the liver is stimulated to produce more protein, including lipoprotein. However, there is less available lipoprotein lipase to break down the additional lipoprotein. This leads to dyslipidemia, which is often underrecognized but nearly universal in patients with nephrotic syndrome.

Infection

Circulating immunoglobulins and complement factors are lost through urine, leading to lower immune function and higher infection risk. Peripheral edema can also predispose the site to infection.[76]

Bone Mineral Density Disease

Vitamin D-binding protein is lost through urine, resulting in lower circulating 1,25-dihydroxyvitamin D levels to promote bone health.[78] Steroid therapy for nephrotic syndrome is also a common contributor to bone mineral density disease.

Causes and Diagnosis

The causes of nephrotic syndrome can be divided into primary causes and secondary causes.[79] Primary causes include intrinsic kidney diseases that can result in kidney damage, such as minimal change nephropathy, focal glomerulosclerosis, and membranous nephropathy. Secondary causes refer to systemic diseases that can affect the kidneys, such as lupus erythematosus, diabetes mellitus, amyloidosis, and human immunodeficiency virus (HIV). The diagnosis of nephrotic syndrome is made upon evaluation of three aspects: heavy proteinuria, hypoalbuminemia, and edema. The diagnosis criteria are presented in **Table 12.12**.

Nutrition Intervention

As previously explained, nephrotic syndrome is characterized by massive protein loss via urine. However, an early clinical trial has shown that a high-protein diet did not replenish the serum albumin level.[80] On

Table 12.12 Diagnostic Criteria for Nephrotic Syndrome

Clinical Parameter	Criteria
Proteinuria	Spot urine: protein-to-creatinine ratio >3–3.5 mg protein/mg creatinine or 300–350 mg/mmol Or 24-hour urine collection >3–3.5 grams protein
Hypoalbuminemia	Serum albumin <2.5 grams/dL
Edema	Clinical evidence of peripheral edema
Hyperlipidemia (not required for diagnosis)	Total cholesterol >350 mg/dL

Data from Kodner C. Diagnosis and management of nephrotic syndrome in adults. *Am Fam Physician*. 2016;93(6):479-485. https://www.aafp.org/pubs/afp/issues/2016/0315/p479.html#afp20160315p479-b1.

the contrary, the high protein diet group (2 grams/ideal body weight/day) resulted in increased proteinuria and serum levels, which may contribute to further kidney damage and disease progression. It is suggested that patients with nephrotic syndrome consume 0.8–1.0 gram/kg/day of protein.[81] To prevent calorie protein malnutrition, 35 kcal/kg/day is recommended, unless the weight loss is desired. Due to the risk of dyslipidemia and cardiovascular disease, saturated fat and cholesterol intake should be limited, if able. Sodium and fluid restriction may be necessary to help control fluid overload based on a patient's clinical status. The limitations in protein and fat bring the necessity of increasing the calorie percentage from carbohydrate to meet elevated calorie needs. Complex carbohydrates are recommended for better glycemic control in this case. It is important to keep in mind that fat and carbohydrate intake should be individually adjusted to best fit the patient's clinical status. For example, if patients are experiencing poor glycemic control, the RD should consider lowering the carbohydrate recommendation and increasing fat recommendation. Iron, zinc, and calcium are commonly deficient in nephrotic syndrome due to the loss of the carrier proteins in the urine. Iron, zinc, calcium, and vitamin D supplementations are important if the patient is found to have a deficiency. **Table 12.13** summarizes nutrition recommendations for nephrotic syndrome.

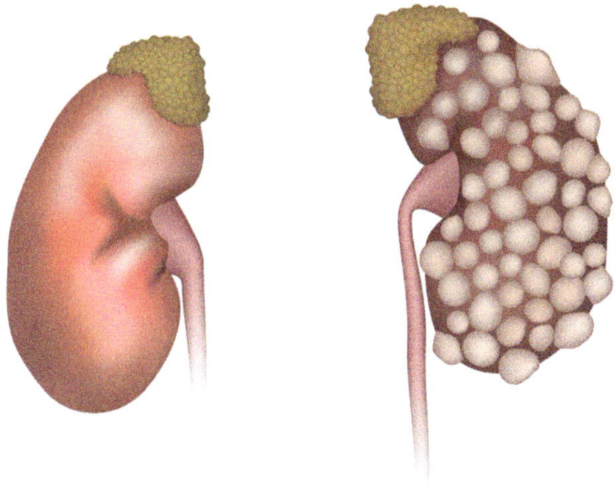

Figure 12.13 Polycystic Kidney Disease

Monitoring and Evaluation

Patients with nephrotic syndrome should be monitored for signs of fluid overload including weight trends and nutrition-focused physical findings of edema. Biochemical assessment should include electrolytes, particularly sodium, albumin, a lipid panel, iron studies, zinc, corrected calcium, and vitamin D levels. Assessment of oral intake is critical to ensure increased energy and moderate protein intake.

PRACTICE POINT

Dietary recommendations should always be individualized for patients with nephrotic syndrome based on other existing clinical conditions, especially conditions that may alter energy and protein requirements, such as cancer, sepsis, and colitis.

Polycystic Kidney Disease

Autosomal dominant polycystic kidney disease (ADPKD), the most common monogenic cause of ESKD, is development of kidney cysts, hypertension, and destruction of the kidney parenchyma (**Figure 12.13**).[82] ADPKD is the most common inherited kidney disorder, occurring in 1 of 400 to 1000 live births, and it is the most common of all hereditary cystic disorders. ADPKD affects all ethnic groups equally, and it has been reported worldwide. It accounts for approximately 5% of the ESKD population in the United States and 10% of those under 60 years of age.[83] ADPKD is a systemic disorder that affects

Table 12.13 Nutrition Recommendations for Nephrotic Syndrome

Category	Recommendation	Notes
Energy	35 kcal/kg/day Unless obese	Adjust based on clinical status. Should be adequate to prevent protein utilization for fuel.
Protein	0.8–1.0 gram/kg/day	High protein intake may result in worsening proteinuria and renal damage.
Fat	<30% of total energy <200 mg/day cholesterol 10% polyunsaturated fatty acids	Adjust based on clinical status and glycemic control.
Carbohydrate	High complex carbohydrate if clinical condition allows	Adjust based on clinical status and glycemic control.
Sodium	1–2 grams/day	Liberalize if clinical status allows.
Phosphorus	<12 mg/kg/day	Restrict only if necessary.
Calcium	1000–1500 mg/day Do not exceed 2000 mg/day Supplement and calcium-containing binders combined	Calcium binds to albumin in blood. Loss of albumin results in lower calcium level. Loss of vitamin D-binding protein also results in lower calcium level.

Data from Academy of Nutrition and Dietetics. *Nutrition Care Manual: Nephrotic syndrome*. Academy of Nutrition and Dietetics; 2024. Accessed September 22, 2024.

almost every organ, resulting in significant extrarenal manifestations; however, its hallmark is the gradual and massive cystic enlargement of the kidneys, ultimately resulting in kidney failure.[84] Autosomal recessive polycystic kidney disease (ARPKD) occurs in 1 in 20,000 live births, and early onset ARPKD is more severe than ADPKD with faster progression of ESKD.[85]

Total kidney volume (TKV) incorporates all the aforementioned clinical and genetic risk factors and is the strongest predictor of future GFR loss. Transplantation is a viable treatment for PKD. The medication tolvaptan (Jynarque, Samsca) may be used for adults at risk of ADPKD to slow cyst growth. However, it increases the risk of liver damage, so close monitoring of liver function is necessary.[86]

Nutrition Intervention

The goal for nutrition recommendations for PKD is to slow cyst growth through sodium restriction, increased hydration, moderate caloric restriction, and moderate protein restriction for patients with declining kidney function.[87]

Recently, time-restricted feeding and a plant-based ketogenic diet with supplementation of beta-hydroxy butyrate (BHB) have demonstrated decreased cyst growth in animal studies[88,89]; however, the results in humans have not been as effective as in animal studies.[90] **Table 12.14** summarizes the most recent dietary recommendations for ADPKD.[91]

Monitoring and Evaluation

Patients with PKD should be monitored for the progression of CKD including eGFR levels, electrolytes such as sodium, potassium, chloride, and bicarbonate, as well as serum creatinine, BUN, phosphorus, and magnesium levels. If kidney function is declining, assessment of oral intake to ensure moderate energy and moderate protein consumption is important. For patients receiving tolvaptan, monitor liver function tests.

PRACTICE POINT

Patients with PKD have different stages of CKD. Diet and fluid recommendations should be based on CKD stage, medication use, and electrolyte balance, especially serum sodium and potassium levels.

Kidney Stones

Kidney stones, or nephrolithiasis, are hard deposits formed by the crystallization of substances like calcium, oxalate, or uric acid in the urine.[92] They can affect the entire urinary system, including the kidney, bladder, and ureters. Small stones often go unnoticed, but passing them can cause severe, sharp abdominal pain that radiates to the side of the back. Additional symptoms may include nausea, vomiting, hematuria, and urinary tract infection. Large stones can lead to urinary obstruction. The prevalence of kidney stones

Table 12.14 Summary of Diet Recommendation for ADPKD

Nutrients	Recommendation	Comments
Water	>2 L/day	Decrease vasopressin, prevent kidney stones Need to be adjusted for medications and minimize hyponatremia
Sodium	<2 grams/day or <5 grams salt	High Na related to kidney volume in ADPKD Avoid processed foods
Protein	0.8–1.0 gram/kg/day	Increase plant-based protein than animal protein Do not exceed protein >1.3 grams/kg/day
Calories	25–35 kcal/kg/day Individualize based on weight status	BMI >25 can be associated with faster progression of ADPKD
Caffeine	<400 mg/day	General recommendation by the World Health Organization
General	Well-balanced foods Increased fruits and vegetables, whole grain, fiber, legumes, plant-based protein, nuts, and less fat Less, processed foods, refined carbohydrates, and sweets	Overall high fruits and vegetable consumption except high starch foods More fiber consumption Dietary Guidelines for Americans 2020–2025

Data from Kidney Disease: Improving Global Outcomes (KDIGO). KDIGO 2023 clinical practice guideline for the evaluation, management, and treatment of autosomal dominant polycystic kidney disease (ADPKD) [public review draft]. 2023.; Chebib FT, Nowak KL, Chonchol MB, et al. Polycystic kidney disease diet: what is known and what is safe. *Clin J Am Soc Nephrol*. 2024;19(5):664-682.

CASE STUDY REVISITED

Dean develops acute onset of severe sharp left-sided abdominal pain that radiates to his back. A CT is obtained and shows a kidney stone in his left kidney. The attending physician and nephrologist think that a calcium stone is the most likely stone type in his situation. Dean reports experiencing anorexia, nausea, and an "unpleasant taste in his mouth" in this admission.

Anthropometric Data:

Weight: 88 kg

Biochemical Data:

Sodium 129 (136–145 mEq/L)
Potassium 5.9 (3.5–5.0 mEq/L)
Chloride 115 (96–106 mEq/L)
Carbon dioxide 19 (22–31 mEq/L)
Blood urea nitrogen 89 (8–20 mg/dL)
Creatinine 4.2 (0.7–1.3 mg/dL)
Glucose 99 (70–139 mg/dL)
Calcium 7.2 (8.5–10.5 mg/dL)
Phosphorus 8.8 (2.5–4.5 mg/dL)

Dietary Data:

24-Hour Dietary Recall:
Breakfast (8 am): 1 banana, 8 oz orange juice
Lunch (12 pm): ½ tuna sandwich on whole wheat bread, 8 oz water
Snack (3 pm): Small coffee with cream and sugar, 3 oatmeal cookies
Dinner (7 pm): 1½ cups pasta with tomato sauce and 1 meatball; 1 cup garden salad with romaine lettuce, carrots, and tomatoes with Italian dressing; 16 oz diet cola

Diet Prescription: 2 grams sodium, 2 grams potassium diet

Questions

1. What are Dean's kidney stone risk factors?
2. The nephrology team is requesting your advice on his diet prescription. What would you recommend?
3. What specific diet changes do you suggest (considering Dean's CKD and kidney stone)?

in the United States is 9.9%.[93] Kidney stones are more common in males, individuals with obesity, and non-Hispanic White people.[94]

Stone Types and Causes

Kidney stones are classified by stone content. Calcium stones, including calcium oxalate stones and calcium phosphate stones, are the two most common stone types. They make up 80% of all kidney stone cases.[92] Uric acid stones are less common, followed by the mineral struvite. Stone formation begins with supersaturation and crystallization.[95] Supersaturation occurs when the concentration of a substance in the urine exceeds its maximum solubility, leading to the formation of crystals. Crystals grow larger over time, aggregate with each other, and eventually leads to stone precipitation.[96] Inadequate fluid intake and concentrated urine significantly contribute to stone formation by promoting supersaturation. Increased urinary calcium, oxalate, or uric acid levels also contribute to stone formation. Additionally, urinary pH plays a crucial role in determining the solubility of substances in the urine. Acidic urine favors calcium oxalate and uric acid stone formation, whereas alkaline urine favors calcium phosphate and struvite stones.[97] Genetic and disease states can also affect the risk of kidney stones. For example, amino acid cystine stones are the result of a genetic disorder that is characterized by cystinuria.[92] Gout may lead to increased urinary uric acid excretion contributing to uric acid stones. Overactive parathyroid activity can cause hypercalciuria, which increases the risk of calcium stones. Individuals who have undergone malabsorptive GI procedures, such as a Roux-en-Y gastric bypass or small bowel resections, may experience fat malabsorption.[98] Fat malabsorption causes more calcium and fatty acids to saponify in the intestine, reducing calcium's availability to bind with oxalate. This increases oxalate's availability for absorption and can lead to hyperoxaluria, promoting calcium oxalate stones.

Nutrition Intervention

Fluid

As mentioned, supersaturation is the direct cause of stone formation. Therefore, increasing fluid intake is essential to reduce kidney stone risk. Fluid intake should be adjusted to produce 2.5 L urine/day.[99,100] However, fluid type matters. Sugar-sweetened soda, artificially sweetened soda, punch, and grapefruit juice are associated with higher stone risk.[101,102] Coffee, tea, beer, wine, and orange juice are found to lower stone risk.

Sodium

A high-sodium diet is known to cause hypercalciuria and contribute to calcium stones.[103] Therefore, sodium restriction is also essential in preventing and treating kidney stones. It is recommended that individuals limit sodium intake to 2300 mg/day.[99]

Protein

Animal protein is rich in sulfur-containing amino acids, which can act as acid precursors in the body. A diet high in animal protein is linked to increased risk of kidney stones, as it promotes chronic low-grade metabolic acidosis that requires the kidneys to excrete more acid via urine leading to lower urinary pH.[104] As mentioned, acidic urine favors the formation of calcium oxalate and uric acid stones. A moderate protein intake of 0.8–1.2 grams/kg is recommended to prevent stone formation.[99,100] Individuals should incorporate a variety of protein sources such as seafood, dairy, and plant-based proteins, and a moderate amount of red meat and limit aged, hard cheeses.

Calcium

Hypercalciuria is an important kidney stone risk factor. Diets high in sodium and animal protein are associated with hypercalciuria.[103,105] As previously mentioned, sodium restriction and keeping a moderate animal protein intake are ways to prevent kidney stone formation by reducing urinary calcium. It is important to know that dietary calcium restriction is not effective in reducing hypercalciuria. On the contrary, adequate dietary calcium intake is associated with a reduction in kidney stone risk.[106] This is because adequate dietary calcium intake binds with dietary oxalate in the GI tract, which lowers oxalate's bioavailability and reduces urinary oxalate excretion. A daily intake of 800–1200 mg calcium is recommended with meals for stone prevention purposes.[99,100] For this reason, in a moderate animal protein diet, dairy foods that are low in sodium should still be allowed.

Oxalate

Hyperoxaluria contributes to calcium oxalate stone formation, and adequate dietary calcium intake is important to reduce hyperoxaluria. High dietary oxalate intake is associated with increased stone risk.[107] Commonly consumed high-oxalate foods are spinach, whole potatoes, rhubarb, and beets, for example. Dietary oxalate restriction might be needed in patients with recurrent kidney stones, but it is not generally recommended. To follow an oxalate-restricted diet, a reliable food oxalate content database is required.

Table 12.15 Dietary Recommendations for Kidney Stones

Nutrients	Recommendation	Notes
Fluid	>3.0 L/day	Adjust based on 24-hour urine volume to produce 2.5 L urine/day.
Protein	0.8–1.2 grams/kg/day	Moderate protein intake for otherwise healthy stone formers. Encourage moderate animal protein, increase plant-based protein.
Calcium	8000–1200 mg/day	Focus on fresh dairy (milk and yogurt) that are lower in sodium. Limit hard, aged cheeses that are high in sodium. Recommend calcium-fortified non-dairy milk for those who need protein restriction.
Sodium	2300 mg/day	Important for all stone types.
Oxalate	Limit foods high in oxalate. Consume oxalate-rich foods with calcium-rich foods at the same time.	
Citrate	Take potassium citrate as directed by doctor. Increase dietary citrate intake: lemon and lime juice. Recommend more fruits and vegetables to produce more alkaline.	
Vitamin C	Adult males: 90 mg/day Adult females: 75 mg/day High dose of vitamin C >1000 mg/day should be avoided.	

Data from Han H, Segal AM, Siefter JL, Dwyer JT. Nutritional management of kidney stones (nephrolithiasis). *Clin Nutr Res*. 2015;4(3):137-152.; Pearle MS, Goldfarb DS, Assimos DG, et al. Medical management of kidney stones: AUA guideline. *J Urol*. 2014;192(2):316-324.; Akram M, Jahrreiss V, Skolarikos A, et al. Urological guidelines for kidney stones: overview and comprehensive update. *J Clin Med*. 2024;13(4).

However, oxalate content may vary in a single food depending on ripeness, cooking method, food processing techniques, and soil quality.[108] Therefore, instead of an oxalate-restricted diet, consuming oxalate-rich foods with calcium-rich foods is recommended to help reduce the availability of oxalate in the GI tract.

Vitamin C

Vitamin C is an important nutrient for normal physiological function. Vitamin C is partially converted to oxalate and excreted in urine. A study has shown that high vitamin C intake (>500 mg/day, foods and supplements combined) was associated with higher kidney stone risk in males.[109] However, dietary vitamin C intake alone exceeding 700 mg/day was not associated with higher stone risk. Multivitamins that contain some vitamin C were also not associated with higher stone risk.[110] It is reasonable to recommend that patients with kidney stones consume vitamin C from foods but not vitamin C supplements and follow the Dietary Reference Intake (DRI) levels (90 mg/day for adult males, 75 mg/day for adult females).[111]

Citrate and Phytates

Citrate is a stone inhibitor. It is abundant in citrus fruits such as lemons, oranges, limes, etc. Citrate can form soluble complexes with calcium ions in the urine to prevent calcium supersaturation and crystal aggregation.[112] Potassium citrate can effectively improve urinary citrate levels and increase urinary pH in patients with kidney stones.[113] Phytate is a substance found in plants, rich in legumes, nuts, seeds, and whole grains. It can bind to multiple minerals in the GI tract to inhibit absorption, including oxalate absorption. It has been found that calcium oxalate stone formers have significantly lower urinary phytate levels compared to healthy controls, and low dietary phytate is associated with a significant reduction in urinary phytate.[114] Females who consume more dietary phytate have significantly lower kidney stone risk.[115] It is reasonable to recommend higher legume, nut, and seed intake for patients with kidney stones, as it will not only help to increase phytate intake but also lower the percentage of animal protein intake. Dietary recommendations for kidney stones are summarized in **Table 12.15**.[99,100,116]

PRACTICE POINT

For patients with kidney stones, increasing fluid intake is the most important recommendation and should always be prioritized.

Monitoring and Evaluation

Monitoring of dietary composition, particularly intake of dietary sodium and calcium, animal protein, fruit, vegetable, and high-oxalate food intake is important for patients with kidney stones. Evaluation of the amount and type of fluid intake is critical. Assess dietary supplement usage, such as vitamin C intake above the DRI. Finally, since kidney stones are more common among those with obesity, weight trends should be followed.

Summary

There are different types of kidney disease including AKI, CKD (non-dialysis), ESKD, nephrotic syndrome, PKD, and kidney stones. Each disease has unique characteristics and each treatment is different. MNT should be based on the causes and work with medical treatment to optimize nutritional status. RDs should consider patients' cultural background and medical management and provide individualized diet education.

Key Terms

nephrons, glomerulus, Bowman's capsule, ultrafiltrate, tubules, ureters, glomerular filtration rate (GFR), adaptive hyperfiltration, antidiuretic hormone (ADH), nitrogenous waste, erythropoietin (EPO), acute kidney injury (AKI), chronic kidney disease (CKD), kidney disease improving global outcomes (KDIGO), estimated glomerular filtration rate (eGFR), urea kinetic modeling (UKM), Kidney Disease Outcome Quality Initiative (KDOQI), renal replacement therapy (RRT), prerenal AKI, intrinsic AKI, postrenal AKI, continuous renal replacement therapy (CRRT), end-stage kidney disease (ESKD), chronic kidney disease (CKD), end-stage renal disease (ESRD), polycystic kidney disease (PKD), standard body weight (SBW), adjusted edema-free body weight (aBW_{ef}), phosphate binders, hemodialysis (HD), kinetic modeling, urea reduction ratio (URR), peritoneal dialysis (PD), continuous ambulatory peritoneal dialysis (CAPD), continuous cycling peritoneal dialysis (CCPD), normalized protein nitrogen appearance (nPNA), intradialytic parenteral nutrition (IDPN), nephrotic syndrome

References

1. Kovesdy CP. Epidemiology of chronic kidney disease: an update 2022. *Kidney Int Suppl (2011)*. 2022;12(1):7–11. doi:10.1016/j.kisu.2021.11.003
2. Francis A, Harhay MN, Ong ACM, et al. Chronic kidney disease and the global public health agenda: an international consensus. *Nat Rev Nephrol*. 2024;20(7):473–485. doi:10.1038/s41581-024-00820-6
3. Centers for Disease Control and Prevention, System KDS. Tracking & Preventing Kidney Disease in America. Accessed July 15, 2024. https://nccd.cdc.gov/CKD/default.aspx
4. Hoenig MP, Hladik GA. 1 - Overview of kidney structure and function. In: Gilbert SJ, Weiner DE, Bomback AS, Perazella MA, Rifkin DE, eds. *National Kidney Foundation's Primer on Kidney Diseases*. 8th ed. Elsevier; 2023:2–18.
5. Skorecki K, Chertow GM, Marsden PA, Taal MW, Yu ASL. *Brenner & Rector's the Kidney*. 10th ed. Elsevier; 2016.
6. Metcalfe W. How does early chronic kidney disease progress? A background paper prepared for the UK Consensus Conference on early chronic kidney disease. *Nephrol Dial Transplant*. 2007;22 Suppl 9:ix26–30. doi:10.1093/ndt/gfm446
7. Helal I, Fick-Brosnahan GM, Reed-Gitomer B, Schrier RW. Glomerular hyperfiltration: definitions, mechanisms and clinical implications. *Nat Rev Nephrol*. 2012;8(5):293–300. doi:10.1038/nrneph.2012.19
8. Fogo AB. Mechanisms of progression of chronic kidney disease. *Pediatr Nephrol*. 2007;22(12):2011–2022. doi:10.1007/s00467-007-0524-0
9. Sands JM, Layton HE. The physiology of urinary concentration: an update. *Semin Nephrol*. 2009;29(3):178–195. doi:10.1016/j.semnephrol.2009.03.008
10. Inker LA, Levey AS. 3 - Assessment of kidney function in acute and chronic settings. In: Gilbert SJ, Weiner DE, Bomback AS, Perazella MA, Rifkin DE, eds. *National Kidney Foundation's Primer on Kidney Diseases*. 8th ed. Elsevier; 2023:26–32.
11. Levin A, Stevens PE. Summary of KDIGO 2012 CKD Guidelines: Behind the scenes, need for guidance, and a framework for moving forward. *Kidney Int*. 2014;85(1):49–61. doi:10.1038/ki.2013.444
12. Inker LA, Eneanya ND, Coresh J, et al. New creatinine- and cystatin c-based equations to estimate GFR without race. *N Engl J Med*. 2021;385(19):1737–1749. doi:10.1056/NEJMoa2102953
13. Bhatraju PK, Zelnick LR, Chinchilli VM, et al. Association between early recovery of kidney function after acute kidney injury and long-term clinical outcomes. *JAMA Netw Open*. 2020;3(4):e202682. doi:10.1001/jamanetwork open.2020.2682
14. Matovinovic MS. 1. Pathophysiology and Classification of Kidney Diseases. *EJIFCC*. 2009;20(1):2–11.
15. National Institute of Diabetes and Digestive and Kidney Disease. Kidney Disease. National Institute of Health. Accessed November 14, 2024. https://www.niddk.nih.gov/health-information/kidney-disease
16. Gonyea JE, Phillips SC, eds. *Nutrition Care in Kidney Disease*. 3rd ed. Academy of Nutrition and Dietetics; 2023.

17. Centers for Disease Control and Prevention. *National Health and Nutrition Examination Survey III: Body Measurements (Anthropometry)*. Accessed November 23, 2024. https://stacks.cdc.gov/view/cdc/53134
18. National Kidney Foundation. K/DOQI clinical practice guidelines for chronic kidney disease: evaluation, classification, and stratification. *Am J Kidney Dis*. 2002;39(2 Suppl 1):S1–266.
19. Ikizler TA, Burrowes JD, Byham-Gray LD, et al. KDOQI Clinical Practice Guideline for Nutrition in CKD: 2020 Update. *Am J Kidney Dis*. 2020;76(3 Suppl 1):S1–S107. doi:10.1053/j.ajkd.2020.05.006
20. Chumlea WC, Roche AF, Steinbaugh ML. Estimating stature from knee height for persons 60 to 90 years of age. *J Am Geriatr Soc*. 1985;33(2):116–20. doi:10.1111/j.1532-5415.1985.tb02276.x
21. Chumlea WC, Roche AF, Mukherjee D. *Nutritional Assessment of the Elderly through Anthropometry*. Ross Laboratories; 1987.
22. Chhabra SK. Using arm span to derive height: impact of three estimates of height on interpretation of spirometry. *Ann Thorac Med*. 2008;3(3):94–99. doi:10.4103/1817-1737.39574
23. World Health Organization. Obesity and Overweight. Accessed February 19, 2025. https://www.who.int/news-room/fact-sheets/detail/obesity-and-overweight#
24. Kaysen GA, Johansen KL, Cheng SC, Jin C, Chertow GM. Trends and outcomes associated with serum albumin concentration among incident dialysis patients in the United States. *J Ren Nutr*. 2008;18(4):323–331. doi:10.1053/j.jrn.2008.04.002
25. Weiner DE, Sarnak MJ. Managing dyslipidemia in chronic kidney disease. *J Gen Intern Med*. 2004;19(10):1045–1052. doi:10.1111/j.1525-1497.2004.40049.x
26. Weiner DE, Sarnak MJ. 54 - Cardiac function and cardiovascular disease in chronic kidney disease. In: Gilbert SJ, Weiner DE, Bomback AS, Perazella MA, Rifkin DE, eds. *National Kidney Foundation's Primer on Kidney Diseases*. 8th ed. Elsevier; 2023:512–521.
27. Hudnall SD. *Hematology: A Pathophysiologic Approach*. 2nd ed. Mosby Physiology Series. Elsevier; 2024.
28. Kraft MD. Phosphorus and calcium: a review for the adult nutrition support clinician. *Nutr Clin Pract*. 2015;30(1):21–33. doi:10.1177/0884533614565251
29. Kidney Disease: Improving Global Outcomes (KDIGO) CKD-MBD Update Work Group. KDIGO 2017 Clinical Practice Guideline Update for the Diagnosis, Evaluation, Prevention, and Treatment of Chronic Kidney Disease-Mineral and Bone Disorder (CKD-MBD). *Kidney Int Suppl (2011)*. 2017;7(1):1–59. doi:10.1016/j.kisu.2017.04.001
30. Burrowes JD, Larive B, Chertow GM, et al. Self-reported appetite, hospitalization and death in haemodialysis patients: findings from the Hemodialysis (HEMO) Study. *Nephrol Dial Transplant*. 2005;20(12):2765–2774. doi:10.1093/ndt/gfi132
31. McCann L. Subjective global assessment as it pertains to the nutritional status of dialysis patients. *Dialysis Transplant*. 1996;25(4):190–202.
32. McCann L, National Kidney Foundation. *Pocket Guide to Nutrition Assessment of Patient with Kidney Disease*. 6th ed. 2011. Accessed November 24, 2024. https://www.kidney.org/sites/default/files/12-85-0946_ica_crn-pocket-guide_v6_chp_0.pdf
33. Fontes D, Generoso Sde V, Toulson Davisson Correia MI. Subjective global assessment: a reliable nutritional assessment tool to predict outcomes in critically ill patients. *Clin Nutr*. 2014;33(2):291–295. doi:10.1016/j.clnu.2013.05.004
34. Kalantar-Zadeh K, Kopple JD, Block G, Humphreys MH. A malnutrition-inflammation score is correlated with morbidity and mortality in maintenance hemodialysis patients. *Am J Kidney Dis*. 2001;38(6):1251–1263. doi:10.1053/ajkd.2001.29222
35. Combe C, Chauveau P, Laville M, et al. Influence of nutritional factors and hemodialysis adequacy on the survival of 1,610 French patients. *Am J Kidney Dis*. 2001;37(1 Suppl 2):S81–88. doi:10.1053/ajkd.2001.20756
36. The National Kidney Foundation. KDOQI History. Accessed August 20, 2024. https://www.kidney.org/kdoqi-history
37. Academy of Nutrition and Dietetics Evidence Analysis Library. *Evidence Analysis Manual: Steps in the Academy Evidence Analysis Process*. Updated April 2016. Accessed February 22, 2023. https://www.andeal.org/vault/2440/web/files/2016_April_EA_Manual.pdf
38. Centers for Disease Control and Prevention. Trends in Incidence Rate of Acute Kidney Injury by Diagnosis Code. Accessed September 13, 2024. https://nccd.cdc.gov/CKD/detail.aspx?Qnum=Q773
39. Goyal A, Daneshpajouhnejad P, Hashmi MF, Bashir K. Acute kidney injury. In: *StatPearls*. StatPearls Publishing; 2024.
40. Manzoor H, Bhatt H. Prerenal kidney failure. In: *StatPearls*. StatPearls Publishing; 2024.
41. Perazella MA, Rosner MH. Drug-induced acute kidney injury. *Clin J Am Soc Nephrol*. 2022;17(8):1220–1233. doi:10.2215/CJN.11290821
42. Khwaja A. KDIGO clinical practice guidelines for acute kidney injury. *Nephron Clin Pract*. 2012;120(4):c179–184. doi:10.1159/000339789
43. McClave SA, Taylor BE, Martindale RG, et al. Guidelines for the Provision and Assessment of Nutrition Support Therapy in the Adult Critically Ill Patient. *JPEN*. 2016;40:159–211. https://doi.org/10.1177/0148607115621863
44. Brown RO, Compher C, American Society for Parenteral and Enteral Nutrition Board of Directors. A.S.P.E.N. clinical guidelines: nutrition support in adult acute and chronic renal failure. *JPEN*. 2010;34(4):366–377. doi:10.1177/0148607110374577
45. Schneeweiss B, Graninger W, Stockenhuber F, et al. Energy metabolism in acute and chronic renal failure. *Am J Clin Nutr*. 1990;52(4):596–601. doi:10.1093/ajcn/52.4.596
46. Saunders H, Rehan A, Hashmi MF, Sanghavi DK. Continuous renal replacement therapy. In: *StatPearls*. StatPearls Publishing; 2024.
47. Stapel SN, de Boer RJ, Thoral PJ, Vervloet MG, Girbes ARJ, Oudemans-van Straaten HM. Amino acid loss during continuous venovenous hemofiltration in critically ill patients. *Blood Purif*. 2019;48(4):321–329. doi:10.1159/000500998
48. Bellomo R, Tan HK, Bhonagiri S, et al. High protein intake during continuous hemodiafiltration: impact on amino acids and nitrogen balance. *Int J Artif Organs*. 2002;25(4):261–268. doi:10.1177/039139880202500403
49. Grams ME, Estrella MM, Coresh J, et al. Fluid balance, diuretic use, and mortality in acute kidney injury. *Clin J Am Soc Nephrol*. 2011;6(5):966–973. doi:10.2215/CJN.08781010
50. Kidney Disease: Improving Global Outcomes CKDWG. KDIGO 2024 Clinical Practice Guideline for the Evaluation and Management of Chronic Kidney Disease. *Kidney Int*. 2024;105(4S):S117–S314. doi:10.1016/j.kint.2023.10.018
51. National Kidney Foundation. Chronic Kidney Disease (CKD). Updated September 11, 2023. Accessed November 23, 2024. https://www.kidney.org/kidney-topics/chronic-kidney-disease-ckd#about-chronic-kidney-disease-ckd

52. Xie Y, Bowe B, Mokdad AH, et al. Analysis of the Global Burden of Disease study highlights the global, regional, and national trends of chronic kidney disease epidemiology from 1990 to 2016. *Kidney Int.* 2018;94(3):567–581. doi:10.1016/j.kint.2018.04.011
53. Kumar M, Dev S, Khalid MU, et al. The bidirectional link between diabetes and kidney disease: mechanisms and management. *Cureus.* 2023;15(9):e45615. doi:10.7759/cureus.45615
54. de Boer IH, Caramori ML, Chan JCN, et al. Executive summary of the 2020 KDIGO Diabetes Management in CKD Guideline: evidence-based advances in monitoring and treatment. *Kidney Int.* 2020;98(4):839–848. doi:10.1016/j.kint.2020.06.024
55. Perkovic V, Jardine MJ, Neal B, et al. Canagliflozin and renal outcomes in type 2 diabetes and nephropathy. *N Engl J Med.* 2019;380(24):2295–2306. doi:10.1056/NEJMoa1811744
56. De Bhailis AM, Kalra PA. Hypertension and the kidneys. *Br J Hosp Med (Lond).* 2022;83(5):1–11. doi:10.12968/hmed.2021.0440
57. Kidney Disease: Improving Global Outcomes Blood Pressure Work G. KDIGO 2021 Clinical Practice Guideline for the Management of Blood Pressure in Chronic Kidney Disease. *Kidney Int.* 2021;99(3S):S1–S87. doi:10.1016/j.kint.2020.11.003
58. Romagnani P, Kitching AR, Leung N, Anders HJ. The five types of glomerulonephritis classified by pathogenesis, activity and chronicity (GN-AC). *Nephrol Dial Transplant.* 2023;38(Supplement_2):ii3–ii10. doi:10.1093/ndt/gfad067
59. Service NH. Glomerulonephritis. National Health Service. Updated April 13, 2023. Accessed November 23, 2024. https://www.nhs.uk/conditions/glomerulonephritis/
60. National Kidney Foundation. Maintaining a Vegetarian Diet with Kidney Disease. Accessed November 24, 2024. https://www.kidney.org/kidney-topics/maintaining-vegetarian-diet-kidney-disease
61. Swiatek L, Jeske J, Miedziaszczyk M, Idasiak-Piechocka I. The impact of a vegetarian diet on chronic kidney disease (CKD) progression - a systematic review. *BMC Nephrol.* 2023;24(1):168. doi:10.1186/s12882-023-03233-y
62. Levey AS, Eckardt KU, Dorman NM, et al. Nomenclature for kidney function and disease: report of a Kidney Disease: Improving Global Outcomes (KDIGO) consensus conference. *Kidney Int.* 2020;97(6):1117–1129. doi:10.1016/j.kint.2020.02.010
63. Liu P, Quinn RR, Lam NN, et al. Progression and regression of chronic kidney disease by age among adults in a population-based cohort in Alberta, Canada. *JAMA Netw Open.* 2021;4(6):e2112828. doi:10.1001/jamanetworkopen.2021.12828
64. Vadakedath S, Kandi V. Dialysis: a review of the mechanisms underlying complications in the management of chronic renal failure. *Cureus.* 2017;9(8):e1603. doi:10.7759/cureus.1603
65. Arasu R, Jegatheesan D, Sivakumaran Y. Overview of hemodialysis access and assessment. *Can Fam Physician.* 2022;68(8):577–582. doi:10.46747/cfp.6808577
66. Andreoli MCC, Totoli C. Peritoneal dialysis. *Rev Assoc Med Bras (1992).* 2020;66Suppl1(Suppl1):s37–s44. doi:10.1590/1806-9282.66.S1.37
67. Misra M. Basic mechanisms governing solute and fluid transport in hemodialysis. *Hemodial Int.* 2008;12 Suppl 2:S25–28. doi:10.1111/j.1542-4758.2008.00320.x
68. Torreggiani M, Piccoli GB, Moio MR, et al. Choice of the dialysis modality: practical considerations. *J Clin Med.* 2023;12(9) doi:10.3390/jcm12093328
69. Weinhandl ED, Liu J, Gilbertson DT, Wetmore JB, Johansen KL. Associations of COVID-19 outcomes with dialysis modalities and settings. *Clin J Am Soc Nephrol.* 2022;17(10):1526–1534. doi:10.2215/CJN.03400322
70. Fishman G, Singer P. Metabolic and nutritional aspects in continuous renal replacement therapy. *J Intensive Med.* 2023;3(3):228–238. doi:10.1016/j.jointm.2022.11.001
71. Kotla SK, Saxena A, Saxena R. A Model to estimate glucose absorption in peritoneal dialysis: a pilot study. *Kidney360.* 2020;1(12):1373–1379. doi:10.34067/KID.0004722020
72. National Institute of Diabetes and Digestive and Kidney Disease. *Hemodialysis Dose and Adequacy.* 2009. Accessed November 24, 2024. https://quality.allianthealth.org/wp-content/uploads/2021/07/Hemo_Dose_Adequacy.pdf
73. National Institute of Diabetes and Digestive and Kidney Disease. *Peritoneal Dialysis Dose and Adequacy.* NIH Publication No. 07–4578. NIH; 2006.
74. Tapia C, Bashir K. Nephrotic syndrome. In: *StatPearls.* StatPearls Publishing; 2024.
75. Damien G Noone KI, Rulan Parekh. Nephrotic syndrome. *Lancet.* 2018. Accessed September 18, 2024. https://www.thelancet.com/clinical/diseases/nephrotic-syndrome
76. McCloskey O, Maxwell AP. Diagnosis and management of nephrotic syndrome. *Practitioner.* 2017;261(1801):11–15.
77. Agrawal S, Zaritsky JJ, Fornoni A, Smoyer WE. Dyslipidaemia in nephrotic syndrome: mechanisms and treatment. *Nat Rev Nephrol.* 2018;14(1):57–70. doi:10.1038/nrneph.2017.155
78. Mittal SK, Dash SC, Tiwari SC, Agarwal SK, Saxena S, Fishbane S. Bone histology in patients with nephrotic syndrome and normal renal function. *Kidney Int.* 1999;55(5):1912–1919. doi:10.1046/j.1523-1755.1999.00413.x
79. Kodner C. Diagnosis and management of nephrotic syndrome in adults. *Am Fam Physician.* 2016;93(6):479–485.
80. Mansy H, Goodship TH, Tapson JS, Hartley GH, Keavey P, Wilkinson R. Effect of a high protein diet in patients with the nephrotic syndrome. *Clin Sci (Lond).* 1989;77(4):445–451. doi:10.1042/cs0770445
81. Academy of Nutrition and Dietetics. Nephrotic syndrome. In: *Nutrition Care Manual.* Academy of Nutrition and Dietetics; 2024.
82. Chebib FT, Torres VE. Recent advances in the management of autosomal dominant polycystic kidney disease. *Clin J Am Soc Nephrol.* 2018;13(11):1765–1776. doi:10.2215/CJN.03960318
83. Chebib FT, Torres VE. Autosomal dominant polycystic kidney disease: core curriculum 2016. *Am J Kidney Dis.* 2016;67(5):792–810. doi:10.1053/j.ajkd.2015.07.037
84. Chapman AB, Rahbari-Oskoui FF, Cook J, Rizk DV. 39 - Polycystic and other cystic kidney diseases. In: Gilbert SJ, Weiner DE, Bomback AS, Perazella MA, Rifkin DE, eds. *National Kidney Foundation's Primer on Kidney Diseases.* 8th ed. Elsevier; 2023:375–386.
85. Dell KM. The spectrum of polycystic kidney disease in children. *Adv Chronic Kidney Dis.* 2011;18(5):339–347. doi:10.1053/j.ackd.2011.05.001
86. Sans-Atxer L, Joly D. Tolvaptan in the treatment of autosomal dominant polycystic kidney disease: patient selection and special considerations. *Int J Nephrol Renovasc Dis.* 2018;11:41–51. doi:10.2147/ijnrd.S125942
87. Chebib FT, Nowak KL, Chonchol MB, et al. Polycystic kidney disease diet: what is known and what is safe. *Clin J Am Soc Nephrol.* 2024;19(5):664–682. doi:10.2215/CJN.0000000000000326

88. Torres JA, Kruger SL, Broderick C, et al. Ketosis ameliorates renal cyst growth in polycystic kidney disease. *Cell Metab*. 2019;30(6):1007–1023 e5. doi:10.1016/j.cmet.2019.09.012
89. Torres JA, Rezaei M, Broderick C, et al. Crystal deposition triggers tubule dilation that accelerates cystogenesis in polycystic kidney disease. *J Clin Invest*. 2019;129(10):4506–4522. doi:10.1172/JCI128503
90. Cukoski S, Lindemann CH, Arjune S, et al. Feasibility and impact of ketogenic dietary interventions in polycystic kidney disease: KETO-ADPKD-a randomized controlled trial. *Cell Rep Med*. 2023;4(11):101283. doi:10.1016/j.xcrm.2023.101283
91. KDIGO. KDIGO 2023 clinical practice guideline for the evaluation, management, and treatment of autosomal dominant polycystic kidney disease (ADPKD) [public review draft. 2023].
92. InformedHealth.org. Overview: Kidney Stones. Institute for Quality and Efficiency in Health Care (IQWiG). Updated March 1, 2023. Accessed September 23, 2024. https://www.ncbi.nlm.nih.gov/books/NBK348937/
93. Chew BHM, Larry E, Eisner B, Bhattacharyya S, Bhojani N. Prevalence, incidence, and determinants of kidney stones in a nationally representative sample of US adults. *JU Open Plus*. 2024;2(1):e00006. doi:10.1097/JU9.0000000000000107
94. Charles D. Scales Jr ACS, Janet M. Hanley, Christopher S. Saigal. Prevalence of kidney stones in the United States. *European Urology*. 2012;62(1):160–165. doi:10.1016/j.eururo.2012.03.052
95. Worcester EM, Coe FL. Nephrolithiasis. *Prim Care*. 2008;35(2):369–391, vii. doi:10.1016/j.pop.2008.01.005
96. Ratkalkar VN, Kleinman JG. Mechanisms of stone formation. *Clin Rev Bone Miner Metab*. 2011;9(3–4):187–197. doi:10.1007/s12018-011-9104-8
97. Frassetto L, Kohlstadt I. Treatment and prevention of k idney stones: an update. *Am Fam Physician*. 2011;84(11):1234–1242.
98. Canales BK, Hatch M. Kidney stone incidence and metabolic urinary changes after modern bariatric surgery: review of clinical studies, experimental models, and prevention strategies. *Surg Obes Relat Dis*. 2014;10(4):734–742. doi:10.1016/j.soard.2014.03.026
99. Han H, Segal AM, Seifter JL, Dwyer JT. Nutritional management of kidney stones (nephrolithiasis). *Clin Nutr Res*. 2015;4(3):137–152. doi:10.7762/cnr.2015.4.3.137
100. Pearle MS, Goldfarb DS, Assimos DG, et al. Medical management of kidney stones: AUA guideline. *J Urol*. 2014;192(2):316–324. doi:10.1016/j.juro.2014.05.006
101. Ferraro PM, Taylor EN, Gambaro G, Curhan GC. Soda and other beverages and the risk of kidney stones. *Clin J Am Soc Nephrol*. 2013;8(8):1389–1395. doi:10.2215/CJN.11661112
102. Curhan GC, Willett WC, Rimm EB, Spiegelman D, Stampfer MJ. Prospective study of beverage use and the risk of kidney stones. *Am J Epidemiol*. 1996;143(3):240–247. doi:10.1093/oxfordjournals.aje.a008734
103. Massey LK, Whiting SJ. Dietary salt, urinary calcium, and kidney stone risk. *Nutr Rev*. 1995;53(5):131–139. doi:10.1111/j.1753-4887.1995.tb01536.x
104. Adeva MM, Souto G. Diet-induced metabolic acidosis. *Clin Nutr*. 2011;30(4):416–421. doi:10.1016/j.clnu.2011.03.008
105. Lemann J, Jr. Relationship between urinary calcium and net acid excretion as determined by dietary protein and potassium: a review. *Nephron*. 1999;81(Suppl 1):18–25. doi:10.1159/000046294
106. Curhan GC, Willett WC, Rimm EB, Stampfer MJ. A prospective study of dietary calcium and other nutrients and the risk of symptomatic kidney stones. *N Engl J Med*. 1993;328(12):833–838. doi:10.1056/NEJM199303253281203
107. Taylor EN, Curhan GC. Oxalate intake and the risk for nephrolithiasis. *J Am Soc Nephrol*. 2007;18(7):2198–2204. doi:10.1681/ASN.2007020219
108. Attalla K, De S, Monga M. Oxalate content of food: a tangled web. *Urology*. 2014;84(3):555–560. doi:10.1016/j.urology.2014.03.053
109. Ferraro PM, Curhan GC, Gambaro G, Taylor EN. Total, dietary, and supplemental vitamin C intake and risk of incident kidney stones. *Am J Kidney Dis*. 2016;67(3):400–407. doi:10.1053/j.ajkd.2015.09.005
110. Thomas LD, Elinder CG, Tiselius HG, Wolk A, Akesson A. Ascorbic acid supplements and kidney stone incidence among men: a prospective study. *JAMA Intern Med*. 2013;173(5):386–388. doi:10.1001/jamainternmed.2013.2296
111. Dietary Reference Intakes (DRIs): Recommended Dietary Allowances and Adequate Intakes, Vitamins (2011). National Academies Press; 2011.
112. Ashby RA, Sleet RJ. The role of citrate complexes in preventing urolithiasis. *Clin Chim Acta*. 1992;210(3):157–65. doi:10.1016/0009-8981(92)90201-z
113. Koff SG, Paquette EL, Cullen J, Gancarczyk KK, Tucciarone PR, Schenkman NS. Comparison between lemonade and potassium citrate and impact on urine pH and 24-hour urine parameters in patients with kidney stone formation. *Urology*. 2007;69(6):1013–1016. doi:10.1016/j.urology.2007.02.008
114. Grases F, March JG, Prieto RM, et al. Urinary phytate in calcium oxalate stone formers and healthy people—dietary effects on phytate excretion. *Scand J Urol Nephrol*. 2000;34(3):162–164. doi:10.1080/003655900750016526
115. Curhan GC, Willett WC, Knight EL, Stampfer MJ. Dietary factors and the risk of incident kidney stones in younger women: Nurses' Health Study II. *Arch Intern Med*. 2004;164(8):885–891. doi:10.1001/archinte.164.8.885
116. Akram M, Jahrreiss V, Skolarikos A, et al. Urological guidelines for kidney stones: overview and comprehensive update. *J Clin Med*. 2024;13(4). doi:10.3390/jcm13041114

CHAPTER 13

Nutrition in Liver Disease

Molly Uebele Harrigan

CHAPTER OUTLINE

Core Concepts
Introduction to the Liver
Metabolic Changes in Liver Disease
Acute Liver Disease
Chronic Liver Disease
Cirrhosis
Nutrition Assessment
Nutrition Intervention
Monitoring and Evaluation

CORE CONCEPTS

1. Significant liver cell damage (approximately 80–90% of liver cells) must occur before physiologic function is impaired. Complete liver failure is incompatible with life and can only be treated with a liver transplant.
2. Many over-the-counter herbal products can be hepatotoxic, including green tea extracts, turmeric, ashwagandha, and some Chinese and Ayurvedic herbal medicines. Take caution regarding multi-ingredient products marketed for weight loss or athletic performance.
3. Patients with acute liver failure may need parenteral glucose administration to prevent hypoglycemia related to the liver's failure to release glucose and metabolize insulin. Metabolic and nutrition support should be provided according to the patient's clinical condition and severity of illness.
4. In the United States, alcohol-related liver disease is now the leading indication for liver transplant and the leading cause of liver-related death. Harmful drinking is defined as greater than 2 servings per day (or 14 per week) in women or greater than 3 servings per day (or 21 per week) in men.
5. Lifestyle modification through diet and exercise is the primary treatment for metabolic dysfunction–associated steatotic liver disease.
6. Malnutrition correlates with severity of liver disease and is nearly universal in patients with end-stage liver disease.
7. Muscle and adipose tissue wasting in patients with liver disease is an independent predictor of mortality. Muscle loss is also associated with hepatic encephalopathy. Nutrition assessment will require measures of muscle mass or function, rather than weight and BMI.
8. Indirect calorimetry should be used to determine energy needs for patients with cirrhosis. Handheld calorimeters are a valid option.
9. Patients with cirrhosis require a minimum 1.2 grams protein/kg/day, up to 2 grams/kg/day depending on their nutritional status and clinical condition. Protein should not be restricted in hepatic encephalopathy.

10. Malnutrition, fat malabsorption, alcohol use disorder, and diuretic therapy increase risk of micronutrient deficiencies. Decisions to supplement micronutrients should be made on an individual basis.
11. Patients with cirrhosis should eat a bedtime snack to avoid the accelerated proteolysis and lipid oxidation that occurs after a short period of fasting.
12. Patients with ascites should follow a reduced-sodium diet, although this should be liberalized for patients who are not meeting their protein and energy requirements. A free water restriction is only indicated in the setting of severe hyponatremia (serum sodium <125 mEq/L).

LEARNING OBJECTIVES

1. Differentiate among acute hepatitis, chronic liver disease, acute liver failure, and fulminant liver failure.
2. Describe the progression of liver disease from hepatitis to cirrhosis.
3. Explain how alterations in metabolism during liver disease lead to muscle wasting, hypoglycemia, hyperglycemia, hypoalbuminemia, and micronutrient deficiencies.
4. List the nutrition and lifestyle recommendations for individuals with metabolic dysfunction–associated steatotic liver disease.
5. Define and briefly explain the pathogenesis of hepatic encephalopathy, coagulopathy, portal hypertension, ascites, and varices.
6. Assess the nutrition status of patients with chronic liver disease.
7. Defend the recommended energy and protein requirements for patients with cirrhosis.
8. Identify micronutrients that should be monitored for deficiency in patients with various types of chronic liver disease.
9. Make dietary recommendations that will benefit patients with cirrhosis.
10. Recommend the timing and route of nutrition support for patients unable to take nutrition by mouth.

Introduction to the Liver

The liver is often considered the nutritional gatekeeper of the body (**Figure 13.1**). It is the only organ capable of all major metabolic pathways in protein, carbohydrate, and lipid metabolism. Through careful regulation, it maintains a constant supply of energy for the body to do work, whether fed, fasting, or starving. It synthesizes important proteins, such as albumin, clotting factors, and transaminases, just to name a few. It is involved in vitamin and mineral metabolism, including vitamins D, B12, B5 (pantothenic acid), and iron. Finally, it metabolizes medications and clears chemicals such as alcohol and ammonia from the blood. The liver's failure to carry out these functions has a detrimental effect on the body's homeostasis.

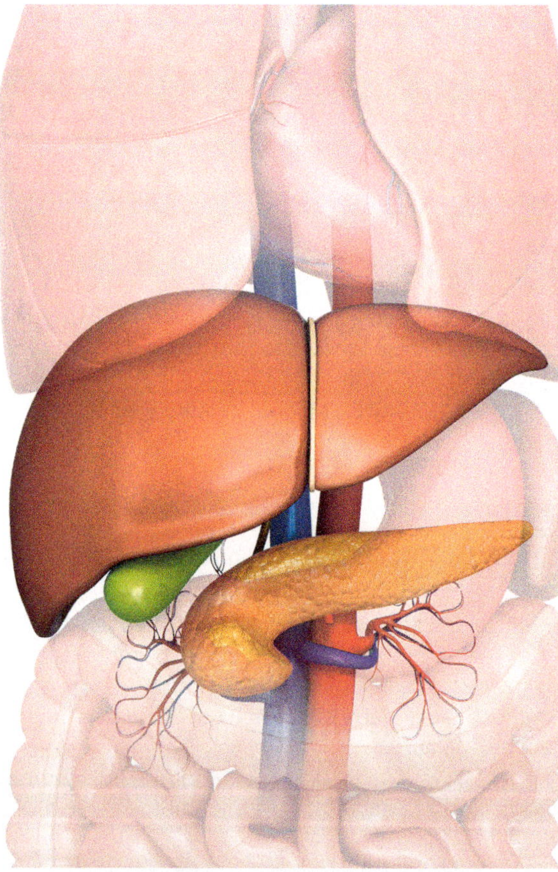

Figure 13.1 The Liver

Liver Structure and Functions

The liver weighs 1–1.5 kg, making it the second-largest organ of the body. Whereas dialysis can replace kidney function and mechanical ventilation can stand in for the lungs, the liver's functions are so vital and complex that there is currently no effective medical or surgical substitute. Frank liver failure is incompatible with life and can only be treated with a liver transplant.

The liver is comprised of hepatocytes, Kupffer cells, stellate cells, endothelial cells, and bile ductular cells. Two-thirds of liver cells are hepatocytes, which perform numerous functions including synthesis of serum proteins, production of bile and its carriers, regulation of nutrients, and metabolism and conjugation of compounds (medications, bilirubin) for excretion via bile or urine. The **Kupffer cells** are macrophages dedicated to the liver. They protect against pathogens arising from the gut, called "endotoxin," by releasing proinflammatory cytokines such as tumor necrosis factor-alpha (TNF-α). **Stellate cells** are hepatic cells responsible for collagen formation and hold 90% of the body's vitamin A stores (**Figure 13.2**). About 80–90% of liver cells must be damaged before a physiologic function is impaired.[1]

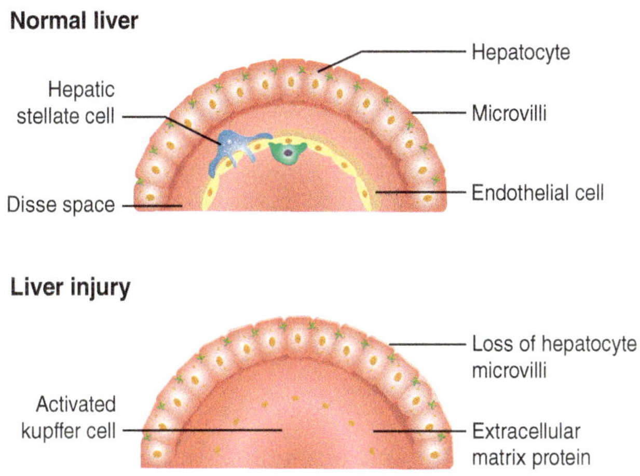

Figure 13.2 Cellular Components of the Liver

CORE CONCEPT 1

Significant liver cell damage (approximately 80–90% of liver cells) must occur before physiologic function is impaired. Complete liver failure is incompatible with life and can only be treated with a liver transplant.

The liver has dual blood supply: about 20% is oxygen-rich blood from the hepatic artery, and about 80% is nutrient-rich blood carried by the portal vein from the stomach, intestines, pancreas, and spleen.[1] Because the liver "sees" most of what we put in our mouth, our diet and gut microbiome affect liver function, and vice versa. The intricate relationship is referred to as the **gut-liver axis**.[2]

CASE STUDY INTRODUCTION

Marisol is a 33-year-old female with a past medical history of prediabetes, obesity, and elevated liver enzymes who is referred by her Primary Care Provider (PCP) to an outpatient RD for the diagnosis of metabolic dysfunction-associated steatotic liver disease (MASLD). Marisol informs the RD that she has not been prescribed any medications, but was told by her PCP that with changes in her diet, her liver disease can be reversed. Marisol is originally from El Salvador and has lived in the United States since she was 10 years old. She lives with her spouse and two children, aged 10 and 15. She works in the cafeteria at the local public school.

Anthropometric Data:

Height: 160 cm
Weight: 80 kg
BMI: 31.2 kg/m^2
Waist circumference: 74 cm

Biochemical Data:

Hemoglobin A1c 5.9% (4.3–5.8%)
LDL-cholesterol 130 (Desirable <100 mg/dL)
HDL-cholesterol 40 (Desirable >40 mg/dL)
Triglycerides 225 (Optimal <150 mg/dL)
Fasting glucose 106 (<100 mg/dL)
Alanine aminotransferase 100 (4–36 units/L)
Aspartate aminotransferase 40 (10–40 units/L)
Alkaline phosphatase 90 (30–120 units/L)
Total bilirubin 0.7 (0.3–1.9 mg/dL)

Clinical Data:

Past Medical History: Prediabetes, obesity, MASLD
Medications: Hormonal intrauterine device (IUD)
Vital Signs: Blood pressure 130/82 mm Hg, Temperature 97.3°F, Heart rate 85 beats/min
Nutrition-Focused Physical Exam: Obese with increased visceral adiposity, no evident muscle wasting or functional deficit.

Dietary Data:

Dietary History: Marisol has a good appetite. She often misses meals or relies on snacks during the day, but has one large meal with her family around 8 pm. She may cook traditional Hispanic food for dinner, but also brings home takeout about 50% of the time.

Alcohol Intake: If she goes out with friends, she will have 2 cocktails. She says she goes out 1–2×/month.

Activity: Marisol is on her feet for 6 hours at work, 5 days/week. At home, she rarely sits down, busy managing the household. She does not do any structured exercise.

Sleep: Marisol states it is hard for her to fall asleep, and she wakes up at 4 am to start her day, so she may sleep 5–6 hours/night.

24-Hour Diet Recall:

Lunch (12 pm): None today

Dinner (9 pm): 1 cup rice, 1/2 cup beans, 3 oz pork with cheese

Snacks: Cinnamon bun from the school cafeteria this morning, chocolate bar last night

Fluids: Water and three 8 oz cans of regular soda

Questions

1. Evaluate Marisol's liver function tests. What do the elevated values mean with respect to hepatocellular function?
2. Assess Marisol's food patterns and intake and write two Problem/Etiology/Signs and Symptoms (PES) statements for Marisol.
3. Identify the nutrition interventions you would like to initiate for Marisol to address the problems identified in your PES statements.
4. What indices are included in your monitoring and evaluation plan? Why?

Overview and Pathophysiology of Liver Disease

With many different and often intersecting etiologies, liver disease can be confusing. Before delving into nutrition research and recommendations regarding specific types of liver disease, it is key to understand the basic categories, terminology, progression of disease, and physiologic complications.

Hepatocellular Versus Cholestatic

Liver disease can be described as either hepatocellular, cholestatic, or mixed. Within each category, there are several possible etiologies (refer to **Table 13.1**).[3]

- **Hepatocellular liver disease** is caused by liver cell injury.
- **Cholestatic liver disease** is caused by inhibition of bile flow.[1] Serum tests help to differentiate between hepatocellular and cholestatic damage.

Acute Versus Chronic Liver Disease

Liver disease is also categorized by duration and severity of injury.

- **Acute hepatitis** is liver inflammation lasting up to 6 months. Some cases of acute hepatitis do not resolve, progressing to chronic hepatitis.
- **Acute liver failure** describes massive hepatic necrosis with the onset of hepatic encephalopathy and coagulopathy (described later in the chapter) within 6 months of known liver disease.
- **Chronic hepatitis** and chronic liver disease both describe liver conditions lasting longer than 6 months.[4] While the liver has significant mechanisms to regenerate after injury, sometimes the regeneration process can be overwhelmed by inflammation and lead to detrimental scarring of the liver. The most nutritionally relevant etiology to understand is steatosis.
  - Steatosis is defined as the accumulation of triglycerides within hepatocytes, which occurs when the liver's production of triglycerides overwhelms its ability to export them. This is reversible.
  - Steatosis can progress to steatohepatitis, where hepatocyte death via lipotoxicity and other inflammatory mediators triggers liver repair mechanisms that produce fibrosis. **Fibrosis** is a buildup of connective tissue (or scar tissue) as a result of hepatocyte regeneration (or wound healing) after injury.
  - The final stage of fibrosis is called **cirrhosis**. At this stage, the liver's attempts at repair are defective and futile. The accumulation of scar

Table 13.1 Liver Function Tests and Their Interpretation

Lab Measure[4]	Description	Possible Diagnosis with Elevated Values
Alanine Aminotransferase (ALT) (4–36 units/L)	Enzyme present primarily in the liver	Hepatocellular damage
Aspartate Aminotransferase (AST) (10–40 units/L)	Enzyme present primarily in the liver, but also in cardiac muscle, skeletal muscle, and other cells	Hepatocellular damage Myocardial infarction
Alkaline Phosphatase (ALP) (30–120 units/L)	Enzyme in the bile canalicular membrane of hepatocytes, but also in the bone, placenta, and small intestine.	Interference with bile flow (cholestasis) Rapid bone growth
Gamma-Glutamyl Transpeptidase (GGT) (9–48 units/L)	Enzyme in the bile duct epithelial cells	Interference with bile flow (cholestasis)
Total Bilirubin (0.3–1.9 mg/dL)	A breakdown product of heme-containing proteins	Cholestasis or hepatocellular damage
Direct Bilirubin (<0.3 mg/dL)	The fraction of bilirubin that is conjugated, meaning it is water soluble	Cholestasis or hepatocellular damage
International Normalized Ratio (INR) (0.8–1.1)	A measure that standardizes PT by using the International Sensitivity Index, which is validated only in patients on warfarin therapy	Increased degree of anticoagulation

Data from Pratt DS, Kaplan MM. Evaluation of liver function. In: Longo DL, Fauci AS, Kasper DL, Hauser SL, Jameson JL, Loscalzo J, eds. *Harrison's Principles of Internal Medicine*. 18th ed. New York, NY: McGraw-Hill; 2012:chap 302.

tissue forms nodules that alter the structure and function of the liver. Individuals with cirrhosis are at risk of developing hepatocellular carcinoma.[5,6]

Hepatocellular Carcinoma

Hepatocellular carcinoma (HCC) accounts for 90% of primary liver cancers. With a high mortality rate, it is the third most common cause of cancer death worldwide. The 5-year survival rate is only 5–15%. The leading risk factor for HCC is cirrhosis of the liver.[7]

Metabolic Changes in Liver Disease

Metabolism is deranged in patients with liver disease, which is not surprising given the prominent role of the liver in regulating nutrient metabolism. Understanding these alterations is key to providing and explaining the rationale of all nutrition recommendations for these patients. **Table 13.2** highlights alterations in metabolism of macronutrients.

Carbohydrate Metabolism

A 70-kg, healthy male can store approximately 100 g of glycogen in the liver and 300–400 g in skeletal muscle. Thus, without eating, glycogen stores can provide the fuel needed for about one day of normal activity. Glycogen stored in muscle cannot be released into circulation. Therefore, only the liver can release stored glucose into the blood for use by the whole body. Once liver glycogen is depleted, blood glucose is maintained via hepatic gluconeogenesis from amino acids, glycerol, and lactate. During prolonged fasting, the body adapts to spare glucose and amino acids by relying on fatty acid oxidation and ketone synthesis. After 14 days of starvation, adipose tissue provides more than 90% of the body's energy.[8]

Patients with cirrhosis have decreased hepatic glycogen storage and increased insulin resistance.[9] As a result, their metabolism after 12 hours of fasting is similar to that of a healthy person after several days of fasting. They rely primarily on lipid oxidation for energy, and proteolysis supplies amino acids for gluconeogenesis.[10] In severe liver failure, inability to metabolize insulin and release glucose via hepatic gluconeogenesis leads to fasting hypoglycemia. The goal

Table 13.2 Metabolic Alterations Due to Cirrhosis

Metabolism	Liver Function	Cirrhotic Liver	Consequences
Carbohydrate	Glycogenolysis Glycogenesis Glycolysis Gluconeogenesis De novo lipogenesis Fructose metabolism	Decreased glycogen stores Impaired gluconeogenesis Insulin resistance	Rapid depletion of glycogen with increased lipolysis and proteolysis while fasting Fasting hypoglycemia Hyperglycemia
Protein	Transamination Urea cycle Synthesis of serum proteins, clotting factors	Increased utilization of BCAA Decreased synthetic function Decreased urea cycle function	Hypoalbuminemia Coagulopathy Hyperammonemia Elevated AAA-to-BCAA ratio
Lipid	Synthesize bile, cholesterol, lipoproteins, phospholipid, ketones Beta oxidation of fatty acid Lipogenesis	Decreased ability to export triglycerides from liver Decreased excretion of bile (derived from cholesterol) Increased reliance on lipid oxidation after short periods of fasting	Steatosis Hyperlipidemia Fat and fat-soluble vitamin malabsorption Adipose and muscle tissue wasting (sarcopenia)

Data from: Bethea ED, Pratt DS. Evaluation of liver function. In: Loscalzo J, Fauci A, Kasper D, Hauser S, Longo D, Jameson J, eds. *Harrison's Principles of Internal Medicine*. 21st ed. McGraw-Hill Education; 2022. Espina S, Casas-Deza D, Bernal-Monterde V, Domper-Arnal MJ, García-Mateo S, Lué A. Evaluation and management of nutritional consequences of chronic liver diseases. *Nutrients*. 2023;15(15). doi:10.3390/nu15153487

of nutrition interventions is to maintain euglycemia and spare lean body mass by preventing early "starvation" metabolism.

Protein Metabolism

A healthy liver is key for protein metabolism as well. The portal vein delivers dietary amino acids to the liver, where they are used to synthesize important transport proteins, such as albumin, prealbumin, transferrin, lipoproteins, fibrinogen, and prothrombin. The breakdown of amino acids (exogenous or endogenous) results in nitrogenous wastes, such as ammonia, which the liver detoxifies via the urea cycle and excretes in urine. Of note, skeletal muscle also participates in removing ammonia via a reaction with glutamate to form glutamine. The muscle supplies glutamate via catabolism of **branched-chain amino acids (BCAAs)**, leucine, isoleucine, and valine.[11]

As liver function fails, the body relies more heavily on muscle to remove ammonia from the blood. With muscle "using up" BCAA to detoxify ammonia, serum BCAA levels become low.[12] There is then a relatively high concentration of aromatic amino acids (AAA). One downstream effect is the increased uptake of AAA in the brain. One of these, tryptophan, is a precursor for 5-hydroxytryptamine, which is a neurotransmitter that can cause lethargy.

The liver's failure to synthesize important proteins, such as albumin and clotting factors, and an altered ratio of BCAA and AAA are implicated in the major complications of severe liver disease. Nutrition therapy focuses on appropriate protein provision and possible supplementation of BCAAs, aiming to prevent skeletal muscle catabolism and treat or prevent complications.

Fat Metabolism

The liver is involved in digestion, metabolism, and transport of fat. It synthesizes and excretes bile, which is required for digestion and absorption of long-chain fatty acids in the lumen of the intestine. About 8–12% of dietary lipids end up in the liver after a meal, where they can be oxidized for energy or used to create cholesterol, phospholipids, lipoproteins, and ketones. The liver also converts excess dietary carbohydrate into triglycerides via de novo lipogenesis.[13]

Due to a decreased ability to store hepatic glycogen, patients with cirrhosis rely heavily on lipid oxidation for energy after brief periods of fasting. This has been demonstrated by measuring the fasting respiratory quotient (RQ) through indirect calorimetry. Generally speaking, an RQ of 1 indicates carbohydrate as the primary substrate, 0.85 indicates protein or mixed substrate metabolism, and 0.7 indicates lipid metabolism. Both stable and hospitalized patients with cirrhosis have significantly lower RQs than healthy controls, averaging an RQ of 0.78 and sometimes presenting with RQs lower than what is generally considered compatible with life (0.69).[14] Lower RQ correlated with lower skeletal muscle mass and lower visceral and subcutaneous fat mass.[15]

CASE STUDY REVISITED

Marisol does not follow up with her PCP or RD. Eight years later, now age 41, she returns to the clinic with complaints of general fatigue and right knee pain. Her PCP finds she now has type 2 diabetes and hypertension. She has been started on medication. The PCP referred her back to the RD and also to a gastroenterologist. In the interview, Marisol states that she stopped working to care for her father, who passed away from cancer 3 years ago. She has not been back to clinic for many reasons: she lost her health insurance for a period of time; she spent a lot of time in El Salvador and avoided seeking medical care due to fear of giving the COVID-19 virus to her father. To help with her grief, isolation, and sleep, she started having a cocktail or two every night. In happier news, her daughter had a healthy baby. She is providing full-time child care.

Anthropometric Data:

Height: 160 cm
Weight: 90 kg
BMI: 35.2 kg/m^2
Waist circumference: 81 cm

Biochemical Data:

Hemoglobin A1c 6.8% (<5.7%)
LDL-cholesterol 125 (Optimal <100 mg/dL)
HDL-cholesterol 41 (Optimal >40 mg/dL)
Triglycerides 289 (Optimal <150 mg/dL)
Fasting glucose 130 (<100 mg/dL)
Alanine aminotransferase 100 (4–36 units/L)
Aspartate aminotransferase 40 (10–40 units/L)
Alkaline phosphatase 90 (30–120 units/L)
Total bilirubin 0.7 (0.3–1.9 mg/dL)

Clinical Data:

Past Medical History: MASLD, type 2 diabetes, hypertension, dyslipidemia, right knee pain
Medications: Hormonal IUD, diclofenac, losartan, metformin, rosuvastatin
Over-the-Counter Medications/Supplements: Omega-3 fish oil 1000 mg daily
Vital Sign: Blood pressure 130/80 mm Hg, Temperature 97.8°F, Heart rate 70 beats/min
Nutrition-Focused Physical Exam: Obese with increased visceral adiposity, no evident muscle wasting or functional deficit.

Nutrition History:

Dietary History: Marisol's diet pattern has not changed, but she has incorporated more vegetables and has cut back on sugar. She typically finishes the food from her grandchild's plate for breakfast and lunch, then eats a traditional large dinner that she cooks for her spouse, two adult children, and grandchild, who still live with her.
Alcohol Intake: 1–2 cocktails on most nights. When asked about her cocktail recipe, she states she uses 2 "shots" of tequila with a low-sugar margarita mix.
Activity: Marisol takes a short walk with her grandchild to the playground when the weather is nice. She rarely sits down at home but has not been able to exercise due to her knee pain.
Sleep: Marisol says her sleep is better because of the cocktails. She can fall asleep and doesn't have to get up as early anymore. She sleeps 7–8 hours. However, she still feels extremely tired in the morning, so she has 2 cups of coffee in the morning.
Fluids: Water, 2 coffees (each with cream and 2 teaspoons of sugar), 1 caffeinated diet soda in the afternoon.

Questions

1. Marisol is diagnosed by the gastroenterologist with MASH. They have ruled out chronic viral infection, autoimmune hepatitis, hemochromatosis, and other rare causes of liver disease. List Marisol's risk factors for progression of her liver disease from MASLD/MASH to cirrhosis. Calculate and evaluate her alcohol intake.
2. Assess Marisol's PES statements from her initial visit. Identify if each statement remains an active issue or if the PES statement has been resolved. If the PES statement remains an active issue, has improvement in the issue been noted? If the issue has been resolved, write a new PES statement.
3. Marisol is overwhelmed by this new diagnosis. If you can only make three nutrition recommendations, what changes would you prioritize?

In severe cirrhosis, lipid digestion and absorption are impaired by the inability of adequate bile to reach the intestinal lumen. Therefore, these patients can have all the consequences of fat malabsorption, including steatorrhea, essential fatty acid and fat-soluble vitamin deficiency, and malnutrition.[16] Of note, this is not only the case for those with cholestatic disease; patients with hepatocellular etiology of liver disease are equally at risk. Vitamin A deficiency is actually more common in hepatocellular liver disease, likely because of decreased storage capacity. Low albumin is a predictor of fat-soluble vitamin deficiency in patients awaiting liver transplant.[17] Deficiencies in vitamins A, D, E, and K are positively correlated with serum bilirubin and disease severity, regardless of the underlying etiology.[18]

Acute Liver Disease

Acute hepatitis and liver failure are most often caused by a viral infection or hepatotoxic medications, resulting in hepatic necrosis. Nutrition interventions are primarily supportive. Acute alcohol-related hepatitis is a unique **"acute-on-chronic"** presentation of a chronic liver disease and will be discussed separately.

Acute Viral Hepatitis

Viral hepatitis is a systemic infection that damages the liver and is almost always caused by one of five viral agents (A, B, C, D, or E) (**Figure 13.3**). Patients present with elevated liver function tests (LFTs), normal or low white blood cell count, malaise, anorexia, nausea, vomiting, fever, jaundice, and tender hepatomegaly. The virus is diagnosed by detecting antibodies and viral nucleic acid in serum. **Table 13.3** describes the different types of hepatitis.[4,19,20]

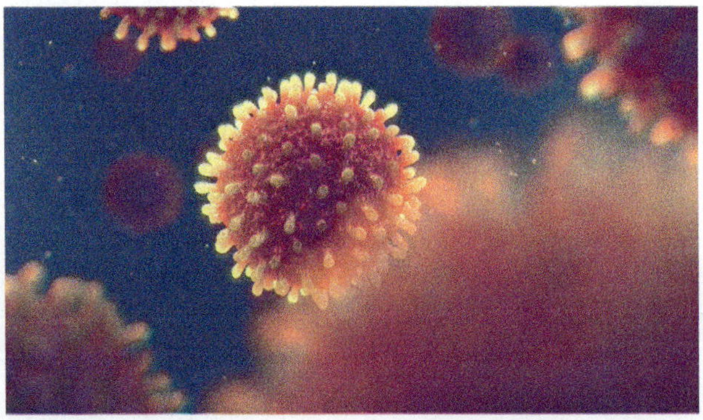

Figure 13.3 Viral Hepatitis Infection

Acute Drug-Induced Liver Injury (DILI)

There are a multitude of medications and herbal and dietary supplements (HDS) that can be hepatotoxic when inhaled, ingested, or given intravenously, either alone or in combination with other drugs. The type of liver injury varies by the medication or supplement. Presentation is often similar to that of viral hepatitis or biliary tract obstruction. DILI can lead to acute liver failure requiring liver transplant or even death. The likelihood of hepatotoxicity leading to liver transplant or death seems to be greater for supplements than for medications. This is perhaps because more is known about hepatotoxicity of drugs, compared to dietary supplements, given minimal federal regulation over supplements in the United States. Since 1995, there has been an eight-fold increase in individuals listed for liver transplant in the United States due to dietary supplement–related liver failure.[21] It is important to note that not all drug-induced liver injuries present with acute hepatitis; some may cause asymptomatic chronic liver inflammation. Furthermore, individuals may have genetic risk factors or preexisting chronic liver disease that, when combined with a hepatotoxic supplement, pushes them into acute liver disease or failure.[22]

The National Institutes of Health has an online database presenting data on hepatotoxicity of medications or herbal supplements at livertox.nih.gov. Examples of hepatotoxic medications include acetaminophen, amoxicillin-clavulanate, trimethoprim-sulfamethoxazole, terbinafine, anti-tuberculosis agents, allopurinol, valproic acid, diclofenac, fenofibrate, and many more. Examples of hepatotoxic dietary and herbal supplements include vitamin A, niacin, heavy metals, anabolic steroids, Chinese skullcap, kratom, green tea extract, turmeric, and ashwagandha.[22] Refer to **Table 13.4** for a more complete list of hepatotoxic herbal supplements.

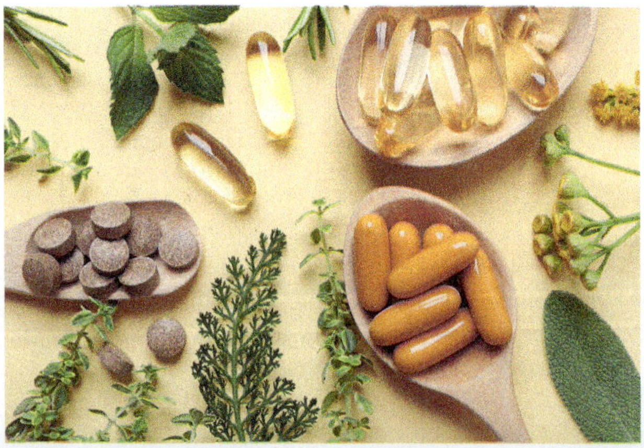

Table 13.3 Categories of Acute Viral Hepatitis

Type	Transmission	Risk Factors	Prognosis
Hepatitis A	Fecal–oral	Travel in underdeveloped countries or regions; exposure to international travelers	Less than 0.6% mortality rate. Recovery from acute illness within 2–3 weeks, with complete recovery within 3 months. Does not lead to chronic hepatitis A.
Hepatitis B	Inoculation of infected blood, sexual contact, maternal–neonatal	Sexual exposure, history of IV drug use, received a blood transfusion before 1986, exposure to infected individuals in health care (needle sticks), incarceration	Less than 1% mortality rate. Greater than 90% recovery within 3–6 months. Between 1% and 2% of immunocompetent adults and 90% of infected infants (maternal–neonatal transmission) develop chronic hepatitis; 40% of patients with chronic HBV develop cirrhosis.
Hepatitis C	Inoculation of infected blood, sexual contact (low risk), maternal–neonatal (low risk)	IV drug use (most common), received a blood transfusion before 1992, tattooing and body piercing, incarceration, multiple sexual partners	Less than 1% mortality rate. After infection, 50–70% develop chronic hepatitis, and 20–25% of those develop cirrhosis. Although this should improve with new treatment options available.
Hepatitis D	Must have hepatitis B to contract; blood and body fluids	Rare in the United States (mostly in South America, West Africa, Russia, Pacific Islands, Central Asia, the Mediterranean)	
Hepatitis E	Waterborne, swine	Exposure to endemic regions (mostly in Central and Southeast Asia, the Middle East, or North Africa)	In endemic regions, 10–20% mortality rate in pregnant women.

Data from Dienstag JL. Chronic hepatitis. In: Loscalzo J, Fauci AS, Kasper DL, Hauser SL, Longo DL, Jameson JL, eds. *Harrison's Principles of Internal Medicine*. 21st ed. New York, NY: McGraw-Hill Education; 2022.

Table 13.4 Hepatotoxic Herbal Supplements

- Aloe vera
- Ashwagandha
- Black cohosh
- Chinese medicines:
  - Ba Jiao Lian
  - Chi R Yun
  - Ephedra
  - Jin Bu Huan
  - Sho Saiko To
- Fenugreek
- Germander
- Ginkgo
- Ginseng
- Glucosamine
- Greater celandine
- Green tea
- Horse chestnut
- Kava
- Milk thistle
- Pennyroyal
- St. John's wort
- Saw palmetto
- Senna
- Skullcap
- Turmeric

Data from Teschke R, Frenzel C, Schulze J, Eickhoff A. Herbal hepatotoxicity: challenges and pitfalls of causality assessment methods. *World J Gastroenterol*. 2013;19(19): 2864-2882.

There are over 100,000 herbal and dietary supplements available over the counter and online.[22] Herbs have been used safely in traditional medicine for centuries. However, today's supplements often contain multiple ingredients marketed for weight loss or sports performance, and it is challenging to determine if each ingredient, or their combination, is safe. Examples include Hydroxycut, Herbalife, and OxyElite Pro. These brands have multiple, frequently changing formulations, making it difficult to determine causality. Green tea extract and *Garcinia cambogia* are known hepatotoxins commonly found in weight loss products.[22] In November 2013, the Food and Drug Administration (FDA) required a recall of OxyELITE Pro, a product advertised to aid in weight loss and muscle building that is believed to have caused over 50 cases of acute hepatitis, some even leading to acute liver failure and death. In 2015, the FDA issued a warning that their reformulated product, OxyELITE Pro Super Thermogenic, contained fluoxetine, a pharmaceutical antidepressant. They reported that dietary supplements including hidden medications is a growing trend. These are being marketed for sexual enhancement, weight loss, and body building. They stated that the "FDA is unable to test and identify all products marketed as dietary supplements. Consumers should exercise caution before purchasing any product in the above categories."[23] These products are still widely available.

CORE CONCEPT 2

Many over-the-counter herbal products can be hepatotoxic, including, but not limited to, green tea extracts, kava, turmeric, ashwagandha, and some Chinese and Ayurvedic herbal medicines. Take extra caution regarding multi-ingredient products marketed for weight loss or athletic performance.

PRACTICE POINT

Ask all patients about their usage of herbal supplements, reviewing the safety of each one with the pharmacist and physician.

Acute Liver Failure

Acute liver failure is a rare critical illness characterized by hepatic necrosis (Figure 13.4) and the onset of impaired hepatic synthetic function (coagulopathy, hypoalbuminemia) and hepatic encephalopathy within 6 months of known hepatic disease. The term **fulminant liver failure** is commonly used to describe onset within 8 weeks of known liver disease. Acute liver failure occurs most often in previously healthy adults in their thirties and carries a poor prognosis, with multi-organ failure and death occurring in up to one-half of cases. Treatment depends on the underlying cause, but is primarily supportive and requires hospitalization, preferably at a facility capable of liver transplantation. Identifying candidates for transplant early is key, because the severity of illness and multi-organ failure can progress rapidly. Only 10% of liver transplants are performed in patients with acute liver failure.

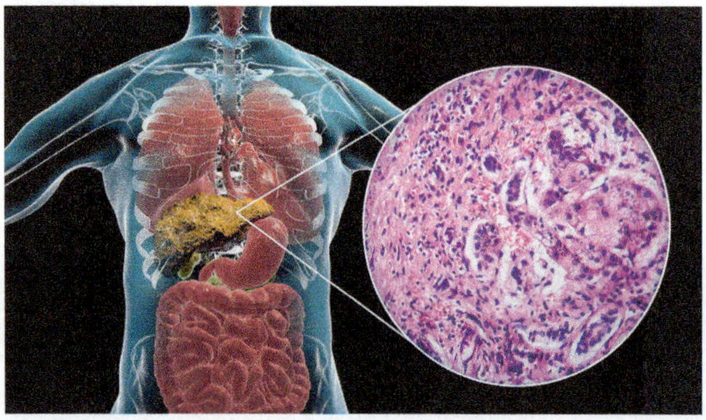

Figure 13.4 Necrosis of Liver Cells

In the United States, DILI is responsible for 50% of all cases of acute liver failure, with acetaminophen toxicity being the number one cause overall. Acute liver failure can occur from ingestion of a single 10- to 15-g dose of acetaminophen, but more often occurs when patients are taking substantial amounts for symptom relief without any intention of self-poisoning. Individuals with malnutrition and alcohol use disorder are at increased risk of this due to a decreased threshold for toxicity. Although viral hepatitis causes only 12% of cases of acute liver failure in the United States, hepatitis A and E are probably the most common causes in low-resource nations where vaccines are less accessible, and sanitation can be poor.

Acute liver failure can be a result of ischemic hepatocellular injury, also called **shock liver**. This can occur in critically ill patients with cardiac, circulatory, or respiratory failure when the liver receives inadequate oxygen perfusion. Other causes of acute liver failure include Budd–Chiari syndrome, heat stroke, mushroom ingestion, undiagnosed Wilson's disease, and, rarely, herpes simplex virus and cytomegalovirus.[24]

Nutrition Management in Acute Liver Disease

There are no data to support nutrition therapy recommendations specifically for patients with acute hepatitis or acute liver failure. Treatment is primarily supportive, which includes ensuring adequate nutritional and metabolic support. Patients with acute liver failure may be unable to maintain adequate intake by mouth due to hepatic encephalopathy and critical illness. Appropriate nutrition should be provided in accordance with the patient's clinical condition and severity of illness. In fulminant liver failure, patients may require parenteral dextrose administration to treat hypoglycemia, caused by the liver's failure to metabolize insulin and release glucose via gluconeogenesis.[25] Energy expenditure is increased but predictive equations are unreliable; thus indirect calorimetry should be utilized when possible.[26] These patients can experience some of the same complications as patients with decompensated chronic liver disease, including hepatic encephalopathy, which will be discussed later in the chapter.

CORE CONCEPT 3

Patients with acute liver failure may need parenteral glucose administration to prevent hypoglycemia related to the liver's failure to release glucose and metabolize insulin. Metabolic and nutrition support should be provided according to the patient's clinical condition and severity of illness.

Chronic Liver Disease

Chronic liver disease has many possible etiologies, both acquired and inherited, and often overlapping. These include chronic viral infection, alcohol and metabolic dysfunction–associated steatohepatitis, and inherited autoimmune and metabolic disorders. Patients with chronic right heart failure can develop "hepatic congestion," called "cardiac cirrhosis." Less common causes of chronic liver disease include hepatotoxic medications and supplements, certain inborn errors of metabolism, kwashiorkor, refeeding syndrome, celiac disease, and long-term parenteral nutrition.

Chronic liver disease can range from benign steatosis to decompensated cirrhosis. Early stages are asymptomatic, evident only by abnormal liver enzymes or imaging. In this section of the chapter, we will review the etiologies of liver disease with important and specific nutrition interventions.

Alcohol-Related Steatotic Liver Disease

Alcohol intake inhibits fatty acid oxidation and increases lipogenesis, causing an accumulation of triglycerides in the liver cells, called **steatosis**. This is benign and can be reversed through abstinence from alcohol. However, approximately 20–30% of patients with chronic increased alcohol intake (>10 years) can develop **steatohepatitis**, or **alcohol-related liver disease (ALD)**. About 10–20% of those will develop cirrhosis. In the United States, ALD is now the leading indication for liver transplant and the leading cause of liver-related death.[27]

Harmful drinking is defined as greater than 2 servings per day (or 14 per week) in women or greater than 3 servings per day (or 21 per week) in men. One "serving" is defined as 14 g pure alcohol. This equates to 12 oz beer (5% alcohol content), 5 oz wine (12% alcohol content), or 1.5 oz liquor (40% or 80 proof) (**Figure 13.5**).[28] It is estimated that 40% of adults globally are considered heavy drinkers.[27] Alcohol use disorder and ALD have increased significantly in the last 10 years, exacerbated by the COVID-19 pandemic. The increase is especially noted in younger people, women, and Black and Hispanic Americans.[28]

One mechanism in the progression of steatosis to steatohepatitis involves the gut–liver axis. Chronic alcohol intake changes the intestinal epithelial barrier and increases gut permeability. This allows bacteria to translocate across the intestinal barrier into portal circulation.[29] Alcohol also promotes the growth of gram negative bacteria in the intestine; these bacteria have a lipopolysaccharide (LPS), called **endotoxin**, in the cell wall. When endotoxin translocates into portal circulation, it stimulates Kupffer cells in the liver to secrete proinflammatory cytokines, such as **tumor necrosis factor-alpha (TNF-α)**, and generate oxidative stress.[30] Additionally, these cytokines can lead to fever, anorexia, and muscle wasting, thereby contributing to poor nutrition. **Table 13.5** lists risk factors for progression of ALD.

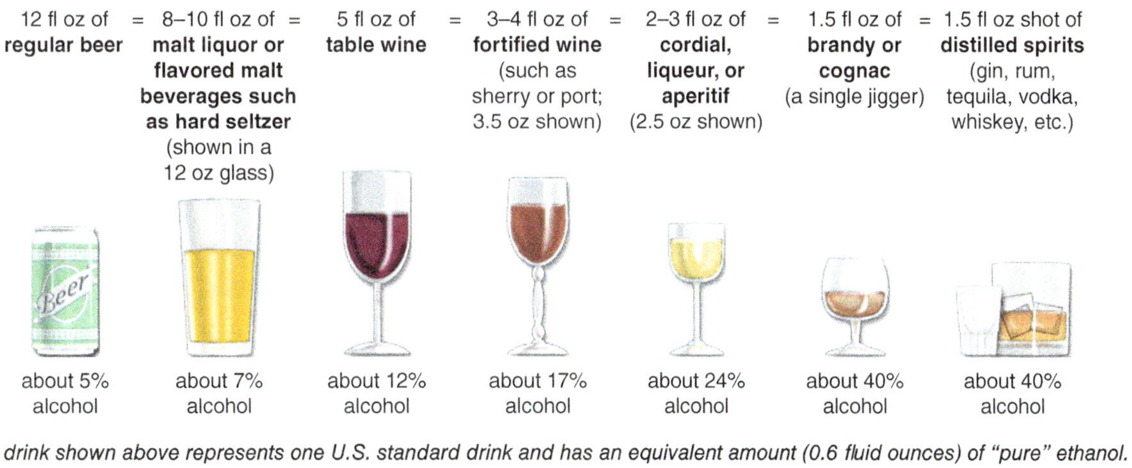

Figure 13.5 Serving Sizes of Alcohol

Reproduced from National Institute on Alcohol Abuse and Alcoholism. Alcohol's effects on health: What is a standard drink? https://www.niaaa.nih.gov/alcohols-effects-health/overview-alcohol-consumption/what-standard-drink. Accessed August 18, 2024.

Table 13.5 Risk Factors for Progression of Alcohol-Related Liver Disease

Obesity (BMI >30 kg/m^2)
Diabetes (6× risk of admission, mortality, HCC)
History of gastric bypass (2–3× risk of AH diagnosis)
Drinking alcohol outside of meals
Drinking liquor rather than wine or beer
Female sex
Heavy daily alcohol use + binge drinking

Heavy daily use

- *Men: 4 drinks on any day or 14 drinks/week*
- *Women: 3 drinks in a day or 7 drinks/week*

Binge drinking

- *Men: 5 drinks within 2 hours*
- *Women: 4 drinks within 2 hours*

Data from Jophlin LL, Singal AK, Bataller R, et al. ACG clinical guideline: alcohol-associated liver disease. *Am J Gastroenterol*. 2024;119(1):30-54. doi:10.14309/ajg.0000000000002572

At any point in the spectrum of ALD, patients can develop an acute form of the disease called **alcohol-related hepatitis (AH)**. These patients will present with jaundice and may have systemic inflammatory response syndrome, fever, hypotension, leukocytosis, and/or mental status changes. AH can be distinguished from other causes of acute hepatitis by a serum AST to ALT ratio (called the **De Ritis ratio**) >2:1 (**Table 13.6**). The suppressed elevation of ALT in comparison to AST is likely secondary to alcohol-induced hepatic mitochondrial damage and deficiency of pyridoxine (vitamin B_6). Severe AH may include complications of decompensated liver failure and increases the risk of developing cirrhosis if not already present. The only treatment with proven efficacy is corticosteroids. The 1-month mortality risk is 25–50%.[28]

Nearly all patients with severe AH have some degree of malnutrition, and the severity of malnutrition closely correlates with development of all serious complications, mortality, and response to treatment.[31] Thiamine should be given empirically for prevention or treatment of possible Wernicke's encephalopathy. Energy needs can be estimated as 35 kcal/kg/day. Protein requirements are 1.2–1.5 g/kg/day. Patients who are unable to take >21 kcal/kg/day will benefit from oral nutrition supplements or nutrition support.[32] When oral or enteral nutrition is not feasible, parenteral nutrition (PN) is indicated in a patient with malnutrition (and nearly all have malnutrition).[25] A meta-analysis on nutritional supplementation (including oral, enteral, and parenteral support) for hospitalized patients with AH found that supplementation provided no benefit in mortality or ascites, but significantly alleviated hepatic encephalopathy.[33]

Table 13.6 Trends in Liver Function Tests in Liver Disease

Laboratory Value	Notable Trends
Alkaline phosphatase	■ Less than 3× normal: Any type of liver disease ■ Greater than 4× normal: Cholestatic liver disease, bone disease ■ Isolated elevation: Early cholestasis, hepatic infiltration by tumor, Hodgkin's disease, diabetes, hyperthyroidism, congestive heart failure, amyloidosis, inflammatory bowel disease
Alanine aminotransferase & aspartate aminotransferase	■ Greater than 1000: Indicates severe injury, likely viral, ischemic, or drug-induced hepatitis ■ AST:ALT ratio <1 Chronic viral hepatitis or MASLD. As cirrhosis develops, this ratio rises to >1. ■ AST:ALT ratio >2:1 or 3:1 = ALD (AST is rarely >300, and the ALT is often normal due to pyridoxal phosphate deficiency)
Bilirubin	■ The higher the bilirubin, the greater the hepatocellular damage

Data from Pratt DS, Kaplan MM. Evaluation of liver function. In: Longo DL, Fauci AS, Kasper DL, Hauser SL, Jameson JL, Loscalzo J, eds. *Harrison's Principles of Internal Medicine*. 18th ed. New York, NY: McGraw-Hill; 2012:chap 302.

CORE CONCEPT 4

In the United States, alcohol-related liver disease is now the leading indication for liver transplant and the leading cause of liver-related death. Harmful drinking is defined as greater than 2 servings per day (or 14 per week) in women or greater than 3 servings per day (or 21 per week) in men.

Metabolic Dysfunction-Associated Steatotic Liver Disease

Metabolic dysfunction-associated steatotic liver disease (MASLD) is hepatic steatosis related to metabolic syndrome, and without significant alcohol consumption. It is the most common liver disease in the world, with a global prevalence of 25%.[34] Diagnosis requires steatosis on imaging, no significant alcohol

Table 13.7 Cardiometabolic Risk Factors in Metabolic Dysfunction–Associated Steatotic Liver Disease

Diagnosis requires hepatic steatosis on imaging and at least 1 out of the 5 criteria below:
BMI ≥25 kg/m² [23 Asians] *OR* WC >94 cm (M)/80 cm (F)
Fasting serum glucose ≥100 mg/dL *OR* HbA1c ≥5.7% *OR* Type 2 diabetes *OR* Treatment for type 2 diabetes
Blood pressure ≥130/85 mm Hg *OR* Antihypertensive drug treatment
Plasma triglycerides ≥150 mg/dL *OR* Lipid-lowering treatment
HDL-cholesterol ≤40 mg/dL (male)/50 mg/dL (female) *OR* Lipid-lowering treatment

Data from Rinella ME, Lazarus JV, Ratziu V, et al. A multisociety Delphi consensus statement on new fatty liver disease nomenclature. *Hepatology*. 2023;78(6):1966. doi:10.1097/HEP.0000000000000520

consumption, and at least 1 out of 5 cardiometabolic risk factors. These are presented in **Table 13.7** and pertain only to adults. MASLD is diagnosed in children and adolescents with differing criteria.[35] The etiology of MASLD is not completely understood, but involves insulin resistance, the gut–liver axis, and obesity as an inflammatory state.[6] Please note that this disease was previously called "non-alcoholic fatty liver disease" (NAFLD), but the nomenclature was changed in 2023 to better capture its pathophysiology and to avoid stigmatizing language.

Simple steatosis from MASLD is benign but should not be ignored because at least 25% of patients with steatosis will progress to steatohepatitis, called **metabolic dysfunction-associated steatohepatitis (MASH)**. It is estimated that 6–8% of U.S. adults have MASH.[6] With MASH, fibrosis can progress rapidly, and approximately 20–25% of patients with MASH develop cirrhosis.[34,36] Progression involves multiple inflammatory insults to the liver, as described in ALD. Obesity is a leading risk factor, implicating proinflammatory cytokines and adipokines secreted by visceral adipose tissue. However, several other factors play a role, including alcohol intake, age, sex, comorbidities, ethnicity/race, and genetics. Identifying MASH is not simple. It cannot be distinguished from MASLD on simple imaging, and although a persistent ALT elevation is common, the degree of elevation does not correlate with severity of injury. In many patients, liver enzymes may even be normal. Biopsy is the gold standard for diagnosis, but no longer always required. Instead, the degree of fibrosis in MASH can be estimated using a Fib-4 score, calculated from readily available labs, and a measure of liver stiffness with advanced imaging modalities.[6] MASH is now the third leading cause of cirrhosis in the United States. Interestingly, HCC can develop in individuals with MASH even in the absence of cirrhosis.[7,37]

Treatment of MASLD/MASH aims to reduce cardiometabolic risk factors and ameliorate inflammation of the liver.[38] There is no current medication therapy specifically approved for MASH, making early identification and intervention with nutrition and lifestyle modification crucial. Current evidence supports the recommendation that patients with obesity should lose 5–10% of their weight through exercise and a reduced-calorie diet.[39–41] For those unable to lose weight through lifestyle modification, bariatric surgery is effective to reduce or resolve MASLD/MASH and should be considered.[39,42] Notably, up to 20% of patients with MASH are not obese. For these and all patients, a Mediterranean-style diet and exercise have been shown to improve liver fibrosis independent of weight loss.[43] A generally accepted recommendation is 150 minutes of moderate exercise per week, or an increase from baseline by 60 minutes/week. The reduction in liver steatosis correlates with the intensity of exercise, so patients should be recommended to exercise as much as they are capable.[39,43] All patients should be advised to avoid alcohol intake.[28]

CORE CONCEPT 5

Lifestyle modification through diet and exercise is the primary treatment for metabolic dysfunction–associated steatotic liver disease. A dietitian should work with the patient alongside an interprofessional team.

Vitamin E 800 IU daily is recommended for MASH in individuals without cirrhosis or diabetes.[25,34,43] In one trial, patients who took 800 IU of vitamin E daily for 96 weeks had a significant improvement in MASH.[44] However, in a 2005 meta-analysis, high-dose (>400 IU/day) vitamin E supplements were associated with increased risk of prostate cancer and a slight increase in all-cause mortality.[45] The majority of the studies involved individuals with chronic diseases. Another meta-analysis in 2014 found no association with supplementation and mortality in healthy adults.[46] Because of this, the recommendation for

CASE STUDY REVISITED

In the nutrition appointment, Marisol informs the RD that obesity runs in her family, and she has been overweight her whole life. She agrees that she needs to decrease her soda consumption and incorporate more vegetables into her diet. She also wants to start exercising and is interested in using natural supplements to heal her liver and help with weight loss.

Questions

1. How might you respond to Marisol's suggestion for taking supplements to improve her liver health?
2. What are the current recommendations for the treatment of MASLD?

vitamin E supplementation should be limited to those with MASH who are otherwise fairly healthy.

Although several other supplements and micronutrients are being studied for treatment of MASLD, most evidence points toward a Mediterranean diet pattern and away from a Western diet pattern.[47,48] Omega-3 fatty acids inhibit proinflammatory cytokines; however, while adequate intake is needed from food sources such as oily fish, walnuts, and olive oil, there is insufficient data to support specific recommendations for supplemental doses.[49,50] Probiotics may be helpful to strengthen the gut mucosal barrier and improve liver health via the gut–liver axis. In one study, taking a symbiotic (prebiotic + probiotic) supplement reduced liver enzymes more than lifestyle intervention alone.[51] While there is insufficient data to recommend a certain supplement, the Mediterranean diet pattern is high in pre/probiotics and antioxidants from fruits, vegetables, yogurt, and whole grains. Coffee, another excellent source of antioxidants, also seems to have an antifibrotic effect. Several studies have shown that those who drink coffee have lower risk of MASLD than those who do not drink coffee.[52,53] Those who have more than 3 cups per day seem to have the greatest benefit.[54] Barring any contraindications, patients should be encouraged to drink 3 or more cups of unsweetened coffee daily.[39] **Table 13.8** summarizes the current nutrition recommendations for MASLD/MASH.

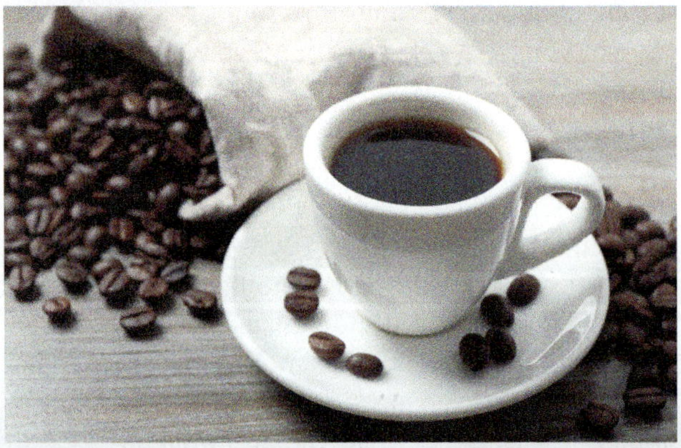

Patients should be discouraged from drinking sugar-sweetened beverages. MASLD is associated with soft drink consumption, even in people without other risk factors. In two studies, 80% of people with MASLD consumed, on average, >50 g added sugar from soft drinks daily. Their intake was five times more than the intake of healthy controls.[55,56] In theory, this may be explained by high intake of fructose, which is metabolized in an unregulated fashion by the liver, unlike glucose. Beverages are sweetened by

Table 13.8 Recommendations for Metabolic Dysfunction–Associated Steatotic Liver Disease

- Follow a Mediterranean-style diet pattern.
- Patients with obesity recommended to achieve a 5–10% weight loss. Consider bariatric surgery if unsuccessful with lifestyle modification alone.
- Engage in moderate to vigorous physical activity. Aim for 150 minutes/week or at least 60 minutes/week increase from baseline.
- Avoid alcohol.
- Drink 3 or more cups of unsweetened coffee daily.
- For those with MASH and no diabetes, take vitamin E 800 IU daily.

Data from Rinella ME, Neuschwander-Tetri BA, Siddiqui MS, et al. AASLD practice guidance on the clinical assessment and management of nonalcoholic fatty liver disease. *Hepatology*. 2023;77(5):1797-1835. doi:10.1097/HEP.0000000000000323; Hassani Zadeh S, Mansoori A, Hosseinzadeh M. Relationship between dietary patterns and nonalcoholic fatty liver disease: a systematic review and meta-analysis. *J Gastroenterol Hepatol*. 2021;36(6):1470-1478. doi:10.1111/jgh.15363; Asrih M, Jornayvaz FR. Diets and nonalcoholic fatty liver disease: the good and the bad. *Clin Nutr*. 2014;33(2):186-190. doi:10.1016/j.clnu.2013.11.003; Gupta V, Mah XJ, Garcia MC, Antonypillai C, Van der Poorten D. Oily fish, coffee and walnuts: dietary treatment for nonalcoholic fatty liver disease. *World J Gastroenterol*. 2015;21(37):10621. doi:10.3748/wjg.v21.i37.10621; de Castro GS, Calder PC. Nonalcoholic fatty liver disease and its treatment with n-3 polyunsaturated fatty acids. *Clin Nutr*. 2018;37(1):37-55. doi:10.1016/j.clnu.2017.01.006; Eslamparast T, Poustchi H, Zamani F, Sharafkhah M, Malekzadeh R, Hekmatdoost A. Synbiotic supplementation in nonalcoholic fatty liver disease: a randomized, double-blind, placebo-controlled pilot study. *Am J Clin Nutr*. 2014;99(3):535-542. doi:10.3945/ajcn.113.068890; Ebadi M, Ip S, Bhanji RA, Montano-Loza AJ. Effect of coffee consumption on nonalcoholic fatty liver disease incidence, prevalence, and risk of significant liver fibrosis: systematic review with meta-analysis of observational studies. *Nutrients*. 2021;13(9):3042. doi:10.3390/nu13093042; Hayat U, Siddiqui AA, Okut H, Afroz S, Tasleem S, Haris A. The effect of coffee consumption on nonalcoholic fatty liver disease and liver fibrosis: a meta-analysis of 11 epidemiological studies. *Ann Hepatol*. 2021;20:100254. doi:10.1016/j.aohep.2020.08.071; Chen YP, Lu FB, Hu YB, Xu LM, Zheng MH, Hu ED. A systematic review and dose-response meta-analysis of coffee dose and nonalcoholic fatty liver disease. *Clin Nutr*. 2019;38(6):2552-2557. doi:10.1016/j.clnu.2018.11.030

sugar or high fructose corn syrup, which are 50% and 55% fructose, respectively, and are the primary dietary sources of fructose. Excess consumption may contribute to MASLD by increasing visceral fat stores, insulin resistance, and postprandial serum triglycerides.[57]

Parenteral Nutrition-Related Liver Disease

Parenteral nutrition-associated liver disease (PNALD), which is also referred to as **intestinal failure-associated liver disease (IFALD)**, is a form of steatotic liver disease that occurs with long-term PN; the etiology is not completely understood. Several factors are likely to contribute, including overfeeding calories and dextrose, resulting in hepatic de novo lipogenesis; inadequate choline intake, inhibiting the liver's ability to make lipoproteins to export triglycerides from the liver; and excess soybean oil–based lipid provision, which promotes inflammation. A proinflammatory "second hit" to the liver, such as a central line infection, can cause steatosis to progress to steatohepatitis. Intestinal failure can also result in biliary sludge and cholestatic liver disease due to lack of enteral stimulation with nutrients; this occurs more often in children and neonates.[58]

Hemochromatosis

Hemochromatosis is an autosomal recessive disease characterized by accumulation of iron in the liver, pancreas, heart, adrenals, testes, pituitary, and kidneys. It is more common in individuals of northwest European ancestry. Hemochromatosis is caused by an inability to downregulate intestinal iron absorption when iron stores are adequate. Most patients are asymptomatic for four to five decades, but elevated liver enzymes and ferritin may lead to a diagnosis much earlier now with increased availability of genetic testing. Patients may develop arthropathy, hepatomegaly, altered skin pigmentation (slate-gray or bronze), cardiac enlargement, or erectile dysfunction. Treatment is phlebotomy, with frequency adjusted to maintain a serum ferritin between 50 and 100 ng/mL.[59]

Patients should be instructed to avoid vitamin C and iron supplements. They should avoid alcohol intake to limit overall liver injury. They should also avoid raw shellfish due to increased risk of infection from siderophilic organisms (bacteria that require free iron) such as *Vibrio vulnificus*. Beyond that, dietary modifications to reduce iron absorption do not have a clinically significant effect. Diet changes may reduce iron absorption by 2–4 mg/day, whereas phlebotomy removes 250 mg.[59] If patients want to be active in their treatment by modifying their diet, they can be encouraged to follow a plant-based diet.[60] They should be monitored to ensure adequate intake of other nutrients typically in an iron-rich diet (zinc, vitamin B_{12}).[61]

> **PRACTICE POINT**
>
> For patients with hemochromatosis, a strict avoidance of dietary iron is not essential; ensure that patients do not develop deficiencies of other nutrients typically in iron-rich foods if they do follow a modified diet.

Wilson's Disease

Wilson's disease is another autosomal recessive disorder characterized by excessive deposition of copper in the liver and brain. The cause of Wilson's disease is excessive copper absorption in the small intestine combined with decreased copper excretion in the liver. The majority of patients present this disease before the age of 40 years. Symptoms include hepatitis; a brownish or gray-green ring at the rim of the cornea, called the **Kayser-Fleischer ring**; and neurologic or psychiatric abnormalities. Labs suggestive of Wilson's disease are a low serum ceruloplasmin and elevated urinary copper excretion. Early treatment with penicillamine, a chelating agent, can remove excess copper via urine before hepatic or neurologic damage is incurred. Pyridoxine (vitamin B6) must be supplemented (50 mg once a week) for patients taking penicillamine, which is an antimetabolite of the vitamin. Side effects are common, and include **dysgeusia** (altered taste perception), anorexia, vomiting, and diarrhea. Dietary copper restriction may be helpful during early treatment; shellfish, organ foods, nuts, mushrooms, and chocolate are high in copper. Zinc acetate or zinc gluconate (50 mg, three times per day) is also used in presymptomatic patients or as maintenance after chelation therapy. Zinc interferes with intestinal absorption by inducing the expression of intestinal metallothionein. **Metallothionein** binds to copper absorbed into the enterocyte, preventing its absorption. As enterocytes turn over, the copper remains bound to the cell and is excreted along with it in feces.[62] Unfortunately, some patients first present with Wilson's disease in acute liver failure; these patients require a liver transplant.[63,64]

Cirrhosis

Cirrhosis is the 10th leading cause of death in the United States.[65] The most common etiologies in the United States are ALD (45%), chronic hepatitis C

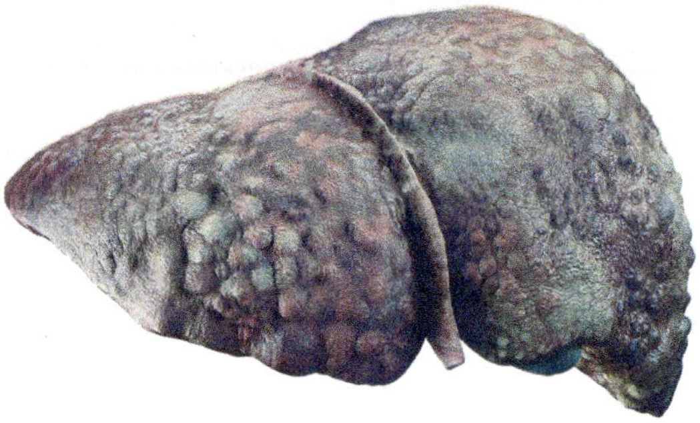

Figure 13.6 Liver Fibrosis

(41%), and MASH (26%).[66] Cirrhosis progresses clinically in three stages: compensated (asymptomatic), compensated with varices, and decompensated. Extensive fibrosis and tissue scarring obstructs blood flow through the liver (**Figure 13.6**). This scarring causes increased blood pressure in the portal vein. This **portal hypertension**, technically defined as venous pressure greater than 10 mm Hg (normal 5–10 mm Hg), causes a cascade of imbalances in the body that contributes to fluid retention and ascites, formation of varices, and progressive kidney disease.[5,67]

When the pressure in the portal vein is high, blood is redirected to veins in the esophagus, stomach, and rectum, which have lower venous pressure. This is called **portosystemic shunting** (**Figure 13.7**). Increased circulation in those veins causes **varices**, or extremely dilated submucosal veins, which are easily susceptible to rupture.[67] Patients are advised to follow a soft diet to prevent rupture of esophageal varices, and to avoid constipation (through adequate fiber and fluid intake, or use of stool softeners) to prevent straining that might rupture rectal varices.

Changes in circulation also cause peripheral arteriolar vasodilation, which triggers the renin–angiotensin–aldosterone system, communicating to the kidneys to increase blood volume by retaining sodium and water. Furthermore, splanchnic vasodilation increases lymph production so much that fluid accumulates in the peritoneal cavity. This is one theory, called the **underfill hypothesis**, for the pathogenesis of **ascites** related to liver disease, although there are other unrelated causes of ascites, such as malignancy, tuberculosis, or abdominal trauma.[5]

The most complex complication of cirrhosis is **hepatic encephalopathy (HE)**, which is a neuropsychiatric disorder characterized by personality changes, altered levels of consciousness, and cognitive impairment. HE can be referred to as "minimal" HE, only identified by neuropsychiatric testing, or "overt" HE with obvious mental status changes. **Table 13.9** provides

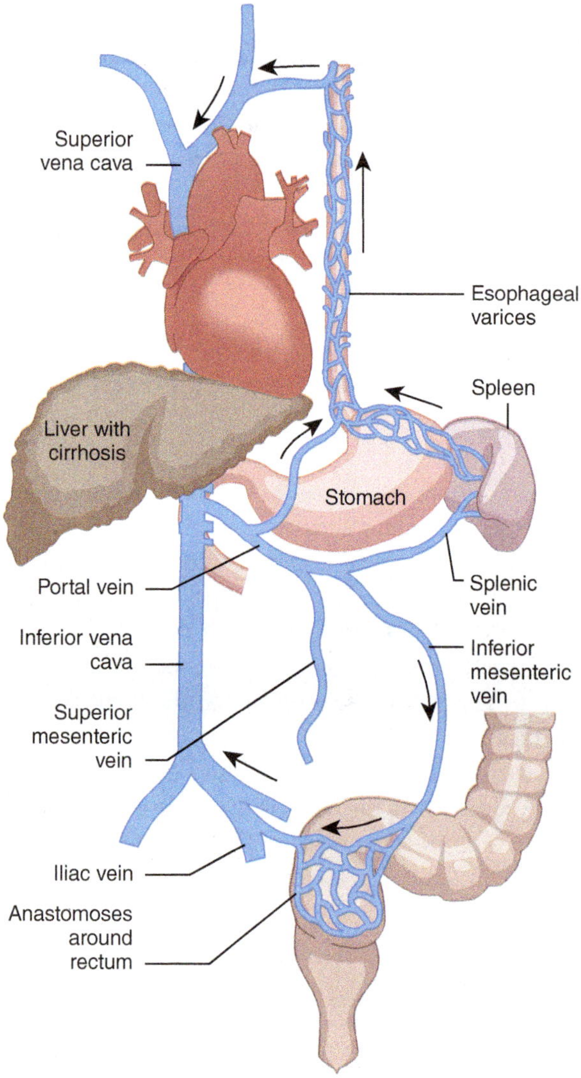

Figure 13.7 High Pressure in the Hepatic Portal Vein Causes an Increase in Varices

the classification and staging of HE. HE also occurs in severe acute hepatitis (AH) and acute liver failure due to cerebral edema, in the absence of cirrhosis.[5] The exact pathogenesis is still unclear, but involves an increase in chemicals that are neurotoxic, such as aromatic amino acids (AAA), ammonia, and TNF-α. HE is a clinical diagnosis, and other causes of mental status changes should be excluded. Serum ammonia is commonly used to aid in identifying HE, but is not actually reliable and does not provide prognostic information.[68] HE is not associated with a particular etiology of cirrhosis, but it is associated with malnutrition, reduced muscle mass, and reduced muscle strength.[69–71] **Table 13.10** gives a brief overview of the theories postulated to lead to HE and potential nutrition interventions being investigated.

In **decompensated cirrhosis**, sometimes called **end-stage liver disease (ESLD)**, the body is unable to compensate for the functional deterioration of the liver, resulting in life-threatening complications.

Table 13.9 Classifications and Related Staging of Hepatic Encephalopathy

Classification		West Haven Stages	
Minimal (MHE)	Subclinical (West Haven Stage 0)	0	Normal consciousness and behavior, impaired psychomotor ability
Persistent	Chronic Never free of overt HE (West Haven Stage 1–4)	1	Mild lack of awareness, shortened attention span, mild asterixis
Episodic	Acute Clinically undetectable (West Haven Stage 0) between overt episodes	2	Lethargic, disoriented, inappropriate behavior, asterixis, slurred speech
		3	Somnolent but arousable, gross disorientation, incoherent speech, bizarre behavior, hyper-reflexia, muscular rigidity
		4	Comatose, decerebrate posturing

Data from Bajaj JS. Review article: the modern management of hepatic encephalopathy. *Aliment Pharmacol Ther.* 2010;31(5):537-547.

Table 13.10 Theories on the Pathogenesis of Hepatic Encephalopathy

	Pathophysiology	Potential Nutrition Intervention
Ammonia	Increased circulating levels of ammonia, derived primarily from the gut; accumulation due to decreased urea cycle function; result depletes glutamate (an excitatory neurotransmitter) and increases glutamine in astrocytes (causing swelling)	Probiotic to decrease bacterial urease activity in the intestinal lumen and decrease ammonia absorption. Correct zinc deficiency.
Manganese	Increased circulating levels of manganese lead to manganese deposition in the brain, causing dopaminergic dysfunction, neuronal loss, and astrocytic changes	Avoid manganese supplement.
False neurotransmitter/ aromatic amino acid (AAA)	Increased circulating levels of AAA and decreased circulating levels of branched-chain amino acid (BCAA) allow enhanced AAA uptake by brain neurotransmitters	BCAA supplementation and/or encourage vegetable proteins, which are high in BCAA
Tumor necrosis factor-alpha (TNF-α)	Circulating levels correlate with severity of encephalopathy in acute and chronic liver disease, which may be neurotoxic. TNF-α is produced in response to intestinal translocation of endotoxin, among other things.	Probiotic/prebiotic to decrease intestinal permeability

Data from Kalaitzakis E, Josefsson A, Bjornsson E. Type and etiology of liver cirrhosis are not related to the presence of hepatic encephalopathy or health-related quality of life: a cross-sectional study. *BMC Gastroenterol.* 2008;8:46.; Bacon BR. Genetic, metabolic, and infiltrative diseases affecting the liver. In: Longo DL, Fauci AS, Kasper DL, Hauser SL, Jameson JL, Loscalzo J, eds. *Harrison's Principles of Internal Medicine.* 18th ed. New York, NY: McGraw-Hill; 2012:chap 309.

The following are complications that may be found in ESLD.

- Bleeding varices: Patients may present with hematemesis or melena secondary to bleeding varices, which can be treated by endoscopic band ligation. **Transjugular intrahepatic portosystemic shunt (TIPS)** placement helps alleviate portal hypertension to prevent recurrent variceal bleeds.
- **Coagulopathy**: The liver's inability to synthesize clotting proteins, along with malnutrition and vitamin K deficiency, causes coagulopathy. Subcutaneous vitamin K and fresh frozen plasma may be given in an effort to improve blood clotting.
- Refractory ascites: Patients may have respiratory distress, early satiety, and abdominal pain due to severe ascites. This can be treated with **paracentesis** (aspiration of fluid from the peritoneal cavity) and parenteral albumin administration. TIPS placement can alleviate refractory ascites as well.

- **Spontaneous bacterial peritonitis (SBP)**: Patients may have fevers and abdominal pain due to SBP, a complication of ascites and paracentesis. This is treated with antibiotics after analysis of peritoneal fluid.
- Jaundice: Patients may notice a yellowing of the skin and eyes, called jaundice or icterus, respectively, due to hyperbilirubinemia.
- **Hepatorenal syndrome (HRS)**: Patients may require hemodialysis due to HRS. HRS is only reversed by liver transplant.
- Hepatic encephalopathy: Patients may present with severe hepatic encephalopathy. Hepatic encephalopathy can be precipitated by gastrointestinal (GI) bleeding, sepsis, dehydration, hyponatremia, surgery, TIPS, constipation, infection (including SBP), paracentesis, and medication noncompliance. Primary treatment includes identifying and treating the precipitant along with a prescription of lactulose, which is a nonabsorbable polysaccharide that acidifies the colon and promotes elimination of ammonia and the bacteria that synthesize ammonia.[5,67]

It is good to be familiar with two scoring systems that are used to classify the severity of disease and prognosis of individuals with cirrhosis: the **Child-Pugh score** and **MELD (Model for End-Stage Liver Disease)** score. The MELD score is now preferred and used in considering patients for liver transplant. Both are calculated using readily available labs (such as bilirubin, albumin, international normalized ratio [INR], and creatinine) and clinical factors (presence of ascites, age, need for dialysis). The Child–Pugh scoring system uses class A, B, or C, with class C being the most severe. The MELD gives a score of 1 to >40. Higher scores predict higher 90-day mortality.[67]

CORE CONCEPT 6

Malnutrition correlates with severity of liver disease and is nearly universal in patients with end-stage liver disease.

Nutrition Assessment

In 2019, the Global Leadership Initiative on Malnutrition (GLIM), a committee comprised of representatives from nutrition associations from the United States, Europe, Latin America, and Asia, published a consensus report for diagnostic criteria for malnutrition. The diagnosis requires at least one "phenotypic criterion" and one "etiologic criterion." Phenotypic criteria include weight loss, low body mass index, and reduced muscle mass. Etiologic criteria include reduced food intake or absorption and inflammation (acute or chronic disease). Severity can then be differentiated into moderate or severe malnutrition based on cut-offs within two of the phenotypic criteria (degree of weight loss, BMI). The committee proposed a two-step process: screening and assessment. Validated screening tools, such as Nutrition Risk Screening-2002 (NRS-2002), the Malnutrition Universal Screening Tool (MUST), and the Mini-Nutrition Assessment–Short Form (MNA-SF), should be used to identify those at risk for malnutrition. Refer to Chapter 1, *Nutrition Assessment,* for more information on nutrition screening tools. Those at risk should then undergo a formal nutrition assessment using the GLIM criteria.[72] **Table 13.11** the general criteria.

Table 13.11 GLIM Categories for Malnutrition

PHENOTYPIC CRITERIA
Weight loss
Low body mass index
Reduced muscle mass
ETIOLOGIC CRITERIA
Reduced food intake or assimilation
Inflammation

Data from Cederholm T, Jensen GL, Correia MITD, et al. ESPEN endorsed recommendation: GLIM criteria for the diagnosis of malnutrition—a consensus report from the global clinical nutrition community. *Clin Nutr.* 2019;38(1):1-9. doi:10.1016/j.clnu.2018.08.002

Historically, the challenge with nutrition screening and assessment tools for patients with liver disease is the reliance on weight, which is hugely confounded by ascites or edema. The GLIM acknowledges this by removing weight loss and BMI as necessary criteria, allowing for reduced muscle mass to qualify as a phenotypic criterion for malnutrition. Next will be a discussion of the application of the GLIM recommendations in this population, as well as a brief introduction to some liver disease–specific tools for screening and assessment.

Nutrition Screening

Using the GLIM criteria for malnutrition diagnosis as the gold standard, both the MNA-SF and the Royal Free Hospital–Nutrition Prioritizing Tool (RFH-NPT) have been found to be accurate screening tools in patients with cirrhosis.[73,74] The RFH-NPT is a liver disease–specific tool that is most widely recommended.[25,66,75,76] This tool classifies nutrition risk as low, moderate, or high. Anyone who is a transplant candidate/recipient, has acute AH, or requires enteral nutrition is automatically high risk. The rest are assessed for fluid overload. Those without fluid overload are scored according to weight change, BMI, and presence of acute illness. Those with fluid overload are scored according to their dietary intake and weight loss.[25,66]

Phenotypic Criteria

As mentioned earlier, the phenotypic criteria using weight can be problematic in patients with ascites and edema. For these patients, an estimated dry weight should be used. Ideally, this is the patient's usual or post-paracentesis weight. If this is not available, subtract a percentage of the actual weight for ascites (5% for mild ascites, 10% for moderate ascites, 15% for severe ascites). Subtract an additional 5% of the actual weight if pedal edema is present.[25,66,75] Since many patients with cirrhosis have obesity, the BMI criteria may not be met in an individual with malnutrition. Therefore, the most important phenotypic criteria in this population will be reduced muscle mass, determined using validated body composition measuring techniques. Functional muscle assessments, such as handgrip strength, may be used as well.[77]

Sarcopenia, which is reduced muscle mass and strength, is associated with mortality in cirrhosis.[66,78] Significant muscle depletion increases the risk of HE.[69] The gold standard for diagnosing sarcopenia is measuring skeletal muscle on a computed tomography (CT) scan at the L3 vertebral level. Other measures of muscle mass use a dual-energy X-ray absorptiometry (DEXA) scan or bioelectrical impedance analysis (BIA), but these may not be readily available and are not reliable in individuals with fluid overload. Mid-arm muscle circumference (MAMC) or calf circumference measures may also be used (**Figure 13.8**). These correlate with severity of disease and are less affected by non-nutritional factors, such as fluid retention.[76] However, they may be more valuable in the outpatient setting to monitor changes in body composition in the same patient over time.

Reduced muscle function correlates with depletion of lean body mass and protein calorie malnutrition.[79] Handgrip strength measured by a handgrip dynamometer is an inexpensive, simple tool for objectively measuring muscle function and can be used to diagnose sarcopenia and satisfy the phenotypic criteria for malnutrition.[76] In a study of patients with compensated liver disease, handgrip dynamometry was significantly reduced in 63% of patients, and these patients had a significantly higher

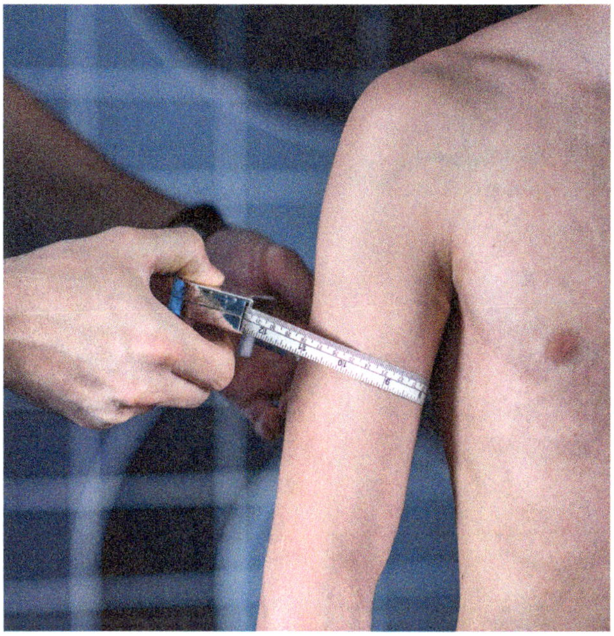

Figure 13.8 Mid-Arm Muscle Circumference (MAMC) That Measures Lean Tissue Stores May Be a Useful Indicator of Nutritional Status in Patients with Liver Disease

morbidity and mortality in the following year.[80] The Liver Frailty Index is a tool to assess frailty specific to this population; it incorporates handgrip strength, a timed chair stand test, and a timed balance test. This calculator, along with detailed instructions for the functional tests, can be found online at https://liverfrailtyindex.uscf.edu/. Frailty, as measured using this tool, is associated with liver disease progression and mortality.[66,81–83]

Unless a CT scan is available to evaluate for sarcopenia, other objective measures of muscle mass and function are challenging in a patient who is bedbound or cannot follow instructions due to mental status or acute illness. This is where a subjective assessment, such as asking the patient or family about their ability to engage in typical activities and a physical exam identifying muscle wasting, may be more practical than objective measurements. It is good to be aware of two global nutrition assessment tools that have been recommended for patients with cirrhosis.[12,75] These include the Subjective Global Assessment (SGA) and the Royal Free Hospital Global Assessment (RFH-GA), which is specifically adapted for liver disease. These have been validated and correlate with disease prognosis.[84,85] However, a study in 2023 comparing the SGA and RFH-GA to the GLIM criteria found that the GLIM criteria more accurately predicted mortality in this population.[86]

CORE CONCEPT 7

Muscle and adipose tissue wasting in patients with liver disease is an independent predictor of mortality. Muscle loss is also associated with hepatic encephalopathy. Nutrition assessment will require measures of muscle mass or function, rather than weight and BMI.

Etiologic Criteria

Any patient with acute illness experiencing complications of hepatic decompensation or an unrelated acute illness (sepsis, trauma) will meet the etiologic criteria for inflammation. Simply having chronic liver disease does not meet this criteria, but a C-reactive protein (CRP) level over 5 mg/dL does.[76,77] Those without inflammation will need an assessment of food intake to determine whether they meet the etiologic criteria for malnutrition.

Evaluating for reduced food intake likely requires the expertise and clinical judgment of a registered dietitian (RD). Identifying energy requirements is difficult in patients with cirrhosis, as described in the next section of the chapter.[76] The RD can also assess chronicity of reduced intake since multiple factors contribute to poor oral intake in patients with liver disease. They may have anorexia and taste changes related to anorexigenic cytokines, zinc deficiency, or elevated brain serotonin levels. Dietary restrictions may make food options limited and less desirable. If ascites is present, early satiety and abdominal discomfort can severely limit intake. Malabsorption of fat and fat-soluble vitamins also contributes to malnutrition for patients with liver disease. Patients with alcohol-related liver disease may ingest a greater percentage of their calories in the form of alcohol and have impaired absorption of thiamine and folic acid. As liver disease progresses, not only are the aforementioned issues compounded, but patients may be frequently hospitalized, where they are often incapable of eating or kept nil per os (NPO) for procedures.[12,66] **Table 13.12** highlights the multiple factors that can contribute to malnutrition in this population.

Nutrition Intervention

Malnutrition predicts complications, patient survival, and outcomes following liver transplant. It is associated with increased risk of bacterial infections, encephalopathy, posttransplant mortality, and longer hospital stays. Muscle and adipose tissue wasting is an independent predictor of mortality. Using the GLIM criteria for diagnosis of malnutrition, 57% of patients awaiting liver transplant were malnourished, and they had 3.79 times increased risk of mortality.[86] The severity of malnutrition correlates with the severity of liver disease and is especially prevalent in alcohol-related liver disease.[87] Thus, preventing and treating malnutrition early should be of utmost importance in this population.

Table 13.12 Causes of Malnutrition in Liver Disease

Factors Contributing to Malnutrition		Etiology
Impaired intake	▪ Anorexia ▪ Abnormal taste ▪ Early satiety ▪ Altered mental status ▪ Frequent hospitalization ▪ Dietary restrictions	▪ Cytokine mediated, zinc deficiency ▪ Ascites ▪ Severe hepatic encephalopathy with dysphagia ▪ Frequent NPO status for procedures ▪ Inappropriate diet orders
Metabolic alterations	▪ Hypermetabolism ▪ Early starvation metabolism ▪ Protein deficiency ▪ Micronutrient deficiency	▪ Cytokine mediated ▪ Decreased hepatic glycogen content ▪ Decreased synthesis of protein/increased protein needs for gluconeogenesis ▪ Impaired nutrient storage
Increased nutrient losses	▪ Treatment related ▪ Malabsorption	▪ Diuretic therapy, paracentesis ▪ Alcohol use disorder, decreased bile flow

Modified from Saunders J, Brian A, Wright M, et al. Malnutrition and nutrition support in patients with liver disease. *Frontline Gastroenterol.* 2010;1:105-111.

CASE STUDY REVISITED

Three years later at a follow-up visit, the RD finds from Marisol's medical record that she has been diagnosed with cirrhosis. She has been following up regularly with her PCP and taking her prescribed medications. Her PCP prescribed a GLP-1 agonist for her, but her insurance would not cover it. She went for a consultation with a bariatric surgeon. She also saw an orthopedist for her knee and was diagnosed with meniscal tear and recommended surgery. Of note, she was hospitalized last year with sepsis and hypoxic respiratory failure due to pneumonia. After this, her pulmonologist diagnosed her with obstructive sleep apnea.

In the interview, Marisol, now 44 years old, states she declined bariatric surgery because it is too extreme. She completed physical therapy, which helped her knee somewhat, but she still cannot do much activity. Since her grandchild is in school and she is now working at a grocery store, she cannot afford to take time off from her job and household duties to have the recommended knee surgery.

Anthropometric Data:

Height: 160 cm
Weight: 90 kg
BMI: 35.2 kg/m^2
Waist circumference: 88 cm

Biochemical Data:

Hemoglobin A1c 6.2% (<5.7%)
LDL-cholesterol 69 (Optimal <100 mg/dL)
HDL-cholesterol 41 (Optimal >40 mg/dL)
Triglycerides 176 (Optimal <150 mg/dL)
Fasting glucose 102 (<100 mg/dL)
Alanine aminotransferase 70 (4–36 units/L)
Aspartate aminotransferase 30 (10–40 units/L)
Alkaline phosphatase 63 (30–120 units/L)
Total bilirubin 0.9 (0.3–1.9 mg/dL)

Clinical Data:

Past Medical History: Obesity, cirrhosis, diabetes, dyslipidemia, hypertension, alcohol dependence, right knee meniscus tear, obstructive sleep apnea

Medications: Chlorthalidone, diclofenac, losartan, metformin, rosuvastatin

OTC Meds/Supplements: Women's multivitamin

Vital Signs: Blood pressure 138/84 mm Hg, Temperature 97.8°F, Heart rate 90 beats/min

Nutrition-Focused Physical Exam: Handgrip strength: two standard deviations below the reference normal. You note an increase in her waist circumference as well as temporal, upper, and lower extremity muscle wasting.

Dietary History:

Due to a decreased appetite and shifting work schedule, Marisol only eats small snacks throughout the day. With her children no longer living with her, she does not prepare meals often so it is easy for her to avoid rice. Working at a grocery store makes it easier to incorporate a fruit and vegetable daily. She has been avoiding meat because she read online that protein is bad for the liver. She was able to cut out coffee and soda, because she sleeps better now with a continuous positive airway pressure (CPAP) machine so does not need caffeine. However, she still enjoys drinking 1 cocktail containing 3 oz of tequila most nights.

Questions

1. What do you interpret Marisol's weight?
2. Assess Marisol's PES statements from her last visit. Identify if each statement remains an active issue or if the PES statement has been resolved. If the PES statement remains an active issue, has improvement in the issue been noted? If the issue has been resolved, write a new PES statement.
3. Are there any micronutrients that you would like to supplement?
4. What socioeconomic factors may have contributed to Marisol's decline in liver function?

Energy Requirements

Predictive equations for energy requirements in people with cirrhosis are not accurate. When comparing predicted to measured energy expenditure, studies have found wide individual variation. Between 5% and 58% of patients are hypermetabolic (measured energy requirement greater than 120% of predicted energy requirement), while 11–36% are hypometabolic (measured energy expenditure less than

90% of predicted). The Harris–Benedict and Schofield equations tend to underestimate energy requirements, while weight-based (kcal/kg) calculations tend to overestimate. People with severe malnutrition, on diuretics, and with more advanced disease are more likely to be hypermetabolic.[88,89] Therefore, guidelines from international organizations all agree that indirect calorimetry should be used to measure resting energy expenditure, especially in patients who are critically ill or in stable patients who experience muscle wasting despite seemingly adequate nutritional intake.[66,88–90] Handheld calorimeters are a less-expensive alternative to the metabolic cart and are valid in hospitalized patients with cirrhosis.[91]

Various organizations provide guidance for estimating energy needs in the absence of available indirect calorimetry. Patients with cirrhosis without obesity can be estimated to need 35–40 kcal/kg/day. The higher end of the range is for those with severe malnutrition or acute illness. For patients with a BMI of 30–40 kg/m^2, use 25–35 kcal/kg/day. For patients with BMI over 40 kg/m^2, use 20–25 kcal/kg/day. If significant edema or ascites is present, the patient's dry weight should be used to estimate needs.[12,66,75,92]

CORE CONCEPT 8

Indirect calorimetry should be used to determine energy needs for patients with cirrhosis. Handheld calorimeters are a valid option.

Protein Requirements

Protein requirements for patients with cirrhosis are increased. This, along with physical activity, should be emphasized for maintenance of lean body mass. Recommended protein intake is 1.2–1.5 g/kg of protein for compensated and decompensated cirrhosis, respectively. For those that are acutely or critically ill, protein requirements are similar to those of patients in the intensive care unit: 1.2–2 g/kg for BMI less than 30 kg/m^2, 2 g/kg ideal body weight for BMI 30–40 kg/m^2, and 2.5 g/kg ideal body weight for BMI over 40 kg/m^2.[25,75,90]

Protein should not be restricted as a strategy to reduce risk of HE. Historically, it was common practice to restrict protein intake in people with HE, thinking that increased protein intake would lead to higher levels of ammonia. This practice is now widely condemned. A prospective study at Veterans Affairs Medical Centers in the 1990s evaluated HE and dietary protein intake in patients with AH. They found that low protein intake was independently associated with worsening HE, whereas those that were less malnourished and had higher protein intake had improved HE.[93] A key trial by Cordoba et al.[94] in 2004 compared a low-protein diet (0.5 g/kg/day) to a higher-protein diet (1.2 g/kg/day) for patients with cirrhosis admitted with an episode of HE. There was no difference in outcomes and higher endogenous protein breakdown in the low-protein diet group compared to the higher-protein diet.[94] Therefore, providing adequate protein is safe and can preserve lean body mass in patients with HE.[95] Furthermore, protein intake <0.8 g/kg/day was found to be an independent predictor of mortality in patients awaiting liver transplant.[96]

A 2017 Cochrane review of 16 trials found high-quality evidence that BCAA supplementation improves HE, although there was no benefit to mortality.[97] Eight trials evaluated oral BCAA supplementation, while seven evaluated intravenous BCAAs.

CORE CONCEPT 9

Patients with cirrhosis require a minimum of 1.2 grams protein/kg/day, up to 2 grams/kg/day depending on their nutritional status and clinical condition. Protein should not be restricted in hepatic encephalopathy.

Micronutrients

There are not enough high-quality studies to be able to make a general recommendation for micronutrient supplementation in cirrhosis. However, there are many situations where supplementation is appropriate based on clinical or suspected deficiencies. Thiamine (vitamin B1) and folic acid (vitamin B9) should be empirically provided to individuals with increased alcohol consumption. High-dose thiamine should be given to patients presenting with altered mental status who have cirrhosis from any etiology (not only ALD), to exclude Wernicke's encephalopathy before assuming HE. Other B vitamin deficiencies (B6, B12) may develop rapidly due to decreased hepatic storage, and empiric supplementation is safe.[12]

Vitamin D deficiency is common and associated with advanced liver disease. People with cirrhosis have increased risk of osteoporosis, called "hepatic osteodystrophy," although this is not well understood.[98] In one study, severe deficiency (25-hydroxyvitamin D [25(OH)D] <7 ng/mL) was present in about one-third of patients and 92% had 25(OH)D levels <30 ng/dL, which is the suggested threshold for vitamin D sufficiency.[99] In patients with ALD, 25(OH)D levels <10 ng/mL have been associated with increased liver damage and mortality.[100] Finally, vitamin D levels <6 ng/mL were identified as a significant predictor of death in patients with advanced liver cirrhosis (Child–Pugh C).[101] There are multiple explanations for why vitamin D serum levels may be low in cirrhosis. It could be actual deficiency from inadequate intake and sun exposure or fat malabsorption. It could also appear low due to decreased serum binding proteins or decreased hydroxylation of vitamin D to 25(OH)D as the first step in converting it to its active form. Although there is no evidence that vitamin D supplementation improves mortality, oral vitamin D supplementation improves 25(OH)D levels,[102] and there are a few small studies showing a benefit in long-term supplementation of 1000 or 2000 IU/day.[103,104] It is reasonable, if not advisable, to monitor and replete vitamin D in patients with cirrhosis and cholestatic liver disease.[25] Empiric supplementation of 1000 IU daily is also reasonable if laboratory studies are not available or too costly.[75]

Clinical Roundtable

Background: Health disparities are plausibly preventable health differences experienced by socially disadvantaged populations. While alcohol use disorder has increased in all demographics, the burden of ALD has disproportionately affected racial and ethnic marginalized communities and people living in economic hardship, particularly women. For MASLD, Hispanic persons, women >50, and people with food insecurity are at highest risk. Racial and ethnic marginalized communities and/or those who are under- or uninsured have greater liver disease related mortality from viral hepatitis and later-stage diagnosis of HCC.

Roundtable Discussion

1. What policy level changes can be implemented to improve health equity for individuals with MASLD and ALD?
2. What health system changes can be implemented?
3. What change can you implement into your daily practice?
4. Can you give an example of a personal advantage you possess that improves your health and explain why?

References

Data from Jones PD, Lai JC, Bajaj JS, Kanwal F. Actionable solutions to achieve health equity in chronic liver disease. *Clin Gastroenterol Hepatol*. 2023;21(8):1992-2000. doi:10.1016/j.cgh.2023.03.043; Kardashian A, Serper M, Terrault N. Health disparities in chronic liver disease. *Hepatology*. 2023;77:1382-1403. doi:10.1002/hep.32743.

PRACTICE POINT

Micronutrient deficiencies are common in chronic liver disease, in particular vitamin D, zinc, and B vitamins. There is insufficient evidence to make a generalized recommendation, but it is reasonable to empirically supplement micronutrients when dietary or clinical deficiencies are suspected.

Zinc deficiency has been implicated in the pathophysiology of HE due to the role of zinc as a coenzyme in pathways that remove ammonia from the blood.[105] However, clear evidence that zinc supplementation improves HE is lacking.[106,107] Many clinical manifestations of zinc deficiency overlap with symptoms of chronic liver disease (**Table 13.13**). If zinc deficiency is the cause of anorexia, taste abnormalities, weight loss, impaired wound healing, increased susceptibility to infection, mental lethargy and emotional disorders, or hyperammonemia, these can be reversed with supplementation.[108] Those taking diuretics or abusing alcohol have especially high urinary zinc excretion and subsequently have higher risk of zinc deficiency.[109–111] Because zinc is bound to albumin in the blood, serum zinc level is not a reliable indicator of zinc status in a patient with low albumin. However, it may be prudent to empirically supplement a patient who has symptoms of zinc deficiency, especially those with severe malnutrition, alcohol use disorder, refractory hyperammonemia, or in those taking diuretics. One concern with zinc supplementation is that it may induce copper deficiency; however, patients with cirrhosis may have increased copper levels due to decreased excretion via bile.[112] Therefore, it is considered safe to give supplementation of 50 mg elemental zinc (220 mg zinc sulfate) orally per day. It should be taken with a meal to avoid potential side effects of nausea or GI distress.[62]

CORE CONCEPT 10

Malnutrition, fat malabsorption, alcohol use disorder, and diuretic therapy increase risk of micronutrient deficiencies. Decisions to supplement micronutrients should be made on an individual basis.

Oral Nutrition

Nutrition counseling by an RD, as part of a multidisciplinary team, has been shown to improve survival and quality of life in patients with cirrhosis.[113] RDs can identify micronutrient deficiencies and help patients to achieve their calorie and protein intake

Table 13.13 Signs and Symptoms of Zinc Deficiency

Zinc Deficiency	Mild	Moderate	Severe
Symptoms	■ Oligospermia ■ Decreased lean body mass ■ Hyperammonemia ■ Hypogeusia ■ Decreased dark adaptation	■ Growth faltering ■ Delayed puberty ■ Hypogonadism ■ Rough skin ■ Poor appetite ■ Mental lethargy ■ Delayed wound healing ■ Taste abnormalities	■ Alopecia ■ Diarrhea ■ Emotional disorders ■ Weight loss ■ Intercurrent infections ■ Hypogonadism ■ Bullous-pustular dermatitis ■ Death

Data from Rode A, Fourlanos S, Nicoll A. Oral vitamin D replacement is effective in chronic liver disease. *Gastroenterol Clin Biol.* 2010;34(11):618-620.; Hayashi M, Ikezawa K, Ono A, et al. Evaluation of the effects of combination therapy with branched-chain amino acid and zinc supplements on nitrogen metabolism in liver cirrhosis. *Hepatol Res.* 2007;37(8):615-619.; Ghany M, Hoofnagle JH. Approach to the patient with liver disease. In: Longo DL, Fauci AS, Kasper DL, Hauser SL, Jameson JL, Loscalzo J, eds. *Harrison's Principles of Internal Medicine.* 18th ed. New York, NY: McGraw-Hill; 2012:chap 301.

requirements in spite of their symptoms (e.g., reduced appetite, early satiety) and sometimes dietary restrictions (sodium, processed foods, simple carbohydrates in the setting of diabetes).

Patients with cirrhosis should be instructed to eat regular meals and a bedtime snack to avoid prolonged fasting.[25,75,114] As described earlier, these patients have accelerated starvation, entering a catabolic state with a low RQ overnight. Having a late evening snack decreases lipid oxidation and proteolysis (increases fasting RQ), improves nitrogen balance, and significantly increases total body protein compared to not having a snack or having the equivalent snack during the day.[115–119] Most studies use a high carbohydrate food containing roughly 200 kcal, but an isocaloric BCAA mixture has been shown to be equally efficacious at ameliorating fasting catabolism.[120] Furthermore, a BCAA-fortified snack increased serum albumin and RQ more than a nonfortified snack after being given for 3 months.[121] A trial in 2018 compared a high protein (1.2 grams/kg/day), high fiber (30 grams/day) diet with and without BCAA supplementation for 6 months in patients with cirrhosis (Child Pugh A and B). The group that was given a BCAA supplement had increased MAMC.[122] Oral nutrition supplements (ONS) are recommended for patients who do not meet their nutrition needs with food alone.[25] Along with dietary advice, use of ONS, particularly in the late evening, improves intake and may improve body composition.[115,123]

CORE CONCEPT 11

Patients with cirrhosis should eat a bedtime snack to avoid the accelerated proteolysis and lipid oxidation that occurs after a short period of fasting.

Oral BCAA supplementation for patients with decompensated cirrhosis is recommended[75] due to the demonstrated benefit on HE.[97] The suggested dose is 0.25 g/kg/day. Trials of long-term oral BCAA supplementation have been shown to improve quality of life, reduce the risk for HCC, and prolong survival in patients with cirrhosis.[12,124–127] The first trial to successfully demonstrate this was in Japan in 2005. The BCAA-supplemented group had significantly reduced occurrence of hepatic failure, variceal bleeding, development of HCC, and death from any cause compared to the control group. These findings were so significant that the study was discontinued 10 months early out of concern for the control group.[125] Challenges to patient compliance with BCAA supplementation are palatability and cost of the supplements. There has been some suggestion that patients should be advised to consume a diet high in vegetable and dairy protein due to its increased BCAA content, but there are remarkably few studies to support this and certainly not enough evidence to discourage animal protein in a population that is already struggling to meet protein requirements.[25,75] In a large study of 630 patients awaiting liver transplant, only 24% met the recommended protein intake of >1.2 g/kg/day.[96]

First-line therapy for patients with ascites or edema has been a 2-gram sodium diet restriction. If they have concurrent severe hyponatremia (serum sodium <125 mEq/L), an oral fluid restriction of 1.5 L/day is indicated. Fluid restriction is not recommended for patients with ascites who only have mild-to-moderate hyponatremia or have hypovolemic hyponatremia.[128] An extremely low sodium diet may be considered unpalatable and can exacerbate malnutrition if overall intake is reduced. Without clear evidence that the benefit of a 2-gram sodium diet outweighs this risk, a more reasonable and practical

CORE CONCEPT 12

Patients with ascites should follow a reduced-sodium diet, although this should be liberalized for patients who are not meeting their protein and energy requirements. A free water restriction is only indicated in the setting of severe hyponatremia (serum sodium <125 mEq/L).

PRACTICE POINT

Long-term oral BCAA supplements (0.25 g/kg/day) are beneficial for patients with cirrhosis.

recommendation is a no added salt diet (which usually equates to 4–6 grams Na/day) with avoidance of pre-prepared meals.[12,75,129]

Enteral Nutrition

Enteral nutrition (EN) support is indicated for patients with a functional GI tract who are unable to meet their nutrition needs orally. Patients with liver disease should be given nutrition support with the same considerations as any other patient. Although there is benefit from giving long-term BCAA for chronic liver disease, there is no evidence that a formula high in BCAAs provides benefit for acute episodic HE or patients who are critically ill. Therefore, a standard polymeric protein formula is recommended.[25,75,90] Patients with severe hyponatremia (<125 mEq/L) will need a concentrated formula.

Nonbleeding esophageal varices are not a contraindication for nasoenteric tube placement or EN. In patients with a variceal bleed, it is recommended to wait 48–72 hours after endoscopic treatment of the bleed before initiating EN or oral nutrition.[130] However, a 2023 meta-analysis of 10 randomized controlled trials found no difference between early EN (initiation of EN within 24 hours of achieving hemostasis after upper GI bleed) or delayed EN (waiting 48–72 hours) in terms of early or late rebleeding risk and mortality.[131] More trials are needed specifically in patients with esophageal varices. If a patient is encephalopathic or withdrawing from alcohol, both oral and enteral nutrition carry a high risk of aspiration. The risk of aspiration must be weighed against the risks associated with parenteral nutrition (PN); there are no studies evaluating this. Percutaneous gastrostomy and jejunostomy feeding tubes are generally contraindicated in patients with ascites, due to risk of bleeding and because leakage of gastric contents into the peritoneum can lead to peritonitis.[25,75]

CASE STUDY REVISITED

Another 3 years later, Marisol's spouse brings her to the emergency department with complaints of bloody emesis and mental status changes. On presentation, Marisol (now 47 years old) is barely arousable and unable to answer questions appropriately. Her husband reports that she stayed home with a stomach flu for the past 5 days and today started having bright-red blood in her vomit. She has been confused and progressively more lethargic. The emergency room provider admits Marisol to the inpatient gastroenterology service, and they have requested a nutrition consultation for nutrition assessment and feeding recommendations.

Anthropometrics:

Height: 160 cm
Weight: 114 kg
BMI: 45 kg/m^2
Waist circumference: 96 cm

Biochemical Data:

Cholesterol 215 (Desirable<200 mg/dL)
Alanine aminotransferase 58 (4–36 units/L)
Aspartate aminotransferase 45 (10–40 units/L)
Alkaline phosphatase 100 (30–120 units/L)
Total bilirubin 2.6 (0.3–1.9 mg/dL)
Albumin 2.9 (3.5–5.5 g/dL)
INR 2.6 (0.8–1.1)
PT 9 (11–13.5 seconds)
Hemoglobin 11.2 (13.5–17.5 g/dL)
Hematocrit 35 (37–47% in females)

Clinical Data:

Past Medical History: Obesity, cirrhosis, diabetes, dyslipidemia, hypertension, alcohol dependence, right knee meniscus tear, obstructive sleep apnea

Medications: Lactulose, regular insulin sliding scale, pantoprazole, prednisone

Vital Signs: Blood pressure 102/60 mm Hg, Temperature 97.8°F, Heart rate 101 beats/min

Nutrition-Focused Physical Exam: Handgrip strength: unable to assess; abdomen is protuberant and tense.Her skin is jaundiced. She has temporal, upper, and lower extremity muscle wasting.

Dietary Data:

Diet History: Per Marisol's spouse, Marisol has had minimal oral intake for the last week, but she has not lost any weight recently. She has not been taking any supplements. She stopped drinking alcohol 6 months ago.

Questions

1. At what point would you advocate for Marisol to be placed on nutrition support? Which route is most appropriate and why?
2. Which signs and symptoms indicate that Marisol has developed HE? What may have precipitated HE?

PRACTICE POINT

In a patient at high risk of aspirating oral feeding due to altered mental status, consider bolus enteral feeding to prevent aspiration on a continuous infusion that may occur if the feeding tube is dislodged. Parenteral nutrition may be required for these patients.

Parenteral Nutrition

PN is indicated for patients who are unable to meet their nutrition needs orally or enterally. For such patients who are malnourished, PN should be started immediately. European guidelines recommend starting PN for patients who will require fasting for procedures, especially if fasting for more than 3 days is expected. If a patient requires to be fasted >12 hours, they recommend providing continuous intravenous fluid with 5% or 10% dextrose, providing a glucose infusion rate of 2–3 mg/kg/min.[25] The latter recommendation is based on evidence that late evening meals ameliorate catabolism during an overnight fast, as described earlier. Certainly, patients with fasting hypoglycemia unable to eat should be given intravenous dextrose infusions. However, many patients with cirrhosis are insulin resistant, and it is unclear whether the benefit of providing short-term intravenous dextrose outweighs the risk of hyperglycemia.[120] Caution against overfeeding via PN is important because excess dextrose and lipid calories can lead to hepatic accumulation of triglycerides, or steatosis, especially in a liver that is incapable of adequately exporting triglycerides in lipoproteins. This is when indirect calorimetry to determine energy requirements is especially important.

⚠ Clinical Controversy

Malnutrition that accompanies end-stage liver failure may prompt clinicians to prescribe nutrition support strategies. Maharshi et al. in a randomized controlled trial, demonstrated improved nutritional status and hospital-related quality of life and reduced symptoms of HE. Findings such as these encourage the use of oral supplementation for improving nutritional status and outcome in advanced stages of liver disease. In contrast, Seguin et al. in their randomized controlled trial, could not demonstrate the benefit of perioperative oral supplementation in patients undergoing hepatic surgery.

Questions

1. How do you interpret the differences in these findings?
2. How might differences in study design impact your results (consider intervention used, sample population, outcomes measured)?
3. Would you use either of these supplement strategies for your patients?

References

Data from Maharshi S, Sharma BC, Sachdeva S, Srivastava S, Sharma P. Efficacy of nutritional therapy for patients with cirrhosis and minimal hepatic encephalopathy in a randomized trial. *Clin Gastroenterol Hepatol*. 2016;14:454-460.; Seguin P, Locher C, Bellissant E, et al. Effect of a perioperative nutritional supplementation with Oral Impact in patients undergoing hepatic surgery for liver cancer: a prospective, placebo-controlled, randomized, double-blind study. *Nutr Cancer*. 2016;68(3):464-472.

Table 13.14 Summary of Nutrition Recommendations for Compensated Cirrhosis

Prescribe a bedtime snack.
Prescribe a high protein diet (1.2–1.5 g/kg body weight). Recommend 0.25 g/kg of daily protein be from a BCAA supplement if possible.
Emphasize physical activity, especially resistance exercise for maintaining muscle.
Supplement micronutrients based on individual patient needs.
If ascites is present, avoid added salt and packaged/prepared meals to limit dietary sodium.

Data from Bischoff SC, Bernal W, Dasarathy S, et al. ESPEN practical guideline: clinical nutrition in liver disease. *Clin Nutr*. 2020;39(12):3533-3562. doi:10.1016/j.clnu.2020.09.001; European Association for the Study of the Liver. EASL clinical practice guidelines on nutrition in chronic liver disease. *J Hepatol*. 2019;70:172-193. doi:10.1016/j.jhep.2018.06.024; McClave SA, Taylor BE, Martindale RG, et al. Guidelines for the provision and assessment of nutrition support therapy in the adult critically ill patient: Society of Critical Care Medicine (SCCM) and American Society for Parenteral and Enteral Nutrition (A.S.P.E.N.). *J Parenter Enteral Nutr*. 2016;40(2):159-211. doi:10.1177/0148607115621863; Ney M, Abraldes JG, Ma M, et al. Insufficient protein intake is associated with increased mortality in 630 patients with cirrhosis awaiting liver transplantation. *Nutr Clin Pract*. 2015;30(4):530-536. doi:10.1177/0884533614567716; Gluud LL, Dam G, Les I, et al. Branched-chain amino acids for people with hepatic encephalopathy. Cochrane Database Syst Rev. 2017;2017(5):CD001939. doi:10.1002/14651858.CD001939.pub4

A parenteral amino acid solution containing a higher amount of BCAA and a lower amount of AAA was developed in the 1980s when studies associated low plasma BCAA and concurrent high plasma AAA with HE. The evidence for parenteral BCAA provision in HE is not convincing. Trials have shown benefit in mental status but no effect on survival.[97] Guidelines recommended using a standard amino acid composition.[25,90]

Patients with cirrhosis may have elevated serum copper and manganese,[112] thus they should have copper and manganese decreased or removed from their PN to avoid toxicity, especially long term. Manganese toxicity is associated with motor and psychiatric disturbances and may also be a factor in the pathogenesis of HE.[132] Intravenous thiamine should be supplemented to all patients with malnutrition to prevent deficiency. These patients should also be closely monitored for refeeding syndrome with the initiation of PN. For patients with severe hyponatremia, parenteral nutrients should be mixed in normal saline (154 mEq/L or 0.9% NaCl) to restrict free water. However, an overall fluid restriction is not always indicated, because patients with ascites can still be intravascularly dry. **Tables 13.14** and **13.15** provide summaries for nutrition recommendations for patients with compensated and decompensated cirrhosis, respectively.

Table 13.15 Summary of Nutrition Recommendations for Decompensated or Acutely Ill Patients with Cirrhosis

EN and PN support is indicated just as it is in any other patient population.
Energy requirements should be determined using indirect calorimetry.
Protein requirements are 1.2–2 g/kg body weight (using estimated dry weight). Do not restrict protein provision in hepatic encephalopathy.
Standard protein formulations (both EN and PN) should be used. Concentrated formulas are necessary if there is severe hyponatremia (<125 mEq/L).
Ensure appropriate micronutrient repletion based on individual patient assessment.
Omit copper and manganese from PN formulation.

Data from Bischoff SC, Bernal W, Dasarathy S, et al. ESPEN practical guideline: clinical nutrition in liver disease. *Clin Nutr*. 2020;39(12):3533-3562. doi:10.1016/j.clnu.2020.09.001; European Association for the Study of the Liver. EASL clinical practice guidelines on nutrition in chronic liver disease. *J Hepatol*. 2019;70:172-193. doi:10.1016/j.jhep.2018.06.024; McClave SA, Taylor BE, Martindale RG, et al. Guidelines for the provision and assessment of nutrition support therapy in the adult critically ill patient: Society of Critical Care Medicine (SCCM) and American Society for Parenteral and Enteral Nutrition (A.S.P.E.N.). *J Parenter Enteral Nutr*. 2016;40(2):159-211. doi:10.1177/0148607115621863; Ney M, Abraldes JG, Ma M, et al. Insufficient protein intake is associated with increased mortality in 630 patients with cirrhosis awaiting liver transplantation. *Nutr Clin Pract*. 2015;30(4):530-536. doi:10.1177/0884533614567716; Gluud LL, Dam G, Les I, et al. Branched-chain amino acids for people with hepatic encephalopathy. Cochrane Database Syst Rev. 2017;2017(5):CD001939. doi:10.1002/14651858.CD001939.pub4

PRACTICE POINT

In patients with ALD, provide 200 mg intravenous or intramuscular thiamine prior to initiation of nutrition support and daily thereafter for 3 days. In any patient with malnutrition with liver disease, provide 100 mg oral thiamine for 5–7 days. Thereafter, recommend a B complex if the patient is not able to take adequate food on a daily basis.

PRACTICE POINT

Work with the healthcare team to avoid prolonged periods of fasting for procedures for patients with cirrhosis. If it is necessary for the patient to be fasted for more than 3 days, consider starting PN for patients with malnutrition.

Monitoring and Evaluation

Monitoring patients with liver disease includes tracking nutritional status, primarily through measures of lean body mass and nutritional intake. Weight and waist circumference can be monitored to assess edema and ascites. Handgrip strength, MAMC, and frailty testing can be used to monitor functional status, a surrogate for lean body mass. For those who are losing lean mass despite seemingly adequate nutritional intake, monitor for energy imbalance and, if possible, measure energy expenditure via indirect calorimetry. Monitor food choices, ensuring a high protein diet that incorporates plant-based proteins, if possible. Evaluate and mitigate barriers to adequate nutritional intake, such as dietary restrictions, early satiety, altered taste, altered mental status, and frequent hospitalizations. Monitor meal patterns, ensuring avoidance of prolonged fasting through regular meals and a bedtime snack. For those who are having difficulty meeting their protein and energy requirements orally, monitor for the need for a liberalized diet or for enteral or parenteral nutrition according to their aspiration risk and GI function. Assess adequacy of micronutrient intake, and supplement empirically when dietary or clinical deficiencies are apparent. Assess for fat and fat-soluble vitamin deficiency. Fluid and sodium intake should be monitored for patients on a fluid restriction. Always ask about patient use of herbal and dietary supplements, to monitor compliance to prescribed supplements (such as vitamin E or BCAA) as well as potentially hepatotoxic supplements they may have started on their own. Ask about alcohol intake, encouraging abstinence from alcohol for all patients with liver disease, regardless of etiology. Ask about physical activity, both to reverse steatosis and to maintain lean body mass in those with more advanced disease. Monitor stool patterns, assessing for adequate fiber to minimize straining from constipation and diarrhea, which can occur as a side effect of lactulose or from malabsorption. Finally, evaluate for socioeconomic challenges (food insecurity, lack of transportation, language barriers) and refer appropriately to resources that may help patient adherence or access to nutrition and medical care.

Summary

Although there are many different types of liver disease, all are affected by malnutrition and its associated complications. The liver has a prominent role in metabolism of nutrients; understanding the derangements in metabolism during liver disease and failure is central to providing medical nutrition therapy. The RD is an essential part of the care team, not only to provide assessment and counseling of the patient, but to guide and educate the healthcare team on what nutrition interventions can or cannot benefit the patient. Nutrition is as important, if not more important, for the outpatient in the early stages of disease, as it is for the patient with decompensated failure. There is much yet to be understood about therapies for MASLD, ascites, and HE, as well as the role of probiotics, zinc, BCAAs, and other nutrients.

Key Terms

Kupffer cells, stellate cells, gut–liver axis, hepatocellular liver disease, cholestatic liver disease, acute hepatitis, acute liver failure, chronic hepatitis, fibrosis, cirrhosis, portal hypertension, portosystemic shunting, varices, underfill hypothesis, ascites, hepatic encephalopathy (HE), decompensated cirrhosis/end-stage liver disease (ESLD), transjugular intrahepatic portosystemic shunt (TIPS), coagulopathy, paracentesis, spontaneous bacterial peritonitis (SBP), hepatorenal syndrome (HRS), Child–Pugh score and MELD (Model for End-Stage Liver Disease), viral hepatitis, fulminant liver failure, shock liver, acute-on-chronic hepatitis, steatosis, alcohol-related liver disease (ALD), steatohepatitis, alcohol-related hepatitis (AH), endotoxin, tumor necrosis factor-alpha (TNF-α), De Ritis ratio, metabolic dysfunction–associated steatotic liver disease (MASLD), metabolic dysfunction–associated steatohepatitis (MASH), parenteral nutrition–associated liver disease (PNALD), intestinal failure–associated liver disease (IFALD), hemochromatosis, Wilson's disease, Kayser–Fleischer ring, dysgeusia, metallothionein, branched-chain amino acids (BCAAs)

References

1. Ghany MG, Hoofnagle JH. Approach to the patient with liver disease. In: Loscalzo J, Fauci A, Kasper D, Hauser S, Longo D, Jameson J, eds. *Harrison's Principles of Internal Medicine*. 21st ed. McGraw-Hill Education; 2022.
2. Tilg H, Adolph TE, Trauner M. Gut-liver axis: pathophysiological concepts and clinical implications. *Cell Metab*. 2022;34(11):1700–1718. doi:10.1016/J.CMET.2022.09.017

3. Bethea ED, Pratt DS. Evaluation of liver function. In: Loscalzo J, Fauci A, Kasper D, Hauser S, Longo D, Jameson J, eds. *Harrison's Principles of Internal Medicine.* 21st ed. McGraw-Hill Education; 2022.
4. Dienstag JL. Chronic hepatitis. In: Loscalzo J, Fauci A, Kasper D, Hauser S, Longo D, Jameson J, eds. *Harrison's Principles of Internal Medicine.* 21st ed. McGraw-Hill Education; 2022.
5. Befeler AS, Bacon BR. Cirrhosis and its complications. In: Loscalzo J, Fauci AS, Kasper DL, Hauser SL, Longo DL, Jameson JL, eds. *Harrison's Principles of Internal Medicine.* 21st ed. New York, NY: McGraw-Hill Education; 2022.
6. Abdelmalek MF, Diehl AM. Nonalcoholic fatty liver diseases and nonalcoholic steatohepatitis. In: Loscalzo J, Fauci A, Kapser D, Hauser S, Longo D, Jameson J, eds. *Harrison's Principles of Internal Medicine.* 21st ed. McGraw-Hill Education; 2022.
7. Phoolchund AGS, Khakoo SI. MASLD and the development of HCC: pathogenesis and therapeutic challenges. *Cancers.* 2024;16(2). doi:10.3390/CANCERS16020259
8. Ling P, McCowen K. Carbohydrate metabolism. In: McClave S, Mueller C, eds. *The A.S.P.E.N. Adult Nutrition Support Core Curriculum.* 2nd ed. The American Society of Enteral and Parenteral Nutrition; 2012:43–46.
9. Mijller MJ, Willmann O, Rieger A, et al. Mechanism of insulin resistance associated with liver cirrhosis. *Gastroenterol.* 1992;102:2033–2943.
10. Verboeket-van de Venne WP, Westerterp KR, Van Hoek B, Swart GR. Energy expenditure and substrate metabolism in patients with cirrhosis of the liver: effects of the pattern of food intake. *Gut.* 1995;36(1):110. doi:10.1136/GUT.36.1.110
11. Young L, Kearns L, Schoefel S, Canon Clark N. Protein. In: McClave S, Mueller C, eds. *The A.S.P.E.N. Adult Nutrition Support Core Curriculum.* 2nd ed. American Society for Parenteral and Enteral Nutrition; 2012:92.
12. Espina S, Casas-Deza D, Bernal-Monterde V, Domper-Arnal MJ, García-Mateo S, Lué A. Evaluation and management of nutritional consequences of chronic liver diseases. *Nutrients.* 2023;15(15). doi:10.3390/nu15153487
13. Lambert JE, Parks EJ. Postprandial metabolism of meal triglyceride in humans. *Biochim Biophys Acta.* 2012;1821(5):721. doi:10.1016/J.BBALIP.2012.01.006
14. Mouzaki M, Ng V, Kamath BM, Selzner N, Pencharz P, Ling SC. Enteral energy and macronutrients in end-stage liver disease. *JPEN.* 2014;38(6):673–681. doi:10.1177/0148607114522488
15. Glass C, Hipskind P, Tsien C, et al. Sarcopenia and a physiologically low respiratory quotient in patients with cirrhosis: a prospective controlled study. *J Appl Physiol.* 2013;114(5):559. doi:10.1152/JAPPLPHYSIOL.01042.2012
16. Send SR. Nutritional management of cholestasis. *Clin Liver Dis.* 2020;15(1):9. doi:10.1002/CLD.865
17. Teriaky A, Mosli M, Chandok N, Al-Judaibi B, Marotta P, Qumosani K. Prevalence of fat-soluble vitamin (A, D, and E) and zinc deficiency in patients with cirrhosis being assessed for liver transplantation *Acta Gastroenterol Belg.* 2017; 80(2):237–241. PMID: 29560688.
18. Abbott-Johnson W, Kerlin P, Clague A, Johnson H, Cuneo R. Relationships between blood levels of fat soluble vitamins and disease etiology and severity in adults awaiting liver transplantation. *J Gastroenterol Hepatol.* 2011;26(9): 1402–1410. doi:10.1111/J.1440-1746.2011.06746.X
19. Castaneda D, Gonzalez AJ, Alomari M, Tandon K, Zervos XB. From hepatitis A to E: a critical review of viral hepatitis. *World J Gastroenterol.* 2021;27(16):1691. doi:10.3748/WJG.V27.I16.1691
20. Dienstag JL. Acute viral hepatitis. In: Loscalzo J, Fauci A, Kapser D, Hausesr S, Longo D, Jameson J, eds. *Harrison's Principles of Internal Medicine.* 21st ed. McGraw-Hill Education; 2022.
21. Ghabril M, Ma J, Patidar KR, et al. Eight-fold increase in dietary supplement–related liver failure leading to transplant waitlisting over the last quarter century in the United States. *Liver Transplant.* 2022;28(2):169–179. doi:10.1002/LT.26246
22. Fontana RJ, Liou I, Reuben A, et al. AASLD practice guidance on drug, herbal, and dietary supplement-induced liver injury. *Hepatol.* 2023;77(3):1036–1065. doi:10.1002/hep.32689
23. U.S. Food and Drug Administration. Public notification: Oxy ELITE Pro Super Thermogenic contains hidden drug ingredient. Published March 3, 2015. Accessed August 16, 2024. https://www.fda.gov/drugs/medication-health-fraud/public-notification-oxy-elite-pro-super-thermogenic-contains-hidden-drug-ingredient.
24. Bernal W, Wendon J. Acute liver failure. *N Eng J Med.* 2013;369(26):2525–2534. doi:10.1056/NEJMRA1208937
25. Bischoff SC, Bernal W, Dasarathy S, et al. ESPEN practical guideline: clinical nutrition in liver disease. *Clin Nutr.* 2020;39(12):3533–3562. doi:10.1016/j.clnu.2020.09.001
26. Walsh T, Wigmore S, Hopton P, Richardson R, Lee A. Energy expenditure in acetaminophen-induced fulminant hepatic failure. *Crit Care Med.* 2000;28(3):6496–6654.
27. Terrault NA, Francoz C, Berenguer M, Charlton M, Heimbach J. Liver transplantation 2023: status report, current and future challenges. *Clin Gastroenterol Hepatol.* 2023;21:2150–2166. doi:10.1016/j.cgh.2023.04.005
28. Jophlin LL, Singal AK, Bataller R, et al. ACG clinical guideline: alcohol-associated liver disease. *Am J Gastroenterol.* 2024;119(1):30–54. doi:10.14309/ajg.0000000000002572
29. Swanson GR, Garg K, Shaikh M, Keshavarzian A. Increased intestinal permeability and decreased resiliency of the intestinal barrier in alcoholic liver disease. *Clin Transl Gastroenterol.* 2024;15(4). doi:10.14309/CTG.0000000000000689
30. Purohit V, Bode JC, Bode C, et al. Alcohol, intestinal bacterial growth, intestinal permeability to endotoxin, and medical consequences: summary of a symposium. *Alcohol.* 2008;42(5):349. doi:10.1016/J.ALCOHOL.2008.03.131
31. Singal AK, Charlton MR. Nutrition in alcoholic liver disease. *Clin Liver Dis.* 2012;16(4):805–826. doi:10.1016/J.CLD.2012.08.009
32. Moreno C, Deltenre P, Senterre C, et al. Intensive enteral nutrition is ineffective for patients with severe alcoholic hepatitis treated with corticosteroids. *Gastroenterol.* 2016;150(4): 903–910.e8. doi:10.1053/j.gastro.2015.12.038
33. Antar R, Wong P, Ghali P. A meta-analysis of nutritional supplementation for management of hospitalized alcoholic hepatitis. *Can J Gastroenterol.* 2012;26(7):463. doi:10.1155/2012/945707
34. Cusi K, Isaacs S, Barb D, et al. American Association of Clinical Endocrinology Clinical Practice Guideline for the Diagnosis and Management of Nonalcoholic Fatty Liver Disease in Primary Care and Endocrinology Clinical Settings: Co-Sponsored by the American Association for the Study of Liver Diseases (AASLD). *Endocr Pract.* 2022; 28(5):528–562. doi:10.1016/j.eprac.2022.03.010

35. Rinella ME, Lazarus J V., Ratziu V, et al. A multisociety Delphi consensus statement on new fatty liver disease nomenclature. *Hepatol*. 2023;78(6):1966. doi:10.1097/HEP.0000000000000520
36. Chan WK, Ida NH, Cheah PL, Goh KL. Progression of liver disease in non-alcoholic fatty liver disease: a prospective clinicopathological follow-up study. *J Dig Dis*. 2014;15(10): 545–552. doi:10.1111/1751-2980.12175
37. Sanyal A, Poklepovic A, Moyneur E, Barghout V. Population-based risk factors and resource utilization for HCC: US perspective. *Curr Med Res Opin*. 2010;26(9):2183–2191. doi:10.1185/03007995.2010.506375
38. Vos MB, Abrams SH, Barlow SE, et al. NASPGHAN Clinical Practice Guideline for the Diagnosis and Treatment of Nonalcoholic Fatty Liver Disease in Children: Recommendations from the Expert Committee on NAFLD (ECON) and the North American Society of Pediatric Gastroenterology, Hepatology and Nutrition (NASPGHAN). *J Pediatr Gastroenterol Nutr*. 2017;64(2):319. doi:10.1097/MPG.0000000000001482
39. Rinella ME, Neuschwander-Tetri BA, Siddiqui MS, et al. AASLD Practice Guidance on the clinical assessment and management of nonalcoholic fatty liver disease. *Hepatol*. 2023; 77(5):1797–1835. doi:10.1097/HEP.0000000000000323
40. (EASL)* EA for the S of the L, (EASD) EA for the S of D, (EASO) EA for the S of O. EASL-EASD-EASO Clinical Practice Guidelines on the Management of Metabolic Dysfunction-Associated Steatotic Liver Disease (MASLD). *Obes Facts*. 2024;17(4):374. doi:10.1159/000539371
41. Koutoukidis DA, Astbury NM, Tudor KE, et al. Association of weight loss interventions with changes in biomarkers of nonalcoholic fatty liver disease: a systematic review and meta-analysis. *JAMA Intern Med*. 2019;179(9):1262. doi:10.1001/JAMAINTERNMED.2019.2248
42. Verrastro O, Panunzi S, Castagneto-Gissey L, et al. Bariatric–metabolic surgery versus lifestyle intervention plus best medical care in non-alcoholic steatohepatitis (BRAVES): a multicentre, open-label, randomised trial. *Lancet*. 2023; 401(10390):1786–1797. doi:10.1016/S0140-6736(23)00634-7
43. Long MT, Noureddin M, Lim JK. AGA Clinical Practice Update: diagnosis and management of non-alcoholic fatty liver disease (NAFLD) in lean individuals: expert review. *Gastroenterol*. 2022;163(3):764. doi:10.1053/J.GASTRO.2022.06.023
44. Sanyal AJ, Chalasani N, Kowdley KV, et al. Pioglitazone, vitamin E, or placebo for nonalcoholic steatohepatitis. *N Engl J Med*. 2010;362(18):1675–1685. doi:10.1056/NEJMOA0907929/SUPPL_FILE/NEJMOA0907929_DISCLOSURES.PDF
45. Miller ER, Pastor-Barriuso R, Dalal D, Riemersma RA, Appel LJ, Guallar E. Meta-analysis: high-dosage vitamin E supplementation may increase all-cause mortality. *Ann Intern Med*. 2005;142(1). doi:10.7326/0003-4819-142-1-200501040-00110/ASSET/IMAGES/110TT3.JPG
46. Curtis AJ, Bullen M, Piccenna L, McNeil JJ. Vitamin E supplementation and mortality in healthy people: a meta-analysis of randomised controlled trials. *Cardiovasc Drugs Ther*. 2014;28(6):563–573. doi:10.1007/S10557-014-6560-7/METRICS
47. Hassani Zadeh S, Mansoori A, Hosseinzadeh M. Relationship between dietary patterns and non-alcoholic fatty liver disease: a systematic review and meta-analysis. *J Gastroenterol Hepatol*. 2021;36(6):1470–1478. doi:10.1111/JGH.15363
48. Asrih M, Jornayvaz FR. Diets and nonalcoholic fatty liver disease: The good and the bad. *Clin Nutr*. 2014;33(2):186–190. doi:10.1016/j.clnu.2013.11.003
49. Gupta V, Mah XJ, Garcia MC, Antonypillai C, Van Der Poorten D. Oily fish, coffee and walnuts: dietary treatment for nonalcoholic fatty liver disease. *World J Gastroenterol*. 2015;21(37):10621. doi:10.3748/WJG.V21.I37.10621
50. de Castro GS, Calder PC. Non-alcoholic fatty liver disease and its treatment with n-3 polyunsaturated fatty acids. *Clin Nutr*. 2018;37(1):37–55. doi:10.1016/J.CLNU.2017.01.006
51. Eslamparast T, Poustchi H, Zamani F, Sharafkhah M, Malekzadeh R, Hekmatdoost A. Synbiotic supplementation in nonalcoholic fatty liver disease: a randomized, double-blind, placebo-controlled pilot study. *Am J Clin Nutr*. 2014; 99(3):535–542. doi:10.3945/AJCN.113.068890
52. Ebadi M, Ip S, Bhanji RA, Montano-Loza AJ. Effect of coffee consumption on non-alcoholic fatty liver disease incidence, prevalence and risk of significant liver fibrosis: Systematic review with meta-analysis of observational studies. *Nutrients*. 2021;13(9). doi:10.3390/nu13093042
53. Hayat U, Siddiqui AA, Okut H, Afroz S, Tasleem S, Haris A. The effect of coffee consumption on the non-alcoholic fatty liver disease and liver fibrosis: a meta-analysis of 11 epidemiological studies. *Ann Hepatol*. 2021;20. doi:10.1016/j.aohep.2020.08.071
54. Chen YP, Lu F Bin, Hu YB, Xu LM, Zheng MH, Hu E De. A systematic review and a dose-response meta-analysis of coffee dose and nonalcoholic fatty liver disease. *Clin Nutr*. 2019;38(6):2552–2557. doi:10.1016/J.CLNU.2018.11.030
55. Abid A, Taha O, Nseir W, Farah R, Grosovski M, Assy N. Soft drink consumption is associated with fatty liver disease independent of metabolic syndrome. *J Hepatol*. 2009;51(5): 918–924. doi:10.1016/j.jhep.2009.05.033
56. Assy N, Nasser G, Kamayse I, et al. Soft drink consumption linked with fatty liver in the absence of traditional risk factors. *Can J Gastroenterol*. 2008;22(10):811. doi:10.1155/2008/810961
57. Vos MB, Lavine JE. Dietary fructose in nonalcoholic fatty liver disease. *Hepatol*. 2013;57(6):2525–2531. doi:10.1002/hep.26299
58. Tillman EM. Review and clinical update on parenteral nutrition–associated liver disease. *Nutr Clin Pract*. 2013;28(1): 30–39. doi:10.1177/0884533612462900
59. Bacon BR, Adams PC, Kowdley KV, Powell LW, Tavill AS. Diagnosis and management of hemochromatosis: 2011 Practice Guideline by the American Association for the Study of Liver Diseases. *Hepatol*. 2011;54(1):328–343. doi:10.1002/HEP.24330
60. Milman NT. Managing genetic hemochromatosis: an overview of dietary measures, which may reduce intestinal iron absorption in persons with iron overload. *Gastroenterology Res*. 2021;14(2):66. doi:10.14740/GR1366
61. Moretti D, Van Doorn GM, Swinkels DW, Melse-Boonstra A. Relevance of dietary iron intake and bioavailability in the management of HFE hemochromatosis: a systematic review. *Am J Clin Nutr*. 2013;98(2):468–479. doi:10.3945/AJCN.112.048264
62. Mohommad MK, Zhou Z, Cave M, Barve A, McClain CJ. Zinc and liver disease. *Nutr Clin Pract*. 2012;27(1):8. doi:10.1177/0884533611433534
63. Schilsky ML, Roberts EA, Bronstein JM, et al. A multidisciplinary approach to the diagnosis and management of

Wilson disease: 2022 Practice Guidance on Wilson Disease from the American Association for the Study of Liver Diseases. *Hepatol*. Published online ahead of print 2022. doi:10.1002/hep.32801

64. Coni P, Pichiri G, Lachowicz JI, et al. Zinc as a drug for Wilson's disease, non-alcoholic liver disease and COVID-19-related liver injury. *Molecules*. 2021;26(21). doi:10.3390/MOLECULES26216614
65. Centers for Disease Control and Prevention. FastStats—Leading Causes of Death. Accessed August 16, 2024. https://www.cdc.gov/nchs/fastats/leading-causes-of-death.htm
66. Lai JC, Tandon P, Bernal W, et al. Malnutrition, frailty, and sarcopenia in patients with cirrhosis: 2021 Practice Guidance by the American Association for the Study of Liver Diseases. *Hepatol*. 2021;74(3):1611–1644. doi:10.1002/hep.32049
67. Friedman LS. Cirrhosis. In: Papadakis MA, Rabow MW, McQuaid KR, Ghandhi M, eds. *Current Medical Diagnosis & Treatment* 2025. New York, NY: McGraw-Hill Education; 2025.
68. Machado MV. Liquid diagnosis of hepatic encephalopathy: are we there already? *GE Port J Gastroenterol*. 2020;27:378–382. doi:10.1159/000510059
69. Merli M, Giusto M, Lucidi C, et al. Muscle depletion increases the risk of overt and minimal hepatic encephalopathy: results of a prospective study. *Metab Brain Dis*. 2013;28(2):281–284. doi:10.1007/S11011-012-9365-Z/METRICS
70. Kalaitzakis E, Josefsson A, Castedal M, et al. Hepatic encephalopathy is related to anemia and fat-free mass depletion in liver transplant candidates with cirrhosis. *Scand J Gastroenterol*. 2013;48(5):577–584. doi:10.3109/00365521.2013.777468
71. Kalaitzakis E, Josefsson A, Björnsson E. Type and etiology of liver cirrhosis are not related to the presence of hepatic encephalopathy or health-related quality of life: a cross-sectional study. *BMC Gastroenterol*. 2008;8:46. doi:10.1186/1471-230X-8-46
72. Cederholm T, Jensen GL, Correia MITD, et al. ESPEN Endorsed Recommendation GLIM criteria for the diagnosis of malnutrition: a consensus report from the global clinical nutrition community. *Clin Nutr*. 2019;38(1):1–9. doi:10.1016/j.clnu.2018.08.002.
73. Casas Deza D, Betoré Glaria ME, Sanz-París A, et al. Mini nutritional assessment - Short form is a useful malnutrition screening tool in patients with liver cirrhosis, using the Global Leadership Initiative for Malnutrition Criteria as the gold Standard. *Nutr Clin Pract*. 2021;36(5):1003–1010. doi:10.1002/NCP.10640
74. Boulhosa RSSB, Lourenço RP, Côrtes DM, Oliveira LPM, Lyra AC, de Jesus RP. Comparison between criteria for diagnosing malnutrition in patients with advanced chronic liver disease: GLIM group proposal versus different nutritional screening tools. *J Hum Nutr Diet*. 2020;33(6):862–868. doi:10.1111/JHN.12759
75. European Association for the Study of the Liver. EASL Clinical Practice Guidelines on nutrition in chronic liver disease. *J Hepatol*. 2019;(70):172193. doi:10.1016/j.jhep.2018.06.024
76. Buchard B, Boirie Y, Cassagnes L, Lamblin G, Coilly A, Abergel A. Assessment of malnutrition, sarcopenia and frailty in patients with cirrhosis: which tools should we use in clinical practice? *Nutrients*. 2020;12:186. doi:10.3390/nu12010186
77. Jensen GL, Cederholm T, Correia MITD, et al. GLIM criteria for the diagnosis of malnutrition: a consensus report from the global clinical nutrition community. *JPEN*. 2019;43(1):32–40. doi:10.1002/JPEN.1440
78. Montano-Loza AJ, Meza-Junco J, Prado CMM, et al. Muscle wasting is associated with mortality in patients with cirrhosis. *Clin Gastroenterol Hepatol*. 2012;10(2):166–173.e1. doi:10.1016/j.cgh.2011.08.028
79. Peng S, Plank LD, McCall JL, Gillanders LK, McIlroy K, Gane EJ. Body composition, muscle function, and energy expenditure in patients with liver cirrhosis: a comprehensive study. *Am J Clin Nutr*. 2007;85(5):1257–1266. doi:10.1093/AJCN/85.5.1257
80. Álvares-Da-Silva MR, Reverbel Da Silveira T. Comparison between handgrip strength, subjective global assessment, and prognostic nutritional index in assessing malnutrition and predicting clinical outcome in cirrhotic outpatients. *Nutrition*. 2005;21(2):113–117. doi:10.1016/J.NUT.2004.02.002
81. Wang CW, Lebsack A, Chau S, Lai JC. The range and reproducibility of the Liver Frailty Index HHS Public Access. *Liver Transpl*. 2019;25(6):841–847. doi:10.1002/lt.25449
82. Lai JC, Covinsky KE, Dodge JL, et al. Development of a novel frailty index to predict mortality in patients with end-stage liver disease. *Hepatol*. 2017;66(2):564–574. doi:10.1002/hep.29219
83. Wang S, Whitlock R, Xu C, et al. Frailty is associated with increased risk of cirrhosis disease progression and death. *Hepatol*. 2022;75(3):600–609. doi:10.1002/HEP.32157
84. Pentiuk N, Motsiuk V. Evaluation of nutritional status in patients with liver cirrhosis. Validity and prognostic value of the Patient-Generated Subjective Global Assessment. *Prz Gastroenterol*. 2023;18(3):327. doi:10.5114/PG.2022.119964
85. Ramachandran G, Pottakkat B, Mohan P, Basu S. Effectiveness of different tools for malnutrition in the assessment of patients with cirrhosis. *Am J Med Sci*. 2024;368(1):61–67. doi:10.1016/j.amjms.2024.03.015
86. Sousa FI da S e., Medeiros LT, Braga RAM, Daltro AFCS, Maia CSC. Power of mortality prediction in patients awaiting liver transplantation according to the Global Leadership Initiative on Malnutrition criteria and Subjective Global Assessment and Royal Free Hospital Global Assessment scores. *Nutrition*. 2023;106:111889. doi:10.1016/J.NUT.2022.111889
87. Mendenhall C, Roselle GA, Gartside P, Moritz T. Relationship of protein calorie malnutrition to alcoholic liver disease: a reexamination of data from two Veterans Administration Cooperative Studies. *Alcohol Clin Exp Res*. 1995;19(3):635–641. doi:10.1111/J.1530-0277.1995.TB01560.X
88. Chapman B, Testro A, Gow P, Whitcher B, Sinclair M. Determining energy requirements in cirrhosis: an update on the role of indirect calorimetry. *Curr Hepatol Rep*. 2021. doi:10.1007/s11901-021-00564-y/
89. Chapman B, Wong D, Whitcher B, et al. Redefining nutritional requirements in end-stage liver disease: towards a personalized approach. *Nutrients*. 2023;15(22):4770. doi:10.3390/nu15224770.
90. McClave SA, Taylor BE, Martindale RG, et al. Guidelines for the Provision and Assessment of Nutrition Support Therapy in the Adult Critically Ill Patient: Society of Critical Care Medicine (SCCM) and American Society for Parenteral and Enteral Nutrition (A.S.P.E.N.). *JPEN*. 2016;40(2):159–211. doi:10.1177/0148607115621863
91. Glass C, Hipskind P, Cole D, Lopez R, Dasarathy S. Handheld calorimeter is a valid instrument to quantify resting energy expenditure in hospitalized cirrhotic patients:

A prospective study. *Nutr Clin Pract.* 2012; 27(5): 677–688. doi:10.1177/0884533612446195
92. Mendez-Guerrero O, Carranza-Carrasco A, Chi-Cervera LA, Torre A, Navarro-Alvarez N. Optimizing nutrition in hepatic cirrhosis: a comprehensive assessment and care approach. *World J Gastroenterol.* 2024;30(10):1313–1328. doi:10.3748/WJG.V30.I10.1313
93. Morgan TR, Moritz TE, Mendenhall CL, Haas R. Protein consumption and hepatic encephalopathy in alcoholic hepatitis. VA Cooperative Study Group #275. *J Am Coll Nutr.* 1995;14(2):152–158. doi:10.1080/07315724.1995.10718487
94. Cordoba J, Lopez-Hellin J, Planas M. Normal protein diet for episodic hepatic encephalopathy: results of a randomized study. *J Hepatol.* 2004;41(1):38–43.
95. Cabral C, Burns D. Low-protein diets for hepatic encephalopathy debunked: let them eat steak. *Nutr Clin Pract.* 2011;26(2):155–159.
96. Ney M, Abraldes JG, Ma M, et al. Insufficient protein intake is associated with increased mortality in 630 patients with cirrhosis awaiting liver transplantation. *Nutr Clin Pract.* 2015;30(4):530–536. doi:10.1177/0884533614567716
97. Gluud LL, Dam G, Les I, et al. Branched-chain amino acids for people with hepatic encephalopathy. *Cochrane Database Syst Rev.* 2017;2017(5). doi:10.1002/14651858.CD001939.PUB4
98. Yadav A, Carey EJ. Osteoporosis in chronic liver disease. *Nutr ClinPract.*2013;28(1):52–64.doi:10.1177/0884533612470145
99. Arteh J, Narra S, Nair S. Prevalence of vitamin D deficiency in chronic liver disease. *Dig Dis Sci.* 2010;55(9):2624–2628. doi:10.1007/S10620-009-1069-9/TABLES/5
100. Trépo E, Ouziel R, Pradat P, et al. Marked 25-hydroxyvitamin D deficiency is associated with poor prognosis in patients with alcoholic liver disease. *J Hepatol.* 2013;59(2):344–350. doi:10.1016/j.jhep.2013.03.024
101. Stokes CS, Krawczyk M, Reichel C, Lammert F, Grünhage F. Vitamin D deficiency is associated with mortality in patients with advanced liver cirrhosis. *Eur J Clin Invest.* 2014;44(2):176–183. doi:10.1111/ECI.12205
102. Rode A, Fourlanos S, Nicoll A. Oral vitamin D replacement is effective in chronic liver disease. *Gastroenterol Clin Biol.* 2010;34(11):618–620. doi:10.1016/J.GCB.2010.07.009
103. Okubo T, Atsukawa M, Tsubota A, et al. Effect of Vitamin D supplementation on skeletal muscle volume and strength in patients with decompensated liver cirrhosis undergoing branched chain amino acids supplementation: a prospective, randomized, controlled pilot trial. *Nutrients.* 2021;13(6):1874. doi:10.3390/NU13061874
104. Savić Ž, Vračarić V, Milić N, et al. Vitamin D supplementation in patients with alcoholic liver cirrhosis: a prospective study. *Minerva Med.* 2018;109(5):352–357. doi:10.23736/S0026-4806.18.05723-3
105. Yoshida Y, Higashi T, Nouso K, et al. Effects of zinc deficiency/zinc supplementation on ammonia metabolism in patients with decompensated liver cirrhosis. *Acta Med Okayama.* 2001;55(6):349–355. doi:10.18926/AMO/32003
106. Chavez-Tapia NC, Cesar-Arce A, Barrientos-Gutiérrez T, Villegas-López FA, Méndez-Sanchez N, Uribe M. A systematic review and meta-analysis of the use of oral zinc in the treatment of hepatic encephalopathy. *Nutr J.* 2013;12(1):74. doi:10.1186/1475-2891-12-74
107. Shen YC, Chang YH, Fang CJ, Lin YS. Zinc supplementation in patients with cirrhosis and hepatic encephalopathy: a systematic review and meta-analysis. *Nutr J.* 2019;18(1):34. doi:10.1186/s12937-019-0461-3
108. Prasad AS. Clinical manifestations of zinc deficiency. *Annu Rev Nutr.* 1985;5:341–363. doi:10.1146/ANNUREV.NU.05.070185.002013
109. Allan JG, Fell GS, Russell RI. Urinary zinc in hepatic cirrhosis. *Scottish Med J.* 1975;20(3):109–111. doi:10.1177/003693307502000308
110. Chiba M, Katayama K, Takeda R, et al. Diuretics aggravate zinc deficiency in patients with liver cirrhosis by increasing zinc excretion in urine. *Hepatol Res.* 2013;43(4):365–373. doi:10.1111/J.1872-034X.2012.01093.X
111. Rodriguez-Moreno F, González-Reimers E, Santolaria-Fernandez F, et al. Zinc, copper, manganese, and iron in chronic alcoholic liver disease. *Alcohol.* 1997;14(1):39–44. doi:10.1016/S0741-8329(96)00103-6
112. Domej W, Krachler M, Goessler W, Maier A, Irgolic KJ, Lang JK. Concentrations of copper, zinc, manganese, and magnesium. *Biol Trace Elem Res.* 2000;78(1–3):53–66. doi:10.1385/BTER:78:1-3:53
113. Iwasa M, Iwata K, Hara N, et al. Nutrition therapy using a multidisciplinary team improves survival rates in patients with liver cirrhosis. *Nutrition.* 2013;29(11–12):1418–1421. doi:10.1016/J.NUT.2013.05.016
114. Liuzzi JP, Leoni L, Valoriani F, et al. Unlocking the power of late-evening snacks: practical ready-to-prescribe chart menu for patients with cirrhosis. *Nutrients.* 2023;15(15):3471. doi:10.3390/nu151
115. Plank LD, Gane EJ, Peng S, et al. Nocturnal nutritional supplementation improves total body protein status of patients with liver cirrhosis: a randomized 12-month trial. *Hepatol.* 2008;48(2):557–566. doi:10.1002/hep.22367
116. Hou W, Li J, Lu J, et al. Effect of a carbohydrate-containing late-evening snack on energy metabolism and fasting substrate utilization in adults with acute-on-chronic liver failure due to Hepatitis B. *Eur J Clin Nutr.* 2013;67(12):1251–1256. doi:10.1038/ejcn.2013.163
117. Yamanaka-Okumura H, Nakamura T, Takeuchi H, et al. Effect of late evening snack with rice ball on energy metabolism in liver cirrhosis. *Eur J Clin Nutr.* 2006;60(9): 1067–1072. doi:10.1038/sj.ejcn.1602420
118. Chang WK, Chao YC, Tang HS, Lang HF, Hsu CT. Effects of extra-carbohydrate supplementation in the late evening on energy expenditure and substrate oxidation in patients with liver cirrhosis. *JPEN.* 1997;21(2):96–99. doi:10.1177/014860719702100296
119. Tsien CD, Mccullough AJ, Dasarathy S. Late evening snack: exploiting a period of anabolic opportunity in cirrhosis. *J Gastroenterol Hepatol.* 2012;27(3):430–441. doi:10.1111/J.1440-1746.2011.06951.X
120. Nakaya Y, Harada N, Kakui S, et al. Severe catabolic state after prolonged fasting in cirrhotic patients: effect of oral branched-chain amino-acid-enriched nutrient mixture. *J Gastroenterol.* 2002;37:531–536.
121. Nakaya Y, Okita K, Suzuki K, et al. BCAA-enriched snack improves nutritional state of cirrhosis. *Nutrition.* 2007;23(2):113–120. doi:10.1016/J.NUT.2006.10.008
122. Ruiz-Margáin A, Macías-Rodríguez RU, Ríos-Torres SL, et al. Effect of a high-protein, high-fiber diet plus supplementation with branched-chain amino acids on the nutritional status of patients with cirrhosis. *Revista de Gastroenterologia de Mexico.* 2018;83(1):9–15. doi:10.1016/J.RGMX.2017.02.005

123. Baldwin C, Weekes CE. Dietary advice with or without oral nutritional supplements for disease-related malnutrition in adults. *Cochrane Database Syst Rev*. 2011;2011(9). doi:10.1002/14651858.CD002008.PUB4
124. Norman K, Valentini L, Lochs H, Pirlich M. Protein catabolism and malnutrition in liver cirrhosis - impact of oral nutritional therapy. *Z Gastroenterol*. 2010;48(7):763–770. doi:10.1055/S-0029-1245388
125. Muto Y, Sato S, Watanabe A, et al. Effects of oral branched-chain amino acid granules on event-free survival in patients with liver cirrhosis. *Clin Gastroenterol Hepatol*. 2005; 3(7):705–713. doi:10.1016/S1542-3565(05)00017-0
126. Hayaishi S, Chung H, Kudo M, et al. Oral branched-chain amino acid granules reduce the incidence of hepatocellular carcinoma and improve event-free survival in patients with liver cirrhosis. *Dig Dis*. 2011;29(3):326–332. doi:10.1159/000327571
127. Kawaguchi T, Taniguchi E, Sata M. Effects of oral branched-chain amino acids on hepatic encephalopathy and outcome in patients with liver cirrhosis. *Nutr Clin Pract*. 2013; 28(5):580–588. doi:10.1177/0884533613496432
128. Johnson TM, Overgard EB, Cohen AE, Dibaise JK. Nutrition assessment and management in advanced liver disease. *Nutr Clin Pract*. 2013;28(1):15–29. doi:10.1177/0884533612469027
129. Chapman B, Sinclair M, Gow PJ, Testro AG. Malnutrition in cirrhosis: more food for thought. *Gastroenterol Hepatol*. 2020;12(11):883–896. doi:10.4254/wjh.v12.i11.883
130. Hébuterne X, Vanbiervliet G. Feeding the patients with upper gastrointestinal bleeding. *Curr Opin Clin Nutr Metab Care*. 2011;14(2):197–201. doi:10.1097/MCO.0B013E3283436DC5
131. Obeidat M, Teutsch B, Floria DE, Veres DS, Hegyi P, Erőss B. Early nutrition is safe and does not increase complications after upper gastrointestinal bleeding-a systematic review and meta-analysis of randomized controlled trials. *Sci Rep*. 2024;14:10725. doi:10.1038/s41598-024-61543-z
132. Rivera-Mancía S, Ríos C, Montes S. Manganese accumulation in the CNS and associated pathologies. *Biometals*. 2011;24(5):811–825. doi:10.1007/S10534-011-9454-1.

CHAPTER 14

Nutrition in Pulmonary Disease

Grace Phelan

CHAPTER OUTLINE

Core Concepts
Introduction
Pulmonary Physiology in Health and Disease
Nutrition Assessment
Nutrition Intervention
Micronutrients
Quality of Life and Psychosocial Support
Monitoring and Evaluation
Acute Respiratory Distress Syndrome
Nutrition Support and Pulmonary Disease
Immunonutrition

CORE CONCEPTS

1. Modest weight loss may improve asthma parameters in people with obesity.
2. Diet can influence inflammation and immunity by altering the gut–lung axis.
3. In chronic obstructive pulmonary disease (COPD), weight status correlates with hospital outcomes.
4. Oxidant–antioxidant imbalance is ubiquitous in many pulmonary diseases, emphasizing the importance of an antioxidant-rich diet.
5. Individuals with COPD who are malnourished have described greater levels of fatigue and score higher on depressive order scales.

LEARNING OBJECTIVES

1. Describe the role of dietary components on asthma parameters.
2. Identify the metabolic changes caused by pulmonary disease and cachexia.
3. Recognize the factors that influence nutritional risk and impact nutrition status in patients with chronic obstructive pulmonary disease.
4. Explain the integral role nutrition plays on quality of life in people with pulmonary disease.
5. State strategies for weight maintenance in end-stage chronic obstructive pulmonary disease.
6. Formulate appropriate enteral and parenteral nutrition recommendations in the setting of pulmonary disease.
7. Identify specialty enteral nutrition and micronutrients in patients with acute respiratory distress syndrome.

Introduction

Pulmonary diseases, such as asthma and chronic obstructive pulmonary disease (COPD), are the third leading cause of death in the United States, with approximately 13% of the adult population carrying a diagnosis of chronic bronchitis, emphysema, or asthma.[1,2] Early nutrition intervention is essential for optimal health in the presence of pulmonary disease. Nutrition strategies play an important role in the treatment of certain pulmonary diseases and conditions.

Pulmonary Physiology in Health and Disease

The primary function of the pulmonary system is gas exchange: delivering oxygen to the bloodstream and removing excess carbon dioxide. During inspiration, air travels through the trachea, bronchi, and bronchioles to the lungs (**Figure 14.1**). Oxygen is then delivered to the heart via pulmonary circulation, while excess carbon dioxide is returned to the lungs for expiration. In health, the diaphragm and intercostal muscles primarily support these functions. However, in cases of pulmonary disease, accessory muscles, namely the sternocleidomastoid, scalene, and abdominal muscles, may be recruited for sufficient gas exchange.[3]

Asthma

Asthma is a chronic inflammatory disease of the lungs characterized by periods of reversible airflow limitation and airway hyperresponsiveness. Symptoms commonly include shortness of breath, wheezing, coughing, and chest tightness. Asthma affects approximately 8.7% of the U.S. population, and is more likely to affect people who are female, over 60 years of age, smoke, have low income, or obesity.[3] There is no cure for asthma, so treatment targets symptom management (**Figure 14.2**).

Obesity

The impact of obesity on asthma is one of great research interest given the well documented increase in systemic inflammation observed in both people with obesity[4,5] and people with asthma.[5–8] When these conditions coexist, the pattern of inflammation is different as compared with asthma without obesity.[9]

The mechanisms by which obesity worsens lung function in the presence or absence of asthma are multifaceted and include the presence of metabolic syndrome, increased circulation of inflammatory markers, response to oxidative stress, dietary factors and the gut microbiome, and mechanical and genetic factors. Each of these may each play a role in symptoms and response to therapies.[10,11] Researchers have observed an obesity phenotype of asthma[12–19] that appears to respond less favorably to standard interventions compared to individuals with lower adiposity. Additionally, common diagnostic tools for asthma tend to be less accurate when obesity is present.[10]

Both abdominal adiposity and overall obesity appear to have a dose–response relationship with asthma.[20,21] Numerous studies have indicated that even modest weight loss of 5–10% body weight can improve metabolic parameters such as insulin sensitivity and blood pressure.[22,23] Weight loss of 5% body weight has been associated with significant

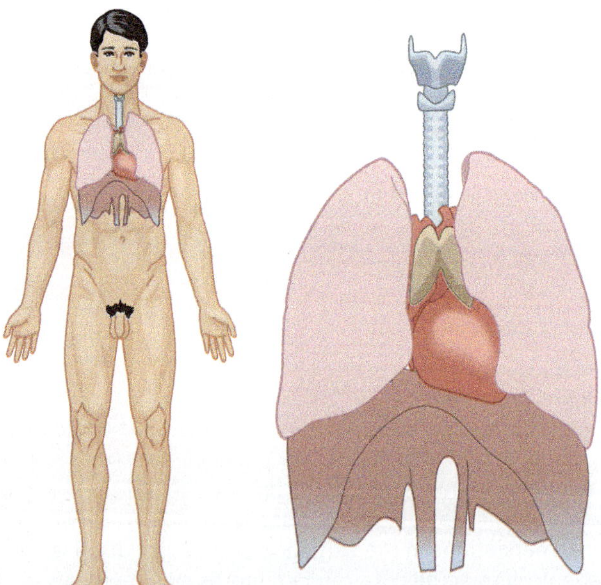

Figure 14.1 Respiratory System

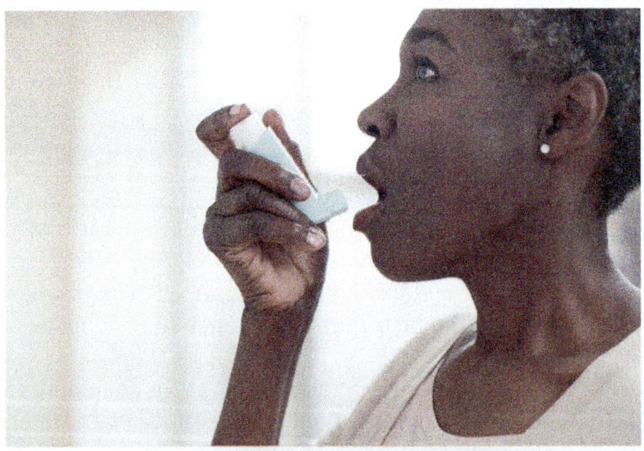

Figure 14.2 Inhalers Are Often Used for Symptom Management in Asthma

improvements in asthma control and quality of life[24] with more consistent improvement when weight loss exceeds 5%.[25–29] Not all studies are in agreement as some indicate only a trend toward benefit.[20]

Bariatric surgery produces greater weight loss and more dependably improves asthma outcomes and reduces medication use compared to non-surgical weight loss methods.[30] However, weight loss and maintenance of lost weight are not realistic goals for all people, and weight loss interventions, particularly surgery, are not without risk. Therefore, care plan decisions should be made collaboratively considering an individual's unique medical and social histories. It is important to acknowledge that improvements in dietary quality may improve lung function and quality of life without weight loss, particularly in individuals with non-obesity–related phenotypes of asthma. Studies observing the effects of weight loss on asthma outcomes do not always control for independent dietary factors, such as fatty acid or fiber intake. Support for individual dietary patterns and nutrients will be discussed in the following sections.

CORE CONCEPT 1

Modest weight loss may improve asthma parameters in people with obesity.

Dietary Patterns

Dietary supplement trials suggest that the benefit of whole foods and overall dietary pattern may offer health benefits that individual nutrients alone do not achieve. Interactions between macronutrients, micronutrients, and phytochemicals within and among foods, bioavailability, and absorption of foods influence the gut microbiome, inflammation, and overall health. The extent to which food groups and dietary patterns can modify asthma risk and related health parameters is not yet conclusive. Data from the National Health and Nutrition Examination Survey (NHANES) reveals that adults with asthma are more likely to have diets that lack alignment with current dietary patterns as compared to those without asthma.[31] This raises questions as to whether or not certain dietary habits, such as the lack of fruits and vegetables, contribute to asthma outcomes and, if so, to what extent.

The contribution of fruit and vegetable consumption to asthma risk in children and adults remains unclear. While some studies looking at these two food groups indicate a protective role, others find no significance.[32] The Mediterranean diet is naturally high in fruits and vegetables as well other sources of fiber in the form of whole grains and legumes. Further, it offers additional anti-inflammatory benefits with the inclusion of nuts, seeds, fish, and oils. Adherence to the Mediterranean diet during childhood has been associated with lower occurrence of childhood asthma in several studies,[33–35] but more rigorous study is needed to confirm this finding. Evidence is also lacking regarding the role of prenatal Mediterranean diet on development of childhood asthma.[36] Other dietary patterns like the Dietary Approaches to Stop Hypertension (DASH) diet, known for its rich content of fruits, vegetables, whole grains, and low-fat dairy products, may reduce proinflammatory markers in adults with asthma; however, more outcome data are necessary to draw definitive conclusions.[37]

Looking at diet overall, one cohort study in adults did not find diet quality to be a strong predictor of adult-onset asthma,[38] although a study in children found that improved diet quality reduced airway inflammation and asthma prevalence in children. While the data on high-quality diets displays favorable trends, they remain equivocal. In contrast, proinflammatory diets like the Western Diet, which is characterized by low intake of fruits and vegetables and higher intake of red meat and other high saturated fat foods, highly processed foods, and refined grains, are associated with adverse asthma outcomes. In particular, there is a positive relationship between sugar-sweetened beverage intakes and asthma diagnosis in children.[39,40]

Additionally, an increase in saturated fatty acid consumption from fast-food and deep fried foods has been linked to an increase in asthma and wheezing in children and adolescents.[41–44] These choices may displace vegetables, in which a low intake is also associated with asthma. In adults, a Western diet has been found to reduce lung function and increase disease exacerbation.[45–47]

Macronutrients

Carbohydrates and the Microbiome. Not all carbohydrates are equal. Diets high in sugar are positively associated with the development of adult-onset asthma and an increase in asthma prevalence in children, whereas diets high in fiber are negatively associated with asthma development.[48,49] Epidemiologic data show reduced inflammatory markers in people with asthma who consume high-fiber diets than those who consume low-fiber diets.[50] Consumers of high-fiber diets are more likely to engage in other health behaviors, which may influence overall health, but there are several mechanisms by which soluble fiber intake can positively impact asthma outcomes.

These include modification of the gut microbiome, modulation of immunity in the host, and short-chain fatty acid production. Fiber consumption can alter gut or lung microbiota, which influences the **gut-lung axis**, a bidirectional exchange of microbiota and their metabolites, the signaling of which is involved in immune modulation. Dysbiosis due to diet, antibiotics, or chronic illness can disrupt this homeostasis resulting in systemic inflammation and an increase in opportunistic infections.[51,52] The altered microbiota in both the lungs[44,53,54] and the intestines in people with asthma is associated with an increase in the development of childhood asthma.[55,56]

The gut microbiome plays a pivotal role in shaping the immune system early in life. Modulation of dysbiosis through fiber intake and pre-, pro- and synbiotics is a growing area of study. Available data show more compelling benefits of high-fiber diets or fiber supplementation in adults than in children, although there is inconsistency among studies as to which biomarkers fiber intake most influences.[33] Factors such as fiber dose, supplementation versus whole diet, and study timing and duration may influence such indicators. Larger, well-designed studies are needed to add clarity to the role that fiber plays on asthma control and lung function.

Probiotic use appears to be safe and may reduce asthma symptoms and exacerbations[57]; however, the variation in particular strains of bacteria, route of administration (oral or intranasal), and severity of disease among the existing data make it difficult to find consensus. There is a paucity of studies on prebiotic or synbiotic use, so firm conclusions on the role of enhancing biodiversity in the prevention or treatment of asthma in children cannot be made at this time.[36,51,58]

CORE CONCEPT 2

Diet can influence inflammation and immunity by altering the gut–lung axis.

Fatty acids. Fatty acids in the body play a role in cell structure and function and energy storage. Short-chain fatty acids, which include acetate, propionate, and butyrate, are a product of fiber fermentation and can influence immune cell growth and function and alleviate inflammation in the gut.[52] Butyrate has also been found to block production of proinflammatory cytokines in the lung.[59] An epigenetic effect of acetate has been demonstrated in a mice model with further study indicating that benefits can be conferred from the maternal diet to a fetus while in utero.[60] Future study in humans looking at the role of prenatal short-chain fatty acids is needed to strengthen this assertion.

Linoleic- and linolenic–omega-6 polyunsaturated fatty acids (PUFAs), along with omega-3 PUFAs, are considered essential fatty acids because the human body cannot synthesize them. Omega-3 fatty acids are known to support anti-inflammation pathways. However, several systematic reviews and meta-analyses have found no relationship between prenatal omega-3 fatty acid supplementation and the development of childhood asthma.[61–64] In children, increased fish consumption[65] and higher blood levels of omega-3 PUFAs[66] may reduce current asthma and the risk of developing asthma, respectively. Due to limited data and variations in study methods, more research is needed to reach a consensus.[67,68] Similarly, omega-3 PUFAs do not appear to improve lung function or asthma control in adults with asthma.[69] Additionally, studies using this hypothesis often use varying doses of supplementation and short durations, which limits the potential for identifying a significant effect.

Amino acids. Arginine metabolism seems to be altered in people with asthma, with variations across different asthma phenotypes.[70] These changes can impact lung function and nitric oxide production and bioavailability due to competition between nitric oxide synthases and arginase I and II.[71] Supplementation of the non-essential amino acid L-citrulline may compensate for some of the dysregulation within this pathway, increasing nitric oxide availability and influencing bronchodilation.[72]

Micronutrients

Vitamin A. Epidemiologic data indicate a positive association between serum vitamin A levels and lung function.[32] Adults with asthma tend to have low vitamin A intakes compared to healthy controls, and asthma severity correlates with lower intakes. Given this association and the increase in production of systemic free radicals in asthma, providing an antioxidant like vitamin A would seem a logical intervention. However, intervention trials have not indicated a benefit of vitamin A supplementation on the improvement of lung function in children.

Vitamin C. Adults with chronic respiratory diseases have low blood levels and dietary intakes of vitamin C, along with more oxidative stress, compared with healthy controls.[73,74] Children with obesity also maintain lower blood levels of vitamin C despite similar supplementation compared to their counterparts of lower body weight.[75] A positive association exists between obesity and vitamin C intakes in children, perhaps due to higher fruit juice consumption. In contrast to children, vitamin C levels do not consistently correlate with asthma risk in adults[76] and support for vitamin C supplementation in the prevention and treatment of asthma are limited. On average, no causal relationship has been identified to support a preventive role of vitamin C and asthma in children.[77,78] Patient selection may be relevant, as there are limited data to support supplementation in people who smoke and others that support an inverse association between vitamin C intake and asthma in people with high C-reactive protein levels.[79–81]

Vitamin D. Vitamin D plays a crucial role in skeletal health and has immunomodulatory effects on the body. Given that vitamin D levels in people with asthma are commonly low,[82] research has focused on benefits of supplementation. While some studies suggest that vitamin D supplementation reduces asthma exacerbation,[83,84] the larger body of work in this area does not support its use to improve asthma control in either adults or children.[82,85,86]

Vitamin E. Vitamin E, a family of fat-soluble nutrients, functions as an antioxidant and as a necessary component in immunity, potentially influencing inflammation and asthma. Various forms of vitamin E naturally occur, including tocopherols and tocotrienols, each with different isomers (α-, β-, γ-, and δ-). Studying vitamin E can be challenging as different forms of vitamin E are absorbed and function differently and may influence tissue levels of other isomers.[87] A predominance of soybean oil in the diet, an oil high in γ-tocopherol, may influence inflammation and tissue concentrations differently than diets high in sunflower or safflower oils, which are lower in γ-tocopherol. Current data do not support vitamin E supplementation for the prevention of childhood asthma, either pre- or postnatally.[32,36] More controlled studies in humans with specific isomer concentrations before and after supplementation are needed to conclude whether or not there is a role for vitamin E in the prevention or treatment of asthma.[88]

Zinc. Zinc is involved in immune function by several mechanisms and also has antioxidant properties. Blood levels of zinc are not significantly different in children with asthma when compared to children without asthma.[89] Similar to other antioxidant trials, there is insufficient evidence to support zinc supplementation for the prevention or treatment of asthma in children.[36]

Dietary Additives

Salicylates. Salicylates are organic compounds found naturally in many plants, as well as some medications such as aspirin (acetylsalicylic acid) and other nonsteroidal anti-inflammatory drugs (NSAIDs). Hypersensitivity to aspirin is more common among people with asthma, which has prompted a research interest in the role of dietary salicylates in asthma control. Generally, the dietary contribution of salicylates is lower compared with that of aspirin. Foods with higher salicylate content include certain herbs and spices, some vegetables, most fruits (particularly dried), coffee, tea, and some condiments.

A small study reported favorable results in asthma control for those who followed a low-salicylate diet, defined as no more than one serving of high salicylate food per day and up to five servings of food containing 0.05 mg of salicylates per serving.[90] Adherence to this restrictive diet was challenging in this study that was only 2–4 weeks duration. Another even smaller crossover trial found symptomatic improvements, but no biomarker improvement among seven participants.[91]

More data are needed to support recommendations for salicylate restriction. The Food Allergy Working Group of the German Society for Allergology and Clinical Immunology currently advises against such diets.[92] The limited data available stems from a small number of patients with known aspirin hypersensitivity lacked studies without blinding or control that relied on subjective evaluation of reactions. Nonetheless, if clients request a trial of a low-salicylate diet, a registered dietitian (RD) should be consulted. This can help identify tolerated foods while ensuring adequate nutrition status and preventing long-term elimination.

Sulfites. Sulfites are compounds found naturally in the body and in certain foods, including beer, wine, vinegar, certain dried fruits, lemon juice, baked goods, and tomato paste. Additionally, sulfites may be added to foods, cosmetics, and some medications as preservatives. People with asthma may experience bronchoconstriction in response to inhaled sulfur dioxide, unlike those without asthma.[93,94] A number of adverse events in the 1980s prompted the United States Food and Drug Administration (FDA) to require labeling for containing more than 10 ppm of sulfites. People who are sensitive to sulfites may manifest dermatological, gastrointestinal, and respiratory symptoms. The estimated prevalence of hypersensitivity to sulfites among people with asthma is around 3–10%,[95] with a higher incidence in people whose asthma is steroid-dependent.[96] However, not all people with asthma are sensitive to sulfites, so dietary exclusion should occur on an individual basis.[96]

Oral Health

Several epidemiologic studies have found associations between asthma and oral health risk.[97,98] Specifically, people with asthma may experience higher tooth loss and are more likely to have dental caries, often with a greater number of untreated caries. This underscores the importance of communication between medical and dental professionals and is relevant to RDs given the nutrition risk associated with poor oral health.

Chronic Obstructive Pulmonary Disease

Chronic obstructive pulmonary disease (COPD) as defined by the Global Initiative for Chronic Obstructive Lung Disease, is "a heterogeneous lung condition characterized by chronic respiratory symptoms (dyspnea, cough, expectoration and/or exacerbations) due to abnormalities of the airways (bronchitis, bronchiolitis) and/or alveoli (emphysema) that cause persistent, often progressive, airflow obstruction."[99] Diagnosis requires confirmation by **spirometry**, a pulmonary function test that measures how well lungs work by quantifying the amount of air inhaled and exhaled at maximal effort.[100] Symptoms commonly include chronic cough with or without sputum production, and **dyspnea** or difficulty breathing on exertion.[99] At advanced stages of the disease, people with COPD tend to experience shortness of breath during basic activities of daily living. In particular, activities engaging upper extremities pose a greater respiratory challenge than those involving lower extremities.[101]

There are several causes of COPD. Over time, genetic, social, and environmental factors can lead to direct damage to the lungs or interfere with normal

CASE STUDY INTRODUCTION

Leigh is a 79-year-old woman with end-stage chronic obstructive pulmonary disease (COPD) who presents to the nutrition clinic with complaints of a 6.8-kg unintentional weight loss due to decreased oral intake in the previous 3-month time period. She is widowed with two adult children. Her daughter and son-in-law live across town and her son lives out of state. She has a history of smoking but quit during her first pregnancy. She denies alcohol use. She appears dyspneic and is unable to speak in complete sentences.

Anthropometric Data:

Weight: 63.6 kg
Height: 170 cm
BMI: 22 kg/m^2

Weight History
Usual body weight: 71 kg (3 months ago)
Weight at diagnosis 3 years ago: 89 kg
Leigh has sustained a gradual decline in weight over the last several years since diagnosis.

Biochemical Data:

Sodium 142 (136–145 mEq/L)
Potassium 4.4 (3.5–5.0 mEq/L)
Chloride 96 (98–106 mEq/L)
Carbon dioxide 33 (22–31 mEq/L)
Blood urea nitrogen 18 (8–20 mg/dL)
Creatinine 1.1 (0.7–1.3 mg/dL)
Fasting glucose 117 (70–99 mg/dL)

Arterial blood gases (ABG)
pH 7.09 (7.35–7.45)
$PaCO_2$ 97 (35–45 mm Hg)
PaO_2 72 (80–100 mm Hg)
HCO_3^- 35 (22–26 mEq/L)

Clinical Data:

Past Medical History: COPD, hypertension
Medications: Budesonide/formoterol inhaled daily, ipratropium/albuterol as needed
Vital Signs: Blood pressure 170/88 mm Hg, Temperature 98.6°F, Heart rate 60 beats/min
Nutrition-focused Physical Exam: Leigh appears pale with mild peripheral muscle wasting, including temporal muscle wasting, and loose skin noted on arms. Oral exam notable for dry oral mucosa and cracked lips, good dentition, and normal tongue. Skin appears dry. Significant shortness of breath at rest and exacerbated with conversation and activity noted.

Dietary Data:

Dietary History: Leigh follows a low-sodium diet but often relies on prepackaged meals due to her decreased functional capacity.

Diet Prescription: Low sodium, small frequent meals, limit fluid to between meals

Questions

1. What are Leigh's nutritional risk factors? What factors explain her weight loss?
2. Does Leigh classify with malnutrition? If so, what type?
3. How would you interpret Leigh's labs, specifically her ABG labs?
4. Write two Problem/Etiology/Signs and Symptoms (PES) statements for Leigh.
5. Identify the nutrition interventions you would like to initiate for Leigh to address the problems identified in your PES statements.
6. What indices are included in your monitoring and evaluation plan? Why?

lung development and aging. Cigarette smoking is the predominant environmental risk factor for the development of COPD, accounting for about half of cases.[102] Occupational exposure and air pollution also increase risk for COPD.[102] Genetic mutations cause COPD less commonly, but may contribute to individual patient risk.[103] Socioeconomic status influences the risk for COPD, although more study is needed to determine the extent to which healthcare access and/or the environment in high-risk areas plays a role.[104,105] Improved socioeconomic status appears to have a disproportionate benefit in White people as compared with people who are Black or Hispanic. Causal factors for this variation are still unknown, but researchers speculate that cultural and lifestyle patterns may account for some racial disparity despite similar socioeconomic improvements.

Comorbid conditions such as hypertension, cardiovascular disease, diabetes mellitus, osteoporosis, and metabolic syndrome are more prevalent in people with COPD than those without COPD, particularly in those who smoke.[102] Cognitive dysfunction frequently parallels COPD and is likely multifactorial in nature owing to poor sleep, increased fatigue, depressive order, and other factors.[106] These comorbidities can influence disease progression and outcomes; early and effective interventions for these diseases as well as COPD are consequential. Treatment focuses on improving symptoms, slowing progression of disease, and improving physical endurance. Strategies to achieve these goals include smoking cessation for smokers and oxygen therapy for individuals with hypoxemia. Pharmacologic therapies are commonly used to alleviate symptoms and are presented in **Table 14.1**. Pulmonary rehabilitation is a strategy effective at improving symptoms and decreasing disease exacerbations and hospital admissions.

In advanced stages of disease and during disease exacerbations, patients with COPD demonstrate a marked increase in basal energy expenditure and catabolism.[107] On average, pulmonary disease increases resting energy expenditure (REE) by 15–25%,[108–110] but has been noted to increase REE by up to 45%.[111] Hypermetabolism is consistently greater in those patients with COPD who have sustained weight loss as compared with those of stable weight.[112–116] In healthy subjects, energy expenditure of respiration usually amounts to <3% of resting energy needs,[116] but the increased work of breathing that is common in people with COPD results in an increase in energy required for respiration. Increased work of breathing does not appear to be solely responsible for the elevation in energy expenditure.[117] Plasma cytokines and other inflammatory markers have correlated with REE independent of airway obstruction or work of breathing, suggesting inflammation as an etiology of hypermetabolism.[118–120] Given the wide variation of REE relative to disease stage and individual body composition, indirect calorimetry (IC) is the recommended energy assessment tool. A number of predictive equations can be used if IC is not available. The Westerterp equation estimates REE the best in this population, although the World Health Organization (WHO) equation omitting height or the Harris–Benedict equation (HBE) provide similar accuracy.[121] Although REE is elevated with pulmonary disease, one study found that total daily energy expenditure (TEE) remained similar to that of healthy controls.[122] TEE was also similar between patients with COPD with and without elevated REE.[123] The likely explanation for these findings is a reduction

Table 14.1 Classes of Drugs Used in the Treatment of Chronic Obstructive Pulmonary Disease

Drug Class	Mechanism of Action	Nutritional Considerations
Antimuscarinics (anticholinergic agents) Examples: ▪ Short-acting: ipratropium bromide ▪ Long-acting: tiotropium	Block the bronchoconstricting effects of acetylcholine on M3 muscarinic receptors in airway smooth muscle	▪ Tiotropium contains lactose, may contain milk proteins ▪ May cause constipation, taste changes, nausea, vomiting, dyspepsia, xerostomia, or hypokalemia ▪ Caffeine may result in tremor or mild heart rate elevation in those taking albuterol
Bronchodilators (β-2 adrenergic agents [agonists]) Examples: ▪ Short-acting: albuterol ▪ Long-acting: salmeterol	Increase FEV_1 and/or change other spirometric variables; relax airway smooth muscle	▪ Albuterol and salmeterol contain lactose, may contain milk proteins ▪ Caffeine may result in tremor or mild heart rate elevation ▪ May influence appetite ▪ May cause taste changes, nausea, or dyspepsia
Inhaled corticosteroids Examples: budesonide, fluticasone Phosphodiesterase-4 (PDE-4) inhibitors Example: roflumilast	Activate glucocorticoid receptors; suppress proinflammatory mediators; reduce immune cell activation Increase cyclic adenosine monophosphate (cAMP) levels in cells	▪ Budesonide and fluticasone contain lactose, may contain milk proteins ▪ May cause taste changes or nausea ▪ Calcium supplements, milk, magnesium hydroxide, or antacids may interfere with enteric coated products due to the influence on pH ▪ Sodium or potassium salts may cause hypernatremia or fluid retention ▪ Echinacea may interact adversely with steroids ▪ May cause nausea, diarrhea, dyspepsia, or abdominal pain ▪ May influence appetite ▪ May cause unexplained weight loss ▪ May cause cough or sore throat
Methylxanthines Examples: aminophylline, theophylline	Act as non-selective PDE inhibitors, which increase cAMP levels; Antagonize adenosine receptors	▪ Some theophylline may be manufactured using corn or corn products ▪ Caffeine may increase symptoms of nausea, irritability, and nervousness ▪ May cause diarrhea, gastroesophageal reflux, hypercalcemia, hypokalemia, and vomiting ▪ Charcoal may decrease drug effectiveness ▪ St. John's wort may increase metabolism of drug

Data from Micromedex [electronic version]. Merative; 2024. https://www.micromedexsolutions.com. Accessed December 12, 2024.

in physical activity resulting from increased fatigue and decreased endurance. Using 30 kcal/kg body weight in people with COPD and without obesity produces a similar estimation of TEE compared with measured values, although with wide variability in accuracy. Protein requirement for people with COPD has not been studied, so clinicians should use clinical judgment to ensure protein adequacy in this population.

PRACTICE POINT

Resting energy expenditure (REE) is elevated by 15–25% in the setting of pulmonary disease.

Body Composition

Weight status correlates with hospital outcomes. When COPD and malnutrition coexist, people are more likely to be readmitted to the hospital and more likely to die prior to hospital discharge. Conversely, people with COPD and obesity are less likely to be readmitted and more likely to survive as compared to their normal weight counterparts.[124,125] Still, it is unlikely that weight has a linear relationship on COPD mortality. Weight is a simple and practical measure that can be trended over time in a variety of home and healthcare settings, but it does not provide any information about body composition.

Underweight and obesity are diagnosed by a simple calculation of body mass index (BMI), a tool also known to have limitations as it does not distinguish fat mass from fat-free mass, nor does it account for normal variation in body composition due to age, sex, or race. More studies are revealing the limitations of weight and BMI as prognostic tools in people with COPD. Rather, fat-free mass index (FFMI) assessed by bioelectrical impedance analysis (BIA) is a predictor of mortality.[126] Low FFMI also correlates with poor pulmonary function and poor functional status. Higher FFMI in people who are underweight results in better exercise capacity.[127] Understanding fat mass is also important, as the distribution of fat mass may be more meaningful than absolute adiposity. For instance, excess abdominal visceral fat has been associated with an increase in all-cause mortality stemming from increased interleukin-6 (IL-6).[128]

Sarcopenia, defined as a loss of muscle mass and function commonly associated with aging, is estimated to be present in 15–34% of people with COPD, more commonly in people with greater disease severity.[129] The coexistence of sarcopenia and COPD is likely multifactorial and includes systemic inflammation, oxidative stress, and mitochondrial dysfunction in muscle cells.[130] The presence of sarcopenia correlates with poor clinical outcomes including pulmonary function, exercise tolerance, and quality of life. Diagnosis commonly involves imaging such as dual energy x-ray absorptiometry (DXA), computed tomography (CT), magnetic resonance imaging (MRI), or BIA and functional measurement such as handgrip dynamometry and assessment of gait speed.

CORE CONCEPT 3

In chronic obstructive pulmonary disease (COPD), fat-free mass index correlates with hospital outcomes.

Obesity is linked to the development of several comorbidities including, but not limited to, cardiovascular disease, diabetes, certain malignancies, and functional and respiratory impairments.[131] In people with obesity who smoke, weight gain has been found to worsen overall health status,[132] and there is strong evidence associating obesity and dyspnea.[133] Further, National Health and Nutrition Examination Survey (NHANES) data have identified an increased risk of death from a respiratory condition in people with extreme obesity.[134] However, when severe airway obstruction is present, overweight and obesity may have a protective effect.[135] This finding likely highlights the value of energy stores in individuals with altered energy metabolism and impaired dietary intake. Lifestyle interventions in people with COPD may result in modest weight loss, but did not improve clinical outcomes in one study.[136] At this time, there are no specific recommendations for intentional weight loss in subpopulations of people with COPD and overweight or obesity and a general healthful diet should be encouraged.

PRACTICE POINT

Given the substantial body of evidence in support of achieving a healthy weight to prevent chronic disease, nutritional management of people with mild-to-moderate COPD should be centered on achieving a healthy weight for that individual.

CASE STUDY REVISITED

After a few minutes, Leigh catches her breath and manages to report the following diet information:

24-Hour Diet Recall:

10 am Breakfast: 12 oz coffee with milk and 1–2 pieces of dry wheat toast, occasionally a banana

1 pm Lunch: 16 oz water and a frozen dinner, usually baked ziti or pasta primavera

7 pm Dinner: 16 oz water and a frozen dinner, usually lasagna or chicken stir fry

Questions

1. How would you assess Leigh's current intake?
2. How does Leigh's weight status impact her COPD outcome?
3. What strategies can you offer Leigh to prevent further weight loss?

Some individuals with COPD may develop cachexia, a syndrome characterized by weight loss and the loss of lean body mass (LBM) and fat mass, that often does not fully respond to nutrition interventions. Inflammation and oxidative and nitrosative stress are the likely mechanisms for muscle wasting in COPD cachexia while adipocytes such as leptin, adiponectin, and zinc alpha-2 glycoprotein may hold the key to fat wasting.[137] While age, sex, and genetic factors may increase risk for cachexia development, a number of modifiable factors can influence the course of disease. Lifestyle factors like smoking cessation, alcohol cessation, and increasing physical activity are important to mitigate protein breakdown and inhibition of protein synthesis and maintain muscle function. Medical treatment of **hypoxemia** and hypercapnia can help to maintain appetite, body weight, and muscle function. Interestingly, overnight noninvasive positive pressure ventilation has been associated with weight gain, perhaps due to a reduction in energy expenditure of respiration.[138]

Researchers have explored various pharmacologic agents aimed at increasing weight and LBM in people with COPD. One example is megestrol acetate, an appetite stimulant with anti-inflammatory effects. This medication reliably increases weight, primarily as additional fat mass.[139] When combined with testosterone, weight stability and LBM gain can be achieved.[140] However, anabolic steroids such as nandrolone or testosterone can achieve these changes in body mass independently.[141] Future studies are needed to determine which population of patients most benefit, the potential adverse effects, and optimal dose and duration of therapy.[142]

Preliminary data support the use of β-hydroxy-β-methylbutyrate (HMB), a metabolite of the branched chain amino acid leucine, to preserve strength and muscle mass in various populations, including patients who are older, critically ill, HIV-positive, and/or have cancer.[143–147] This research provides a framework for the use of HMB in pulmonary disease. Limited evidence suggests that HMB supplementation may reduce inflammation and muscle catabolism and improve pulmonary function.[148] When included as part of a calorie-dense supplement drink, HMB might also improve strength and reduce mortality risk.[149] However, further study is needed to substantiate the efficacy and clinical significance of HMB in patients with pulmonary disease.

Nutrition Assessment

Individuals with compromised respiratory performance face several challenges that can hinder their ability to consume adequate food and drink. Frequently, these barriers result in early satiety or physical exhaustion. For example, using continuous positive airway pressure machines, eating too quickly, and consuming carbonated beverages can cause **aerophagia**, or excessive swallowing of air. This can create the sensation of fullness that diminishes appetite and overall food intake. Likewise, any exertion at or around mealtimes can impact total consumption for those with low pulmonary reserve. Nutrition assessment will depend upon the stage of illness, but includes measuring anthropometrics (height and weight), identifying weight trends (gains or losses), assessing body composition, food and fluid intake, micronutrient and supplement intake, eating and meal patterns including hunger and satiety trends, respiratory status including oxygen dependence and evaluation of dyspnea with meals or on exertion, laboratory values, and functional status, especially related to the ability to shop and cook. Nutrition-focused physical examination should include evaluation of fat and muscle wasting for individuals with weight loss or cachexia.

Nutrition Intervention

Nutrition therapy interventions can improve body composition and weight, enhance quality of life, and boost functional status. In addition, implementation of dietary strategies may improve respiratory symptoms as reflected by dyspnea scores. However, objective parameters of lung function are not consistently influenced by these interventions.[121] Multidisciplinary care is crucial,[150] as nutrition interventions alone are insufficient to improve exercise capacity. Economically, this translates into reduced hospital admissions and healthcare costs overall.

Diet composition may influence clinical outcomes in patients with COPD. Higher energy intakes are associated with improved dyspnea scores whereas higher protein intakes may improve respiratory symptoms, quality of life, and functional status. Although greater protein and leucine intake have increased muscle mass in some patients with sarcopenia, results are not consistent across all individuals.[151] Baseline nutrition status and other factors may play a critical role in choosing effective interventions. Carbohydrate intake may also improve body strength and performance on a 6-minute walk test, although evidence supporting this is quite limited. Ultimately, the macronutrient distribution of the diet should be tailored to each individual, taking into account their nutrition status, COPD diagnosis, and related comorbid conditions.

Improving diet quality as a whole may be beneficial. For instance, one study evaluating the effect of medical nutrition therapy including a diet enriched with whey protein, omega-3 fatty acids, and vitamin D found improved exercise fatigue and dyspnea at 12 weeks in patients with COPD and cachexia.[152]

Dietary counseling by a RD can increase dietary intake, support the maintenance of weight and lean body mass, and improve quality of life in people with COPD.[150,153,154] Additionally, when nutrition supplementation is combined with a rehabilitation program it can lead to greater gains in weight and fat-free mass, helping to offset the increased energy expenditure associated with increased physical activity.[155,156] Generally, patients with COPD who are physically active tend to have greater LBM compared to those who are inactive.[157]

Oral nutrition supplements (ONS) are often recommended to both inpatients and outpatients to enhance protein and calorie intake. For people with COPD, these supplement drinks have been found to improve body weight and anthropometric measurements such as triceps skinfold thickness, mid-arm muscle circumference,[158] and hand grip strength.[149] The benefits are especially pronounced in those with preexisting malnutrition, particularly among those with adhere closely to recommended consumption of ONS.[159]

There are strategies that can address the challenges of poor oral intake, aerophagia, early satiety, and mealtime fatigue in this population. One approach is to ensure adequate fluid intake, which can thin mucus associated with COPD. Timing is also important; for some, ingesting liquids during meals satisfies hunger quickly, displacing calorie- and protein-dense foods. In such cases, drinking between meals might be more beneficial. Eating small frequent meals (four to six times a day) can help those who feel full with larger volumes, and this strategy may also reduce mealtime fatigue. Resting before meals can boost mealtime endurance, and consuming more food earlier in the day may be useful for those who tire easily later in the day. Some individuals may find softer foods and liquids less demanding than those that require extensive chewing, making modified consistencies and/or ONS worthwhile options.

Accessing groceries and preparing meals can also be significant challenges for some people. Community food programs and social support systems are valuable resources to help bridge the nutrition gap created by impaired functional status and endurance. The services available, along with eligibility criteria (e.g., age, income) can vary by state and community.

Micronutrients

Antioxidants

Cigarette smoking increases oxidative damage, thereby increasing the demand for vitamin C. As such, the Dietary Reference Intake for vitamin C is set at an additional 35 mg/day for smokers.[160] It is well established that people with COPD have low blood levels of antioxidants.[161–163] Higher blood levels of vitamin C have been observed to have a protective effect on **forced expiratory volume (FEV_1)**, or the amount of air a person can exhale during forced breathing, in some,[164–167] but not all,[168] studies. Evidence in support of vitamin E to preserve FEV_1 is less, with higher vitamin E levels positively associated in one study,[168] but not others.[165,167,169] Vitamin A and several carotenoids also have been found to protect FEV_1.[168–170]

Recognizing that an oxidant–antioxidant imbalance is ubiquitous in a number of pulmonary diseases, the hypothesis that antioxidant supplementation can influence respiratory outcomes is an area of interest for researchers. Negative associations between COPD and vitamin C, E, and beta-carotene levels have been observed,[171] but intervention trials have rendered less-than-compelling results. A few small trials found positive effects of vitamins A, C, and/or E,[161,172,173] while others have not.[174–180] More study is needed to determine whether supplementation of a particular antioxidant or combination of nutrients at a certain dose and duration can positively affect clinically relevant respiratory parameters.

The importance of high-quality diets to pulmonary health cannot be understated (**Figure 14.3**). Even though intensive supplementation does not appear to prevent or improve respiratory outcomes, a diet

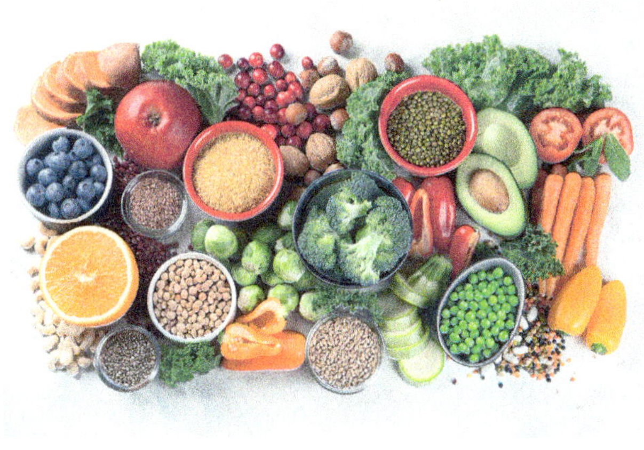

Figure 14.3 Foods High in Antioxidants Are Beneficial to Pulmonary Health

high in antioxidants improves levels of vitamin E and beta-carotene[172] and may be associated with better lung function.[181] Considering that oxidative damage from smoking and environmental exposures occurs over time, the significance of healthful dietary patterns over the course of a lifetime may produce more meaningful benefit, although this has yet to be investigated.

CORE CONCEPT 4

Oxidant–antioxidant imbalance is ubiquitous in many pulmonary diseases, emphasizing the importance of an antioxidant-rich diet.

Vitamins and Minerals

The high prevalence of malnutrition in people with COPD also increases the risk for refeeding syndrome. Therefore, it is advisable to achieve normal blood concentrations of potassium, magnesium, and phosphate to sustain normal blood levels in the presence of nutrition support. In particular, phosphorus and magnesium support lung function. Refer to Chapter 2, *Biochemical Assessment*, for more information on refeeding syndrome.

Phosphorus

Phosphorus is of particular significance to the patient with pulmonary disease due to its role in the production of adenosine triphosphate (ATP) and 2,3-diphosphoglycerate (2,3-DPG). Severe hypophosphatemia diminishes contractility of the diaphragm and leads to subnormal pulmonary function.[182]

Magnesium

Like phosphorus, magnesium is required for ATP. Magnesium also plays a direct role in the relaxation of bronchial smooth muscle (bronchodilation) and has anticholinergic effects. Given these functions, deficiency of magnesium may result in bronchoconstriction. Hypomagnesemia has also been associated with low vitamin D levels given the role that magnesium plays on calcium ion transport and cell signaling. Low magnesium levels have been observed in patients with asthma in some,[183,184] but not all, studies.[185–187] Further study is required to inform magnesium supplementation, but patients with magnesium poor diets may benefit from consumption of high magnesium foods.

Iron

Studies have presented that people with COPD often experience higher rates of iron deficiency,[188] which is more pronounced in prevalence as the disease progresses.[189] Mechanisms by which this may occur include both inadequate dietary intake and blood loss, as well as a functional iron deficiency. In COPD, inflammation can lead to the sequestration of iron by macrophages, which makes it less available for red blood cell production. Iron supplementation has been found to improve exercise capacity in a small pilot study of people with COPD,[190] but there are no standard recommendations for iron replacement in people with COPD.

B Vitamins

Low intakes of various B vitamins have been reported in patients with COPD,[191] but they are not well studied. One study found an association of low pyridoxine (Vitamin B6) and frailty, but this association was not true for other B vitamins studied. Another study observed an improvement in cycle ergometer endurance when vitamin B12 was added to exercise regimens in a group of people with advanced COPD.[192] However, there is not enough research to inform the need for supplementation of any B vitamin in the COPD population.

Vitamin D

According to epidemiologic data, it is common for vitamin D deficiency to parallel COPD[193–195]; however, intervention trials have yet to find a link with mortality or frequency of disease exacerbation in patients who are vitamin D replete.[196–198] Supplementation in people with vitamin D deficiency has reduced COPD exacerbations in some studies,[199,200] and had no benefit in others.[201]

Poor vitamin D status has been implicated in the development of osteoporosis due to the role that vitamin D plays in bone mineralization. Poor oral intake, underweight, and malnutrition all play a role in the development of bone disease associated with vitamin D deficiency. Some individuals with COPD specifically avoid milk, a significant source of calcium and vitamin D in the American diet, due to the belief that it enhances mucus production; however, this has not been scientifically proven.[202] Medication and lifestyle factors such as glucocorticoid use, immobility, and smoking are also contributors to poor vitamin D status. In addition to maintaining calcium homeostasis, the role of vitamin D in maintaining serotonin levels and reducing inflammation has been proposed to influence the development of depressive order in deficient persons.[203] There is no recommendation for routine supplementation of vitamin D in this at-risk population, but correction of deficiency may mitigate or prevent some of the comorbidities commonly associated with COPD.

Quality of Life and Psychosocial Support

COPD has a significant negative impact on quality of life. Low FEV_1 is associated with a decreased ability to perform daily activities, leading to greater impairments in energy levels, physical mobility, and social interaction as lung function declines.[204] Mild disease exacerbations can diminish quality of life; however, an increase in frequency, to three or more exacerbations per year, along with increased severity, is linked to even greater impairments in quality of life.[205] The exacerbations also contribute to a decreased capacity for daily living and exercise, with depressive order and anxiety disorder being more prevalent among patients experiencing them. The psychological impact of these exacerbations is likely underappreciated. Additionally, a study found that underweight individuals with COPD reported compromised physical function, emotional well-being, bodily pain, and overall health, highlighting the critical importance of weight maintenance in this vulnerable population.[206] Individuals with malnutrition also experienced higher levels of fatigue and scored worse on depressive order scales.[207] Key factors affecting BMI in these patients include lung diffusion capacity, early satiety, and active cigarette smoking.

CORE CONCEPT 5

Individuals with COPD who are malnourished have described greater levels of fatigue and score higher on depressive order scales.

Monitoring and Evaluation

Monitoring patients with COPD would include trending weight, laboratory values, evaluating diet records and meal patters to assess food and fluid intake behaviors, as well as physical functioning to assess barriers to adequate intake. It would be important to monitor hydration status as well as lean body and fat mass wasting through nutrition-focused physical examination.

Acute Respiratory Distress Syndrome

Acute respiratory distress syndrome (ARDS) is a type of hypoxemic respiratory failure that accounts for at least 10% of inpatient admissions to the intensive care unit and carries a high in-hospital mortality rate.[208] Per the Berlin Definition, ARDS is characterized by several criteria: acute development of bilateral lung infiltrates on imaging that occurs within 1 week of clinical insult or new respiratory symptoms (**Figures 14.4** and **14.5**), edema that is non-cardiogenic in nature and not

Clinical Roundtable

Topic: Weight status in COPD

Background: The role of obesity in COPD is complex. The correlation between weight and hospital outcomes in these patients is well established. In the early stages of COPD, obesity can increase risk of comorbidities, such as diabetes and cardiovascular disease. In the later stages of the disease, patients with obesity may have improved outcomes such as lower rates of hospital readmissions and death, although unintended weight loss is associated with higher mortality. Despite this, there are no weight recommendations for individuals with obesity and COPD. When treating patients with COPD, clinicians are tasked with weighing the advantages and disadvantages of current weight status.

Roundtable Discussion

Consider the relationship of weight in COPD.

1. What would be the advantages and disadvantages of recommending weight loss in patients with COPD?
2. What factors would you consider when deciding to prioritize weight management in this population?
3. How might you monitor a patient with COPD who is losing weight?

References

Zapatero A, Barba R, Ruiz J, et al. Malnutrition and obesity: influence on mortality and readmissions in chronic obstructive pulmonary disease patients. *J Hum Nutr Diet.* 2013;26(Suppl 1):16-22.; Putcha N, Anzueto AR, Calverley PMA, et al. Mortality and exacerbation risk by body mass index in patients with COPD in TIOSPIR and UPLIFT. *Ann Am Thorac Soc.* 2022;19(2):204-213. doi:10.1513/AnnalsATS.202006-722OC.

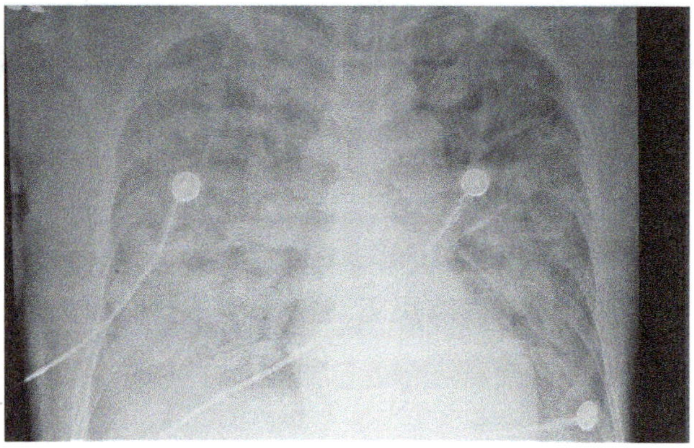

Figure 14.4 Chest X-ray of a Patient with ARDS

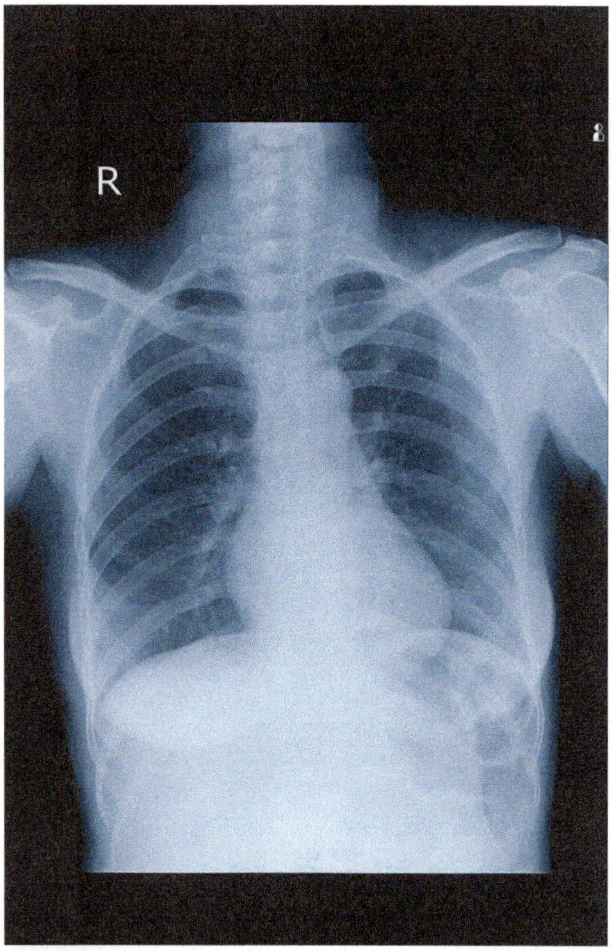

Figure 14.5 Normal Chest X-ray

explained by fluid overload, and an arterial oxygen tension to fraction of inspired oxygen ratio (PaO_2/FiO_2 or "P:F ratio") less than 300 mm Hg with positive end-expiratory pressure (PEEP) or continuous positive airway pressure (CPAP) ≥5 cm H_2O.[209,210] Common causes of ARDS are listed in **Table 14.2**. Severity of disease is stratified into mild,

Table 14.2 Causes of Acute Respiratory Distress Syndrome

Direct Lung Injury
Aspiration of gastric contents
Inhalation of toxic substances
Near drowning
Pneumonia
Pulmonary contusion
Viral infection
Indirect Lung Injury
Cardiopulmonary bypass
Drug overdose
Pancreatitis
Repeated blood transfusions
Sepsis
Severe trauma

Data from: Gorman EA, O'Kane CM, McAuley DF. Acute respiratory distress syndrome in adults: diagnosis, outcomes, long-term sequelae, and management. *Lancet.* 2022;400(10358): 1157–1170. doi:10.1016/s0140-6736(22)01439-8

moderate, and severe, with PaO_2/FiO_2 ranges of 200 to ≤300 mm Hg, 100 to ≤200 mm Hg, and ≤100 mm Hg, respectively.[211] Treatment for ARDS includes lung protective mechanical ventilation and oxygenation strategies to address hypoxemia, or low blood oxygen; fluid restriction and diuretic therapy to control edema; and management of acidosis. Steroids may be appropriate for some patients, such as those with ARDS due to COVID-19. Refer to Chapter 6, *Nutrition in Critical Illness*, for more information on nutrition assessment, nutrition intervention, and monitoring and evaluation during critical illness.

Patients intubated for ARDS are likely to need enteral nutrition (EN) support. Current critical care guidelines advise initiation of EN within 24–48 hours of admission to the intensive care unit, increasing to goal over the first 7 days.[212] In cases of severe hypoxemia, hypercapnia, or acidosis,[213] a delay in feeding may be warranted. While general guidelines recommend feeding 12–25 kcal/kg over the first 7–10 days,[214] clinicians should use caution in the population with ARDS as there is evidence to suggest that delivering full energy requirements over the first week of critical illness in this subgroup could be harmful.[215–217] The patient with critical illness and ARDS often

CASE STUDY REVISITED

Leigh is admitted to the hospital 6 months later with a COPD exacerbation. Upon admission, she reports that her weight has been stable for the previous 6 months. After a brief stay, she is discharged home only to be readmitted a month later with another COPD exacerbation. During this admission, she is intubated for respiratory failure requiring ventilatory support and transferred to the intensive care unit. A nasoenteric tube is placed and the medical team requests enteral nutrition recommendations.

Anthropometrics:

Weight: 60.2 kg
Last admission weight (6 months ago): 63.6 kg

Questions

1. Describe Leigh's nutrition risk and current nutrition status?
2. How would you assess her energy needs?
3. What type of formula would you recommend for Leigh while she is intubated?
4. Write two Problem/Etiology/Signs and Symptoms (PES) statements for Leigh.

experience other comorbidities and organ failures. Secondary diagnoses, along with medications used to treat these conditions, make estimating energy needs challenging. IC should be used to measure energy expenditure when available; however, respiratory instability often limits the feasibility of obtaining good quality studies. Mechanical ventilation set to a FiO_2 greater than 60% and/or PEEP greater than 10 cm H_2O will reduce study accuracy.[218] Additionally, hyper- and hypoventilation will prevent attainment of a "steady state," thereby yielding indeterminable results. The Penn State equation has been validated for use in patients who are critically ill and mechanically ventilated and is an appropriate substitution when IC cannot be performed. Energy delivery between 12 and 25 kcal/kg may also be appropriate.[214] Recommended protein intakes for patients with critical illness with a BMI <30 kg/m^2 is between 1.2 and 2.0 g/kg actual body weight.[212]

PRACTICE POINT

Indirect calorimetry is the gold standard for determining energy requirements. When unavailable, the Penn State equation or 12–25 kcal/kg should be used.

Nutrition Support and Pulmonary Disease

According to the 2016 Clinical Guidelines from the American Society for Parenteral and Enteral Nutrition (ASPEN), using a concentrated enteral formula is advised for patients with acute respiratory failure who require nutrition support and could benefit from fluid restriction.[212] This patient group often experiences fluid buildup and pulmonary edema, which are linked to poor clinical outcomes. Additionally, the buildup of carbon dioxide in diseased lungs can further impair pulmonary function making it more difficult for individuals to wean off mechanical ventilation. Historically there has been a focus on restricting carbohydrate since carbohydrates metabolism results in more carbon dioxide than protein and fat. However, studies indicate that carbohydrate restriction does not significantly improve ventilation when compared to a normal distribution of macronutrients within calorie needs.

Carbon dioxide is a by-product of energy substrate metabolism, so it is crucial to avoid overfeeding. Evidence includes an elevated $PaCO_2$ in arterial blood gas (ABG) tests.[219] When planning nutrition support, it is also important to consider the caloric contributions of medications commonly used in intensive care, such as propofol and dextrose infusions, to help mitigate the risk of overfeeding.

PRACTICE POINT

Because carbon dioxide is a by-product of energy substrate metabolism, it is important to avoid overfeeding.

Typically, hospitalized patients are fed enterally while resting in the supine position with standard aspiration precautions in place. These include elevating the head of bed, confirming proper tube placement by x-ray, and monitoring for signs of respiratory and abdominal intolerance. In select cases, ARDS treatment may incorporate prone positioning—lying face down—to alleviate pressure put on the dorsal lungs by ventral organs to improve gas exchange.[220,221] Use of prone therapy, and enteral feeding in the prone position, increased dramatically during the COVID-19 pandemic due to the rise in cases of acute lung injury that progressed to ARDS.

Enteral nutrition (EN) is safe in the prone patient,[222–224] and does not significantly increase vomiting, pneumonia, or gastric residuals when compared to supine feeding.[223–225] Elevating the head of bed by reverse Trendelenburg positioning (**Figure 14.6**), where the body is flat but the head is 15–30 degrees higher than the feet; prokinetic agents; and postpyloric feeding with or without gastric decompression may be used to optimize success of EN. Institutional protocols may be helpful to standardize provision and monitoring of EN for patients in the prone position.

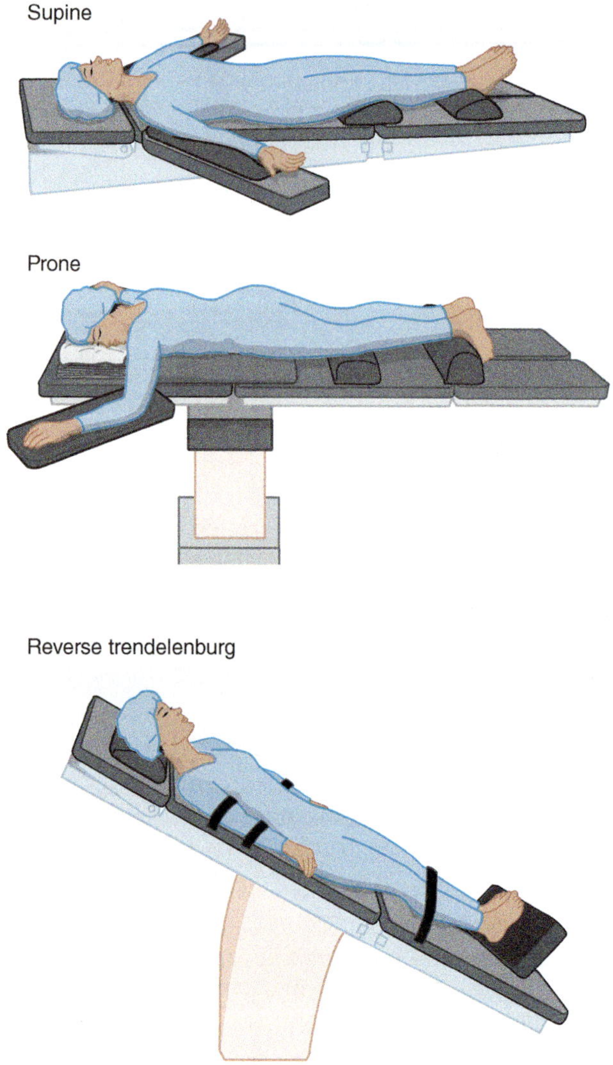

Figure 14.6 Supine Position/Prone Position/Reverse Trendelenburg Position

Immunonutrition

Immune-modulating enteral formulations contain greater quantities of anti-inflammatory ingredients such as antioxidants, omega-3 fatty acids, and amino acids, and have been found to influence clinical outcomes in some critical care populations.[212] Conceptually, an enteral formula high in omega-3 fatty acids sourced from fish or borage oil, such as eicosapentaenoic acid (EPA) and docosahexaenoic acid (DHA), can work to reduce the inflammatory response through production of resolvins and protectins. Omega-3 fatty acids may also help to reduce synthesis of proinflammatory eicosanoids by displacing proinflammatory omega-6 fatty acids such as arachidonic acid.

Despite several studies in support of immune-modulating EN,[226–229] controversy exists over its use in the population of patients with ARDS. Two recent systematic reviews found that these formulas do not influence mortality in patients with ARDS, and whether or not there is a role for improvement of other clinical outcomes is inconclusive.[230,231] Owing to the heterogeneity of study design and confounding influence of mechanical ventilation strategies on outcome parameters, optimal dosing, timing, method of administration, and duration of enteral supplementation, or efficacy at all, remain unclear. It is likely safe to use these formulas in patients with ARDS,[232] but they cannot be recommended over standard polymeric formulas at this time.[212]

⚠ Clinical Controversy

Optimal Macronutrient Content of Enteral Feeding in COPD

Manipulation of macronutrients in the management of pulmonary disease has been a topic of discussion for several years. Pulmonary-specific enteral formulas have been designed to provide a higher fat and lower carbohydrate ratio due to the potential impact of carbon dioxide generation by carbohydrate. In one study of patients on mechanical ventilators, a high-fat, low-carbohydrate diet resulted in decreased arterial carbon dioxide tension, improved minute volume, and fewer days on ventilation. However, this result is not a consistent finding, and research exists showing no clear benefit for the use of disease-specific enteral formulas in patients who are critically ill with hyperglycemia. Excessive fat intake can have implications for gastrointestinal tolerance, inflammation, and cell dynamics. In addition, patients with critical illness may also be receiving lipid-based sedatives, such as propofol, which further increases fat intake. These factors should be weighed against the strength of evidence in support of a high-fat, low-carbohydrate diet.

Questions

1. Based upon this research, discuss the potential risks and benefits of providing a high-fat, low-carbohydrate enteral formula to patients with pulmonary dysfunction.
2. What factors might you consider in determining if a patient would benefit from a higher-fat diet?

References

Faramawy MA, Allah AA, Batrawy SL, Amer H. Impact of high-fat, low-carbohydrate enteral feeding on weaning from mechanical ventilation. Egypt *J Chest Dis Tuberc*. 2014;63:931-938.; Mesejo A, Acosta JA, Ortega C, et al. Comparison of a high-protein disease-specific enteral formula with a high-protein enteral formula in hyperglycemic critically ill patients. *Clin Nutr*. 2003;22(3):295-305.; Hsieh MJ, Yang TM, Tsai YH. Nutritional supplementation in patients with chronic obstructive pulmonary disease. *J Formos Med Assoc*. 2016;115(8):595-601. doi:10.1016/j.jfma.2015.10.008

Chapter Summary

Medical nutrition therapy is essential for managing patients with pulmonary disease. Adequate nutrient intake and effective weight management significantly influence the progression of both asthma and COPD, its response to therapies, and patients' quality of life. Early interventions that combine a healthful diet with exercise strategies can provide important benefits to patients with COPD. In cases of acute respiratory distress syndrome (ARDS), ensuring sufficient energy intake—potentially along with key micronutrients—can optimize patient and hospital outcomes. Future research is essential to better understand the specific roles that individual nutrients or their combinations can play in the effective treatment of pulmonary disease.

Key Terms

asthma, gut–lung axis, chronic obstructive pulmonary disease (COPD), spirometry, dyspnea, aerophagia, acute respiratory distress syndrome (ARDS), hypoxemia, forced expiratory volume (FEV_1)

References

1. CDC/National Center for Health Statistics. Asthma. Accessed October 5, 2024. http://www.cdc.gov/nchs/fastats/asthma.htm
2. CDC/National Center for Health Statistics. Chronic obstructive pulmonary disease (COPD) includes: Chronic bronchitis and emphysema. Accessed October 5, 2024. http://www.cdc.gov/nchs/fastats/copd.htm
3. Swed S, Sawaf B, Al-Obeidat F, et al. Asthma prevalence among United States population insights from NHANES data analysis. *Sci Rep*. 2024;14(1):8059. doi:10.1038/s41598-024-58429-5
4. Dandona P, Ghanim H, Monte SV, et al. Increase in the mediators of asthma in obesity and obesity with type 2 diabetes: reduction with weight loss. *Obesity (Silver Spring)*. 2014;22(2):356–62. doi:10.1002/oby.20524
5. Fantuzzi G. Adipose tissue, adipokines, and inflammation. *J Allergy Clin Immunol*. 2005;115(5):911-9; quiz 920. doi:10.1016/j.jaci.2005.02.023
6. Lambrecht BN, Hammad H, Fahy JV. The Cytokines of Asthma. *Immunity*. 2019;50(4):975–991. doi:10.1016/j.immuni.2019.03.018
7. Wood LG, Baines KJ, Fu J, Scott HA, Gibson PG. The neutrophilic inflammatory phenotype is associated with systemic inflammation in asthma. *Chest*. 2012;142(1):86–93. doi:10.1378/chest.11-1838
8. Olafsdottir IS, Gislason T, Thjodleifsson B, et al. C reactive protein levels are increased in non-allergic but not allergic asthma: a multicentre epidemiological study. *Thorax*. 2005;60(6):451–454. doi:10.1136/thx.2004.035774
9. Scott HA, Ng SH, McLoughlin RF, et al. Effect of obesity on airway and systemic inflammation in adults with asthma: a systematic review and meta-analysis. *Thorax*. 2023;78(10):957–965. doi:10.1136/thorax-2022-219268
10. Mohan A, Grace J, Wang BR, Lugogo N. The effects of obesity in asthma. *Curr Allergy Asthma Rep*. 2019;19(10):49. doi:10.1007/s11882-019-0877-z

11. Dixon AE, Que LG. Obesity and asthma. *Semin Respir Crit Care Med*. 2022;43(5):662–674. doi:10.1055/s-0042-1742384
12. Haldar P, Pavord ID, Shaw DE, et al. Cluster analysis and clinical asthma phenotypes. *Am J Respir Crit Care Med*. 2008;178(3):218–224. doi:10.1164/rccm.200711-1754OC
13. Moore WC, Meyers DA, Wenzel SE, et al. Identification of asthma phenotypes using cluster analysis in the Severe Asthma Research Program. *Am J Respir Crit Care Med*. 2010;181(4):315–323. doi:10.1164/rccm.200906-0896OC
14. Dixon AE, Poynter ME. Mechanisms of asthma in obesity. Pleiotropic aspects of obesity produce distinct asthma phenotypes. *Am J Respir Cell Mol Biol*. 2016;54(5):601–608. doi:10.1165/rcmb.2016-0017PS
15. Sutherland ER, Goleva E, King TS, et al. Cluster analysis of obesity and asthma phenotypes. *PloS One*. 2012;7(5):e36631. doi:10.1371/journal.pone.0036631
16. Carr TF, Kraft M. Use of biomarkers to identify phenotypes and endotypes of severeasthma. *Ann Allergy Asthma Immunol*. 2018;121(4):414–420. doi:10.1016/j.anai.2018.07.029
17. Bates JHT, Poynter ME, Frodella CM, Peters U, Dixon AE, Suratt BT. Pathophysiology to phenotype in the asthma of obesity. *Ann Am Thorac Soc*. 2017;14(Supplement_5): S395–s398. doi:10.1513/AnnalsATS.201702-122AW
18. Bates JH. Physiological mechanisms of airway hyperresponsiveness in obese asthma. *Am J Respir Cell Mol Biol*. 2016;54(5):618–623. doi:10.1165/rcmb.2016-0019PS
19. Holguin F, Bleecker ER, Busse WW, et al. Obesity and asthma: an association modified by age of asthma onset. *J Allergy Clin Immunol*. 2011;127(6):1486–1493.e2. doi:10.1016/j.jaci.2011.03.036
20. Parasuaraman G, Ayyasamy L, Aune D, et al. The association between body mass index, abdominal fatness, and weight change and the risk of adult asthma: a systematic review and meta-analysis of cohort studies. *Sci Rep*. 2023;13(1):7745. doi:10.1038/s41598-023-31373-6
21. Jiang D, Wang L, Bai C, Chen O. Association between abdominal obesity and asthma: a meta-analysis. *Allergy Asthma Clin Immunol*. 2019;15:16. doi:10.1186/s13223-019-0333-6
22. Ashtary-Larky D, Ghanavati M, Lamuchi-Deli N, et al. Rapid weight loss vs. slow weight loss: which is more effective on body composition and metabolic risk factors? *Int J Endocrinol Metab*. 2017;15(3):e13249. doi:10.5812/ijem.13249
23. Mertens IL, Van Gaal LF. Overweight, obesity, and blood pressure: the effects of modest weight reduction. *Obes Res*. 2000;8(3):270–278. doi:10.1038/oby.2000.32
24. Johnson O, Gerald LB, Harvey J, et al. An online weight loss intervention for people with obesity and poorly controlled asthma. *J Allergy Clin Immunol Pract*. 2022;10(6):1577–1586.e3. doi:10.1016/j.jaip.2022.02.040
25. Ma J, Strub P, Xiao L, et al. Behavioral weight loss and physical activity intervention in obese adults with asthma. A randomized trial. *Ann Am Thorac Soc*.2015;12(1):1–11. doi:10.1513/AnnalsATS.201406-271OC
26. Stenius-Aarniala B, Poussa T, Kvarnström J, Grönlund EL, Ylikahri M, Mustajoki P. Immediate and long term effects of weight reduction in obese people with asthma: randomised controlled study. *BMJ*. 2000;320(7238): 827–832. doi:10.1136/bmj.320.7238.827
27. Özbey Ü, Balaban S, Sözener Z, Uçar A, Mungan D, Mısırlıgil Z. The effects of diet-induced weight loss on asthma control and quality of life in obese adults with asthma: a randomized controlled trial. *J Asthma*. 2020;57(6):618–626. doi:10.1080/02770903.2019.1590594
28. Pakhale S, Baron J, Dent R, Vandemheen K, Aaron SD. Effects of weight loss on airway responsiveness in obese adults with asthma: does weight loss lead to reversibility of asthma? *Chest*. 2015;147(6):1582–1590. doi:10.1378/chest.14-3105
29. Hakala K, Stenius-Aarniala B, Sovijärvi A. Effects of weight loss on peak flow variability, airways obstruction, and lung volumes in obese patients with asthma. *Chest*. 2000;118(5):1315–1321. doi:10.1378/chest.118.5.1315
30. Hossain N, Arhi C, Borg CM. Is bariatric surgery better than nonsurgical weight loss for improving asthma control? a systematic review. *Obes Surg*. 2021;31(4):1810–1832. doi:10.1007/s11695-021-05255-7
31. Zhang P, Lopez R, Arrigain S, Rath M, Khatri SB, Zein JG. Dietary patterns in patients with asthma and their relationship with asthma-related emergency room visits: NHANES 2005–2016. *J Asthma*. 2022;59(10):2051–2059. doi:10.1080/02770903.2021.1984529
32. Williams EJ, Berthon BS, Stoodley I, Williams LM, Wood LG. Nutrition in asthma. *Semin Respir Crit Care Med*. 2022;43(5):646–661. doi:10.1055/s-0042-1742385
33. Papamichael MM, Itsiopoulos C, Susanto NH, Erbas B. Does adherence to the Mediterranean dietary pattern reduce asthma symptoms in children? A systematic review of observational studies. *Public Health Nutr*. 2017;20(15): 2722–2734. doi:10.1017/s1368980017001823
34. Koumpagioti D, Boutopoulou B, Moriki D, Priftis KN, Douros K. Does adherence to the Mediterranean diet have a protective effect against asthma and allergies in children? A systematic review. *Nutrients*. 2022;14(8). doi:10.3390/nu14081618
35. Antonogeorgos G, Kogias C, Douros K, Panagiotakos D. Greater fruit and vegetables consumption, and adherence to a Mediterranean type of diet reduces the risk for asthma in children; a systematic review and meta-analysis. *Int J Food Sci Nutr*. 2024;75(1):4–30. doi:10.1080/09637486.2023.2276033
36. Takkinsatian P, Mairiang D, Sangkanjanavanich S, Chiewchalermsri C, Tripipitsiriwat A, Sompornrattanaphan M. Dietary factors associated with asthma development: a narrative review and summary of current guidelines and recommendations. *J Asthma Allergy*. 2022;15:1125–1141. doi:10.2147/jaa.S364964
37. Nygaard UC, Xiao L, Nadeau KC, et al. Improved diet quality is associated with decreased concentrations of inflammatory markers in adults with uncontrolled asthma. *Am J Clin Nutr*. 2021;114(3):1012–1027. doi:10.1093/ajcn/nqab063
38. Visser E, de Jong K, Pepels JJS, Kerstjens HAM, Ten Brinke A, van Zutphen T. Diet quality, food intake and incident adult-onset asthma: a Lifelines Cohort Study. *Eur J Nutr*. 2023;62(4):1635–1645.
39. Al-Zalabani AH, Noor Elahi I, Katib A, et al. Association between soft drinks consumption and asthma: a systematic review and meta-analysis. *BMJ Open*. 2019;9(10):e029046. doi:10.1136/bmjopen-2019-029046
40. Xie L, Atem F, Gelfand A, Delclos G, Messiah SE. Association between asthma and sugar-sweetened beverage consumption in the United States pediatric population. *J Asthma*. 2022;59(5):926–933. doi:10.1080/02770903.2021.1895210
41. von Ehrenstein OS, Aralis H, Flores ME, Ritz B. Fast food consumption in pregnancy and subsequent asthma symptoms in young children. *Pediatr Allergy Immunol*. 2015;26(6): 571–577. doi:10.1111/pai.12433
42. Carey OJ, Cookson JB, Britton J, Tattersfield AE. The effect of lifestyle on wheeze, atopy, and bronchial

hyperreactivity in Asian and white children. *Am J Respir Crit Care Med*. 1996;154(2 Pt 1):537–540. doi:10.1164/ajrccm.154.2.8756835

43. Huang YJ, Nelson CE, Brodie EL, et al. Airway microbiota and bronchial hyperresponsiveness in patients with suboptimally controlled asthma. *J Allergy Clin Immunol*. 2011;127(2):372–381.e1-3. doi:10.1016/j.jaci.2010.10.048
44. Wickens K, Barry D, Friezema A, et al. Fast foods - are they a risk factor for asthma? *Allergy*. 2005;60(12):1537–1541. doi:10.1111/j.1398-9995.2005.00945.x
45. Varraso R, Kauffmann F, Leynaert B, et al. Dietary patterns and asthma in the E3N study. *Eur Respir J*. 2009;33(1):33–41. doi:10.1183/09031936.00130807
46. Brigham EP, Kolahdooz F, Hansel N, et al. Association between Western diet pattern and adult asthma: a focused review. *Ann Allergy Asthma Immunol*. 2015;114(4):273–280. doi:10.1016/j.anai.2014.11.003
47. Wood LG, Garg ML, Gibson PG. A high-fat challenge increases airway inflammation and impairs bronchodilator recovery in asthma. *J Allergy Clin Immunol*. 2011;127(5):1133–1140. doi:10.1016/j.jaci.2011.01.036
48. Zhang H, Zhang X, Yang H, et al. Dietary carbohydrate types, genetic predisposition, and risk of adult-onset asthma: a longitudinal cohort study. *Int J Biol Macromol*. 2024;261(Pt 1):129824. doi:10.1016/j.ijbiomac.2024.129824
49. DeChristopher LR, Tucker KL. Excess free fructose, apple juice, high fructose corn syrup and childhood asthma risk - the National Children's Study. *Nutr J*. 2020;19(1):60. doi:10.1186/s12937-020-00578-0
50. Saeed MA, Gribben KC, Alam M, Lyden ER, Hanson CK, LeVan TD. Association of dietary fiber on asthma, respiratory symptoms, and inflammation in the Adult National Health and Nutrition Examination Survey population. *Ann Am Thorac Soc*. 2020;17(9):1062–1068. doi:10.1513/AnnalsATS.201910-776OC
51. Meirlaen L, Levy EI, Vandenplas Y. Prevention and management with pro-, pre and synbiotics in children with asthma and allergic rhinitis: a narrative review. *Nutrients*. 2021;13(3). doi:10.3390/nu13030934
52. Ashique S, De Rubis G, Sirohi E, et al. Short chain fatty acids: fundamental mediators of the gut-lung axis and their involvement in pulmonary diseases. *Chem Biol Interact*. 2022;368:110231. doi:10.1016/j.cbi.2022.110231
53. Huang YJ, Boushey HA. The microbiome in asthma. *J Allergy Clin Immunol*. 2015;135(1):25–30. doi:10.1016/j.jaci.2014.11.011
54. Hilty M, Burke C, Pedro H, et al. Disordered microbial communities in asthmatic airways. *PloS One*. 2010;5(1):e8578. doi:10.1371/journal.pone.0008578
55. Hufnagl K, Pali-Schöll I, Roth-Walter F, Jensen-Jarolim E. Dysbiosis of the gut and lung microbiome has a role in asthma. *Semin Immunopathol*. 2020;42(1):75–93. doi:10.1007/s00281-019-00775-y
56. Liu C, Makrinioti H, Saglani S, et al. Microbial dysbiosis and childhood asthma development: integrated role of the airway and gut microbiome, environmental exposures, and host metabolic and immune response. *Front Immunol*. 2022;13:1028209. doi:10.3389/fimmu.2022.1028209
57. Ciprandi G, Tosca MA. Probiotics in children with asthma. *Children (Basel)*. 2022;9(7). doi:10.3390/children9070978
58. Kleniewska P, Pawliczak R. Can probiotics be used in the prevention and treatment of bronchial asthma? *Pharmacol Rep*. 2024;76(4):740–753. doi:10.1007/s43440-024-00618-0
59. Lewis G, Wang B, Shafiei Jahani P, et al. Dietary fiber-induced microbial short chain fatty acids suppress ILC2-dependent airway inflammation. *Front Immunol*. 2019;10:2051. doi:10.3389/fimmu.2019.02051
60. Thorburn AN, McKenzie CI, Shen S, et al. Evidence that asthma is a developmental origin disease influenced by maternal diet and bacterial metabolites. *Nat Commun*. 2015;6:7320. doi:10.1038/ncomms8320
61. Vahdaninia M, Mackenzie H, Dean T, Helps S. ω-3 LCPUFA supplementation during pregnancy and risk of allergic outcomes or sensitization in offspring: a systematic review and meta-analysis. *Ann Allergy Asthma Immunol*. 2019;122(3):302–313.e2. doi:10.1016/j.anai.2018.12.008
62. Lin J, Zhang Y, Zhu X, Wang D, Dai J. Effects of supplementation with omega-3 fatty acids during pregnancy on asthma or wheeze of children: a systematic review and meta-analysis. *J Matern Fetal Neonatal Med*. 2020;33(10):1792–1801. doi:10.1080/14767058.2018.1529161
63. Gunaratne AW, Makrides M, Collins CT. Maternal prenatal and/or postnatal n-3 long chain polyunsaturated fatty acids (LCPUFA) supplementation for preventing allergies in early childhood. *Cochrane Database Syst Rev*. 2015;2015(7):Cd010085. doi:10.1002/14651858.CD010085.pub2
64. Venter C, Agostoni C, Arshad SH, et al. Dietary factors during pregnancy and atopic outcomes in childhood: a systematic review from the European Academy of Allergy and Clinical Immunology. *Pediatr Allergy Immunol*. 2020;31(8):889–912. doi:10.1111/pai.13303
65. Papamichael MM, Shrestha SK, Itsiopoulos C, Erbas B. The role of fish intake on asthma in children: a meta-analysis of observational studies. *Pediatr Allergy Immunol*. 2018;29(4):350–360. doi:10.1111/pai.12889
66. Magnusson J, Ekström S, Kull I, et al. Polyunsaturated fatty acids in plasma at 8 years and subsequent allergic disease. *J Allergy Clin Immunol*. 2018;142(2):510–516.e6. doi:10.1016/j.jaci.2017.09.023
67. Muley P, Shah M, Muley A. Omega-3 fatty acids supplementation in children to prevent asthma: is it worthy?-a systematic review and meta-analysis. *J Allergy (Cairo)*. 2015;2015:312052. doi:10.1155/2015/312052
68. Yang H, Xun P, He K. Fish and fish oil intake in relation to risk of asthma: a systematic review and meta-analysis. *PloS One*. 2013;8(11):e80048. doi:10.1371/journal.pone.0080048
69. van Brakel L, Mensink RP, Wesseling G, Plat J. Nutritional interventions to improve asthma-related outcomes through immunomodulation: a systematic review. *Nutrients*. 2020;12(12). doi:10.3390/nu12123839
70. Althoff MD, Peterson R, McGrath M, et al. Phenotypic characteristics of asthma and morbidity are associated with distinct longitudinal changes in L-arginine metabolism. *BMJ Open Respir Res*. 2023;10(1). doi:10.1136/bmjresp-2023-001683
71. Scott JA, Maarsingh H, Holguin F, Grasemann H. Arginine therapy for lung diseases. *Front Pharmacol*. 2021;12:627503. doi:10.3389/fphar.2021.627503
72. Holguin F, Grasemann H, Sharma S, et al. L-Citrulline increases nitric oxide and improves control in obese asthmatics. *JCI Insight*. 2019;4(24). doi:10.1172/jci.insight.131733
73. Abuhajar SM, Taleb MH, Ellulu MS. Vitamin C deficiency and risk of metabolic complications among adults with chronic respiratory diseases: a case-control study. *Clini Nutr ESPEN*. 2021;43:448–455. doi:10.1016/j.clnesp.2021.03.007
74. Hu J, Sang J, Hao F, Liu L. Association between vitamin A and asthma: a meta-analysis with trial sequential analysis.

Front Pharmacol. 2023;14:1100002. doi:10.3389/fphar.2023.1100002

75. Bird JK, Feskens EJ, Melse-Boonstra A. A systematized review of the relationship between obesity and vitamin C requirements. *Curr Dev Nutr*. 2024;8(5):102152. doi:10.1016/j.cdnut.2024.102152
76. Wang K, Zhao L, Luo H, Deng C, Gong L, Chen Z. Association of serum vitamin C levels with asthma in adults: results of NHANES 2003–2006 and Mendelian randomization study. *BMC Pulm Med*. 2024;24(1):4. doi:10.1186/s12890-023-02821-w
77. Beckhaus AA, Garcia-Marcos L, Forno E, Pacheco-Gonzalez RM, Celedón JC, Castro-Rodriguez JA. Maternal nutrition during pregnancy and risk of asthma, wheeze, and atopic diseases during childhood: a systematic review and meta-analysis. *Allergy*. 2015;70(12):1588–1604. doi:10.1111/all.12729
78. Nurmatov U, Devereux G, Sheikh A. Nutrients and foods for the primary prevention of asthma and allergy: systematic review and meta-analysis. *J Allergy Clin Immunol*. 2011;127(3):724–733.e1-30. doi:10.1016/j.jaci.2010.11.001
79. Shorey-Kendrick LE, McEvoy CT, O'Sullivan SM, et al. Impact of vitamin C supplementation on placental DNA methylation changes related to maternal smoking: association with gene expression and respiratory outcomes. *Clin Epigenetics*. 2021;13(1):177. doi:10.1186/s13148-021-01161-y
80. García-García C, Kim M, Baik I. Associations of dietary vitamin A and C intake with asthma, allergic rhinitis, and allergic respiratory diseases. *Nutr Res Pract*. 2023;17(5):997–1006. doi:10.4162/nrp.2023.17.5.997
81. McEvoy CT, Schilling D, Clay N, et al. Vitamin C supplementation for pregnant smoking women and pulmonary function in their newborn infants: a randomized clinical trial. *JAMA*. 2014;311(20):2074–2082. doi:10.1001/jama.2014.5217
82. Nitzan I, Mimouni FB, Nun AB, Kasirer Y, Mendlovic J. Vitamin D and asthma: a systematic review of clinical trials. *Curr Nutr Rep*. 2022;11(2):311–317. doi:10.1007/s13668-022-00411-6
83. Jaura J, Kelsberg G, Safranek S. Does vitamin D supplementation reduce asthma exacerbations? *J Fam Pract*. 2020;69(4):E4–E6.
84. Chen Z, Peng C, Mei J, Zhu L, Kong H. Vitamin D can safely reduce asthma exacerbations among corticosteroid-using children and adults with asthma: a systematic review and meta-analysis of randomized controlled trials. *Nutr Res*. 2021;92:49–61. doi:10.1016/j.nutres.2021.05.010
85. Williamson A, Martineau AR, Sheikh A, Jolliffe D, Griffiths CJ. Vitamin D for the management of asthma. *Cochrane Database Syst Rev*. 2023;2(2):Cd011511. doi:10.1002/14651858.CD011511.pub3
86. Forno E, Bacharier LB, Phipatanakul W, et al. Effect of vitamin D3 supplementation on severe asthma exacerbations in children with asthma and low vitamin D levels: The VDKA randomized clinical trial. *JAMA*. 2020;324(8):752–760. doi:10.1001/jama.2020.12384
87. Jiang J, Mehrabi Nasab E, Athari SM, Athari SS. Effects of vitamin E and selenium on allergic rhinitis and asthma pathophysiology. *Respir Physiol Neurobiol*. 2021;286:103614. doi:10.1016/j.resp.2020.103614
88. Cook-Mills JM, Averill SH, Lajiness JD. Asthma, allergy and vitamin E: current and future perspectives. *Free Radic Biol Med*. 2022;179:388–402. doi:10.1016/j.freeradbiomed.2021.10.037
89. Ghaffari J, Alizadeh-Navaei R, Dabaghzadeh A, Ghaffari N. Serum zinc level and children`s asthma: a systematic and meta-analysis review article. *Caspian J Intern Med*. 2021;12(3):236–242. doi:10.22088/cjim.12.3.236
90. Kęszycka PK, Lange E, Gajewska D. Effectiveness of personalized low salicylate diet in the management of salicylates hypersensitive patients: interventional study. *Nutrients*. 2021;13(3). doi:10.3390/nu13030991
91. Sowerby LJ, Patel KB, Schmerk C, Rotenberg BW, Rocha T, Sommer DD. Effect of low salicylate diet on clinical and inflammatory markers in patients with aspirin exacerbated respiratory disease—a randomized crossover trial. *J Otolaryngol Head Neck Surg*. 2021;50(1):27. doi:10.1186/s40463-021-00502-4
92. Dölle-Bierke S, Plank-Habibi S, Schäfer C, et al. Dietary implications in acetylsalicylic acid intolerance. *Allergo J Int*. 2020;29(Suppl 1):93–96. doi:10.1007/s40629-020-00125-7
93. Sheppard D, Wong WS, Uehara CF, Nadel JA, Boushey HA. Lower threshold and greater bronchomotor responsiveness of asthmatic subjects to sulfur dioxide. *Am Rev Respir Dis*. 1980;122(6):873–878. doi:10.1164/arrd.1980.122.6.873
94. Bethel RA, Epstein J, Sheppard D, Nadel JA, Boushey HA. Sulfur dioxide-induced bronchoconstriction in freely breathing, exercising, asthmatic subjects. *Am Rev Respir Dis*. 1983;128(6):987–990. doi:10.1164/arrd.1983.128.6.987
95. Vally H, Misso NL. Adverse reactions to the sulphite additives. *Gastroenterol Hepatol Bed Bench*. 2012;5(1):16–23.
96. Skypala IJ, Williams M, Reeves L, Meyer R, Venter C. Sensitivity to food additives, vaso-active amines and salicylates: a review of the evidence. *Clin Transl Allergy*. 2015;5:34. doi:10.1186/s13601-015-0078-3
97. Shah PD, Badner VM, Rastogi D, Moss KL. Association between asthma and dental caries in US (United States) adult population. *J Asthma*. 2021;58(10):1329–1336. doi:10.1080/02770903.2020.1784196
98. Shah PD, Badner VM. Association between asthma and severe tooth loss in the adult population of the United States. *J Asthma*. 2022;59(3):462–468. doi:10.1080/02770903.2020.1856868
99. Venkatesan P. GOLD COPD report: 2024 update. *Lancet Respir Med*. 2024;12(1):15–16. doi:10.1016/s2213-2600(23)00461-7
100. Graham BL, Steenbruggen I, Miller MR, et al. Standardization of Spirometry 2019 Update. An Official American Thoracic Society and European Respiratory Society Technical Statement. *Am J Respir Crit Care Med*. 2019;200(8):e70–e88. doi:10.1164/rccm.201908-1590ST
101. Castagna O, Boussuges A, Vallier JM, Prefaut C, Brisswalter J. Is impairment similar between arm and leg cranking exercise in COPD patients? *Respir Med*. Mar 2007;101(3):547–553. doi:10.1016/j.rmed.2006.06.019
102. Yang IA, Jenkins CR, Salvi SS. Chronic obstructive pulmonary disease in never-smokers: risk factors, pathogenesis, and implications for prevention and treatment. *Lancet Respir Med*. 2022;10(5):497–511. doi:10.1016/s2213-2600(21)00506-3
103. Cho MH, Hobbs BD, Silverman EK. Genetics of chronic obstructive pulmonary disease: understanding the pathobiology and heterogeneity of a complex disorder. *Lancet Respir Med*. 2022;10(5):485–496. doi:10.1016/s2213-2600(21)00510-5
104. Beran D, Zar HJ, Perrin C, Menezes AM, Burney P. Burden of asthma and chronic obstructive pulmonary disease and

access to essential medicines in low-income and middle-income countries. *Lancet Respir Med.* 2015;3(2):159–170. doi:10.1016/s2213-2600(15)00004-1

105. Gershon AS, Warner L, Cascagnette P, Victor JC, To T. Lifetime risk of developing chronic obstructive pulmonary disease: a longitudinal population study. *Lancet (London, England).* 2011;378(9795):991–996. doi:10.1016/s0140-6736(11)60990-2
106. Dodd JW, Getov SV, Jones PW. Cognitive function in COPD. *Eur Respir J.* 2010;35(4):913–922. doi:10.1183/09031936.00125109
107. Creutzberg EC, Schols AM, Bothmer-Quaedvlieg FC, Wouters EF. Prevalence of an elevated resting energy expenditure in patients with chronic obstructive pulmonary disease in relation to body composition and lung function. *Eur J Clinl Nutr.* 1998;52(6):396–401. doi:10.1038/sj.ejcn.1600571
108. Kao CC, Hsu JW, Bandi V, Hanania NA, Kheradmand F, Jahoor F. Resting energy expenditure and protein turnover are increased in patients with severe chronic obstructive pulmonary disease. *Metabolism.* 2011;60(10):1449–1455. doi:10.1016/j.metabol.2011.02.013
109. Donahoe M, Rogers RM, Wilson DO, Pennock BE. Oxygen consumption of the respiratory muscles in normal and in malnourished patients with chronic obstructive pulmonary disease. *Am Rev Respir Dis.* 1989;140(2):385–391. doi:10.1164/ajrccm/140.2.385
110. Goldstein SA, Thomashow BM, Kvetan V, Askanazi J, Kinney JM, Elwyn DH. Nitrogen and energy relationships in malnourished patients with emphysema. *Am Rev Respir Dis.* 1988;138(3):636–644. doi:10.1164/ajrccm/138.3.636
111. Rao ZY, Wu XT, Wang MY, Hu W. Comparison between measured and predicted resting energy expenditure in mechanically ventilated patients with COPD. *Asia Pac J Clin Nutr.* 2012;21(3):338–346.
112. Schols AM, Fredrix EW, Soeters PB, Westerterp KR, Wouters EF. Resting energy expenditure in patients with chronic obstructive pulmonary disease. *Am J Clin Nutr.* 1991;54(6):983–987. doi:10.1093/ajcn/54.6.983
113. Schols AM, Soeters PB, Mostert R, Saris WH, Wouters EF. Energy balance in chronic obstructive pulmonary disease. *Am Rev Respir Dis.* 1991;143(6):1248–1252. doi:10.1164/ajrccm/143.6.1248
114. Wilson DO, Donahoe M, Rogers RM, Pennock BE. Metabolic rate and weight loss in chronic obstructive lung disease. *JPEN.* 1990;14(1):7–11. doi:10.1177/014860719001400107
115. Sahebjami H, Sathianpitayakul E. Influence of body weight on the severity of dyspnea in chronic obstructive pulmonary disease. *Am J Respir Crit Care Med.* 2000;161(3 Pt 1):886–890. doi:10.1164/ajrccm.161.3.9905023
116. Barret K, Barman SM, Boitano S, Brooks H. Introduction to pulmonary structure and mechanics. In: *Ganong's Review of Medical Physiology*. 25th ed. McGraw Hill; 2016:634–652.
117. Nguyen LT, Bedu M, Caillaud D, et al. Increased resting energy expenditure is related to plasma TNF-alpha concentration in stable COPD patients. *Clin Nutr.* 1999;18(5):269–274. doi:10.1016/s0261-5614(98)80023-x
118. Cohen RI, Marzouk K, Berkoski P, O'Donnell CP, Polotsky VY, Scharf SM. Body composition and resting energy expenditure in clinically stable, non-weight-losing patients with severe emphysema. *Chest.* 2003;124(4):1365–1372. doi:10.1378/chest.124.4.1365
119. Broekhuizen R, Wouters EF, Creutzberg EC, Schols AM. Raised CRP levels mark metabolic and functional impairment in advanced COPD. *Thorax.* 2006;61(1):17–22. doi:10.1136/thx.2005.041996
120. Schols AM, Buurman WA, Staal van den Brekel AJ, Dentener MA, Wouters EF. Evidence for a relation between metabolic derangements and increased levels of inflammatory mediators in a subgroup of patients with chronic obstructive pulmonary disease. *Thorax.* 1996;51(8):819–824. doi:10.1136/thx.51.8.819
121. Hanson C, Bowser EK, Frankenfield DC, Piemonte TA. Chronic obstructive pulmonary disease: a 2019 evidence analysis center evidence-based practice guideline. *J Acad Nutr Diet.* 2021;121(1):139–165.e15. doi:10.1016/j.jand.2019.12.001
122. Hugli O, Schutz Y, Fitting JW. The daily energy expenditure in stable chronic obstructive pulmonary disease. *Am J Respir Crit Care Med.* 1996;153(1):294–300. doi:10.1164/ajrccm.153.1.8542132
123. Baarends EM, Schols AM, Westerterp KR, Wouters EF. Total daily energy expenditure relative to resting energy expenditure in clinically stable patients with COPD. *Thorax.* 1997;52(9):780–785. doi:10.1136/thx.52.9.780
124. Cao C, Wang R, Wang J, Bunjhoo H, Xu Y, Xiong W. Body mass index and mortality in chronic obstructive pulmonary disease: a meta-analysis. *PloS One.* 2012;7(8):e43892. doi:10.1371/journal.pone.0043892
125. Zapatero A, Barba R, Ruiz J, et al. Malnutrition and obesity: influence in mortality and readmissions in chronic obstructive pulmonary disease patients. *J Hum Nutr Diet.* 2013;26 Suppl 1:16–22. doi:10.1111/jhn.12088
126. Raad S, Smith C, Allen K. Nutrition Status and Chronic Obstructive Pulmonary Disease: Can We Move Beyond the Body Mass Index? *Nutr Clin Pract.* 2019;34(3):330–339. doi:10.1002/ncp.10306
127. Machado FVC, Vogelmeier CF, Jörres RA, et al. Differential impact of low fat-free mass in people with COPD based on BMI classifications: results from the COPD and Systemic Consequences-Comorbidities Network. *Chest.* 2023;163(5):1071–1083. doi:10.1016/j.chest.2022.11.040
128. van den Borst B, Gosker HR, Koster A, et al. The influence of abdominal visceral fat on inflammatory pathways and mortality risk in obstructive lung disease. *Am J Clin Nutr.* 2012;96(3):516–526. doi:10.3945/ajcn.112.040774
129. Sepúlveda-Loyola W, Osadnik C, Phu S, Morita AA, Duque G, Probst VS. Diagnosis, prevalence, and clinical impact of sarcopenia in COPD: a systematic review and meta-analysis. *J Cachexia Sarcopenia Muscle.* 2020;11(5):1164–1176. doi:10.1002/jcsm.12600
130. Nan Y, Zhou Y, Dai Z, et al. Role of nutrition in patients with coexisting chronic obstructive pulmonary disease and sarcopenia. *Front Nutr.* 2023;10:1214684. doi:10.3389/fnutr.2023.1214684
131. Schelbert KB. Comorbidities of obesity. *Prim Care.* 2009;36(2):271–285. doi:10.1016/j.pop.2009.01.009
132. Sood A, Petersen H, Meek P, Tesfaigzi Y. Spirometry and health status worsen with weight gain in obese smokers but improve in normal-weight smokers. *Am J Respir Crit Care Med.* 2014;189(3):274–281. doi:10.1164/rccm.201306-1060OC
133. Sin DD, Jones RL, Man SF. Obesity is a risk factor for dyspnea but not for airflow obstruction. *Arch Intern Med.* 2002;162(13):1477–1481. doi:10.1001/archinte.162.13.1477

134. Jordan JG, Jr., Mann JR. Obesity and mortality in persons with obstructive lung disease using data from the NHANES III. *SouthMedJ*.2010;103(4):323–330.doi:10.1097/SMJ.0b013e3181d394b4
135. Spelta F, Fratta Pasini AM, Cazzoletti L, Ferrari M. Body weight and mortality in COPD: focus on the obesity paradox. *Eat Weight Disord*. 2018;23(1):15–22. doi:10.1007/s40519-017-0456-z
136. Au DH, Gleason E, Hunter-Merrill R, et al. Lifestyle intervention and excess weight in chronic obstructive pulmonary disease (COPD): INSIGHT COPD randomized clinical trial. *Ann Am Thorac Soc*. 2023;20(12):1743–1751. doi:10.1513/AnnalsATS.202305-458OC
137. De Brandt J, Beijers R, Chiles J, et al. Update on the etiology, assessment, and management of COPD cachexia: considerations for the clinician. *Int J Chron Obstruct Pulmon Dis*. 2022;17:2957–2976. doi:10.2147/copd.s334228
138. Budweiser S, Heinemann F, Meyer K, Wild PJ, Pfeifer M. Weight gain in cachectic COPD patients receiving noninvasive positive-pressure ventilation. *Respir Care*. 2006;51(2):126–132.
139. Weisberg J, Wanger J, Olson J, et al. Megestrol acetate stimulates weight gain and ventilation in underweight COPD patients. *Chest*. 2002;121(4):1070–1078. doi:10.1378/chest.121.4.1070
140. Casaburi R, Nakata J, Bistrong L, Torres E, Rambod M, Porszasz J. Effect of megestrol acetate and testosterone on body composition and hormonal responses in COPD cachexia. *Chronic Obstr Pulm Dis*. 2015;3(1):389–397. doi:10.15326/jcopdf.3.1.2015.0128
141. Jenkins AR, Gaynor-Sodeifi K, Lewthwaite H, et al. Efficacy of interventions to alter measures of fat-free mass in people with COPD: a systematic review and meta-analysis. *ERJ Open Res*. 2023;9(4). doi:10.1183/23120541.00102-2023
142. Pan L, Wang M, Xie X, Du C, Guo Y. Effects of anabolic steroids on chronic obstructive pulmonary disease: a meta-analysis of randomised controlled trials. *PloS One*. 2014;9(1):e84855. doi:10.1371/journal.pone.0084855
143. Molfino A, Gioia G, Rossi Fanelli F, Muscaritoli M. Beta-hydroxy-beta-methylbutyrate supplementation in health and disease: a systematic review of randomized trials. *Amino Acids*. 2013;45(6):1273–1292. doi:10.1007/s00726-013-1592-z
144. Kuhls DA, Rathmacher JA, Musngi MD, et al. Beta-hydroxy-beta-methylbutyrate supplementation in critically ill trauma patients. *J Trauma*. 2007;62(1):125–131; discussion 131–132. doi:10.1097/TA.0b013e31802dca93
145. May PE, Barber A, D'Olimpio JT, Hourihane A, Abumrad NN. Reversal of cancer-related wasting using oral supplementation with a combination of beta-hydroxy-beta-methylbutyrate, arginine, and glutamine. *Am J Surg*. 2002;183(4):471–479. doi:10.1016/s0002-9610(02)00823-1
146. Clark RH, Feleke G, Din M, et al. Nutritional treatment for acquired immunodeficiency virus-associated wasting using beta-hydroxy beta-methylbutyrate, glutamine, and arginine: a randomized, double-blind, placebo-controlled study. *JPEN*. 2000;24(3):133–139. doi:10.1177/0148607100024003133
147. Rathmacher JA, Nissen S, Panton L, et al. Supplementation with a combination of beta-hydroxy-beta-methylbutyrate (HMB), arginine, and glutamine is safe and could improve hematological parameters. *JPEN*. 2004;28(2):65–75. doi:10.1177/014860710402800265
148. Hsieh LC, Chien SL, Huang MS, Tseng HF, Chang CK. Anti-inflammatory and anticatabolic effects of short-term beta-hydroxy-beta-methylbutyrate supplementation on chronic obstructive pulmonary disease patients in intensive care unit. *Asia Pac J Clin Nutr*. 2006;15(4):544–550.
149. Deutz NE, Ziegler TR, Matheson EM, et al. Reduced mortality risk in malnourished hospitalized older adult patients with COPD treated with a specialized oral nutritional supplement: sub-group analysis of the NOURISH study. *Clin Nutr*. 2021;40(3):1388–1395. doi:10.1016/j.clnu.2020.08.031
150. Mancin S, Khadhraoui S, Starace E, et al. Prevention and management of malnutrition in patients with chronic obstructive pulmonary disease: a scoping review. *Adv Respir Med*. 2024;92(5):356–369. doi:10.3390/arm92050034
151. Ganapathy A, Nieves JW. Nutrition and sarcopenia-what do we know? *Nutrients*. 2020;12(6). doi:10.3390/nu12061755
152. Calder PC, Laviano A, Lonnqvist F, Muscaritoli M, Öhlander M, Schols A. Targeted medical nutrition for cachexia in chronic obstructive pulmonary disease: a randomized, controlled trial. *J Cachexia Sarcopenia Muscle*. 2018;9(1):28–40. doi:10.1002/jcsm.12228
153. Nguyen HT, Pavey TG, Collins PF, Nguyen NV, Pham TD, Gallegos D. Effectiveness of tailored dietary counseling in treating malnourished outpatients with chronic obstructive pulmonary disease: a randomized controlled trial. *J Acad Nutr Diet*. 2020;120(5):778–791.e1. doi:10.1016/j.jand.2019.09.013
154. Weekes CE, Emery PW, Elia M. Dietary counselling and food fortification in stable COPD: a randomised trial. *Thorax*. 2009;64(4):326–331. doi:10.1136/thx.2008.097352
155. Sugawara K, Takahashi H, Kasai C, et al. Effects of nutritional supplementation combined with low-intensity exercise in malnourished patients with COPD. *Respir Med*. 2010;104(12):1883–1889. doi:10.1016/j.rmed.2010.05.008
156. Gurgun A, Deniz S, Argın M, Karapolat H. Effects of nutritional supplementation combined with conventional pulmonary rehabilitation in muscle-wasted chronic obstructive pulmonary disease: a prospective, randomized and controlled study. *Respirology*. 2013;18(3):495–500. doi:10.1111/resp.12019
157. Monteiro F, Camillo CA, Vitorasso R, et al. Obesity and physical activity in the daily life of patients with COPD. *Lung*. 2012;190(4):403–410. doi:10.1007/s00408-012-9381-0
158. Bernardes S, Eckert IDC, Burgel CF, Teixeira PJZ, Silva FM. Increased energy and/or protein intake improves anthropometry and muscle strength in chronic obstructive pulmonary disease patients: a systematic review with meta-analysis on randomised controlled clinical trials. *Br J Nutr*. 2022:1–18. doi:10.1017/s0007114522000976
159. Conway V, Hukins C, Sharp S, Collins PF. Nutritional support in malnourished outpatients with chronic obstructive pulmonary disease (COPD): a randomized controlled pilot study. *Nutrients*. 2024;16(11). doi:10.3390/nu16111696
160. Institute of Medicine Panel on Dietary Antioxidants and Related Compounds. *Dietary Reference Intakes for Vitamin C, Vitamin E, Selenium, and Carotenoids*. National Academies Press; 2000.
161. Agacdiken A, Basyigit I, Ozden M, et al. The effects of antioxidants on exercise-induced lipid peroxidation in patients with COPD. *Respirology*. 2004;9(1):38–42. doi:10.1111/j.1440-1843.2003.00526.x

162. Nicks ME, O'Brien MM, Bowler RP. Plasma antioxidants are associated with impaired lung function and COPD exacerbations in smokers. *COPD*. 2011;8(4):264–269. doi:10.3109/15412555.2011.579202
163. Ahmad A, Shameem M, Husain Q. Altered oxidant-antioxidant levels in the disease prognosis of chronic obstructive pulmonary disease. *Int J Tuberc Lung Dis*. 2013;17(8):1104–1109. doi:10.5588/ijtld.12.0512
164. McKeever TM, Lewis SA, Smit HA, Burney P, Cassano PA, Britton J. A multivariate analysis of serum nutrient levels and lung function. *Respir Res*. 2008;9(1):67. doi:10.1186/1465-9921-9-67
165. Kelly Y, Sacker A, Marmot M. Nutrition and respiratory health in adults: findings from the health survey for Scotland. *Eur Respir J*. 2003;21(4):664–671. doi:10.1183/09031936.03.00055702
166. Hu G, Zhang X, Chen J, Peto R, Campbell TC, Cassano PA. Dietary vitamin C intake and lung function in rural China. *Am J Epidemiol*. 1998;148(6):594–599. doi:10.1093/oxfordjournals.aje.a009685
167. Pearson P, Britton J, McKeever T, et al. Lung function and blood levels of copper, selenium, vitamin C and vitamin E in the general population. *Europ J Clin Nutr*. 2005;59(9):1043–1048. doi:10.1038/sj.ejcn.1602209
168. Schünemann HJ, Freudenheim JL, Grant BJ. Epidemiologic evidence linking antioxidant vitamins to pulmonary function and airway obstruction. *Epidemiol Rev*. 2001;23(2):248–267. doi:10.1093/oxfordjournals.epirev.a000805
169. Grievink L, de Waart FG, Schouten EG, Kok FJ. Serum carotenoids, alpha-tocopherol, and lung function among Dutch elderly. *Am J Respir Crit Care Med*. 2000;161(3 Pt 1):790–795. doi:10.1164/ajrccm.161.3.9904040
170. Chuwers P, Barnhart S, Blanc P, et al. The protective effect of beta-carotene and retinol on ventilatory function in an asbestos-exposed cohort. *Am J Respir Crit Care Med*. 1997;155(3):1066–1071. doi:10.1164/ajrccm.155.3.9116988
171. Zheng L, Yu X, Xia Z, Guo Y, Dai Y. The associations between serum vitamins and carotenoids with chronic obstructive pulmonary disease: Results from the NHANES. *Int J Chron Obstruct Pulmon Dis*. 2023;18:2985–2997. doi:10.2147/copd.s432995
172. Paiva SA, Godoy I, Vannucchi H, Fávaro RM, Geraldo RR, Campana AO. Assessment of vitamin A status in chronic obstructive pulmonary disease patients and healthy smokers. *Am J Clin Nutr*. 1996;64(6):928–934. doi:10.1093/ajcn/64.6.928
173. Tecklenburg SL, Mickleborough TD, Fly AD, Bai Y, Stager JM. Ascorbic acid supplementation attenuates exercise-induced bronchoconstriction in patients with asthma. *Respir Med*. 2007;101(8):1770–1778. doi:10.1016/j.rmed.2007.02.014
174. Rautalahti M, Virtamo J, Haukka J, et al. The effect of alpha-tocopherol and beta-carotene supplementation on COPD symptoms. *Am J Respir Crit Care Med*. 1997;156(5):1447–1452. doi:10.1164/ajrccm.156.5.96-11048
175. MRC/BHF Heart Protection Study of antioxidant vitamin supplementation in 20,536 high-risk individuals: a randomised placebo-controlled trial. *Lancet*. 2002;360(9326):23–33. doi:10.1016/s0140-6736(02)09328-5
176. Nadi E, Tavakoli F, Zeraati F, Goodarzi MT, Hashemi SH. Effect of vitamin C administration on leukocyte vitamin C level and severity of bronchial asthma. *Acta Med Iran*. 2012;50(4):233–238.
177. Fogarty A, Lewis SA, Scrivener SL, et al. Oral magnesium and vitamin C supplements in asthma: a parallel group randomized placebo-controlled trial. *Clin Exp Allergy*. 2003;33(10):1355–1359. doi:10.1046/j.1365-2222.2003.01777.x
178. Pearson PJ, Lewis SA, Britton J, Fogarty A. Vitamin E supplements in asthma: a parallel group randomised placebo controlled trial. *Thorax*. 2004;59(8):652–656. doi:10.1136/thx.2004.022616
179. Lattanzi G, Lelli D, Antonelli Incalzi R, Pedone C. Effect of macronutrients or micronutrients supplementation on nutritional status, physical functional capacity and quality of life in patients with COPD: a systematic review and meta-analysis. *J Am Nutr Assoc*. 2024;43(5):473–487. doi:10.1080/27697061.2024.2312852
180. Li M, Zhao L, Hu C, et al. Improvement of lung function by micronutrient supplementation in patients with COPD: a systematic review and meta-analysis. *Nutrients*. 2024;16(7). doi:10.3390/nu16071028
181. Keranis E, Makris D, Rodopoulou P, et al. Impact of dietary shift to higher-antioxidant foods in COPD: a randomised trial. *Eur Respir J*. 2010;36(4):774–780. doi:10.1183/09031936.00113809
182. Aubier M, Murciano D, Lecocguic Y, et al. Effect of hypophosphatemia on diaphragmatic contractility in patients with acute respiratory failure. *N Engl J Med*. 1985;313(7):420–424. doi:10.1056/nejm198508153130705
183. Alamoudi OS. Hypomagnesaemia in chronic, stable asthmatics: prevalence, correlation with severity and hospitalization. *Eur Respir J*. 2000;16(3):427–431. doi:10.1034/j.1399-3003.2000.016003427.x
184. Oladipo OO, Chukwu CC, Ajala MO, Adewole TA, Afonja OA. Plasma magnesium in adult asthmatics at the Lagos University Teaching Hospital, Nigeria. *East Afr Med J*. 2003;80(9):488–491. doi:10.4314/eamj.v80i9.8748
185. de Valk HW, Kok PT, Struyvenberg A, et al. Extracellular and intracellular magnesium concentrations in asthmatic patients. *Eur Respir J*. 1993;6(8):1122–1125.
186. Fantidis P, Ruiz Cacho J, Marín M, Madero Jarabo R, Solera J, Herrero E. Intracellular (polymorphonuclear) magnesium content in patients with bronchial asthma between attacks. *J R Soc Med*. 1995;88(8):441–445.
187. Kazaks AG, Uriu-Adams JY, Albertson TE, Stern JS. Multiple measures of magnesium status are comparable in mild asthma and control subjects. *J Asthma*. 2006;43(10):783–788. doi:10.1080/02770900601031870
188. Pizzini A, Aichner M, Sonnweber T, Tancevski I, Weiss G, Löffler-Ragg J. The significance of iron deficiency and anemia in a real-life COPD cohort. *Int J Med Sci*. 2020;17(14):2232–2239. doi:10.7150/ijms.46163
189. Hardang IM, Søyseth V, Kononova N, Hagve TA, Einvik G. COPD: Iron deficiency and clinical characteristics in patients with and without chronic respiratory failure. *Chronic Obstr Pulm Dis*. 2024;11(3):261–269. doi:10.15326/jcopdf.2023.0477
190. Grasmuk-Siegl E, Urban MH, Scherrer S, Funk GC. Effect of intravenous ferric carboxymaltose on exercise capacity and quality of life in patients with COPD: a pilot study. *Wien Klin Wochenschr*. 2023;135(1–2):35–44. doi:10.1007/s00508-022-02073-4
191. Chambaneau A, Filaire M, Jubert L, Bremond M, Filaire E. Nutritional intake, physical activity and quality of life in COPD patients. *Int J Sports Med*. 2016;37(9):730–737. doi:10.1055/s-0035-1569368

192. Paulin FV, Zagatto AM, Chiappa GR, Müller PT. Addition of vitamin B12 to exercise training improves cycle ergometer endurance in advanced COPD patients: a randomized and controlled study. *Respir Med*. 2017;122:23–29. doi:10.1016/j.rmed.2016.11.015
193. Black PN, Scragg R. Relationship between serum 25-hydroxyvitamin d and pulmonary function in the third national health and nutrition examination survey. *Chest*. 2005;128(6):3792–3798. doi:10.1378/chest.128.6.3792
194. Persson LJ, Aanerud M, Hiemstra PS, Hardie JA, Bakke PS, Eagan TM. Chronic obstructive pulmonary disease is associated with low levels of vitamin D. *PloS One*. 2012;7(6):e38934. doi:10.1371/journal.pone.0038934
195. Janssens W, Bouillon R, Claes B, et al. Vitamin D deficiency is highly prevalent in COPD and correlates with variants in the vitamin D-binding gene. *Thorax*. 2010;65(3):215–220. doi:10.1136/thx.2009.120659
196. Holmgaard DB, Mygind LH, Titlestad IL, et al. Serum vitamin D in patients with chronic obstructive lung disease does not correlate with mortality—results from a 10-year prospective cohort study. *PloS One*. 2013;8(1):e53670. doi:10.1371/journal.pone.0053670
197. Berg I, Hanson C, Sayles H, et al. Vitamin D, vitamin D binding protein, lung function and structure in COPD. *Respir Med*. 2013;107(10):1578–1588. doi:10.1016/j.rmed.2013.05.010
198. Puhan MA, Siebeling L, Frei A, Zoller M, Bischoff-Ferrari H, Ter Riet G. No association of 25-hydroxyvitamin D with exacerbations in primary care patients with COPD. *Chest*. 2014;145(1):37–43. doi:10.1378/chest.13-1296
199. Martineau AR, James WY, Hooper RL, et al. Vitamin D3 supplementation in patients with chronic obstructive pulmonary disease (ViDiCO): a multicentre, double-blind, randomised controlled trial. *Lancet Respir Med*. 2015;3(2):120–130. doi:10.1016/s2213-2600(14)70255-3
200. Lehouck A, Mathieu C, Carremans C, et al. High doses of vitamin D to reduce exacerbations in chronic obstructive pulmonary disease: a randomized trial. *Ann Int Med*. 2012;156(2):105–114. doi:10.7326/0003-4819-156-2-201201170-00004
201. Rafiq R, Aleva FE, Schrumpf JA, et al. Vitamin D supplementation in chronic obstructive pulmonary disease patients with low serum vitamin D: a randomized controlled trial. *Am J Clin Nutr*. 2022;116(2):491–499. doi:10.1093/ajcn/nqac083
202. Wüthrich B, Schmid A, Walther B, Sieber R. Milk consumption does not lead to mucus production or occurrence of asthma. *J Am Coll Nutr*. 2005;24(6 Suppl):547s–555s. doi:10.1080/07315724.2005.10719503
203. Berridge MJ. Vitamin D and depressive order: cellular and regulatory mechanisms. *Pharmacol Rev*. 2017;69(2):80–92. doi:10.1124/pr.116.013227
204. Monsó E, Fiz JM, Izquierdo J, et al. Quality of life in severe chronic obstructive pulmonary disease: correlation with lung and muscle function. *Respir Med*. 1998;92(2):221–227. doi:10.1016/s0954-6111(98)90099-3
205. Hurst JR, Skolnik N, Hansen GJ, et al. Understanding the impact of chronic obstructive pulmonary disease exacerbations on patient health and quality of life. *Eur J Intern Med*. 2020;73:1–6. doi:10.1016/j.ejim.2019.12.014
206. Katsura H, Yamada K, Kida K. Both generic and disease specific health-related quality of life are deteriorated in patients with underweight COPD. *Respir Med*. 2005;99(5):624–630. doi:10.1016/j.rmed.2004.09.017
207. Cochrane WJ, Afolabi OA. Investigation into the nutritional status, dietary intake and smoking habits of patients with chronic obstructive pulmonary disease. *J Hum Nutr Diet*. 2004;17(1):3–11; quiz 13–15. doi:10.1046/j.1365-277x.2003.00478.x
208. Bellani G, Laffey JG, Pham T, et al. Epidemiology, patterns of care, and mortality for patients with acute respiratory distress syndrome in intensive care units in 50 countries. *Jama*. 2016;315(8):788–800. doi:10.1001/jama.2016.0291
209. Lee W, Slutsky, A. Acute respiratory distress syndrome. In: Mason R, Broaddus, V, Martin T, et al, ed. *Murray and Nadel's Textbook of Respiratory Medicine*. 5th ed. Saunders; 2010:2104–2129.
210. Gorman EA, O'Kane CM, McAuley DF. Acute respiratory distress syndrome in adults: diagnosis, outcomes, long-term sequelae, and management. *Lancet*. 2022;400(10358):1157–1170. doi:10.1016/s0140-6736(22)01439-8
211. Ranieri VM, Rubenfeld GD, Thompson BT, et al. Acute respiratory distress syndrome: the Berlin Definition. *JAMA*. 2012;307(23):2526–2533. doi:10.1001/jama.2012.5669
212. McClave SA, Taylor BE, Martindale RG, et al. Guidelines for the Provision and Assessment of Nutrition Support Therapy in the Adult Critically Ill Patient: Society of Critical Care Medicine (SCCM) and American Society for Parenteral and Enteral Nutrition (A.S.P.E.N.). *JPEN*. 2016;40(2):159–211. doi:10.1177/0148607115621863
213. Singer P, Blaser AR, Berger MM, et al. ESPEN guideline on clinical nutrition in the intensive care unit. *Clin Nutr (Edinburgh, Scotland)*. 2019;38(1):48–79. doi:10.1016/j.clnu.2018.08.037
214. Compher C, Bingham AL, McCall M, et al. Guidelines for the provision of nutrition support therapy in the adult critically ill patient: The American Society for Parenteral and Enteral Nutrition. *JPEN*. 2022;46(1):12–41. doi:10.1002/jpen.2267
215. Peterson SJ, McKeever L, Lateef OB, Freels S, Fantuzzi G, Braunschweig CA. Combination of high-calorie delivery and organ failure increases mortality among patients with acute respiratory distress syndrome. *Crit Care Med*. 2019;47(1):69–75. doi:10.1097/ccm.0000000000003476
216. Braunschweig CA, Sheean PM, Peterson SJ, et al. Intensive nutrition in acute lung injury: a clinical trial (INTACT). *JPEN*. 2015;39(1):13–20. doi:10.1177/0148607114528541
217. Casaer MP, Wilmer A, Hermans G, Wouters PJ, Mesotten D, Van den Berghe G. Role of disease and macronutrient dose in the randomized controlled EPaNIC trial: a post hoc analysis. *Am J Respir Crit Care Med*. 2013;187(3):247–255. doi:10.1164/rccm.201206-0999OC
218. Oshima T, Berger MM, De Waele E, et al. Indirect calorimetry in nutritional therapy. A position paper by the ICALIC study group. *Clin Nutr*. 2017;36(3):651–662. doi:10.1016/j.clnu.2016.06.010
219. Canada T, Lord LM. Fluid, electrolytes, and acid-base disorders. In: Chan LN ed. *ASPEN Adult Nutrition Support Core Curriculum*. 4th ed. The American Society for Parenteral and Enteral Nutrition; 2025:159–192.
220. Rampon GL, Simpson SQ, Agrawal R. Prone positioning for acute hypoxemic respiratory failure and ARDS: a review. *Chest*. 2023;163(2):332–340. doi:10.1016/j.chest.2022.09.020
221. Scholten EL, Beitler JR, Prisk GK, Malhotra A. Treatment of ARDS with prone positioning. *Chest*. 2017;151(1):215–224. doi:10.1016/j.chest.2016.06.032
222. Savio RD, Parasuraman R, Lovesly D, et al. Feasibility, tolerance and effectiveness of enteral feeding in critically ill patients in prone position. *J Intensive Care Soc*. 2021;22(1):41–46. doi:10.1177/1751143719900100

223. Al-Dorzi HM, Arabi YM. Enteral nutrition safety with advanced treatments: extracorporeal membrane oxygenation, prone positioning, and infusion of neuromuscular blockers. *Nutr Clin Pract*. 2021;36(1):88–97. doi:10.1002/ncp.10621
224. Saez de la Fuente I, Saez de la Fuente J, Quintana Estelles MD, et al. Enteral nutrition in patients receiving mechanical ventilation in a prone position. *JPEN*. 2016;40(2):250–255. doi:10.1177/0148607114553232
225. Linn DD, Beckett RD, Foellinger K. Administration of enteral nutrition to adult patients in the prone position. *Intensive Crit Care Nurs*. 2015;31(1):38–43. doi:10.1016/j.iccn.2014.07.002
226. Gadek JE, DeMichele SJ, Karlstad MD, et al. Effect of enteral feeding with eicosapentaenoic acid, gamma-linolenic acid, and antioxidants in patients with acute respiratory distress syndrome. Enteral Nutrition in ARDS Study Group. *Crit Care Med*. 1999;27(8):1409–1420. doi:10.1097/00003246-199908000-00001
227. Singer P, Theilla M, Fisher H, Gibstein L, Grozovski E, Cohen J. Benefit of an enteral diet enriched with eicosapentaenoic acid and gamma-linolenic acid in ventilated patients with acute lung injury. *Crit Care Med*. 2006;34(4):1033–1038. doi:10.1097/01.ccm.0000206111.23629.0a
228. Pontes-Arruda A, Aragão AM, Albuquerque JD. Effects of enteral feeding with eicosapentaenoic acid, gamma-linolenic acid, and antioxidants in mechanically ventilated patients with severe sepsis and septic shock. *Crit Care Med*. 2006;34(9):2325–2333. doi:10.1097/01.ccm.0000234033.65657.b6
229. Pontes-Arruda A, Demichele S, Seth A, Singer P. The use of an inflammation-modulating diet in patients with acute lung injury or acute respiratory distress syndrome: a meta-analysis of outcome data. *JPEN*. 2008;32(6):596–605. doi:10.1177/0148607108324203
230. Dushianthan A, Cusack R, Burgess VA, Grocott MP, Calder PC. Immunonutrition for acute respiratory distress syndrome (ARDS) in adults. *Cochrane Database Syst Rev*. 2019;1(1):Cd012041. doi:10.1002/14651858.CD012041.pub2
231. Langlois PL, D'Aragon F, Hardy G, Manzanares W. Omega-3 polyunsaturated fatty acids in critically ill patients with acute respiratory distress syndrome: a systematic review and meta-analysis. *Nutrition*. 2019;61:84–92. doi:10.1016/j.nut.2018.10.026
232. Singer P, Blaser AR, Berger MM, et al. ESPEN guideline on clinical nutrition in the intensive care unit. *Clin Nutr*. 2019;38(1):48–79. doi:10.1016/j.clnu.2018.08.037

CHAPTER 15

Nutritional Management of Food Allergies and Food Intolerances

Jingwen Wu
Shibani Mallik
John Leung

CHAPTER OUTLINE

CORE CONCEPTS

1. Adverse reactions to food are classified into immunologically mediated food allergies (IgE-mediated, non-IgE-mediated, and mixed) and non-immunologically mediated food intolerances, as well as their respective pathophysiological mechanisms. Understanding the differences between these reactions is crucial to nutritional and clinical management.
2. The most common food allergies in the United States are the "Big 9": peanuts, tree nuts, milk, eggs, wheat, soy, fish, shellfish, and sesame.
3. Most food allergies typically develop in childhood and are more likely to occur in patients with atopic comorbidities.
4. The range of symptoms in IgE-mediated food allergic reactions varies widely, from patients experiencing mild cutaneous symptoms to severe, life-threatening anaphylaxis.
5. The diagnostic tools for identifying IgE-mediated food allergies include skin prick tests, serum-specific IgE tests, and oral food challenges. A detailed clinical history is critical for proper diagnosis. Patients with suspected food allergies should consult with an allergist, and if required, undergo testing to avoid unnecessary dietary restriction.

6. Patients with confirmed food allergies should always carry an epinephrine autoinjector or nasal spray in case of an emergency. Management of food allergies also includes patient and caretaker education on allergen avoidance, and therapeutic measures such as oral immunotherapy, or omalizumab, a biologic for the reduction of IgE-mediated food allergic reactions.
7. Unlike food allergies, food intolerances predominantly affect the digestive system, are dose-dependent, and typically have a delayed onset.

LEARNING OBJECTIVES

1. Outline the key differences between food allergies and food intolerances, including their clinical manifestations, diagnosis, and treatment.
2. Identify the symptoms associated with IgE-mediated food allergies, as well as the diagnostic criteria for anaphylaxis.
3. Assess the indications, risks, and benefits of therapeutic approaches for food allergies, including oral immunotherapy and biologic treatments like omalizumab, and determine their role in improving patient outcomes.
4. Develop nutritional management plans for patients with food allergies to ensure a nutritionally balanced diet.

Introduction

Adverse reactions to food (ARF) are defined as any abnormal physiological responses that occur following the ingestion of food. Up to one-fifth of the population in industrialized nations modifies their diet due to ARF, which can lead to significant nutritional deficiencies without proper guidance and supervision.[1] ARF can be classified into immunologically mediated (food allergy) and non-immunologically mediated (food intolerance). **Food allergy** is characterized by an adverse immunological response to a food protein, which can be immunoglobulin E (IgE)-mediated, non-IgE-mediated, or a mix of IgE/non-IgE-mediated mechanisms. These reactions have the potential to escalate into severe, life-threatening conditions such as anaphylaxis. Non-IgE-mediated immune responses include conditions such as **celiac disease (CD)** and **food protein-induced enterocolitis syndrome (FPIES)**. Additionally, conditions like **eosinophilic esophagitis (EoE)** may involve both IgE-mediated and non-IgE-mediated mechanisms. **Food intolerance** refers to undesirable physiological responses to specific foods or food components that do

CORE CONCEPT 1

Adverse reactions to food are classified into immunologically-mediated food allergies (IgE-mediated, non-IgE-mediated, and mixed) and non-immunologically-mediated food intolerances, as well as their respective pathophysiological mechanisms. Understanding the differences between these reactions is crucial to nutritional and clinical management.

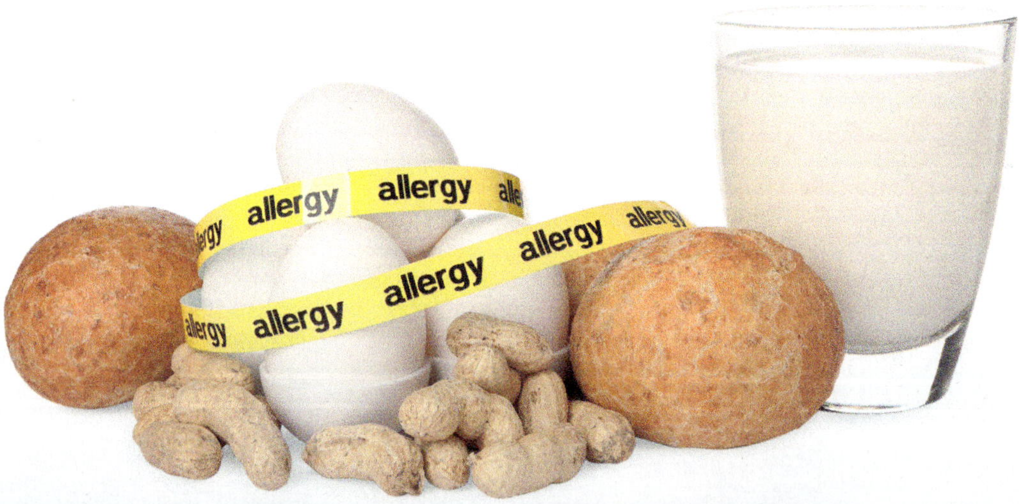

not involve the immune system and typically manifest with less severe symptoms. In clinical practice, distinguishing between food allergy and food intolerance is crucial due to the substantial differences in their nutritional management. This chapter will focus on pathophysiology, diagnosis, clinical manifestations, and dietary management of food allergy and food intolerance.

Prevalence

In the United States, the prevalence of diagnosed food allergies is estimated to affect approximately 8% of children and 11% of adults.[2] This trend is correlated with a rise in hospitalizations, ambulatory care visits, and outpatient visits over the past two decades in pediatric patients.[3] Self-reported rates of food allergy are consistently higher, with approximately 19% of U.S. adults believing they have a food allergy, potentially leading to unnecessary dietary restrictions.[4]

The spectrum of food allergy includes reactions to over 170 identified foods, although the "Big 9" allergens in the United States are milk, eggs, peanuts, tree nuts, soy, wheat, fish, shellfish, and sesame.[5,6] These allergens account for the majority of food allergy reactions, with variations observed across different geographical and cultural contexts. For instance, milk, egg, peanut, and tree nut allergies are more prevalent in the Americas, Australia, and Western Europe, while fish and shellfish allergies are more common in Asian countries.[5] Additionally, the most common food allergies vary between adults and children. In adults, the most prevalent food allergies are to peanuts, tree nuts, and finned fish.[4,7] In children, the primary triggers are milk, eggs, and peanuts.[7] Research demonstrates distinct patterns in the resolution of food allergies among children. Approximately 79% of children are likely to outgrow their milk allergy by the age of 16.[8] Similarly, egg allergies are commonly outgrown, with about 89% of children overcoming this allergy by the age of 6.[8] However, peanut allergies present a more persistent challenge. Studies indicate that only about 22% of children with peanut allergies develop tolerance as they mature into adulthood.[8]

CORE CONCEPT 2

The most common food allergies in the United States are the "Big 9": peanuts, tree nuts, milk, eggs, wheat, soy, fish, shellfish, and sesame.

CORE CONCEPT 3

Most food allergies typically develop in childhood and are more likely to occur in patients with atopic comorbidities.

Pathophysiology of IgE-Mediated Food Allergy

IgE-mediated allergic reactions are the most prevalent and recognizable form of food allergy, notable for their rapid onset—symptoms can emerge within minutes to an hour following exposure to the allergen. These reactions can vary from mild, localized symptoms affecting the skin and mucous membranes, to severe systemic responses that culminate in anaphylaxis. Anaphylaxis is characterized by widespread effects on multiple organ systems, is potentially fatal, and is a primary cause of urgent visits to emergency departments.

Mechanism

In individuals with food allergies, there is an absence of both immunologic and clinical tolerance to specific foods. These allergies manifest through mechanisms mediated by immunoglobulin E antibodies (IgE-ab) or less commonly non-IgE antibodies.[1] **Sensitization** to food allergens can occur through various routes including the gastrointestinal (GI) tract, compromised skin barriers, or through airway mucosa.[9,10] Normally, the immune system of healthy individuals recognizes food antigens as non-pathogenic. In individuals with food allergies, food antigens trigger the activation and proliferation of T-helper type 2 cells, or Th2 cells, as shown in **Figure 15.1**. These cells facilitate the class switching of plasma cells to produce IgE-ab. IgE-ab bind to mast cells and basophils to trigger the release of inflammatory mediators, such as histamine. This release leads to symptoms including increased mucus production, vasodilation, and enhanced vascular permeability, which can manifest as acute allergic reactions like edema, stomach pain, vomiting, diarrhea, urticaria (hives), and in severe cases, bronchial obstruction and anaphylaxis.[9,10] The likelihood of severe reactions is notably higher in patients with poorly controlled asthma. Moreover, individuals with food allergies often experience other atopic conditions such as **atopic dermatitis** and **allergic rhinitis**, suggesting a shared underlying atopic predisposition.[10]

Environmental interactions, particularly with the skin and gut microbiome, also play a significant role

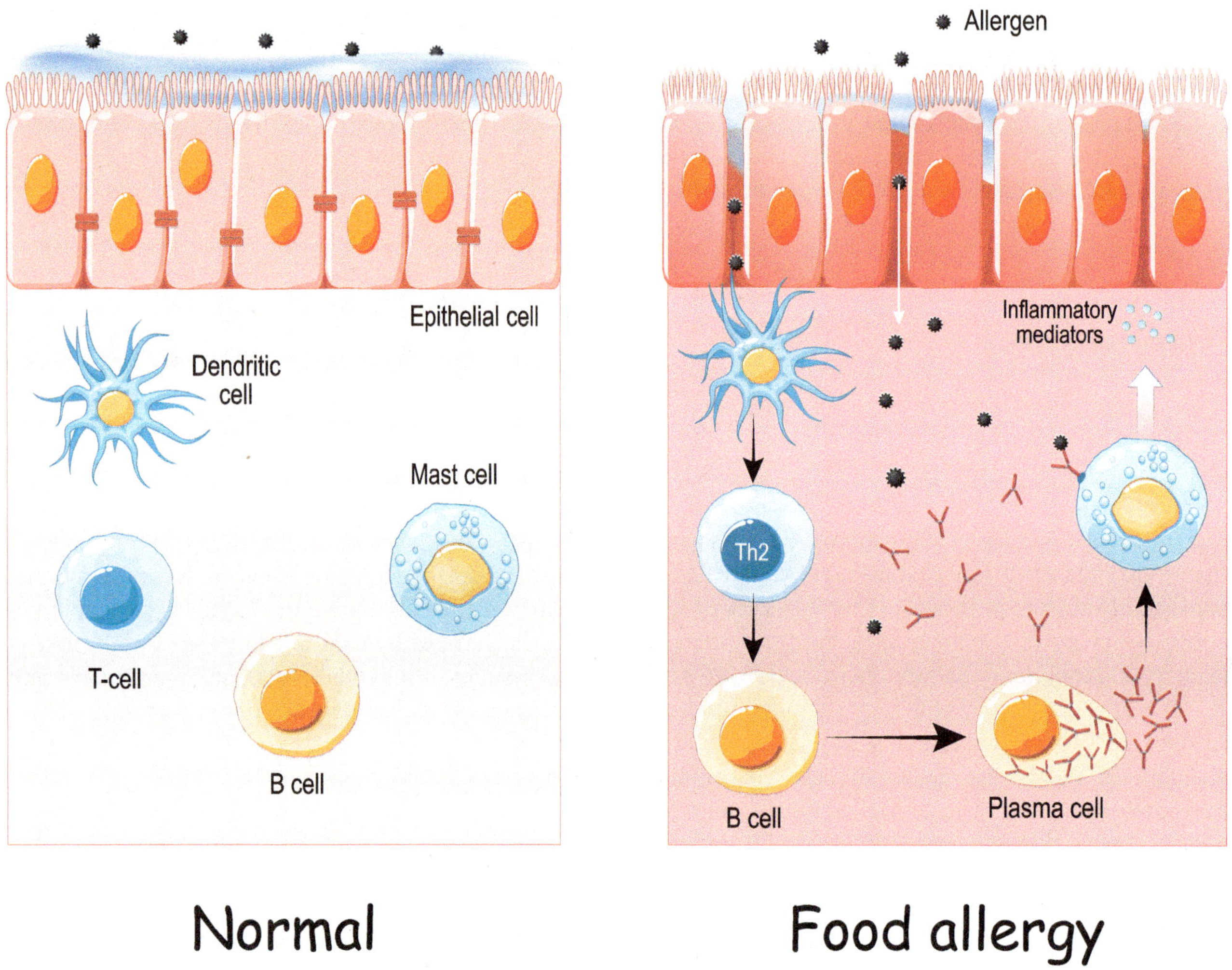

Figure 15.1 Phases of IgE-Mediated Allergic Response

in the pathogenesis of food allergies. The skin microbiome, especially the presence of *Staphylococcus aureus*, and the gut microbiome's specific compositions can influence the development of food allergies.[11] Local cytokines from skin and gut barrier sites, such as Th2-inducing cytokines (TSLP, IL-33, and IL-25), can significantly contribute to the development of food allergies.[11] These cytokines help in the proliferation of Th2 cells. Interventions that alter these cytokine levels can mitigate allergic responses and are potential targets for treating food allergies.[11]

Etiology

IgE-mediated allergies are influenced by a complex interplay of genetic, environmental, immune, and microbial factors. Understanding these contributors is crucial for diagnosing and managing these conditions effectively.

Genetic Predisposition

Genetic factors play a significant role in the susceptibility to IgE-mediated allergies. Research has shown that the familial incidence of allergies is high, suggesting a heritable component. Specific genetic loci, especially those within the HLA-DR and HLA-DQ gene regions, have been identified as critical in the development of food allergies.[12] Studies involving twins further underscore this genetic link, with identical twins displaying higher concordance rates for allergies such as peanut allergy compared to fraternal twins.[12,13]

Environmental Influences

The environment also significantly impacts the development of allergies. Factors such as the timing and mode of exposure to allergens can dictate whether tolerance or sensitization occurs.[10,11] Early life exposure to allergens through the GI tract, skin, or respiratory mucosa is particularly critical.[11] The conditions under which children are raised, ranging from dietary habits to microorganism exposure, can affect immune system development and function, influencing the likelihood of developing allergies.[13]

Microbiome and Immune Interactions

Emerging research has highlighted the role of the gut microbiome in modulating immune responses and potentially influencing allergy development and resolution. The interactions between gut microbiota and the immune system during early life are critical. A diverse microbiome can promote a more balanced immune response, potentially reducing the risk of allergies.[12,13] For example, certain microbiome signatures are associated with the resolution of milk allergies and are characterized by an enrichment of *Clostridia* and *Firmicutes*, suggesting a protective role of these bacteria against food allergies.[11] Conversely, a less diverse microbiome might predispose individuals to allergic conditions by failing to establish proper immune tolerance.[9] Lastly, there is evidence to support that vitamin D sufficiency in infancy (largely within the first year of life) may protect against the development of food allergy.[14]

Dual Allergen Exposure Hypothesis

Recent insights suggest that the dual allergen exposure hypothesis could play a vital role in allergy development. This theory proposes that the route of initial allergen exposure is key: oral exposure may promote tolerance, while accidental cutaneous exposure, particularly through a damaged skin barrier, might lead to sensitization.[11] This hypothesis is supported by observations that disruptions in the skin barrier, such as those caused by atopic dermatitis, enhance the risk of developing food allergies, potentially through increased transcutaneous sensitization.[11]

Clinical Manifestations

The timing of reactions in IgE-mediated food allergy can vary widely, from minutes to several hours after ingesting the allergenic food. These reactions encompass a spectrum of symptoms, detailed in **Table 15.1**, which range from mild and bothersome to severe and potentially fatal. It is important to note that not every individual with an IgE-mediated food allergy experiences all listed symptoms, and symptom presentation can differ with each occurrence.[5] The severity and nature of reactions may depend on the quantity of food consumed and the duration since last exposure. For example, a person may experience only minor oral irritation initially but could face more severe reactions in subsequent exposures, particularly if the allergen is not consistently avoided.

Skin

Common cutaneous reactions include **erythematous rashes**, **pruritus**, **urticaria** (**Figure 15.2**), and **angioedema** (**Figure 15.3**).[1] Such cutaneous symptoms are frequently the most prevalent indications of an IgE-mediated allergic response to food and are often reproducible. The mildest forms of these reactions may manifest as scratching, with or without visible hives.[5] Hives (urticaria) are characterized by well-defined areas of dermal edema and erythema that typically blanches with pressure and is distinctly pruritic.[5] These reactions commonly occur minutes after the ingestion of an allergenic food and can persist for several hours if untreated.[5] Chronic urticaria (defined as urticaria >6 weeks) is rarely caused by food allergy.[15] Angioedema is another manifestation, often presenting as swelling of the eyelids, face, or lips, causing

Table 15.1 Signs and Symptoms of Food Allergy

Integumentary	Respiratory	Gastrointestinal	Cardiovascular
Erythema*	Rhinorrhea	Oral/throat pruritus	Tachycardia
Pruritus*	Congestion	Nausea/vomiting*	Hypotension
Urticaria	Coughing	Abdominal pain*	Syncope
Angioedema	Wheezing	Diarrhea*	
	Shortness of breath		
	Laryngeal edema		

**Denotes symptoms that may also present in non-IgE-mediated food allergic reactions*

Data from Waserman S, Bégin P, Watson W. IgE-mediated food allergy. *Allergy Asthma Clin Immunol.* 2018;14(Suppl 2):2.

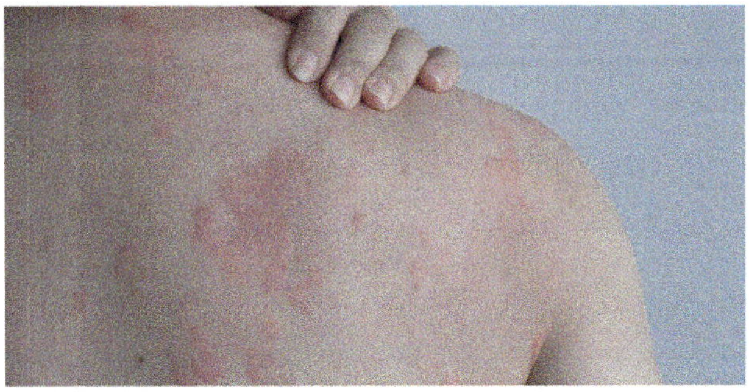

Figure 15.2 Urticaria

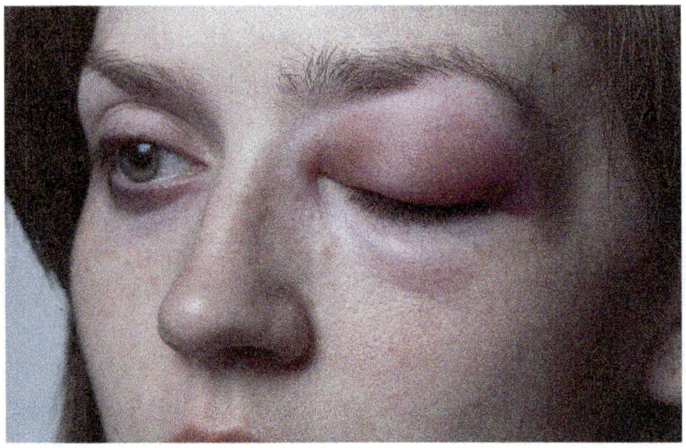

Figure 15.3 Angioedema

significant discomfort.[5] The severity of these cutaneous symptoms can often be assessed by the extent of skin involvement, which reflects the severity of the allergic reaction.[5] Such cutaneous symptoms are frequently the most prevalent indications of an IgE-mediated allergic response to food.

Respiratory

Respiratory symptoms associated with IgE-mediated food allergies might affect both upper and lower airways. Mild respiratory reactions are characterized by sporadic sniffing or nose rubbing, whereas more severe symptoms manifest as persistent **rhinorrhea** or nasal congestion, including complete blockage of the nares.[2] Ocular symptoms, such as tearing, redness, and itching, may also present alone or accompany upper airway symptoms. Severe respiratory reactions, such as asthma and laryngeal edema, can be life-threatening.

Gastrointestinal

In terms of GI involvement, symptoms range from subjective (itching in the mouth or throat, nausea, abdominal pain) to objective (vomiting, intermittent or persistent diarrhea).[5,6,9] Typically, these symptoms

CASE STUDY INTRODUCTION

Chase is a 26-year-old male who was referred to the allergy clinic by his primary care physician due to symptoms suggestive of food allergies. He reports an overall decreased appetite and states that he experiences itching of the mouth and swelling of the lips and throat after consuming peaches and apples. Additionally, he reports bloating and diarrhea after eating dairy products, as well as severe reactions including facial bloating, hives, stomach pain, and difficulty swallowing after consuming nuts, particularly pistachios and cashews.

Anthropometric Data:

Weight: 70 kg
Height: 180 cm
BMI: 21.6 kg/m^2

Weight History
Usual body weight 72 kg 6 months ago

Biochemical Data:

Sodium 149 (136–145 mEq/L)

Serum osmolality 320 (275–295 mOsm/kg)

Clinical Data:

Past Medical History: Eczema, gastroesophageal reflux disease
Medications: Imodium, omeprazole
Vital Signs: Blood pressure 120/80 mm Hg, Temperature 98.6°F

Questions

1. What are your concerns regarding Chase's nutritional status?
2. Which specific diagnostic tests should be performed to confirm suspected food allergies and intolerances?

appear almost immediately post-ingestion, generally not exceeding a few hours, and are typically characteristic of anaphylactic reactions. In contrast, non-IgE-mediated food allergies typically manifest with delayed reactions. Signs like failure to thrive/growth faltering bloody diarrhea, and weight loss are indicative of non-IgE-mediated mechanisms and are associated with cellular immune responses.[5,9]

Cardiovascular

The cardiovascular symptoms represent the most severe manifestations of IgE-mediated food allergies, potentially leading to tachycardia, hypotension, or even fatal cardiovascular collapse.[2] These severe reactions often occur in conjunction with symptoms affecting other organ systems like the respiratory or integumentary systems.

CORE CONCEPT 4

The range of symptoms in IgE-mediated food allergic reactions varies widely, from patients experiencing mild cutaneous symptoms to severe, life-threatening anaphylaxis.

PRACTICE POINT

It is important to work closely with an allergist in nutritional management to ensure that the patient is safely avoiding allergenic foods to prevent complications from severe reactions.

Oral Allergy Syndrome (OAS)

A specific localized IgE-mediated reaction is known as **oral allergy syndrome (OAS)** characterized by a hypersensitivity reaction to certain plant-based foods, typically manifesting as itching, tingling, or swelling in the oropharyngeal region.[1,3,5] OAS is the most common form of food allergy, affecting approximately 5–8% of the population.[1] This syndrome is typically triggered in individuals who are allergic to pollen and experience cross-reactivity between the IgE antibodies to certain pollens and proteins found in fresh produce like bananas, melons, carrots, celery, and apples.[1,6,9] Fortunately, these reactions are eliminated by the heat-labile nature of the allergenic proteins, which means cooking these foods can denature the proteins, thus preventing the allergic reaction.[1] This distinction is a key diagnostic indicator of OAS, which is particularly common in individuals with allergies to birch tree, ragweed, or grass pollen.[1] Although systemic progression of OAS is rare, it can occur and should be monitored closely.

Food-Dependent Exercise-Induced Anaphylaxis (FDEIA)

Food-dependent exercise-induced anaphylaxis (FDEIA) represents a unique category within immediate hypersensitivity reactions to foods. These reactions are mediated by allergen-specific IgE-ab and occur specifically when certain foods are consumed prior to or during physical activity.[17] The most common trigger is wheat, but others include seafood, shellfish, and grains.[16] The symptoms of FDEIA are as varied as those associated with other types of food allergies, and in some cases, exercise alone can provoke allergic symptoms without the ingestion of food.[17] The pathophysiological mechanisms underlying these reactions are not fully understood. With the growing public health focus on increasing physical activity, the incidence of reported cases of exercise-induced food allergies may rise.

PRACTICE POINT

Collect a detailed dietary and medical history to identify potential food allergens, considering factors such as timing, frequency, and nature of reactions. Pay special attention to the circumstances of a reaction to identify conditions like OAS or FDEIA.

Alpha-Gal Syndrome (AGS)

Alpha-gal syndrome (AGS) is characterized by an immune response to galactose-alpha-1,3-galactose (alpha-gal), a carbohydrate found in the glycolipids and glycoproteins of mammals but absent in poultry, humans, and higher primates.[18] Mammalian products that trigger reactions include meat, milk, and gelatin.[18] Alpha-gal is primarily introduced through tick bites, particularly the Lone Star tick in the United States. IgE antibodies are produced against alpha-gal, resulting in a delayed allergic response that typically manifests 2–24 hours post-consumption of mammalian meats, often during nighttime.[18] The prevalence of AGS is challenging to determine due to insufficient research; however, studies suggest a notable incidence in areas with high tick populations.[19] Symptoms of AGS range from mild, such as urticaria and GI discomfort, to severe reactions like anaphylaxis.

Individuals with AGS do not consistently react to every exposure to mammalian products; thus, diagnosing this allergy can be complex. Serum IgE testing for alpha-gal is preferred over traditional skin prick tests using mammalian meat extracts.[20] Reactions may also occur with cooked meats as alpha-gal is heat stable.[18] Management of AGS centers on avoiding mammalian meats and products containing alpha-gal. This includes certain medications, vaccines, and medical devices derived from mammals that may trigger reactions. For ongoing symptomatic control, antihistamines and mast cell stabilizers are commonly employed.[18] In terms of emergent therapies, oral immunotherapy using mammalian meat or dairy products is explored, alongside biologics targeting IgE.[18] Managing AGS also involves avoiding tick bites, as new bites can exacerbate the condition, and the disease may improve with minimized tick exposure.[18]

Anaphylaxis

Anaphylaxis is the most critical and severe form of IgE-mediated hypersensitivity reaction that rapidly affects multiple organ systems and poses a potential threat to life if untreated. It is the leading cause of food allergy–related emergency room visits, with over 50% of anaphylaxis cases in this setting linked to food triggers.[21] According to clinical guidelines, a patient must exhibit specific symptoms following exposure to an allergen to be diagnosed with anaphylaxis. Symptoms can affect multiple organ systems and can include skin reactions, cardiovascular instability, GI discomfort, and respiratory difficulty.[22] Foods such as peanuts, tree nuts, shellfish, fish, cow's milk, and eggs are commonly associated with anaphylactic reactions; however, virtually any food has the potential to trigger such a response.[22] Timely administration of epinephrine is critical and markedly reduces the likelihood of a fatal outcome.

The diagnostic criteria for anaphylaxis, developed by the National Institute of Allergy and Infectious Diseases (NIAID) and the Food Allergy and Anaphylaxis Network (FAAN) in 2006, serve as guidelines for identifying and diagnosing anaphylactic episodes, as outlined in **Table 15.2**.[5] These guidelines, which have been validated for their high sensitivity and specificity, are still widely used despite the World Allergy Organization (WAO) proposing slight modifications in 2020 to include more specific respiratory and GI symptoms.[23] These criteria continue to guide healthcare providers in the accurate identification and management of suspected anaphylactic episodes.[23,24] Anaphylactic reactions can also exhibit biphasic characteristics, where an initial response is followed by a delayed phase occurring in approximately 10% of cases.[25] Clinical manifestations of anaphylaxis can vary by age group. Infants often present with vomiting and hives, while preschool-aged children may exhibit symptoms like wheezing and stridor.[25] Teenagers commonly report difficulty breathing or swallowing as primary symptoms. Notably, a small percentage of children may present with hypotension.[25]

Table 15.2 Clinical Criteria for Diagnosing Anaphylaxis

Patient must meet one of the following criteria for anaphylaxis:
1. **Acute Onset of Allergic Reaction** Symptoms manifest within minutes to hours involving skin/mucosal tissue AND any of the following: respiratory symptoms, decreased BP, or signs of end-organ dysfunction.
2. **Multiple Rapid Symptoms Following Allergen Exposure** At least two of the following occurr swiftly after exposure to a potential allergen: skin/mucosal involvement, respiratory symptoms, decreased BP, or GI symptoms.
3. **Blood Pressure Reduction Post Allergen Exposure** A marked reduction in BP subsequent to allergen exposure, serving as a direct indicator of an allergic reaction.

BP, blood pressure; GI, gastrointestinal

Data from Waserman S, Bégin P, Watson W. IgE-mediated food allergy. *Allergy Asthma Clin Immunol*. 2018;14(Suppl 2):2.

PRACTICE POINT

Support pediatric patients and caregivers in developing emergency action plans for managing anaphylactic reactions at school. A common emergency action plan used by food-allergic patients is the FARE (Food Allergy Research & Education) Food Allergy & Anaphylaxis Emergency Care Plan.

Diagnosis

The diagnosis of a food allergy involves a comprehensive evaluation that includes a detailed history and physical examination, supplemented by diagnostic tests such as skin prick tests (SPT) and serum-specific IgE assessments. In some cases, an oral food challenge (OFC) may be necessary (**Table 15.3**). Patients with

Table 15.3 Available Diagnostic Tests for Food Allergy

Diagnostic Test	Description	Advantages	Disadvantages
Oral food challenge	Administers increasing doses of the allergen orally until a response is observed	Gold standard for diagnosis; highly accurate	Costly; time-consuming; risk of severe allergic reactions
Skin prick test	Introduces allergen subcutaneously to check for an allergic reaction by observing skin response	High sensitivity; quick results	Low specificity; low positive predictive value
Serum-specific IgE	Uses a fluorescent enzyme-labeled antibody assay to measure specific IgE antibodies in the blood	Can correlate strongly with clinical reactions	More expensive; variability across different test assays

Data from Onyimba F, Crowe SE, Johnson S, Leung J. Food allergies and intolerances: a clinical approach to the diagnosis and management of adverse reactions to food. *Clin Gastroenterol Hepatol*. 2021;19(11):2230-2240.e1.

suspected food allergies should be referred to an allergist to confirm the diagnosis. It is advisable for these patients to avoid the suspected food(s) and to have an epinephrine auto-injector or nasal spray available, even if the diagnosis has not yet been confirmed.

An effective diagnosis begins with a comprehensive collection of patient history, focusing on potential allergenic foods, their preparation methods (whether raw, cooked, or seasoned), and the timing and severity of symptoms relative to food intake.[1,9] It is also important to note the reproducibility of symptoms with repeated exposure. Identifying factors that might amplify allergic reactions, such as exercise, intake of nonsteroidal anti-inflammatory drugs, or alcohol consumption, is crucial.[9] Some individuals may only experience reactions when the allergen is ingested alongside these factors.

Diagnostic Tests

While validated testing and procedures are available to aid in diagnosing food allergy (detailed below), many food allergy tests are available online and marketed to consumers. These tests are often costly and are supported by little to no evidence. Therefore, it is important to educate patients on these differences.

Skin Prick Tests (SPTs)

The **skin prick test (SPT)** (Figure 15.4) is a rapid, safe, and sensitive diagnostic tool for identifying IgE-mediated food allergies and can be administered in an office setting.[5,26] During this test, the skin is pricked with a small amount of the suspected allergen, and a positive reaction typically appears as a wheal (raised, itchy bump) and flare on the skin. Although SPTs are highly sensitive, with a sensitivity

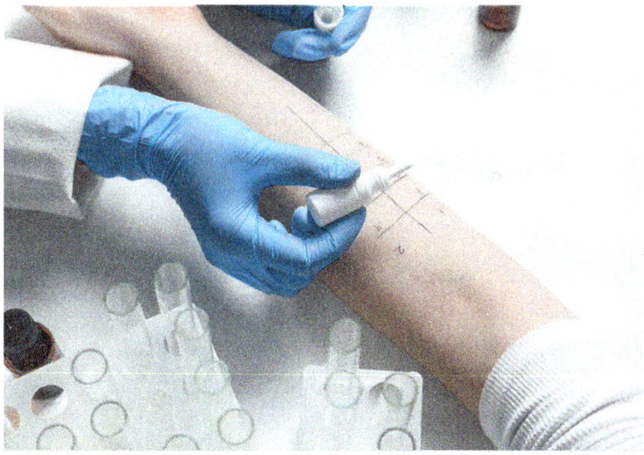

Figure 15.4 Skin Prick Test

rate of approximately 90%, their specificity is relatively low at around 50%.[26] This means that while a positive SPT indicates a likely allergy, it cannot confirm it independently without corroborative clinical history. To reduce the incidence of false positives, it is advisable to limit SPT to allergens suggested by the patient's history. A negative result on the SPT, which has a predictive value of over 95%, generally indicates the absence of an IgE-mediated reaction.[26]

Serum-Specific IgE Testing

Serum-specific IgE testing offers a quantitative assessment of food-specific IgE antibodies and is particularly useful when SPTs cannot be performed, such as in cases of extensive skin disease, dermatographia, or ongoing antihistamine therapy.[13,26] This test, although less sensitive and more costly than SPTs, measures the amount of IgE antibodies specific to particular foods in the blood.[26] While higher specific IgE levels often correlate with clinical reactivity, their predictive value varies depending on factors such as age, ethnicity, and time elapsed since the last allergen exposure.[9,26] Additionally, the predictive value of specific IgE tests is influenced by the total serum IgE levels, which are often elevated in individuals with other atopic conditions. This testing can assist in managing the long-term outlook of the allergy and determining the appropriateness of an oral food challenge in combination with SPT.

Oral Food Challenges (OFC)

When results from SPT and serum-specific IgE testing are inconclusive, but there is still a suspicion of food allergy, an **oral food challenge (OFC)** may be necessary. The OFC may be conducted openly, with a placebo control for patient blinding, or under double-blind, placebo-controlled conditions (DBPCFC)—the latter being the diagnostic standard mainly used in research settings.[27] This test involves the gradual introduction of the suspected food under strict medical supervision to monitor for adverse reactions. In an OFC, the allergenic food is administered in gradually increasing amounts over a set period, typically given 15–20 minutes apart until an appropriate serving is reached.[5,27] If symptoms develop, the test is discontinued, and immediate treatment is provided. For situations where patient anxiety or subjective symptoms could influence the results, a single-blind or DBPCFC approach may be preferable.[27]

CORE CONCEPT 5

The diagnostic tools for identifying IgE-mediated food allergies include skin prick tests, serum-specific IgE tests, and oral food challenges. A detailed clinical history is critical for proper diagnosis. Patients with suspected food allergies should consult with an allergist, and if required, undergo testing to avoid unnecessary dietary restriction.

Management of IgE-Mediated Food Allergy

Pharmacotherapy

The first step in initial management is the identification of anaphylaxis. If anaphylaxis is confirmed, the primary treatment is the administration of epinephrine, with dosing based on patient weight. For epinephrine autoinjectors, dosing is as follows: 0.1 mg for <16 kg, 0.15 mg for <30 kg, or 0.30 mg for ≥30 kg.[9] In August 2024, an epinephrine nasal spray (Neffy®) was approved by the FDA as another form of emergency epinephrine in patients who weigh ≥30 kg. Epinephrine should be administered immediately upon recognizing anaphylaxis, as delayed or absent administration at the onset of symptoms is associated with increased fatalities.[9,21] If the patient does not respond to the first dose of epinephrine, additional injections or nasal spray administrations may be necessary.

Following epinephrine administration, antihistamines (e.g., diphenhydramine) and glucocorticoids (e.g., prednisone) can be used as secondary treatments for symptomatic relief in the event of anaphylaxis.[9] After the acute event, the patient should be discharged with a prescription for epinephrine and referred to an allergist for further evaluation and management. The allergist will confirm or rule out a food allergy diagnosis and further educate the patient on the proper use of epinephrine.

Avoidance

Once a diagnosis is established, long-term management includes avoidance of the allergen, patient education, and maintaining a prescription for emergency epinephrine. Patients should work with their allergist to develop an Emergency Action Plan and ensure they always carry their prescribed medications. Strict avoidance of the allergenic food is essential to prevent allergic reactions. A well-planned elimination diet, managed by a registered dietitian (RD), can help maintain the individual's symptom-free status while ensuring nutritional adequacy. Reintroduction of the eliminated food should only be considered when there is clinical evidence indicating that the allergy has resolved.

Despite best efforts, accidental ingestion is common, with studies indicating that as many as 50% of children with peanut allergies experience an accidental reaction within a 2-year period, and up to 75% experience such reactions over the course of 10 years.[28] Effective management involves careful reading of ingredient labels, preventing cross-contact with allergens, clear communication with restaurant staff when dining out, and being prepared to administer emergency treatment in case of a reaction.[5,28]

In the United States, food labeling laws require that the nine most common allergens (milk, eggs, peanuts, tree nuts, wheat, soy, fish, crustacean shellfish, and sesame) be identified on packaged food labels. However, individuals allergic to less common foods may face challenges when interpreting ingredient labels. Additionally, voluntary precautionary statements like "may contain [allergen]" or "manufactured on shared equipment with [allergen]" are not regulated.[28] It is typically recommended that individuals with allergies avoid products with these precautionary labels to minimize risk.

Children with food allergies, particularly those allergic to milk or with multiple food allergies, are at a higher risk of experiencing growth deficiencies.[5] Nutritional counseling from an RD is strongly encouraged for these patients. An RD can provide education on allergen avoidance strategies while also advising on appropriate nutrient supplementation to prevent deficiencies.

PRACTICE POINT

It is critical to educate patients about cross-contamination risks in home, school, and restaurant settings, emphasizing the importance of properly cleaning dining utensils and food preparation areas.

Oral Immunotherapy (OIT)

Oral immunotherapy (OIT) involves administering progressively larger doses of an allergenic food, starting from a small quantity that does not trigger an allergic reaction.[29,30] This phase, known as the "buildup phase," often extends over several months. After reaching a maintenance dose, the patient continues to consume this dose daily for a prolonged period to maintain desensitization.[5,30] **Desensitization** refers to a temporary elevation in the threshold of allergen required to provoke an allergic reaction, contingent upon continuous allergen exposure.[5] The goal of OIT is to protect against severe reactions from accidental exposures to allergens.

In clinical trials, significant desensitization has been achieved through OIT in a majority of participants who can tolerate the regimen. The largest OIT study reported that 67.2% of participants achieved desensitization after 6 months of daily intake of 300 mg of peanut protein, compared to only 4% in the placebo group.[30] Severe reactions, including anaphylaxis, can occur. GI symptoms and anaphylaxis are the primary reasons for withdrawal from OIT studies, with EoE also being occasionally reported.[30] Some pediatric patients have been shown to reach **sustained unresponsiveness (SU)**, a longer-lasting state of tolerance that persists even after OIT maintenance treatment is discontinued. A 2014 study showed that 50% of subjects achieved SU to peanuts following OIT, confirmed by oral challenge.[31] SU has also been shown in children following egg OIT.[32]

This treatment process should be individualized based on the patient's allergy severity and timeline. Due to its individualized nature and novelty, there is significant variability in OIT maintenance doses and duration. In 2020, the U.S. Food and Drug Administration (FDA) approved a peanut allergen oral immunotherapy powder (Palforzia® or peanut [*Arachis hypogaea*] Allergen Powder-dnfp) for use by Risk Evaluation and Mitigation Strategy (REMS)-certified clinicians in treating peanut-allergic children aged 4 and older.[33] There are concerns about safety, as data indicate an increased risk of reactions during OIT, including a higher likelihood of anaphylactic reactions. Despite this, OIT can improve the quality of life for patients by providing protection against accidental exposures in the long term.

Omalizumab (XOLAIR®)

Omalizumab, marketed as Xolair®, was approved by the FDA on February 16, 2024, for the reduction of IgE-mediated food allergies in individuals aged 1 year and older. This treatment, which has been approved for the treatment of allergic asthma, chronic spontaneous urticaria, and chronic rhinosinusitis with nasal polyps, is now the first approved treatment option for reducing the risks associated with accidental exposure to multiple food allergens.[34] Omalizumab functions by decreasing free circulating IgE levels and reducing the expression of FcεR1 on mast cells and basophils, which diminishes their capacity to release inflammatory mediators when exposed to allergens.[34]

The findings from the OUtMATCH trial highlighted omalizumab's effectiveness in raising the threshold for allergic reactions to various foods (peanut, milk, egg, wheat, cashew, hazelnut, and walnut) when consumed alone or with other confirmed food allergens, thereby offering protection against accidental exposures.[35] The trial showed that omalizumab could be effectively used as monotherapy, but also in conjunction with patients undergoing OIT. The broad application of omalizumab, in contrast to Palforzia®, which is limited to treating peanut allergies, significantly enhances the management of food allergies. However, it is not a cure for food allergies and does not permit the unrestricted consumption of allergenic foods.[34]

Patients likely to benefit from omalizumab are those with a definitive history of IgE-mediated allergic reactions and who have demonstrated specific IgE sensitization.[34] The use of omalizumab must be carefully considered, in terms of eligibility, dosage, and the potential need for reevaluation of food allergy status.[34] However, the outcome of a successful oral food challenge in pediatric patients may be confusing, as it is unclear whether tolerance is due to omalizumab or if the allergy was outgrown. Moreover, serum-specific IgE testing and SPT may become less reliable for reevaluation as omalizumab counteracts IgE. Therefore, the use of omalizumab in clinical practice requires a careful approach such that the patient does not experience allergic reaction or anaphylaxis during treatment.

CORE CONCEPT 6

Patients with confirmed food allergies should always carry an epinephrine autoinjector or nasal spray in case of an emergency. Management of food allergies also includes patient and caretaker education on allergen avoidance, and therapeutic measures such as oral immunotherapy, or omalizumab, a biologic for the reduction of IgE-mediated food allergic reactions.

PRACTICE POINT

RDs can help patients identify alternatives to allergic foods to ensure a nutritionally balanced diet, which is especially crucial for pediatric patients.

Prevention

Early exposure to antigens plays a crucial role in developing the immune system's response to foods. Primary oral exposure to antigens typically encourages a tolerogenic response, which may promote immune tolerance.[24] Conversely, initial exposure through the skin has been associated with an increased risk of sensitization in infants with atopic dermatitis.[36] Epidemiological evidence supports the beneficial effects of early oral exposure, particularly with peanuts.[37] Studies in various cultural groups that introduce peanuts early in life demonstrate a lower prevalence of peanut allergies.

Notably, research shows that high-risk infants—those with severe atopic dermatitis or an egg allergy—can significantly reduce their risk of developing peanut allergies if they start consuming peanuts regularly between the ages of 4 and 11 months and continue until about 60 months.[37] This practice is now widely recommended internationally, and guidelines in Australia and the United Kingdom also advocate for the early introduction of eggs into the diets of high-risk infants to prevent egg allergies. While there is a lack of data on the preventive effects of introducing other allergenic foods early, there is no evidence to suggest that delaying the introduction of allergenic solids has any benefits. Further research is ongoing to determine if reducing the risk of atopic dermatitis can also prevent the development of food allergies.

Finally, the importance of educating caregivers of children with food allergies is imperative for the prevention of food allergic reactions. These include parents, legal guardians, and in some cases, babysitters or second-degree relatives who care for the child. These parties should be properly educated by an allergist and RD on avoidance measures and indications for epinephrine administration.

CASE STUDY REVISITED

Upon interviewing Chase further, you obtain the following dietary history:

Dietary Data:

Dietary History: Chase reports he has avoided suspected food allergens (most fruit and nuts) and acidic and spicy foods for the past few weeks to help manage his condition and reduce discomfort.

Usual Diet Recall:

Breakfast: 1 slice of toast with almond butter, 6 oz of herbal tea

Lunch: 1 grilled cheese sandwich on whole wheat bread

Dinner: 4 oz of baked salmon, 1/3 cup of mashed sweet potatoes, 1/2 cup of boiled spinach, 16 oz water

Questions

1. Write two Nutrition Diagnosis statements for Chase identifying the Problem/Etiology/Signs and Symptoms (PES) of Chase's active nutrition issues.
2. Identify the nutrition interventions you would like to initiate for Chase to address the problems identified in your PES statements.
3. What should be included in your monitoring and evaluation plan? Why?

Nutritional Management of IgE-Mediated Food Allergy

Nutrition Assessment

Nutrition assessment should include anthropometric evaluation of growth in children and weight trending in adults to assess for weight loss. Since GI side effects can lead to fluid imbalance, biochemical assessment should include evaluation of a basic metabolic panel to assess for dehydration. A detailed dietary history should include a timeline for breastfeeding or formula consumption and food introduction for children, description of physical symptoms, onset of symptoms, correlation of physical symptoms with timing and type of food and activity, past and current food patterns, foods restricted, and vitamin and mineral supplementation. Nutrition-focused physical examination should include evaluation of skin for rashes, signs of fat and/or muscle wasting for those with a history of weight loss or significant food restriction, and signs of micronutrient deficiencies.

Nutrition Intervention

Cow's Milk Allergy

Cow's milk allergy (CMA) is one of the most common food allergies observed in early childhood, affecting approximately 2.5% of children by the age of 1 in industrialized nations. While up to 14% of young children are reported by parents to have CMA, the prevalence confirmed by oral food challenge is significantly lower.[38] Although CMA typically decreases with age and is rare in adults, it can persist or even first appear during adulthood. Adolescents and adults with this allergy often experience severe symptoms and are sensitive to small quantities of milk proteins.

Management of CMA primarily involves the avoidance of cow's milk (CM) and its derivatives, which are found in numerous food products such as baked goods, cereals, chocolates, processed meats, and many types of prepared dishes. Milk from other mammalian species is often not tolerated due to cross-reactivity.[10,39] While milk from donkeys and mares may be more tolerable, it is not widely available commercially.[38,39] CM is a rich source of protein, fat, calcium, vitamins D, B12, A, pantothenic acid, and riboflavin. Its widespread presence makes elimination challenging, potentially impacting nutrition and quality of life.

For adults, most nutrients found in CM can be replaced with alternative dietary sources such as soy milk, almond milk, and oat milk. However, meeting calcium and vitamin D needs can be challenging without dairy, and sometimes supplementation is recommended to mitigate the risk of osteoporosis and fractures.

For breastfed infants diagnosed with CMA, it is recommended to continue breastfeeding as long as the mothers can effectively exclude dairy products from their diet. Mothers on a dairy-free diet should supplement with 1,000 mg/day of calcium and a dairy-free prenatal vitamin to ensure adequate nutrient intake.[7,39] For formula-fed infants with CMA, extensively hydrolyzed formulas (eHFs) such as Similac® Alimentum®, Enfamil Nutramigen®, and Pregestimil® are recommended over soy formulas or partially hydrolyzed CM formulas.[39] These eHFs are designed to minimize allergen exposure and are preferable for managing CMA.

As infants transition from formula to other milk sources around the age of 1, enriched alternative milk beverages (EAMB) such as rice milk, soymilk, and potato milk often do not provide nutrition comparable to whole CM or formula.[39] Breast milk and/or eHF remain superior options during this transition. For older toddlers, enriched soymilk is an appropriate alternative if soy is tolerated. For those with concurrent milk and soy allergies, enriched oat milk is a viable option. It is crucial to ensure that the entire protein requirement is met through solid foods before transitioning to EAMB due to their lower protein content.[39] Additional fat may be added in the form of vegetable oils if needed. Generally, plant-based EAMB are preferred over mammalian milk due to their wide availability and reduced risk of cross-reactivity with CM.

Approximately 75% of patients with CMA can tolerate extensively heated or baked forms of milk, such as those found in muffins, cookies, and cakes.[38] Regular consumption of these products may help to accelerate the development of tolerance to CM. For successful desensitization to CMA through baked milk, it is recommended that baked milk be consumed at least three times per week, if tolerated. However, about a quarter of CMA patients react to these forms of milk, with a third of those potentially experiencing anaphylaxis.[38,39] Thus, a supervised OFC following diagnostic testing to extensively heated milk is essential to confirm tolerance before incorporating baked milk products into the diet of individuals with CMA.

Egg Allergy

Egg allergies are seen most commonly in young children, affecting 1.3% of children under 5 years old.[40] Although eggs are rich sources of protein, vitamin B12, riboflavin, pantothenic acid, biotin, and selenium, their omission from the diet is generally not associated with nutritional deficiencies because these nutrients are abundantly available in other foods. Individuals diagnosed with an allergy to chicken eggs should also avoid eggs from other birds like ducks, turkeys, geese, and quails, due to cross-reactivity among avian eggs.[41]

Effective management of egg allergy necessitates comprehensive education on avoiding egg products, crucially facilitated by RDs. Essential aspects of this education include understanding food labeling—both ingredients and precautionary allergen labeling (PAL).[41] When dining out, effective communication with restaurant staff is also vital to prevent egg cross-contact.

The allergenic potential of egg varies with its preparation; raw and cooked eggs are highly allergenic, whereas baking (extensive heating) reduces this allergenicity significantly.[41] Studies indicate that approximately 70% of children with egg allergy can tolerate baked forms of egg, which enhances their dietary variety and improves their overall quality of life by reducing dietary restrictions.[41] The introduction of baked egg, however, is not without controversy. While some observational studies suggest benefits, such as accelerated allergy resolution through regular consumption of baked egg, definitive evidence from randomized controlled trials remains scant. Research reveals that children who initially react to baked egg tend to have a more persistent allergy.[41] However, those who can tolerate and regularly consume baked egg may develop tolerance to cooked egg. In clinical practice, the introduction of baked egg should be carefully considered, weighing the potential nutritional and social benefits against the risks of allergic reactions.

Peanut and Tree Nuts Allergy

Peanuts and tree nuts are among the leading causes of severe food-related allergic reactions, including fatal anaphylaxis. Peanut allergies affect approximately 1–4.5% of the population in Western countries, while tree nut allergies range from 0.05% to 4.9%.[3,42] These allergies usually manifest early in life and are seldom outgrown. Only about 9–20% of cases show transient sensitization over time, and nearly all individuals who lose sensitization initially had low levels of specific IgE antibodies (sIgE-ab) to peanuts and tree nuts.[43]

Recent studies have highlighted the preventative potential of early peanut consumption in avoiding the development of peanut allergies. Consequently, updated guidelines in many countries now advocate for the introduction of peanuts into the diet of infants before the age of 1 year.[44]

Patients may also experience OAS to peanuts and tree nuts. OAS is primarily triggered by the cross-reactivity between pollen proteins and similar proteins found in various foods.[45] In the case of nuts, individuals sensitized to tree pollens like birch may experience OAS symptoms upon consuming nuts due to similar protein structures shared between the pollen and nuts.[45]

Despite common beliefs among many nut-allergic patients, research indicates that airborne or skin exposure to peanuts or tree nuts alone does not cause severe allergic reactions; there have been no fatalities solely from airborne exposure to peanuts.[44] Studies have shown that only minute amounts of peanut proteins are detectable in the air, insufficient to trigger severe reactions. However, oral ingestion of even small amounts of peanuts can still be fatal.[44]

Given the risks of cross-contamination, complete avoidance of peanuts and all tree nuts is generally advised for young children with peanut allergies. For older children and adults, a supervised OFC may be considered before introducing other tree nuts into their diets to assess tolerance and safety. This approach helps manage the risks associated with potential cross-contamination and the difficulty in distinguishing between different nuts.

Fish Allergy

Prevalence rates for fish allergy range from 0.5% to 2.9% based on clinical history and sensitization.[46] After peanuts and tree nuts, fish ranks as one of the most frequent allergens responsible for fatal anaphylactic reactions to foods.[46] In the United States, the fish species most commonly reported to elicit allergic reactions include salmon, tuna, catfish, and cod, followed by flounder, halibut, trout, and bass.[46] Sensitization typically begins in childhood and often persists into adulthood.

The primary allergen in fish is **parvalbumin**, a protein found across various species and known for its stability even when heated or cooked.[46,47] Diagnosis of fish allergy primarily relies on SPT or detection of sIgE-ab to cod or other fish proteins, combined with the patient's clinical history.[47]

To manage fish allergy, it is noteworthy that some individuals may exhibit allergic reactions to specific fish species while tolerating others.[46] To prevent unnecessary dietary restrictions, an OFC is recommended. With these results, an RD can develop a tailored diet plan that enables the safe inclusion of certain fish species, eliminating the need for a complete avoidance of all fish. It is important to note that fish and shellfish are not cross-reactive, and therefore patients with fish allergy are likely able to tolerate shellfish if they do not report a history of clinical reaction.

Shellfish Allergy

Shellfish allergy impacts up to 10.3% of the global population and is more prevalent than fish allergy, with estimates suggesting up to 3% of adults are affected, particularly in the Asia Pacific region.[48] Shellfish are categorized into crustaceans (shrimp, crab, and lobster) and mollusks, and it is a common misconception that individuals allergic to one subgroup must avoid all shellfish.[48] However, some may react only to crustaceans but can tolerate mollusks, or they may have species-specific allergies.

The major allergen in shellfish is tropomyosin, which shows high homology (90%) among shrimp, crab, crayfish, and lobster, indicating strong cross-reactivity.[48,49] Cross-reactivity between shellfish and mites or insects is also significant due to similar protein structures. For example, there is 80% homology between shrimp and house dust mites, leading to potential sensitization to both.[48] Patients diagnosed with a crustacean allergy are generally advised to avoid all crustaceans due to the high risk of cross-reactivity. However, they do not need to avoid fish, and vice versa, as these groups do not cross-react.[49]

Wheat Allergy

There are three distinct types of IgE-mediated wheat allergy: wheat allergy in children, **wheat-dependent exercise-induced anaphylaxis (WDEIA)**, and baker's asthma. Wheat allergy in children is among the top three most prevalent allergies in some countries, following milk and egg, with a prevalence just below 1%.[50] IgE sensitization to wheat is more common than clinical wheat allergy, often due to cross-reactions with grass pollen.[51]

Most children outgrow their wheat allergy, but those who retain it into adolescence or young adulthood often suffer from severe reactions, potentially leading to anaphylaxis upon ingestion of wheat-containing food.[7] The level of sIgE-ab to wheat during the first year of life can predict the duration of the allergy, where low levels (<2 kUA/L) often resolve early and high levels (>50 kUA/L) tend to persist.[52]

WDEIA, also known as "omega-5-gliadin allergy," is a rare condition affecting adults and is typically triggered by the consumption of wheat accompanied by exercise, but may also be induced by acetylsalicylic acid and other NSAIDS, alcohol, and infections.[51,52] Diagnosis of WDEIA significantly relies on clinical history and often involves sIgE-ab testing for ω-5-gliadin, identified as the major allergen.[52]

Baker's asthma or rhinitis results from repeated exposure to inhaling wheat flour and represents another form of IgE-mediated wheat allergy.[51] Given the close relationship between wheat and other cereals like rye and barley, avoidance of these grains may also be recommended in managing wheat allergy.

Wheat is prevalent in numerous processed products like crackers, cookies, cakes, pasta, bread, and cereal, as well as minor ingredients in condiments, marinades, cold cuts, soy sauce, hard candies, and low-fat products. The primary derivative of wheat, wheat flour, is an excellent source of carbohydrate, iron, thiamine, riboflavin, niacin, folic acid, pyridoxine (vitamin B6), magnesium, and fiber. Alternatively, a broad array of wheat-free and gluten-free products is available, made from alternative flours such as rice, corn, oat, barley, buckwheat, rye, amaranth, millet, and quinoa. Although these alternative flours are widely accessible, they are rarely fortified. To boost nutritional value, a fortified infant cereal made from grains that the patient is not allergic to can be added to these alternative flours. It's crucial to recognize that up to 20% of individuals with an allergy to one grain may also react to other grains, hence the use of these alternative grain products should be customized based on tolerance as assessed by an allergist.[51,52] Note that CD is not considered a grain allergy in this context.

Soy Allergy

Soy allergy ranks among the prevalent food allergies during childhood.[52] Soy is a source of several nutrients, including protein, thiamine, riboflavin, pyridoxine, folic acid, calcium, phosphorus, magnesium, iron, and zinc. It is not a staple in Western diets, and its exclusion generally does not cause nutritional deficiencies unless the individual has additional dietary restrictions or allergies, such as to milk, or follows a vegetarian or vegan diet.[52] Soy proteins are prevalent in many vegetarian products and are also found in a diverse range of other food items, including baked goods, cereals, crackers, canned tuna, soups, reduced-fat peanut butter, cold cuts, and hot dogs. Most individuals with a soy allergy can safely consume highly refined soy oil and soy lecithin, which are commonly used in processed and manufactured foods.[52] However, soy fibers, a by-product of soybean processing, may retain soy proteins and should be avoided by those with soy allergies to prevent allergic reactions.[53]

Sesame Allergy

Sesame was recognized as the ninth major food allergen in the United States in 2021 due to its rising prevalence. This increase is partly due to sesame's growing popularity in Western diets. It appears as seeds on breads, bagels, and sushi; as oil in Asian cuisine; and as tahini or sesame paste in Middle Eastern dishes like hummus and baba ghanoush.[54] Sesame is also found in some desserts, such as halva, and in certain cookies and candies.

Recognizing its significance as an allergen, the United States enacted the Food Allergy Safety, Treatment, Education, and Research (FASTER) Act in 2021, mandating clear labeling of sesame on packaged products.[53] Despite these regulations, avoiding sesame remains challenging due to its widespread use and the complexities of food labeling. The introduction of the FASTER Act led to some unintended consequences, such as manufacturers adding sesame to products or altering labels to include precautionary statements like "may contain sesame" or "made in a facility with sesame."[54] These changes can sometimes reflect adjustments in recipe formulations or a legal precaution, adding complexity for consumers trying to avoid sesame.

The cornerstone of managing sesame allergy involves rigorous avoidance of sesame in all its forms. This includes sesame seeds, oil, paste, and any derivative products. Given the widespread use of sesame in various cuisines, individuals with this allergy must be adept at reading ingredient labels and inquiring about food preparation methods when dining out to avoid accidental exposure guided by RDs.

Table 15.4 outlines potential nutritional deficiencies as well as substitute food options for each of the most common 9 IgE-mediated food allergies.

Table 15.4 Potential Nutritional Deficiencies and Alternatives for Common Food Allergies

Allergen	Potential Deficiencies	Substitute Food
Cow's Milk	Calcium, vitamin D, protein, phosphorus, magnesium, potassium, vitamin B12, zinc	Almond milk, oat milk, coconut milk, rice milk, cashew milk, hemp milk, macadamia milk
Egg	Retinol (vitamin A), riboflavin, thiamine, vitamin B6, vitamin B12, biotin, folate, pantothenic acid, potassium, magnesium, phosphorus, iron, selenium, zinc, iodine	Tofu, mashed banana, yogurt, buttermilk, chia seeds
Tree Nuts	Protein, fat, monounsaturated fatty acids, polyunsaturated fatty acids, linoleic acid, carbohydrate, fiber, calcium, iron, magnesium, phosphorus, potassium, sodium, selenium, zinc, copper, vitamin C, thiamine, riboflavin, niacin, pantothenic acid, vitamin B6, folate, vitamin B12, vitamin A, β-carotene, lycopene, lutein, zeaxanthin, vitamin E	Pumpkin seeds, sunflower seeds, chickpeas, sesame seeds, olives, avocado
Peanut	Protein, fat, fiber, magnesium, folate, vitamin E, copper, arginine	Sunflower seeds, sesame seeds, flax seeds, tree nuts (almonds, cashews, walnuts)
Fish	Omega-fatty acids, proteins, iron, zinc, copper, vitamin B12, vitamin D	Walnuts, flaxseed oil, soy oil, canola oil, egg, sesame butter, leafy green vegetables (spinach)
Shellfish	Omega-fatty acids, proteins, irons, zinc, copper, vitamin B12	Coldwater fish (salmon, tuna, mackerel, sardines), egg, nuts, seeds
Wheat	Fiber, folate, vitamin B12, selenium, manganese, phosphorus, copper	Rice, quinoa, millet, amaranth, buckwheat, sorghum, teff
Soy	Protein, fat, fiber, vitamin C, vitamin K, thiamine, riboflavin, folate, iron, magnesium, phosphorus, potassium, zinc, manganese, copper, vitamin E, niacin, vitamin B6, pantothenic acid	Fresh vegetables, plant proteins, grains
Sesame	Calcium, magnesium, iron, zinc, copper, thiamine	Sunflower seeds, pumpkin seeds, flaxseeds, chia seeds, hemp seeds, poppy seeds

Data from Gargano D, Appanna R, Santonicola A, De Bartolomeis F, Stellato C, Cianferoni A, et al. Food allergy and intolerance: a narrative review on nutritional concerns. *Nutrients*. 2021;13(5):1638.

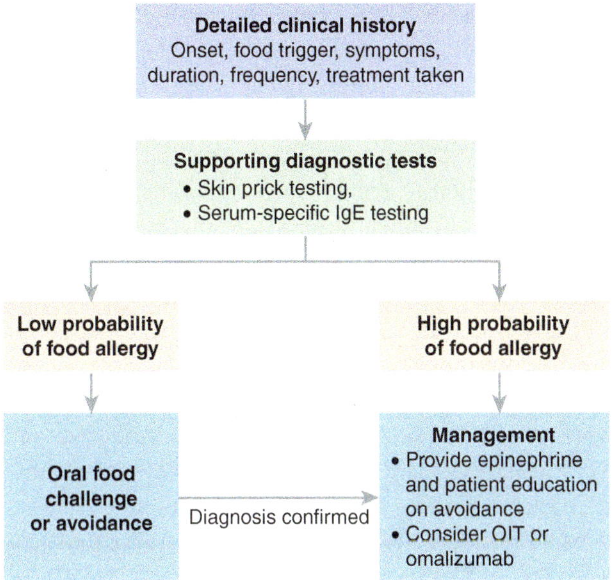

Figure 15.5 Algorithms for the Diagnosis and Management of IgE-Mediated Food Allergy.

Data from Waserman S, Bégin P, Watson W. IgE-mediated food allergy. *Allergy Asthma Clin Immunol.* 2018;14(Suppl 2):2.

PRACTICE POINT

Adapt dietary recommendations to accommodate cultural preferences, such as managing sesame allergies in East Asian diets or milk allergies in regions with high dairy consumption. It is also important to provide the family or caretakers with these recommendations to avoid cross-contamination.

Figure 15.5 provides an algorithm for the diagnosis and management of IgE-mediated food allergy.

Non-IgE-Mediated and Mixed IgE/Non-IgE Food Allergy

Non-IgE-mediated food allergies encompass a spectrum of disorders marked by subacute to chronic inflammatory responses primarily within the GI system but may involve the skin.[55] These conditions differ significantly from IgE-mediated food allergy, which is known for its potential to trigger rapid anaphylactic reactions. The principal conditions within this group include **food protein–induced enterocolitis syndrome** (FPIES), **food protein-induced allergic proctocolitis (FPIAP)**, and **eosinophilic gastrointestinal disorders (EGIDs)** including eosinophilic esophagitis (EoE). These conditions are less common than IgE-mediated food allergy and are distinguished by different immune mechanisms.

The diagnosis of non-IgE-mediated food allergies typically relies on clinical history rather than specific tests, as there are no definitive biomarkers for these conditions.[55] This reliance on clinical evaluation stems from the complex nature of these allergies, which do not involve the typical IgE antibodies that are present in more common allergic responses. Instead, other components of the immune system are implicated, and understanding these pathways remains a significant challenge in the field of allergy and immunology.

Food Protein-Induced Enterocolitis Syndrome (FPIES)

FPIES represents one of the non-IgE-mediated ARF. It typically manifests within the first year of life, typically following the introduction of the first foreign food protein in the infants' diet.[19] Symptoms include severe, repeated projectile vomiting, often accompanied by diarrhea. These episodes can lead to dehydration, lethargy, and failure to thrive for the younger population.[56] Notably, these reactions do not involve cutaneous or respiratory symptoms typical of IgE-mediated reactions.

Recent studies have identified that FPIES is not confined to early childhood and can also emerge in older children and adults, although it remains less commonly recognized in this age group.[19] Unlike children, adults with FPIES are less likely to exhibit vomiting and are more likely to exhibit acute GI symptoms such as abdominal pain, cramping, nausea, and diarrhea within 1–6 hours after ingesting the triggering food.[19] The emphasis on vomiting as a major diagnostic criterion in the existing guidelines may lead to underdiagnosis in adults if healthcare providers are not aware of these distinctions.[19]

The most common food allergen triggers are CM for infants and shellfish and finned fish for adults, but others like rice, dairy, egg, wheat, beef, poultry, fruit, and vegetables are also potential allergens.[19] Symptoms generally appear around 4–7 months of age, coinciding with the introduction of solid foods.[56] It is shown that approximately 28% of affected children overcome their trigger by age 2 years, 53% by age 3 years, 65% by age 4 years, and 72% by age 5 years.[19]

The presentation of FPIES can be divided into acute and chronic phases:

- **Acute Phase:** Triggered by infrequent ingestion of the allergen or when an allergen is introduced for the first time or reintroduced after a period of avoidance. Symptoms such as vomiting and diarrhea appear 1–3 hours post-ingestion and can last several hours. In severe cases, symptoms may escalate to shock, pallor, hypertonia, and hypothermia.[56]

- **Chronic Phase:** Occurs when the trigger food is ingested regularly, leading to intermittent, chronic symptoms like diarrhea, vomiting, and poor weight gain. Over time, this can result in nutritional deficiencies such as hypoproteinemia and hypoalbuminemia.[56]

Diagnosis of FPIES is primarily based on a detailed clinical history and the resolution of symptoms upon the elimination of the trigger food. An OFC may be conducted to confirm the diagnosis, but given that approximately 15–20% of FPIES reactions result in shock, this must be performed under strict medical supervision with appropriate emergency resources available.[57]

Post-diagnosis, the offending allergen is eliminated from the patient's diet. For those triggered by CM or soy, a switch to a casein hydrolysate-based formula is recommended, and less commonly, an amino acid-based formula may be necessary. Breastfeeding mothers may need to eliminate dairy and soy from their diets as well. Improvement is typically observed within 3–10 days of eliminating the trigger.[56,58] It is crucial not to delay the introduction of solid foods beyond 6 months of age. Introducing a variety of low-risk vegetables and fruits initially, followed by meats, grains, and other potentially allergenic foods, can help identify tolerable foods and those that provoke reactions.[58] Foods are introduced one at a time, with careful monitoring for any adverse effects. Management of FPIES requires ongoing collaboration with healthcare professionals, including allergists and RDs, to ensure safe introduction of new foods and to meet the patient's nutritional needs effectively. For infants, regular monitoring of growth parameters and careful introduction of a variety of food textures and flavors are essential to prevent restrictive eating patterns and ensure overall dietary balance.

PRACTICE POINT

Most children outgrow FPIES by age 3. Reintroduction should be carefully evaluated by an allergist and RD to avoid reaction.

Food Protein-Induced Allergic Protocolitis (FPIAP)

FPIAP is a self-limiting and generally benign condition that manifests primarily in infants during the first 6 months of life.[59] It is characterized by the presence of blood in the stool of an otherwise healthy infant. This condition is predominantly observed in breastfed infants, with about 60% of cases occurring in this group.[59,60] Although FPIAP can affect formula-fed infants, it is often triggered by proteins ingested by the breastfeeding mother, notably CM or soy.[60] Less commonly, proteins from corn and eggs have also been identified as triggers.

Diagnosing FPIAP involves ruling out other potential causes of rectal bleeding, such as anal fissures and infections.[59] Once other causes are excluded, management typically involves dietary modifications. For breastfed infants, the offending allergen is eliminated from the mother's diet. For formula-fed infants, a switch to a casein hydrolysate formula is usually effective.[60] Symptoms generally show marked improvement or complete resolution within 72 hours of these dietary changes. If the infant is on formula, the allergenic food is eliminated for at least 6 months before any reintroduction is attempted. The majority of infants with FPIAP will develop tolerance to the allergens by the age of 3 years. The reintroduction of allergenic foods should be carefully managed to monitor for any recurrence of symptoms and to ensure the safe reintegration of these foods into the child's diet.[60]

Eosinophilic Gastrointestinal Disorders (EGIDs)–EoE

EGIDs are a group of inflammatory conditions characterized by an increased presence of eosinophils in the GI tract. Diagnosis is confirmed through endoscopic biopsies of mucosal tissue, with the disorders classified based on the site of eosinophilic infiltration, such as the esophagus, stomach, small bowel, or colon.[61] Of all EGIDs, EoE is the most extensively researched. This condition is diagnosed when a patient exhibits symptoms of esophageal dysfunction, and esophageal biopsies reveal 15 or more eosinophils per high-power field.[61–64] The symptomatology varies between pediatric and adult populations; children commonly present with vomiting, abdominal pain, heartburn, and failure to thrive, whereas adults frequently experience dysphagia, heartburn, and food impaction, with dysphagia reported in over 60% of adult cases.[62–66] There is a notable association between atopic conditions and EoE, with a significant percentage of both adult and pediatric patients with EoE also suffering from conditions such as allergic rhinitis, food allergies, asthma, and dermatitis.[65] Family history of EoE also slightly increases the risk. Over recent decades, the prevalence and incidence of EoE have risen. Currently, an estimated 1 in 700 patients in the United States have a diagnosis of EoE.[67]

Upon diagnosis, several first-line therapies are available, including food elimination diets, swallowed topical corticosteroids, and proton pump inhibitors (PPIs).[65] Three primary types of elimination diets are used: empirical elimination, testing-guided elimination, and elemental or amino-acid based diet.[65] Notably, the testing-guided approach has declined due to lower efficacy and higher costs compared to empirical diets.[65]

After achieving histological and symptomatic remission with an elimination diet, specific trigger food groups are identified through serial reintroduction and monitored by subsequent histological and symptom assessments. The empirical elimination approach generally yields an efficacy rate of about 55–85%.[65] It is imperative for patients undergoing a food elimination diet consult with RDs for nutritional counseling. This ensures the diet remains balanced and palatable while meeting all nutritional needs. RDs play a crucial role in educating patients about hidden sources of trigger foods and providing suitable dietary alternatives, such as replacing cow's milk with oat milk for those avoiding dairy products. Overall, managing EoE and other EGIDs requires a comprehensive approach that combines dietary management, regular monitoring, and interdisciplinary care to ensure effective treatment and maintenance of patient health and quality of life.

In 2022, dupilumab injection, a monoclonal antibody, was approved for the treatment of EoE, and is now used in patients 1 year of age or older. Many patients have been able to resume a normal diet on dupilumab, despite following food elimination diets prior to treatment. Budesonide, an oral corticosteroid, was released in 2024, becoming the first and only FDA-approved oral treatment for EoE in patients 11 years and older.

Food Intolerance

Most adverse food reactions do not have an immunological basis and are classified as food intolerances. These reactions commonly affect multiple organ systems, with GI symptoms being particularly predominant. Individuals with food intolerance may experience abdominal pain, bloating, abdominal distension, flatulence, and diarrhea.[68,69] Unlike food allergy, which can be triggered by even trace amounts of allergens, the reactions associated with food intolerance are dose-dependent.[69] This correlation indicates that the severity of symptoms in food intolerance is closely related to the amount of the trigger food consumed, and symptoms typically worsen as more of the trigger food is ingested. Additionally, food intolerance reactions often have a delayed onset and a prolonged symptomatic phase compared to the immediate responses typically seen with food allergy.[1,69]

Prevalence

Food intolerance is considerably more common than food allergies, affecting an estimated 20% of the population.[68] In this chapter, we will discuss lactose intolerance more in depth. Lactose intolerance is the most prevalent food intolerance, predominantly resulting from a genetically regulated reduction in intestinal lactase activity occurring in late childhood or early adolescence.

CORE CONCEPT 7

Unlike food allergies, food intolerances predominantly affect the digestive system, are dose-dependent, and typically have a delayed onset.

PRACTICE POINT

Food intolerances are more common than food allergies, with the most common food intolerance being lactose intolerance.

FODMAP Intolerance

FODMAP intolerance refers to adverse effects from consuming FODMAPs (fermentable oligo-, di-, monosaccharides, and polyols), which are short-chain carbohydrates that include fructose, lactose, polyols, fructan, and galacto-oligosaccharides. These compounds are naturally present in a wide array of foods, such as fruits, vegetables, cereals, dairy products, and sweeteners, as detailed in Chapter 11, *Nutritional Management of Gastrointestinal Malabsorption*.

The consumption of high amounts of FODMAPs can lead to excessive production of short-chain fatty acids and gases like carbon dioxide, hydrogen, and methane, due to fermentation by intestinal bacteria.[68,70] This process results in luminal distension and water retention, triggering symptoms such as bloating, abdominal pain, flatulence, and diarrhea in affected individuals.[68,70] To manage these symptoms, the first-line therapy typically involves a low-FODMAP diet, which has been shown to reduce symptoms by 50–80%.[68]

CASE STUDY REVISITED

After a workup, Chase is diagnosed with an allergy to tree nuts, lactose intolerance, and oral allergy syndrome.

1. What are the key considerations for Chase to manage his condition effectively?
2. Provide five specific dietary recommendations for Chase to address these new dietary restrictions.

Phases of a low-FODMAP diet implementation are as follows:

1. **Elimination Phase:** This initial phase involves removing all high-FODMAP foods from the diet for typically 4–6 weeks.[70] During this period, it is crucial to educate patients about the role of FODMAPs in GI symptoms and counsel them on which foods have high FODMAP contents and how to avoid them.
2. **Reintroduction Phase:** After the elimination phase, the diet progresses to carefully reintroduce FODMAPs to assess individual tolerance levels. This phase involves a structured reintroduction of foods, monitoring each for 3 days to identify specific triggers of symptoms.[70]
3. **Maintenance Phase:** The final phase is the development of a long-term, customized diet that accommodates the patient's specific FODMAP tolerance levels. The goal is to maintain a flexible diet that ensures nutritional adequacy and controls symptoms.

A low-FODMAP diet can lead to nutritional deficiencies if not properly managed, due to restrictions that may reduce intake of fiber, calcium, and other important nutrients. Fiber supplements and careful dietary planning are essential to avoid complications such as constipation and ensure a balanced nutritional intake.[68] It is recommended that patients collaborate with an RD to develop and maintain a long-term dietary plan. This ensures careful monitoring to prevent the onset of eating disorders and other complications associated with dietary restrictions, which can significantly impact a patient's emotional well-being and overall quality of life.

Lactose Intolerance

Lactose intolerance is characterized by a range of symptoms that arise due to difficulties in digesting and absorbing lactose, the primary sugar found in dairy products. This condition is typically caused by diminished activity or production of lactase, the enzyme essential for lactose breakdown. Globally, the confirmed prevalence of lactose intolerance is approximately 57%, but estimates suggest that the actual prevalence could exceed 65%, with significant geographical variations—about 50% in the United States, 70% in Asia, and nearly 100% in Africa.[71] In the United States, prevalence rates vary among ethnic groups: 15% among White people, 53% among Mexican Americans, and 80% among Black Americans.[7]

Mechanism

The symptoms of lactose intolerance include abdominal pain, bloating, flatulence, diarrhea, borborygmi (rumbling sounds caused by gas movement in the intestines), nausea, and sometimes vomiting.[72] These symptoms typically manifest about 1 hour after consuming lactose-containing foods. The deficiency of lactase impairs the absorption of lactose present in the GI tract, leading to symptom onset depicted in **Figure 15.6**. Under normal lactose digestion, lactase enzymes in the small intestine cleave lactose into two simple sugars, glucose and galactose, which are then absorbed into the bloodstream.[72] In the absence of sufficient lactase, lactose remains undigested as it moves into the large intestine. This undigested lactose causes an osmotic effect, drawing water into the intestine and increasing the intestinal water content, which can lead to symptoms like bloating and diarrhea.[72] Subsequently, the colonic microbiome ferments the undigested lactose, producing gases such as hydrogen (H_2), carbon dioxide (CO_2), and methane (CH_4), along with short-chain fatty acids.[71,72] These gases contribute to the typical symptoms of lactose intolerance, including flatulence and abdominal pain. Symptoms generally manifest when lactase activity is less than 50%.[72] However, some individuals may develop tolerance over time, particularly if they gradually expose their intestinal flora to small amounts of lactose. Most people with lactase non-persistence are able to tolerate small amounts of lactose when it is consumed as part of a mixed meal.

Diagnostic Test

The **hydrogen breath test (HBT)** (**Figure 15.7**), commonly coupled with methane measurement, is

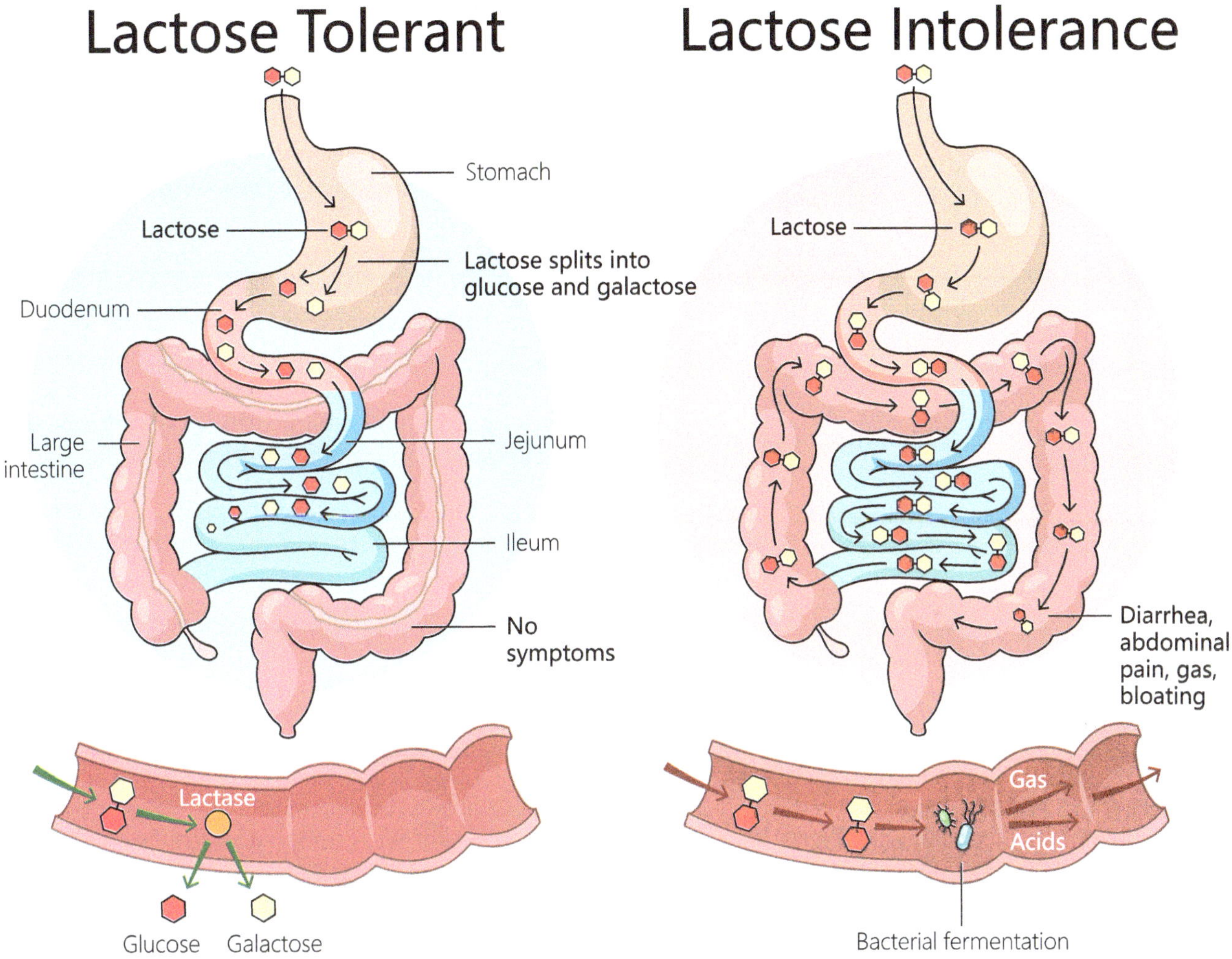

Figure 15.6 Normal Digestion of Lactose in Presence of Lactase; Lactose Intolerance Due to Lactase Deficiency

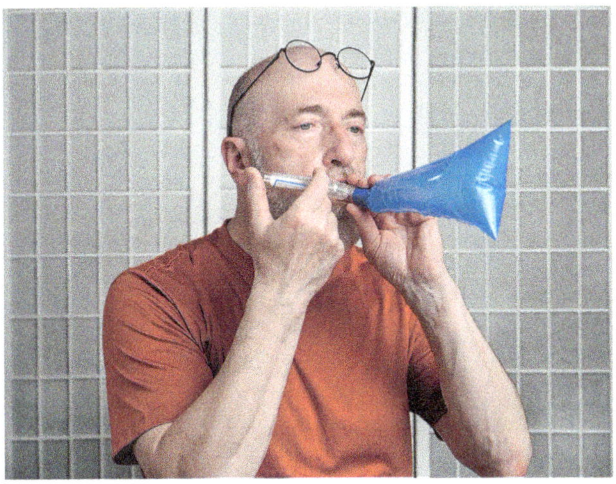

Figure 15.7 Hydrogen Breath Test

the most prevalent diagnostic tool for lactose intolerance due to its cost-effectiveness, non-invasiveness, and high sensitivity and specificity.[71,72] The HBT operates on the principle that undigested lactose fermented by intestinal bacteria produces gas, including hydrogen.[72] During the test, the patient's exhaled hydrogen is measured after fasting, followed by the ingestion of a lactose dose ranging from 25 to 50 grams.[72] Subsequent hydrogen levels are then measured at 15-minute intervals over a period of 3–6 hours. An increase in hydrogen concentration of more than 20 parts per million (ppm) from the baseline suggests lactase deficiency, commonly known as "hypolactasia."[71,72] Exhaled methane may also be measured for improved sensitivity of intolerance testing. Lactase deficiency is defined by an increase in methane concentration of more than 10 ppm from baseline.[73] Disaccharidase testing via biopsy is the gold standard for diagnosing disaccharidase deficiency.[74] This involves obtaining biopsies from the duodenum during an endoscopy.[74] These biopsies are then analyzed for the activity levels of specific enzymes like lactase, sucrase, maltase, and isomaltase, which are crucial for the digestion of carbohydrates.[74]

Nutritional Management

Lactose intolerance may impact nutrition, particularly due to the potential restrictions on dairy consumption. Dairy products are important dietary sources of protein, calcium, magnesium, potassium, zinc, and vitamin D.[75] The majority of individuals with lactose intolerance can consume adequate dairy products to meet their daily calcium requirement. Research indicates that most people with lactose intolerance can tolerate up to 100 mL of milk per serving without worsening their symptoms.[75] Consequently, complete avoidance of dairy products is generally unnecessary and not recommended, as dairy is one of the most bioavailable sources of calcium and vitamin D. Among dairy products, milk and ice cream contain the highest concentrations of lactose, whereas cheeses and live culture yogurts have significantly lower lactose content.[75] These low or no lactose dairy products are generally well tolerated by individuals with lactose intolerance and provide excellent sources of protein and calcium. To manage lactose intolerance, commercially available lactase enzymes can be added to lactose-containing foods or taken with meals to alleviate symptoms.[75] Additionally, lactose-free dairy products are widely available in grocery stores, offering viable alternatives for maintaining dairy intake. Given that individuals with lactose intolerance often have lower calcium intake, supplementation with calcium and vitamin D is recommended to reduce the risk of osteoporosis and fractures.

Clinical Controversy

Histamine Intolerance and Dietary Management

Histamine intolerance (HIT) is an emerging clinical concern characterized by an adverse reaction to histamine-rich foods, hypothesized to be due to impaired histamine degradation. This proposed intolerance can lead to a variety of symptoms, including digestive issues, headaches, and skin rashes. The intolerance is thought to be caused by the reduction of diamine oxidase (DAO) and histamine-*N*-methyltransferase activity. However, HIT is controversial due to the lack of association between these biomarkers and symptoms. A 2023 study detailed a placebo-controlled histamine challenge in which about two-thirds of the study cohort reacted to placebo. Moreover, serum DAO, while somewhat reduced in patients with proposed HIT, varied widely in those without HIT.

The primary treatment approach for managing suspected histamine intolerance involves adhering to a low-histamine diet. The lack of standardized food lists for those with histamine intolerance contributes to significant confusion and controversy. Different healthcare providers and dietary guidelines suggest varying lists of foods to avoid, which can be perplexing for patients seeking clear guidance. For example, some sources recommend avoiding all fermented foods, which are typically high in histamine, while others suggest that only certain types, such as specific cheeses or processed meats, should be excluded. This inconsistency not only makes dietary compliance challenging but also raises questions about the scientific basis of these recommendations.

Histamine levels in foods can also vary widely depending on numerous factors such as the method of food preparation, storage conditions, and the maturation process of fermented foods. For instance, the histamine content in cheese can differ significantly between batches and brands, depending on how the cheese is aged and stored. Such variations make it problematic to label specific foods as "safe" or "unsafe," leading to discrepancies in dietary advice and potential mismanagement of HIT.

Patient responses to a low-histamine diet can vary greatly. While some individuals report significant improvement in their symptoms when following a strict low-histamine diet, others notice little to no effect. This variability in effectiveness may be due to individual differences in histamine threshold. Additionally, strict dietary restrictions can lead to poor compliance, especially when patients do not perceive a direct benefit from following the diet. This raises questions about the practicality and sustainability of long-term dietary management of HIT.

There is a critical lack of evidence investigating the diagnoses of HIT and the effectiveness of low-histamine diets for those with proposed HIT. Most of the existing evidence supporting the use of these diets comes from small studies or anecdotal reports. Clinical trials are necessary to establish clear diagnostic and dietary guidelines and to understand the mechanisms by which histamine in foods affects individuals with suspected HIT. Without this information, healthcare providers face challenges in recommending evidence-based dietary interventions.

Questions:

1. What criteria should be used to standardize the classification of foods as high or low in histamine to aid in dietary recommendations for histamine intolerance?
2. How does individual variability in histamine metabolism influence the effectiveness of

low-histamine diets, and should personalized dietary plans be considered?

3. What are the long-term nutritional implications of adhering to a low-histamine diet, and how can these potential deficiencies be mitigated?

References

Sánchez-Pérez S, Comas-Basté O, Veciana-Nogués MT, Latorre-Moratalla ML, Vidal-Carou MC. Low-histamine diets: is the exclusion of foods justified by their histamine content? *Nutrients*. 2021;13(5):1395. doi:10.3390/nu13051395; Bent RK, Kugler C, Faihs V, Darsow U, Biedermann T, Brockow K. Placebo-controlled histamine challenge disproves suspicion of histamine intolerance. *J Allergy Clin Immunol Pract*. 2023;11(12):3724-3731.e11. doi:10.1016/j.jaip.2023.08.030.

Wheat Intolerance

Wheat, a staple in many diets, contains complex proteins and carbohydrates that can induce food intolerance. The protein component primarily consists of gluten, a mixture of gliadin and glutenin proteins.[76] Gluten is not only prevalent in wheat but also in rye, barley, and oats, contributing to dough quality and consistency in products like pasta, cakes, pastries, and biscuits. Gluten may also act as a binding agent in various processed foods. Additionally, wheat contains α-amylase/trypsin inhibitors (ATIs) and wheat germ agglutinin, which are less prominent but can impact health due to their respective enzymatic inhibition and sugar-binding properties.[77,78] The carbohydrate fraction mainly includes fructans, discussed in the FODMAP section due to their role in digestive discomfort.

Beyond CD (as discussed previously in Chapter 11, *Nutritional Management of Gastrointestinal Malabsorption*) and wheat allergy, gluten consumption is linked with **non-celiac gluten sensitivity (NCGS)**. NCGS is a clinical condition characterized by both GI and extraintestinal symptoms that manifest after the ingestion of gluten-containing foods in individuals without CD-related antibodies or elevated specific IgE levels.[77,78] The prevalence of NCGS varies widely, reported between 0.6% and 6%, likely due to the absence of specific biomarkers for its diagnosis.[78] NCGS predominantly affects females in their third to fourth decade of life.[78] Symptoms, which can appear within hours to days after gluten consumption, include abdominal pain, bloating, diarrhea, and nausea, along with extraintestinal manifestations such as fatigue, eczema-like rashes, and neurological disturbances like gluten ataxia and "foggy mind."[76,78] Unlike CD, individuals with NCGS do not exhibit intestinal damage or autoantibodies typical of CD and generally lack the HLA-DQ2 or HLA-DQ8 genotypes associated with CD.[78]

The pathophysiology behind wheat-related intolerances is not fully understood due to inconsistent clinical responses. Potential mechanisms include the activation of both innate and adaptive immune responses, alterations in intestinal permeability, and shifts in gut microbiota.[76,78] ATIs may exacerbate these responses by activating immune cells through toll-like receptor 4, leading to inflammation that could potentially affect other bodily systems.[78] Wheat germ agglutinin has also been shown to increase intestinal permeability and contribute to immune-mediated damage at the epithelial level.[76]

The dietary management of NCGS typically incorporates a gluten-reduced diet complemented by a low-FODMAP and ATI-free regimen to alleviate symptoms.[78] This approach addresses the complexities involved with the simultaneous presence of fructans and gluten in wheat, which often obscures the identification of the primary irritant. Recent studies suggest that fructans may exert a more significant role in triggering NCGS symptoms than gluten, underscoring the importance of a low-FODMAP diet in managing this condition effectively.[78]

Monitoring and Evaluation

Monitoring patients with food allergy or food intolerance would include following growth trends and developmental evaluation of feeding skills in children, evaluating weight/body mass index in adults, and assessing diet records and meal patterns to assess for appropriate energy, protein, and micronutrient consumption. Identifying the continuation, resolution, or reemergence of physical symptoms associated with food intake can provide data about the success of any interventions. It is important to evaluate patient and/or caretaker knowledge to reduce the risk of unintentional exposure. Since previous negative experiences with food reactions can decrease nutrition quality of life, it is critical to identify

Clinical Roundtable

Racial and Socioeconomic Barriers to Diagnosing and Managing Food Allergies

The diagnosis and management of food allergies can be extremely challenging. These challenges are often compounded by various racial and socioeconomic disparities. Racial disparities can be found in food allergy prevalence. Black children have higher rates of food allergies[1] with more severe outcomes and higher rates of anaphylaxis.[2] Challenges with diagnosis of skin-related conditions in people of color can lead to underdiagnosis. For example, "redness" is often described as an identifying symptom associated with atopic dermatitis, eczema, and skin rashes but this may present as variable color shades (dark brown or gray) in darker skin. Economic disparities can impact allergy testing and treatment, which is often associated with greater out-of-pocket costs which can be burdensome for the financially constrained. Allergy management can be challenging for some since medications may be expensive and not covered by health insurance. Additionally, the Special Supplemental Nutrition Program Women, Infant, and Children (WIC) and Supplemental Nutrition Assistance Programs (SNAP) provide coverage of only certain foods that can be a barrier for the food insecure. Finally, there has been limited research on food allergies in people of color, which may impact treatment efficacy.

Roundtable Discussion

1. How can you as a clinician minimize the impacts of racial and economic disparities related to food allergy diagnosis and management in your patient population?
2. What questions can you pose to your patients to address these disparities?

References

Gupta RS, Warren CM, Smith BM, Blumenstock JA, Jiang J, Davis MM, Nadeau KC. The public health impact of parent-reported childhood food allergies in the United States. *Pediatrics*. 2018;142(6):e20181235. doi:10.1542/peds.2018-1235. Erratum in: *Pediatrics*. 2019;143(3):e20183835. doi:10.1542/peds.2018-383; Warren CM, Jiang J, Gupta RS. Epidemiology and burden of food allergy. *Curr Allergy Asthma Rep*. 2020;20(2):6. doi:10.1007/s11882-020-0898-7; American College of Allergy, Asthma & Immunology; Allergy & Asthma Network. *Eczema in skin of color*. Accessed March 7, 2025. https://eczemainskinofcolor.org/

any unnecessary overrestriction or signs of disordered eating. It is vital to assess for any barriers to adequate intake in children due to school food availability, caretaker knowledge, or food insecurity (see Clinical Roundtable).

Additional Information and Resources

Additional resources related to food allergies:

American College of Allergy, Asthma & Immunology: https://acaai.org/

Allergy and Asthma Network: https://allergyasthmanetwork.org/food-allergies/

Food Allergy Research and Education: https://www.foodallergy.org/

Food and Drug Administration: https://www.fsis.usda.gov/food-safety/safe-food-handling-and-preparation/food-safety-basics/food-allergies-big-9

National Eczema Association: https://nationaleczema.org/

Chapter Summary

Understanding food allergies is crucial for effective management and improving patient outcomes. Food allergies can trigger a range of symptoms from mild to severe, including life-threatening anaphylaxis, primarily mediated through IgE antibodies. Accurate diagnosis of IgE-mediated food allergy is confirmed through various methods such as SPTs, serum-specific IgE testing, and OFCs. Management strategies consist of allergen avoidance, pharmacological interventions, and potentially oral immunotherapy. Non-IgE-mediated and mixed IgE/non-IgE food allergies such as FPIES and EoE affect the GI tract, often presenting with delayed symptoms that require careful clinical management. RDs play a significant role in helping patients navigate safe dietary practices. This includes educating them on how to read food labels carefully and providing allergen-free alternatives to ensure nutritional balance.

Key Terms

Adverse reactions to food (ARF), food allergy, celiac disease (CD), food protein–induced enterocolitis syndrome (FPIES), eosinophilic esophagitis (EoE), food intolerance, sensitization, atopic dermatitis, allergic rhinitis, erythematous rashes, pruritus, urticaria, angioedema, rhinorrhea, oral allergy syndrome (OAS), alpha-gal syndrome (AGS), skin prick test (SPT), serum-specific IgE testing, oral food challenge (OFC), oral immunotherapy (OIT), desensitization, sustained unresponsiveness (SU), cow's milk allergy (CMA), parvalbumin, wheat-dependent exercise-induced anaphylaxis (WDEIA), baker's asthma, food protein–induced allergic proctocolitis (FPIAP), eosinophilic gastrointestinal disorders (EGIDs), hydrogen breath test (HBT), non-celiac gluten sensitivity (NCGS)

References

1. Onyimba F, Crowe SE, Johnson S, Leung J. Food allergies and intolerances: a clinical approach to the diagnosis and management of adverse reactions to food. *Clin Gastroenterol Hepatol*. 2021;19(11):2230–2240.e1.
2. Sindher SB, Long A, Chin AR, et al. Food allergy, mechanisms, diagnosis and treatment: innovation through a multi-targeted approach. *Allergy*. 2022;77(10):2937–2948.
3. Sicherer SH, Sampson HA. Food allergy: a review and update on epidemiology, pathogenesis, diagnosis, prevention, and management. *J Allergy Clin Immunol*. 2018;141(1):41–58.
4. Gupta RS, Warren CM, Smith BM, et al. Prevalence and severity of food allergies among US adults. *JAMA Netw Open*. 2019;2(1):e185630.
5. Waserman S, Bégin P, Watson W. IgE-mediated food allergy. *Allergy Asthma Clin Immuno*. 2018;14(Suppl 2):55. doi:10.1186/s13223-018-0284-3
6. Bird JA, Burks AW. Food allergy. In: Rich RR, Fleisher TA, Schroeder HW, Weyand CM, Corry DB, Puck JM, eds. *Clinical Immunology: Principles and Practice*. 6th ed. Elsevier; 2023:623–629.
7. Radlović N, Leković Z, Radlović V, Simić D, Ristić D, Vuletić B. Food allergy in children. *Srp Arh Celok Lek*. 2016;144(1–2):99–103.
8. Jeong K, Lee S. Natural course of IgE-mediated food allergy in children. *Clin Experiment Pediatr.* 2023;66(12):504–511.
9. Anvari S, Miller J, Yeh C-Y, Davis CM. IgE-mediated food allergy. *Clin Rev Allergy Immunol*. 2019;57(2):244–260.
10. Tedner SG, Asarnoj A, Thulin H, Westman M, Konradsen JR, Nilsson C. Food allergy and hypersensitivity reactions in children and adults—A review. *J Intern Med*. 2021;291(3):283–302.
11. Ramsey N, Berin MC. Pathogenesis of IgE-mediated food allergy and implications for future immunotherapeutics. *Pediatr Allergy Immunol*. 2021;32(7):1416–1425.
12. Wang J, Zhou Y, Zhang H, et al. Pathogenesis of allergic diseases and implications for therapeutic interventions. *Signal Transduct Target Ther*. 2023;8(1):1–30.
13. Zellweger F, Eggel A. IgE-associated allergic disorders: recent advances in etiology, diagnosis, and treatment. *Allergy*. 2016;71(12):1652–1661.
14. Allen KJ, Koplin JJ, Ponsonby AL, et al. Vitamin D insufficiency is associated with challenge-proven food allergy in infants. *J Allergy Clin Immunol*. 2013;131(4):1109–1116.e6. doi:10.1016/j.jaci.2013.01.017
15. Jaros J, Shi VY, Katta R. Diet and Chronic urticaria: dietary modification as a treatment strategy. *Dermatol Pract Concept*. 2019;10(1):e2020004. doi:10.5826/dpc.1001a04
16. Jeong K. Food-dependent exercise-induced anaphylaxis: the need for better understanding and management of the disease. *Allergy Asthma Immunol Res*. 2022;14(4):345.
17. Taylor SL, Baumert JL. Food allergies and intolerances. In: Erdman JW, Macdonald IA, Zeisel SH, eds. *Present Knowledge in Nutrition*. Wiley-Blackwell; 2012.
18. Macdougall JD, Thomas KO, Iweala OI. The meat of the matter: understanding and managing Alpha-Gal syndrome. *ImmunoTargets Ther.* 2022;11:37–54.
19. Anvari S, Ruffner MA, Nowak-Wegrzyn A. Current and future perspectives on the consensus guideline for food protein-induced enterocolitis syndrome (FPIES). *Allergol Int*. 2024;73(2):188–195. doi:10.1016/j.alit.2024.01.006
20. Commins SP. Diagnosis and management of alpha-gal syndrome. Lessons from 2,500 patients. *Expert Rev Clin Immunol*. 2020;16(7):667–677.
21. Shaker MS, Wallace DV, Golden DBK, et al. Anaphylaxis—a 2020 practice parameter update, systematic review, and grading of recommendations, assessment, development and evaluation (GRADE) analysis. *J Allergy Clin Immunol*. 2020;145(4):1082–1123.
22. Cardona V, Ansotegui IJ, Ebisawa M, et al. World Allergy Organization Anaphylaxis Guidance 2020. *World Allergy Organ J*. 2020;13(10):100472. doi:10.1016/j.waojou.2020.100472
23. Turner PJ, Worm M, Ansotegui IJ, et al. Time to revisit the definition and clinical criteria for anaphylaxis? *World Allergy Organ J*. 2019;12(10):100066. doi:10.1016/j.waojou
24. Loprinzi Brauer CE, Motosue MS, Li JT, et al. Prospective validation of the NIAID/FAAN criteria for emergency department diagnosis of anaphylaxis. *J Allergy Clin Immunol Pract*. 2016;4(6):1220–1226.
25. Grabenhenrich LB, Dölle S, Moneret-Vautrin A, et al. Anaphylaxis in children and adolescents: the European Anaphylaxis Registry. *J Allergy Clin Immunol*. 2016;137(4):1128–1137.e1.
26. Santos AF, Riggioni C, Agache I, et al. EAACI guidelines on the diagnosis of IgE-mediated food allergy. *Allergy*. 2023;78(12):3057–3076. doi:10.1111/all.15902
27. Calvani M, Bianchi A, Reginelli C, Peresso M, Testa A. Oral food challenge. *Medicina*. 2019;55(10):651. doi:10.3390/medicina55100651
28. De Almeida Kotchetkoff EC, De Oliveira LCL, Sarni ROS. Elimination diet in food allergy: friend or foe? *Jornal De Pediatria*. 2023;100:S65–S73.
29. Brotons-Canto A, Martín-Arbella N, Gamazo C, Irache JM. New pharmaceutical approaches for the treatment of food allergies. *Expert Opin Drug Deliv*. 2018;15(7):675–686.
30. Pouessel G, Lezmi G. Oral immunotherapy for food allergy: translation from studies to clinical practice? *World*

Allergy Organ J. 2023;16(2):100747. doi:10.1016/j.waojou.2023.100747
31. Vickery BP, Scurlock AM, Kulis M, et al. Sustained unresponsiveness to peanut in subjects who have completed peanut oral immunotherapy. *J Allergy Clin Immunol*. 2014;133(2):468–475. doi:10.1016/j.jaci.2013.11.007
32. Jones SM, Burks AW, Keet C, et al. Long-term treatment with egg oral immunotherapy enhances sustained unresponsiveness that persists after cessation of therapy. *J Allergy Clin Immunol*. 2016;137(4):1117–1127.e10. doi:10.1016/j.jaci.2015.12.1316
33. Hise K, Rabin RL. Oral immunotherapy for food allergy—a US regulatory perspective. *Curr Allergy Asthma Rep*. 2020;20(12):77.
34. Casale TB, Fiocchi A, Greenhawt M. A Practical guide for implementing omalizumab therapy for food allergy. *J Allergy Clin Immunol*. 2024;153(6):1510–1517. doi:10.1016/j.jaci.2024.03.01
35. Wood RA, Chinthrajah RS, Spergel AKR, et al. Protocol design and synopsis: omalizumab as monotherapy and as adjunct therapy to multiallergen OIT in children and adults with food allergy (OUtMATCH). *J Allergy Clin Immunol Global*. 2022;1(4):225–232.
36. Du Toit G, Tsakok T, Lack S, et al. Prevention of food allergy. *J Allergy Clin Immunol*. 2016;137(4):998–1010. doi:10.1016/j.jaci.2016.02.005.
37. Du Toit G, Katz Y, Sasieni P, et al. Early consumption of peanuts in infancy is associated with a low prevalence of peanut allergy. *J Allergy Clin Immunol*. 2008;122:984–991.
38. Warren CM, Agrawal A, Gandhi D, Gupta RS. The US population-level burden of cow's milk allergy. *World Allergy Organ J*. 2022;15(4):100644. doi:10.1016/j.waojou.2022.100644
39. Robert E, Al-Hashmi HA, Al-Mehaidib A, et al. Symptoms and management of cow's milk allergy: perception and evidence. *Front Allergy*. 2024;5. doi.10.3389/falgy.2024.1348769
40. Samady W, Warren C, Wang J, Das R, Gupta RS. Egg allergy in US children. *J Allergy Clin Immunol Pract*. 2020;8(9):3066–3073.e6.
41. Anagnostou A. Optimizing patient care in egg allergy diagnosis and treatment. *J Asthma Allergy*. 2021;14:621–628.
42. McWilliam V, Koplin J, Lodge C, Tang M, Dharmage S, Allen K. The prevalence of tree nut allergy: a systematic review. *Curr Allergy Asthma Rep*. 2015;15(9):54.
43. Liu M, Burks AW, Green TD. Tree nut allergy: risk factors for development, mitigation of reaction risk and current efforts in desensitization. *Expert Rev Clin Immunol*. 2015;11:673–679.
44. Togias A, Cooper SF, Acebal ML, et al. Addendum guidelines for the prevention of peanut allergy in the United States: report of the National Institute of Allergy and Infectious Diseases–sponsored expert panel. *J Allergy Clin Immunol*. 2017;139:29–44.
45. Kashyap RR, Kashyap RS. Oral allergy syndrome: an update for stomatologists. *J Allergy*. 2015;2015:1–6.
46. Leung ASY, Fusayasu N, Álvarez LA, Gu Y, Ebisawa M, Wong GWK. Fish allergy management: should fish be completely avoided? The pros and cons debate. *J Allergy Hypersensitivity Dis*. 2024;2:100008.
47. Dijkema D, Emons JAM, Van de Ven AAJM, Elberink JNGO. Fish allergy: fishing for novel diagnostic and therapeutic options. *Clin Rev Allergy Immunol*. 2020;62(1):64–71.
48. Davis CM, Gupta RS, Aktas ON, Diaz V, Kamath SD, Lopata AL. Clinical management of seafood allergy. *J Allergy Clin Immunol Pract*. 2020;8(1):37–44.
49. Wai CYY, Leung NYH, Chu KH, et al. Overcoming shellfish allergy: how far have we come? *Int J Molecul Sci*. 2020;21(6):2234.
50. Liu W, Wu Y, Wang J, et al. A meta-analysis of the prevalence of wheat allergy worldwide. *Nutrients*. 2023;15(7):1564.
51. Scherf KA, Brockow K, Biedermann T, Koehler P, Wieser H. Wheat-dependent exercise-induced anaphylaxis. *Clin Exp Allergy*. 2016;46:10–20.
52. Cianferoni A. Wheat allergy: diagnosis and management. *J Asthma Allergy*. 2016;9:13–25.
53. Savage JH, Kaeding AJ, Matsui EC, Wood RA. The natural history of soy allergy. *J Allergy Clin Immunol*. 2010;125(3):683–686.
54. Oriel RC, Elizur A, Sicherer SH. Comprehensive diagnosis, management, and treatment of sesame allergy. *J Allergy Clin Immunol Pract*. 2023;12(3):590–597.
55. Zhang S, Sicherer S, Berin MC, Agyemang A. Pathophysiology of non-IgE-mediated food allergy. *ImmunoTargets Ther*. 2021;10:431–446.
56. Leonard SA, Pecora V, Fiocchi AG, Nowak-Wegrzyn A. Food protein-induced enterocolitis syndrome: a review of the new guidelines. *World Allergy Organ J*. 2018;11(1):4. doi:10.1186/s40413-017-0182-z
57. Cherian S, Varshney P. Food Protein-Induced Enterocolitis Syndrome (FPIES): review of recent guidelines. *Curr Allergy Asthma Rep*. 2018;18(4):28.
58. Agyemang A, Nowak-Wegrzyn A. Food protein-induced enterocolitis syndrome: a comprehensive review. *Clin Rev Allergy Immunol*. 2019;57(2):261–271.
59. Nowak-Węgrzyn A. Food protein-induced enterocolitis syndrome and allergic proctocolitis. *Allergy Asthma Proc*. 2015;36(3):172–184.
60. Mennini M, Fiocchi AG, Cafarotti A, et al. Food protein-induced allergic proctocolitis in infants: literature review and proposal of a management protocol. *World Allergy Organ J*. 2020;13(10):100471.
61. Collins MH, Capocelli K, Yang G-Y. Eosinophilic gastrointestinal disorders pathology. *Front Med*. 2018;4:261. doi:10.3389/fmed.2017.00261
62. Dellon ES, Liacouras CA, Molina-Infante J, et al. Updated international consensus diagnostic criteria for eosinophilic esophagitis: proceedings of the AGREE conference. *Gastroenterol*. 2018;155(4):1022–1033.e10.
63. Reed CC, Dellon ES. Eosinophilic esophagitis. *Med Clin North Am*. 2019;103(1):29–42.
64. Dellon ES, Kim HP, Sperry SLW, Rybnicek DA, Woosley JT, Shaheen NJ. A phenotypic analysis shows that eosinophilic esophagitis is a progressive fibrostenotic disease. *Gastrointest Endosc*. 2014;79(4):577–585.e4.
65. Muir A, Falk GW. Eosinophilic esophagitis. *JAMA*. 2021;326(13):1310.
66. Biedermann L, Straumann A. Mechanisms and clinical management of eosinophilic oesophagitis: an overview. *Nature Rev Gastroenterol Hepatol*. 2022;20(2):101–119.
67. Thel HL, Anderson C, Xue AZ, Jensen ET, Dellon ES. Prevalence and costs of eosinophilic esophagitis in the United States. *Clin Gastroenterol Hepatol*. 2025;23(2):272–280.e8. doi:10.1016/j.cgh.2024.09.031.

68. Tuck CJ, Biesiekierski JR, Schmid-Grendelmeier P, Pohl D. Food intolerances. *Nutrients*. 2019;11(7):1684.
69. Gargano D, Appanna R, Santonicola A, et al. Food allergy and intolerance: a narrative review on nutritional concerns. *Nutrients*. 2021;13(5):1638.
70. Zingone F, Bertin L, Maniero D, et al. Myths and facts about food intolerance: a narrative review. *Nutrients*. 2023;15(23):4969.
71. Szilagyi A, Ishayek N. Lactose intolerance, dairy avoidance, and treatment options. *Nutrients*. 2018;10(12):1994.
72. Catanzaro R, Sciuto M, Marotta F. Lactose intolerance: an update on its pathogenesis, diagnosis, and treatment. *Nutr Res*. 2021;89:23–34.
73. De Geyter C, Van de Maele K, Hauser B, Vandenplas Y. Hydrogen and methane breath test in the diagnosis of lactose intolerance. *Nutrients*. 2021;13(9):3261.
74. Viswanathan L, Rao SS. Intestinal disaccharidase deficiency in adults: evaluation and treatment. *Current Gastroenterol Rep*. 2023;25(6):134–139.
75. Facioni MS, Raspini B, Pivari F, Dogliotti E, Cena H. Nutritional management of lactose intolerance: the importance of diet and food labelling. *J Translation Med*. 2020;18(1):260. doi:10.1186/s12967-020-02429-2.
76. Roszkowska A, Pawlicka M, Mroczek A, Bałabuszek K, Nieradko-Iwanicka B. Non-celiac gluten sensitivity: a review. *Medicina*. 2019;55(6):222.
77. Barbaro MR, Cremon C, Stanghellini V, Barbara G. Recent advances in understanding non-celiac gluten sensitivity. *F1000Research*. 2018;7:1631. doi:10.12688/f1000research.15849.1
78. Singla D, Malik T, Singh A, Thakur S, Kumar P. Advances in understanding wheat-related disorders: a comprehensive review on gluten-free products with emphasis on wheat allergy, celiac and non-celiac gluten sensitivity. *Food Chemistry Advances*. 2024;4:100627.

CHAPTER 16

Nutrition in Solid Organ Transplantation

Lauren Parsly Read-Button
Jessica Seltz Porto
Lily Lichtenstein-Swain

CHAPTER OUTLINE

Core Concepts
Introduction
Background
Indications and Contraindications for Transplantation
Medical Treatment
Nutritional Assessment
Nutrition Intervention
Monitoring and Evaluation

CORE CONCEPTS

1. Medical advances have made solid organ transplants a viable option for many people with end-stage organ failure.
2. Recipients of organ transplants are those who are deemed to be able to survive the rigors of surgery and recovery and go on to lead productive, higher-quality lives for many years following the transplant.
3. As recipients of organ transplants live longer, there is an increased risk of chronic issues from long-term use of immunosuppressants.
4. Postoperative nutritional management should be individualized according to the patient's nutritional status, the organ transplanted, and any complications that may arise during or after surgery.

LEARNING OBJECTIVES

1. Describe indications and contraindications for solid organ transplants.
2. Recognize complications that can arise from solid organ transplantation.
3. Identify immunosuppressant medications and their nutritional implications.
4. Estimate short-term and long-term nutritional needs for patients who have undergone solid organ transplants.

Introduction

The number of recipients awaiting solid organ transplants, which include kidney, heart, liver, lung, pancreas, and small bowel transplantation, continues to increase each year. Organ transplantation is considered life-saving surgery or a last stage intervention to improve one's quality of life. Medical nutrition therapy has an important role throughout all phases of the transplantation process. Early preoperative nutrition intervention is essential to optimize surgery outcomes, while long-term postoperative monitoring is vital to prevent the development of chronic disease.

Background

The act of transplanting one part of the body, or part of someone else's body, onto another has been around for several millennia. Hindu texts dating from 2500 to 3000 BCE describe skin grafts taken from the buttocks and chin and molded to make new noses on criminals who had lost theirs to punishment.[1] A graft is any tissue or organ used for implantation or transplantation, while a host is the recipient of the organ or tissue. There has been evidence from the Bronze Age of both autograft transplantation and allograft transplantation of bone, skin, and teeth.[1] Autograft transplantation, also known as "autotransplantation," is defined as transplantation of a tissue or an organ from one site onto another one or in the body of the same individual. Allograft transplantation, also known as "allotransplantation" or "allogenic transplantation," describes a graft of tissue transplanted between individuals of the same species but of disparate genotype; types of donors can be cadaveric, living related, and living unrelated. Some solid organ transplants are characterized as **orthotopic**, which describes something that occurs in the usual place in the body, such as tissue or an organ that is transplanted into its usual place in the body.

It was not until the early 1900s that advances in surgical and clinical skills allowed solid organ transplantation experimentation to garner attention. In 1902, French surgeon Alexis Carrel wrote a paper detailing successful kidney reimplantation in the neck of the same dog and later, between two dogs.[1] Through his experiments, Dr. Carrel noted that unsuccessful organ transplants were due to host rejection of the transplant.[1] Rejection is an immune reaction against grafted tissue that results in failure of the graft to survive. In 1954, successful kidney transplants were achieved in monozygotic twins.[1] The surgeries were performed by Dr. Joseph Murray and Dr. John Merrill at the Peter Bent Brigham Hospital, and they identified that genetic matching of the allograft transplantation donor and recipient was necessary.

In lieu of genetic matching, it was soon discovered that **immunosuppression**, or suppression of the immune response by medications or radiation, could decrease the rate of host rejection of the transplanted organ.[1] By suppressing the immune system, the organ recipient has a decreased risk of immune cells identifying the transplanted organ as an invading body and attacking it. Blunt irradiation of the organ recipient led to premature deaths, not from host rejection, but from the effects of the radiation.[1] The discovery of using a combination of immunosuppressive medications to eliminate organ rejection from nongenetically matched donors opened the door to organ transplantation with both live and deceased donors as a viable option to save lives.[1] Today, many immunosuppressive medications such as tacrolimus and mycophenolate mofetil are widely used in organ transplantation. They are so effective in suppressing the immune system that 90–95% of recipients of kidney transplants and 85% of recipients of heart transplants survive 1 year after their surgery.[2,3]

As recipients of organ transplants live longer, additional problems occur due to the effects of the immunosuppressive medications. Recipients of organs face increased risk of viral, bacterial, and other pathogenic infections that their bodies are no longer able to resist. As organ transplantation moves into the 21st century and antibiotic development advances, organ transplantation and immunosuppression have the highest success rate thus far. Doctors can successfully transplant hearts, kidneys, lungs, livers, intestines, and pancreas. According to the Organ Procurement and Transplantation Network, more than 105,000 candidates on the U.S. organ transplant waiting list await one or more solid organ(s).[4] An individual's placement on the organ waitlist varies by organ, but allocation involves many considerations, including degree of illness and medical urgency, blood type, waiting time, donor/recipient immune system compatibility, pediatric status, height or weight, and distance from the donor hospital.[5]

In 2023, there were 46,632 transplants performed based on data from the United Network for Organ Sharing (UNOS).[4] Specifically, 10,824 Black patients received transplants last year, more than any year prior.[6] The demand for organs continues to exceed the supply available. Survival rates vary according to recipient sex, age, diagnosis, organ, blood type, age, and vital status (deceased versus living) of the

CASE STUDY INTRODUCTION

George is a 59-year-old male with ischemic cardiomyopathy, an ejection fraction (EF) of 15%, type 2 diabetes mellitus, and hypertension (HTN). He presents for a nutrition assessment as part of an interprofessional pretransplant evaluation for a heart transplant. His cardiovascular history includes a myocardial infarction 5 years ago, requiring percutaneous coronary intervention (PCI); a cardiac arrest 2 years ago; and an implantable cardioverter defibrillator (ICD) placement last year. George has had several hospital admissions over the last year due to decompensated heart failure and recently started on home milrinone. George had been working in construction but has been unable to work over the previous few months due to progressive shortness of breath (SOB) and fatigue. He is divorced and currently lives alone.

Anthropometric Data:

Weight: 115 kg
Height: 178 cm
Body mass index (BMI): 36 kg/m^2

Weight History
Usual body weight (UBW): 126 kg, 6 months ago
Recent highest weight: 132 kg, 3 months ago, in the setting of volume overload
Estimated dry weight: 113 kg

Biochemical Data:

Sodium 132 (136–145 mEq/L)
Potassium 4.2 (3.5–5.0 mEq/L)
Blood urea nitrogen 23 (8–20 mg/dL)
Creatinine 1.0 (0.7–1.3 mg/dL)
Blood glucose 169 (70–139 mg/dL)

Total cholesterol 140 (Desirable <200 mg/dL)
Low-density lipoprotein 69 (Desirable <100 mg/dL)
High-density lipoprotein 19 (Desirable ≥40 mg/dL)
Triglycerides: 200 (Desirable <150 mg/dL)
HbA1c 7.5% (4.3–5.6%)

Clinical Data:

Past Medical History: Ischemic cardiomyopathy with EF 15%, MI, s/p PCI, ICD placement, type 2 diabetes mellitus, left leg deep vein thrombosis, obstructive sleep apnea, obesity, hypertension, dyslipidemia, and depressive order

Medications: atorvastatin, carvedilol, furosemide, insulin glargine 18 units at bedtime, insulin lispro 8 units three times daily, losartan, milrinon, potassium chloride 20 mEq, warfarin

Vital Signs: Blood pressure: 98/70 mm Hg; Temperature 98.6° F; Heart rate 100 beats/min

Nutrition-Focused Physical Exam: Appears obese with central adiposity. Skin feels warm to touch, appears slightly dry. There is evidence of pitting edema on legs bilaterally. Good dentition noted with normal mouth and tongue. No wounds or skin breakdown noted. No obvious SOB noted when in conversation. Evidence of mild muscle mass loss observed in biceps and quadriceps.

Dietary Data:

Dietary History: George reports decreased appetite in comparison to baseline over the last 1–2 months. He continues to eat three meals per day, but portion sizes are smaller than he usually eats. He does not count carbohydrates but has been trying to follow a low-sodium diet by not adding salt to foods. Due to SOB and fatigue, he has been eating more prepared/take-out foods lately.

Diet Prescription: low sodium, 1.5-L fluid restriction, consistent carbohydrate

Questions

1. Is George an appropriate candidate for heart transplant? Why or why not?
2. Should weight loss be encouraged?
3. Does George have any nutrition-related contraindications to transplant?
4. Write two Problem/Etiology/Signs and Symptoms (PES) statements for George.
5. Identify the nutrition interventions you would like to initiate for George to address the problems identified in your PES statements.
6. What indices are included in your monitoring and evaluation plan? Why?

donor. For example, the median survival period for recipients of heart transplants ranges from 11 to 14 years.[3] Median survival for deceased donor transplants increased from 8.2 years during 1995–1999 to an estimated 11.7 years in the most recent era. Living kidney donor transplant median survival increased from 12.1 years during 1995–1999 to an estimated 19.2 years for transplants during 2014–2017.[7]

CORE CONCEPT 1

Medical advances have made solid organ transplants a viable option for many people with end-stage organ failure.

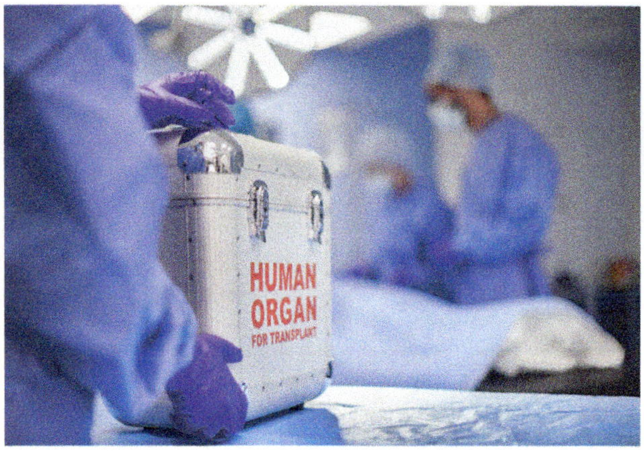

Indications and Contraindications for Transplantation

Who is a candidate for organ transplant? Individuals with decompensated end-stage organ failure are eligible to be placed on the organ waitlist. This is a life-saving surgery for individuals who need heart, liver, and lung transplants. While dialysis, insulin therapy, and parenteral nutrition (PN) are alternative treatments for patients with kidney, pancreatic, and intestinal failure, respectively, life-threatening complications may lead to loss of intravenous (IV) access for PN or dialysis, necessitating alternative options. The benefits of transplantation must outweigh the risks associated with major surgery and long-term immunosuppression.

Kidney Transplant Indications

There are a number of diseases and etiologies leading to end-stage kidney disease (ESKD), such as glomerulonephritis, hypertension, diabetes, congenital abnormalities, polycystic kidney disease, or urinary tract obstruction.[8] Diabetic nephropathy and hypertensive nephrosclerosis are the most common causes of ESKD.[9] In the absence of contraindications, kidney transplantation is indicated when a patient reaches ESKD, which is demonstrated by either requiring dialysis or having a GFR of ≤20 mg/dL (**Figure 16.1**).[10]

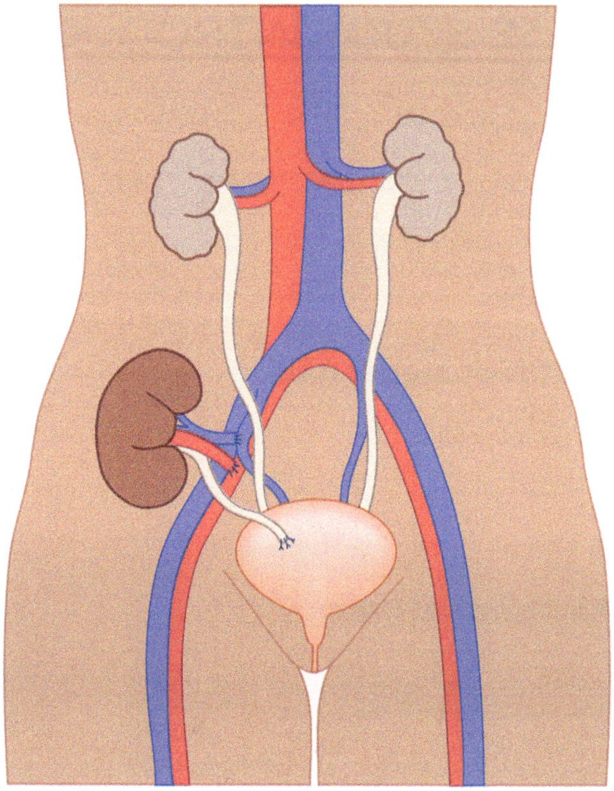

Figure 16.1 Kidney Post Transplant

Pancreas Transplant Indications

The most common indication for pancreas transplantation is type 1 diabetes, to produce independence from injected insulin. Pancreas transplants are typically done in conjunction with a kidney transplant due to the underlying etiology of diabetes-related ESKD. It is not life-saving surgery, but rather completed as a means of improving quality of life. A small percentage of pancreas transplants are performed for other reasons, such as after a pancreatectomy in the setting of chronic pancreatitis.[11]

Liver Transplant Indications

Alcohol-related liver disease (ALD) is now the number one indication for liver transplantation in the United States, followed closely by metabolic dysfunction–associated steatohepatitis (MASH), which was formerly known as nonalcoholic steatohepatitis (NASH).[12] Hepatitis C virus–related chronic liver disease was previously the most common indication for liver transplantation in the United States until 2015, following the development of direct-acting antiviral (DAA) agents in 2013. Other common etiologies include hepatic malignancy, hepatitis B virus–related chronic liver disease, cholestatic cirrhosis, such as primary biliary cirrhosis, and metabolic diseases, such as Wilson's disease or cystic fibrosis.[13] Acute liver failure is a less common etiology but is a strong indication for transplantation. Prompt transplantation has been found to have good outcomes and therefore supersedes all other etiologies on the waiting list.[13,14] Patients with ALD must abstain from drinking alcohol for at least 6 months prior to placement on the waiting list at most programs.[2]

The Model of End-stage Liver Disease (MELD) score is a validated predictor of 3-month survival with liver disease via a mathematical calculation that incorporates serum levels of creatinine, bilirubin, INR, and now sodium.[15] In most cases, an increasing MELD score would be associated with an increased mortality risk. A MELD score–based allocation system is now used and has been found to reduce waitlist mortality compared with a waiting time allocation system.[15]

Heart Transplant Indications

Chronic heart failure from cardiomyopathy of various etiologies and ischemic heart disease are the most common reasons for a heart transplant (**Figure 16.2**).[2] Patients who are critically ill with heart failure may require placement of a ventricular assist device, a surgically implanted mechanical pump that supports heart function by pumping blood to circulate oxygen-rich blood throughout the body until a donor heart is available. Refer to Chapter 9, *Nutrition in Cardiovascular Disease and Heart Failure*, for additional information about ventricular assist devices.

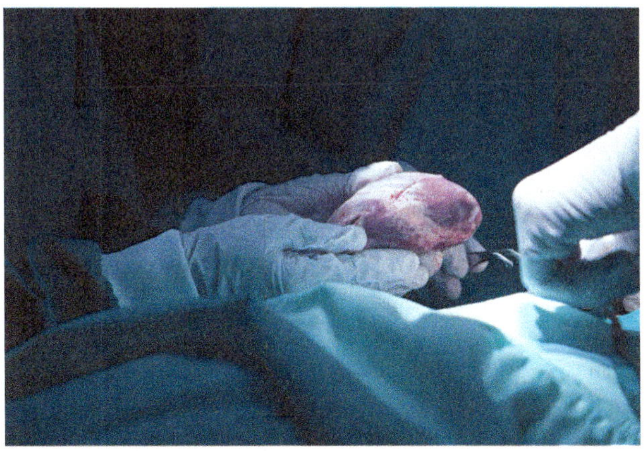

Figure 16.2 Surgeon Performing Heart Transplant

Lung Transplant Indications

The most common diseases requiring lung transplantation are cystic fibrosis, chronic obstructive pulmonary disease (COPD), pulmonary fibrosis, and pulmonary hypertension.[2] Bilateral lung transplants tend to take place more frequently than unilateral lung transplants. Some patients may require both heart and lung transplantation if lung failure precipitated heart failure.[2]

Small Bowel Transplant Indications

Short bowel syndrome, dysmotility syndrome, impaired enterocyte absorption, and failure of PN are common reasons for small bowel transplantation. Medicare usually approves intestinal transplantation in patients with irreversible intestinal failure who have failed PN.[16]

Contraindications to Transplantation

Contraindications for an organ transplant include advanced age, poor posttransplant prognosis, sepsis, malignancies, infections (both active or latent), poor social support, active substance misuse, multisystem organ failure, active psychiatric or psychological pathologies, or inability to adhere to a complex medical regimen, which may be demonstrated by lack of insight or medication nonadherence.[17] Proper evaluation for transplant candidacy requires an interprofessional approach. Registered dietitians (RDs), pharmacists, social workers, medical doctors, surgeons, and financial coordinators collaborate to bring their unique expertise to produce a thorough assessment of participants. Nutritionally, malnutrition and obesity may be contraindications to transplant due to risk for poor surgical outcomes and significantly higher morbidity and mortality compared with other groups.[18] While not an absolute contraindication, obesity has been found to increase a patient's risk of wound complications.[19,20] Patients with obesity must be evaluated by the transplant team for associated comorbidities such as infection, uncontrolled diabetes, uncontrolled blood pressure, or other organ dysfunction to determine transplant recipient candidate suitability.[19]

CORE CONCEPT 2

Recipients of organ transplants are those who are deemed to be able to survive the rigors of surgery and recovery and go on to lead productive, higher-quality lives for many years following the transplant.

Nutritional Considerations

Obesity

In simultaneous pancreas/kidney transplants, obesity (BMI 30–40 kg/m^2) has been found to delay kidney graft function and increase rates of 1-year acute kidney rejection, pancreas graft thrombosis, and patient death.[21] **Graft thrombosis**, or obstruction of blood flow to a graft, can lead to graft rejection. A BMI of >27 kg/m^2 has been associated with increased pancreas and kidney graft loss.[21,22] Obesity has also been associated with a greater risk of graft dysfunction and decreased short- and long-term survival in recipients of lung transplants with the BMI cut off of <27 kg/m^2, as well.[19,23]

Studies have demonstrated a protective effect of overweight and obesity in the heart failure population.[24] The best heart failure outcomes occur in patients who are overweight followed by patients who are obese, while the worst outcomes occur in patients with heart failure who are underweight followed by those with a BMI in the normal range.[24] Patients with obesity who undergo open heart surgery have higher risk for poor wound healing, infection, pulmonary complications, and lower extremity thrombosis. However, having a BMI <18.5 kg/m^2 and BMI of >35 kg/m^2 have been found to increase morbidity and mortality.[18] Despite the uncertainties regarding the impact of obesity on survival in heart failure, there are several potential benefits of weight loss, such as improvement in insulin sensitivity, blood pressure, and lipid profile, for example. It is important to keep in mind that meaningful weight loss may be challenging for patients with limited exercise capacity due to their end-stage organ failure. Additionally, it is crucial to limit loss of lean muscle loss, which can be an unintentional side effect of weight loss.

The protective effect of obesity is not evident in recipients of kidney transplants; however, it has been noticed among those with ESKD specifically on dialysis. In 2011, more than one-third of the recipients of kidney transplants in the United States were categorized as obese.[25] Of these, 23% had a BMI of 30–34.9 kg/m^2, 9.4% had a BMI 35–39.9 kg/m^2, and 2.1% had a BMI ≥40 kg/m^2.[25] A retrospective review of all recipients in the UNOS database from 2004 to 2009 revealed a significantly increased risk for delayed graft function among patients with obesity, with odds ratios rising in parallel with degree of obesity.[25] Overall, the risk of surgical site complications, delayed graft function, and increased hospital length of stay is associated with obesity in recipients of kidney transplants. Recipients with an underweight BMI have poorer graft survival as well as poorer overall survival. While studies appear to support a neutral impact of obesity on long-term graft and patient survival, there is an increased risk of new-onset diabetes.[25] A study that reviewed the U.S. Renal Data System database from 1995 to 1999 found that the survival benefit of kidney transplantation versus remaining on dialysis was lost above a BMI of 41 kg/m^2.[26]

The 2013 American Association for the Study of Liver Disease practice guidelines state that class 3 obesity (BMI ≥40 kg/m^2) is a relative contraindication in liver transplantation.[27] This guideline is based on a 2002 Nair et al.[28] study that reported that 1-, 2-, and 3-year mortality rates were significantly higher in patients with BMI >40 kg/m^2. Underweight status is associated with higher perioperative mortality and poorer patient and graft survival among patients post liver transplant as well.[29]

The use of weight loss medications has become increasingly popular, especially to help those become eligible for a transplant and meet their weight loss goals. The role of the RD in this capacity is to help optimize balanced oral intake, avoid muscle mass loss, and help manage symptoms like nausea or early satiety due to delayed gastric emptying.

Although current literature regarding weight loss prior to transplantation is limited, it is generally recommended to encourage weight loss in the patient with obesity before transplantation.[17] Some studies suggest that bariatric surgery may be a safe and symptomatically beneficial procedure at experienced centers for patients with heart or kidney failure who are obese.[30,31] Overall BMI cutoffs may vary depending on the organ and transplant center.

Malnutrition

Malnutrition can be a complicating factor in solid organ transplantation and has been found to compromise posttransplant survival as well as increase length of hospital stay and wound healing times.[32–36] It is common for individuals with end-stage organ failure to have a degree of malnutrition; for example, 70–79% of patients undergoing liver transplantation are malnourished.[11] Patients must be assessed carefully for signs of deficiencies related to weight loss or malabsorption caused by their end-stage organ disease. Efforts must be made to reverse malnutrition before the patient undergoes transplant surgery to decrease risks of posttransplant complications and comorbidities. Oral nutrition therapy is the preferred method of correcting malnutrition, but enteral nutrition (EN) may be considered to increase caloric intake for patients who are unable to meet their needs orally.

Cachexia

Cachexia is defined by unintentional weight loss caused by catabolism.[37] Cardiac cachexia is associated with increased mortality, but it remains unclear whether nutritional supplementation or other interventions can reverse wasting or improve outcomes.[37] At this time, it is recommended to improve and treat the underlying disease that is driving the catabolic state. Implantation of a mechanical circulatory support device (MCSD), including ventricular assist devices, has been associated with reversing cachexia associated with heart failure as well as improving functional status.[37–39] Some institutions may provide transplants to patients with low-end BMIs or cachexia if they are not eligible for MCSDs.

Frailty

Frailty is a pathobiological process characterized by loss of physiological reserve and increased vulnerability to stressors.[39] It is common in patients with end-stage organ disease who are awaiting organ transplantation. Specifically, it affects mortality on the waitlist and in the posttransplant period. There are a variety of tools to screen for frailty. While some frailty measurements have been validated in certain populations, the best frailty tool to use in other populations remains unclear. Fried Frailty Phenotype (FFP) is the most studied in the kidney transplant population, while the Liver Frailty Index is utilized most frequently for liver transplants. Other screening tools include the 6-minute walk test or hand grip strength test.

Decreased functional status and frailty status are often observed in those with end-stage organ disease. For example, 52% of patients on dialysis were identified as frail using the FFP parameters.[40] Specifically, frailty at the time of transplantation was associated with significantly higher odds of mortality, delayed graft function, longer lengths of stay, and decreased quality of life.[39] Recommended interventions to optimize frail candidates are physical therapy or center-based rehabilitation programs, nutrition supplementation, and targeted protein intake. Frailty does not have to limit access to transplantation, but the goal is to intervene to improve outcomes. Identifying potential reversible components contributing to frailty allows for ways to intervene, optimize timing for transplantation, and improve outcomes.

Medical Treatment

Organ Donation and Matching

Once an organ donor has been evaluated for **brain death**, where irreversible cessation of all brain activity over a period of time has been acknowledged, organs are then evaluated for possible donation. To meet the increasing demand for donated organs, additional avenues are explored to increase organ donation among deceased donors. Donation of organs can also occur after a patient is deceased by means of cardiac death, referred to as **donation after cardiac death (DCD)**. When a deceased organ donor is identified, the UNOS system creates a ranked list of candidates who are appropriate to receive each organ based on blood type, tissue type, body size, medical urgency, waiting time, and geography, as well as other criteria.[5] Heart and lung organs can only survive outside a body for 4–6 hours, so these organs are first offered based on proximity to the donor's hospital.[5] Organ size is also an important consideration because the heart or lung(s) must be able to fit inside the recipient's rib cage. Livers can survive outside the body for 8–12 hours, while kidneys can survive for 24–36 hours.[5] This longer time frame allows patients from a wider geographical area to be considered as recipients of the organ, pending matching blood type and waitlist time. Living kidney and liver donors (**Figure 16.3**) require an assessment by the interprofessional transplant team. Past medical history, social support, and donation intentions are reviewed. Many centers have BMI cutoffs for living donors to minimize surgical complications and infection postoperatively. It has been found that obesity significantly increases the risk of ESKD among living kidney donors.[41]

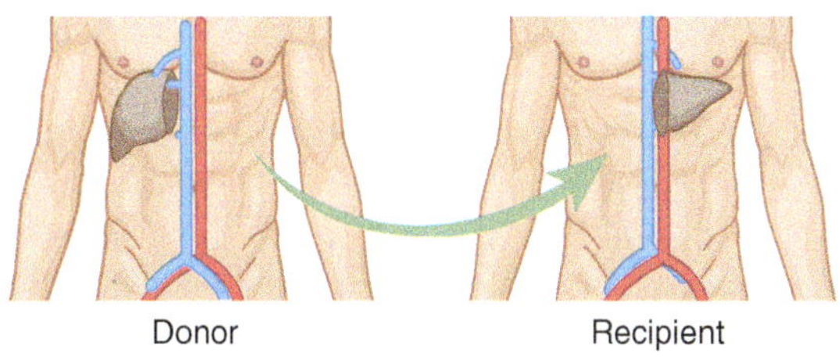

Figure 16.3 Liver Transplantation from Living Donor

Clinical Roundtable

Topic: Weight Loss Prior to Transplantation

Background: The current literature regarding weight loss in end-stage organ failure, especially prior to transplantation, is limited. There is evidence to support that having a BMI in the overweight or obese range may be protective for patients with heart failure and for patients requiring renal replacement therapy. Conversely, there are significant data demonstrating that obesity can increase risk of complications like wound infections or delayed graft function among all transplant candidates. Many patients struggle and often fail to achieve the requested weight loss. Achieving a BMI <30 kg/m^2 is usually the recommended weight loss goal for the general population. It has also been demonstrated that modest weight loss of 5–10% can help with insulin resistance, cholesterol, and blood pressure in healthy individuals. One study has indicated that <10% of potential kidney recipients lose weight when recommended for listing, while <5% reach the goal BMI of <30 kg/m^2. Moreover, many of the patients who lost weight to become eligible on the waiting list had a high risk for quickly regaining weight in the early posttransplant period without significant benefit to transplant outcomes (i.e., survival or graft outcomes). The long-term sustainability of weight maintenance is also a common issue.

Roundtable Discussion

1. Should BMI cutoffs be an absolute contraindication to transplant?
2. Should weight loss be recommended in patients with end-stage organ failure who are overweight or obese despite their compromised medical condition? Why or why not?
3. Should bariatric surgery be considered and, if so, when?

Reference

1. Chan G, Garneau P, Hajjar R. The impact and treatment of obesity in kidney transplant candidates and recipients. *Can J Kidney Health Dis.* 2015;2:26. doi:10.1186/s40697-015-0059-4

Complicating Factors

Rejection

Organ rejection can occur after a transplant. **Rejection** is the body's response to the transplanted organ's foreign proteins, resulting in the body trying to attack the new organ. Acute rejection usually occurs within the first few months, while chronic rejection happens slowly over the years, which can contribute to organ damage. Taking the prescribed immunosuppression medication is the most effective method to avoid rejection, although rejection can still occur.[42]

Immunosuppression

Although patients need to be adequately immunosuppressed for rejection prevention, a balance needs to be maintained to avoid other life-threatening infections and complications. Suppression of the natural immune system of the organ recipient increases the vulnerability of organ recipients to infection and malignancies as they are less able to resist bacteria and viruses or destroy rogue cells that have the potential to become malignant.[2] Induction immunosuppression, an intense prophylactic therapy, is usually administered as a short course during the immediate pre- and postoperative transplant periods to prevent or delay the onset of rejection. This is followed by a long-term immunosuppression regimen, which usually consists of two or more medications from different drug classes with varying mechanisms of action (**Figure 16.4**). Most patients will require a calcineurin inhibitor, such as tacrolimus or cyclosporine, and a DNA synthesis inhibitor, such as mycophenolate mofetil, and some will also require steroids, such as prednisone. Patients will need to take immunosuppressive medications for the rest of their lives, as long as the transplanted organ is still functioning.[2]

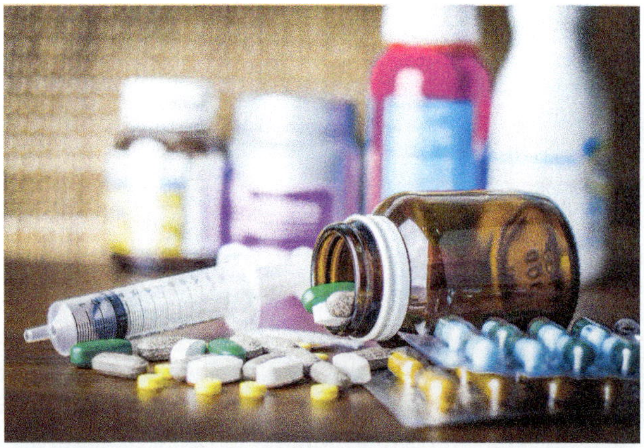

Figure 16.4 There Is a Complex Medication Regimen After Transplantation

The amount of immunosuppression may be tapered to a lower maintenance level 3–6 months after the transplant. The immune system must always be kept in check to avoid rejection of the graft, even years later. Different organs may require varying amounts and combinations of immunosuppressive medications.[2] Immunosuppressive medications come with a variety of side effects that can have nutritional consequences. **Table 16.1** details common side effects and nutrition interventions for immunosuppressive medications.

Table 16.1 Transplant Immunosuppressive Medications, Side Effects, and Interventions

Common Drug Brands and Class	Potential Nutrition Side Effects	Nutrition Intervention
Azathioprine *(Imuran)* ■ Antimetabolite	■ Nausea, vomiting, diarrhea, steatorrhea ■ Stomatitis, esophagitis ■ Anorexia	■ Monitor for adequate nutrient intake. Encourage small, frequent bland meals; consider antiemetic agents; ensure adequate fluid intake; decrease fat in diet for steatorrhea ■ Avoid spicy and acidic foods; consider soft-food diet ■ Monitor oral intake; consider appetite stimulants
Cyclosporine *(Neoral, Sandimmune, Gengraf)* ■ Calcineurin inhibitors	■ Anorexia ■ Gum hyperplasia ■ Hyperglycemia ■ Hyperkalemia ■ Hyperlipidemia ■ Hypertension ■ Hypomagnesemia	■ Avoid grapefruit products ■ Monitor oral intake; consider appetite stimulants ■ Emphasize good oral hygiene; consider soft diet ■ Monitor blood sugar and need for carbohydrate-controlled diet ■ Restrict high-potassium foods ■ Encourage a heart-healthy diet* and maintenance of healthy weight ■ Avoid high-sodium foods and maintain healthy weight ■ Increase high-magnesium foods or consider magnesium supplements
Mycophenolate mofetil *(Cellcept)*, mycophenolic acid *(Myfortic)* ■ Antimetabolite/DNA synthesis inhibitor	■ Nausea, vomiting, constipation, diarrhea ■ Dyspepsia ■ Oral candidiasis, stomatitis ■ Hypomagnesemia ■ Hypercholesterolemia	■ Monitor for adequate nutrient intake. Encourage small, frequent bland meals; consider antiemetic agents; ensure adequate fluid intake; add more fiber and fluid for constipation. Consider nutrition support if oral intake remains suboptimal ■ Avoid caffeine, acidic foods, carbonated beverages ■ Monitor oral intake; emphasize good oral hygiene; consider soft-food diet ■ Increase high-magnesium foods or consider magnesium supplements (supplementation should be taken separately from drug) ■ Encourage heart-healthy diet* and maintenance of healthy weight
Prednisone *(deltasone)*, methylprednisolone *(solumedrol)* ■ Corticosteroid	■ Increased appetite, weight gain ■ Slow wound healing, increased protein catabolism ■ Hyperglycemia ■ Osteoporosis due to calcium wasting ■ Altered fluid and sodium retention, hypertension	■ Educate on balanced meals, portion control, and mindful eating behaviors ■ Ensure adequate protein intake; maintain good blood glucose control; consider need for vitamin/mineral supplements ■ Monitor blood sugar and need for carbohydrate-controlled diet ■ Ensure adequate calcium and vitamin D intake; consider need for bone-building medications ■ Avoid high-sodium foods, maintain a healthy weight
Sirolimus *(Rapamune)*, everolimus *(Zortress)* ■ mTOR inhibitors	■ Nausea, vomiting, diarrhea, constipation ■ Hyperlipidemia	■ Monitor for adequate nutrient intake. Encourage small, frequent bland meals; consider antiemetic agents; ensure adequate fluid intake; add fiber and fluid for constipation ■ Encourage heart-healthy diet* and maintenance of healthy weight

(continues)

Table 16.1 Transplant Immunosuppressive Medications, Side Effects, and Interventions *(continued)*

Common Drug Brands and Class	Potential Nutrition Side Effects	Nutrition Intervention
Tacrolimus *(Prograf)* ■ Calcineurin inhibitor)	■ GI adverse effects such as abdominal pain, dyspepsia, nausea, vomiting, diarrhea, constipation, gastritis ■ Hyperglycemia ■ Hypertension ■ Oral candidiasis, stomatitis, dysphagia ■ Hyperkalemia ■ Hypomagnesemia	■ Avoid grapefruit products ■ Monitor for adequate nutrient intake. Encourage small, frequent bland meals; consider antiemetic agents; ensure adequate fluid intake; add fiber and fluid for constipation. Avoid caffeine, acidic foods, and carbonated beverages with gastritis ■ Monitor blood sugars and need for long-term carbohydrate-controlled diet ■ Avoid high-sodium foods and maintain healthy weight ■ Emphasize good oral hygiene; consider soft diet ■ Avoid high-potassium foods ■ Increase high-magnesium foods or consider magnesium supplements

*A heart-healthy diet is characterized as a diet low in saturated fat and added sugars and high in fiber from whole grains, fruits, and vegetables.
Data from Pronsky ZM, Elbe D, Ayoob K. Food–Medication Interactions. 18th ed. Birchrunville, PA: *Food-Medication Interactions*; 2015.

CORE CONCEPT 3

As recipients of organ transplants live longer, there is an increased risk of chronic issues from long-term use of immunosuppressants.

Nutritional Assessment

As previously mentioned, the transplant RD is an important member of the interprofessional transplant team. In fact, CMS requires that an RD plays a part in transplant evaluation and care. The transplant RD participates in the transplant planning process throughout all phases of donation and transplantation. Before a patient can be placed on the organ transplant waiting list, they must be assessed by the transplant RD, who plays a key role in ensuring optimal nutritional status prior to transplant to allow for adequate healing after surgery. Specifically, medical nutrition therapy is provided to transplant candidates, especially to address modifiable nutritional risks and barriers like malnutrition, obesity, or diabetes management preoperatively as well as medication side effects, which can cause gastrointestinal (GI) issues and electrolyte abnormalities posttransplant. The transplant RD provides education to both candidates and caregivers and, at a minimum, completes nutrition assessments during the transplant evaluation period prior to surgery and then again postoperatively. In addition, living donors are assessed or screened prior to surgery and then again after the surgery.

Pretransplant Phase

Both subjective and objective nutrition status measures can be used in completing nutrition assessments in the transplant population. Objective measures include a weight history based on past medical records; patient's current weight, height, BMI, and percentage weight loss; and laboratory values. It may be difficult to obtain accurate weights on patients pretransplant due to fluid retention and fluid shifts. Body composition is important to evaluate because standard calculations like BMI do not take frame size or lean body mass into consideration. The waist-to-hip ratio (WHR), which is calculated by dividing the waist circumference by the hip (or gluteal) circumference, can be a helpful tool that assesses the proportion of fat stored at the waist and hips.[42] It is preferred that the waist circumference is less than the hip circumference; therefore, a WHR <1 is ideal.[43] There is an increased risk of diabetes, cardiovascular disease, and hypertension with increased abdominal fat.[35] Hemoglobin A1c (HbA1c) is another objective measure used to assess a patient's long-term glycemic control as corticosteroids are often a part of the immunosuppression regimen following transplant. This metric is usually more reflective than diet history but can be skewed if a patient received blood products, erythropoietin-enhancing products, or has history of ESKD. A full subjective global assessment should be performed, and a diet recall/history should be completed to assess adequacy of calorie, fluid, protein, and micronutrient intake.[44] As there are advantages and drawbacks to a variety of methods, it is important to use a combination of objective and subjective measures when assessing a patient's nutritional status.[17]

CASE STUDY REVISITED

George has been approved and placed on the waiting list for a heart transplant. After 9 months on the list, George receives a heart transplant and is now postoperative day (POD) #3. His transplant was uncomplicated. He has been extubated and no longer requires ventilatory support but remains in the ICU for volume overload and hyperglycemia requiring an intravenous insulin infusion.

Anthropometric Data:

Preoperative weight: 115 kg

Current weight: 118 kg

Biochemical Data:

Sodium 139 (136–145 mEq/L)
Potassium 4.1 (3.5–5.0 mEq/L)
Blood urea nitrogen 26 (8–20 mg/dL)
Creatinine 1.6 (0.7–1.3 mg/dL)
Glucose 112 (70–139 mg/dL)

Dietary Data:

Diet Prescription: low bacteria, carbohydrate-controlled diet

Questions

1. What factors should you consider when developing a nutrition plan?
2. What are his acute postop nutrition requirements?
3. Assess George's PES statements from his initial visit. Identify if each statement remains an active issue or if the PES statement has been resolved. If the PES statement remains an active issue, has improvement in the issue been noted? If the issue has been resolved, write a new PES statement.
4. Identify the nutrition interventions you would like to initiate for George to address the problems identified in your PES statements.
5. What indices are included in your monitoring and evaluation plan? Why?

It is also important to inquire about food access, financial vulnerabilities, and food preparation area access since this can limit food availability, influence food security, or play a role in food selection. The RD can partner with the social worker to provide resources like meal delivery services options or food pantries to increase food availability.

Acute Posttransplant Phase

The acute posttransplant period is usually defined as the first few months after surgery. Posttransplant nutrition goals focus on achieving adequate nutrient intake for the patient, providing increased nutrition during the process of healing, and preventing infection and complications of acute rejection. Proper nutrition can help the body resist infections, heal surgical wounds, and enhance strength to participate in physical therapy.[17] Depending on the organ transplanted and any other comorbidities, the patient may be able to start eating within a few days of surgery. For example, following orthotopic heart transplantation, most patients are able to start an oral diet within the first 2–5 days if there are no complications. If the patient is unable to consume an oral diet by this duration, EN or PN may be considered based on the patient's diagnosis. Many medications used to prevent or treat rejection and infection, including antibiotics and antifungal drugs, can cause nausea, vomiting, diarrhea, and changes in taste, and ultimately can impact dietary intake.[45] The side effects of mycophenolate mofetil, a common immunosuppressive agent, are primarily GI issues such as nausea, esophageal reflux, and diarrhea, which can be reduced by decreasing the dosage or substituting with a different medication.[11]

Overall nutrient requirements during the posttransplant period are not well defined and are mostly based on other guidelines, such as critical care nutrition guidelines, or clinical judgment.

Energy

The stress of surgery and side effects from immunosuppressive medications can cause changes in the patient's metabolism posttransplant.[17] If secondary conditions, such as sepsis, are not present, the patient is unlikely to be significantly hypermetabolic posttransplant, so calorie needs are similar to those of other patients postsurgery.[11,17] It is necessary to consider factors such as pretransplant nutritional status and other medical conditions when estimating needs. Studies assessing energy needs among patients post liver transplant during the first posttransplant month found that resting energy expenditure (REE) was 7–42% above predicted values, based on indirect calorimetry results.[17]

Protein

Although not necessarily hypermetabolic, patients posttransplant may have increased protein catabolism, protein losses, and protein oxidation, which can acutely increase protein requirements after surgery.[17,46] Surgical stress and high corticosteroid use in addition to losses from wounds, surgical drains, stomas, dialysis, malnutrition, infection, or acute rejection can contribute to elevated protein needs.[5,46,47] It has been demonstrated in recipients of liver transplants that protein catabolism is increased postoperatively as evidenced by excretion of large quantities of urinary nitrogen.[47] The use of steroids is a main cause of increased protein oxidation; higher steroid doses are given during the acute phase, which leads to increased protein needs.[17,46] As the steroid dose is tapered, protein needs will also likely decrease.[17] Additionally, recipients of heart and lung transplants that require sternotomy will have increased protein needs of 1.5–2 g/kg.[48,49]

Fluid

Fluid needs may be increased due to fluid losses from diarrhea, wounds, surgical drains, and urine and ostomy output. Fluid status must be monitored closely because excess fluid administration and/or decreased urine output can lead to fluid overload. Adequate hydration is usually encouraged to avoid nephrotoxic effects of some medications, such as tacrolimus.

Additional Metabolic Abnormalities

It is common to observe electrolyte abnormalities after transplantation. In the acute setting, serum potassium, phosphorus, and magnesium levels may be depleted due to diuretic use or refeeding syndrome and require close monitoring.[47] In liver transplantation, many of these electrolyte shifts are attributed to GI losses from abdominal drains and other sources, as well as fluid overload.[47] Hyperkalemia is a frequent side effect of the immunosuppressive agent tacrolimus, often requiring a low-potassium diet restricting potassium to 1–3 g/day.[50] Hypophosphatemia has been documented to occur in up to 90% of recipients of kidney transplants during the acute posttransplant phase, which has been attributed to renal phosphate wasting.[51] Hypomagnesemia is another common electrolyte abnormality observed due to calcineurin inhibitors, such as tacrolimus or cyclosporine, often requiring additional magnesium supplementation to maintain levels.[50] Because high doses of magnesium oxide may exacerbate diarrhea, the provision of magnesium-rich foods may be a better choice to mitigate low serum levels.

Hyperglycemia is common immediately posttransplant, with a frequency reported at 80% or more for recipients of kidneys in the first days to weeks following transplant.[52] Research has indicated that hyperglycemia postoperatively can lead to an increased risk of kidney transplant rejection.[17] There is also an increased risk for infection with uncontrolled hyperglycemia.[52] Even in patients with no history of diabetes, it may be prudent to use insulin to control blood glucose after a transplant until serum glucose levels improve. If PN is warranted, an intravenous insulin infusion or insulin in the PN may be needed to tightly manage blood glucose levels. For patients who were obese before transplantation, it is important to consider strategies to safely lower the amount of corticosteroids, if possible, to help reduce weight gain after surgery.[17] Refer to **Table 16.2** for additional nutritional recommendations for patients recovering from organ transplantation.

General diet education should focus on the adequacy of oral intake and the importance of meeting increased protein needs for wound healing and infection prevention. The use of oral supplements may be indicated to help meet energy and protein requirements. Be mindful of choosing an appropriate type of oral supplement postoperatively. For example, consideration of potassium or carbohydrate content may be warranted for those patients with elevated serum levels. Many recipients follow a much more restricted diet prior to the transplant, so it is necessary to review changes for short-term and long-term dietary goals.

CORE CONCEPT 4

Postoperative nutritional management should be individualized according to the patient's nutritional status, the organ being transplanted, and any complications that may arise during or after surgery.

Table 16.2 Estimated Nutrient Needs Posttransplant (Use Estimated Dry or Ideal Body Weight)

Energy
- Measure via indirect calorimetry (IC)
- If IC unavailable, recommend REEX 1.2–1.5 or 15–35 kcal/kg

Protein
- Provide between 1.5 and 2.5 g/kg

Factors that may increase both energy and protein requirements:
- Malnutrition
- Dialysis
- Wounds
- Inflammatory state due to sepsis or surgery
- Malabsorption

Factors that may increase protein requirements:
- High-output surgical drains

Carbohydrate
- Provide about 40–50% of calories as carbohydrates

Fat
- Provide about 30% of calories

Fluid
- Adjust based on fluid status
  - Fluid resuscitation may be needed with hypovolemia
  - Dialysis, renal replacement therapy, and/or fluid restriction may be needed with hypervolemia

Medications
- Lipid-containing medications may decrease needed caloric provision and require monitoring triglycerides
- Dextrose-containing medications or intravenous or dialysate fluids may decrease needed caloric provision and can worsen hyperglycemia
- High-dose corticosteroids may increase protein requirements and can cause hyperglycemia and/or hyperlipidemia
- Calcineurin inhibitors can cause hyperglycemia
- Epinephrine can cause hyperglycemia
- Pancreatic enzyme replacement may be needed for patients with exocrine pancreatic insufficiency

Data from Hahn M, Wood A, Hasse JM. Nutrition support management of organ transplant recipients in the acute posttransplant phase. *Nutr Clin Pract.* 2024;39(1):45-58. doi:10.1002/ncp.11104

PRACTICE POINT

Recipients of organs should be encouraged to limit added sugar and sodium, choose heart-healthy fats and oils and lean proteins, and increase fiber.

Nutrition Intervention

Pretransplant Phase

Prior to solid organ transplantation, nutrition intervention would mirror care provided in end-stage organ failure. Refer to Chapters 9, 11, 12, 13, and 14 for nutrition interventions related to care in heart, intestinal, kidney, liver, and pulmonary failure, respectively.

Acute Posttransplant Phase

Nutrition Support

Following solid organ transplantation, nutrition support should be considered in cases when oral nutrition may not be feasible or sufficient. Chronicity of disease, frailty/nutritional status pretransplantation, and other transplant-specific complications should be considered when determining appropriate nutrition intervention.[53] If the patient requires ventilation for a prolonged period of time, EN via an orogastric or nasogastric tube may be indicated.[54] Early EN (started within 48 hours of surgery) has been found to reduce infection rates in patients post liver transplantation.[53] Other indications for EN include the inability of a patient to tolerate an oral diet due to chewing and/or swallowing issues or the inability of the patient to meet their nutrient needs orally, possibly related to extended sedation after surgery, or in cases of severe malnutrition and/or frailty. In patients posttransplant with a functioning GI tract, EN over PN is the preferred modality of feeding.[53,55] In patients post liver transplant, EN has been associated with decreased postoperative infection rates and fewer metabolic complications in comparison to PN.[47] PN may be indicated in cases with prolonged GI bleeding, ileus, high-output intestinal fistula, or in cases of inadequate provision of EN.[17] Infection risk of PN may be decreased through proper line care, avoidance of overfeeding, and tight glycemic management.[55]

Patients who have undergone a small bowel transplant have unique nutritional concerns. These recipients need to delay oral intake until the transplanted graft is functioning.[56] Although each transplant center's protocol may vary, PN is usually reinitiated posttransplant, but with a lower volume needed to maintain adequate hydration.[17] PN may be provided for the first 4 weeks, transitioning to EN as tolerated after the first few weeks, depending on observation of allograft motility.[57] Some centers may start EN at a rate of 5–10 mL/hour and slowly taper PN as EN tolerance improves and the rate increases.[17]

For patients who may have had a gastrostomy tube prior to surgery, especially those with a history of cystic fibrosis, it is recommended to delay the removal of the tube until a BMI >19 kg/m^2 is achieved and maintained for 3 months without supplementary nutrition.[45]

For those patients who may have inadequate intake posttransplant, oral nutrition supplements may be recommended to help meet energy and/or protein requirements. Since there are various products available, it is important to consider the calorie, protein, fluid, fat, and carbohydrate content as well as micronutrients or other additives like phosphorus, caffeine, or herbal supplements, depending upon the needs of the patient. If a patient requires a fluid restriction, protein bars or protein chips can also be helpful.

Food Safety Guidelines

Patients posttransplant receive high doses of immunosuppressive medications that minimize rejection of the new organ(s), but also increase infection risk due to reduced immunity. **Neutropenia** is defined as an abnormally low level of neutrophils in the blood.[58] Neutrophils are white blood cells produced in the bone marrow that protect the body against infectious disease or foreign invaders by engulfing bacteria. Neutropenia is a serious disorder because it makes the body vulnerable to bacterial and fungal infections. A low-microbial diet, also known as a "low-bacteria diet" or "neutropenic diet," is designed to prevent food-borne illnesses in immunocompromised patients (**Figure 16.5**). There are no published guidelines constituting what should be considered a low-bacteria diet, and published studies have determined no benefit of this diet.[59] Many institutions independently determine which foods may or may not be given to patients following a transplant as well as the length of time the patient must comply with the low-bacteria diet. Some institutions may recommend a patient follow the low-bacteria diet for as long as they are taking immunosuppressants (which may be the entire duration of the patient's life) or they may allow a patient to follow a regular diet after discharge.

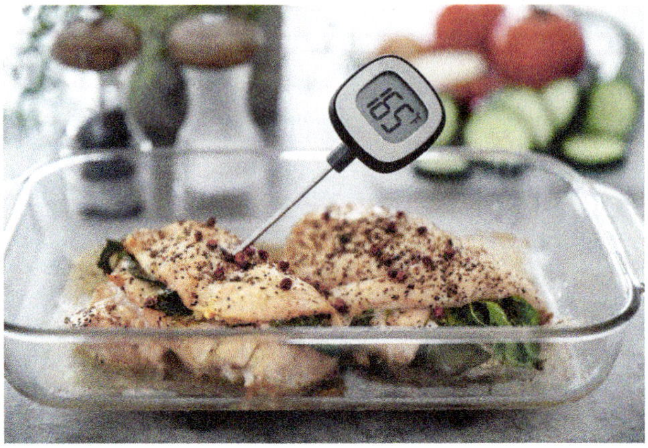

Figure 16.5 Transplant Recipients Are at High Risk for Food-Borne Illnesses

A low-microbial diet follows food safety basics and emphasizes the importance of hand washing before touching food, avoiding cross-contamination of raw food, sanitizing cooking areas, washing fruits and vegetables, heating foods to the proper temperature, and cooling foods to the proper temperature in a timely manner.[60] **Cross-contamination** is the passage of pathogens indirectly from one source to another due to the improper use of sterilization procedures, unclean instruments, or recycling of products. In general, most patients are advised to avoid higher risk foods, which include unpasteurized dairy products, undercooked or raw meats, poultry, eggs, seafood, soft or moldy cheeses, leftovers or deli meats that have not been heated to the proper temperature, water from a well, and buffets or salad bars.[60] The main goal is to limit the risk of getting food-borne illnesses like *Listeria, Salmonella, or Escherichia coli.*

CASE STUDY REVISITED

George's condition improves, and he is transferred out of the ICU. His appetite is slow to return, so oral nutrition supplements are recommended. On POD #7, George's appetite has improved significantly, and he continues to drink high-calorie/high-protein supplements with all of his meals. The medical team is worried about his hyperkalemia and hyperglycemia.

Anthropometric Data:

Current weight: 114.5 kg

Biochemical Data:

Sodium 141 (136–145 mEq/L)
Potassium 5.3 (3.5–5.0 mEq/L)
Blood urea nitrogen 22 (8–20 mg/dL)
Creatinine 1.3 (0.7–1.3 mg/dL)
Glucose 296 (70–139 mg/dL)

Clinical Data:

Medications (include): insulin, mycophenolate mofetil, prednisone, tacrolimus

Dietary Data:

Diet Order: Low bacteria, consistent carbohydrate with high-calorie oral nutrition supplement three times daily with meals (provides 350 kcal, 30 g protein, 41 g carbohydrate, 470 mg K+ per 8 oz bottle)

Questions

1. What adjustment could be made to his diet order?
2. How might his medication regimen influence his nutritional status and diet prescription?
3. What diet education could be provided for the acute phase as well as with consideration for the chronic (long-term) phase?

PRACTICE POINT

Following basic food safety rules and guidelines can prevent immunosuppressed patients from contracting food-borne illnesses.

Food-Drug Interactions and Supplement Use

There are significant drug–nutrient interactions observed with grapefruit and grapefruit products. Cyclosporine and tacrolimus, as well as other medications, are metabolized by the cytochrome P450 system in the GI tract.[11] Research suggests that flavonoids and other substances in grapefruit juice act by inhibiting the cytochrome P450 enzymes, which can increase the bloodstream concentration, activity, and potential toxicity of these drugs.[11] It is recommended that grapefruit products be avoided.[11] Most herbal and alternative supplements are discouraged due to concern for interactions with immunosuppressive medications or the potential to damage organs.[58]

There are increasing reports of probiotic-associated infections, calling into question the safety of using these products. One case study looked at a recipient post cardiothoracic transplant who received *Lactobacillus rhamnosus GG* and developed an empyema.[61] The same strain of *Lactobacillus* that the patient was taking in supplement form was found in the pleural fluid. Alternatively, in the liver transplant population, probiotics, specifically *Lactobacillus* spp, in combination with prebiotics, may be effective in reducing infection complications.[62,63] Special caution should be exercised when using these supplements in patients who are immunocompromised.[61,64]

Chronic Posttransplant Phase

Prevention of chronic disease is the main long-term goal of nutrition therapy in the chronic posttransplant phase. There are currently no guidelines, and research is limited on long-term dietary interventions posttransplant.[65] Emphasizing and reinforcing dietary compliance to recommended diets, particularly those treating comorbidities such as diabetes

Clinical Controversy

Is a low-bacteria diet beneficial posttransplant?

Background: A low-bacteria or neutropenic diet is one intervention that has been used to reduce the risk of developing life-threatening infections among immunocompromised patients. The intended purpose is to limit the intake of bacteria into a host's GI tract to reduce the risk of infection. Limited evidence exists to support this cause-and-effect relationship or determine whether a restricted diet is beneficial. One group of researchers conducted a study that evaluated 46 patients undergoing allogenic stem cell transplants and found that there were no significant differences between infection rates or nutritional status among patients who received the neutropenic diet or an unrestricted diet.

Another study assessed the outcomes of patients undergoing induction for acute myeloid leukemia who were randomly assigned to a diet containing raw fresh fruits and vegetables (raw diet, $n = 75$) or one that excluded raw fresh fruits and vegetables (cooked diet, $n = 78$). There appeared to be a trend toward fewer fevers of unknown origin in the cooked-diet group, while the incidence of bacteremia was higher in the raw-diet group.

Another study looked at the microbiological profile and nutritional quality of a regular diet compared to a neutropenic diet in a pediatric oncology unit in Brazil. There was no statistical difference observed between the diets, but the neutropenic diet was noted to be lower in vitamin C and fiber.

Questions

1. What are potential advantages and disadvantages of the low-microbial diet in the transplant population?
2. Can the results of the studies referenced above, which were conducted with patients with cancer, be applied to solid organ transplant recipients?
3. Would you recommend a low-microbial diet to a solid organ transplant recipient?

References

1. Lassiter M, Schneider SM. A pilot study comparing the neutropenic diet to a non-neutropenic diet in the allogeneic hematopoietic stem cell transplantation population. *Clin J Oncol Nurs.* 2015;19(3):273–278.
2. Gardner A, Mattiuzzi G, Faderl S, et al. Randomized comparison of cooked and noncooked diets in patients undergoing remission induction therapy for acute myeloid leukemia. *J Clin Oncol.* 2008;26:5684–5688.
3. Maia JE, da Cruz LB, Gregianin LJ. Microbiological profile and nutritional quality of a regular diet compared to a neutropenic diet in a pediatric oncology unit. *Pediatr Blood Cancer.* 2018;65:e26828.

or hypertension that led to the original organ failure, is of utmost importance. A transplant does not eradicate the preexisting condition. A healthy diet such as a heart-healthy diet, Mediterranean diet, and the American Heart Association (AHA) Step 1 diet will likely benefit the recipient posttransplant and can help with some of the common chronic posttransplant metabolic conditions, such as diabetes, obesity, hypertension, and dyslipidemia.[17,65] Surgical complications or infections, particularly those that prompt multiple hospitalizations or procedures, may compromise a recipient's nutritional status, requiring more aggressive nutrition intervention to prevent or reverse malnutrition or replete losses. Individualized diet recommendations continue to benefit the patient and can help to manage nutritional issues that arise over time.

Long-Term Metabolic and Nutritional Consequences

Organ transplantation is designed to help people lead longer, healthier lives. The screening process for recipients of organs helps ensure that those who receive an organ will be healthy enough not only to survive the transplant, but to continue to live many productive years. By correctly matching organ donors to recipients and using immunosuppressive medication, recipients of organs are living longer than ever. Acknowledgment of nutrition-related impacts of specific immunosuppression regimens is vital for appropriate posttransplant management.

Weight Gain. Posttransplant weight gain is common among recipients. Weight gain after transplantation has been associated with increased postoperative complications, worsening of metabolic syndrome, increased graft loss, and reduced patient and graft survival (**Figure 16.6**).[26] Corticosteroids may play a significant role in weight gain, but other factors may include a less-restricted diet and overall improved appetite and well-being. It has been found that the greatest weight gain occurs 6 months after liver transplantation,[47] possibly related to a reduction in energy expenditure following liver transplantation that can lead to increased fat mass and obesity.[66–68] Another study found that for each 5 kg/m^2 increment increase in BMI during the first

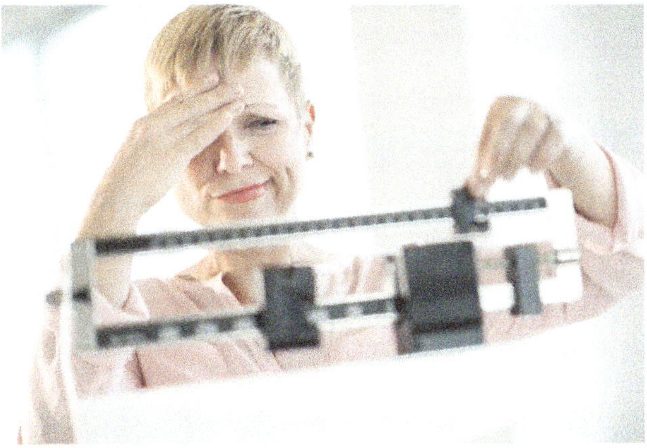

Figure 16.6 Weight Gain Can Be a Complicating Factor Posttransplant

year after kidney transplantation, there was a 1.23 additional relative risk for death.[25]

Diabetes. Recipients of transplants may require long-term management of blood glucose. **New-onset diabetes after transplantation (NODAT)** has been reported to occur in 4–25% of recipients of kidney transplants, 4–40% of recipients of heart transplants, 2.5–25% of recipients of liver transplants, and 30–35% of recipients of lung transplants.[69] Immunosuppression regimens contribute to hyperglycemia. About 5% of patients on long-term cyclosporine will develop diabetes, despite careful monitoring of blood levels.[2] Tacrolimus has an even higher incidence of neurotoxicity and diabetes.[2] Corticosteroid dose reduction has been found to improve glucose tolerance during the first year after transplant.[69] Studies assessing the impact of NODAT on patient and allograft outcomes have generated a variety of results, yet substantial research suggests that recipients of kidney transplants who develop NODAT are at two- to threefold increased risk of cardiovascular events compared to patients without diabetes.[69] The development of NODAT is also associated with an increased risk for graft rejection and infectious complications. Nutrition intervention for NODAT includes diabetes diet education, modest weight loss of 5–10% of total body weight if overweight, and physical activity.[69] Additional pharmacological management, such as insulin, may be needed if hyperglycemia persists. Increased risk of NODAT appears to be associated with increased age, BMI, and waist circumference among recipients of kidney transplants.[25] Early detection and routine monitoring for hyperglycemia are important in both acute and chronic postoperative phases.

Hypertension. The prevalence of hypertension also remains an issue among recipients of kidney transplants, affecting up to 90% of recipients.[70] Immunosuppressive medications like corticosteroids and calcineurin inhibitors contribute to high blood pressure through vasoconstriction, sodium retention, and vasodilation inhibition.[70] A study completed in Japan found that short-term dietary counseling on sodium intake among recipients of kidney transplants can be effective in reducing blood pressure and perhaps the quantity of antihypertensive medications needed.[70]

Dyslipidemia. Impaired lipid metabolism, which has been observed among many transplant recipients, is associated with some immunosuppressive medications. Up to 45% of recipients of liver transplants develop hyperlipidemia.[71] Cyclosporine and steroids are associated with hyperlipidemia.[11] Cyclosporine can bind to the low-density lipoprotein (LDL) cholesterol receptor and can inhibit hepatic clearance of LDL, leading to an increase in circulating LDL.[71] Dietary restrictions and modifications, such as following a Mediterranean diet or the AHA Step 1 diet, have been found to help improve dyslipidemia in patients after kidney transplants.[65] Reducing saturated fat, balancing carbohydrate at 50–60% of calories, and increasing plant sterols have been found to be effective diet therapies for recipients of kidney and heart transplants with dyslipidemia or uncontrolled weight gain.[65] Some studies have found that hyperlipidemia may persist despite dietary modifications and weight reduction, so more aggressive pharmacological interventions, such as a statin, may also be necessary in conjunction with diet modification.[71]

Cancer. The success of immunosuppression in recipients of transplants has led to an increased rate of malignancy in this population. There is a threefold increased risk for cancer in those who have received an organ compared to the general population.[72] Most of the cancer types that tend to afflict recipients of organs have a known or suspected infectious cause, such as Kaposi sarcoma; Hodgkin's lymphoma; hepatobiliary and liver cancer; melanoma; colorectal cancer; and cancers of the cervix, anus, vulva, penis, oral cavity, and pharynx.[72–75] The higher incidence of cancers among the transplant population may be the result of years on immune suppression therapy, with a smaller percentage stemming from prior disease risk from their end-stage organ failure.[72]

Bone Health and Osteoporosis. **Osteoporosis** can arise from both pretransplant bone disease and immunosuppressive agent use after transplantation.[76] Osteodystrophy, or abnormal development of bone, is frequently observed. Specifically, renal **osteodystrophy** from kidney disease, decreased bone mineral density in end-stage heart disease, hepatic osteodystrophy and malabsorption in liver disease, and the use of steroids in COPD can all contribute to osteoporosis and increased risk of fractures before transplant occurs.[76,77] After transplant, the reported prevalence of vitamin D insufficiency ranges from 51% to 97% and severe deficiency can range from 26% to 33%.[77] Recipients of transplants are at risk for vitamin D deficiency due to compromised health status postoperatively, which may lead to reduced dietary intake of vitamin D–containing foods. There is also an increased risk of skin cancer in this population, leading to a decrease in intentional sun exposure.[77] Some studies demonstrate that glucocorticoids can increase catabolism of 25-hydroxyvitamin D.[77] Impaired absorption or increased excretion of calcium is also observed in the setting of corticosteroids.[56] It has been reported that bone loss can occur within the first 3–6 months after liver transplantation, but then becomes more stable over the next 12 months.[47] Vitamin D deficiency should be corrected whenever possible, and patients should be encouraged to take at least the recommended dietary allowance for both calcium and vitamin D before and after their transplant to counteract the bone mineral–depleting effects of their medications.[76] Based on the 2017 American College of Rheumatology guidelines for the prevention and treatment of glucocorticoid-induced osteoporosis, calcium intake of 1000–1200 mg/day, vitamin D intake of 600–900 IU/day, and serum vitamin D levels ≥20 ng/mL are recommended.[78] Weight-bearing activities are also encouraged.

Monitoring and Evaluation

Monitoring patients post solid organ transplant includes tracking side effects from medications such as diabetes, hyperlipidemia, hypertension, and weight gain. It would be critical to follow anthropometrics such as weight and waist circumference, as well as evaluate dietary choices including carbohydrate for NODAT, protein intake due to wound healing and increased needs related to steroid administration, saturated fat consumption due to impaired lipid metabolism, sodium intake due to hypertension risk, and calcium and vitamin D intake for bone health. Identifying behaviors related to food safety, supplement intake (such as probiotics), and grapefruit juice consumption would be vital to reduce risk of food-borne illnesses and drug–nutrient interactions. It would be important to monitor lab values, especially glucose and HbA1c for NODAT, lipid panel for dyslipidemia, and vitamin D levels for bone health. Finally, it is important to assess lifestyle choices including physical activity and weight-bearing activities to help manage weight gain and bone health as well as sun exposure to reduce skin cancer risk.

PRACTICE POINT

Long-term nutrition therapy is recommended to manage long-term side effects from medications such as diabetes, hyperlipidemia, hypertension, and weight gain.

Chapter Summary

Solid organ transplantation has evolved since the beginning of the 20th century. As medical technology improves, an increase in both organ donation and survival of recipients is evident. Advances in immunosuppressive medications have improved the health and longevity of recipients of organs. Medical nutrition therapy plays an important role both pre- and posttransplant to reverse malnutrition and assist with weight loss for potential transplant candidates with obesity. Postoperative medical nutrition therapy is critical to optimize outcomes by supporting wound healing and managing nutritional consequences and/or side effects of immunosuppressive medications. Long-term medical nutrition therapy can optimize the health and productivity of recipients of transplants, decrease the risk of food-borne illness, and promote a well-balanced diet and lifestyle.

Key Terms

New-onset diabetes after transplantation (NODAT), orthotopic, rejection, immunosuppression, graft thrombosis, cachexia, brain death, donation after cardiac death (DCD), neutropenia, cross-contamination, osteoporosis, osteodystrophy

References

1. Linden PK. History of solid organ transplantation and organ donation. *Crit Care Clin.* 2009;25(1):165–184.
2. Watson CJ, Dark JH. Organ transplantation: historical perspective and current practice. *Br J Anaesth.* 2012;108 (suppl 1):29–42.
3. Anand J, Singh SK, Antoun DG, et al. Durable mechanical circulatory support versus organ transplantation: past, present, and future. *Biomed Res Int.* 2015;2015:849571. doi:10.1155/2015/849571
4. United Network for Organ Sharing. Data and trends. Accessed August 6, 2024. https://www.unos.org/data
5. United Network for Organ Sharing. Facts about organ donation. Accessed August 6, 2024. https://www.unos.org/donation/facts
6. United Network for Organ Sharing. Innovations and policy updates drive equity and a record number of lifesaving organ transplants in 2023. Published January 11, 2024. Accessed August 6, 2024. https://unos.org/media-resources/releases/innovations-policy-updates-drive-equity-and-record-organ-transplants-2023
7. Poggio ED, Augustine JJ, Arrigain S, Brennan DC, Schold JD. Long-term kidney transplant graft survival—making progress when most needed. *Am J Transplant.* 2021;21(8): 2824–2832. doi:10.1111/ajt.16463
8. Wolk R, Foulks C. Renal disease. In: Mueller C, McClave S, Kuhn JM, eds. *The A.S.P.E.N. Adult Nutrition Support Core Curriculum.* 2nd ed. American Society for Parenteral and Enteral Nutrition; 2012:491–510.
9. Ghaderian SB, Beladi-Mousavi SS. The role of diabetes and hypertension in chronic kidney disease. *J Renal Inj Prev.* 2014;3(4):109–110. doi:10.12861/jrip.2014.31
10. National Kidney Foundation. The kidney transplant waitlist. Last updated April 3, 2024. Accessed November 20, 2024. https://www.kidney.org/atoz/content/transplant-waitlist
11. Hasse JM, Blue LS. *Comprehensive Guide to Transplant Nutrition.* American Dietetic Association; 2002.
12. Cholankeril G, Ahmed A. Alcoholic liver disease replaces hepatitis C virus infection as the leading indication for liver transplantation in the United States. *Clin Gastroenterol Hepatol.* 2018;16(8):1356–1358. doi:10.1016/j.cgh.2017.11.045
13. Farkas S, Hackl C, Schlitt HJ. Overview of the indications and contraindications for liver transplantation. *Cold Spring Harb Perspect Med.* 2014;1;4(5):a015602. doi:10.1101/cshperspect.a015602
14. Dababneh Y, Mousa OY. Liver transplantation. In: *StatPearls.* StatPearls Publishing; 2023. https://www.ncbi.nlm.nih.gov/books/NBK559161/
15. Ruf A, Dirchwolf M, Freeman RB. From Child-Pugh to MELD score and beyond: taking a walk down memory lane. *Ann Hepatol.* 2022;27(1):100535. doi:10.1016/j.aohep.2021.100535
16. Sudan D. The current state of intestine transplantation: indications, techniques, outcomes and challenges. *Am J Transplant.* 2014;14(9):1976–1984. doi:10.1111/ajt.12812
17. Hasse JM, Matarese LE. Solid organ transplantation. In: Mueller C, McClave S, Kuhn JM, eds. *The A.S.P.E.N. Adult Nutrition Support Core Curriculum.* 2nd ed. American Society for Parenteral and Enteral Nutrition; 2012:523–535.
18. Russo MJ, Hong KN, Davies RR, et al. The effect of body mass index on survival following heart transplantation: do outcomes support consensus guidelines? *Ann Surg.* 2010;251(1):144–152.
19. Hasse J. Pretransplant obesity: a weighty issue affecting transplant candidacy and outcomes. *Nutr Clin Pract.* 2007;22(5):494–504.
20. Potluri K, Hou S. Obesity in kidney transplant recipients and candidates. *Am J Kidney Dis.* 2010;56(1):143–156.
21. Sampaio MS, Reddy PN, Kuo HT, et al. Obesity was associated with inferior outcomes in simultaneous pancreas kidney transplant. *Transplantation.* 2010;89(9):1117–1125.
22. Bumgardner GL, Henry ML, Elkhammas E, et al. Obesity as a risk factor after combined pancreas/kidney transplantation. *Transplantation.* 1995;60(12):1426–1430.
23. Lederer DJ, Kawut SM, Wickersham N, et al. Obesity and primary graft dysfunction after lung transplantation: the lung transplant outcomes group obesity study. *Am J Respir Crit Care Med.* 2011;184(9):1055–1061.
24. Lavie CJ, Milani RV, Ventura HO. Obesity and cardiovascular disease: risk factor, paradox, and impact of weight loss. *J Am Coll Cardiol.* 2009;53:1925–1932.
25. Tran M-H, Foster CE, Kalantar-Zadeh K, Ichii H. Kidney transplantation in obese patients. *World J Transplant.* 2016;6(1):135–143. doi:10.5500/wtj.v6.i1.135
26. Chan G, Garneau P, Hajjar R. The impact and treatment of obesity in kidney transplant candidates and recipients. *Can J Kidney Health Dis.* 2015;2:26. doi:10.1186/s40697-015-0059-4
27. Martin P, DiMartini A, Feng S, Robert Brown J, Fallon M. Evaluation for liver transplantation in adults: 2013 practice guideline by the AASLD and the American Society of Transplantation. *Hepatology.* 2014;59(3):1144–1165. doi:10.1002/hep.26972
28. Nair S, Verma S, Thuluvath PJ. Obesity and its effect on survival in patients undergoing orthotopic liver transplantation in the United States. *Hepatology.* 2002;35(1):105–109.
29. Ayloo S, Hurton S, Cwinn M, Molinari M. Impact of body mass index on outcomes of 48281 patients undergoing first time cadaveric liver transplantation. *World J Transplant.* 2016;6(2):356–369. doi:10.5500/wjt.v6.i2.356
30. Vest AR, Patel P, Schauer PR, et al. Clinical and echocardiographic outcomes after bariatric surgery in obese patients with left ventricular systolic dysfunction. *Circ Heart Fail.* 2016;9:e002260. doi:10.1161/circheartfailure.115.002260
31. Shimada YJ, Tsugawa Y, Brown DFM, Hasegawa K. Bariatric surgery and emergency department visits and hospitalizations for heart failure exacerbation: population-based, self-controlled series. *J Am Coll Cardiol.* 2015;67:895–903.
32. Hasse JM. Nutrition assessment and support of organ transplant recipients. *JPEN J Parenter Enteral Nutr.* 2001;25(3):120–131.
33. Lowell JA. Nutritional assessment and therapy in patients requiring liver transplantation. *Liver Transpl Surg.* 1996;2 (5 suppl 1):79–88.
34. Molnar MZ, Kovesdy CP, Bunnapradist S, et al. Associations of pretransplant serum albumin with post-transplant outcomes in kidney transplant recipients. *Am J Transplant.* 2011;11(5):1006–1015.
35. ter Wee PM. Protein energy wasting and transplantation. *J Ren Nutr.* 2013;23(3):246–249. doi:10.1053/j.jrn.2013.02.004
36. Merli M, Giusto M, Gentili F, et al. Nutritional status: its influence on the outcome of patients undergoing liver transplantation. *Liver Int.* 2010;30(2):208–214.
37. Ilonze OJ, Parsly Read-Button L, Cogswell R, et al. Controversies and conundrums in cardiac cachexia: key questions

about wasting in patients with HFrEF. *JACC Heart Fail.* 2024;12(10):1645–1660. doi:10.1016/j.jchf.2024.03.003
38. Maurer MS, Horn E, Reyentovich A, et al. Can a left ventricular assist device in individuals with advanced systolic heart failure improve or reverse frailty? *J Am Geriatr Soc.* 2017;65(11):2383–2390. doi:10.1111/jgs.15124
39. Kobashigawa J, Dadhania D, Bhorade S, et al. Report from the American Society of Transplantation on frailty in solid organ transplantation. *Am J Transplant.* 2019;19(4):984–994. doi:10.1111/ajt.15198
40. Fitzpatrick J, Sozio SM, Jaar BG, et al. Frailty, body composition and the risk of mortality in incident hemodialysis patients: the Predictors of Arrhythmic and Cardiovascular Risk in End Stage Renal Disease study. *Nephrol Dial Transplant.* 2019;1;34(2):346–354. doi:10.1093/ndt/gfy124
41. MedlinePlus. Transplant rejection. Accessed November 11, 2024. https://medlineplus.gov/ency/article/000815.htm
42. Lee RD, Nieman DC. *Nutritional Assessment.* 6th ed. McGraw-Hill Education; 2013.
43. Hammad A, Kaido T, Uemoto S. Perioperative nutritional therapy in liver transplantation. *Surg Today.* 2015;45(3):271–283.
44. Hirche TO, Knoop C, Hebestreit H, et al. Practical guidelines: lung transplantation in patients with cystic fibrosis. *Pulm Med.* 2014;2014:621342. doi:10.1155/2014/621342
45. Martins C, Pecoits-Filho R, Riella MC. Nutrition for the post-renal transplant recipients. *Transplant. Proc.*2004; 36(6):1650–1654.
46. Sanchez AJ, Aranda-Michel J. Nutrition for the liver transplant patient. *Liver Transpl.* 2006;12(9):1310–1316.
47. Tynan C, Hassee J. Current nutrition practices in adult lung transplantation. *Nutr Clin Pract.* 2004;19(6):587–596. doi:10.1177/0115426504019006587
48. Aggarwal A, Kimar A, Gregory M, et al. Nutrition assessment in advanced heart failure patients evaluated for ventricular assist devices or cardiac transplantation. *Nutr Clin Pract.* 2013;28(1):112–119.
49. Pronsky ZM, Elbe D, Ayoob K. *Food-Medication Interactions.* 18th ed. Food-Medication Interactions; 2015.
50. Kanaan N, Claes K, Devogelaer J-P, et al. Fibroblast growth factor-23 and parathyroid hormone are associated with post-transplant bone mineral density loss. *Clin J Am Soc Nephrol.* 2010;5(10):1887–1892. doi:10.2215/CJN.00950110
51. Boerner B, Shivaswamy V, Goldner W, Larsen J. Management of the hospitalized transplant patient. *Curr Diab Rep.* 2015;15(4):19. doi:10.1007/s11892-015-0585-6
52. Hahn M, Wood A, Hasse JM. Nutrition support management of organ transplant recipients in the acute posttransplant phase. *Nutr Clin Pract.* 2024;39(1):45–58. doi:10.1002/ncp.11104
53. Cresci G, ed. *Nutrition Support for the Critically Ill Patient: A Guide to Practice.* Taylor & Francis Group/CRC Press; 2005.
54. Compher C, Bingham AL, McCall M, et al. Guidelines for the provision of nutrition support therapy in the adult critically ill patient: the American Society for Parenteral and Enteral Nutrition. *JPEN J Parenter Enteral Nutr.* 2022;46:12–41. doi:10.1002/jpen.2267
55. Nutrition Care Manual. Organ transplant-practice related guidelines: nutrition support. Accessed November 21, 2024. https://www.nutritioncaremanual.org
56. Weseman RA, Gilroy R. Nutrition management of small bowel transplant patients. *Nutr Clin Pract.* 2005;20:509–516.
57. National Cancer Institute. NCI dictionary of cancer terms. Accessed December 2, 2024. https://www.cancer.gov/publications/dictionaries/cancer-terms/def/neutropenia
58. Jubelirer SJ. The benefit of the neutropenic diet: fact or fiction? *Oncologist.* 2011;16(5):704–707.
59. U.S. Food and Drug Administration. Food safety for older adults and people with cancer, diabetes, HIV/AIDS, organ transplants, and autoimmune diseases. Published 2020. Accessed November 21, 2024. https://www.fda.gov/food/people-risk-foodborne-illness/food-safety-older-adults-and-people-cancer-diabetes-hivaids-organ-transplants-and-autoimmune
60. Luong M-L, Sareyyupoglu B, Nguyen MH, et al. Lactobacillus probiotic use in cardiothoracic transplant recipients: a link to invasive *Lactobacillus* infection? *Transpl Infect Dis.* 2010;12:561–564.
61. Jorgenson MR, Descourouez JL, Siodlak M, Tjugum S, Rice JP, Fernandez LA. Efficacy and safety of probiotics and synbiotics in liver transplantation. *Pharmacotherapy.* 2018;38(7):758–768. doi:10.1002/phar.2130
62. Sawas T, Al Halabi S, Hernaez R, Carey WD, Cho WK. Patients receiving prebiotics and probiotics before liver transplantation develop fewer infections than controls; a systematic review and meta-analysis. *Clin Gastroenterol Hepatol.* 2015;13(9):1567–1574.e3; quiz e143–e144. doi:10.1016/j.cgh.2015.05.027
63. Twombley KE, Seikaly MG. New paradigms for the use of prebiotics, probiotics, and synbiotics in renal disease. *Dial Transplant.* 2011;40:200–204. doi:10.1002/dat.20568
64. Zeltzer SM, Taylor DO, Tang WH. Long-term dietary habits and interventions in solid-organ transplantation. *J Heart Lung Transplant.* 2015;34(11):1357–1365.
65. Richardson RA, Garden OJ, Davidson HI. Reduction in energy expenditure after liver transplantation. *Nutrition.* 2001;17(7–8):585–589.
66. Ferreira LG, Santos LF, Anastacio LR, Lima AS, Correia MI. Resting energy expenditure, body composition, and dietary intake: a longitudinal study before and after liver transplantation. *Transplantation.* 2013;96(6):579–585.
67. Giusto M, Lattanzi B, Di Gregorio V, Giannelli V, Lucidi C, Merli M. Changes in nutritional status after liver transplantation. *World J Gastroenterol.* 2014;20(31):10682–10690.
68. Pham P-TT, Pham P-MT, Pham SV, Pham P-AT, Pham P-CT. New onset diabetes after transplantation (NODAT): an overview. *Diabetes Metab Syndr Obes.* 2011;4:175–186. doi:10.2147/DMSO.S19027
69. Asai K, Kobayashi T, Miyata H, et al. The short-term impact of dietary counseling on sodium intake and blood pressure in renal allograft recipients. *Prog Transplant.* 2016;26(4)365–371.
70. Charlton M. Obesity, hyperlipidemia, and metabolic syndrome. *Liver Transpl.* 2009;15(S2):S83–S89. doi:10.1002/lt.21914
71. Vajdic CM, van Leeuwen MT. Cancer incidence and risk factors after solid organ transplantation. *Int J Cancer.* 2009;125(8):1747–1754.
72. Safaeian M, Robbins HA, Berndt SI, Lynch CF, Fraumeni JF Jr, Engels EA. Risk of colorectal cancer after solid organ transplantation in the United States. *Am J Transplant.* 2016; 16(3):960–967. doi:10.1111/ajt.13549
73. Robbins HA, Clarke CA, Arron ST, et al. Melanoma risk and survival among organ transplant recipients. *J Invest Dermatol.* 2015;135(11):2657–2665.

74. Koshiol J, Pawlish K, Goodman MT, McGlynn KA, Engels EA. Risk of hepatobiliary cancer after solid organ transplant in the United States. *Clin Gastroenterol Hepatol.* 2014;12(9): 1541–1549.e3.
75. Lan GB, Xie XB, Peng LK, Liu L, Song L, Dai HL. Current status of research on osteoporosis after solid organ transplantation: pathogenesis and management. *Biomed Res Int.* 2015;2015:10.
76. Stein EM, Shane E. Vitamin D in organ transplantation. *Osteoporos Int.* 2011;22(7):2107–2118. doi:10.1007/s00198-010-1523-8
77. Buckley L, Guyatt G, Fink HA, et al. 2017 American College of Rheumatology guideline for the prevention and treatment of glucocorticoid-induced osteoporosis. *Arthritis Care Res.* 2017;69(8):1095–1110. doi:10.1002/acr.23279

CHAPTER 17

Nutrition in Oncology and Hematopoietic Stem Cell Transplantation

Deena Altschwager

CHAPTER OUTLINE

CORE CONCEPTS

1. Almost half of new cancer diagnoses are caused by modifiable factors, including obesity, suboptimal nutrition, physical inactivity, tobacco use, and heavy alcohol consumption.
2. Cancer is the second most common cause of death in the United States, surpassed only by heart disease.
3. Medical treatment of cancer can lead to nutrition impact symptoms that may impair a patient's nutritional status.
4. Weight loss and malnutrition are well documented in patients with cancer and may influence disease prognosis, treatment tolerance, quality of life, and be predictive of early mortality.
5. Dietary counseling by a registered dietitian results in improved outcomes, including fewer treatment-related side effects, improved quality of life, and better dietary intake.
6. Nutrition impact symptoms and energy requirements differ based on the specific type of cancer or solid tumor present.
7. Cancer cachexia can lead to progressive functional impairment in advanced cancers. Proinflammatory cytokines may play a role in mediating alterations in metabolism found in cancer cachexia and may also affect other gastrointestinal processes.
8. Cancer cachexia results in preferential loss of skeletal muscle mass and may contribute to an increase in resting energy expenditure.

9. Because no evidence-based treatments are available for cancer cachexia, focus should be placed on early nutrition interventions to prevent the onset and acceleration of cancer cachexia.
10. Patients with head and neck cancer have the highest risk for malnutrition compared to other malignancies due to the physical location of the tumor and likelihood of dysphagia.
11. The allogeneic hematopoietic stem cell transplant (HSCT) is considered one of the most intense treatments in the oncology population and puts patients at increased nutrition risk due to prolonged neutropenia, gastrointestinal side effects, and risk of graft versus host disease (GVHD).
12. Patients undergoing HSCT have increased energy needs due to increased catabolism and treatment-related complications.
13. Nutrition is critical following HSCT because impaired nutritional status can lead to longer engraftment time and a greater likelihood of developing infection.
14. Graft versus host disease can occur following allogeneic HSCT and places patients at increased nutrition risk due to impaired function of the gastrointestinal tract, including the oral mucosa.
15. Nutrition support in the patient with advanced cancer should be assessed on a case-by-case basis with consideration of goals of care.

LEARNING OBJECTIVES

1. Describe the magnitude and etiology of cancer today.
2. Explain the medical treatment of cancer, including the nutrition impact symptoms related to the treatment.
3. Describe the prevalence of malnutrition among the cancer population and the types of tools used to screen for malnutrition.
4. Assess nutrition status and develop nutrition care plans for people with cancer diagnoses.
5. Describe cancer cachexia, including the changes in metabolism associated with cachexia, and appropriate nutritional management.
6. Determine optimal enteral and parenteral feeding practices for patients with cancer.
7. Identify high-risk cancer types based on tumor sites and their associated nutritional management.
8. Assess the unique nutrition needs of patients with hematological cancers undergoing hematopoietic stem cell transplant.
9. Develop care plans for patients undergoing hematopoietic stem cell transplants, including management and treatment of graft versus host disease.
10. Compare appropriate diet recommendations for patients who are immunosuppressed versus patients who are non-immunosuppressed.
11. Select optimal nutrition support practices for patients with advanced cancer.

Background/Etiology

Cancer is a term used to describe a group of more than 100 diseases characterized by uncontrolled growth of abnormal cells, with the ability to invade other tissues.[1] All cancer starts as a single cell that has lost control of its normal growth and replication process. Cancer is caused by both external factors (such as tobacco, alcohol, and chemicals) and internal factors (such as inherited mutations and immune conditions). These factors may act together or in sequence to imitate or promote the development of cancer.[1] Only about 5–10% of cancers are strongly hereditary, as most cancers result from the damage to genes occurring during a person's lifetime.[2] Inherited factors are known to play a larger role in determining risk for some cancers, including colorectal, breast, and prostate cancers.[3] It is estimated that 42% of men and 40% of women will develop cancer in their lifetime.[4]

A substantial portion of cancers can be prevented (**Table 17.1**). According to the National Cancer Institute (NCI) and American Cancer Society (ACS), the cause of 42% of newly diagnosed cancers is modifiable, related in part to smoking or other tobacco

Table 17.1 Exogenous Cancer Risk Factors

Risk Factor	Cancers with Increased Risk
Alcohol	Colorectal, gastrointestinal, liver, oral
High fat intake	Lymphoma, prostate
Low fruit/ vegetable intake	Most cancers
Obesity	Biliary, colorectal, gallbladder, gynecologic, liver, pancreatic, prostate, renal, thyroid
Tobacco	Bladder, cervical, gastrointestinal, liver, lung, oral, pancreatic, renal

Data from American Cancer Society. Cancer risk and prevention. Accessed November 9, 2025. https://www.cancer.org/cancer/risk-prevention.html

CASE STUDY INTRODUCTION

Seth is a 65-year-old male with newly diagnosed acute myelogenous leukemia (AML). He has completed two cycles of high-dose chemotherapy complicated by weight loss, nausea, anorexia, mucositis, and febrile neutropenia. He will eventually require an allogeneic hematopoietic stem cell transplant. Seth is a retired banker; he is currently married.

Anthropometric Data:

Height: 178 cm
Weight: 86 kg
BMI: 27 kg/m^2

Weight history
Usual body weight (UBW): 95.5 kg 6 months ago
Weight 1 month ago: 92 kg

Biochemical Data:

Sodium 137 (136–145 mEq/L)
Potassium 3.7 (3.5–5.0 mEq/L)
Chloride 103 (96–110 mEq/L)
Carbon dioxide 25 (21–31 mEq/L)
Blood urea nitrogen 20 (8–20 mg/dL)

Creatinine 0.9 (0.7–1.3 mg/dL)
Glucose 134 (70–139 mg/dL)
Phosphorus 3.1 (2.5–4.5 mg/dL)
Magnesium 1.8 (1.5–2.7 mg/dL)
Albumin 3.0 (3.5–5.5 g/dL)

Clinical Data:

Past Medical History: AML s/p two cycles of high-dose chemotherapy, hypertension, dyslipidemia, pre-diabetes, obesity
Medications: metoprolol, multivitamin with minerals, pravastatin
Vital Signs: Blood pressure 130/85 mm Hg, Temperature 99°F, Heart rate 80 beats/min
Nutrition-Focused Physical Exam: Appears tired. Central adiposity noted. Skin intact, no edema or wounds noted. Evident muscle loss of upper extremities. Oral exam notable for dry mucosa, intact dentition, normal tongue.

Dietary Data:

Dietary History: Seth follows a low-sodium, low-saturated fat diet. Prior to starting chemotherapy, he had decreased intake due to fatigue and poor appetite. Since starting chemotherapy, Seth's oral intake and appetite have decreased even more significantly to 50% of his typical intake due to treatment-related side effects. He has intermittently relied on a soft-solid/full-liquid diet due to pain with eating. He is not currently supplementing his diet with an oral nutritional supplement drink.

Usual Diet Recall:

Breakfast (9 am): 12 oz coffee, ½ cup oatmeal
Lunch (12 pm): Chicken sandwich with 3 oz chicken and fat-free mayonnaise, 12 oz diet ginger ale
Dinner (5 pm): 1 cup pasta with tomato sauce, ½ cup green beans, 12 oz water
Diet Prescription: Regular diet with high calorie high protein liquid oral nutrition supplement

Questions

1. Describe Seth's weight status, rate of weight loss, and current intake. Does Seth meet the criteria for malnutrition?
2. Write two Problem/Etiology/Signs and Symptoms (PES) statements for Seth.
3. Identify the nutrition interventions you would like to initiate for Seth to address the problems identified in your PES statements. What strategies can you offer Seth to prevent further weight loss?
4. What indices are included in your monitoring and evaluation plan? Why?

use, heavy alcohol consumption, excess body weight, suboptimal nutrition, or physical inactivity.[1,4] Certain cancers caused by infectious agents (such as human papillomavirus, hepatitis B and C viruses, and *Helicobacter pylori*) could be avoided by preventing infection through behavioral change, vaccination, or treatment of infection. Greater than five million skin cancer cases diagnosed annually could be prevented by protecting skin from excessive sun exposure and avoiding indoor tanning.[4]

Endogenous causes can occur through inherited germ-line mutations, oxidative stress from reactive oxygen species, and inflammation. Chronic inflammation can produce cytokines, growth factors, reactive oxygen, and nitrogen species, which can increase proliferation and differentiation, inhibit apoptosis (programmed cell death), and induce angiogenesis.[5] In addition to inflammation and stress, lifetime exposure to estrogen has been shown to raise the risk of breast, ovarian, and endometrial cancers.[5]

CORE CONCEPT 1

Almost half of new cancer diagnoses are caused by modifiable factors, including obesity, suboptimal nutrition, physical inactivity, tobacco use, and heavy alcohol consumption.

Epidemiology

According to the ACS, lifetime risk of cancer development is one in two for men and one in three for women; however, risk changes with exposure and genetic susceptibility. Cancer risk is known to increase with age, with 88% of cancer diagnosed in people 50 years or older.[4] In addition, more than 600,000 Americans are expected to die of cancer annually (about 1680 people per day), making cancer the second most common cause of death in the United States, surpassed only by heart disease.[4]

More than 100 types of cancer exist; they occur as a solid or hematologic malignancy and are named primarily for the organ or type of cell in which they originate. Solid malignancies present as an abnormal mass of tissue that is typically not cystic or liquid. Types of solid malignancies include **carcinomas** (beginning in the skin or tissues that line or cover internal organs) and **sarcomas** (cancers that begin in the bone, cartilage, fat, muscle, blood vessels, or connective or supportive tissue) (**Figure 17.1**). **Hematologic malignancies** are defined as cancers that begin in the blood-forming tissue, such as bone marrow (leukemias) or in the cells of the immune system (lymphomas and myelomas), and can be classified as acute or chronic in nature.

CORE CONCEPT 2

Cancer is the second most common cause of death in the United States, surpassed only by heart disease.

Cancer Staging

When cancer is diagnosed, it must be staged to determine the most effective treatment plan and offer prognosis. Staging describes the severity of a cancer based on the location of the primary tumor, tumor size, involvement of lymph nodes, and whether the primary tumor has spread to other areas of the body.[6] There are four different types of cancer staging, according to the American Joint Commission on Cancer (AJCC)[6]:

- Clinical staging: Determines how much cancer is present using physical exam, image testing, and biopsies
- Pathologic staging: Uses the clinical staging and surgical results following surgical removal of a tumor
- Post-therapy or post-neoadjuvant therapy staging: Determines how much cancer remains after a patient is first treated with systemic (chemotherapy) and/or radiation therapy; assessed by clinical and/or pathologic staging guidelines
- Recurrence: Used to determine the extent of disease if cancer returns following treatment

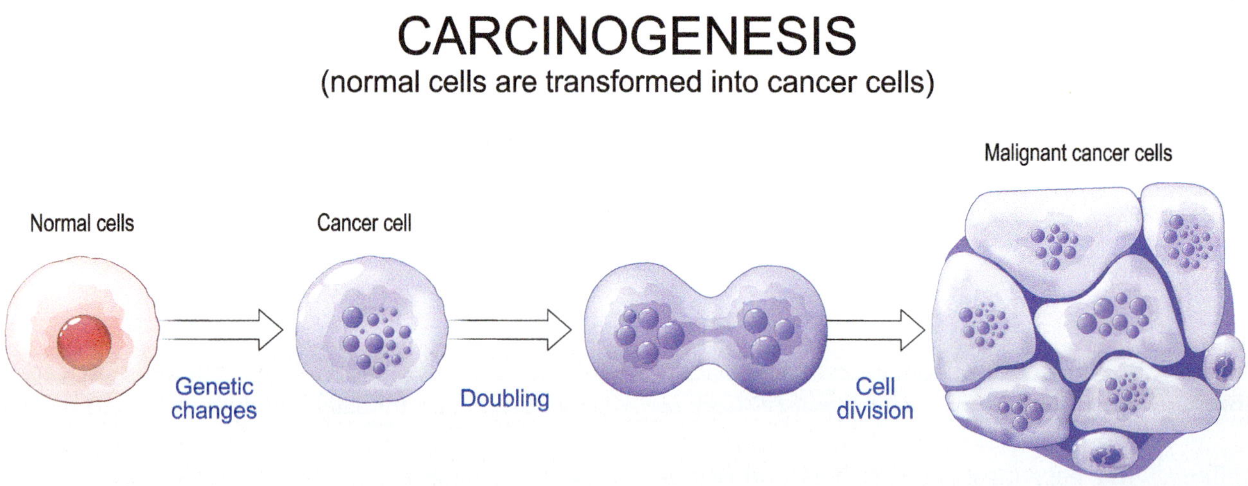

Figure 17.1 Stages of Carcinogenesis

The Tumor, Lymph Node, and Metastasis (TNM) Staging System was developed and is maintained by the AJCC and the Union for International Cancer Control (UICC)[6] and is a tool for staging different types of cancers based on standardized criteria. This is the most widely used staging tool among physicians. In this staging tool, T (description of the original tumor) is described as Tx (primary tumor cannot be evaluated; for example, it might not be seen on a scan), T0 (primary tumor cannot be found), Tis (carcinoma in situ or pre-cancer that has not spread to a nearby tissue), or T1–T4 (describes the size and extent of the primary tumor) with a larger number meaning a larger tumor. The N explains if the cancer has reached the nearby lymph nodes with Nx (lymph nodes cannot be assessed), N0 (nearby lymph nodes do not have cancer), or N1–N3 (cancer has spread to lymph nodes) with a higher number indicating a great spread of cancer to the lymph nodes. The final category, M, shows if cancer has spread to other distant parts of the body (M1) or not (M0).

Restaging may be assessed after completion of treatment to determine the extent to which the cancer responded to treatment or if a cancer has recurred and may require further treatments.

Medical Treatment of Cancer

Once the medical team determines the cancer stage, the patient and team decide on a treatment plan, which may include chemotherapy, radiation therapy, surgery, or a combination of therapies. Anticancer treatments may impact the patient's appetite and ability to ingest/digest food, placing patients at increased nutrition risk. Each cancer has its own unique set of nutrition-related side effects called **nutrition impact symptoms**. **Table 17.2** outlines typical nutrition impact symptoms related to specific cancers and anticancer treatments and their management.

Table 17.2 Nutrition Impact Symptoms and Their Nutritional Management

Nutrition Impact Symptom	Description	Associated Cancers	Nutritional Management
Anorexia	Lack of appetite, possibly due to delayed gastric emptying	All	▪ Maximize intake when appetite is present ▪ Limit fluid with meals to avoid feeling of fullness ▪ Eat small, frequent meals
Constipation	Infrequent or hard-to-pass bowel movements	All	▪ Ensure adequate fiber and fluid intake
Diarrhea	Frequent, loose, and watery stools	All; especially intestinal, pancreatic	▪ Avoid highly concentrated sweets, sip electrolyte-fortified beverages, eat soluble fiber
Dumping syndrome	Rapid movement of food, especially sugar, into the small bowel that results in cramps, diarrhea, and hypoglycemia	Esophageal, gastric, intestinal, pancreatic	▪ Avoid drinking beverages with meals ▪ Consume soluble fiber ▪ Follow a lactose-free diet ▪ Eat small, frequent meals
Dysgeusia	Alterations in taste	Head and neck, esophageal, gastric, lung	▪ *Metallic taste*: Use plastic utensils; eat nuts, cheese, and poultry for protein as red meats are often not tolerated ▪ *Sweet sensitivity*: Drink flavorless supplements or diluted juices ▪ *Impaired taste*: Use spiced or very flavorful foods
Dysphagia	Difficulty swallowing	Head and neck, esophageal, gastric, lung	▪ Change textures of foods based on level of dysphagia ▪ Thickening agents may be indicated for fluids

(continues)

Table 17.2 Nutrition Impact Symptoms and Their Nutritional Management (continued)

Nutrition Impact Symptom	Description	Associated Cancers	Nutritional Management
Esophagitis/ gastritis	Inflammation of the esophageal and gastric mucosa	Esophageal, gastric, lung	■ Eat bland, pureed, or soft foods ■ Avoid alcohol, coffee, or spicy and acidic foods
Mucositis (Figure 17.4)/ stomatitis	Inflammation of mucosal membranes, often in oral cavity	Head and neck, esophageal, gastric, lung	■ Consume soft, nonfibrous, nonacidic foods ■ Avoid hot foods and beverages
Nausea	Uneasiness or queasiness of the stomach	All	■ Avoid noxious odors by using microwaves or opening windows when cooking
Radiation enteritis	Inflammation of the small and/or large intestine caused by radiation	Intestinal, pancreatic	■ Follow a lactose-free and low-fat diet ■ Drink electrolyte-fortified beverages for hydration
Steatorrhea	Frequent, loose, and watery stools that contain excess fat	All; especially intestinal, pancreatic	■ Take pancreatic replacement enzymes, follow a low-fat diet, supplement with medium-chain triglyceride oil
Vomiting	Emptying of stomach contents through the mouth	All	■ Avoid greasy foods the day of treatment ■ Drink electrolyte-fortified beverages after vomiting
Xerostomia	Diminished or loss of saliva production	Head and neck, esophageal, gastric, lung	■ Chew sugar-free gum or suck on tart candies ■ Use sauces and gravies to moisten foods

Data from Grosvenor M, Bulcavage L, Chlebowski RT. Symptoms potentially influencing weight loss in a cancer population: correlations with primary site, nutritional status, and chemotherapy administration. *Cancer*. 1989;63(2):330–334. doi:10.1002/1097-0142(19890115)63:2<330::AID-CNCR2820630224>3.0.CO;2-3.

Chemotherapy

Chemotherapy involves the use of antineoplastic medications, used as a single agent or in combination with other agents, that disrupt the reproductive cycle of cancer cells. The goal of chemotherapy is to shrink cancer cells, control tumor growth, and palliate symptoms related to cancer, such as pain. Chemotherapy is utilized as a primary treatment for hematological cancers, as an adjuvant treatment after surgery, as a neo-adjuvant treatment before surgery, or as a concurrent treatment with radiation therapy. Chemotherapy acts by targeting rapidly dividing cells, such as cancer cells, but it may also attack healthy cells, such as those that line the gastrointestinal (GI) tract, resulting in unwanted GI side effects such as nausea, vomiting, diarrhea, and mucositis that may place patients at increased nutrition risk.

Radiation Therapy

Radiation therapy is the use of high-energy radiation from x-rays, gamma rays, or other sources used to kill cancer cells and shrink tumors (**Figure 17.2**). It can be external or systemic, which uses a radioactive substance that circulates throughout the body. Side effects of radiation therapy typically start 2 weeks after the beginning of treatment, with the type and severity dependent on the location of the radiation treatment. Common side effects include fatigue, skin changes, nausea, and anorexia. **Odynophagia** (pain with swallowing), dysphagia, and pneumonitis are more commonly found in patients with head and neck cancer. Radiation enteritis and diarrhea are more common in cancers of the lower GI tract and pelvic region.

Proton therapy, or protein beam therapy, is a type of radiation therapy that delivers a beam of protons to disrupt and destroy tumor cells, whereas traditional radiation uses photons. The ability to kill cancer cells while saving the surrounding healthy tissue makes this treatment ideal for brain, esophageal, liver, and pediatric cancers. Additionally, greater control of the treatment allows for reduced toxicity and increased quality of life. However, concern has been raised about the clinical efficacy of this treatment in addition to the significant cost.[7]

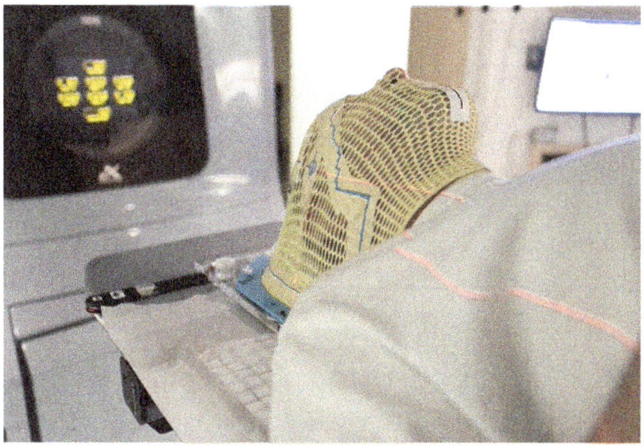

Figure 17.2 Patient Receiving Radiation Therapy
© John Panella/Shutterstock

Further research is needed on this treatment modality as <1% of patients with cancer are treated using proton therapy.

Surgery

Surgery is used in solid tumors as both a palliative and curative regimen with a goal to remove a localized tumor or limit the local regional spread by removal of cancer cells. It may be used as primary, adjuvant, or combination treatment or as a salvage therapy, which is an extensive surgery to treat local recurrence after a less-extensive primary approach has been implemented. When resection cannot be performed, other treatment modalities may be used in an attempt to reduce the size of the cancer and allow for future surgical removal. The nutritional status of patients should be monitored both pre- and postoperatively because surgical interventions can lead to nutritional deterioration due to changes in metabolism, tissue function, and body composition.

Biotherapy

Biotherapy, also known as "biological therapy," is a cancer therapy that may stimulate or suppress the body's immune system to kill cancer cells. It is used in the treatment of many types of cancer, such as lymphoma, to prevent or slow tumor growth and spread with fewer side effects than other cancer treatments. Biotherapy works by either inducing the immune system to attack cancer cells or making cancer cells easier for the immune system to recognize. Biotherapy is an extremely active area of cancer research and predominantly available in clinical trials.

Hormone Therapy

Hormone therapy is a treatment aimed at slowing or stopping the growth of certain hormone-sensitive cancers (such as breast and prostate) through synthetic hormones. These hormones may be given to block the body's natural hormones to treat the cancer or improve patient cancer symptoms.

CORE CONCEPT 3

Medical treatment of cancer can lead to nutrition impact symptoms that may impair a patient's nutritional status.

Nutrition Screening and Assessment in Patients with Cancer

Patients with cancer are at elevated risk of malnutrition given disease burden, treatment-related side effects, and metabolic and physiological side effects related to cancer. Weight loss and malnutrition, the most common secondary diagnosis for patients with advanced cancers, have been documented in more than 30–90% of patients, often at the time of diagnosis, depending on disease severity, treatment regimen, and associated side effects.[8–10] As many as 20% of patients with cancer die from the effects of malnutrition rather than malignancy.[10] Nutritional status may influence disease prognosis, treatment tolerance, and quality of life (QOL) and may hasten the onset of cancer cachexia. As little as a 5% weight loss before initiation of chemotherapy is predictive of early mortality and can predict a reduction in response to treatment, survival, and QOL.[11] Weight loss associated with cancer treatment can be highly distressing to the patient and caregiver and may further impair QOL.

CORE CONCEPT 4

Weight loss and malnutrition are well documented in patients with cancer and may influence disease prognosis, treatment tolerance, and quality of life and be predictive of early mortality.

Nutrition Screening

Screening patients newly diagnosed with cancer and those undergoing therapy is key to preventing and identifying malnutrition at the earliest phase in an attempt to prevent or halt negative outcomes. According to the Academy of Nutrition and Dietetics Evidence Analysis Library, "all adult patients should be screened for malnutrition risk on entry into oncology services; early identification and management of malnutrition risk improves and protects nutrition

Table 17.3 Nutrition Screening Tools Validated in the Oncology Population

Tool	Summary	Advantages	Disadvantages
Malnutrition Screening Tool (MST)	Short-form (only 2 questions) screening tool that assesses recent weight loss and recent poor intake	▪ Can be used in inpatient and outpatient settings ▪ Suitable screening tool for both radiation and chemotherapy outpatients ▪ Quick and easy to calculate	▪ Poor sensitivity for oncology inpatients ▪ Does not include times frame for weight loss ▪ Does not include triage recommendations
Malnutrition Screening Tool for Cancer Patients (MSTC)	Identifies inpatient patients with cancer who are at risk of malnutrition based on intake change, weight loss, BMI, and the Eastern Cooperative Oncology Group performance status	▪ High validity compared with other available screening tools	▪ Valid and reliable only for inpatients ▪ Specifically tailored for Korean patients with cancer
Malnutrition Universal Screening Tool (MUST)	5-step tool that uses BMI, weight loss percentage, and acute disease effect to identify patients who are malnourished, at risk of malnutrition, or obese	▪ Consistent and reliable screening tool ▪ Quick and easy ▪ Can be used by any care professional ▪ Management guidelines for care plan included	▪ Valid and reliable only for inpatients ▪ Evaluation of appetite and intake is limited ▪ Not designed to identify vitamin or mineral deficiencies or excess intake
Patient Generated Subjective Global Assessment (PG-SGA)	Assesses nutrition risk based on anthropometrics, intake, symptoms, activity, age, and metabolic stress	▪ Allows patients to become involved ▪ Highlights nutrition impact symptoms ▪ Includes nutrition triage recommendations ▪ Can predict direction and magnitude of change in QOL	▪ Associated with large costs in terms of time and manpower ▪ Reliability influenced by experience of facilitator ▪ Misinterpretation of questions is common

Data from Bauer J, Capra S, Ferguson M. Use of the scored patient-generated subjective global assessment (PG-SGA) as a nutrition assessment tool in patients with cancer. *Eur J Clin Nutr.* 2002;56(8):779-785.; Isenring E, Bauer J, Capra S. The scored patient-generated subjective global assessment (PG-SGA) and its association with quality of life in ambulatory patients receiving radiotherapy. *Eur J Clin Nutr.* 2003;57(2):305-309; Shaw C, Fleuret C, Pickard M, et al. Comparison of novel screening tools for adult oncology patients. *Support Care Cancer.* 2015;23:47-54. doi:10.1007/s00520-041-2319-8.; Boléo-Tomé C, Monteiro-Grillo I, Camilo M, et al. Validation of the Malnutrition Universal Screening Tool (MUST) in cancer. *Br J Nutr.* 2012;108(2):343-348. doi:10.1017/S000711451100571X.; Chao P, Chuang H, Tsao L, et al. The Malnutrition Universal Screening Tool (MUST) and a nutrition education program for high-risk cancer patients: strategies to improve dietary intake in cancer patients. *Biomedicine (Taipei).* 2015;5(3):17. doi:10.7603/s40681-015-0017-6.; Isenring EA, Bauer JD, Capra S. Nutrition support using the American Dietetic Association medical nutrition therapy protocol for radiation oncology patients improves dietary intake compared with standard practice. *J Am Diet Assoc.* 2007;107(3):404-412

status and QOL, which leads to improved outcomes. Re-screening should be repeated routinely throughout treatment to facilitate referral as needed."[12]

A variety of nutrition screening tools are recommended for use in ambulatory cancer centers; unfortunately, there is a lack of implementation of consistent screening, triage, and assessment tools that are evidence-based in the oncology population.[13] Appropriate screening tools should be validated for use in the oncology population and be able to identify malnutrition risk in patients with cancer. The current screening tools validated for use in the oncology population include the Patient Generated Subjective Global Assessment (PG-SGA), the Malnutrition Screening Tool (MST), the Malnutrition Screening Tool for Cancer Patients (MSTC), and the Malnutrition Universal Screening Tool (MUST).[6] **Table 17.3**

PRACTICE POINT

All patients with cancer should be screened early and often for nutrition risk given that early identification and management of malnutrition risk can lead to improved outcomes. Patients identified at nutritional risk should be referred to a registered dietitian for nutrition assessment.

provides a summary of the validated screening tools along with their advantages and disadvantages.[14–19] Patients identified as malnourished or at nutrition risk should be referred to a registered dietitian (RD) for evaluation, nutrition assessment, and, if indicated, medical nutrition therapy to manage nutrition risk. It is important to remember to re-screen patients often throughout treatment to monitor nutritional changes.

Nutrition Assessment

Nutrition assessment of the patient with cancer should include a thorough assessment of the patient's baseline and current oral food and fluid intake, including the addition of medical food supplements, vitamin/mineral and herbal supplements, and enteral nutrition (EN) and parenteral nutrition (PN). The patient's current treatment regimen with assessment of current and predicted nutrition impact symptoms should be included in the nutrition assessment. Weight trends, including pre-diagnosis weight and degree of unintentional weight loss, should be assessed in conjunction with a nutrition-focused physical examination of fluid retention/edema, muscle wasting, and decline in functional status. A nutrition care plan is then developed by the RD and shared with the interprofessional care team. During active cancer treatment, the overall goals of nutrition care that guide the care plan are to prevent or reverse nutrition deficiencies, to preserve lean body mass, to minimize nutrition-related side effects, and to maximize QOL. There is a significant benefit of dietary counseling during cancer treatment for improving outcomes, such as fewer treatment-related side effects, improved QOL, and better dietary intake.[19]

CORE CONCEPT 5

Dietary counseling by a registered dietitian (RD) results in improved outcomes, including fewer treatment-related side effects, improved quality of life, and better dietary intake.

Estimating Nutrition Needs in Patients with Cancer

Energy requirements differ depending on the type of tumor present. Normal resting energy expenditure (REE) has been reported in patients with gastric or colorectal cancers, while those with pancreatic cancer usually have higher energy expenditures. Previous nutrition recommendations for all patients with cancer were to provide 30–35 kcal/kg and 1.2–2.0 g protein/kg body weight.[20] More recently, the calorie recommendation has been estimated to be 25–30 kcal/kg, or more similar to the needs of healthy individuals.[21] This change helps to reflect the likely decrease in physical activity and the need to avoid hypercaloric feeding, which can lead to undesired metabolic effects.

Individual nutrition needs of patients with cancer vary greatly and are based upon tumor type, treatment regimen, presence of stressors (such as infection), and need for weight gain. For example, weight loss of >10% is associated with an increased REE when compared to patients with cancer who are weight-stable.[22] Additionally, the metabolic effects of the tumor and proinflammatory cytokines may alter energy expenditure as a result of altered macronutrient metabolism and the progressive syndrome of cancer cachexia.

A universal REE of patients with cancer has been deemed inconsistent in research as **hypermetabolism**, or the physiological state of increased rate of metabolic activity characterized by an abnormal increase in the body's basal metabolic rate and is not uniformly present in patients with cancer. The Harris–Benedict equation (HBE), along with a stress factor, has been utilized in practice as an estimation equation in this population, but it has been shown to both over- and underestimate calorie needs in the cancer population. Indirect calorimetry remains the ideal method of determining energy needs in this patient population; however, it is not always accessible. Estimated energy requirements should be reassessed based on weight trends, treatment plan, and changes in the patient's clinical picture, and should always be individualized to each patient.

PRACTICE POINT

Energy needs assessment should be individualized and based on clinical judgment, as hypermetabolism is not uniformly present in patients with cancer.

PRACTICE POINT

Weight loss of >10% is associated with increased energy expenditure.

CORE CONCEPT 6

Nutrition impact symptoms and energy requirements differ based on the specific solid tumor present.

Cancer Cachexia and Metabolic Changes Associated with Cancer

Cancer Cachexia

The term *cachexia* comes from the Greek word for "poor condition" and is a clinical syndrome of debilitation and weight loss associated with the end stage of numerous chronic conditions. **Cancer cachexia** is a multifactorial syndrome characterized by an ongoing loss of skeletal muscle mass that cannot be fully reversed by conventional nutrition support.[23–27] It reduces cardiac mass and influences cardiac muscle contraction and may subsequently lead to progressive functional impairment in up to 80% of progressive cancers.[24,28] The degree of cachexia can vary according to tumor type, site, mass, and anatomical position. Clinical characteristics can include anorexia, early satiety, weakness, and weight loss (**Figure 17.3**). The mechanisms of cancer cachexia are poorly understood but are thought to be tumor induced and driven by proinflammatory cytokines. **Cytokines** are cell-signaling molecules that aid in cell-to-cell communication in immune responses and stimulate the movement of cells toward sites of inflammation, infection, and trauma. Cancer-related cytokines include tumor necrosis factor, interleukin-1, and interleukin-6. These proinflammatory cytokines play a large role in metabolic alterations, as observed in advanced cancer and cancer cachexia, and also can affect other physiologic processes, including altered gastric emptying, decreases in intestinal blood flow, and changes in bowel motility. The tumor-induced factors are further confounded by the effects of cancer treatment, such as GI side effects, reduced appetite, and reduced or loss of taste, which may further impair nutrition intake.

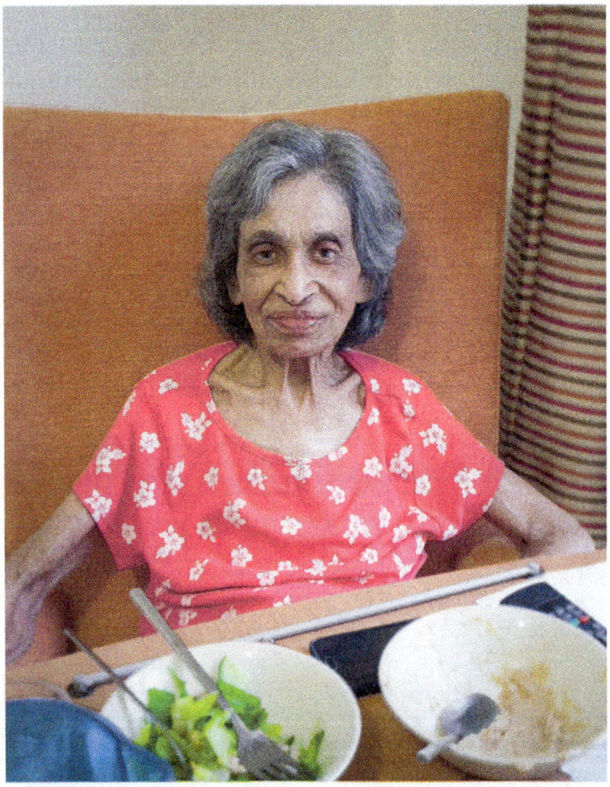

Figure 17.3 A Patient with Wasting Associated with Cancer Cachexia

CORE CONCEPT 7

Cancer cachexia can lead to progressive functional impairment in advanced cancers. Proinflammatory cytokines may play a role in mediating alterations in metabolism observed in cancer cachexia and may also affect other gastrointestinal processes.

The metabolic effect of cancer cachexia has been shown to be similar to severe sepsis or injury, since nutrients move from the periphery to the liver, resulting in increased gluconeogenesis and breakdown in fat stores.[26] In contrast to severe sepsis, there is a preferential loss of skeletal muscle associated with decreased protein synthesis and increased protein degradation in the presence of proinflammatory cytokines (**Table 17.4**).[28,29] Unlike the mechanism of starvation, where REE is conserved, it is unclear whether patients with cancer have elevated energy expenditure. The proposed mechanism of presumed hypermetabolism in patients with cachexia seems to be due to systemic inflammation, high rates of glycolysis, and the result of adrenergic state, not reversed by feeding alone.[23,24] Studies indicate that overall glucose fluctuation between gluconeogenesis and glycogenolysis increases in patients with cancer who are weight-losing, which contributes up to 40% of increased REE in metastatic cancer.[22]

CORE CONCEPT 8

Cancer cachexia results in preferential loss of skeletal muscle mass and may contribute to an increase in resting energy expenditure.

Table 17.4 Changes in Macronutrient Metabolism Associated With Cancer/Cancer Cachexia

Macronutrient	Metabolism in Cancer/Cachexia	Proposed Mechanism
Carbohydrates	■ Increased rate of anaerobic glycolysis leading to increased consumption rate of glucose, resulting in lactate production ■ Elevated Cori cycle activity converting lactate back to glucose via gluconeogenesis, resulting in net consumption of adenosine triphosphate	■ Presence of proinflammatory cytokines ■ High rate of anaerobic glycolysis in malignant cells
Lipids	■ Enhanced lipolysis via proinflammatory cytokines further induced by hyperlipidemia ■ Decreased/inhibited lipogenesis ■ Increased mobilization of lipids, specifically triglycerides, hydrolyzed to free fatty acids resulting in fat atrophy	■ Effect of proinflammatory cytokines, adrenergic activation, and tumor-related lipolytic factor
Protein	■ Increased protein degradation and skeletal muscle breakdown ■ Amino acids diverted to synthesis of acute phase reactants, resulting in muscle degradation and decreased muscle protein synthesis ■ Increased turnover of whole-body protein and amino acids	■ Presence of proinflammatory cytokines ■ Increased metabolic demands by tumor

Data from Arends J, Bachmann P, Baracos V, et al. ESPEN guidelines on nutrition in cancer patients. *Clin Nutr.* 2017;36(1):11-48. doi:10.1016/j.clnu.2016.07.015

Nutrition Interventions in the Patient with Cancer

Approaches to Management in Cancer Cachexia

No evidence-based treatments are available for the treatment of cancer cachexia, and standard nutrition support may not necessarily improve outcomes in this group. Early identification of patients at risk of cachexia is crucial to prevent the onset of this syndrome, but this remains challenging as the mechanisms of cancer cachexia remain poorly understood. Early nutrition intervention plays a significant role in delaying the progression of weight loss, which may further delay the onset and acceleration of cancer cachexia.[30] Although research has been conducted on multiple medications and feeding strategies to mitigate the effects of cancer cachexia, current treatment strategies remain inadequate and fail to improve clinical outcomes. An overview of researched medical treatment strategies for cancer cachexia can be found in **Table 17.5**.[31–42]

The use of hypercaloric feeding via nutrition support in the form of oral supplements and/or EN and PN is often encouraged in patients with cancer cachexia but may not be associated with a measurable clinical benefit. Studies have failed to show that there are improvements in lean body mass when providing patients with a hypercaloric feeding regimen; in fact, loss of lean body mass persists and weight gain is observed in the form of fat mass.[24,27,30] Feeding regimens do not come without risk, and the use of PN support in particular is not associated with a measurable clinical benefit but may be associated with increased risk of catheter-related sepsis.[24] The timing of nutrition support in the cancer population remains controversial due to a lack of rigorous randomized, controlled trials.

PRACTICE POINT

Nutrition support and hypercaloric feeding in patients with cancer cachexia is not associated with a measurable clinical benefit.

CORE CONCEPT 9

Because no evidence-based treatments are available for cancer cachexia, focus should be placed on early nutrition interventions to prevent the onset and acceleration of the condition.

Overview of Nutrition Support in Patients with Cancer

Although nutrition support may not provide clinical benefit to the patient with cancer cachexia, nutrition support interventions with EN or PN may be important in optimizing the patient's nutrition status to achieve the best possible outcomes. Nutrition support should

Table 17.5 Medical Management of Cancer Cachexia

Medical Treatment	Proposed Benefit	Potential Disadvantages and Research Limitations
β-Hydroxy-β-methylbutyrate (HMB)	Leucine metabolite thought to preserve lean muscle mass	▪ Supplements studied contained arginine and glutamine, which may confound results ▪ Exact reason HMB may promote fat-free mass gain remains unknown
Branch chain amino acids (BCAA)	Associated with increased protein synthesis and decreased protein degradation due to integral role in skeletal muscle proteins	▪ Results have only been demonstrated in rats with cachexia also using leucine and valine (not replicated in human studies) ▪ Supplements also contained fish oil/omega-3 fatty acids
Glucocorticoids	Associated with increased appetite and improved quality of life in short-term setting	▪ Inconclusive effects on lean body mass ▪ Adverse side effects associated with long-term use, including insulin resistance, water retention, adrenal insufficiency
Omega-3 fatty acids	Associated with profound anti-inflammatory effects, potential to stabilize weight loss, and attenuate lean tissue wasting	▪ Lack of consistent data supporting the dose, duration, timing, and route of administration ▪ Larger randomized controlled trials have not demonstrated a clear benefit in maintaining weight, lean body mass, survival, or QOL
Progesterones (megesterol acetate)	Associated with increased appetite and weight gain	▪ Weight gain remains largely fat mass and edema with limited improvements in lean body mass, performance status, or QOL ▪ Insufficient evidence to define optimal dose

Data from Aapro M, Arends J, Bozzetti F, et al. Early recognition of malnutrition and cachexia in the cancer patient: a position paper of a European School of Oncology Task Force. *Ann Oncol*. 2014;25(8):1492-1499. doi:10.1093/annonc/mdu085; Kuhn KS, Muscaritoli M, Wischmeyer P, Stehle P. Glutamine as an indispensable nutrient in oncology: experimental and clinical evidence. *Eur J Nutr*. 2010;49(4):197-210. doi:10.1007/s00394-010-0091-4; Eley HL, Russell ST, Tisdale MJ. Effect of branched-chain amino acids on muscle atrophy in cancer cachexia. *Biochem J*. 2007;407:113-120. doi:10.1042/BJ20070651

be initiated if it is expected that a patient will be unable to eat for a minimum of 7 days. Additionally, patients with severe nutrition risk (>10% weight loss in 6 months or body mass index [BMI] <18.5 kg/m^2) benefit from nutrition support 10–14 days prior to major surgery, even if the surgery has to be delayed. PN should only be initiated when patients cannot be fed through the enteral route. This can occur from radiation enteritis, ileus, bowel obstruction, or other severe intestinal insufficiency.[20,21]

PRACTICE POINT

Nutrition support is important for malnourished patients with cancer or those who may not be able to eat for 7 days. Patients with severe nutrition risk benefit from nutrition support 10–14 days prior to major surgery.

Enteral Nutrition

Nasogastric tubes (NGT) are placed for the short term, while percutaneous endoscopic gastrostomy

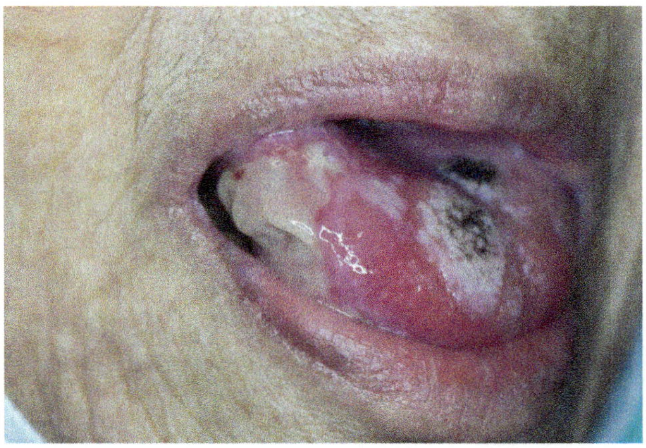

Figure 17.4 Mucositis

(PEG) tubes are for longer term use. A PEG tube may have a decreased chance of tube displacement compared to an NGT, but the cancer may metastasize to the gastrostomy itself. If a patient is experiencing ulcerative mucositis (**Figure 17.4**), the presence of an

NGT may exacerbate irritation, and thus a PEG may be a more ideal choice.[43]

Standard enteral formulas are generally recommended for EN; however, immunonutrition (IN) formulas are becoming increasingly used in GI cancers. **Immunonutrition** is the effect of nutrients, including macronutrients, vitamins, minerals, and trace elements, on inflammation, the formation of antibodies, and the resistance to disease. Common immune-modulating formulas contain higher amounts of omega-3 fatty acids, arginine, nucleic acids, glutamine, and antioxidants, which may improve GI mucosal integrity and enhance cell-mediated immune response. Some controversy exists regarding the use of glutamine in patients with cancer given in vitro evidence of glutamine being a primary fuel source for tumor cells. However, clinical studies show that glutamine benefits host metabolism, mucosal integrity, and immune function without enhancing tumor cell growth.[42] The European Society of Clinical Nutrition and Metabolism (ESPEN) guidelines recommend using IN for patients diagnosed with GI or head and neck cancer for 5–7 days prior to abdominal surgery, independent of their nutrition status.[20,21]

When initiating EN in patients who have had decreased oral intake, slow advancement over several days is recommended to avoid refeeding syndrome. If there is a concern for refeeding, it is vital to provide daily thiamine along with potassium, phosphate, and magnesium as needed.[22]

PRACTICE POINT

Immune-modulating formulas may provide clinical benefit to patients with GI or head and neck cancer when used for 5–7 days prior to abdominal surgery, independent of nutrition status.

Parenteral Nutrition

When oral intake and enteral intake are not sufficient, PN may be indicated. Despite widespread central line access, PN should not be routinely used with cancer treatment. Instead, PN should be reserved for patients with moderate to severe malnutrition who are not tolerating oral or enteral feeds, and those with postoperative ileus, malignant bowel obstruction, high output GI fistula, or large volume diarrhea/high output ostomy.[44] When initiating PN, it is important to slowly increase to goal nutrition over several days while closely monitoring laboratory values to avoid refeeding syndrome.[21]

Nutritional Management of Specific Solid Tumors

Head and Neck Cancers

Head and neck cancers (HNC) make up about 3% of all new cancer cases in the United States.[45,46] HNC include those of the sinus cavity and oropharyngeal region.[45] New cases occur most frequently in Black men, aged 50 years or older, who have a history of alcohol and tobacco use. Other risk factors are poor oral hygiene and history of human papillomavirus infection.[45] Those with early, localized HNC are managed by surgery and/or radiation. If the cancer is more advanced, aggressive multimodal therapies including surgery, chemotherapy, and radiation may be indicated.[47]

Patients with HNC are the most at risk for malnutrition compared to any other malignancy. In fact, around 25% of patients face impaired nutrition status at the time of diagnosis, prior to any treatment.[48] Dysphagia secondary to the physical obstruction of the tumor and a history of alcohol and tobacco use are the biggest predictors of malnutrition observed in this population.[46,49] Additionally, nutrition intake is often limited during treatment due to mucositis and xerostomia, causing difficulty chewing and swallowing.[44]

Early nutrition intervention is needed to help patients navigate these symptoms. If a patient is experiencing dry mouth, interventions may include staying hydrated, consuming moist and soft foods, adding sauces, gravy, oil, and butter, and choosing tart foods (to increase saliva). For patients with mouth and throat sores, drinking through a straw, consuming bland room temperature foods, and moistening foods can be beneficial. Patients who are experiencing taste changes may require herbs, spices, and seasonings to be added to food. Adding sugar to salty foods and salt to sugary foods can also be helpful. For patients experiencing metallic tastes, plastic utensils and lemon juice can be helpful.[44] Patients with dysphagia should be referred to a speech language pathologist to identify the appropriate diet consistency that can be safely consumed.

Surgical interventions in HNC usually demand nutrition support. EN is preferred and generally well tolerated given the GI tract is typically functional. The use of NGT and PEG feedings helps to maintain body weight 6 months after treatment; however, each route poses its own unique benefits and risks.[50] Prophylactic PEG placement (prior to the start of treatment) is an acceptable practice with patients with HNC to reduce treatment-induced weight loss, although there

Clinical Controversy

Do patients with head and neck cancer (HNC) benefit from prophylactic percutaneous endoscopic gastrostomy (PEG) placement?

Patients with HNC are at increased risk of malnutrition due to impaired swallowing function and odynophagia, impacting their ability to eat and drink. Inadequate intake can lead to weight loss, malnutrition, dehydration, increased risk of hospitalization, poor treatment tolerance, lower quality of life, and increased mortality. Silander et al. randomized 134 patients with advanced HNC to receive a PEG tube or no PEG tube. The results of the study revealed that there was no difference in hospital stay between the two groups. The healthcare-related quality of life was significantly better, and weight loss was significantly less in the PEG group. Madhoun et al. evaluated characteristics of 143 patients with HNC with prophylactic PEGs and concluded that there was a high rate of unnecessary PEG placement when done prophylactically in HNC due to the fact that almost half of the patients never used the PEG or used it for less than 2 weeks. Finally, Fong et al. assessed 49 patients with HNC and found prophylactic PEG placement to be relatively safe, although some complications were noted.

Questions

1. What are the potential advantages and disadvantages of prophylactic PEG placement in patients with HNC?
2. How would you assess a patient with HNC for a prophylactic PEG placement?
3. Would you recommend a prophylactic PEG for your patient with HNC?

References

Silander E, Nyman J, Bove M, Johansson L, Larsson S, Hammerlid E. Impact of prophylactic percutaneous endoscopic gastrostomy on malnutrition and quality of life in patients with head and neck cancer: a randomized study. *Head Neck*. 2012;34(1):1-9.; Madhoun MF, Blankenship MM,Blankenship DM, Krempl GA, Tierney WM. Prophylactic PEG placement in head and neck cancer: how many feeding tubes are unused (and unnecessary)? *World J Gastroenterol*. 2011;17(8):1004-1008.; Fong SC, Pandey R, Rajaretnam M, Delaibatiki M, Peel DNY. Routine prophylactic percutaneous endoscopic gastrostomy in head and neck cancers with bilateral neck irradiation: a regional cancer experience in New Zealand. *J Med Radiat Sci*. 2023;70(3):292-300. doi:10.1002/jmrs.699

is little evidence to support that their use actually increases body weight.[46] Use of PN in this population is rare given the lower GI tract is generally functional.

PRACTICE POINT

Food textures may require modification if dysphagia is present. In patients with head and neck cancer, prophylactic PEG placement is an accepted practice to reduce treatment-induced weight loss.

CORE CONCEPT 10

Patients with head and neck cancer have the highest risk for malnutrition compared to other malignancies due to the physical location of the tumor and likelihood of dysphagia.

Esophageal Cancer

Esophageal cancer (EC) (**Figure 17.5**) is relatively uncommon in the United States.[45] Most patients are often asymptomatic until late in the disease process, thus a poor long-term survival rate (around 22%) remains.[45] History of tobacco/alcohol use and Barrett's esophagus, a complication of long-term gastroesophageal reflux, are the major risk factors for EC. Some attribute the obesity epidemic, a risk factor of reflux, to a rise in incidence of esophageal cancers.[51]

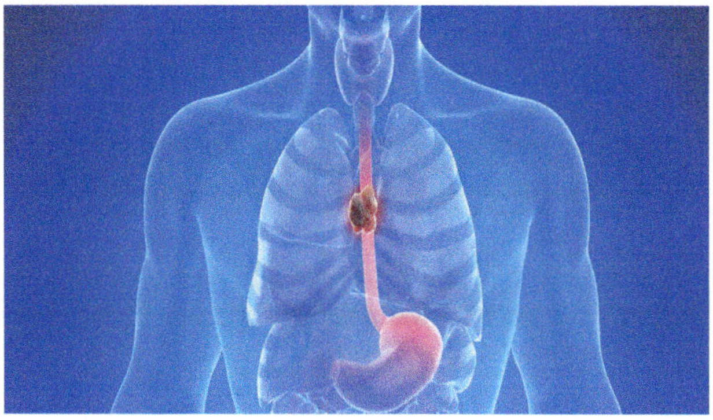

Figure 17.5 Esophageal Cancer

Esophageal resection is the treatment of choice if the cancer is detected early. Surgical options include esophagectomy (resection of part of the esophagus) and esophagogastrectomy (a procedure where the

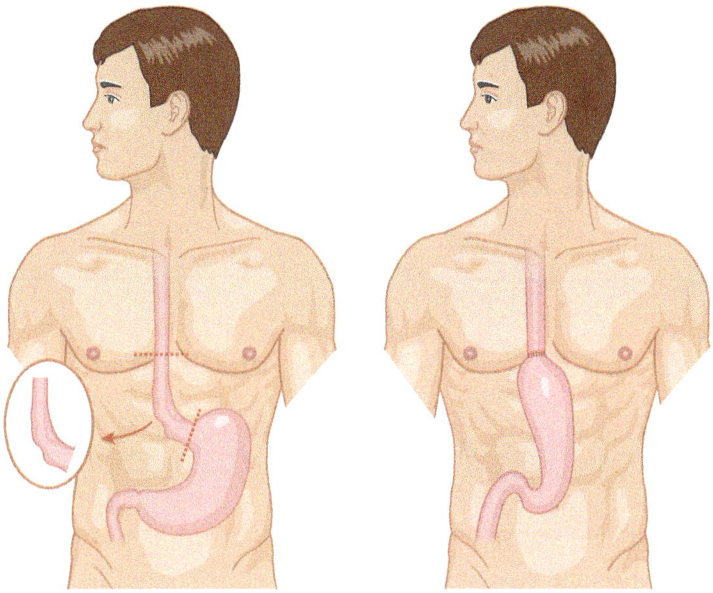

Figure 17.6 Surgery for Treatment of Esophageal Cancer

stomach is used to replace the resected esophagus; **Figure 17.6**). For advanced stages, multimodal therapy including radiation, chemotherapy, and surgery is utilized.[51]

As with patients with HNC, those with EC may benefit from modifying food textures if dysphasia is present. If the stomach was used to reconstruct the esophagus, patients may experience dumping syndrome. Dumping syndrome results from rapid delivery of nutrients into the proximal small bowel characterized by sweating, tachycardia, GI symptoms, and hypoglycemia. To avoid dumping syndrome, patients should limit concentrated sweets, lactose, and high-fat foods. Patients should also avoid drinking beverages until 30–60 minutes after eating to minimize rapid gastric emptying during mealtimes.[52] Refer to Chapter 10, *Nutritional Management of Gastrointestinal Maldigestion*, for more information on nutritional therapy for dumping syndrome. For patients postsurgery who require nutrition support, jejunostomy tubes (J tubes) are the preferred enteral route to bypass the fresh anastomoses in the esophagus or stomach. Most patients can tolerate jejunal feeding as early as 48–72 hours postoperatively.[52–54]

PRACTICE POINT

Food textures may require modification if dysphagia is present in patients with esophageal cancer. Jejunostomy tubes are often used and can be tolerated early after surgery.

Gastric Cancer

Gastric cancer is relatively rare; however, it is more common in men than women and among other races and ethnicities than White people.[45] Common risk factors include *Helicobacter pylori* infection and male sex. If caught early, the 5-year survival rate for localized gastric cancer is 67%.[45]

The primary treatment for GC is surgery, either a total or subtotal gastrectomy (80–85% removal of the stomach). Chemotherapy and radiation are adjuvant therapies.[55] Postgastrectomy syndrome predisposes the patient with GC to micronutrient deficiencies, fat malabsorption, and dumping syndrome. Decreased gastric acid and intrinsic factor production may result in iron, calcium, and vitamin B12 deficiencies. Patients are encouraged to take a daily multivitamin, 1000 mcg sublingual vitamin B12 daily (or 1000 mcg intramuscular injection once monthly), and 500 mg calcium citrate twice daily to prevent such deficiencies. If fat malabsorption occurs, at least 1000 units of vitamin D should be supplemented daily and fat-soluble vitamins should be monitored routinely.[56] Because patients postgastrectomy are also at risk for dumping syndrome, patients should limit concentrated sweets, lactose, and high-fat foods.

For patients requiring nutrition support, J tubes are often placed at the time of the gastrectomy surgery to help patients reach their caloric goals. However, J tubes in this population are associated with increased risk of postoperative infection and anastomotic leak that may lead to re-operation.[57]

PRACTICE POINT

Micronutrient supplementation, including vitamin B12, vitamin D, iron, and calcium, may be necessary after gastric surgery, depending on the amount of stomach resected. Small, frequent, low-fat meals limited in concentrated sweets should be recommended to prevent dumping syndrome after gastric surgery.

Intestinal Cancers

Small bowel malignancies are rare, about 0.5% of all malignancies, and the most common are carcinoid tumors.[45] Conversely, colorectal cancer (CRC) is the third most common cancer diagnosed in the United States.[45] Age is the main risk factor for CRC, with 90% of new cases occurring after age 50 years. Screening for CRC by fecal occult blood testing or routine colonoscopy beginning at 50 years has significantly decreased mortality rates.[58] Surgical intervention is the initial mode of treatment for intestinal cancers, with radiation to the abdomen or pelvis serving as a standard adjuvant therapy.

Abdominal and pelvic radiation may induce enteritis accompanied by diarrhea and malabsorption of fat, electrolytes, and lactose.[59] Nutritional management data for radiation enteritis is limited; however, a low-residue, low-fat, and lactose-free diet with emphasis on hydration is well tolerated in most patients.[60] A low-residue diet is also used after bowel resection with progression to a regular diet as tolerated is recommended. Those who require colostomies or ileostomies after surgery should eat foods with soluble fiber to thicken stool (such as bananas and applesauce) and avoid gas- and odor-producing foods (such as broccoli and beans). If massive resection of the bowel should take place, the patient is at risk for short bowel syndrome (SBS), a malabsorptive state of macro- and micronutrients. Most of these patients often require nutrition support. If an oral diet is tolerated, then small, frequent meals high in protein and low in fat, fiber, and lactose are encouraged. Micronutrient supplementation depends on what portion of the bowel remains, but most require additional vitamin B12 supplements.[61]

For patients requiring nutrition support, continuous NGT feedings of intact protein formulas increase absorption of macronutrients and reduce osmotic diarrhea compared to elemental formulas in patients with SBS.[62] PN may be indicated after bowel resection if SBS occurs, or if obstructions, fistulae, or anastomotic leaks should occur.[61]

PRACTICE POINT

Bowel resection after intestinal surgery requires diet progression from low residue with advancement to a regular diet. If short bowel syndrome should occur, nutrition support is often indicated to maintain nutrition and hydration.

Pancreatic Cancer

Pancreatic cancer is an extremely aggressive malignancy. Despite being the 10th most common cancer in the United States, it is the third leading cause of cancer death.[45] The etiology of pancreatic cancer is poorly understood, but some risk factors include cigarette smoking, increased BMI, and high dietary fat intake.[45] Local surgical resection of the tumor is the primary treatment; however, only 15–20% of patients present with disease than can be resected.[63] Pancreaticoduodenectomy (Whipple procedure; Figure 17.7) and distal or total pancreatectomy are the most commonly performed procedures. Chemotherapy and radiation may be used as well.

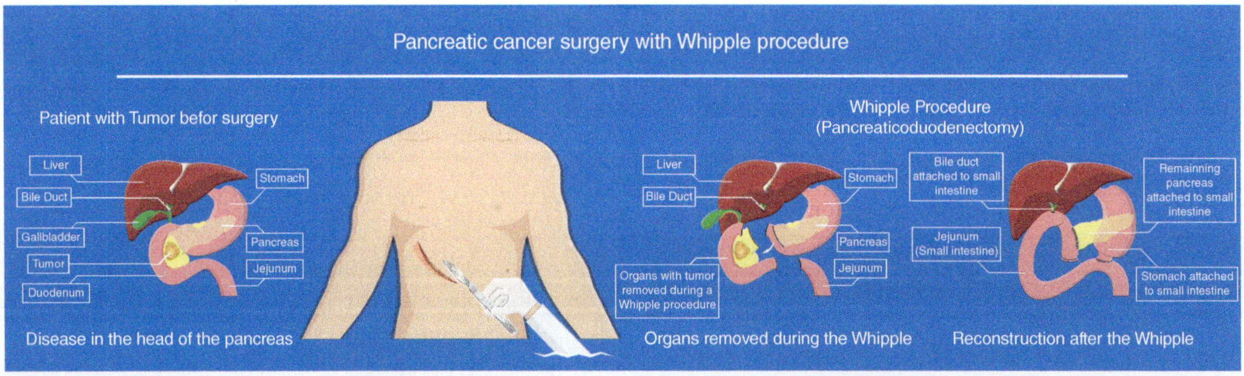

Figure 17.7 Whipple Procedure or Pancreaticoduodenectomy Is a Treatment of Cancer in the Head of the Pancreas

CASE STUDY REVISITED

Seth was readmitted to the hospital 2 months after his initial chemotherapy for a matched unrelated donor allogeneic HSCT (allo-HSCT). His conditioning regimen for transplant includes high-dose chemotherapy and radiation therapy.

Anthropometric Data:

Weight: 82 kg

Biochemical Data:

Sodium 145 (136–145 mEq/L)
Potassium 5.0 (3.5–5.0 mEq/L)
Blood urea nitrogen 29 (8–20 mg/dL)
Creatinine 1.0 (0.7–1.3 mg/dL)
Glucose 95 (70–139 mg/dL)
Albumin 2.8 (3.5–5.5 g/dL)

Dietary Data:

Dietary History: Reports poor appetite.

Diet Prescription: High-calorie/high-protein diet.

Questions

1. What do you think of Seth's current nutrition status?
2. What nutrition risks does Seth face as he prepares for an allo-HSCT?
3. How would you assess Seth's nutrition needs during allo-HSCT? What calorie and protein goals would you set for Seth?

Pancreatic exocrine insufficiency after resection can lead to extreme weight loss secondary to fat malabsorption. Pancreatic enzyme replacement therapy (PERT) can ease steatorrhea, or stool that contains excess fat, and weight loss.[64] Delayed gastric emptying due to the attenuation of the exocrine hormones motilin and cholecystokinin is another common morbidity. The use of small, frequent, low-fat meals helps aid digestion and absorption. Fat-soluble vitamins should be monitored routinely and supplemented as indicated due to increased risk of deficiency with fat malabsorption. Total pancreatectomy, although a rare procedure, results in new-onset diabetes and requires consistent carbohydrate intake in addition to exogenous insulin therapy to achieve glycemic control.[64]

For patients requiring nutrition support, feeding past the pancreas using a nasojejunal or jejunal tube may be warranted in this population if a patient is refractory to PERT. The use of an elemental formula may also be helpful. If a patient develops a pancreatic fistula, the use of PN will be required.[63]

PRACTICE POINT

Pancreatic replacement enzyme supplementation and low-fat meals are usually indicated after pancreatic surgery to prevent weight loss secondary to fat malabsorption due to pancreatic exocrine insufficiency. Fat-soluble vitamins should be monitored routinely and supplemented as indicated.

Lung Cancer

Lung cancer (LC) is the leading cause of death from cancer for both men and women, with the most common diagnosis being nonsmall cell lung cancer.[45] Cigarette smoking remains the primary risk factor for LC, accounting for 90% of all cases. Common symptoms include coughing with or without blood, shortness of breath, and weight loss.[65] Many patients present at advanced stages of the disease, meaning the tumors typically cannot be resected. If it is caught early, patients may have a segmentectomy, lobectomy, or pneumonectomy.[66] The majority of patients undergo radiation and chemotherapy.

Limited evidence exists on effective lung cancer–specific nutrition interventions, despite their significant nutrition risk.[67] Individuals with LC often have increased energy needs secondary to increased work of breathing and have decreased intake from becoming easily fatigued during mealtimes. There is no evidence to support the routine use of nutrition support in patients with LC. Appropriate utilization should be evaluated on an individual basis.

PRACTICE POINT

Small, frequent meals may help patients who easily tire during mealtimes due to increased work of breathing.

Nutritional Management of Hematological Cancers Undergoing Hematopoietic Stem Cell Transplant

Patients with hematological cancers such as leukemia and lymphoma may undergo an autologous or allogeneic **hematopoietic stem cell transplant (HSCT)** in hopes of causing an antitumor effect.[68,69] The stem cells for this treatment are collected from bone marrow (**Figure 17.8**), peripheral blood, or umbilical cord blood from the patient's own stem cells, known as an **autologous HSCT**, or from a related or matched unrelated donor, known as an **allogeneic HSCT**. Prior to transplantation, patients undergo various high-dose chemotherapy and radiation regimens, placing patients at nutrition risk due to treatment-related side effects, including nausea, vomiting, anorexia, malabsorption, and increased metabolic requirements.[70]

Generally, patients undergoing autologous HSCT have shorter periods of neutropenia, or a low neutrophil count, resulting in quicker resolution of GI side effects and less frequent use of nutrition support.[71] Patients undergoing allogeneic HSCT are at increased nutrition risk due to prolonged periods of neutropenia and the risk of developing graft versus host disease (GVHD). During allogeneic HSCT, a patient's immune system is eroded to prevent graft rejection, which may result in prolonged GI side effects necessitating nutrition support. The allogeneic HSCT is considered to be one of the most intense regimens in oncology treatment.[72] Studies indicate that higher BMI (>30 kg/m^2) in patients who are well-nourished may have a protective effect on survival as patients in this category may be more prepared to withstand catabolic stages following transplant than other weight groups.[73]

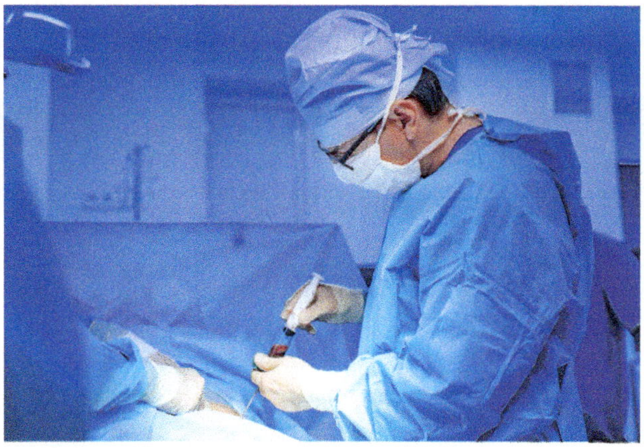

Figure 17.8 Surgeons Harvesting Stem Cells

CASE STUDY REVISITED

Seth has completed his conditioning regimen and has received his allogeneic HSCT today. He has been in the hospital for 1 week with continued poor appetite and has now developed mucositis and vomiting. He is receiving intravenous (IV) fluids and multiple IV medications.

Anthropometric Data:

Current weight: 78 kg

Biochemical Data:

Albumin 2.1 g/dL (3.5–5.5 g/dL)

Clinical Data:

Nutrition-Focused Physical Exam: Appears pale, tired; hollowed appearance under eyes, prominent clavicle bone, depressed interosseous muscle.

Questions

1. Would you provide Seth with nutrition support?
2. If so, what type and why? Provide nutrition support recommendations for Seth.

CORE CONCEPT 11

The allogeneic hematopoietic stem cell transplant (HSCT) is considered one of the most intense treatments in the oncology population and puts patients at increased nutrition risk due to prolonged neutropenia, gastrointestinal side effects, and risk of graft versus host disease.

Estimating Energy Needs

Energy needs in patients undergoing HSCTs are increased due to the catabolic stress associated with radiation and chemotherapy prior to transplant, GVHD, and the need for blood count reconstitution.[70] A patient who is well-nourished with mild complications requires approximately 30 kcal/kg of body weight and 1.5–1.8 g protein/kg body weight.[74] For a patient who is malnourished with severe side effects following transplant, 35–45 kcal/kg may be needed along with 1.8–2.5 g protein/kg.[74] It is important to continuously monitor these patients and adjust their needs accordingly based on any complications that may develop.

Malnutrition can be difficult to estimate in these patients because body weight may not be reflective of nutritional status. Many patients experience edema in the month following transplant due to the use of corticosteroids, nephrotoxic medications, and intravenous hydration, along with the presence of hypoalbuminemia.[68] Albumin and prealbumin levels are not markers of malnutrition given that they are negative acute phase proteins and can be falsely low in the presence of inflammation during transplant. Midarm circumference and handgrip strength may be better tools to assess changes to nutritional or functional status in this population.

CORE CONCEPT 12

Patients undergoing HSCT have increased energy needs due to increased catabolism and treatment-related complications.

PRACTICE POINT

Body weight and serum albumin and prealbumin are not reliable markers of nutritional status in the immediate posttransplant period.

Nutrition Support During Acute Phase of HSCT

Nutrition support is often needed for patients during the acute, hospital phase of transplant, but this remains controversial. The American Society for Parenteral and Enteral Nutrition (ASPEN) states that nutrition support therapy is appropriate for patients with malnutrition undergoing HSCT or those who are anticipated to be unable to ingest or absorb nutrients for at least 7 days.[72] Today, acute nutrition support is more routine in treatment centers for patients following an allogeneic HSCT due to increased nutrition needs and treatment-associated complications that affect nutritional status.[75] Nutrition is critical following transplant, as impaired nutritional status can lead to longer engraftment time and a greater likelihood of developing infection.[76]

Historically, providing PN to patients undergoing HSCT was preferred due to availability of central venous access, reluctance to use NGTs that were perceived as aggressive and hazardous due to NGT placement in the setting of thrombocytopenia (low platelet count), and the high risk of mucositis and enterocolitis in these patients.[68,72] Early studies also demonstrated prolonged survival, decreased incidence of recurrence, and longer recurrence-free survival with PN use in this population.[77]

EN has been associated with improved nitrogen balance and weight gain with a lower risk of infection than PN (**Figure 17.9**).[72,78] After HSCT, EN has been shown to limit gut atrophy and bacterial translocation, which may decrease the risk of sepsis and acute GVHD.[68] However, nausea, vomiting, GI mucositis, and the increased risk of bleeding after tube placement in patients with thrombocytopenia may make EN difficult to implement.[74,76] Patients with continuous GI

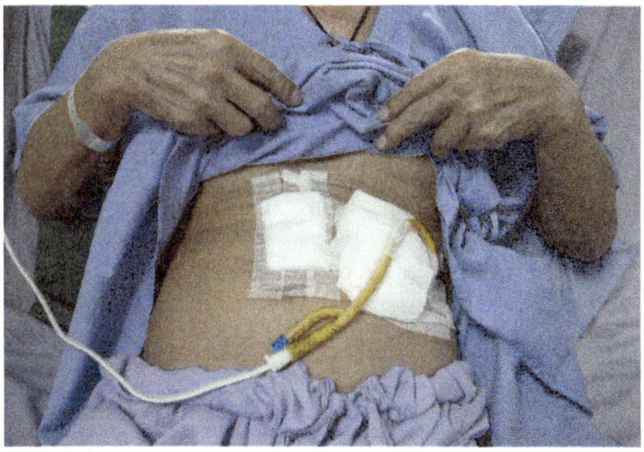

Figure 17.9 Patient Receiving Enteral Nutrition

side effects, such as vomiting, should not receive EN due to the increased risk of aspiration.[79]

Patients who are unable to utilize EN should receive PN if they require nutrition support. Many patients will require PN for nutrition repletion due to significant nitrogen losses from diarrhea and rapid fluid shifts induced by chemotherapy.[77] As patients recover and are able to increase oral or enteral intake, PN should be tapered down in accordance with the amount they can consume orally or enterally and discontinued when patients are able to consistently consume or receive 50–70% of their needs orally or enterally.[70,74,79]

While nutrition support is beneficial in the acute care setting, patients may still have difficulty maintaining adequate nutrition in the long term. The majority of patients are unable to return to their pretransplant weight 1-year posttransplant due to impaired oral intake.[80] In addition, a rapid decline in bone mineral density is observed within 1 year following HSCT as a result of steroid use, and decreased oral intake, and additional calcium and vitamin D supplementation is often required.[81]

PRACTICE POINT

Nutrition support during HSCT is indicated in patients who are malnourished and patients unable to ingest or absorb nutrition for 7 days.

CORE CONCEPT 13

Nutrition is critical following transplant as impaired nutritional status can lead to longer engraftment time and a greater likelihood of developing infection.

Graft Versus Host Disease

Graft versus host disease (GVHD) is a condition that can occur after allogeneic HSCT, when the donor's cells recognize the host's cells as foreign, causing an immune response designed to eliminate the foreign tissue in the recipient. Organs become vulnerable to infections and their functions are disrupted. Donor compatibility, the patient age, and immunosuppressive therapy are a few of the factors that influence GVHD development.[82] Despite advances in medicine, GVHD incidence remains high, likely related to the increased use of allogeneic HSCT.[72] There are two kinds of GVHD: acute, which occurs within 100 days

Clinical Roundtable

Topic: Use of Enteral Nutrition in Allogeneic HSCT

Parenteral nutrition (PN) is a common nutrition support option in clinical practice post-allogeneic HSCT despite studies that show the feasibility and tolerance of enteral nutrition (EN). Preference for PN may be related to the prevalence of GI side effects such as nausea, vomiting, and mucositis potentially impacting EN tolerance, as well as the concern with placing a nasogastric tube in patients with thrombocytopenia due to increased risk of bleeding. There are no guidelines for the specific use of EN in the allogeneic HSCT population, although it is well understood that EN is more physiologic, safer, easier to use, and less costly than PN. In addition, gut mucosal atrophy and dysbiosis, which can worsen with PN use, have been speculated to contribute to HSCT complications. EN has been found to significantly improve patient outcomes by reducing early posttransplant mortality and GVHD incidence and has been associated with a lower risk of infection.

Roundtable Discussion

1. How do you balance the potential risks of administering EN with the outcome benefits of using EN in the HSCT population?
2. What parameters would you use in determining the suitability of and to monitor tolerance to EN?
3. Would you recommend using EN in clinical practice when caring for your HSCT patient?

References

1. Guieze R, Lemal R, Cabrespine A, et al. Enteral versus parenteral nutrition support in allogenic haematopoietic stem-cell transplantation. *Clin Nutr*. 2014;33(3):533–538. doi:10.1016/j.clnu.2013.07.012
2. Seguy D, Duhmael A, Rejeb MB, et al. Better outcomes of patients undergoing enteral tube feeding after myeloablative conditioning for allogeneic stem cell transplantation. *Transplantation*. 2012;94(3):287–294. doi:10.1097/TP.0b013e3182558f60
3. Zama D, Gori D, Muratore E, et al. Enteral versus parenteral nutrition as nutritional support after allogeneic hematopoietic stem cell transplantation: a systematic review and meta-analysis. *Transplant Cell Ther*. 2021;27(2):180.e1–180.e8. doi:10.1016/j.jtct.2020.11.006

CASE STUDY REVISITED

Seth has developed acute GI GVHD resulting in large volumes of diarrhea (approximately 2 L/day). He is now receiving high-dose steroids and is NPO (*nil per os*/nothing by mouth).

Questions

1. How would Seth's diagnosis of GI GVHD change your nutrition management?
2. How would GI GVHD change Seth's nutrition needs?
3. How would you provide Seth nutrition support while he is NPO?
4. What additional biochemical markers would you closely monitor?
5. Should you provide Seth with glutamine?

of transplant, and chronic, which occurs after 100 days posttransplant. Acute GVHD affects approximately 50% of allogeneic HSCT patients, targeting the skin, liver, and GI tract.[68,72] One-third of the patients with acute GVHD will develop chronic GVHD that can involve the skin, oral mucosa, GI tract, eyes, musculoskeletal system, liver, lungs, and vagina.[68,72]

Patients with GVHD may have increased energy and protein needs related to hypermetabolism, infections, protein losses from skin and GI involvement, and use of high-dose corticosteroids.[74,82] Energy needs may increase by 10% in patients with chronic GVHD, requiring 35–45 kcal/kg and 1.8–2.5 g protein/kg/day.[74,82,83] Increased serum concentrations of norepinephrine and glucagon in patients with chronic GVHD may also be responsible for this increase in REE.[83]

PRACTICE POINT

Energy and protein needs are increased in patients with GVHD due to hypermetabolism, protein loss, and use of high-dose corticosteroids.

The metabolic and physiologic burden of GVHD results in a high rate of malnutrition, impacting nearly one-half of patients with GVHD.[84] Patients with GI involvement may experience weight loss due to malabsorption and/or inability to ingest adequate nutrition due to dysphagia, anorexia, odynophagia, mucositis, nausea, and vomiting contributing to weight loss and progressive cachexia.[74,85]

Diminished oral intake and nutrient malabsorption in patients with GVHD place patients at risk for multiple micronutrient deficiencies, including folic acid, zinc, and vitamin B12. A multivitamin supplement (without iron) can be considered for patients with chronic poor oral intake to prevent deficiencies.[82]

Nutrition support is often indicated in patients with GVHD when oral intake is impaired. The type of nutrition support for patients with oral and GI GVHD is decided on a case-by-case basis. In cases of GI dysfunction and severe diarrhea (>1 L/day), bowel rest is indicated with initiation of PN for full nutrition support until stool volume and frequency is controlled and diet can be advanced.[86]

CORE CONCEPT 14

GVHD can occur following allogeneic HSCT and places patients at increased nutrition risk due to impaired function of the gastrointestinal tract, including the oral mucosa.

PRACTICE POINT

Nutrition support is indicated in GI GVHD due to interruption of normal GI function. PN is utilized in cases of severe GI GVHD necessitating bowel rest until stool volume and frequency decrease.

Glutamine and Nutrition Support

Glutamine is the most abundant nonessential amino acid in the body and has been researched in the acute HSCT population for its role in fueling immune and GI cells and reducing the severity of mucositis and GVHD. Despite its status as a nonessential amino acid, needs for glutamine are increased during critical illness and catabolism.[87]

Research related to glutamine in the HSCT population indicates conflicting results. Some studies suggest that administration of parenteral glutamine

CASE STUDY REVISITED

Seth's diarrhea has become more manageable, with less than 500 mL of stool output per day. The plan is to send Seth home within the next week.

Questions

1. What type of diet should Seth follow at home?
2. Should Seth adhere to a low-microbial diet?

to patients post-HSCT may preserve nitrogen loss following transplant, reduce rates of infection, and reduce duration of diarrhea compared to patients given a standard PN formula. Use of parenteral glutamine has also been associated with longer duration of opioid use, longer hospital stays, higher rates of recurrence, and death.[88] Glutamine is not included in standard PN formulas because it is nonessential, has a shorter shelf-life than other amino acids, and is a costly intervention.[89]

Due to conflicting research and potential for poor outcomes, there is no standard practice for the use of glutamine supplementation in the HSCT population. More randomized, controlled trials are needed to learn about the effects of glutamine on clinical outcomes following HSCT.

PRACTICE POINT

Research related to glutamine supplementation in the HSCT population remains controversial. There is no standard practice for the use of glutamine supplementation, and more randomized controlled trials are needed.

Low-Microbial Diets

Patients who can maintain an oral diet status post-HSCT have historically followed a low-microbial diet, also referred to as the "low-bacteria diet" or "neutropenic diet." This diet emerged and gained popularity due to concerns that ingesting food-borne pathogens could increase infection rates in patients post-HSCT. There is no evidence to show the benefit of the low-microbial diet in this population. In fact, research has demonstrated that patients who followed a low-microbial diet after HSCT had no difference in infection rates as compared to patients with no diet restrictions after HSCT.[90,91]

The low-microbial diet lacks consistent dietary definition and implementation parameters, creating variability among institutions that continue to use it.[91] The significant dietary limitations of the low-microbial diet may further limit adequate caloric intake in a population at high nutrition risk. Despite the lack of evidence and consistency in this diet, many institutions continue to utilize the low-microbial diet in their patients post-HSCT. Patients post-HSCT should focus on food safety by utilizing the Food and Drug Administration's published guidelines for patients who have undergone transplants.[92,93]

PRACTICE POINT

The low-microbial diet lacks consistent definition and implementation parameters and has no evidence-based benefit for use after HSCT. Individuals should follow food safety guidelines for transplant patients published by the Food and Drug Administration.

Nutrition Support in the Patient with Advanced Cancer

The role of nutrition support in patients with advanced stage cancer remains controversial as the timeline for initiating, withholding, and/or withdrawing nutrition support in the patient who is terminally ill remains unclear. The notion that providing nutrition support will provide comfort and reduce suffering is not evidence-based. Evidence suggests that the provision of nutrition support in patients who are terminally ill may not enhance a patient's QOL and may, in fact, increase suffering.[72,84–98] There are instances along the spectrum of advanced disease where nutrition support may provide benefit, including improving fluid status and nutrient intake thus improving QOL. However, it is important to remember that nutrition and hydration are considered life-sustaining measures and should be in line with the patient's wishes. Nutrition support should be considered on a case-by-case basis, with the patient's best interest in mind and assessment of multiple factors, including the patient's goals of care (palliation versus end-of-life care), treatment plan, estimated need for nutrition support, and estimated lifespan. If nutrition support will be used outside of a medical facility, the ability of patient and/or caregiver to perform nutrition support tasks, and a safe and clean home environment are needed.[99,100] The assessment of potential risks, including the need for routine blood work, risk of infection, mobility limitations during feeding, bladder and bowel incontinence, edema, and negative GI symptoms, such as nausea, vomiting, and diarrhea, as well as the therapy's perceived futility should also be considered in this decision.[97]

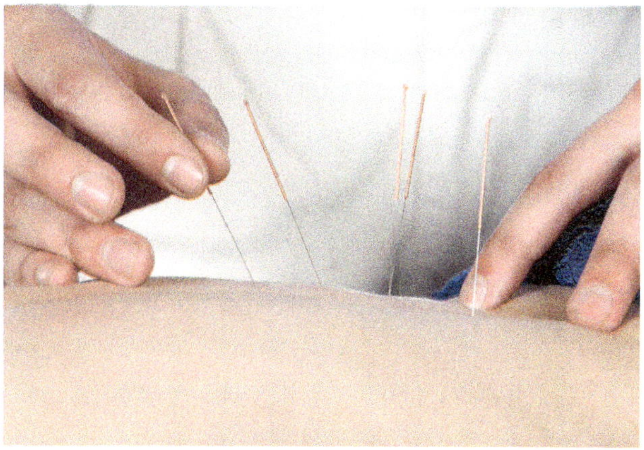

Figure 17.10 Acupuncture Is a Type of Complementary Medicine that Can Be Used in Oncology Treatment

CORE CONCEPT 15

Nutrition support in the patient with advanced cancer should be assessed on a case-by-case basis with consideration of goals of care.

Complementary and Alternative Medicine, Integrative Medicine, and the Patient with Cancer

Complementary and alternative medicine (CAM) refers to medical products and practices that are not part of standard medical care (**Figure 17.10**). **Complementary medicine** (such as acupuncture) is used along with standard medicine, **alternative medicine** (such as botanicals/herbals) is used instead of standard medicine treatment to treat cancer, and **integrative medicine** is a total approach to medicine that combines standard medicine with CAM practices. Integrative medicine has been considered to be a safe and effective practice and is aimed at treating the patient's mind, body, and spirit. A national survey conducted in 2007 showed that 4 out of 10 adults use a CAM therapy, with nearly 50% of patients most commonly using prayer and spiritual practice, relaxation, faith and spiritual healing, and nutritional supplements and vitamins.[101–103] While many CAM therapies have been evaluated and found to be safe and effective, some have been found to be potentially harmful for the patient. Less is known about many CAM therapies as a result of limitations in research due to lack of careful research practices such as those used in standard cancer treatments. The RD should be aware of any botanicals and nutritional products, including dietary supplements, herbal supplements, and vitamins, that a patient is using, as they may be harmful to the patient or interact with the patient's current treatment. Patients are recommended to inform their clinician if they are using or considering using any CAM therapy to evaluate the safety and efficacy of the product. Reliable organizations to find out more about CAM therapies include the National Center for Complementary and Integrative Health,[104] the NCI Office of Cancer Complementary and Alternative Medicine,[105] and the Office of Dietary Supplements.[106]

Monitoring and Evaluation in the Patient with Cancer

Monitoring patients with cancer would include tracking weight to assess weight loss or fluid shifts. Monitoring would also include evaluating nutrition impact symptoms and especially those which can interfere with oral intake, including anorexia, nausea, vomiting, mucositis, dysgeusia, and dysphagia and following GI symptoms, such as diarrhea, steatorrhea, constipation, and dumping syndrome. RDs should check biochemical measures including electrolytes as part of a basic metabolic panel, particularly potassium, magnesium, and phosphorus, especially in those at risk for refeeding syndrome. Fluid intake should be monitored to watch for dehydration, particularly in those patients with poor intake, nausea, and vomiting. Asking about alternative and complementary therapies such as herbal and dietary supplement use is critical. It is also important to monitor for lean body and fat mass wasting through nutrition-focused physical examination for those patients with cachexia and for edema for those undergoing cancer treatment at risk for fluid shifts and patients post-HSCT. Finally, assessing functional status will help to evaluate the ability of patients to shop and prepare meals and identify behaviors related to food safety to reduce risk of food-borne illnesses for patients who are immunosuppressed.

Chapter Summary

Cancer is a complex disease caused by environmental, genetic, and lifestyle factors that is the second most common cause of death in the United States. Medical management of cancer can lead to significant nutrition impact symptoms that may lead to weight loss and malnutrition. Symptoms and their nutritional management can vary greatly based on cancer type and tumor location. Head and neck as well as GI cancers are associated with high rates of malnutrition due to their negative impact on the ability of the patient to ingest and absorb food. Cancer cachexia, a complicating factor in advanced cancer, leads to a loss of lean body mass and can contribute to increased resting energy expenditure. Hematopoietic stem cell transplants, a treatment for hematological cancers, are considered one of the most intense medical treatments and can have significant nutrition implications, including increased energy needs and GI side effects. Nutrition interventions during and after cancer treatments can improve nutrition status, influencing treatment tolerance, quality of life, prognosis, and mortality.

Key Terms

carcinomas, sarcomas, hematologic malignancies, nutrition impact symptoms, radiation therapy, odynophagia, biotherapy, chemotherapy, hypermetabolism, cancer cachexia, cytokines, immunonutrition, hematopoietic stem cell transplant (HSCT), autologous HSCT, allogeneic HSCT, glutamine, graft versus host disease (GVHD), complementary medicine, alternative medicine, integrative medicine

Acknowledgments

The author acknowledges Alicia Romano and Jennifer Mayer for contributions to the previous version of this chapter.

References

1. National Institutes of Health (US); Biological Sciences Curriculum Study. Understanding cancer. In: *NIH Curriculum Supplement Series* [Internet]. National Institutes of Health (US); 2007.
2. Anand P, Kunnumakara AB, Sundaram C, et al. Cancer is a preventable disease that requires major lifestyle changes. *Pharm Res.* 2008;25(9):2097–2116. doi:10.1007/s11095-008-9661-9
3. American Cancer Society. Genes and cancer. Updated November 2, 2023. Accessed November 26, 2024. https://www.cancer.org/cancer/understanding-cancer/genes-and-cancer.html
4. American Cancer Society. *Cancer Facts and Figures 2024.* American Cancer Society; 2024.
5. Reuter S, Gupta SC, Chaturvedi MM, Aggarwal BB. Oxidative stress, inflammation, and cancer: how are they linked? *Free Radic Biol Med.* 2010;49(11):1603–1616. doi:10.1016/j.freeradbiomed.2010.09.006
6. Data from American Joint Committee on Cancer. What is cancer staging? Accessed November 26, 2024. https://www.facs.org/quality-programs/cancer-programs/american-joint-committee-on-cancer/cancer-staging-systems/
7. Mohan R, Grosshans D. Proton therapy- present and future. *Adv Drug Deliv Rev.* 2017;109:26–44.
8. Nitenberg G, Raynard B. Nutritional support of the cancer patient: issues and dilemmas. *Crit Rev Oncol Hematol.* 2000;(34):137–168.
9. Hebuterne X, Lemarie E, Michallet M, et al. Prevalence of malnutrition and current use of nutrition support in patients with cancer. *JPEN J Parenter Enteral Nutr.* 2014;38(2):196–204. doi:10.1177/0148607113502674
10. Bauer JD, Capra S. Nutrition intervention improves outcomes in patients with cancer cachexia receiving chemotherapy: pilot study. *Support Care Cancer.* 2005;13:270–274. doi:10.1007/s00520-004-0746-7
11. Dewys WD, Begg C, Lavin PT, et al. Prognostic effect of weight loss prior to chemotherapy in cancer patients. *Am J Med.* 1980;69:491–497.
12. Reproduced from Academy of Nutrition and Dietetics Evidence Analysis Library. Oncology: executive summary of

recommendations. Published 2013. Accessed November 26, 2024. https://www.andeal.org/topic.cfm?menu=5291&cat=5067

13. Kim JY, Wie G-A, Cho Y-A, et al. Development and validation of screening tool for adult hospitalized cancer patients. *Clin Nutr.* 2011;30:724–729. http://www.cancer.be/sites/default/files/1-article-original-Clinical-Nutrition-2011.pdf
14. Bauer J, Capra S, Ferguson M. Use of the scored patient-generated subjective global assessment (PG-SGA) as a nutrition assessment tool in patients with cancer. *Eur J Clin Nutr.* 2002;56(8):779–785.
15. Isenring E, Bauer J, Capra S. The scored patient-generated subjective global assessment (PG-SGA) and its association with quality of life in ambulatory patients receiving radiotherapy. *Eur J Clin Nutr.* 2003;57(2):305–309.
16. Shaw C, Fleuret C, Pickard M, et al. Comparison of novel screening tools for adult oncology patients. *Support Care Cancer.* 2015;23:47–54. doi:10.1007/s00520-041-2319-8
17. Boléo-Tomé C, Monteiro-Grillo I, Camilo M, et al. Validation of the Malnutrition Universal Screening Tool (MUST) in cancer. *Br J Nutr.* 2012;108(2):343–348. doi:10.1017/S000711451100571X
18. Chao P, Chuang H, Tsao L, et al. The Malnutrition Universal Screening Tool (MUST) and a nutrition education program for high risk cancer patients: strategies to improve dietary intake in cancer patients. *Biomedicine (Taipei).* 2015;5(3):17. doi:10.7603/s40681-015-0017-6
19. Isenring EA, Bauer JD, Capra S. Nutrition support using the American Dietetic Association medical nutrition therapy protocol for radiation oncology patients improves dietary intake compared with standard practice. *J Am Diet Assoc.* 2007;107(3):404–412.
20. Arends J, Bodoky G, Bozzetti F, et al. ESPEN guidelines on enteral nutrition: non-surgical oncology. *Clin Nutr.* 2006;25:245–259.
21. Arends J, Bachmann P, Baracos V, et al. ESPEN guidelines on nutrition in cancer patients. *Clin Nutr.* 2017;36:11–48.
22. Mattox TW. Treatment of unintentional weight loss in patients with cancer. *Nutr Clin Prac.* 2005;20(4):400–410.
23. Fearon KCH, Glass DJ, Guttridge DC. Cancer cachexia: mediators, signaling, and metabolic pathways. *Cell Metab.* 2012;16(2):153–166.
24. Gullett NP, Mazurak V, Hebbar G, Ziegler TR. Nutritional interventions for cancer-induced cachexia. *Curr Probl Cancer.* 2011;35(2):58–90. doi:10.1016/j.currproblcancer.2011.01.001
25. Baracos VE. Regulation of skeletal muscle protein turnover in cancer associated cachexia. *Nutrition.* 2000;16(10):1015–1018.
26. Tisdale MJ. Mechanisms of cancer cachexia. *Physio Rev.* 2009;89(2):381–410.
27. McCreery E, Costello J. Providing nutritional support for patients with cancer cachexia. *Int J Palliat Nurs.* 2013;19(1):32–37.
28. Donohue CL, Ryan AM, Reynolds JV. Cancer cachexia: mechanisms and clinical implications. *Gastroenterol Res Pract.* 2011;2011:601434.
29. Matthews CM. Cancer cachexia: Athophysiology and approaches to management. *Support Line.* 2010;32(4):5–8.
30. Aapro M, Arends J, Bozzetti F, et al. Early recognition of malnutrition and cachexia in the cancer patient: a position paper of a European School of Oncology Task Force. *Ann Oncol.* 2014;25(8):1492–1499. doi:10.1093/annonc/mdu085
31. Loprinzi CL, Ellison NM, Schaid DJ, et al. Controlled trial of megestrol acetate for the treatment of cancer anorexia and cachexia. *J Natl Cancer Inst.* 1998;82:1127–1132.
32. Loprinzi CL, Kugler JW, Sloan JA, et al. Randomized comparison of megestrol acetate versus dexamethasone versus fluoxymesterone for the treatment of cancer anorexia/cachexia. *J Clin Oncol.* 1999;17:32993306.
33. Jatoi A, Windschitl HE, Loprinzi CL, et al. Dronabinol versus megestrol acetate versus combination therapy for cancer associated anorexia: a North Central Cancer Treatment Group study. *J Clin Oncol.* 2002;20:567–573.
34. Moertel CG, Schutt AJ, Reitemeier RJ, Hahn RG. Corticosteroid therapy of preterminal gastrointestinal cancer. *Cancer.* 1974;33:1607–1609.
35. Willox JC, Corr J, Shaw J, et al. Prednisolone as an appetite stimulant in patients with cancer. *Br Med J (Clin Res Ed).* 1984;288:27.
36. Fearon KC, Von Meyenfeldt MF, Moses AG, et al. Effect of a protein and energy dense N–3 fatty acid enriched oral supplement on loss of weight and lean tissue in cancer cachexia: a randomised double blind trial. *Gut.* 2003;52:1479–1486.
37. Jatoi A, Rowland K, Loprinzi CL, et al. An eicosapentaenoic acid supplement versus megestrol acetate versus both for patients with cancer-associated wasting: a North Central Cancer Treatment Group and National Cancer Institute of Canada collaborative effort. *J Clin Oncol.* 2004;22:2469–2476.
38. Fearon KC, Barber MD, Moses AG, et al. Double-blind, placebo-controlled, randomized study of eicosapentaenoic acid diester in patients with cancer cachexia. *J Clin Oncol.* 2006;24:3401–3407.
39. Dewey A, Baughan C, Dean T, Higgins B, Johnson I. Eicosapentaenoic acid (EPA, an omega-3 fatty acid from fish oils) for the treatment of cancer cachexia. *Cochrane Database Syst Rev.* 2007;2007:CD004597.
40. Laviano A, Muscaritoli M, Cascino A, et al. Branched-chain amino acids: the best compromise to achieve anabolism? *Curr Opin Clin Nutr Metab Care.* 2005;8:408–414.
41. Eley HL, Russell ST, Tisdale MJ. Effect of branched-chain amino acids on muscle atrophy in cancer cachexia. *Biochem J.* 2007;407:113–120.
42. Kuhn KS, Muscaritoli M, Wischmeyer P, Stehle P. Glutamine as indispensable nutrient in oncology: experimental and clinical evidence. *Eur J Nutr.* 2010;49(4):197–210. doi:10.1007/s00394-009-0082-2
43. Nugent B, Lewis S, O'Sullivan JM. Enteral feeding methods for nutritional management in patients with head and neck cancers being treated with radiotherapy and/or chemotherapy (review). *Cochrane Database Syst Rev.* 2013;2013:CD007904.
44. Academy of Nutrition and Dietetics. Nutrition care manual. Accessed September 8, 2024. http://www.nutritioncaremanual.org
45. National Cancer Institute. Surveillance, epidemiology, and end results program. Accessed August 4, 2024. https://seer.cancer.gov/statfacts/
46. Languis JA, Zandbergen MC, Eerenstein SE, et al. Effect of nutritional interventions on nutritional status, quality of life and mortality in patients with head and neck cancer receiving chemoradiotherapy: a systematic review. *Clin Nutr.* 2013(32):671–678.
47. Furness S, Glenny AM, Worthington HV, et al. Interventions for the treatment of oral cavity and oropharyngeal cancer: chemotherapy. *Cochrane Database Syst Rev.* 2010;(9):CD006386.
48. Martinovic D, Tokic D, Mladinic E, et al. Nutritional management of patients with head and neck cancer—a comprehensive review. *Nutrients.* 2023;15(8):1864.
49. Dechaphunkul T, Martin L, Alberda C, Olson K, Baracos V, Gramlich L. Malnutrition assessment in patients with cancers

of the head and neck: a call to action and consensus. *Crit Rev Oncol Hematol*. 2013;88:459–476.
50. Corry J, Poon W, McPhee N, et al. Randomized study of percutaneous endoscopic gastrostomy versus nasogastric tubes for enteral feeding in head and neck cancer patients receiving chemoradiation. *J Med Imaging Radiat Oncol*. 2008;52:503–510.
51. Rubenstein JH, Shaheen NJ. Epidemiology, diagnosis, and management of esophageal adenocarcinoma. *Gastroenterology*. 2015;149:302–317.
52. Ukleja A. Dumping syndrome: pathophysiology and treatment. *Nutr Clin Pract*. 2005;20(5):517–525.
53. Gupta V. Benefits versus risks: a prospective audit. Feeding jejunostomy during esophagectomy. *World J Surg*. 2009;33:1432–1438.
54. Ryan AM, Rowley SP, Healy LA, et al. Post-oesophagectomy early enteral nutrition via a needle catheter jejunostomy: 8-year experience at a specialist unit. *Clin Nutr*. 2006;25:386–393.
55. Allum WH, Blazeby JM, Griffin M, Cunningham D, Jankowski JA, Wong R. Guidelines for the management of oesophageal and gastric cancer. *Gut*. 2011;60:1449–1472.
56. Brolin RE, Gorman RC, Milgrim LM, Kenler HA. Multivitamin prophylaxis in prevention of post-gastric bypass vitamin and mineral deficiencies. *Int J Obes*. 1991;15(10):661–667.
57. Dann GC, Squires MH, Postlewait LM, et al. An assessment of feeding jejunostomy tube placement at the time of resection for gastric adenocarcinoma: a seven-institution analysis of 837 patients from the U.S. gastric cancer collaborative. *J Surg Oncol*. 2015;112:195–202.
58. Siegel RL, Miller DK, Jemal A. Cancer statistics, 2016. *Can J Clin*. 2016;66–67.
59. Hauer-Jensen M, Wang J, Denham J. Bowel injury: current and evolving management strategies. *Semin Radiat Oncol*. 2013;13:357–371.
60. Andreyev HJ. Gastrointestinal problems after pelvic radiotherapy: the past, the present and the future. *Clin Oncol*. 2007;19:790–799.
61. Wall EA. An overview of short bowel syndrome management: adherence, adaptation, and practical recommendations. *J Acad Nutr Diet*. 2013;113:1200–1208.
62. Joly F, Dray X, Corcos O, et al. Tube feeding improves intestinal absorption in short bowel syndrome patients. *Gastroenterology*. 2009;136:824.
63. Afaneh C, Gerszber D, Slatter E, Seres DS, Chabot JA, Kluger MD. Pancreatic cancer surgery and nutrition management: a review of the current literature. *HepatoBiliary Surg Nutr*. 2015;4(1):59–71.
64. Berry AJ. Pancreatic surgery: indications, complications, and implications for nutrition intervention. *Nut Clin Pract*. 2013;28:330–357.
65. Gift A, Stommel M, Jablonski A, Given W. A cluster of symptoms over time in patients with lung cancer. *Nurs Res*. 2003;52:393–400.
66. Jagoe RT, Goodship THJ, Gibson GJ. The influence of nutritional status on complications after operations for lung cancer. *Ann Thorac Surg*. 2001;71:936–943.
67. Kiss NKK, Krishnasamy M, Isenring EA. The effect of nutrition intervention in lung cancer patients undergoing chemotherapy and/or radiotherapy: a systematic review. *Nutr Canc*. 2014;66(1):45–56.
68. Buhl ND, Seguy D. Nutritional support in adult patients undergoing allogeneic stem cell transplantation following myeloablative conditioning. In: Rajendram R, Preedy VR, Patel V, eds. *Diet and Nutrition in Critical Care*. Springer Science+Business Media; 2015:593–605.
69. Lemal R, Cabrespine A, Pereira B, et al. Could enteral nutrition improve the outcome of patients with haematological malignancies undergoing allogeneic haematopoietic stem cell transplantation? A study protocol for a randomized controlled trial (the NEPHA study). *Trials*. 2015;16(136):1–9. doi:10.1186/s13063-015-0663-8
70. Zatarain L, Savani BN. The role of nutrition and effects on the cytokine milieu in allogeneic hematopoietic stem cell transplantation. *Cell Immunol*. 2012;276:6–9. doi:10.1016/j.cellimm.2012.05.003
71. Andersen S, Brown T, Kennedy G, Banks M. Implementation of an evidenced based nutrition support pathway for haematopoietic progenitor cell transplant patients. *Clin Nutr*. 2015;34:536–540. doi:10.1016/j.clnu.2014.06.006
72. August DA, Huhmann MB, American Society of Parenteral and Enteral Nutrition Board of Directors. A.S.P.E.N. clinical guidelines: nutrition support therapy during adult anticancer treatment and in hematopoietic cell transplantation. *JPEN J Parenter Enteral Nutr*. 2009;33(5):472–500. doi:10.1177/0148607109341804
73. Jaime-Pérez JC, Colunga-Pedraza PR, Gutiérrez-Gurrola B, et al. Obesity is associated with higher overall survival in patients undergoing an outpatient reduced-intensity conditioning hematopoietic stem cell transplant. *Blood Cells Mol Dis*. 2013;51:61–65. doi:10.1016/j.bcmd.2013.01.010
74. Martin-Salces M, de Paz R, Canales MA, Mesejo A, Hernandez-Navarro F. Nutritional recommendations in hematopoietic stem cell transplantation. *Nutrition*. 2008;24:769–775. doi:10.1016/j.nut.2008.02.021
75. Muscaritoli M, Conversano L, Torelli GF, et al. Clinical and metabolic effects of different parenteral nutrition regimens in patients undergoing allogeneic bone marrow transplantation. *Transplantation*. 1998;66(5):610–616.
76. Wilson S, Kohli-Seth R, Aldeguer Y, et al. Parenteral nutrition utilization in bone marrow transplant recipients. *J Nutr Heal Sci*. 2014;1(1):1–4. doi:10.15744/2393-9060.1.102
77. Weisdorf S, Lysne J, Wind D, et al. Positive effect of prophylactic total parenteral nutrition on long-term outcome of bone marrow transplantation. *Transplantation*. 1987;43(6):276–279.
78. Guieze R, Lemal R, Cabrespine A, et al. Enteral versus parenteral nutritional support in allogeneic haematopoietic stem-cell transplantation. *Clin Nutr*. 2014;33:533–538. doi:10.1016/j.clnu.2013.07.012
79. Williams-Hooker R, Adams M, Havrilla D, Leung W, Roach R, Mosby T. Caregiver and health care provider preferences of nutritional support in a hematopoietic stem cell transplant unit. *Pediatr Blood Cancer*. 2015;62:1473–1476. doi:10.1002/pbc
80. Iestra JA, Fibbe WE, Zwinderman AH, van Staveren WA, Kromhout D. Body weight recovery, eating difficulties and compliance with dietary advice in the first year after stem cell transplantation: a prospective study. *Bone Marrow Transplant*. 2002;29(5):417–424. doi:10.1038/sj.bmt.1703375
81. Schulte CMS, Beelen DW. Bone loss following hematopoietic stem cell transplantation: a long-term follow-up. *Blood*. 2004;103(10):3635–3643. doi:10.1182/blood-2003-09-3081
82. Roberts S, Thompson J. Clinical observations graft-vs-host disease: nutrition therapy in a challenging condition. *Nutr Clin Pract*. 2005;20:440–450.
83. Zauner C, Rabitsch W, Schneeweiss B, et al. Energy and substrate metabolism in patients with chronic extensive graft-versus-host disease. *Transplantation*. 2001;71:524–528.

84. Jacobsohn D, Margolis J, Doherty J, Anders V, Vogelsang G. Weight loss and malnutrition in patients with chronic graft-versus-host disease. *Bone Marrow Transplant*. 2002;29:231–236.
85. Akpek G, Chinratanalab W, Lee LA, et al. Gastrointestinal involvement in chronic graft-versus-host disease: a clinicopathologic study. *Biol Blood Marrow Transplant*. 2003;9(1):46–51. doi:10.1053/bbmt.2003.49999
86. Szeluga DJ, Stuart RK, Brookmeyer R, Szeluga DJ, Utermohlen V, Santos GW. Nutritional support of bone marrow transplant recipients: a prospective randomized clinical trial comparing total parenteral nutrition to an enteral feeding program nutritional support of bone marrow transplant recipients. *Cancer Res*. 1987;47:3309–3316.
87. Oudemans-van Straaten HM, Bosman RJ, Treskes M, Van der Spoel HJI, Zandstra DF. Plasma glutamine depletion and patient outcome in acute ICU admissions. *Intensive Care Med*. 2001;27(1):84–90. doi:10.1007/s001340000703
88. Pytlík R, Benes P, Patorková M, et al. Standardized parenteral alanyl-glutamine dipeptide supplementation is not beneficial in autologous transplant patients: a randomized, double-blind, placebo controlled study. *Bone Marrow Transplant*. 2002;30(12):953–961. doi:10.1038/sj.bmt.1703759
89. Zeigler T, Young L, Benfell K, et al. Clinical and metabolic efficacy of glutamine supplemented parenteral nutrition after bone marrow transplantation. *Ann Intern Med*. 1992;116:821–828.
90. van Dalen EC, Mank A, Leclercq E, et al. Low bacterial diet versus control diet to prevent infection in cancer patients treated with chemotherapy causing episodes of neutropenia. *Cochrane Database Syst Rev*. 2012;(9):CD006247. doi:10.1002/14651858.CD006247.pub2
91. Lassiter M, Schneider SM. A pilot study comparing the neutropenic diet to a non-neutropenic diet in the allogeneic hematopoietic stem cell transplantation population. *Clin J Oncol Nurs*. 2015;19(3):273–278. doi:10.1188/15.CJON.19-03AP
92. Laird K. New and emerging bacterial food pathogens. In: Ricke SC, Donaldson JR, Phillips C, eds. *Food Safety*. Academic Press; 2015:309–316.
93. U.S. Food and Drug Administration. Food safety for older adults and people with cancer, diabetes, HIV/AIDS, organ transplants, and autoimmune diseases. Published July 2020. Accessed November 26, 2024. https://www.fda.gov/food/people-risk-foodborne-illness/food-safety-older-adults-and-people-cancer-diabetes-hivaids-organ-transplants-and-autoimmune
94. Easson AM, Hinshaw DB, Johnson DL. The role of tube feeding and total parenteral nutrition in advanced illness. *J Am Coll Surg*. 2002;194(2):225–229. doi:10.1016/S1072-7515(01)01154-1
95. ASPEN Board of Directors and the Clinical Guidelines Task Force. Guidelines for the use of parenteral and enteral nutrition in adult and pediatric patients. Section I : Introduction. *JPEN J Parenter Enteral Nutr*. 2001;26(1):1SA-138SA.
96. Nitenberg G, Raynard B. Nutritional support of the cancer patient: issues and dilemmas. *Crit Rev Oncol Hematol*. 2000;34(3):137–168. doi:10.1016/S1040-8428(00)00048-2
97. Fuhrman MP, Herrmann VM. Bridging the continuum: nutrition support in palliative and hospice care. *Nutr Clin Pract*. 2006;21(2):134–141.
98. Klein S, Koretz RL. Nutrition support in patients with cancer: what do the data really show? *Nutr Clin Pract*. 1994;9(3):91–100.
99. Mirhosseini N, Fainsinger RL, Baracos V. Parenteral nutrition in advanced cancer: Indications and clinical practice guidelines. *J Palliat Care*. 2005;8(5):914–918.
100. Gavrin JR. Ethical considerations at the end of life in the intensive care unit. *Crit Care Med*. 2007;35(2 suppl): S85–S94.
101. Barnes PM, Bloom B, Nahin RL. Complementary and alternative medicine use among adults and children: United States, 2007. *Natl Health Stat Report*. 2009;12:1–23.
102. Gansler T, Kaw C, Crammer C, et al. A population-based study of prevalence of complementary methods use by cancer survivors: a report from the American Cancer Society's studies of cancer survivors. *Cancer*. 2008;113(5): 1048–1057.
103. Keene M, Heslop I, Sabesan S, Glass B. Complementary and alternative medicine use in cancer: a systemic review. *Compliment Ther Clin Pract*. 2019;35:33–47.
104. U.S. Department of Health and Human Services. National Institute of Health. National Center for Complementary and Integrative Health. Updated November 27, 2024. Accessed November 28, 2024. https://www.nccih.nih.gov
105. National Institute of Health, Division of Cancer Treatment and Diagnosis. Office of Cancer Complementary and Alternative Medicine. Accessed November 28, 2024. https://cam.cancer.gov
106. National Institute of Health, Office of Dietary Supplements. Accessed November 28, 2024. https://ods.od.nih.gov/

CHAPTER 18

Nutrition in Neurology

Sora M Johnson
Kathy Prelack

CHAPTER OUTLINE

CORE CONCEPTS

1. Insult to the central nervous system can result in the dysregulation of nutrient intake and utilization, the severity of which typically depends on the magnitude and acuity of the damage.
2. Dysphagia of any degree is a common occurrence following stroke injury; all patients should be screened for dysphagia prior to initiation of an oral diet.
3. Energy needs following acute stroke may vary according to the type of stroke with subarachnoid hemorrhagic strokes resulting in higher energy needs than ischemic strokes.
4. Secondary brain insult can occur following traumatic brain injury leading to hypoxemia and a systemic inflammatory response.
5. The high energy demand of the brain explains the elevated energy expenditure that follows traumatic brain injury, reaching levels up to 200% of resting energy expenditure.
6. Textured modified diets can reduce the risk of aspiration pneumonia in patients with dysphagia.
7. Malnutrition and dysphagia are closely related; each one posing the risk for the other.
8. Weight loss frequently occurs in persons with dementia prior to formal diagnosis.
9. Malnutrition is widespread among persons with dementia residing in long-term care facilities.
10. Providing a pleasant eating environment for patients with dementia can improve food intake during mealtimes.
11. Parkinson's disease is characterized by dysbiosis and disruption of the blood–brain barrier, which can lead to neuroinflammation.
12. Individuals with amyotrophic lateral sclerosis have increased energy expenditure resulting in negative energy balance, weight loss, and malnutrition.
13. Common symptoms of neurodegenerative disease such as mood changes, altered cognition, dysphagia, impaired vision, inability to self-feed, and fatigue are nutritional risk factors.
14. Dietary patterns that are anti-inflammatory may help slow the progression and improve symptoms of neurodegenerative diseases that are characterized by oxidative stress and neuroinflammation.

LEARNING OBJECTIVES

1. Describe the pathophysiology associated with acute neurotraumatic injury.
2. Describe appropriate medical nutrition therapy interventions following acute neurotraumatic injury.
3. Identify risk factors for malnutrition during the acute and chronic phase of recovery from stroke and traumatic brain injury.
4. Apply the International Dysphagia Diet Standardization Initiative (IDDSI) guidelines for managing dysphagia.
5. Compare and contrast pathophysiology and clinical manifestations of the major neurodegenerative diseases.
6. Identify nutrition risk factors for patients living with neurodegenerative diseases such as dementia and Alzheimer's disease.
7. List aspects of Parkinson's disease that may impact nutritional status.
8. Describe the impact of amyotrophic lateral sclerosis on energy balance and nutritional status.
9. Describe the role of diet and specific nutrients in neurodegenerative disease.
10. Identify the basic principles of the ketogenic diet and how it may be beneficial in neurodegenerative disease.

Introduction

The nervous system includes the brain, spinal cord, and a network of nerves operating through a complex signaling system that controls bodily functions, including movement, regulatory processes, cognition, and more. The nervous system is made up of two parts: the **central nervous system (CNS)** and the peripheral nervous system (PNS). The CNS includes the brain and spinal cord while the PNS is made up of the nerves that branch off the spinal cord and extend to all parts of the body.[1] The basic unit of the nervous system is a nerve cell called a **neuron** (**Figure 18.1**). There are many different types of neurons throughout the body that control functions. These include sensory neurons that detect light, sound, odor, taste, and heat, and motor neurons that send messages to the muscles to generate movement. Neurons also control involuntary movements such as breathing, heartbeat, hormone function, and digestive processes. The human brain contains about 100 billion neurons.[1] Insult to the neurons within the CNS can result in the dysregulation of nutrient intake and utilization, the severity of which typically depends on the magnitude and acuity of the damage. While acute neurological injury often produces immediate consequences on nutrition and metabolic parameters that may resolve, chronic injury or neurodegeneration can result in long-lasting nutritional impacts that remain present as the condition progresses.[2–5]

In this chapter, the pathophysiology, clinical manifestations, and medical nutrition therapy in the two major categories of neurological disease: **neurotraumatic injury**, which includes stroke and traumatic brain injury (TBI), and **neurodegenerative disease** including dementia, Alzheimer's disease (AD), Parkinson's disease (PD), amyotrophic lateral sclerosis (ALS), and multiple sclerosis (MS) will be examined.

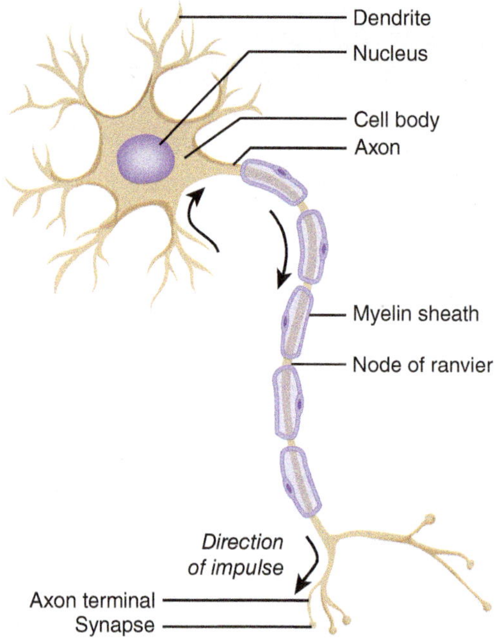

Figure 18.1 The Neuron. The neuron is the basic unit of the nervous system. It has a cell body which contains a nucleus and extensions called axons and dendrites.

Reproduced from U.S. National Institutes of Health, National Institute of Child Health and Human Development. *What are parts of the nervous system?* Accessed January 27, 2026. https://www.nichd.nih.gov/health/topics/neuro/conditioninfo/parts

CORE CONCEPT 1

Insult to the central nervous system can result in the dysregulation of nutrient intake and utilization, the severity of which typically depends on the magnitude and acuity of the damage.

CASE STUDY INTRODUCTION

Paulina is a 41-year-old female who lives in a three-story house with her spouse and two high school–aged children. She works 5 days a week as a systems engineer, travels once or twice a month for work, and has a comfortable work–life balance. As a retired D1 tennis player, Paulina stays active two to three times a week by playing tennis with her partner or going to the gym when traveling. At home, Paulina's partner usually cooks as she works remotely, and they mostly eat a mix of Italian, Malaysian, and American food. Paulina has a family history of cardiovascular disease, dyslipidemia, type 2 diabetes mellitus, and arthritis. Paulina experiences migraine headaches as a residual symptom of two previous sports-related concussions.

Paulina presented to the emergency department with a severe headache and dizziness, reporting that she repeatedly dropped her daughter's plate and cup while washing the dishes earlier that day. After admission, Paulina's condition quickly worsens with unilateral weakness of the left side of her body with numbness in her face and arm. She is diagnosed with a subarachnoid hemorrhagic stroke and admitted to the intensive care unit. A nutrition consult is placed for enteral nutrition support.

Anthropometric Data:

Height: 166 cm
Current Weight: 72 kg
Waist circumference: 104 cm

Biochemical Data:

Sodium 138 (136–145 mEq/L)
Potassium 4.1 (3.5–5.0 mEq/L)
Chloride 111 (96–106 mEq/L)
Carbon dioxide 20 (22–31 mEq/L)
Blood urea nitrogen 18 (8–20 mg/dL)
Creatinine 0.8 (0.7–1.3 mg/dL)
Glucose 235 (70–139 mg/dL)
Serum osmolality 280 (275–295 mOsm/kg)
Magnesium 1.2 (1.5–2.7 mg/dL)
Calcium 8.0 (8.5–10.5 mg/dL)
Phosphorus 3.8 (2.5–4.5 mg/dL)
Albumin 4.4 (3.5–5.5 g/dL)
Hemoglobin 15.1 (14–18 g/dL)
Hematocrit 46.4 (40–50%)
Mean corpuscular volume 90 (80–100 fL)

Clinical Data:

Past Medical History: Hypertension, migraines, concussion × 2 (10 years ago)
Medications: Angiotensin-converting enzyme (ACE) inhibitor, almotriptan
Vital Signs: Blood pressure 159/99 mm Hg, Temperature 99.5°F
Nutrition-Focused Physical Exam: Patient appears well nourished. No evidence of muscle wasting or fat loss.

Dietary Data:

Diet History: N/A

Questions

1. What are Paulina's nutritional risk factors?
2. Describe the possible pathophysiologic etiology associated with her presenting illness.
3. Provide an estimated energy and protein goal for Paulina.
4. Write two Nutrition Diagnosis statements for Paulina identifying the Problem/Etiology/Signs and Symptoms (PES) of her active nutrition issues.
5. Identify the nutrition interventions you would like to initiate for Paulina to address the problems identified in your PES statements. Include a tube feeding recommendation for Paulina.
6. What should be included in your monitoring and evaluation plan? Why?

Each of these conditions presents unique challenges in clinical management, rehabilitation, and recovery, with nutrition playing a critical role in enhancing patient outcomes and facilitating the recovery process.

In managing neurotraumatic injuries and neurodegenerative diseases, several primary issues arise. **Dysphagia**, a frequent complication in this demographic, necessitates careful management to prevent **aspiration** and ensure safe nutritional intake, often requiring modifications to texture and fluid consistency. The complexities of dysphagia management using the **International Dysphagia Diet Standardization**

Initiative (IDDSI) framework will be addressed.[6,7] Furthermore, the chapter will discuss the specific considerations for developing nutrition interventions, particularly in the context of **neuroinflammation** and the role of anti-inflammatory diets and antioxidant nutrients. Current understanding of the impact that specific eating patterns and diets such as the ketogenic diet have on disease progression will be discussed.

Timing of medical nutrition therapy is critical, as early intervention can prevent weight loss and malnutrition. Pharmacological treatments, while essential in managing symptoms of neurological diseases, can be influenced by nutrient intake and lead to impaired gastrointestinal (GI) tolerance, complicating nutrition interventions. Thus, effective nutrition support and planning must integrate a thorough understanding of the patient's medical treatment regimen, drug–nutrient interactions, individual dietary needs, and the physiological changes associated with the patient's condition. Tailored nutrition strategies can significantly improve patient outcomes, addressing both short-term and long-term health recovery in this patient population.

Neurotraumatic Injuries

Acute Ischemic and Hemorrhagic Stroke

Acute strokes can typically be classified into two major types, **ischemic stroke** and **hemorrhagic stroke**. Each requires specific medical and nutritional care. Ischemic strokes account for about 87% of all strokes and are characterized by a blockage of blood flow to the brain either by a clot or plaque in the arteries. Hemorrhagic strokes, which make up approximately 10% of all strokes, are caused by bleeding within the brain due to a ruptured blood vessel, leading to pressure and damage to brain tissues.[8] Acute strokes cause an interruption of oxygen and nutrient supply to brain cells, causing damage that varies in severity, affecting motor skills, speech, and cognitive functions.[9] Stroke is the fourth leading cause of death for Americans (**Figure 18.2**). The risk of stroke is nearly twice as great in non-Hispanic Black adults as for White adults, followed by Pacific Islander adults and non-Hispanic Black adults. The risk of stroke increases with age; however, it can occur at any age.[10] While some risk factors such as race and age are nonmodifiable, there are several modifiable risk factors such as hypertension, smoking, physical inactivity, alcohol consumption, hyperlipidemia, and diet (**Figure 18.3**).[11]

Stroke treatment and mitigation primarily aims to promptly restore blood flow or control bleeding. For ischemic strokes, this will involve use of thrombolytics such as tissue plasminogen activator (tPA) to break up blood clotting and/or endovascular thrombectomy. The latter procedure involves inserting a catheter into an artery in the groin or wrist, which is then guided to the site of the occlusion.[9,12,13] Thereafter, the mainstay of intensive care management includes controlling

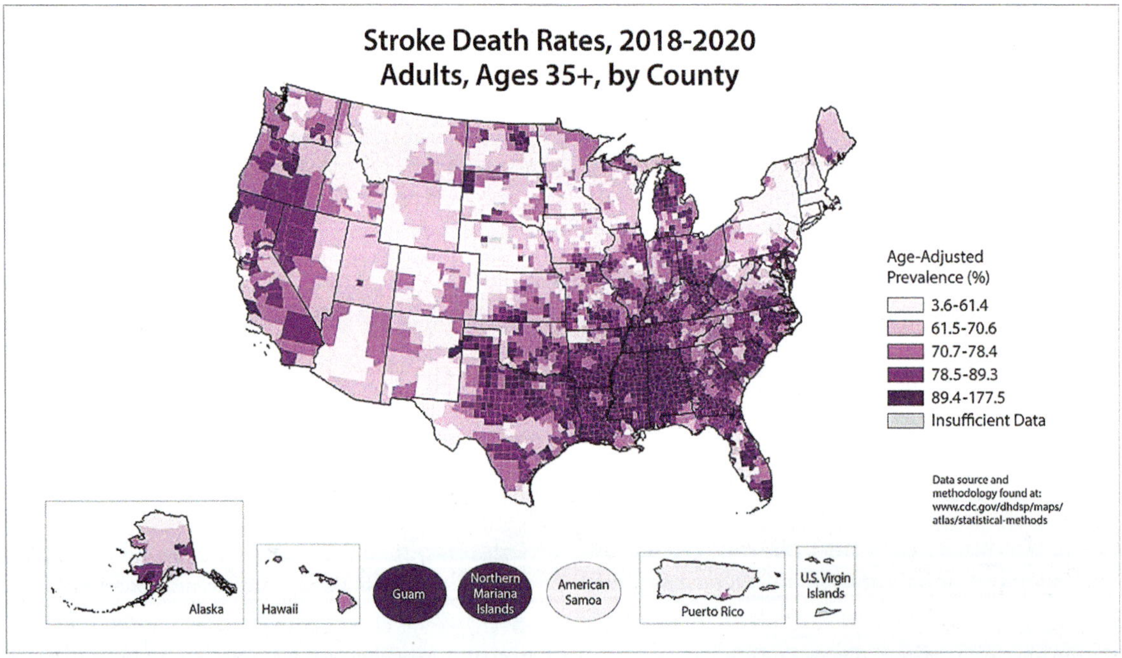

Figure 18.2 Stroke Death Rates for 2018 Through 2020 for Adults Aged 35 Years and Older by County

Reproduced from Centers for Disease Control and Prevention. *Stroke: stroke facts*. Updated October 24, 2024. Accessed January 27, 2025. https://www.cdc.gov/stroke/data-research/facts-stats/index.html

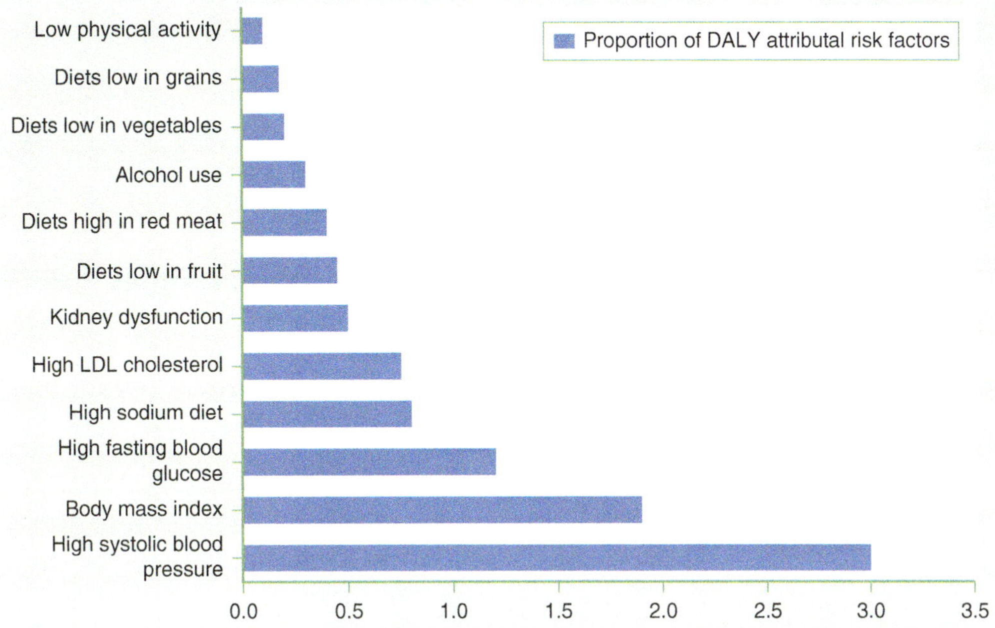

Figure 18.3 Nutritional, Metabolic, and Behavioral Risk Factors Associated with Stroke

DALY (disability-adjusted life years) is the sum of the number of years lost due to premature deaths plus the number of years lived in a state of less than full health adjusted for the severity of disability. Data refer to all types of strokes reported globally.

Data from GBD 2019 Stroke Collaborators. Global, regional, and national burden of stroke and its risk factors, 1990–2019: a systematic analysis for the Global Burden of Disease Study 2019. *Lancet Neurol*. 2021;20(10):795-820. doi:10.1016/S1474-4422(21)00252-0

damage due to reperfusion and minimizing brain edema. Some patients will need hemodynamic stabilization and ventilatory support.[12] This is followed by subsequent nutrition management to maximize functional recovery and prevent lasting complications.

Nutritional Assessment

The risk of malnutrition is high following stroke injury.[7,14] According to European Society of Clinical Nutrition and Metabolism (ESPEN) guidelines, all patients should have a nutrition screen using the Malnutrition Universal Screening Tool (MUST) within the first 48 hours of acute stroke.[7] In studies where this tool has been applied, high versus low scores were associated with an increase in mortality of 6–42%, respectively.[7,15] Furthermore, length of stay and cost significantly increase with malnutrition diagnosis in this population.[15] In the early stages of stroke, depending on the type and severity of stroke, patients may be in a stressed state, similar to that observed following any traumatic injury. Cytokine release will result in inflammation, oxidative stress, and hemodynamic instability.[2] Many patients experience hyperglycemia concurrent with a negative nitrogen balance.[12,16,17] During this stage, nutrition assessment should include anthropometric measurements along with biochemical monitoring of electrolytes, including glucose. Once the patient is stabilized, the primary nutrition-related issue for which to screen is oral pharyngeal function and dysphagia.[7,18] Patients post stroke often experience dysphagia, which can pose other dangers such as **aspiration pneumonia**, malnutrition, or dehydration, if not managed properly. It should be noted that because of these swallowing difficulties, the risk of malnutrition is even greater in the recovery phase as opposed to the acute phase of stroke.[7] While most patients regain full function of their swallowing capability within weeks of the stroke, other patients may experience a longer recovery time or may not regain full swallow capability, requiring long-term adjustments.[18,19]

PRACTICE POINT

All patients with acute stroke injury should have a nutrition screen within the first 48 hours.

CORE CONCEPT 2

Dysphagia of any degree is a common occurrence following stroke injury; all patients should be screened for dysphagia prior to initiation of oral diet.

Assessment of Energy and Protein Requirements. There is not a specific equation for estimating energy requirements in patients who have had a stroke. The degree of hypermetabolism and its effect on energy expenditure may vary depending on type of stroke as well as phase of recovery.[15,19–23] In one study of patients with subarachnoid hemorrhagic (SAH) stroke, measured resting energy expenditure (REE) ranged between 146% and 198% of estimated basal energy expenditure. This was accompanied by negative nitrogen balance and a rise in inflammatory markers.[17] In another study of patients in a neurocritical care unit, weight-based estimates of energy needs using 25 kcal/kg were comparable to measured REE in acute ischemic stroke, whereas patients with SAH had higher energy needs, approximating 35 kcal/kg.[20] These findings suggest that when comparing changes in metabolic demands following either a hemorrhagic or an ischemic stroke, that there is a greater hypermetabolic response following a hemorrhagic stroke.[17,20] The suggested reason for this is because a hemorrhagic stroke has pathophysiology that is more like a TBI than an ischemic stroke, which typically involves less of a stress-induced response throughout the body. While the approach to nutrition intervention following a hemorrhagic stroke will typically involve a large provision of calories, general findings for energy demand following an ischemic stroke suggest that the requirements are more like basal metabolic needs.[17] However, use of weight-based formulas may result in energy intakes that are lower than actual needs in some patients, regardless of type of stroke, suggesting indirect calorimetry (IC)-guided therapy as best practice.[21] Protein intake during the acute phase of stroke should be like that in other critical care environments, ranging from 1.2 to 1.5 g/kg.[22]

CORE CONCEPT 3

Energy needs following acute stroke may vary according to the type of stroke with subarachnoid hemorrhagic strokes resulting in higher energy needs than ischemic strokes.

In the post-acute phase of stroke, measures of REE by IC were 14% lower than REE as predicted by the Mifflin–St Jeor equation. This was accompanied by a decline in measured lean body mass, suggesting that muscle atrophy associated with stroke was the cause of lower energy expenditure.[23] When considering total energy requirements, keep in mind that they may actually be increased due to the energy cost associated with activities of daily living and rehabilitation.[24,25] Although energy needs of patients are not significantly increased following a stroke, a majority of them do not meet their energy requirement due to obstacles with eating and poor intake.[7,19] Protein needs are increased to support rehabilitative efforts with intakes ranging between 0.8 and 1.1 g/kg suggested for better outcomes.[26]

Nutrition Intervention. Medical nutrition therapy provided by a registered dietitian (RD) is recommended for patients following a stroke. Individualized nutrition care plans may include a typical diet for patients without malnutrition, use of oral nutrition supplements for patients with malnutrition (without swallowing problems), and/or enteral nutrition (EN) support by tube feeding. Up to 30% of patients require EN following stroke. These patients include those with severe dysphagia, those who may require mechanical ventilation, and/or are critically ill. EN within 72 hours has been recommended in these instances.[7] Studies have shown use of early enteral nutrition (EEN) to be associated with improved outcomes including a decrease in stroke-associated pneumonia, common in this population,[27] improved neurologic function and recovery,[28–30] and decreased peri-hemorrhagic edema.[31] In addition, EEN decreased the risk of malnutrition and was not associated with GI intolerance such as diarrhea, vomiting, or aspiration.[30,32,33] Use of probiotics combined with EEN may also have a positive influence on outcome. It has been shown that the intestinal microbiome may be altered following stroke, and use of probiotics may help regulate intestinal flora and decrease intestinal permeability, while reducing GI intolerance.[34,35]

Route of enteral access following stroke is frequently deliberated. Current methods include nasogastric, nasojejunal, intermittent feeding tube placement, and percutaneous endoscopic jejunostomy. Factors for consideration with each of these methods include frequency of displacement, risk of aspiration pneumonia, compatibility with dysphagia therapy, and overall progress with rehabilitative efforts.[36–40] Nasogastric feeding tube allows for earlier initiation of tube feedings and should not interfere with therapy for dysphagia.[7] Conversely, use of nasogastric tubes can be associated with increased risk of failed insertions, wrong positioning, aspiration pneumonia, and removal of tube by patient.[36–38] Nasal bridles may be used to help keep feeding tubes in place.[7] Use of intermittent tube feeding placement, which involves placement and removal of feeding tube into the stomach either through the nose or mouth when the patient needs to receive feeding, can be successful

Clinical Roundtable

Topic: Use of Oral Nutrition Supplements and Enteral Tube Feedings in Patients Following Stroke

In 2005, a large, multicenter, randomized controlled trial looked at the timing and route of enteral feeding in patients with dysphagia following stroke. Known as the FOOD (Feed or Ordinary Diet) trial, the researchers aimed to answer three questions: (1) do oral nutrition supplements (ONS) versus a typical hospital diet improve outcomes in patients with stroke; (2) do early enteral feedings improve outcomes in patients who have had strokes and; (3) does enteral feeding via percutaneous endoscopic gastrostomy (PEG) versus nasogastric (NG) tubes result in improved outcomes? The results of this study showed that ONSs did not improve clinical outcomes and that early enteral NG tube feeding enhanced survival. Patients fed by PEG versus NG demonstrated increased mortality and poor outcomes.[1] Decades later, this study continues to be referenced and has helped shape practice for feeding patients who have had a stroke. However, the use of ONS has been shown to improve markers of nutritional status in patients with other neurologic conditions such as dementia and Alzheimer's disease. Current ESPEN guidelines for clinical nutrition in patients with neurologic disease including stroke injury, recommend use of ONS, and initiation of NG feeding in patients who have prolonged dysphagia. In cases where dysphagia persists beyond 28 days, a PEG is recommended.[2]

Roundtable Discussion

1. What are the strengths and limitations of the FOOD study?
2. What are the pros and cons of ONS and enteral tube feeding practice in this population?
3. What might guide your decision making?

References

Dennis MS, Lewis SC, Warlow C; FOOD Trial Collaboration. Effect of timing and method of enteral tube feeding for dysphagic stroke patients (FOOD): a multicentre randomized controlled trial. *Lancet*. 2005;365(9461):764-772. doi:10.1016/S0140-6736(05)17983-5; Burgos R, Bretón I, Cereda E, et al. ESPEN guideline: clinical nutrition in neurology. *Clin Nutr*. 2018;37(1):354-396. doi:10.1016/j.clnu.2017.09.003

for maintaining nutritional status while allowing time away from the bedside for rehabilitation. This approach has also been associated with improved swallowing function during rehabilitation.[39,40] For those patients expected to have long-term EN requirement, placement of a percutaneous endoscopic gastrostomy (PEG) tube may be needed.[7] This approach, however, has been associated with increased disability at discharge and need for institutionalization when compared with nasogastric tube.[41–43]

Traumatic Brain Injury

With approximately 69 million cases globally each year, TBI affects people of all ages and contributes more to death and disability than any other traumatic insult.[44,45] In terms of common unintentional causes, motor vehicle accidents (MVAs) and falls contribute the highest number of TBIs, at over 50% of all cases, across all levels of TBI severity.[45–47] TBIs are structural injuries to the brain along with physiological brain function impairments caused by an external force. These are accompanied by acute onset or gradual worsening of one or more clinical symptoms following the primary insult. TBIs include both penetrating (open) and nonpenetrating (closed head or blunt) injuries, and are generally classified into three categories: mild, moderate, and severe based on clinical factors (**Table 18.1**).[45] Classification of TBI has evolved over time and may be based on numerous factors including causal, pathoanatomic, symptoms/severity, and outcome or prognosis. The **Glasgow Coma Scale (GCS)** is one of the most established scoring systems in a hospital setting. GCS scores of 13–15, 9–12, or <9 represent mild, moderate, and severe TBI respectively.[47] Scoring is based on eye opening, verbal response, degree of confusion and orientation, and motor response to command or painful stimulus. The results of structural brain imaging such as computed tomography (CT) or magnetic resonance imaging (MRI) are used to determine pathologic or anatomic changes and the presence or absence of intracranial lesions.[45,47] While TBIs of all severities can have negative outcomes both acutely and long term, studies have repeatedly shown an increase in the prevalence of negative outcomes and increasing mortality rates with increasing severity of TBI. Compared to mild and moderate TBI, the mortality risk for patients with severe TBI are 2.47 and 7.19 times higher, respectively.[48] The high cost associated with the acute medical treatment and the potential need for long-term rehabilitation indicate that comprehensive and effective acute treatment is crucial in mitigating long-term adverse outcomes and preventing death.[49]

Table 18.1 Characteristics of Traumatic Brain Injury

	Mild (Concussion)	Moderate/Severe
Causes	■ Bump, hit, or jolt to the head ■ Sports injuries ■ Vehicle-related injuries ■ Rapid movement of brain within skull (such as with shaking)	■ Falls ■ Vehicle-related injuries ■ Blunt trauma injuries ■ Fire-arm wounds
Symptoms	■ Headache ■ Nausea/vomiting ■ Confusion/disorientation ■ Concentration/memory problems ■ Problem solving ■ Sensitivity to light or sound ■ Balance problems	In addition to mild symptoms: ■ Minimally conscious state ■ Unresponsive Wakefulness Syndrome (generally unconscious or unaware with occasional periods of wakefulness) ■ Coma ■ Brain death
Diagnosis	■ Neurological exam ■ Neurocognitive tests ■ Neurological tests	■ Glasgow Coma Score ■ CT (computed tomography) scan ■ MRI (magnetic resonance imaging)
Treatment	■ Rest ■ Connect with healthcare provider without travel if possible (telehealth suggested) ■ Over-the-counter or prescribed pain medications	■ Immediate treatment to stabilize and prevent death ■ Ensure proper energy delivery and breathing ■ Control blood pressure ■ Prevent secondary damage: • Hemorrhagic progression of contusion (lesion enlarges/bleeding) • Disruption of blood–brain barrier • Increased intracranial pressure
Comments	■ Multiple concussions (second hit phenomenon) can lead to more severe symptoms and prolonged recovery	■ Leads to long-term or life-long management ■ Rehabilitation often needed to address cognitive, physical, occupational, and emotional difficulties

Data from Centers for Disease Control and Prevention. *Traumatic brain injury and concussion: moderate and severe TBI.* May 16, 2024. Accessed February 9, 2025. https://www.cdc.gov/traumatic-brain-injury/about/moderate-severe-tbi.html

TBI-related injuries may be localized to one area or more widespread or diffuse. The type of brain damage with TBI can include bleeding, swelling, tearing, and inflammation. This initial impact is often compounded by a **secondary brain insult** that leads to hypoxemia, hypercarbia (excessive CO_2 in bloodstream), seizures, alterations in cerebral blood flow, and metabolism. This pathophysiology also elicits a substantial systemic inflammatory and metabolic response, similar to that observed in other types of major trauma and critical illness. Following TBI, there is a release of proinflammatory cytokines and subsequent excretion of counterregulatory hormones including corticosteroids, glucagon, and catecholamines. These, in turn, elicit a cascade of metabolic changes leading to stress-induced hyperglycemia, increased energy demand, and protein wasting. This state of hypermetabolism and hypercatabolic state can quickly lead to the deterioration of the patient's nutritional status.[50–55] Fortunately, initiation of targeted and appropriate nutrition therapy has been implicated as a beneficial therapeutic approach both in isolation and in synergy with the primary medical treatments for modulating these processes. While expert organizations have published recommendations for nutrition therapy for TBI, many of these recommendations lack strong evidence or are nonspecific to TBI; they are instead framed for general critical care patients. Current research has highlighted the importance and potential impact of nutrition in maintaining cerebral homeostasis, reducing mortality, combatting mechanisms of the secondary brain insult, and reducing the incidence of infection-related complications. **Figure 18.4** illustrates the pathophysiology following TBI and its metabolic consequences.

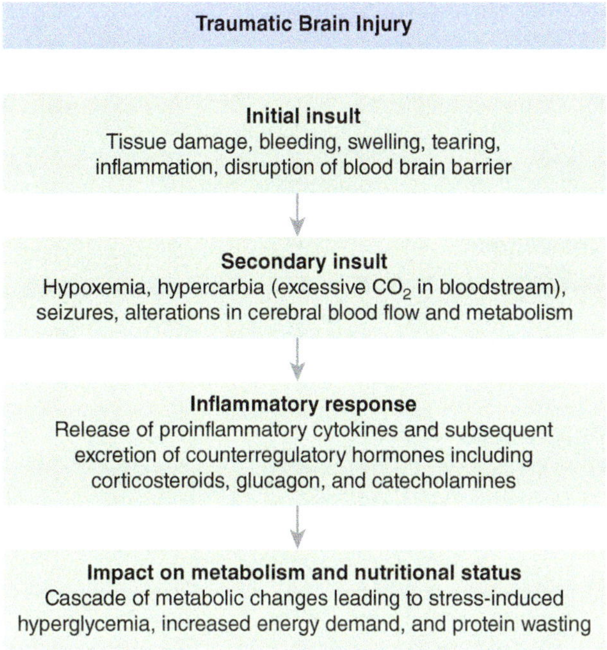

Figure 18.4 Schematic Representation of Traumatic Brain Injury

TBI causes primary and secondary injury. The primary injury results from the initial mechanical insult and is characterized by tissue damage, axonal shearing, and blood–brain barrier (BBB) dysfunction. The secondary response is initiated minutes to hours after TBI and is characterized by increased inflammatory cytokines, brain edema, excitotoxicity, reactive oxygen species (ROS), and immunosuppression. These alterations promote a hypermetabolic and hypercatabolic state that increases morbidity and mortality post-TBI. Optimal nutritional support post-TBI is a potential strategy to meet the increased metabolic demand associated with TBI.

Data from Nwafor D, Goeckeritz J, Hasanpour Z, Davidson C, Lucke-Wold B. Nutritional support following traumatic brain injury: a comprehensive review. *Explor Res Hypothesis Med.* 2023;8(3):236-247. doi:10.14218/ERHM.2022.00086

CORE CONCEPT 4

Secondary brain insult can occur following traumatic brain injury leading to hypoxemia and a systemic inflammatory response.

Nutrition Assessment

Patients presenting with TBI often develop malnutrition, with reports of malnutrition occurring in up to 78% of patients with severe TBI.[50–53] Consequently, malnutrition in patients with TBI can negatively impact pathophysiology and recovery, leading to worsening outcomes.[52] Guidelines for nutritional screening include use of a validated screening tool such as the Nutrition Risk Screening (NRS) 2002 or the Malnutrition Universal Screening Tool (MUST).[56,57] Nutritional screening should be done for all patients in the intensive care unit within 24–48 hours.[55,56] Patients with a GCS of <9 are at greater risk for malnutrition and should be prioritized.[52] Biochemical assessment should include monitoring for electrolyte imbalances and glycemia. Both hypoglycemia and hyperglycemia can occur in this population. Nitrogen balance or urinary urea nitrogen (UUN) measures can be useful to determine degree of nitrogen losses.[53] Reassessment of nutritional status is important following the acute phase of TBI. Many patients may experience severe lean body mass losses. Given the risk of dysphagia with TBI, repeated screening and evaluation of swallowing abnormalities should also be completed.[7]

PRACTICE POINT

Validated screening tools such as the NRS 2002 or MUST are recommended in patients following TBI.

Assessment of Energy and Protein Needs

As mentioned, patients with TBI enter an inflammatory, hypermetabolic state, like most traumatic injuries in the ICU setting. Somewhat unique to patients with TBI, however, are increased cerebral energy requirements, disruption of the **blood-brain barrier (BBB)**, neuroinflammation, and imbalance of energy formation in brain-injured tissues.[52,57] The high energy demand of the brain explains the elevated energy expenditure in TBI, reaching levels up to 200% of REE in an otherwise comparable, healthy individual.[58,59] This sudden increase in energy expenditure peaks within 4–5 days post-trauma and may persist for several weeks or months depending on the extent of neurotrauma.[50,54,58] The impact is a significant loss of lean body mass with a prolonged negative nitrogen balance if energy needs are not met.[59,60] In patients with TBI specifically, this can result in muscle wasting of up to 1000 g/day. Intakes for protein should range between 1.5 and 2 g/kg.[53,57,59–62]

Such a profound metabolic response is the basis for earlier recommendations from the Brain and Trauma Foundation (BTF) for energy intakes of 50 kcal/kg in patients with TBI. In the TBI population, there was a 30–40% decrease in risk of death for every 10 kcal/kg/day after the first 2 weeks, plateauing at 25 kcal/kg/day.[63–65] These findings should be contrasted with more current recommendations suggesting that permissive underfeeding providing approximately 50% of energy goal may be beneficial for some patients post TBI, especially in those where strict glycemic control is crucial.[50,61–63] Another factor to consider in the TBI population is the concurrent medical management such as mechanical ventilation, or the administration of medications that can decrease metabolic demand. Some of these commonly used medications include muscle relaxants, paralytic

Clinical Controversy

Topic: Management: Permissive Versus Strict Glycemic Control in Traumatic Brain Injury

A cornerstone of critical care management following traumatic brain injury (TBI) is to prevent or minimize damage associated with secondary injury, which refers to neuronal damage that occurs as a result of hypoxemia, ischemia, and excitotoxicity. These consequences are mediated by a complex network of inflammatory cytokines and an endocrine response that accelerate gluconeogenesis and hyperglycemia. Stress hyperglycemia is associated with greater severity of secondary insult, including greater neuroinflammation and proliferation of ROS, and poorer outcomes.[1] Despite this, variations in practice exist. The most common approach is intermediate glycemic control using continuous insulin infusion titrated to maintain blood glucose between 140 and 180 mg/dL. This is largely based on the fact that tight glycemic control has not been shown to improve mortality. Furthermore, because neurons are obligate consumers of glucose, hypoglycemia can be more damaging to the brain than other tissues.[1] A meta-analysis by Wang et al. showed that tight versus conventional glycemic control improved neurologic outcomes, reduced infection rates, and decreased length of study in the ICU.[2] Conversely, in a study by Smith et al., tight glucose did not significantly improve the Glasgow Coma Scale score or mortality. Furthermore, severe hypoglycemia occurred in 12% of patients.[3]

Questions

1. Read these studies and compare their findings.
2. Which of the studies has more power?
3. How might the findings of these papers guide your practice in TBI?

References

Garcia-Ballestas E, Villafañe J, Nuñez-Baez K, Perdomo WA, Duran MA, Janjua T, Moscote-Salazar LR, Agrawal A. A systematic review and meta-analysis on glycemic control in traumatic brain injury. *Clin Neurol Neurosurg*. 2024;238:108504.; Wang J, Li J, Yu K, et al. Glycaemic control targets after traumatic brain injury: a systematic review and meta-analysis. *Crit Care*. 2017;21(1):171. doi:10.1186/s13054-017-1883-y; Smith JR, Patel M, Lee A, et al. Intensive versus standard glycemic control in patients with traumatic brain injury: a randomized controlled trial. *Trials*. 2022;23(1):105.

agents, barbiturates, and mechanical ventilation.[57] The advantage and benefit of actual measurement of REE by IC is obvious, and recommended as the gold standard.[56,57] However, in the absence of IC, critical thinking is imperative when assessing energy needs in this population. Consideration should be given to the severity and duration of acute illness as well as clinical condition and medical management. As a general guideline, given the hypercatabolic nature of TBI, progression to 100% of energy targets using weight-based formulas such as 25–30 kcal/kg, the Penn State equation, or other empiric equations should occur within 2 weeks of injury.[63]

CORE CONCEPT 5

The high energy demand of the brain explains the elevated energy expenditure that follows traumatic brain injury, reaching levels up to 200% of resting energy expenditure.

Nutrition Interventions

Timing and Mode of Nutritional Therapy. The key factors considered when addressing nutrition intervention in patients presenting with TBI include optimizing nutrition support to prevent protein-calorie malnutrition, maximally preserving gut motility and function, as well as modulating the severity and intensity of the immune response. Current research has highlighted the importance and potential impact of nutrition in maintaining cerebral homeostasis and neuronal recovery, reducing mortality, combatting mechanisms of the secondary brain insult, and reducing the incidence of infection-related complications.[50,52] Due to lack of studies specific to TBI, recommendations for nutrition support are largely based on general nutrition therapy guidelines for patients who are critically ill. In this respect, both ASPEN and ESPEN recommend the early initiation of medical nutrition therapy in the form of EN or parenteral nutrition (PN) during the first week of therapy.[56,66] While EN is considered preferable, no difference in clinical outcome or harm has been found between the two modes of therapy in patients who are critically ill, and neither is presumed superior during the first week of care.[67] Therefore, timing, rather than route, should be the key consideration with respect to nutrition support in early critical care management of these patients.[56,57,67] Both ASPEN and ESPEN recommend initiation of feeding within the first 24–28 hours in critically ill patients.[56,57,67] At a minimum, the BTF recommends that patients with TBI achieve their basal energy requirement within 5 days, and at most by the seventh day post-injury to lower the risk of death.[64]

Specific to patients with TBI, EEN has been associated with lower risk of infections, and improved endocrine response, including downregulation of thyroid-stimulating hormone, testosterone, and cortisol, which in turn attenuated catabolism.[61,62] Initiation of EEN within 24–48 hours after TBI resulted in maintenance of cerebral homeostasis, reduced inflammatory responses, and lower risk of mortality.[67–69] One large prospective cohort study reported higher survival rates, TBI recovery scores, and better outcomes 1-month post-injury in patients receiving EEN compared to those receiving PN.[69] Systematic literature reviews that pooled results from trials comparing outcomes of patients post TBI provided EEN versus PN also found that patients receiving EN had lower rates of infection, reduced risk of hyper/hypoglycemia, increased mucosal flow, and reduced risk of catheter-related complications.[51,61,70] The implications of TBI on the gut–brain axis and the consequent disruption that occurs in many patients is another compelling reason to promote use of EEN.[71] Small bowel feedings for patients with TBI are generally recommended to improve feeding tolerance and avoid reflux.[63,70]

PRACTICE POINT

Small bowel feedings for patients with TBI are generally recommended to improve feeding tolerance and avoid reflux.

A common barrier to EN in TBI relates to the plethora of pharmaceuticals used as listed in **Table 18.2**. Vasopressors are crucial in TBI management, as the constriction of vessels to maintain cerebral homeostasis is imperative to prevent further damage during the secondary insult; this impacts the gut as it decreases vascular perfusion, which results in reduced gut motility. Additionally, the use of narcotics such as pentobarbital can induce nausea, vomiting, diarrhea, and GI intolerance. Lastly, although TBIs range in terms of location of trauma, many cases of TBI have some degree of impact on the enteric nervous system as well as the autonomic nervous system, which can severely impact the GI tract. These all come together to potentially interfere with feedings that utilize any portion of the GI tract and can cause frequent interruptions and suboptimal delivery of feeds. While EN may be the preferred method of delivery under optimal conditions, given these additional factors, in a patient where these challenges are present and interfere with their ability to achieve adequate intake, PN may be indicated.[62,64,65,70]

Table 18.2 Medications Used in Traumatic Brain Injury and Their Implications

Medications	Nutrition Implications
Barbiturates	▪ Reduces energy requirements ▪ Constipation; combine with bowel regimen
Carbamazepine	▪ Avoid combining suspension with water or other medication diluents (forms rubbery precipitate) ▪ Hyponatremia
Corticosteroids	▪ Hyperglycemia
Demeclocycline	▪ Avoid combination for divalent cations (e.g., magnesium, calcium) or EN
Mannitol	▪ Monitor for hypokalemia, hypomagnesemia, and hypovolemia
Neuromuscular Blocking Agents	▪ Reduces energy requirements
Phenytoin	▪ Caution combining suspension with EN ▪ Hold EN 1–2 hours prior/post administration)
Propofol	▪ 10% lipid emulsion provides 1.1 kcal/Ml ▪ Omit lipid infusion with PN
Propranolol	▪ Reduces energy requirements

Data from Tani J, Wen YT, Hu CJ, Sung JY. Current and potential pharmacologic therapies for traumatic brain injury. *Pharmaceuticals* (Basel). 2022;15(7):838. doi:10.3390/ph15070838

Immune-Modulating Formulations. Use of immune-modulating formulations may be beneficial in patients with TBI. While the overall body of literature is small, formulations high in arginine, glutamine, omega-3 fatty acids, nucleotides, and antioxidants have been proposed to offer neuroprotection from secondary brain insult.[50,56] As a key substrate for glutathione, an important antioxidant used in the brain to scavenge ROS, glutamine is known to provide oxidative defenses. Low levels of glutamine have been thought to be related to the rapid production of ROS and free radicals during the ischemic phase of TBI.[72] In one study, an immunomodulating formula high in omega-3 fatty acids and glutamine significantly reduced interleukin-6

(IL-6) levels, a key inflammatory response regulator in cerebrospinal fluid.[73] Following TBI, increased levels of **glutamate** may also promote rapid calcium influx resulting in excitotoxicity, which is a significant contributor to neuronal death during secondary injury. Because glutamine is a precursor to glutamate, caution is advised, particularly given the disruption of the BBB that follows TBI.[74] Interest in the role of the gut microbiota in regulating glutamate is growing. Studies have postulated that disruption of the **gut-brain axis** is a factor promoting increased glutamate uptake in the brain. It is possible that gut modulation through dietary interventions can reduce neurotoxic glutamate levels following insult. The implications of this extend beyond severe TBI and may benefit patients with other neurologic diseases, including Alzheimer's and Parkinson's diseases, which will be discussed later in this chapter.[75–77] Similarly, use of omega-3 fatty acids has gained support, including in milder cases of TBI and other neurologic disease. Docosahexaenoic acid (DHA) is highly

CASE STUDY REVISITED

After 14 days in the ICU, Paulina is transferred to a general medical floor. She is tolerating her tube feedings at the goal rate. Upon a bedside evaluation from a speech pathologist, Paulina demonstrated choking and coughing with a variety of food and liquid textures. A VFSS or modified barium swallow was done and she was diagnosed with dysphagia. She is cleared for a level 4 IDDSI diet. She will remain on her tube feeding until she can meet 85% of her energy goal. You meet with Paulina and her partner to establish a plan.

Anthropometric Data:

Height: 166 cm
Current Weight: 69 kg
Usual Body Weight: 72 kg (2 weeks ago)

Biochemical Data:

Sodium 140 (136–145 mEq/L)
Potassium 4.4 (3.5–5.0 mEq/L)
Chloride 101 (96–106 mEq/L)
Carbon dioxide 25 (22–31 mEq/L)
Blood urea nitrogen 14 (8–20 mg/dL)
Creatinine 0.7 (0.7–1.3 mg/dL)
Glucose 88 (70–139 mg/dL)
Serum osmolality 285 (275–295 mOsm/kg)
Magnesium 1.8 (1.5–2.7 mg/dL)
Calcium 8.9 (8.5–10.5 mg/dL)
Phosphorus 3.9 (2.5–4.5 mg/dL)
Albumin 3.0 (3.5–5.5 g/dL)
Hemoglobin 16.1 (14–18 g/dL)
Hematocrit 48.3 (40–50%)
Mean corpuscular volume 99 (80–100 fL)

Clinical Data:

Past Medical History: Subarachnoid hemorrhagic stroke, hypertension, migraines, concussion × 2 (10 years ago)
Medications: Clopidogrel, propranolol, warfarin
Vital Signs: Blood pressure 140/79 mm Hg, Temperature 98.6°F
Nutrition-Focused Physical Exam: Patient appears pale. Abdominal exam reveals a non-distended, non-tender abdomen. Mild temporal wasting noted. Patient appears to have adequate fat stores. Hair, skin, nails appear normal. No edema noted.

Dietary Data:

Diet History: Paulina typically follows a diet with no restrictions, "she tries to keep a healthy diet." Her food preferences include chicken, tofu, rice, pasta, peanut butter, oat milk, fruits, and vegetables.

Questions

1. Reassess Paulina's nutritional status and energy and protein goals. Is Paulina malnourished?
2. Provide a tube feeding recommendation that will enable Paulina to attempt her diet while still receiving her tube feedings.
3. Based on Paulina's diet history, what challenges to you see for her to adjust to her new diet order.
4. Assess Paulina's original PES statements. Identify if each statement remains an active issue or if the PES statement has been resolved. If the PES statement remains an active issue, has improvement in the issue been noted? If the issue has been resolved, write a new PES statement.

concentrated in the brain. DHA and eicosapentaenoic acid (EPA) are known for their anti-inflammatory effects and ability to attenuate neuroinflammation.[78] More research is needed for their use, as well as other immunomodulating nutrients following TBI.

Monitoring and Evaluation

Monitoring and evaluation for patients following neurotraumatic injury such as stroke and TBI will proceed according to the stage of injury. During the acute phase, monitoring will be similar to that during critical illness.[50,53,56] Weekly parameters for weight and circumference measures (as appropriate) should be completed. GI tolerance to EN should be assessed daily; given that gastroparesis may occur with neurotrauma, attention to gastric emptying and the need for postpyloric feedings should occur early on. Assessment of adequacy of enteral intake according to estimated or measured energy needs should be completed at least weekly with adjustment in the nutrition plan to assure adequate intake, particularly after the first week of care. Biochemical assessment of electrolytes for hemodynamic stability, hydration, and glycemic control should occur daily until the patient is stabilized. Nitrogen balance may also be performed to assure sufficient protein intake, particularly in patients with TBI who are known to have significant nitrogen losses.[17]

Once the patient enters the rehabilitative phase of care, reassessment of nutrition risk factors is extremely important. Swallowing function should be reassessed by the speech therapist as this can improve over time.[18,19] Fewer restrictions on texture modifications can improve adherence to diet and decrease the risk of malnutrition.[7] Continue monitoring weekly weights and hydration by means of biochemical assessment and intake and output data. A nutrition-focused physical examination (NFPE) is also recommended at least every 3 months.[7] Given that impairment of speech and cognition may be present, patients may not be able to communicate issues related to hunger, appetite, and tolerance. Reassessment using formalized screening tools can help clinicians identify nutrition risk factors as they may arise, particularly in patients that are not able to be interviewed.[79]

Nutritional Management of Dysphagia

The word dysphagia is derived from the Greek term *dys*, meaning disordered, and *phago*, meaning eat or swallow.[80] Dysphagia, characterized by difficulty swallowing, is estimated to affect one in six adults in the United States, and is the 10th leading cause of GI problems leading to ambulatory care visits.[81] Dysphagia may be categorized as oropharyngeal and esophageal dysphagia. **Oropharyngeal dysphagia (OD)** is defined as "the difficulty or inability to move a bolus safely and effectively from the oral cavity to the esophagus, and can include aspirations, choking, and residue."[82] Aspiration, a common manifestation of dysphagia, occurs when food or liquid enters the airway and lungs. **Figure 18.5** represents the abnormal movement of food into the trachea as a result of dysphagia. While many factors contribute to OD, the highest prevalence of dysphagia is found in older adults (10–33%) labeling it as a geriatric syndrome.[83] In addition to older adults, dysphagia can be experienced by adults following stroke, as well as those with neurologic conditions such as PD, MS, and ALS.[18,83–85] Esophageal dysphagia is often the cause of localized neuromuscular disorders or obstructive lesions. Examples include achalasia (a condition where the lower esophageal sphincter does not relax properly), gastroesophageal reflux (GERD), esophageal strictures, obstruction, and carcinomas.[86]

Stages of Swallowing

Swallowing requires multiple levels of the CNS, from the cerebral cortex to the medulla oblongata, to coordinate muscles from the respiratory, oropharyngeal, and GI tract to allow the transit of a bolus of food or liquid from the mouth to the stomach. The first phase of swallowing involves mastication and preparation of a bolus. This requires adequate saliva and the aid of muscles of mastication that are innervated by the mandibular branch of the trigeminal nerve.[87] In the next phase, known as the **oral propulsive phase**, the tongue facilitates the movement of the bolus (or liquid) through the oral cavity into the oropharynx. Next is the **pharyngeal phase** during which the bolus moves through the oropharynx into the esophagus. This phase begins with the elevation of the soft palate to seal the nasopharynx, preventing food from entering the nasal cavity. The pharyngeal phase also serves to protect the airway. This is a well-coordinated physiologic response by which respiration stops (between 0.5 and 1.5 seconds) to allow for swallowing. One of the primary mechanisms of this phase is the closing of the vocal cords. The bolus then moves in peristaltic-like contractions into the esophagus. Finally, during the esophageal stage, the bolus moves down the esophagus into the stomach.[88] **Table 18.3** details the stages of swallowing, examples of swallowing impairment, and resulting consequences. It is during the pharyngeal phase

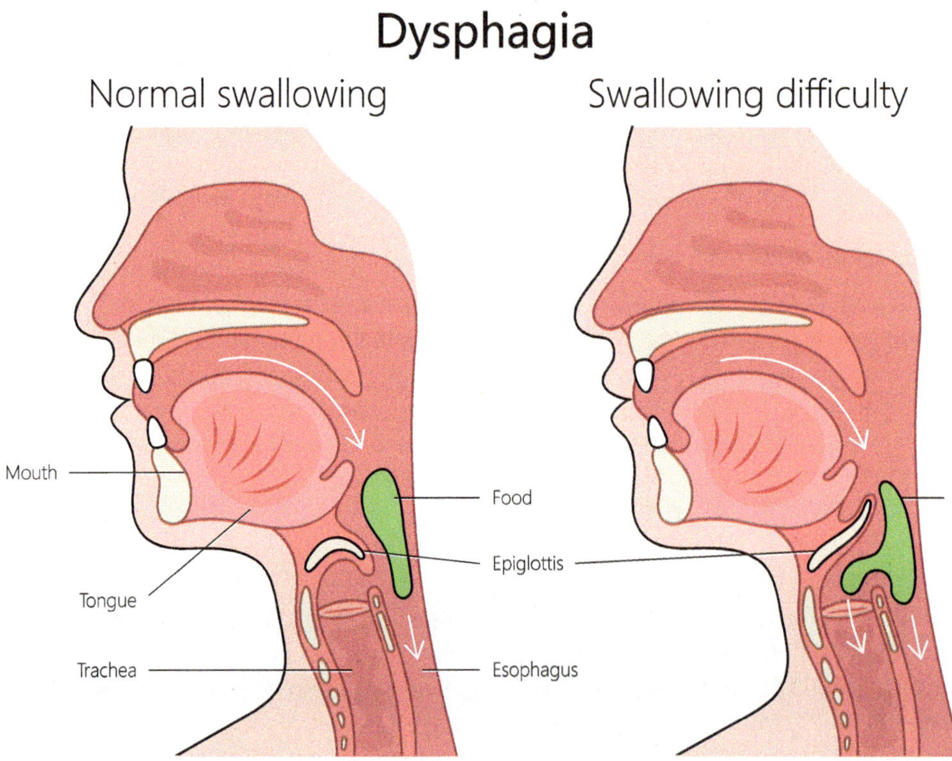

Figure 18.5 Example of Normal and Oropharyngeal Dysphagia During Swallow

Table 18.3 Stages of Swallowing Following Ingestion of Food

Stage	Function	Impairments	Consequence
Oral preparatory	Prepare bolus for propulsion into pharynx	■ Improper mouth closure ■ Lack of oral sensory involvement	■ Food spillage from mouth
Oral propulsive	Tongue pushes bolus through oral cavity into oropharynx	■ Weakness of tongue and other muscles of oral cavity	■ Inadequate bolus formation ■ Inadequate bolus positioning
Pharyngeal	Pharyngeal structures move bolus through the upper esophageal sphincter	■ Failure of sensory information ■ Weakness of pharyngeal muscles	■ Slowed bolus transit across the oropharynx ■ Food residue remaining in oropharynx
Esophageal	Esophageal peristalsis and gravity move the bolus through the lower esophageal sphincter into the stomach		

Data from Sasegbon A, Hamdy S. The anatomy and physiology of normal and abnormal swallowing in oropharyngeal dysphagia. *Neurogastroenterol Motil*. 2017; 29:e13100. https://doi.org/10.1111/nmo.13100

where food slows in transit or food residue remains in the oropharynx that aspiration risk is the highest.

Screening Tools for Dysphagia

As previously described, dysphagia is diagnosed through a combination of clinical assessment, physical examination, and instrumental evaluation. A speech–language pathologist (SLP) typically performs a dysphagia screening to evaluate the patient's ability to swallow safely. This can be done at the bedside and may involve examination of cognitive, behavioral, and language abilities as well as a feeding trial, where the therapist evaluates the patient's swallow to various textures (**Figure 18.6**).

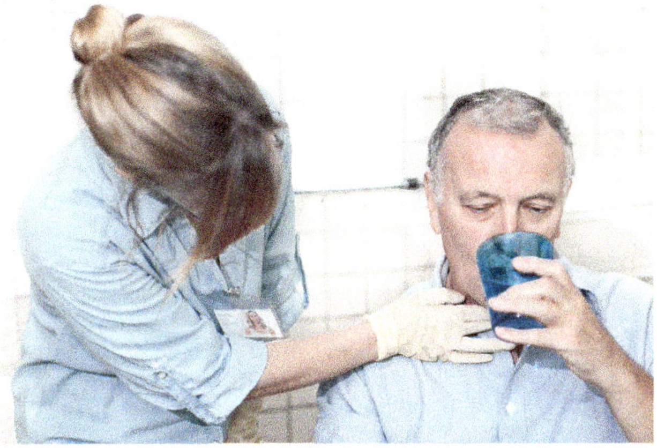

Figure 18.6 Image of a Swallowing Assessment Done at the Bedside

A bedside swallowing examination includes observation of the mouth including movement of the tongue and soft palate using a tongue blade. Observing the patient's ability to mix food with saliva and transfer a food bolus to the pharynx can also be done to identify swallowing problems. Movement of jaw during mastication can be used to detect chewing problems. A variety of liquid textures and foods are often used to determine what type of dysphagia exists.[89] If the dysphagia screening is significant, or in patients demonstrating signs of dysphagia such as coughing, choking, or a "**wet voice**," which suggests long-term laryngeal aspiration, a formal assessment of swallow should be completed.[7] This may include a **videofluorographic swallowing study (VFSS)**, also known as a "modified barium swallow (MBS)," or a **fiberoptic endoscopic evaluation of swallow (FEES)**.[18] **Figure 18.7** shows the results of a VFSS. In this image, the food bolus penetrates the patient's airway.

PRACTICE POINT

A wet voice may indicate long-term laryngeal aspiration and should precipitate a formal evaluation of swallowing.

The relationship between dysphagia and malnutrition is well documented.[90–93] Dysphagia is an independent risk factor for malnutrition.[90] Likewise, malnutrition can lead to dysphagia.[91,92] This phenomenon is commonly observed in older populations with frailty and sarcopenia.[93,94] Dehydration is also associated with dysphagia, which can contribute to cognitive decline.[95,96] This underscores the importance of screening for dysphagia alongside malnutrition screening, particularly in high-risk populations.

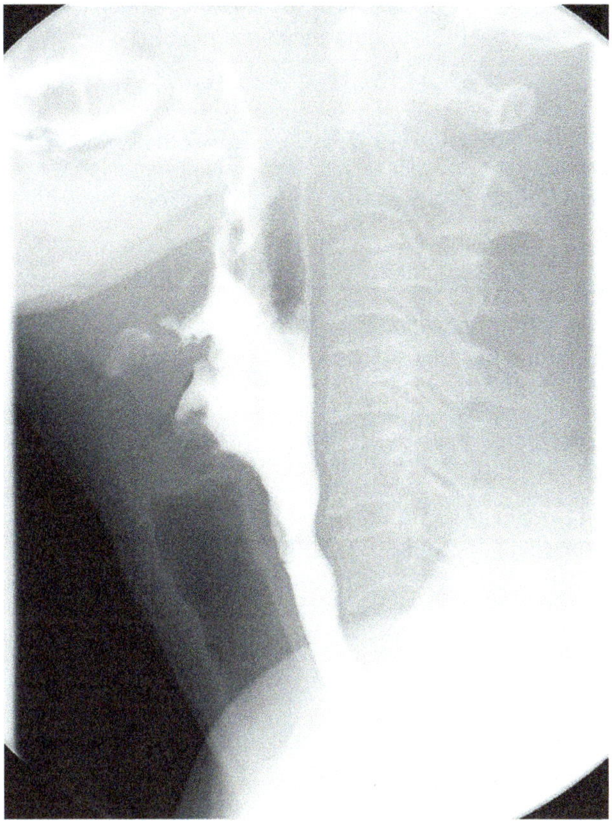

Figure 18.7 Results of a Videofluoroscopic Swallow Study (VFSS) Show Abnormal Transport of Food Bolus Causing It to Penetrate into the Airway

Several screening tools exist for this purpose. A common tool included among these is the Eating Assessment Tool (EAT-10), a 10-item patient self-assessment tool that clinicians can easily administer to describe swallowing function. EAT-10 has proven to be reliable and validated against measures of aspiration by VFSS and FEES.[97] In addition, the Bedside Swallowing Assessment, the Gugging Swallow Screen, and the Toronto Bedside Screening test have all been shown to perform well when compared to VFSS and FEES.[98–101] Several tools simultaneously assess cognition and quality of life such as the Yale Swallow Screen.[102] **Table 18.4** shows the various screening tools that can be used to identify dysphagia.

Texture-Modified Diets

Texture-modified diets (TMDs) are used to prevent the risk of aspiration pneumonia.[7] Uniform terminology and standardization of TMDs is important for communication among health professionals and for the safety of the patient.[103] Founded in 2013, the International Dysphagia Diet Standardization Initiative (IDDSI) was established to develop internationally standardized terms and definitions to characterize

Table 18.4 Dysphagia Screening Tools

Screening Tool	Methodology	Clinical Use
Bedside Swallowing Assessment (Clinical Swallow Evaluation—CSE)[101]	Observation of oral motor function, pharyngeal phase, and signs of aspiration (e.g., coughing, choking, wet voice)	General assessment performed by speech–language pathologists (SLPs) or trained clinicians
3-Ounce Water Swallow Test[98]	Patient drinks 3 oz of water without stopping; failure is indicated by coughing, choking, or wet vocal quality	Quick bedside screening for aspiration risk
Gugging Swallowing Screen (GUSS)[100]	Stepwise assessment of direct and indirect swallowing function	Primarily used for stroke patients to assess aspiration risk
Toronto Bedside Swallowing Screening Test (TOR-BSST)[101]	Cognitive screening, tongue movement assessment, and 10 mL water swallow test	Stroke-specific tool for dysphagia screening
Mann Assessment of Swallowing Ability (MASA)[99]	Comprehensive scoring system evaluating swallowing, respiration, and neurological components	Stroke and neurological patients; determines dysphagia severity
Eating Assessment Tool-10 (EAT-10)[97]	Patient-reported questionnaire assessing dysphagia severity and its impact on quality of life	Self-assessment tool for dysphagia patients
Yale Swallow Protocol[102]	Includes cognitive screening, oral motor exam, and a 3-oz water swallow test	Standardized bedside screening for aspiration risk

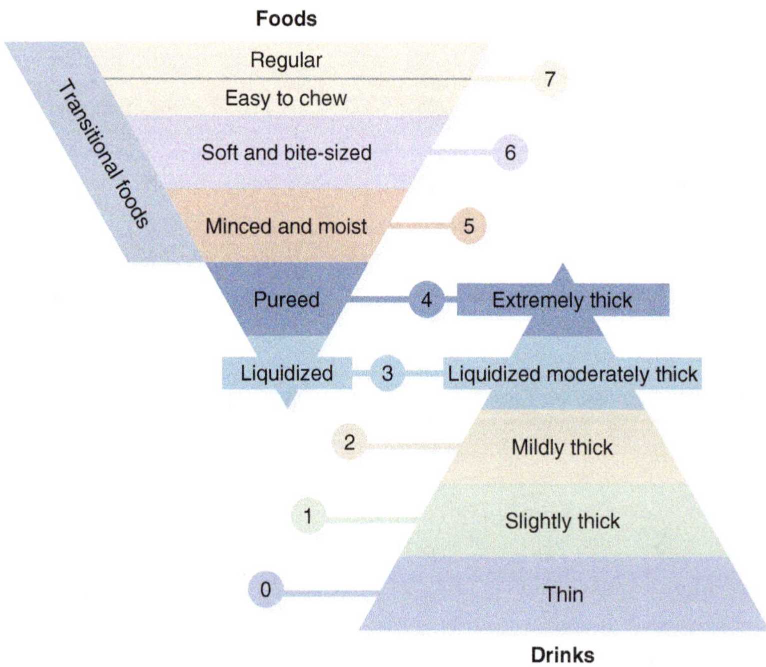

Figure 18.8 IDDSI Framework

thickened liquids and texture-modified foods commonly used for individuals with dysphagia. The most updated version from 2019 categorizes thickened liquids and texture-modified foods into eight levels, identifiable by number, color, and text (**Figure 18.8**). The levels range from zero through seven, describing drinks with levels zero "thin" through four "extremely thick," and food products starting at level

Table 18.5 Description of Levels within IDDSI Framework

Level		Indications	Description
0	Thin liquids	Able to swallow fluid safely and without difficulty	No texture modifications >10 mL passes via syringe in <10 seconds
1	Slightly thick	Able to swallow fluid, but require some modification to prevent choking or aspiration	Slower flow rate but remain drinkable, nectar consistency
2	Mildly thick	Recommended for individuals with more pronounced swallowing difficulties	Thicker than level 1, but still pourable
3	Moderately thick	Recommended for individuals who need greater control over flow as they swallow. Often recommended if there is poor tongue control	Liquids cannot move quickly through the mouth or throat
4	Pureed foods	Safe option for individuals who cannot chew solid foods or who are at high risk for choking	Smooth, lump free; thickened to the extent that it cannot be sipped from a cup or bowl or through a straw; requires use of a utensil such as a spoon
5	Minced and moist foods	Provides a manageable texture for individuals with some ability to chew but who have difficulty with harder, chunkier foods	Foods are finely chopped into small, soft pieces. Soft enough that can be mashed with the tongue
6	Soft and bite-sized foods	Suitable for individuals who can chew but may need softer textures to avoid complications during swallowing	Foods are tender and easy to break down with minimal chewing. Bite-sized pieces ensure foods can be managed safely without overwhelming person's ability to chew or swallow effectively
7	Regular food	Suitable for individuals who have no significant issues with chewing or swallowing	Foods at this level are of any texture allowing the widest range of dietary choices

Data from International Dysphagia Diet Standardisation Initiative. *Framework: The IDDSI Framework (the Standard).* Accessed January 13, 2026. https://www.iddsi.org/standards/framework

three "liquidized" to seven "regular/easy to chew" (**Table 18.5**).[6] The IDDSI framework provides clear, consistent guidelines to improve safety and quality of life for individuals with dysphagia. By offering standardized levels of food textures and liquid consistencies, it helps healthcare providers, caregivers, and individuals better manage the challenges of dysphagia while ensuring that nutritional needs are met in a standardized, safe, and practical manner.[104] A variety of testing methods are used including the flow test, which measures the timing of flow of a liquid through a syringe, and the spoon and fork test, which describes the appropriate consistency of a food using these utensils (**Figure 18.9**). IDDSI guidelines are currently utilized in many countries including the United States, Canada, the United Kingdom, Israel, New Zealand, and Australia.[6]

CORE CONCEPT 6

Textured-modified diets can reduce the risk of aspiration pneumonia in patients with dysphagia.

Many healthcare settings use commercially available modified thickeners, typically starch-based. The thickener-to-liquid or thickener-to-food ratios are categorized using IDSSI guidelines. While this modification of food and beverage viscosity can reduce dysphagia-associated risks related to food consumption, it also lowers the palatability and enjoyment of these food products.[105,106] Adult patients have been found to report negative perceptions of thickened foods based on their texture and taste, which has been associated with poor adherence to diets and risk for

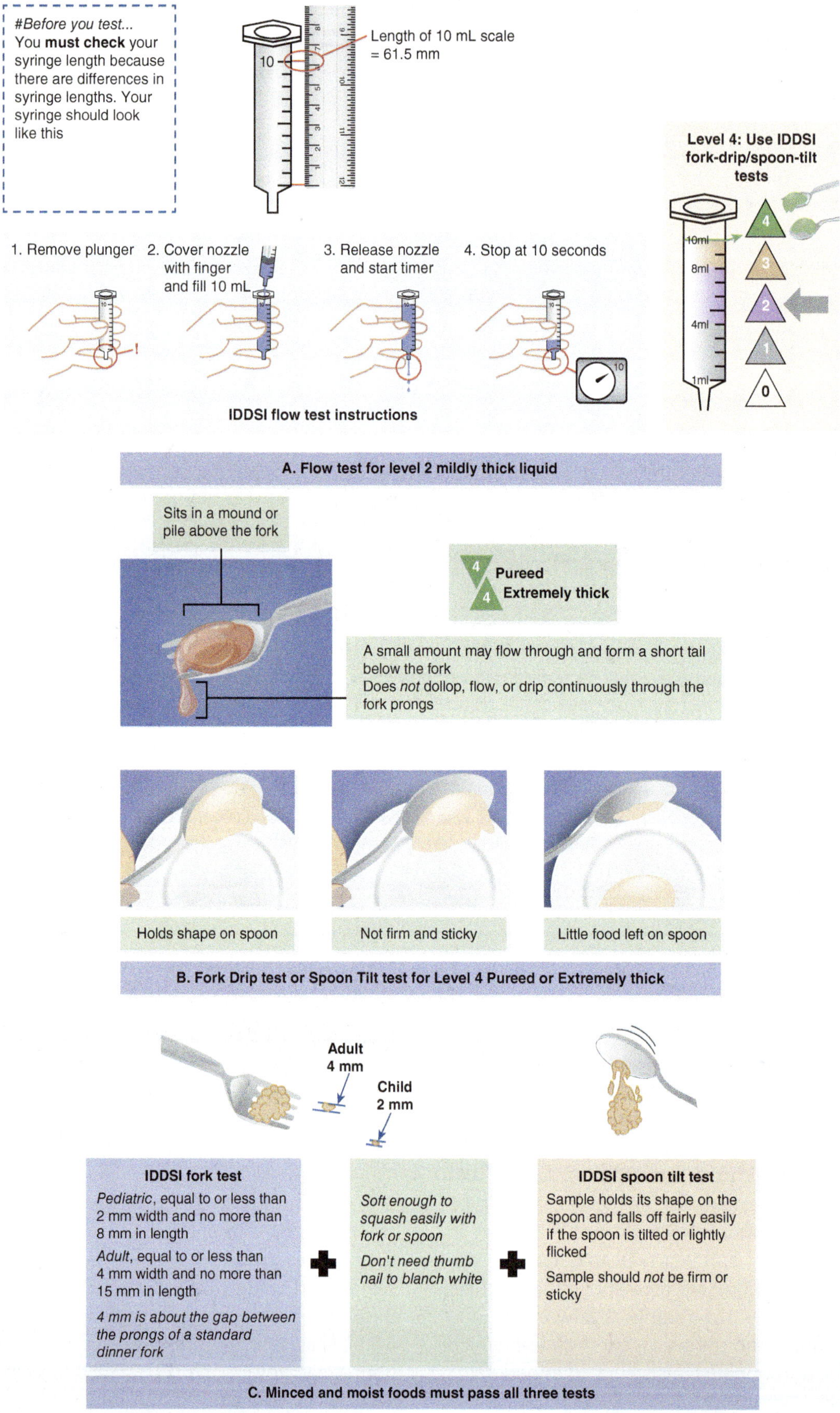

Figure 18.9 Examples of IDDSI Testing Methods

Table 18.6 Strategies for Improving the Appeal of Dysphagia Diets

Flavor enhancement	■ Use herbs and spices (e.g., basil, rosemary, cinnamon) ■ Add broths, soy sauce, nutritional yeast ■ Use citrus or vinegar for brightness (e.g., lemon juice, balsamic vinegar)
Texture and consistency	■ Blend thoroughly for smooth purees ■ Use natural thickeners (e.g., mashed potatoes, yogurt, avocado) ■ Layer soft textures (e.g., mousse with puree) for variety
Presentation and visual appeal	■ Use food molds to shape purees into recognizable forms (e.g., carrot-shaped pureed carrots) ■ Layer colorful purees (e.g., sweet potato, spinach, and chicken casserole) ■ Garnish with smooth sauces or grated cheese for appeal
Temperature control	■ Serve foods at optimal temperatures (e.g., soups hot, fruit purees chilled) ■ Avoid lukewarm foods for better taste and comfort
Variety and familiarity	■ Include familiar and favorite flavors from the individual's regular diet ■ Rotate menus to prevent boredom ■ Offer multiple options within a meal (e.g., savory puree with a sweet fruit puree)
Nutritional enrichment	■ Boost nutrients by adding powdered milk, protein powders, or nut butters ■ Use high-calorie ingredients (e.g., butter, cream, coconut milk) for those needing extra energy
Sweet options and desserts	■ Offer smooth desserts like custards, puddings, or fruit compotes ■ Include cold options like frozen fruit or yogurt parfaits

Data from Chefs for Seniors. *Nutritious foods for dysphagia: tasty solutions for swallowing difficulties*. Published February 12, 2024. Accessed February 23, 2025.; Senior Services of America. *Soft foods for seniors with swallowing issues*. Accessed December 19, 2025. https://seniorservicesofamerica.com/blog/soft-foods-for-seniors-with-swallowing-issues/

malnutrition and dehydration.[107] Inadequate intake is not uncommon in patients prescribed a TMD, which can pose difficulties in clinical settings, as patients with a TMD can only be provided with foods that are compliant with their dysphagia diagnosis. To make changes, patients must be re-evaluated by an SLP to determine their functional capacity before other diet options can be provided. In cases where patients are unable to progress to more palatable diets, alternative methods of ensuring that energy needs are met must be explored. As such, it is important for practitioners to understand the different levels of IDDSI guidelines for modifying food textures as well as the different kinds of thickeners available. While the texture may be difficult to alter, researchers and practitioners can try to improve foods by adding seasonings to combat the negative perceptions of taste and improve intake. **Table 18.6** provides methods that can increase the palatability of TMDs.[106]

Recent advances in food technology have improved thickening agents and ready-to-feed thickened products. Use of xanthum gum, pre-thickened liquids, and naturally occurring nectar-like beverages has improved the palatability of liquid beverages.[108] One emerging trend is the use of 3D food printing. This innovative technology offers a means of providing foods with both the proper nutrient content and texture that is safe to swallow and aesthetically pleasing. This process is evolving as a means for improving appetite and intake of patients with dysphagia.[109] **Figure 18.10** shows an example of 3D printing of a texture-modified food.

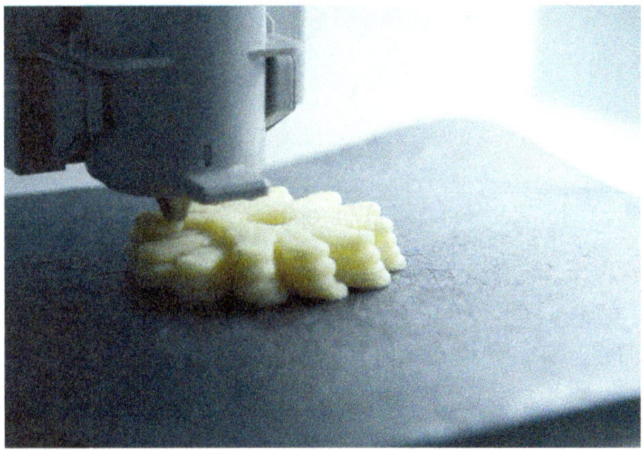

Figure 18.10 3D Printing of Mashed Potatoes

CORE CONCEPT 7

Malnutrition and dysphagia are closely related; each one posing the risk for the other.

PRACTICE POINT

Practitioners can try to improve foods by adding seasoning to combat the negative perceptions of taste to improve intake.

Neurodegenerative Diseases

Dementia and Alzheimer's Disease

Dementia is an umbrella term that describes loss of memory, language, problem-solving, and other thinking abilities that are severe enough to impact activities of daily living. Alzheimer's disease (AD) describes changes within the brain that can lead to dementia. AD accounts for 60–80% of all diagnosed dementia cases. Vascular dementia, which is the result of reduced blood flow to the brain, is the second most common type of dementia. This can result due to microscopic bleeding and blockage of blood vessels that may occur following a stroke.[110]

It is estimated that 6.9 million Americans are currently living with AD, a number that is expected to grow to 13.8 million by 2060.[111] AD can be categorized as sporadic, which makes up most of the cases, or familial, which make up less than 1% of all Alzheimer's cases.[112] Sporadic AD has no specific genetic link but is believed to be the result of the interactions between an individual's genes, environment,

CASE STUDY REVISITED

One month after admission, Paulina is ready for discharge. Her dysphagia has resolved. She was able to achieve adequate intake prior to discharge, and her feeding tube was removed. Paulina was told that there could be risk of cognitive impairment due to her stroke. She has been reading on the internet about diets for improved cognition and is asking about nutrition recommendations. A typical diet recall was obtained and is shown below.

Anthropometric Data:

Height: 166 cm
Current Weight: 72 kg
Usual Body Weight: 72 kg (1 month ago)

Clinical Data:

Past Medical History: Subarachnoid hemorrhagic stroke, hypertension, migraines, concussion × 2 (10 years ago)
Medications: ACE inhibitor, almotriptan
Vital Signs: Blood pressure 120/69 mm Hg, Temperature 98.6°F
Nutrition-Focused Physical Exam: No evidence of muscle wasting or fat loss. Hair, skin, nails appear normal. No edema noted.

Typical 24-Hour Diet Recall:

Breakfast (6:30): Corn flakes with 2% milk or 2 slices of whole grain toast with jam or peanut butter, breakfast sausage with mustard; 1 mug of coffee with 2% milk or oatmilk
AM Snack: Grapefruit juice, granola bar
Lunch (12:30 pm): Hainanese chicken and rice with ginger garlic sauce and soy dipping sauces (leftover)
spicy cucumber and ginger salad, sliced nectarines
Dinner (6:30 pm): Spaghetti Puttanesca with canned tuna; simple salad with citrus vinaigrette
whole wheat bread roll with olive oil
PM Snack: Ice cream (1–2 scoops) every Friday

Questions

1. How would you describe Paulina's current nutritional status?
2. What are your diet recommendations for Paulina upon discharge?
3. Assess Paulina's previous PES statements. Identify if each statement remains an active issue or if the PES statement has been resolved. If the PES statement remains an active issue, has improvement in the issue been noted? If the issue has been resolved, write a new PES statement.

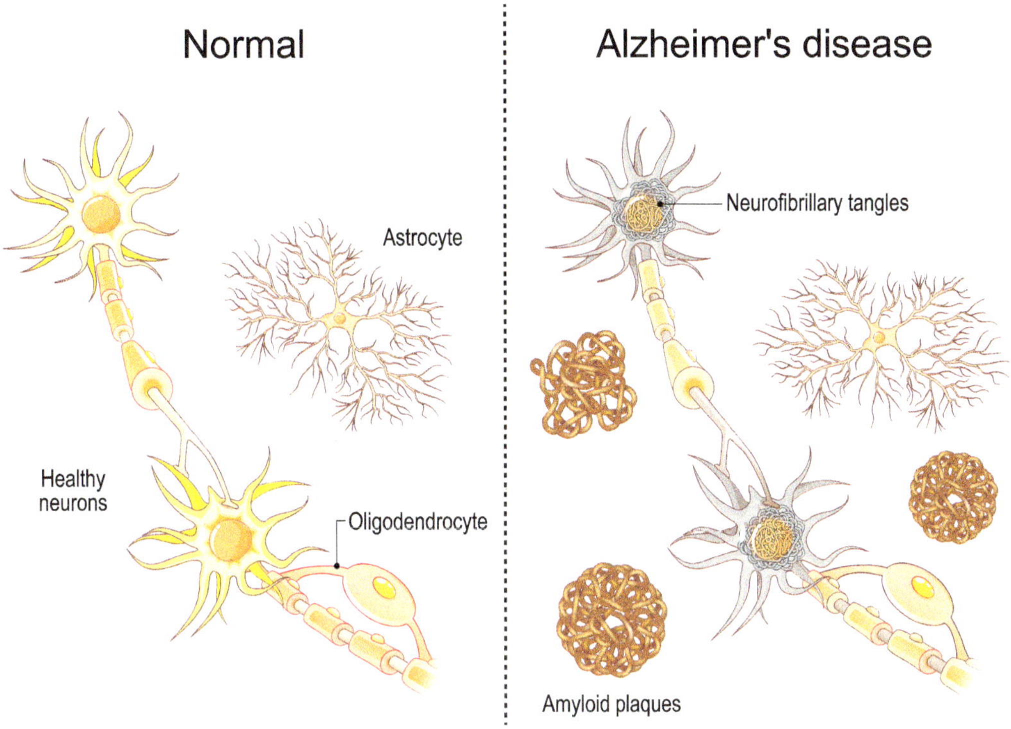

Figure 18.11 Image of a Healthy Neuron and a Neuron During Alzheimer's Disease

and lifestyle. Familial AD, on the other hand, is due to the hereditary mutations of three genes that have been identified thus far: the PSEN1, PSEN2, and APP genes.[112] In both forms of AD, the disease is often first characterized with the loss of cognitive functions such as short-term memory, learning, and critical thinking skills. As the disease progresses, individuals begin to exhibit severe disruptions of basic functions such as walking, swallowing, and the ability to perform daily functions.[110] Although the diagnosis of AD typically occurs after characteristic symptoms begin to arise, the neurological changes observed in the development of AD are believed to begin 20 or more years before any of these behavioral symptoms surface.[113] This gap between the onset of cellular changes and the onset of cognitive symptoms suggests that the neurological changes take time to accumulate and cause significant damage. This in turn points to the importance of determining the inter- and intracellular interactions within the brain to understand AD pathology and treatments that are effective before the neurological changes are too severe.[114] Currently, individuals typically live for 8–10 years after diagnosis; however, there have been cases where individuals live for decades. Lifespan in persons with AD decreases with increasing age.[115]

AD is categorized into two main pathological hallmarks: (1) the aggregation of phosphorylated **tau proteins** and (2) the aggregation of **amyloid-β (Aβ) peptides**. Both the tau and the Aβ pathologies coincide with increased activation of microglia and consequent neuroinflammation.[114,115] Tau proteins act as reinforcing compounds that bind to microtubules, a class of structural proteins, that ultimately act to maintain the structural integrity of cells. They also facilitate a network for the transport of necessary molecules throughout the cell. In AD, tau proteins are hyperphosphorylated, causing the tangling and eventual loss of structural integrity, collapse of the microtubule network, disruption of various cellular communications, and consequent cell death.[116] In healthy brains, soluble Aβ peptides are present in lower amounts throughout the lifespan. However, these peptides are identified as a hallmark of AD when overexpressed, resulting in the formation of dense, insoluble Aβ plaques. These are pathogenic, as they are typically associated with neuritic and synaptic dystrophy, cell signaling disruptions, and eventual cell death.[117] **Figure 18.11** shows amyloid plaque and neurofibrillary tangles due to clumping of tau proteins in the neuron during AD.

Role of Diet in Cognitive Decline and Alzheimer's Disease

Our understanding of the role that nutrition plays in the prevention and care for patients with dementia and AD is limited. This is due to the multimodal aspects of diet, lifestyle, and cognitive function. While a healthy dietary pattern can reduce the risk of diseases that are associated with dementia such as hypertension, dyslipidemia, and diabetes, it is difficult to discern whether diet is an independent factor related to brain health or if its effects are indirect.[118] Likely it is a combination of eating patterns, lifestyle, metabolic, genetic, and brain physiology that contribute to cognitive health (**Figure 18.12**). Healthy eating patterns, which include fruits and vegetables, whole grains, nuts and seeds, and fish, while avoiding ultra-processed foods, sodium, and unhealthy fats, are associated with good cognitive health. In support of this, studies show that the Mediterranean diet, which represents a healthy eating pattern, is associated with lower risk of cognitive decline and dementia.[118] Like the Mediterranean diet, the Dietary Approaches to Stop Hypertension (DASH) diet through its effect on cardiovascular risk factors such as hypertension and low-density lipoprotein (LDL) cholesterol can indirectly decrease risk factors for dementia.[118] The Mediterranean-DASH Intervention for Neurodegenerative Delay (MIND) diet is unique in its strong emphasis on specific foods and nutrients that are theorized to improve brain health such as berries and leafy green vegetables. It also encourages limits on red and processed meats, saturated fats, full fat cheeses, refined grains, and dessert-like products. The MIND diet has been shown to decrease the risk of AD by greater than 50% if strongly adhered to, and over 30% with moderate adherence.[119] **Table 18.7** describes the basic elements of the MIND diet.

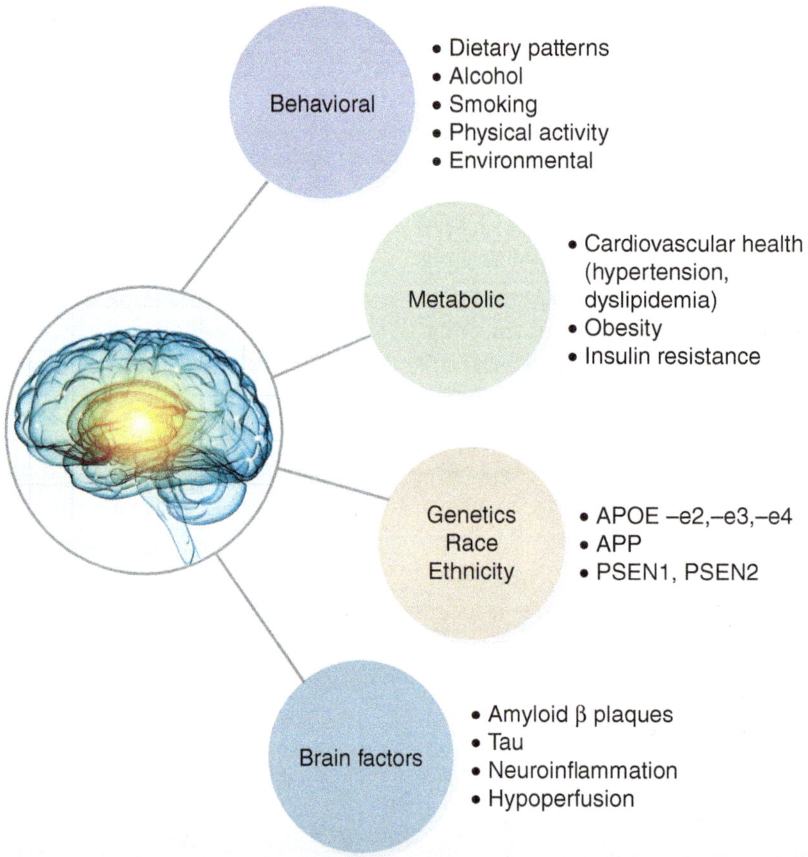

Figure 18.12 Factors that May Contribute to Dementia and Alzheimer's Disease

A: © Sergey Nivens/Shutterstock; B: Created by kprelack.

Table 18.7 Characteristics of the Mind Diet

Food	Servings	Description
Poultry	2 servings/day	Choose light meat without skin
Fish	1 or more servings/week	Focus on fatty fish such as salmon, mackerel, herring, or sardines
Beans	4 or more meals/week	This includes all beans, lentils, and soybeans
Nuts and seeds	5 servings/week	Includes peanuts
Whole grains	3 or more servings/day	Focus on grains that minimally processed
Vegetables	2 or more servings/day	Choose at least 1 leafy green daily
Berries	3–5 servings/week; minimum	Does not include dried berries
Extra-virgin olive oil	2 tablespoons/day	Specifically extra-virgin olive oil; not other olive oil or types of oils

Data from Eat Right PRO. Academy of Nutrition and Dietetics. *What is the MIND diet?* Published December 20, 2023. Accessed March 3, 2025. https://www.eatrightpro.org/news-center/practice-trends/what-is-the-mind-diet

Nutrition Assessment

Weight loss is often observed in patients with AD or dementia. In fact, weight loss often occurs before the diagnosis of dementia is made. This weight loss is likely due to a decrease in caloric intake as loss of smell, taste, and appetite often accompany decreased consumption of food and weight loss. Studies have also pointed to changes within the appetite control centers in the hypothalamus and medial temporal lobe.[120,121] As dementia progresses, decreased attention and orientation may negatively impact the patient's ability to procure food. The ability to socialize and/or concentrate on eating during mealtimes may also occur. Swallowing difficulty, which accompanies many neurologic conditions, creates an additional barrier to eating and ultimately amplifies the risk of malnutrition as well as dehydration.[121]

Malnutrition is widespread among persons with dementia (PWD) residing in long-term care facilities. In one systematic review, diagnosis of malnutrition ranged from 6.8% to 75%.[122] Clinical progression of dementia is increased with malnutrition, emphasizing the importance of nutrition screening in these facilities.[123,124] Nutrition screening tools for the older population, which include questions related to cognition and dementia, should be used in this residential population.[123] A number of such tools have been validated, which include the Edinburgh Feeding Evaluation in Dementia Scale,[125] Mini Nutritional Assessment (MNA),[126] and the Eating Behavior Scale.[127]

Assessment of cognition, feeding difficulties, and mealtime behaviors should be included in nutrition assessment along with changes in weight status. NFPE should be conducted to look for signs of muscle loss and/or fat wasting, as well as decrease in function.[124] Skin turgor should be assessed for signs of dehydration. Oral examination should inspect for dentition and saliva production. Angular stomatitis and glossitis may indicate B vitamin micronutrient deficiencies that are common in the aging population in general.[128]

CORE CONCEPT 8

Weight loss frequently occurs in persons with dementia prior to formal diagnosis.

PRACTICE POINT

An NFPE in PWD should be conducted to look for signs of muscle loss, fat wasting, decrease in function, dehydration, and B vitamin deficiencies.

CORE CONCEPT 9

Malnutrition is widespread among PWD residing in long-term care facilities.

Nutrition Intervention in Dementia and Alzheimer's Disease

Nutritional care in patients with dementia and AD requires the knowledge and skills to ensure that nutrition and fluid needs are met. In long-term care facilities, cooking staff should be competent in providing the proper textures for liquid beverages and foods. Adequate numbers of trained personnel are needed to identify feeding difficulties and manage daily challenges faced by PWD. Direct training of PWD and interventions such as hand exercises can improve intake and promote independence at mealtimes.[129] Provision of attractive foods and snacks with available options helps to support adequate intake. Family and informal caregivers should be educated to help meet nutrient requirements as well as to promote a positive eating experience. Modifications to support a pleasant eating environment such as music, proper lighting, changes in meal service style, shared meals, and home-like features can improve intake at mealtimes.[121]

CORE CONCEPT 10

Providing a pleasant eating environment for patients with dementia can improve food intake during mealtimes.

Oral nutritional supplements (ONS) are an effective way for improving nutritional status and maintaining hydration in patients with AD. Providing a variety of flavors, offering supplements between meals, dispersed throughout the day, and removing them prior to the next meal improves adherence.[120] A systematic review of several randomized controlled trials demonstrated weight gain, improved body mass index, increased mid-arm muscle circumference, as well as increased levels of vitamin B12, thiamine, folic acid, and vitamin D with the use of ONS in patients with dementia and AD. Intakes from ONS ranging between 200 and 780 calories per day were provided with no inhibitory impact on appetite during regular mealtime.[130]

PRACTICE POINT

Provision of a variety of ONS between meals and throughout the day can improve caloric intake without inhibiting appetite at mealtimes.

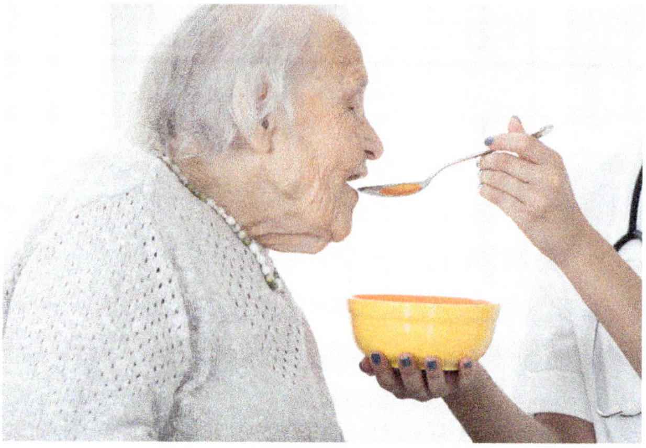

Figure 18.13 Image of Hand Feeding in an Aging Patient

In patients with advanced dementia, research has consistently shown that provision of enteral tube feedings leads to increased tube-related complications with no improvement in survival.[131,132] Use of hand feeding, or giving patients small amounts of food and drink when they can no longer independently feed themselves, may be more effective in maintaining intake without the risk factors associated with tube feeding complications, which may include aspiration (**Figure 18.13**).[133] When compared to hand feeding, tube feedings did not improve overall intake. One study showed that careful hand feeding enabled patients to sustain their intake for over 12 months.[134] While hand feeding may be more comfortable for the patient, it can be associated with increased burden and stress for caregivers.[133]

Parkinson's Disease

Parkinson's Disease (PD) is a fast-growing neurodegenerative disorder that causes uncontrollable movements such as shaking, stiffness, and difficulty with balance and movement. It is the second most common neurodegenerative disorder following AD. The disease is more prominent in men than women. Age is a risk factor; most cases of PD are diagnosed after the age of 60.[134,135] Approximately 3–5% of PD cases are linked to specific PD genes. These cases are known as monogenic PD. The remaining 16–36% of PD cases are explained by a collection of genetic risk variants, referred to as non-monogenic PD. PD is diagnosed based on clinical and historical data as well as neurological exam. Red flag findings may prompt an MRI scan of the brain that can identify cerebrovascular lesions (**Figure 18.14**). Findings of such lesions are associated with manifestations often observed in PD such as gait disturbances and cognitive decline.[134] PD occurs when

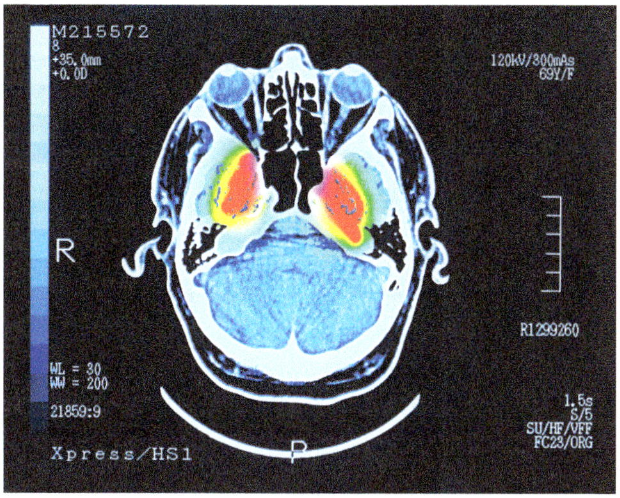

Figure 18.14 MRI of the Human Brain in Parkinson's Disease

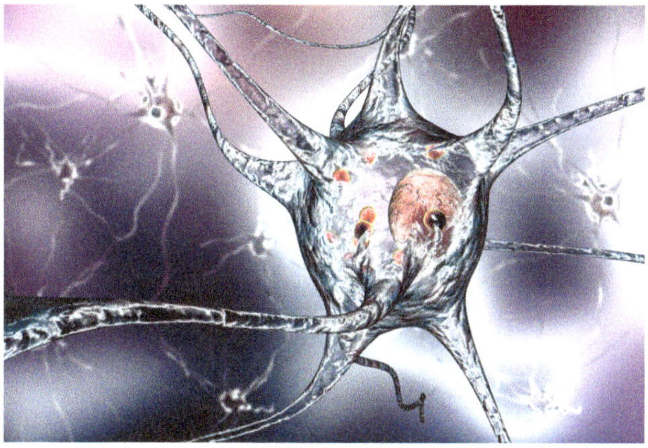

Figure 18.15 A Nerve Cell Affected by Lewy Bodies in Patients With Parkinson's Disease. Lewy Bodies Appear as Small Red Spheres Within the Neuron

the nerve cells in the basal ganglia become impaired or die. The nerve cells of many people with PD contain **Lewy bodies**, which are unusual clumps of proteins called "alpha-synuclein" that develop inside the neuron (**Figure 18.15**). Lewy body dementia can also occur in other neurological diseases. It is unclear why abnormal functioning of these proteins occur.

The neurons impacted in PD are responsible for the release of dopamine. Decreased levels of dopamine are what cause problems with movement and other symptoms of PD. **Table 18.8** shows the four main categories of symptoms in PD. Patients with PD also lose nerve endings that produce norepinephrine, which controls functions including blood pressure and heart rate. These patients may experience fatigue, irregular blood pressure, and slow movement of food down the digestive tract.[134]

Table 18.8 Main Symptoms of Parkinson's Disease

Four Main Symptoms
Tremor in hands, arms, legs, and jaw
Muscle stiffness
Slowness of movement
Loss of balance and impaired coordination
Additional Symptoms
Depression and emotional changes
Difficulty swallowing, chewing, and speaking
Constipation
Urinary problems

Data from National Institutes of Health, National Institute on Aging. *Parkinson's disease: causes, symptoms, and treatment.* Content reviewed April 14, 2022. Accessed February 23, 2025. https://www.nia.nih.gov/health/parkinsons-disease/parkinsons-disease-causes-symptoms-and-treatments

The mainstay of treatment in PD is centered around compensating for lack of dopamine. A common dopaminergic drug, levodopa, can help ease symptoms associated with PD.[134,135] Levodopa is commonly administered along with a dopamine decarboxylase inhibitor, which prevents the peripheral breakdown of levodopa and increases its bioavailability. Unfortunately, over time, desensitization to levodopa can occur, while higher doses lead to undesirable side effects such as unpredictable fluctuation in motor function, and a "wearing off" phase where periods of stiffness and rigidity occur. Interestingly, several nutritional factors can help improve levodopa absorption including protein redistribution diets (where the majority of protein is eaten later in the day), increased fiber, vitamin C, and caffeine. In addition, supplementation of vitamins D, B6, B12, and folate is recommended to reduce the metabolic side effects associated with levodopa therapy.[7,136]

PRACTICE POINT

Protein redistribution diets, fiber, vitamin C, and caffeine can improve bioavailability of dopaminergic drugs such as levodopa.

PRACTICE POINT

Supplementation of vitamins D, B6, B12, and folate can reduce metabolic side effects to levodopa therapy in patients with PD.

Alterations in the microbiome in patients with PD have been well established.[137–139] The interplay between alpha-synuclein proteins from the enteric nervous system, intestinal permeability, and inflammation, and gut microbes and their metabolic production have been linked to the development and progression of PD.[138] Longitudinal analysis of the microbiome in patients with PD demonstrate a persistent underrepresentation of short-chain fatty acids (SCFA)-producing bacteria when compared to individuals without PD. This can lead to a decrease in production of butyrate, a fatty acid that contains properties that supports gut barrier function and regulates inflammatory pathways.[139] Consuming a high-fiber, low-added-sugar diet improves the levels of butyrate-producing favorable bacteria in individuals with PD.[140,141]

This described **dysbiosis** is a major factor in the proinflammatory processes that occur in many neurodegenerative disease states such as PD, where oxidative brain damage and neuroinflammation are involved in the pathogenesis of disease.[142] Gathering evidence suggests that GI symptoms, due to alterations in the microbiome, occur well before changes in the brain occur in individuals with PD. These prodromal symptoms in patients with PD can lead to earlier diagnosis and improved therapy for patients with PD.[143] Use of both prebiotics in the form of fiber and probiotics have been shown to effectively decrease symptoms of PD.[139,144,145] Supplementation of antioxidant nutrients such as vitamins A and E, along with polyunsaturated fatty acids that include a combination of EPA, DHA, and linoleic fatty acids, have also been shown to improve symptoms of PD. The mechanism by which this occurs is, again, postulated to be due to alterations in the microbiome.[146] Likewise, studies incorporating the Mediterranean and MIND diets attribute their beneficial impact on PD symptoms to be mediated through improvement within the microbiome.[146–149] **Figure 18.16** demonstrates the role of microbiota in progression of PD.

CORE CONCEPT 11

Parkinson's disease is characterized by dysbiosis and disruption of the blood–brain barrier, which can lead to neuroinflammation.

PRACTICE POINT

Healthy eating patterns such as the Mediterranean and MIND diets and antioxidant nutrients can improve microbiota and symptoms in patients with Parkinson's disease.

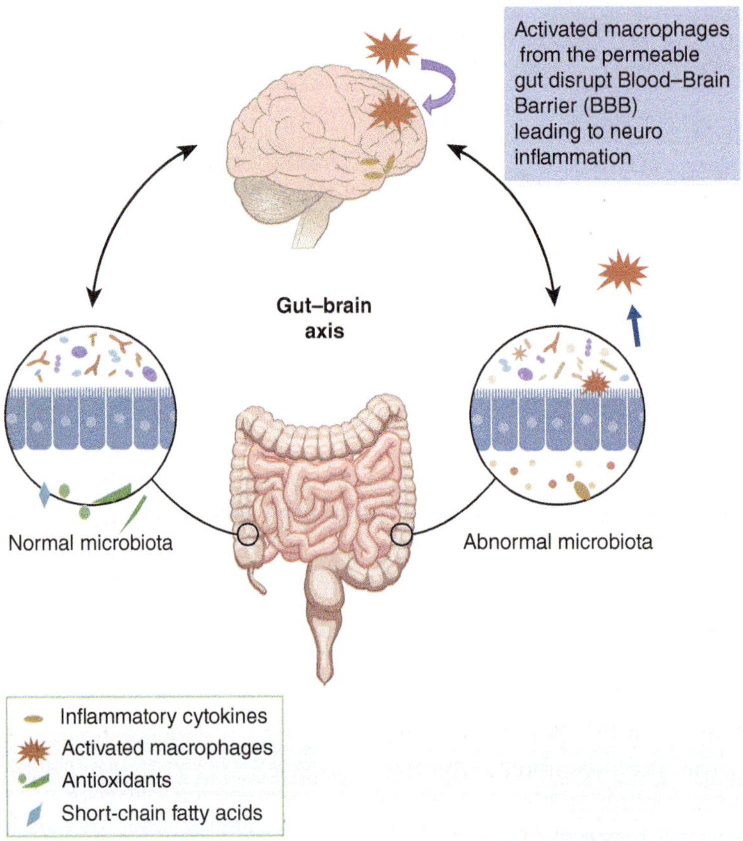

Figure 18.16 The Gut–Brain Axis and the Influence of Abnormal Microbiota in the Development of Neuroinflammation

Amyotrophic Lateral Sclerosis

Amyotrophic lateral sclerosis (ALS) is a neurodegenerative disorder effecting motor neurons within the brain and spinal cord that control voluntary movement and breathing. As these neurons worsen and die, they can no longer send messages to the muscle. ALS has two common presentations. The spinal form of the disease effects approximately 70% of patients. This form is associated with motor neurons effecting the muscles within the limbs and trunk. As the motor neurons become damaged, muscles begin to weaken, twitch, and atrophy. The remaining patients present with the bulbar form, which refers to motor neuron impairment within the corticobulbar region of the brainstem.[150] **Bulbar neurons** are responsible for speech and swallow. This form of ALS is the most devastating form. Moreover, nearly 85% of patients with the spinal form of ALS will have bulbar changes with disease progression.[150] Patients with ALS ultimately lose the ability to walk, talk, eat, and perform the basic activities of daily living. Later symptoms include paralysis and inability to breathe on their own, and eventual death. Mean survival is 3–5 years; patients with older age and bulbar onset ALS have the shortest life expectancy.[7]

The etiology of ALS is multifactorial. Like other neurological diseases, increased oxidative stress, glutamate toxicity, mitochondrial dysfunction, and apoptosis (cell death) play a role in the progression of disease. Diet quality, which includes antioxidant nutrients and limits on proinflammatory foods, as well as glutamate, can lower the risk of developing ALS.[151,152] Studies have also found vitamins D and E to be protective against ALS.[153] Similar to other neurodegenerative disease states, ALS is associated with malnutrition, changes in cognition, anorexia, and significant dysphagia.[7]

Nutritional concerns unique to patients with ALS include impaired energy and substrate metabolism. Patients with ALS, particularly those who are spontaneously breathing (versus ventilated) are hypermetabolic. This hypermetabolic state, combined with poor intake, can quickly result in muscle wasting and worsening atrophy.[154–156] Losses in fat mass occur as well.[156] Rapid decline in body composition leads to decreased survival time in this population.[157] Glucose homeostasis is also impaired in ALS, with evidence showing there is diminished glucose uptake in the frontal lobe and cortex.[152] Disorders in lipid metabolism, which include hypercholesterolemia, increased LDL cholesterol, and hypertriglyceridemia, are common. The CNS relies on a certain amount and variety of lipids to assure membrane fluidity and transmission of electrical impulses. It is theorized that dyslipidemia disturbs mitochondrial function, contributing to the pathogenesis of ALS. What is interesting, however, is that patients with higher versus lower LDL/HDL ratios had improved survival. Furthermore, patients having dyslipidemia had longer survival rates than those with normal lipid metabolism. The understanding of this finding and mechanisms of survival are unclear.[152]

Increased levels of **adipokines** are also found in ALS.[158] Adipokines are cell-signaling proteins that are released by adipose tissue. They can impact many organ systems and play an important role in regulating metabolism, cardiac function, and immunity (**Figure 18.17**). By stimulating the production of immune cells, adipokines can modulate the inflammatory response, leading to both pro- and anti-inflammatory functions. Adipokines can cross the BBB, enabling them to modulate mood, cognition, and stress response through various neurotransmitters including serotonin, dopamine, norepinephrine, and glutamate.[159] Serum levels of adipokines correlate with disease severity in ALS and may help explain neuroinflammation and pathophysiology observed in the population. Evidence to control glucose and lipid metabolism is yet to be confirmed, with no recommendations at this time.[152,158]

CORE CONCEPT 12

Individuals with amyotrophic lateral sclerosis have increased energy expenditure resulting in negative energy balance, weight loss, and malnutrition.

Multiple Sclerosis

Multiple sclerosis (MS) is an autoimmune-mediated neurodegenerative disease. In MS, immune cells attack **myelin** within the central nervous system. Myelin is a combination of proteins and fatty acids that cover and protect the nerve fibers. As this myelin sheath becomes compromised, damage occurs to the nerve fibers. Eventually the outermost layer of the brain (the cerebral cortex) shrinks, also known as "cortical atrophy."[160] MS can be viewed as a two-stage disease, with early inflammation resulting in remitting–elapsing disease, and delayed neurodegeneration being responsible for non-relapsing progression.[161]

The etiology behind MS is not entirely clear. A number of genes can increase susceptibility, most notably the histocompatibility complex (HLA-DRB1 locus). Several

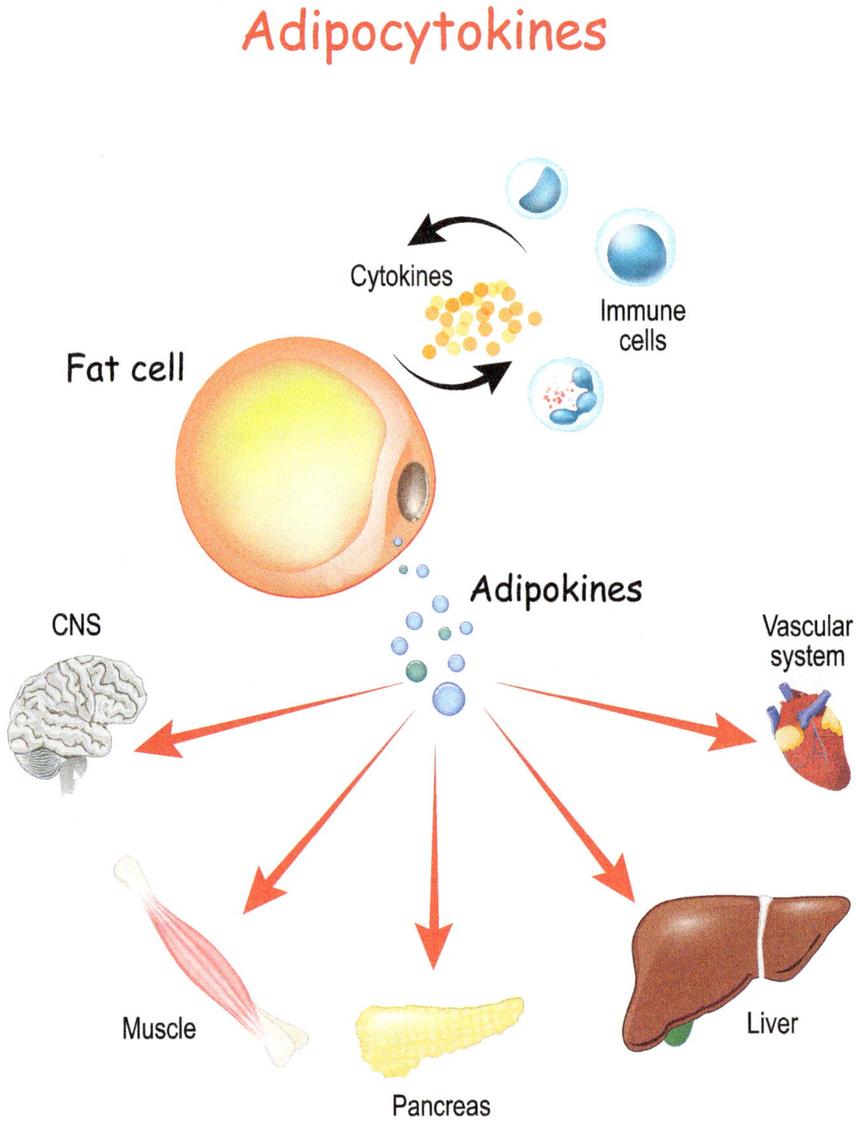

Figure 18.17 Adipokines Modulate Many Processes Impacting Organs Throughout the Body

environmental factors have been associated with the onset of MS including Epstein–Barr virus, infection, ambient UV radiation, and tobacco smoking. Individuals living farther away from the equator are at higher risk of getting MS. Hence, sunshine and vitamin D seem to be protective and reduce the risk of MS. MS generally impacts young adults (mean age at onset 20–30 years). Women are more likely to get MS than men.[160–162]

MS is generally diagnosed according to clinical findings, imaging, and laboratory data, using the current diagnostic criteria known as the "revised McDonald criteria." The revised criteria have improved MS diagnosis particularly by providing clarity on how to interpret the dissemination of white lesions within the brain.[162,163] Classic presentation often begins with blurry vision and pain with eye movement due to optic neuritis (inflammation of the optic nerve), followed by muscle weakness, tingling, numbness or pain in the arms, and difficulty with balance.[160,162] Other symptoms can occur including mood and cognitive changes and mental and physical fatigue.[160]

Like other neurodegenerative diseases, much of the research related to nutrition and diet in MS centers on reducing inflammation.[164–166] During MS, inflammatory cytokines and ROS damage myelin and axons. Furthermore, the clinical course of MS has been associated with markers of oxidative stress including several types of interleukins and tumor necrosis factors.[167] The Mediterranean diet is one of the main eating patterns that has been investigated in patients with MS, along with nutrient factors such as vitamin E and polyunsaturated fatty acids.[64,165] Conversely, the Western diet that includes higher intakes of saturated fats, red meat, and sugar may activate proinflammatory immune activities, negatively impacting the progression of MS.[164] Vitamin D is one nutrient of interest due to its ability to counteract neurodegeneration and oxidative stress in patients with MS.[168] Sunlight and adequate dietary vitamin D intake is recommended, with supplementation as indicated.[7] Fatigue is a debilitating aspect of MS, and several studies have looked at the impact of diet and lifestyle on fatigue and quality of life in persons with MS.[169–171] In this regard, the Mediterranean diet and physical activity have demonstrated a trend toward reduced fatigue in patients with MS.[169]

PRACTICE POINT

Dietary supplementation of vitamin D is recommended in patients with MS who have insufficient intake and/or lack of sunlight.

Nutritional Assessment in Neurodegenerative Diseases: PD, ALS, MS

There are numerous similarities as well as differences in the etiology and clinical manifestations of PD, ALS, and MS. As presented in **Table 18.9**, each of these disease states has marked differences in pathophysiology and disease progression.[172–178] Despite their differences, all three ultimately lead to common, well-known, nutrition risk factors including dysphagia, impaired movement, and altered cognition. Currently, there is no cure for any of these disorders, making symptom management and delay in progression a primary focus of research. Nutrition assessment should include routine anthropometric assessment and screening for early weight loss, as this can occur before other symptoms are occur. Diet history should be conducted with a focus on identifying

Table 18.9 Comparison of Clinical Manifestations and Disease Progression in Amyotrophic Lateral Sclerosis, Parkinson's Disease, and Multiple Sclerosis

Feature	Amyotrophic Lateral Sclerosis	Parkinson's Disease	Multiple Sclerosis
Cause	Motor neuron degeneration	Dopamine-producing neuron loss	Autoimmune attack on myelin sheath
Primary effect	Muscle atrophy, paralysis	Tremors, muscle rigidity, disruption of blood–brain barrier	Muscle weakness, vision problems, numbness
Symptoms	Muscle weakness, twitching, speech and swallowing difficulties, respiratory failure	Uncontrollable movement, tremors, stiffness, balance issues	Vision problems, muscle weakness, fatigue, numbness
Progression	Rapid (death usually within 2–5 years)	Slow, but progressive over decades	▪ Relapsing-remitting or progressive ▪ Can vary greatly between individuals
Cognitive impact	Usually limited, but some may experience frontotemporal dementia	Mild cognitive decline in later stages	Cognitive impairment can occur, but not always severe
Treatment	▪ No cure ▪ Medications may slow progression	▪ No cure ▪ Levodopa to ease symptoms	▪ No cure ▪ Disease-modifying therapies (DMTs) help slow progression
Life expectancy	Shortened (2–5 years post-diagnosis)	Can be near normal with treatment	▪ Variable ▪ Near normal with treatment

Data from Brown RH, Al-Chalabi A. Amyotrophic lateral sclerosis. *N Engl J Med*. 2017;377(2):162-172. doi:10.1056/NEJMra1603471; Kalia LV, Lang AE. Parkinson's disease. *Lancet*. 2015;386(9996):896-912. doi:10.1016/S0140-6736(14)61393-3; Dobson R, Giovannoni G. Multiple sclerosis: a review. *Eur J Neurol*. 2019;26(1):27-40. doi:10.1111/ene.13819; Turner MR, Swash M. The expanding syndrome of amyotrophic lateral sclerosis: a clinical and molecular perspective. *J Neurol Neurosurg Psychiatry*. 2015;86(6):667-673. doi:10.1136/jnnp-2014-308946; Poewe W, Seppi K, Tanner CM, et al. Parkinson disease. *Nat Rev Dis Primers*. 2017;3:17013. doi:10.1038/nrdp.2017.13; Thompson AJ, Baranzini SE, Geurts J, Hemmer B, Ciccarelli O. Multiple sclerosis. *Lancet*. 2018;391(10130):1622-1636. doi:10.1016/S0140-6736(18)30481-1; Ó Breasail M, Smith MD, Tenison E, Henderson EJ, Lithander FE. Parkinson's disease: the nutrition perspective. *Proc Nutr Soc*. 2022;81(1):12-26.

the impact of CNS symptoms on nutritional status. These may include changes in mood and mental status, cognition, fatigue, and difficulties chewing and swallowing. The impact of tremor and paralysis on self-feeding capabilities such as that observed with ALS and patients with PD should also be identified so that the appropriate supports can be put into place (**Figures 18.18** and **18.19**). Biochemical assessment of vitamin D status, electrolyte abnormalities, and hydration may be routinely needed. Nutrient–drug reactions such as that observed in PD with levodopa should be screened for. Constipation related to medications, muscle weakness, and decreased physical activity in all these conditions must also be assessed.

CORE CONCEPT 13

Common symptoms of neurodegenerative disease such as mood changes, altered cognition, dysphagia, impaired vision, inability to self-feed, and fatigue are nutritional risk factors.

Nutrition Interventions Neurodegenerative Diseases: PD, ALS, MS

Table 18.10 displays common nutritional problems and recommended nutrition interventions.[179–184] Given the risk of malnutrition in these disease states, the need for a high-calorie, high-protein diet should be considered. This is particularly true for patients with ALS. Modified textures should also be provided as needed based on dysphagia in these patients. As described in previous sections, most of the nutrition-related research in neurodegenerative disease centers around reducing oxidative stress and neuroinflammation. This can be accomplished by including a combination of diet patterns and specific nutrients including antioxidant nutrients such as omega-3 fatty acids, vitamins A and E, and nutrients that support immune function such as vitamin D. While there is still not enough evidence to make specific recommendations, the typical Mediterranean diet represents a general healthy eating plan that is relatively easy to follow and may improve scores on mental health, quality of life, anxiety, depression, and fatigue.[185] Adherence to this type of healthy eating pattern that emphasizes lean proteins, fish, fruits and vegetables, and whole grains in place of red meat, saturated fats, and processed foods will improve the general health of most patients. Use of the MIND diet initially prescribed for patients with dementia are also recommended for most neurodegenerative disease where cognition is at risk of impairment.[186] **Table 18.11** shows general eating patterns and nutrients that may prevent cognitive decline in neurodegenerative disease.

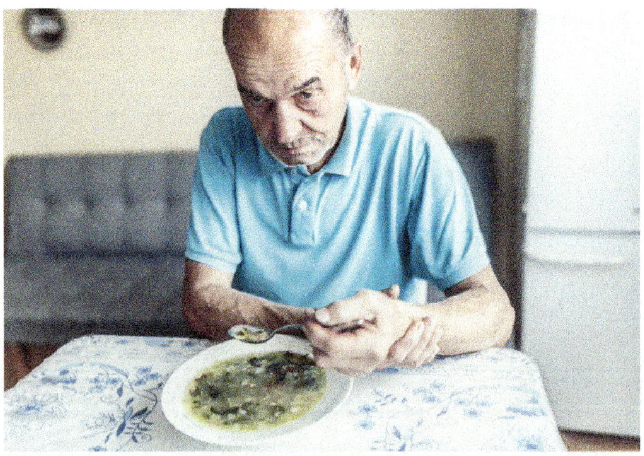

Figure 18.18 Image of a Man With Parkinson's Disease Holding His Hand Steady While Eating Soup

CORE CONCEPT 14

Dietary patterns that are anti-inflammatory may help slow the progression and improve symptoms of neurodegenerative diseases, which are characterized by oxidative stress and neuroinflammation.

The **ketogenic diet (KD)** is a high-fat, low-carbohydrate, low-protein diet which, due to its macronutrient distribution, induces a metabolic state that mimics starvation. Its origins date back to ancient times, where starvation was used to treat epilepsy. In the early 1920s, the KD was implemented as a way

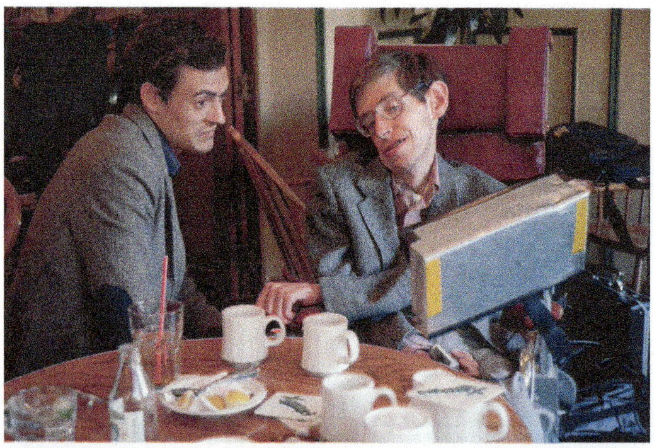

Figure 18.19 Famous Physicist Stephen Hawking Was Diagnosed with Early-Onset ALS. He Gradually Became Paralyzed and Lost His Speech, Using a Computerized Voice Synthesizer to Communicate

Table 18.10 **Comparison of Nutrition Interventions for Individuals with Amyotrophic Lateral Sclerosis, Parkinson's Disease, and Multiple Sclerosis**

Feature	Amyotrophic Lateral Sclerosis	Parkinson's Disease	Multiple Sclerosis
Key nutrition goals	Prevent weight loss, maintain muscle function, support swallowing ability	Reduce inflammation, manage dysbiosis	Reduce inflammation, support immune function, maintain energy levels
Challenges	Dysphagia, muscle wasting, high metabolic rate, altered glucose and lipid metabolism	Constipation, medication interactions, dysphagia, difficulty eating due to tremors	Fatigue, inflammation
Recommended diets	High-calorie, high-protein, modified texture (soft or pureed)	Mediterranean, MIND, high fiber	Mediterranean
Key nutrients	**Antioxidant nutrients** (vitamins A, E, polyunsaturated fatty acids) **Vitamin D** (immune modulation)	**Antioxidant nutrients** (vitamins A, E, polyunsaturated fatty acids) **B6, B12, folate** (improve levodopa side effects) **Probiotics, fiber** (gut health, constipation)	**Antioxidant nutrients** (vitamins A, E, polyunsaturated fatty acid) **Vitamin D** (immune modulation) **B vitamins** (nerve health)
Foods to emphasize	Soft, easy-to-swallow, high-calorie foods (smoothies, nut butters, avocados)	Leafy greens, berries, nuts, whole grains, fatty fish	Colorful vegetables, whole grains, healthy fats (olive oil, nuts, seeds)
Foods to avoid	Hard-to-swallow foods, processed/low-nutrient foods	Processed foods, excess sugar, fried foods (which may worsen inflammation)	Ultra-processed foods, high-sugar foods, dairy (for some individuals)

Data from Wills AM, Hubbard J, Macklin EA, et al. Hypercaloric enteral nutrition in patients with amyotrophic lateral sclerosis: A randomised, double-blind, placebo-controlled phase 2 trial. *Lancet.* 2014;383(9934):2065-2072. doi:10.1016/S0140-6736(14)60222-1.; Mischley LK, Lau RC, Bennett RD. Role of diet and nutritional supplements in Parkinson's disease progression. *Oxid Med Cell Longev.* 2017;2017:6405278. doi:10.1155/2017/6405278.; Zeng C, Yang Y, Feng Y, et al. Diet and nutrition for Parkinson's disease: A review of the literature. *Front Aging Neurosci.* 2022;14:852668. doi:10.3389/fnagi.2022.852668.; Tamtaji OR, Taghizadeh M, Daneshvar Kakhaki R, et al. The effects of omega-3 fatty acids and vitamin E co-supplementation on clinical and metabolic status in patients with Parkinson's disease: A randomized, double-blind, placebo-controlled trial. Neurochem Int. 2019;131:104539. doi:10.1016/j.neuint.2019.104539.; Riccio P, Rossano R. Nutrition facts in multiple sclerosis. ASN Neuro. 2015;7(1):1-20. doi:10.1177/1759091414568185.; Hedstrom AK, Olsson T, Alfredsson L. The role of diet in multiple sclerosis: A review of the literature. *Autoimmun Rev.* 2022;21(2):102927. doi:10.1016/j.autrev.2022.102927.

Table 18.11 **Dietary Eating Patterns May Be Helpful in Managing Cognitive Decline in Neurodegenerative Disease**

Diet Intervention	Description
Healthy eating patterns	▪ Diets include the Mediterranean, DASH, and MIND that emphasize high intakes of fruits, vegetables, nuts, cereal, and fish ▪ Low intakes of meat and dairy products, moderate consumption of alcohol
Low intake of saturated fats and increased intake of mono and polyunsaturated fats	▪ Increased intake of omega-3 fatty acids through fish, seeds, nuts, beans, and green leafy vegetables ▪ Decreased intake of saturated fats common in processed meat, milk, yogurt, cheese, butter
Increased consumption of fruits and vegetables	Increased consumption of fruits and vegetables provides intake of vitamins and minerals, dietary fiber, and nonnutritive substances such as plant sterols, flavonoids, and antioxidants
Increased Vitamin D Intake	▪ Sunlight exposure ▪ Increased consumption of fish and fish products, eggs, fat/oils, bread, and bakery products
Modified Mediterranean-ketogenic diet	Diet includes 60–65% fat, 30% protein, and 15–30% carbohydrate, with emphasis on healthy fats, lean meats and fish, and extra-virgin olive oil.

Data from Ellouze I, Sheffler J, Nagpal R, Arjmandi B. Dietary patterns and Alzheimer's disease: an updated review linking nutrition to neuroscience. *Nutrients.* 2023;15(14):3204. doi:10.3390/nu15143204 of treating epilepsy in children without the need for severe caloric restriction. Even after discovery of anticonvulsant medications, KD remained successful in reducing seizures for refractory epilepsy, eliminating it entirely in some children after 1 year of therapeutic intervention.[187]

Ketosis occurs when there is a shift in the proportion of macronutrients to a high-fat, low-carbohydrate distribution, thereby inducing a glucose-sparing effect. Excessive production of acetyl CoA that cannot be used by the Krebs cycle converts to acetoacetate (AcAC) and other ketone bodies, namely 3-beta hydroxy-butyrate (3HB) and acetone. These ketone bodies can cross the BBB and serve as an important energy source for the brain (**Figure 18.20**). Many types of brain cells including neurons, astrocytes, and oligodendrocytes can take up ketone bodies directly as an energy source.[187,188]

In more recent years, the KD has been researched for its efficacy in treating neurological conditions such as AD, PD, MS, spinal cord injury, and stroke. In addition to being an energy source, ketone bodies have neuroprotective qualities and can have direct effect on inflammatory proteins, transcription factors, and ROS.[189] In vitro studies have shown that KDs enhance free radical scavenging, reduce levels of inflammatory cytokines, and reduce cell death. Hence, they can be effective in alleviating symptoms often experienced in neurologic disease.[187] For example, adherence to a KD may decrease fatigue and depression as well as reduce inflammatory adipokines in patients with MS.[190] In animal studies, the KD improved behavioral and motor function abnormalities by suppressing oxidative pathways that lead to demyelination, demonstrating a potential mechanism to their efficacy in MS.[191] KD has also been investigated among patients with AD. Studies have shown that ketone bodies can protect against amyloid-beta plaque formation by modulating proteins that promote their formation.[188] Clinically, studies have shown that KD can improve cognitive function in mild AD.[192] The KD may be effective in protecting against cell death and improving motor function in patients with PD.[193] Some studies indicate that KD can improve the bioavailability of levodopa. A KD combined with levodopa therapy can halt PD symptoms in some cases.[194]

The main characteristic defining the KD is the ketogenic ratio that defines the ratio of fat to protein plus carbohydrate. The most common ratio is 4:1, which is 4 g of fat to 1 g of protein plus carbohydrate.[192] Numerous variations of the KD have been developed to improve palatability and other health aspects. For example, the addition of MCT oil has been used as a way of increasing ketone bodies while allowing a higher carbohydrate intake and potentially minimizing GI intolerance such as vomiting, diarrhea, and abdominal pain.[195] The MCT-KD is effective in improving cognition

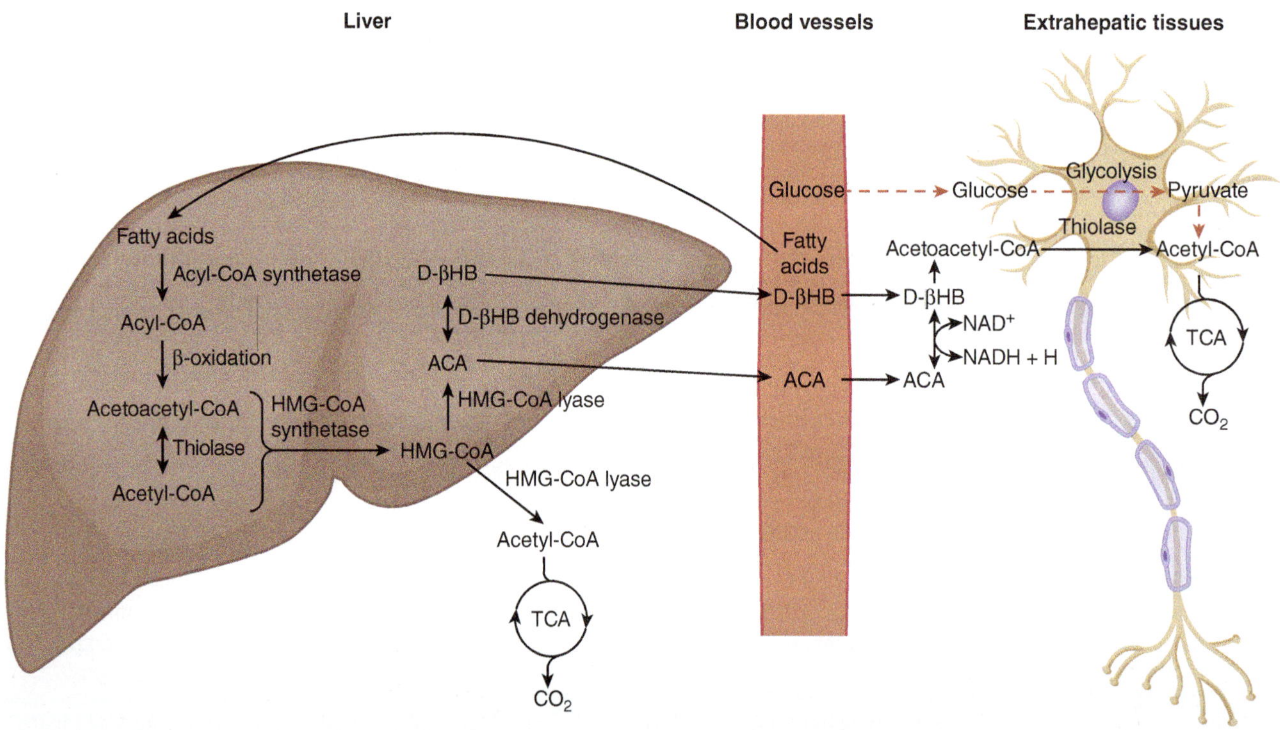

Figure 18.20 Ketogenesis: Fatty acids undergo the process of β-oxidation in the liver, resulting in the formation of ketone bodies. These are then transported to the blood vessels and then to the neurons where, after conversion to acetyl-CoA, they enter the TCA cycle

in AD.[196] Interestingly, use of MCT without inducing deep ketosis has also been shown to improve cognitive function in AD.[197] Some components of MCT oils can cross the BBB and are processed slightly differently than ketone bodies. Caprylic acid ester, a major component of MCT, is utilized by astrocytes, and may be useful in effecting memory and learning processes.[198]

Monitoring and Evaluation

Monitoring and evaluation of nutritional status in patients with neurodegenerative disease is similar to that previously described in this chapter during rehabilitative stages of neurotrauma. A novel approach to monitoring and evaluation in patients with neurological conditions involves recent developments in monitoring technologies within the healthcare sector. Given that AD, PD, and dementia are the leading causes of disability and mortality worldwide, such technologies are being explored in these populations. One example, the Internet of Things (IoT), represents a network of interconnected physical devices equipped with sensors and software technologies allowing for monitoring patients afflicted with neurological disease (Figure 18.21).[199] IoT enables the monitoring of physical activity, dietary intake, and nutritional deficiencies. Devices can also be used to provide nutritional recommendations to patients and their caregivers. Weight can be monitored for patients living at home. Smart sensors in refrigerators and food pantries can be used to monitor food intake. Figure 18.22 illustrates how IoT can be used for monitoring of patients with neurodegenerative disease.[200]

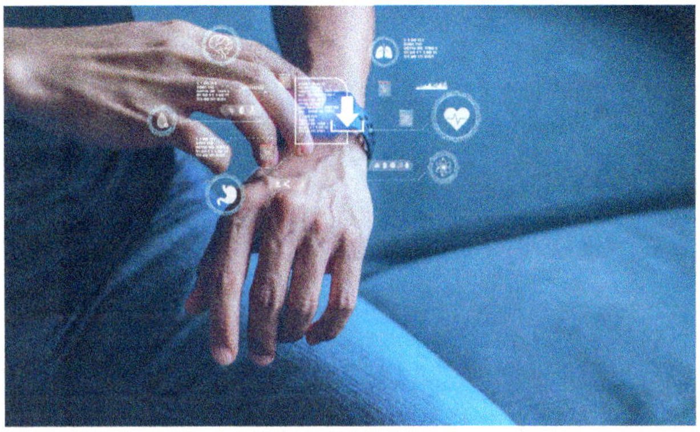

Figure 18.21 Use of IoT to Monitor Health Conditions

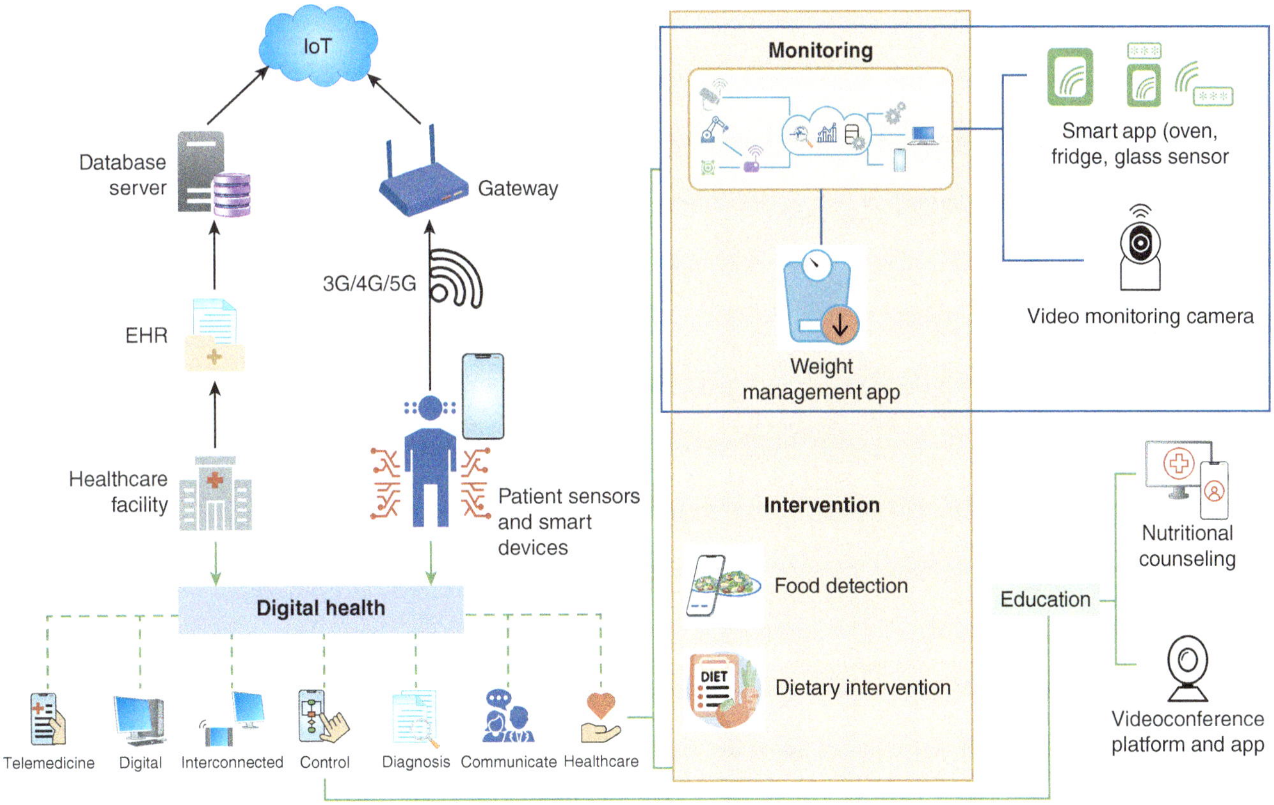

Figure 18.22 Use of IoT for Nutrition Monitoring

Chapter Summary

Neurological disease encompasses a broad spectrum of conditions involving both acute and chronic disease states. Their pathophysiology involves significant oxidative injury and neuronal damage leading to severe impairment, which may or may not be reversed. Neurotraumatic injury includes stroke and traumatic brain injury, often representing an acute condition. Medical nutrition therapy in the initial stages may be quite similar to that in critical care. Nutrition support strategies including parenteral and enteral nutrition therapy may be needed. As patients progress into their rehabilitative phase of care, nutrition interventions depend on the patient's cognitive and physical ability to eat and receive nutrition. Dysphagia is commonly observed in this phase of recovery, necessitating texture-modified diets. Neurodegenerative diseases include (but are not limited to) dementia and Alzheimer's disease, Parkinson's disease, amyotrophic lateral sclerosis, and multiple sclerosis. While these conditions have distinct etiologies, clinical manifestations can be similar and include dysphagia, difficulty eating, and in the case of ALS, hypermetabolism. The role of anti-inflammatory diets including the Mediterranean diet, the MIND diet, and specific antioxidant nutrients such as omega-3 fatty acids and vitamins A, E, and D may play a role in slowing the progression of these disease states. Similarly, ketogenic diets producing ketone bodies that can cross the blood–brain barrier and modulate energy and inflammatory pathways can also have a therapeutic role.

Key Terms

central nervous system, neuron, neurotraumatic injury, neurodegenerative disease ischemic stroke, hemorrhagic stroke, dysphagia, International Dysphagia Diet Standardization Initiative (IDDSI), neuroinflammation, aspiration pneumonia, Glasgow Coma Scale (GCS), secondary brain insult, blood–brain barrier (BBB), glutamate, gut–brain axis, oropharyngeal dysphagia, aspiration, oral propulsive phase, pharyngeal phase, wet voice, videofluorographic swallowing study (VFSS), fiberoptic endoscopic evaluation, texture-modified diets (TMDs), dementia, tau proteins, amyloid-β (Aβ) peptides, Lewy bodies, dysbiosis, bulbar neurons, adipokines, myelin, ketogenic diet

References

1. Eunice Kennedy Shriver National Institute of Child Health and Human Development. What are the parts of the nervous system? Last Reviewed October 10, 2018. Accessed March 6, 2025. https://www.nichd.nih.gov/health/topics/neuro/conditioninfo/parts
2. Kunz A, Dirnagl U, Mergenthaler P. Acute pathophysiological processes after ischaemic and traumatic brain injury. *Best Pract Res Clin Anaesthesiol*. 2010;24(4):495–509.
3. Cadilhac DA, Mahal A. Costs of neurological disorders. *Neuroepidemiol*. 2024;58(6):409–411. doi:10.1159/000539370
4. Stevens AR, Belli A, Ahmed Z. Neurotrauma-from injury to repair: clinical perspectives, cellular mechanisms and promoting regeneration of the injured brain and spinal cord. *Biomedicines*. 2024;12(3):643. doi:10.3390/biomedicines12030643
5. GBD 2021 Nervous System Disorders Collaborators. Global, regional, and national burden of disorders affecting the nervous system, 1990–2021: a systematic analysis for the Global Burden of Disease Study. *Lancet Neurol*. 2021;23(4):344–381.
6. International Dysphagia Diet Standardization Initiative. Framework: the IDDSI framework (the Standard). Accessed January 26, 2025. https://www.iddsi.org/standards/framework
7. Burgos R, Bretón I, Cereda E, et al. ESPEN guideline clinical nutrition in neurology. *Clin Nutr*. 2018;37(1):354–396. doi:10.1016/j.clnu.2017.09.003
8. Virani SS, Alonso A, Aparicio HJ, et al; American Heart Association Council on Epidemiology and Prevention Statistics Committee and Stroke Statistics Subcommittee. Heart disease and stroke statistics 2021 update: a report from the American Heart Association. *Circulation*. 2021;143:e254–e743.
9. Bathla G, Ajmera P, Mehta PM, et al. Advances in acute ischemic stroke treatment: current status and future directions. *AJNR Am J Neuroradiol*. 2023;44(7):750–758. doi:10.3174/ajnr.A7872
10. Centers for Disease Control and Prevention. Stroke: stroke facts. Updated October 24, 2024. Accessed January 27, 2025. https://www.cdc.gov/stroke/data-research/facts-stats/index.html
11. GBD 2019 Stroke Collaborators. Global, regional, and national burden of stroke and its risk factors, 1990–2019: a systematic analysis for the Global Burden of Disease Study 2019. *Lancet Neurol*. 2021;20(10):795–820. doi:10.1016/S1474-4422(21)00252-0
12. Bevers MB, Taylor Kimberly W. Critical care management of acute ischemic stroke. *Curr Treat Options Cardiovasc Med*. 2017;19:41.
13. Papanagiotau P, Ntaios G. Endovascular thrombectomy in acute ischemic stroke. *Circ Cardiovasc Interv*. 2018;11(1):e005362.
14. Huppertz V, Guida S, Holdoway A, et al. Impaired nutritional condition after stroke from the hyperacute to the chronic phase: a systematic review and meta-analysis. *Front Neurol*. 2022;12:780080. doi:10.3389/fneur.2021.780080
15. Gomes F, Emery PW, Weekes CE. Risk of malnutrition is an independent predictor of mortality, length of hospital stay, and hospitalization costs in stroke patients. *J Stroke Cerebrovasc Dis*. 2016;25(4):799–806.

16. Shen D, Cai X, Zhu Q, et al. Increased stress hyperglycemia ratio at hospital admission in stroke patients are associated with increased in-hospital mortality and length of stay. *Diabetol Metabol Syndrome*. 2024;16(1):69.
17. Kasuya H, Kawashima A, Namiki K, Shimizu T, Takakura K. Metabolic profiles of patients with subarachnoid hemorrhage treated by early surgery. *J Neurosurg*. 1998;42(6):1268–1275. doi:10.1097/00006123-199806000-00038
18. González-Fernández M, Ottenstein L, Atanelov L, Christian AB. Dysphagia after stroke: an overview. *Curr Phys Med Rehabil Rep*. 2013;1(3):187–196. doi:10.1007/s40141-013-0017-y
19. Lieber AC, Hong E, Putrino D, Nistal DA, Pan JS, Kellner CP. Nutrition, energy expenditure, dysphagia, and self-efficacy in stroke rehabilitation: a review of the literature. *Brain Sci*. 2018;8(12):218. doi:10.3390/brainsci8120218
20. Smetana KS, Hannawi Y, May CC. Indirect calorimetry measurements compared with guideline weight-based energy calculations in critically ill stroke patients. *JPEN J Parenter Enteral Nutr*. 2021;45(7):1484–1490.
21. Massimo P. Nutritional dietary recommendations for acute ischemic stroke and their outcomes. *J Nutr Disord Ther*. 2023;13:247.
22. Dube SK, Roy H, Jena BR, Rath GP, Mishra N, Prasad K. Comparison of indirect calorimetry versus standard weight-based formula in ischemic stroke patients. *J Neuroanaesthesiol Crit Care*. 2024;11(02):107–113.
23. Serra MC, Hafer-Macko CE, Ryan AS. Reduced resting metabolic rate in adults with hemiparetic chronic stroke. *J Neurol Neurophysiol*. 2015;6(6):1000341. doi:10.4172/2155-9562.1000341
24. Kramer S, Johnson L, Bernhardt J, Cumming T. Energy expenditure and cost during walking after stroke: a systematic review. *Arch Phys Med Rehab*. 2016;97(4):619–632.
25. Serra MC, Treuth MS, Hafer-Macko CE, Ryan AS. Increased energy cost of mobility in chronic stroke. *J Gerontol Geriatr Res*. 2016;5:356. doi:10.4172/2167-7182.1000356.
26. Sato Y, Yoshimura Y, Abe T. Nutrition in the first week after stroke is associated with discharge to home. *Nutrients*. 2021;13(3):943. doi:10.3390/nu13030943
27. Mizuma A, Netsu S, Sakamoto M, Yutani S, Nagata E, Takizawa S. Effect of early enteral nutrition on critical care outcomes in patients with acute ischemic stroke. *J Int Med Res*. 2021;49(11):3000605211055829.
28. Wang J, Yu K, Zeng Y. Early enteral nutrition intervention promotes multiple functional recovery in patients with traumatic intracerebral hemorrhage: a prospective randomized controlled study. *Clin Neurol Neurosurg*. 2023;234:108010.
29. Shabaan G, Abdelwarith M, Diab M. Enteral feeding protocol to improvement functional outcome in stroke patient. *Egyptian J Health Care*. 2021;12(1):735–745.
30. Zheng T, Zhu X, Liang H, Huang H, Yang J, Wang S. Impact of early enteral nutrition on short term prognosis after acute stroke. *J Clin Neurosci*. 2015;22(9):1473–1476. doi:10.1016/j.jocn.2015.03.028
31. Peng J, Volbers B, Sprügel MI, et al. Influence of early enteral nutrition on clinical outcomes in neurocritical care patients with intracerebral hemorrhage. *Front Neurol*. 2021;12:665791.
32. Suzuki K, Sugiyama R, Katano T, et al. The safety of rapid administration of enteral nutrition in acute stroke patients. *J Neurol Sci*. 2022;437:120270.
33. Suzuki K, Sato H, Mori H, et al. Early enteral nutrition with high-protein whey peptide digestive nutrients may improve prognosis in subarachnoid hemorrhage patients. *Medicina*. 2022;58(9):1264.
34. Chen X, Hu Y, Yuan X, et al. Effect of early enteral nutrition combined with probiotics in patients with stroke: a meta-analysis of randomized controlled trials. *Eur J Clin Nutr*. 2022;76:592–603. doi:10.1038/s41430-021-00986-3
35. Tian X, Xia G, Zhang M, et al. Effect of enteral nutrition on the intestinal microbiome and risk of death in ischemic stroke patients. *JPEN J Parenter Enteral Nutr*. 2022;46(8):1847–1858.
36. Wang S, Zeng X, Zhang Q, Li H. Effectiveness of different feeding techniques for post-stroke dysphagia: an updated systematic review and meta-analysis. *Intensive Care Res*. 2022;2(3):108–116.
37. Rabaut J, Thirugnanachandran T, Singhal S, et al. Clinical outcomes and patient safety of nasogastric tube in acute stroke patients. *Dysphagia*. 2022;37(6):1732–1739.
38. Ikenaga Y, Kusunoki T, Yamaguchi H. Percutaneous endoscopic gastrostomy reduces aspiration pneumonia rate in stroke patients with enteral feeding in convalescent rehabilitation wards. *Prog Rehabil Med*. 2021;6:20210031.
39. Yamasaki T, Mori N, Hayami Y, et al. Complications and risk factors of intermittent nasogastric/intermittent orogastric tube feeding in the rehabilitation ward: a retrospective study. *Clin Nutr Open Sci*. 2024;55:205–214.
40. Wu C, Zhu X, Zhou X, et al. Intermittent tube feeding for stroke patients with dysphagia: a meta-analysis and systematic review. *Ann Palliat Med*. 2021;10(7):7406–7415.
41. Joundi RA, Saposnik G, Martino R, Fang J, Porter J, Kapral MK. Outcomes among patients with direct enteral vs nasogastric tube placement after acute stroke. *Neurology*. 2018;90(7):e544–e552. doi:10.1212/WNL.0000000000004962
42. Dennis MS, Lewis SC, Warlow C; FOOD Trial Collaboration. Effect of timing and method of enteral tube feeding for dysphagic stroke patients (FOOD): a multicentre randomised controlled trial. *Lancet*. 2005;365(9461):764–772. doi:10.1016/S0140-6736(05)17983-5
43. Welbank T, Kurien M. To PEG or not to PEG that is the question. *Proc Nutr Soc*. 2021;80(1):1–8. doi:10.1017/S002966512000703X
44. Dewan MC, Rattani A, Gupta S, et al. Estimating the global incidence of traumatic brain injury. *J Neurosurg*. 2018;130(4):1080–1097. doi:10.3171/2017.10.JNS17352
45. National Institute of Neurological Disorders and Stroke. Traumatic brain injury (TBI). Updated October 15, 2024. Accessed February 9, 2025. https://www.ninds.nih.gov/health-information/disorders/traumatic-brain-injury-tbi
46. Peterson AB, Thomas KE. Incidence of nonfatal traumatic brain injury–related hospitalizations—United States, 2018. *MMWR Morb Mortal Wkly Rep*. 2021;70:1664–1668. doi:10.15585/mmwr.mm7048a3
47. Hawryluk GW, Manley GT. Classification of traumatic brain injury: past, present, and future. *Handb Clin Neurol*. 2015;127:15–21.
48. Amare AT, Tesfaye TD, Ali AS, et al. Survival status and predictors of mortality among traumatic brain injury patients in an Ethiopian hospital: a retrospective cohort study. *Afr J Emerg Med*. 2021;11(4):396–403. doi:10.1016/j.afjem.2021.06.003
49. Centers for Disease Control and Prevention. Traumatic brain injury & concussion: about moderate and severe TBI. Published May 16, 2024. Accessed February 9, 2025.

https://www.cdc.gov/traumatic-brain-injury/about/moderate-severe-tbi.html

50. Lee HY, Oh BM. Nutrition management in patients with traumatic brain injury: a narrative review. *Brain Neurorehabil.* 2022;15(1):e4. doi:10.12786/bn.2022.15.e4
51. Kurtz P, Rocha EEM. Nutrition therapy, glucose control, and brain metabolism in traumatic brain injury: a multimodal monitoring approach. *Front Neurosci.* 2020;14:190. doi:10.3389/fnins.2020.00190
52. Poblete RA, Yaceczko S, Aliakbar R, et al. Optimization of nutrition after brain injury: mechanistic and therapeutic considerations. *Biomedicines*. 2023;11(9):2551. doi:10.3390/biomedicines11092551
53. Ganesh S, Ibrahim NA. Nutrition therapy in critically ill patients with traumatic brain injury. *Hum Nutr Metab.* 2023;34:1–5. doi:10.1016/j.hnm.2023.200219
54. Tavarez T, Roehl K, Koffman L. Nutrition in the neurocritical care unit: a new frontier. *Curr Treat Options Neurol.* 2021;23(5):16. doi:10.1007/s11940-021-00670-8
55. Quintard H, Ichai C. Nutritional and metabolic supplementation for the injured brain: an update. *Curr Opin Crit Care.* 2019;25(2):126–131. doi:10.1097/MCC.0000000000000588
56. McClave SA, Taylor BE, Martindale RG, et al. Guidelines for the provision and assessment of nutrition support therapy in the adult critically ill patient: Society of Critical Care Medicine (SCCM) and American Society for Parenteral and Enteral Nutrition (A.S.P.E.N.) [Published correction appears in *JPEN J Parenter Enteral Nutr.* 2016;40(8):1200]. *JPEN J Parenter Enteral Nutr.* 2016;40(2):159–211. doi:10.1177/0148607115621863
57. Singer P, Blaser AR, Berger MM, et al. ESPEN practical and partially revised guideline: clinical nutrition in the intensive care unit. *Clin Nutr.* 2023;42(9):1671–1689. doi:10.1016/j.clnu.2023.07.011
58. Krakau K, Omne-Pontén M, Karlsson T, Borg J. Metabolism and nutrition in patients with moderate and severe traumatic brain injury: a systematic review. *Brain Inj.* 2006;20(4): 345–367. doi:10.1080/02699050500487571
59. Brooks GA, Martin NA. Cerebral metabolism following traumatic brain injury: new discoveries with implications for treatment. *Front Neurosci.* 2015;8:408. doi:10.3389/fnins.2014.00408
60. Maxwell J, Gwardschaladse C, Lombardo G, et al. The impact of measurement of respiratory quotient by indirect calorimetry on the achievement of nitrogen balance in patients with severe traumatic brain injury. *Eur J Trauma Emerg Surg.* 2017;43(6):775–782. doi:10.1007/s00068-016-0724-z
61. Chourdakis M, Kraus MM, Tzellos T, et al. Effect of early compared with delayed enteral nutrition on endocrine function in patients with traumatic brain injury: an open-labeled randomized trial. *JPEN J Parenter Enteral Nutr.* 2012; 36(1):108–116. doi:10.1177/0148607111039787
62. Perel P, Yanagawa T, Bunn F, Roberts I, Wentz R, Pierro A. Nutritional support for head-injured patients. *Cochrane Database Syst Rev.* 2006;2006(4):CD001530. doi:10.1002/14651858.CD001530.pub2
63. Institute of Medicine (US) Committee on Nutrition, Trauma, and the Brain; Erdman J, Oria M, Pillsbury L, eds. Energy and protein needs during early feeding following traumatic brain injury. In: *Nutrition and Traumatic Brain Injury: Improving Acute and Subacute Health Outcomes in Military Personnel.* National Academies Press (US); 2011.
64. Hartl R, Gerber LM, Ni Q, Ghajar J. Effect of early nutrition on deaths due to severe traumatic brain injury. *J Neurosurg.* 2008;109(1):50–56.
65. Carney N, Totten AM, O'Reilly C, et al. Guidelines for the management of severe traumatic brain injury. *Neurosurgery.* 2017;80:6–15. doi:10.1227/NEU.0000000000001432
66. Compher C, Bingham A, McCall M, et al. Guidelines for the provision of nutrition support therapy in the adult critically ill patient. *JPEN J Parenter Enteral Nutr.* 2022;46:12–41.
67. Wang X, Dong Y, Han X, Qi XQ, Huang CG, Hou LJ. Nutritional support for patients sustaining traumatic brain injury: a systematic review and meta-analysis of prospective studies. *PLoS One.* 2013;8(3):e58838. doi:10.1371/journal.pone.0058838
68. Pierre JF. Gastrointestinal immune and microbiome changes during parenteral nutrition. *Am J Physiol Gastrointest Liver Physiol.* 2017;312(3):G246–G256. doi:10.1152/ajpgi.00321.2016
69. Nwafor D, Goeckeritz J, Hasanpour Z, Davidson C, Lucke-Wold B. Nutritional support following traumatic brain injury: a comprehensive review. *Explor Res Hypothesis Med.* 2023;8(3):236–247. doi:10.14218/ERHM.2022.00086
70. Chiang YH, Chao DP, Chu SF, et al. Early enteral nutrition and clinical outcomes of severe traumatic brain injury patients in acute stage: a multi-center cohort study. *J Neurotrauma.* 2012;29(1):75–80. doi:10.1089/neu.2011.1801
71. Weaver JL. The brain-gut axis: a prime therapeutic target in traumatic brain injury. *Brain Res.* 2021;1753:147225. doi:10.1016/j.brainres.2020.147225
72. Al Balushi RM, Paratz JD, Cohen J, Banks M. Glutamine supplementation in multiple trauma of critical care. In: Rajendram R, Preedy VR, Patel VB, eds. *Diet and Nutrition in Critical Care.* Springer; 2015. doi:10.1007/978-1-4614-7836-2_141
73. Rai VRH, Phang LF, Sia SF, et al. Effects of immunonutrition on biomarkers in traumatic brain injury patients in Malaysia: a prospective randomized controlled trial. *BMC Anesthesiol.* 2017;17(1):81. doi:10.1186/s12871-017-0369-4
74. Tehse J, Taghibiglou C. The overlooked aspect of excitotoxicity: glutamate-independent excitotoxicity in traumatic brain injuries. *Eur J Neurosci.* 2019;49(9):1157–1170. doi:10.1111/ejn.14307
75. Gruenbaum BF, Merchant KS, Zlotnik A, Boyko M. Gut microbiome modulation of glutamate dynamics: implications for brain health and neurotoxicity. *Nutrients.* 2024;16(24):4405. doi:10.3390/nu16244405
76. George AK, Behera J, Homme RP, et al. Rebuilding microbiome for mitigating traumatic brain injury: importance of restructuring the gut-microbiome-brain axis. *Mol Neurobiol.* 2021;58:3614–3627. doi:10.1007/s12035-021-02357-2
77. McGeown JP, Hume PA, Theadom A, Quarrie KL, Borotkanics R. Nutritional interventions to improve neurophysiological impairments following traumatic brain injury: a systematic review. *J Neurosci Res.* 2021;99(2):573–603.
78. Poblete RA, Yaceczko S, Aliakbar R, et al. Optimization of nutrition after brain injury: mechanistic and therapeutic considerations. *Biomedicines.* 2023; 11(9):2551. doi:10.3390/biomedicines11092551
79. Tsalamandris G, Hadjivassiliou M, Zis P. The role of nutrition in neurological disorders. *Nutrients.* 2023;15(22):4713. doi:10.3390/nu15224713
80. Gallegos C, Brito-De La Fuente E, Clavé P, Costa A, Assegehegn G. Nutritional aspects of dysphagia management. *Adv Food Nutr Res.* 2017;81:271–318.

81. Adkins C, Takakura W, Spiegel BMR, et al. Prevalence and characteristics of dysphagia based on a population-based survey. *Clin Gastroenterol Hepatol*. 2020;18(9):1970–1979.e2. doi:10.1016/j.cgh.2019.10.029
82. Ortega O, Martín A, Clavé P. Diagnosis and management of oropharyngeal dysphagia among older persons, state of the art. *J Am Med Dir Assoc*. 2017;18(7):576–582. doi:10.1016/j.jamda.2017.02.015
83. Thiyagalingam S, Kulinski AE, Thorsteinsdottir B, Shindelar KL, Takahashi PY. Dysphagia in older adults. *Mayo Clin Proc*. 2021;96(2):488–497. doi:10.1016/j.mayocp.2020.08.001
84. Mirmosayyeb O, Ebrahimi N, Shekarian A, et al. Prevalence of dysphagia in patients with multiple sclerosis: a systematic review and meta-analysis. *J Clin Neurosci*. 2023;108:84–94.
85. Lee J, Madhavan A, Krajewski E, Lingenfelter S. Assessment of dysarthria and dysphagia in patients with amyotrophic lateral sclerosis: review of the current evidence. *Muscle Nerve*. 2021;64(5):520–531.
86. Kruger D. Assessing esophageal dysphagia. *JAAPA*. 2014;27(5):23–30.
87. Sasegbon A, Hamdy S. The anatomy and physiology of normal and abnormal swallowing in oropharyngeal dysphagia. *Neurogastroenterol Motil*. 2017;29:e13100. doi:10.1111/nmo.13100
88. Panara K, Ramezanpour Ahangar E, Padalia D. Physiology, swallowing. In: *StatPearls*. StatPearls Publishing; 2023.
89. Panebianco M, Marchese-Ragona R, Masiero S, Restivo D. Dysphagia in neurological diseases: a literature review. *Neurol Sci*. 2020;41:3067–3073. doi:10.1007/s10072-020-04495-2
90. Nishida T, Yamabe K, Honda S. The Influence of dysphagia on nutritional and frailty status among community-dwelling older adults. *Nutrients*. 2021;13(2):512. doi:10.3390/nu13020512
91. Taguchi K, Wakabayashi H, Fujimoto M, et al. Association between malnutrition severity and swallowing function in convalescent rehabilitation wards: a multi-center cohort study in malnourished patients with sarcopenic dysphagia. *J Nutr Health Aging*. 2022;26(5):469–476.
92. Nishioka S, Wakabayashi H. Interaction between malnutrition and physical disability in older adults: is there a malnutrition-disability cycle? *Nutr Rev*. 2023;81(2):191–205.
93. Fırat Ozer F, Akın S, Soysal T, et al. Relationship between dysphagia and sarcopenia with comprehensive geriatric evaluation. *Dysphagia*. 2021;36:140–146. doi:10.1007/s00455-020-10120-3
94. Özsürekci C, Kara M, Güngör AE, et al. Relationship between chewing ability and malnutrition, sarcopenia, and frailty in older adults. *Nutr Clin Pract*. 2022;37(6):1409–1417.
95. Leira J, Maseda A, Lorenzo-López L, et al. Dysphagia and its association with other health-related risk factors in institutionalized older people: a systematic review. *Arch Gerontol Geriatr*. 2023;110:104991.
96. Tanrıverdi M, Heybeli C, Çalım ÖF, Durna M, Özturan O, Soysal P. The relationship between oropharyngeal dysphagia and dehydration in older adults. *BMC Geriatr*. 2024;24(1):885.
97. Zhang PP, Yuan Y, Lu DZ, et al. Diagnostic accuracy of the Eating Assessment Tool-10 (EAT-10) in screening dysphagia: a systematic review and meta-analysis. *Dysphagia*. 2023;38:145–158. doi:10.1007/s00455-022-10486-6
98. Audag N, Goubau C, Toussaint M, Reychler G. Screening and evaluation tools of dysphagia in adults with neuromuscular diseases: a systematic review. *Ther Adv Chronic Dis*. 2019;10:2040622318821622. doi:10.1177/2040622318821622
99. Kwon S, Sim J, Park J, et al. Assessment of aspiration risk using the Mann assessment of swallowing ability in brain-injured patients with cognitive impairment. *Front Neurol*. 2019;10:1264. doi:10.3389/fneur.2019.01264
100. Trapl M, Enderle P, Nowotny M, et al. Dysphagia bedside screening for acute-stroke patients: the Gugging Swallowing Screen. *Stroke*. 2007;38(11):2948–2952. doi:10.1161/STROKEAHA.107.483933
101. Kiekens C, Tognonato C. Which screening tool should be used for identifying aspiration risk associated with dysphagia in acute stroke? A Cochrane review summary with commentary. *NeuroRehabilitation*. 2022;51(3):533–535.
102. Leder SB, Suiter DM, Green BG. Development and validation of the Yale Swallow Protocol. *Dysphagia*. 2011;26(2):125–132. doi:10.1007/s00455-010-9281-6
103. Ueshima J, Shimizu A, Maeda K, et al. Nutritional management in adult patients with dysphagia: position paper from Japanese working group on integrated nutrition for dysphagic people. *J Am Med Direct Assoc*. 2022;23(10):1676–1682.
104. Cichero JAY, Lam P, Steele CM, et al. Development of international terminology and definitions for texture-modified foods and thickened fluids used in dysphagia management: the IDDSI Framework. *Dysphagia*. 2017;32:293–314. doi:10.1007/s00455-016-9758-y
105. Azizan AA, Shahar S, Manaf ZA, Haron H, Rivan NFM, Razalli NH. An assessment of knowledge, attitudes and practices on pureed diet preparation (KAP DYS-PUREE) among Food Handlers in Malaysian Hospitals for Dysphagia Management. *Healthcare*. 2023;11(14):2026. doi:10.3390/healthcare11142026
106. Brooks A. Dysphagia and aspiration during a Parkinson's hospitalization: a care partner's perspective and recommendations for improving standards of care. *Front Aging Neurosci*. 2023;15:1258979. doi:10.3389/fnagi.2023.1258979
107. Giura L, Urtasun L, Belarra A, Ansorena D, Astiasarán I. Exploring tools for designing dysphagia-friendly foods: a review. *Foods*. 2021;10(6):1334. doi:10.3390/foods10061334
108. Samargia SA. Clinical nutrition: improve compliance in dysphagia patients. *Today's Dietitian*. 2016;18(4):12.
109. Liu Z, Chen X, Li H, et al. 3D printing of nutritious dysphagia diet: status and perspectives. *Trends Food Sci Technol*. 2024;147:104478.
110. Alzheimer's Association. What is dementia? Accessed February 21, 2025. https://www.alz.org/alzheimers-dementia/what-is-dementia
111. 2024 Alzheimer's disease facts and figures. *Alzheimers Dement*. 2024;20(5):3708–3821. doi:10.1002/alz.13809
112. Bekris LM, Yu CE, Bird TD, Tsuang DW. Genetics of Alzheimer disease. *J Geriatr Psychiatry Neurol*. 2010;23(4):213–227. doi:10.1177/0891988710383571
113. Blömeke L, Rehn F, Kraemer-Schulien V, et al. Aβ oligomers peak in early stages of Alzheimer's disease preceding tau pathology [published correction appears in *Alzheimers Dement (Amst)*. 2024;16(2):e12599. doi:10.1002/dad2.12599]. *Alzheimers Dement (Amst)*. 2024;16(2):e12589. doi:10.1002/dad2.12589
114. National Institute on Aging. What happens to the brain in Alzheimer's disease? Updated January 19, 2024. Accessed February 21, 2025. https://www.nia.nih.gov/health/alzheimers-causes-and-risk-factors/what-happens-brain-alzheimers-disease

115. Alzheimer's Association. 2024 Alzheimer's disease facts and figures. Accessed February 21. 2025. https://www.alz.org/getmedia/76e51bb6-c003-4d84-8019-e0779d8c4e8d/alzheimers-facts-and-figures.pdf
116. Iqbal K, Liu F, Gong CX, Grundke-Iqbal I. Tau in Alzheimer disease and related tauopathies. *Curr Alzheimer Res.* 2010;7(8):656–664. doi:10.2174/156720510793611592
117. Murphy MP, LeVine H 3rd. Alzheimer's disease and the amyloid-beta peptide. *J Alzheimers Dis.* 2010;19(1): 311–323. doi:10.3233/JAD-2010-1221
118. Yassine HN, Samieri C, Livingston G, et al. Nutrition state of science and dementia prevention: Recommendations of the nutrition for dementia prevention working group. *Lancet Healthy Longevity*. 2022;3(7):e501–e512.
119. Eatright PRO. What is the MIND diet? Academy of Nutrition and Dietetics. Published December 20, 2023. Accessed March 3, 2025. https://www.eatrightpro.org/news-center/practice-trends/what-is-the-mind-diet
120. Izquierdo Delgado E, Gutiérrez Ríos R, Andrés Calvo M, et al. Nutritional status assessment in Alzheimer disease and its influence on disease progression. *Neurologia (Engl Ed)*. 2022;37(9):735–747. doi:10.1016/j.nrleng.2019.11.006
121. Volkert D, Beck AM, Faxén-Irving G, et al. ESPEN guideline on nutrition and hydration in dementia–update 2024. *Clin Nutr*. 2024;43(6):1599–1626.
122. Perry E, Walton K, Lambert K. Prevalence of malnutrition in people with dementia in long-term care: a systematic review and meta-analysis. *Nutrients*. 2023;15(13):2927.
123. Le HT, Dang AK, Le LTT, et al. Nutritional status, dietary quality and eating disturbance issues among people with dementia in Vietnam: evidence of a cross-sectional study. *J Health Popul Nutr.* 2024:43;107.
124. Doorduijn AS, de van der Schueren MAE, van de Rest O, et al. Nutritional status is associated with clinical progression in Alzheimer's disease: the NUDAD Project. *J Am Med Dir Assoc*. 2023;24(5):638–644.e1. doi:10.1016/j.jamda.2020.10.020
125. Stockdell R, Amella EJ. The Edinburgh feeding evaluation in dementia scale: determining how much help people with dementia need at mealtime. *Am J Nurs*. 2008;108(8):46–54.
126. Vellas B, Guigoz Y, Garry PJ, et al. The Mini Nutritional Assessment (MNA) and its use in grading the nutritional state of elderly patients. *Nutrition*. 1999;15(2):116–122. doi:10.1016/s0899-9007(98)00171-3
127. Tully MW, Matrakas KL, Muir J, Musallam K. The Eating Behavior Scale: a simple method of assessing functional ability in patients with Alzheimer's disease. *J Gerontol Nurs*. 1997;23(7):9. doi:10.3928/0098-9134-19970701-08
128. Martin C. Detect nutrient deficiencies with NFPE. *Today's Dietitian*. 2018;20(3):41.
129. Chang HR, Spencer JC, Ho MH, et al. Effectiveness of interventions on feeding difficulties among people with dementia: a systematic review and meta-analysis. *Australas J Ageing*. 2023;42(2):280–292. doi:10.1111/ajag.13192
130. Tangvik RJ, Bruvik FK, Drageset J, Kyte K, Hunskår I. Effects of oral nutrition supplements in persons with dementia: a systematic review. *Geriatr Nurs*. 2021;42(1):117–123. doi:10.1016/j.gerinurse.2020.12.005
131. Hartford A, Li W, Qureshi D, et al. Use of feeding tubes among hospitalized older adults with dementia. *JAMA Netw Open*. 2025;8(2):e2460780. doi:10.1001/jamanetworkopen.2024.60780
132. Lee YF, Hsu TW, Liang CS, et al. The efficacy and safety of tube feeding in advanced dementia patients: a systemic review and meta-analysis study. *J Am Med Direct Assoc*. 2021;22(2):357–363.
133. Yuen JK, Chan FHW, Chan TC, et al. Hospital careful hand feeding program reduced feeding tube use in patients with advanced dementia. *J Nutr Health Aging*. 2023;27:432–437. doi:10.1007/s12603-023-1926-9
134. National Institutes of Health. National Institute on Aging. Parkinson's disease: causes, symptoms, and treatment. Reviewed April 14, 2022. Accessed February 23, 2025. https://www.nia.nih.gov/health/parkinsons-disease/parkinsons-disease-causes-symptoms-and-treatments
135. Bloem BR, Okun MS, Klein C. Parkinson's disease. *Lancet*. 2021;397(10291):2284–2303.
136. Boelens Keun JT, Arnoldussen IA, Vriend C, van de Rest O. Dietary approaches to improve efficacy and control side effects of levodopa therapy in Parkinson's disease: a systematic review. *Adv Nutr.* 2021;12(6):2265–2287. doi:10.1093/advances/nmab060
137. Lubomski M, Xu X, Holmes AJ, et al. The gut microbiome in Parkinson's disease: a longitudinal study of the impacts on disease progression and the use of device-assisted therapies. *Front Aging Neurosci*. 2022;14:875261. doi:10.3389/fnagi.2022.875261
138. Tan AH, Lim SY, Lang AE. The microbiome–gut–brain axis in Parkinson's disease—from basic research to the clinic. *Nat Rev Neurol*. 2022;18(8):476–495.
139. Cantu-Jungles TM, Rasmussen HE, Hamaker BR. Potential of prebiotic butyrogenic fibers in Parkinson's disease. *Front Neurol*. 2019;10:663. doi:10.3389/fneur.2019.00663
140. Kwon D, Zhang K, Paul KC, et al. Diet and the gut microbiome in patients with Parkinson's disease. *NPJ Parkinsons Dis*. 2024;10(1):89.
141. Palavra NC, Lubomski M, Flood VM, Davis RL, Sue CM. Increased added sugar consumption is common in Parkinson's disease. *Front Nutr*. 2021;8:628845.
142. Romano S, Savva GM, Bedarf JR, Charles IG, Hildebrand F, Narbad A. Meta-analysis of the Parkinson's disease gut microbiome suggests alterations linked to intestinal inflammation. *NPJ Parkinsons Dis*. 2021;7(1):27.
143. Yemula N, Dietrich C, Dostal V, Hornberger M. Parkinson's disease and the gut: symptoms, nutrition, and microbiota. *J Parkinsons Dis*. 2021;11(4):1491–1505. doi:10.3233/JPD-212707
144. Lu CS, Chang HC, Weng YH, Chen CC, Kuo YS, Tsai YC. The add-on effect of *Lactobacillus plantarum* PS128 in patients with Parkinson's disease: a pilot study. *Front Nutr.* 2021;8:650053. doi:10.3389/fnut.2021.650053
145. Van-Wehle T, Vital M. Investigating the response of the butyrate production potential to major fibers in dietary intervention studies. *NPJ Biofilms Microbiomes*. 2024;10:63. doi:10.1038/s41522-024-00533-5
146. Pantzaris M, Loukaides G, Paraskevis D, Kostaki EG, Patrikios I. Neuroaspis PLP10™, a nutritional formula rich in omega-3 and omega-6 fatty acids with antioxidant vitamins including gamma-tocopherol in early Parkinson's disease: a randomized, double-blind, placebo-controlled trial. *Clin Neurol Neurosurg*. 2021;210:106954.
147. Bianchi VE, Rizzi L, Somaa F. The role of nutrition on Parkinson's disease: a systematic review. *Nutr Neurosci*. 2023;26(7):605–628.
148. Bisaglia M. Mediterranean diet and Parkinson's disease. *Int J Mol Sci*. 2023;24(1):42. doi:10.3390/ijms24010042

149. Metcalfe-Roach A, Yu AC, Golz E, et al. MIND and Mediterranean diets associated with later onset of Parkinson's disease. *Mov Disord*. 2021;36:977–984. doi:10.1002/mds.28464
150. Shellikeri S, Karthikeyan V, Martino R, et al. The neuropathological signature of bulbar-onset ALS: a systematic review. *Neurosci Biobehav Rev*. 2017;75:378–392. doi:10.1016/j.neubiorev.2017.01.045
151. Ludolph A, Dupuis L, Kasarskis E, Steyn F, Ngo S, McDermott C. Nutritional and metabolic factors in amyotrophic lateral sclerosis. *Nat Rev Neurol*. 2023;19(9):511–524.
152. D'Amico E, Grosso G, Nieves JW, Zanghì A, Factor-Litvak P, Mitsumoto H. Metabolic abnormalities, dietary risk factors and nutritional management in amyotrophic lateral sclerosis. *Nutrients*. 2021;13(7):2273. doi:10.3390/nu13072273
153. Xia K, Wang Y, Zhang L, et al. Dietary-derived essential nutrients and amyotrophic lateral sclerosis: a two-sample Mendelian randomization study. *Nutrients*. 2022;14(5):920.
154. Li JY, Sun XH, Cai ZY, et al. Correlation of weight and body composition with disease progression rate in patients with amyotrophic lateral sclerosis. *Sci Rep*. 2022;12:13292. doi:10.1038/s41598-022-16229-9
155. Kurihara M, Bamba S, Yasuhara S, et al. Factors affecting energy metabolism and prognosis in patients with amyotrophic lateral sclerosis. *Ann Nutr Metabol*. 2021;77(4):236–243.
156. Fayemendy P, Marin B, Labrunie A, et al. Hypermetabolism is a reality in amyotrophic lateral sclerosis compared to healthy subjects. *J Neurolog Sci*. 2021;420:117257.
157. López-Gómez JJ, Ballesteros-Pomar MD, Torres-Torres B, et al. Malnutrition at diagnosis in amyotrophic lateral sclerosis and its influence on survival: using GLIM criteria. *Clin Nutr*. 2021;40(1):237–244.
158. Li JY, Cui LY, Sun XH, et al. Alterations in metabolic biomarkers and their potential role in amyotrophic lateral sclerosis. *Ann Clin Translation Neurol*. 2022;9(7):1027–1038.
159. Clemente-Suárez VJ, Redondo-Flórez L, Beltrán-Velasco AI, et al. The role of adipokines in health and disease. *Biomedicines*. 2023;11(5):1290. doi:10.3390/biomedicines11051290
160. National Institute of Neurological Disorders and Stroke. Multiple sclerosis. Last updated January 21, 2025. Accessed February 25, 2025. https://www.ninds.nih.gov/health-information/disorders/multiple-sclerosis
161. Dobson R, Giovannoni G. Multiple sclerosis—a review. *Eur J Neurol*. 2019;26:27–40. doi:10.1111/ene.13819
162. McGinley MP, Goldschmidt CH, Rae-Grant AD. Diagnosis and treatment of multiple sclerosis: a review. *JAMA*. 2021;325(8):765–779.
163. Schwenkenbecher P, Wurster U, Konen FF, et al. Impact of the McDonald criteria 2017 on early diagnosis of relapsing-remitting multiple sclerosis. *Front Neurol*. 2019;10:188. doi:10.3389/fneur.2019.00188
164. Stoiloudis P, Kesidou E, Bakirtzis C, et al. The role of diet and interventions on multiple sclerosis: a review. *Nutrients*. 2022;14(6):1150.
165. Fanara S, Aprile M, Iacono S, et al. The role of nutritional lifestyle and physical activity in multiple sclerosis pathogenesis and management: a narrative review. *Nutrients*. 2021;13(11):3774.
166. Di Majo D, Cacciabaudo F, Accardi G, et al. Ketogenic and modified Mediterranean diet as a tool to counteract neuroinflammation in multiple sclerosis: nutritional suggestions. *Nutrients*. 2022;14(12):2384.
167. Miller E, Dziedzic A, Saluk-Bijak J, Bijak M. A review of various antioxidant compounds and their potential utility as complementary therapy in multiple sclerosis. *Nutrients*. 2019;11:1528.
168. Sangha A, Quon M, Pfeffer G, Orton SM. The role of vitamin D in neuroprotection in multiple sclerosis: an update. *Nutrients*. 2023;15(13):2978.
169. Ertaş Öztürk Y, Helvaci EM, Sökülmez Kaya P, Terzi M. Is Mediterranean diet associated with multiple sclerosis related symptoms and fatigue severity? *Nutr Neurosci*. 2022;26(3):228–234. doi:10.1080/1028415X.2022.2034241
170. Aznar G, Guerrero G, Ramos C, et al. Efficacy of diet on fatigue, quality of life and disability status in multiple sclerosis patients: rapid review and meta-analysis of randomized controlled trials. *BMC Neurol*. 2022;22:388. doi:10.1186/s12883-022-02913-w
171. Bohlouli J, Namjoo I, Borzoo-Isfahani M, et al. Modified Mediterranean diet v. traditional Iranian diet: efficacy of dietary interventions on dietary inflammatory index score, fatigue severity and disability in multiple sclerosis patients. *Br J Nutr*. 2022;128(7):1274–1284. doi:10.1017/S000711452100307X
172. Brown RH, Al-Chalabi A. Amyotrophic lateral sclerosis. *N Engl J Med*. 2017;377(2):162–172. doi:10.1056/NEJMra1603471
173. Kalia LV, Lang AE. Parkinson's disease. *Lancet*. 2015;386(9996):896–912. doi:10.1016/S0140-6736(14)61393-3
174. Dobson R, Giovannoni G. Multiple sclerosis—a review. *Eur J Neurol*. 2019;26(1):27–40. doi:10.1111/ene.13819
175. Turner MR, Swash M. The expanding syndrome of amyotrophic lateral sclerosis: a clinical and molecular perspective. *J Neurol Neurosurg Psychiatry*. 2015;86(6):667–673. doi:10.1136/jnnp-2014-308946
176. Poewe W, Seppi K, Tanner CM, et al. Parkinson disease. *Nat Rev Dis Primers*. 2017;3:17013. doi:10.1038/nrdp.2017.13
177. Thompson AJ, Baranzini SE, Geurts J, Hemmer B, Ciccarelli O. Multiple sclerosis. *Lancet*. 2018;391(10130):1622–1636. doi:10.1016/S0140-6736(18)30481-1
178. Breasail MÓ, Smith MD, Tenison E, Henderson EJ, Lithander FE. Parkinson's disease: the nutrition perspective. *Proc Nutr Soc*. 2022;81(1):12–26.
179. Wills AM, Hubbard J, Macklin EA, et al. Hypercaloric enteral nutrition in patients with amyotrophic lateral sclerosis: a randomised, double-blind, placebo-controlled phase 2 trial. *Lancet*. 2014;383(9934):2065–2072. doi:10.1016/S0140-6736(14)60222-1
180. Mischley LK, Lau RC, Bennett RD. Role of diet and nutritional supplements in Parkinson's disease progression. *Oxid Med Cell Longev*. 2017;2017:6405278. doi:10.1155/2017/6405278
181. Zeng C, Yang Y, Feng Y, et al. Diet and nutrition for Parkinson's disease: a review of the literature. *Front Aging Neurosci*. 2022;14:852668. doi:10.3389/fnagi.2022.852668
182. Tamtaji OR, Taghizadeh M, Daneshvar Kakhaki R, et al. The effects of omega-3 fatty acids and vitamin E co-supplementation on clinical and metabolic status in patients with Parkinson's disease: a randomized, double-blind, placebo-controlled trial. *Neurochem Int*. 2019;131:104539. doi:10.1016/j.neuint.2019.104539
183. Riccio P, Rossano R. Nutrition facts in multiple sclerosis. *ASN Neuro*. 2015;7(1):1–20. doi:10.1177/1759091414568185

184. Hedstrom AK, Olsson T, Alfredsson L. The role of diet in multiple sclerosis: a review of the literature. *Autoimmun Rev.* 2022;21(2):102927. doi:10.1016/j.autrev.2022.102927
185. Marck CH, Probst Y, Chen J, et al. Dietary patterns and associations with health outcomes in Australian people with multiple sclerosis. *Eur J Clin Nutr.* 2021;75:1506–1514. doi:10.1038/s41430-021-00864-y
186. Ellouze I, Sheffler J, Nagpal R, Arjmandi B. Dietary patterns and Alzheimer's disease: an updated review linking nutrition to neuroscience. *Nutrients.* 2023;15(14):3204. doi:10.3390/nu15143204
187. Pietrzak D, Kasperek K, Rękawek P, Piątkowska-Chmiel I. The therapeutic role of ketogenic diet in neurological disorders. *Nutrients.* 2022;14(9):1952. doi:10.3390/nu14091952
188. Shahpasand S, Khatami SH, Ehtiati S, et al. Therapeutic potential of the ketogenic diet: a metabolic switch with implications for neurological disorders, the gut-brain axis, and cardiovascular diseases. *J Nutr Biochem.* 2024:109693.
189. Gough SM, Casella A, Ortega KJ, Hackam AS. Neuroprotection by the ketogenic diet: evidence and controversies. *Front Nutr.* 2021;8:782657.
190. Brenton JN, Banwell B, Bergqvist AGC, et al. Pilot study of a ketogenic diet in relapsing-remitting MS. *Neurol Neuroimmunol Neuroinflamm.* 2019;6(4):e565. doi:10.1212/NXI.0000000000000565
191. Liu C, Zhang N, Zhang R, et al. Cuprizone-induced demyelination in mouse hippocampus is alleviated by ketogenic diet. *J Agric Food Chem.* 2020;68(40):11215–11228. doi:10.1021/acs.jafc.0c04604
192. S Pavón, E Lázaro, O Martínez, et al. Ketogenic diet and cognition in neurological diseases: a systematic review. *Nutr Rev.* 2021;79(7):802–813. doi:10.1093/nutrit/nuaa113
193. Thickbroom GW. The therapeutic potential of ketone bodies in Parkinson's disease. *Expert Rev Neurother.* 2021;21(3):255–257.
194. López-Ojeda W, Hurley RA. Ketone bodies and brain metabolism: new insights and perspectives for neurological diseases. *J Neuropsychiatry Clin Neurosci.* 2023;35(2):104–109.
195. Ferraris C, Guglielmetti M, Neri LD, et al. A review of ketogenic dietary therapies for epilepsy and neurological diseases: a proposal to implement an adapted model to include healthy Mediterranean products. *Foods.* 2023;12(9):1743.
196. Grochowska K, Przeliorz A. The effect of the ketogenic diet on the therapy of neurodegenerative diseases and its impact on improving cognitive functions. *Dement Geriatr Cogn Dis Extra.* 2022;12(2):100–106. doi:10.1159/000524331
197. Ota M, Matsuo J, Ishida I, et al. Effects of a medium-chain triglyceride-based ketogenic formula on cognitive function in patients with mild-to-moderate Alzheimer's disease. *Neurosci Lett.* 2019;690:232–236. doi:10.1016/j.neulet.2018.10.048
198. Harvey C, Schofield GM, Williden M, McQuillan JA. The effect of medium chain triglycerides on time to nutritional ketosis and symptoms of keto-induction in healthy adults: a randomized controlled clinical trial. *J Nutr Metab.* 2018;2018:2630565. doi:10.1155/2018/2630565
199. Mouha RA. Internet of things (IoT). *J Data Analysis Info Process.* 2021;9(02):77.
200. Sguanci M, Mancin S, Gazzelloni A, et al. The internet of things in the nutritional management of patients with chronic neurological cognitive impairment: a scoping review. *Healthcare (Basel).* 2024;13(1):23. doi:10.3390/healthcare13010023

SECTION 3

Medical Nutrition Therapy in the Pediatric Patient

CHAPTER 19

Nutritional Management of the Preterm Infant

Antoinette Maraglino

CHAPTER OUTLINE

CORE CONCEPTS

1. Infants that do not complete their full gestation are more susceptible to many physiological conditions that can impact their ability to feed, grow, and thrive, putting them at increased nutritional risk.
2. Compared to term infants, premature infants have higher calorie needs.
3. Protein needs of premature infants are nearly 1.5–2 times higher than protein needs of term infants.
4. Carbohydrate is a major energy source for infants, accounting for 30–40% of their calorie intake.
5. Fat is the primary energy source for preterm infants, with 40–60% of their daily calories coming from fat.
6. Neonates born prior to completing their third trimester are born relatively calcium deficient and are at higher risk of developing osteopenia.
7. Parenteral nutrition is a critical element of neonatal care in terms of the survival and development of premature infants.
8. Carbohydrate in the form of dextrose, providing 3.4 kcal/g, is the major energy source in parenteral nutrition.
9. Provision of amino acids within the first hours of life prevents postnatal growth failure, reduces complications and morbidities, and promotes neurodevelopment, even at low calorie intake.
10. Feeding the gastrointestinal tract early has been shown to promote endocrine adaptation and to accelerate early motility patterns. Premature infants also have better tolerance of feeds, achieve full feeding volume sooner, and have a reduced risk of feeding aversion when fed early, all of which may lead to decreased length of hospital stay.
11. Human milk is the ideal choice for enterally feeding premature infants.

LEARNING OBJECTIVES

1. Recognize the factors that contribute to the increased nutritional risk of premature infants.
2. Identify and explain the anthropometrics used in assessing a neonate's size at birth.
3. Assess the calorie and protein needs of neonates when receiving enteral and parenteral nutrition.
4. Define the initial, advancement rate, and goal of macronutrient provision for neonatal parenteral nutrition support.
5. Identify the enteral feeding selection options for premature neonates.
6. Explain the benefits of feeding human milk to premature infants.
7. Describe the ways in which preterm infant formula differs from term infant formula.
8. State the criteria necessary for a neonate to be discharged from the hospital.

Introduction

Preterm neonates are one of the most medically and nutritionally fragile populations. Premature birth is one of the leading causes of mortality in infancy, and over 10% of infants born in the United States are born prematurely.[1] Black and Indigenous women are 54% more likely to deliver their infants prematurely when compared to the premature birth rates of White women.[1] Additionally, infant mortality rates are more than 2 times higher for babies born to Black and Indigenous biological mothers compared to White and Hispanic mothers.[1] Maternal health factors that increase the risk of preterm birth include pre-pregnancy diabetes, hypertension, smoking, underweight/overweight, and history of a previous preterm delivery. Although technological advances in the care of premature infants have improved outcomes, preterm infants have unique nutritional needs and often require complex interventions. Providing nutrition care to this group is often challenging, but vital to improve survival. Medical nutrition therapy is key to ensuring optimal growth and development.

Background

Neonatology and neonatal nutrition are subspecialties of pediatrics and pediatric nutrition, respectively, which primarily focus on the care of infants born prematurely. Full-term is defined as 40 weeks gestational age (WGA), but a range of 37–42 weeks is considered to be term.[2] Term is further delineated into early term (37 0/7 to 38 6/7 weeks), full term (39 0/7 to 40 6/7 weeks), late term (41 0/7 to 41 6/7 weeks), and postterm (42 0/7 weeks and beyond) to reflect the heterogeneity of outcomes within the 5-week span.[2] Any neonate born prior to 37 weeks gestation is considered to be a preterm infant. The earlier an infant is born, the greater the nutrition risk because infants will be smaller and less developed. The weeks and days of gestation that have elapsed when the preterm infant is born become the neonate's gestational age (GA). Each day and week following birth becomes the neonate's chronological age. The GA plus chronological age is considered the postmenstrual age (PMA) until the infant reaches 40 0/7 weeks PMA or the biological mother's previously assigned due date.[3] For example, a neonate born at 30 weeks gestation is considered to have a GA of 30 weeks. One week later, the neonate has a chronological age of 1 week and is considered to be 31 weeks' PMA.

Table 19.1 Birth Weight Classifications

Classification	Acronym	Birth Weight
Low birth weight	LBW	<2500 g
Very low birth weight	VLBW	<1500 g
Extremely low birth weight	ELBW	<1000 g

Data from ACOG Committee on Obstetric Practice. *Guidelines for Perinatal Care*. AAP Books. 2012.

The immediate nutrition risk of an infant can be assessed just after birth based on weight (**Table 19.1**). Infants born less than 2500 g are considered to be **low birth weight (LBW)**, infants born less than 1500 g are considered to be **very low birth weight (VLBW)**, and infants born less than 1000 g are considered to be **extremely low birth weight (ELBW)**.[4]

Weight for gestational age is also an important factor to consider when assessing a neonate's nutrition risk. Size for gestational age can be assessed by using premature growth curves for intrauterine and extrauterine growth.[5–9] Infants that are born with weights that chart less than the 10th percentile are **small-for-gestational-age (SGA)**.[5–9] Birth weights that chart greater than the 90th percentile are **large-for-gestational-age (LGA)**.[5–9] All infants with birth

CASE STUDY INTRODUCTION

A female infant (Quinn) was born at 30 5/7 weeks gestational age to a 28-year-old biological mother with 1 other child (G_2P_2). The pregnancy was complicated by preeclampsia, placental insufficiency, and **oligohydramnios** (insufficient amniotic fluid). The biological mother's obstetrician had been monitoring the pregnancy closely because Quinn was diagnosed with intrauterine growth restriction (IUGR) at 27 weeks gestation. Quinn was born via induced vaginal delivery due to her biological mother's worsening preeclampsia and Quinn's IUGR status. She was admitted to the neonatal intensive care unit (NICU) on her day of birth or day of life 0 (DOL 0).

Birth Anthropometrics:

Length: 36 cm (9th percentile on Fenton preterm growth chart)
Weight: 965 g (8th percentile on Fenton preterm growth chart)
Head circumference: 27 cm (33rd percentile on Fenton preterm growth chart)

Clinical Data:

Past Medical History: none
Medications: D10W with heparin at 80 mL/kg/day
Vital Signs: Blood pressure 54/33 mmHg, Temperature 97.7°F, Heart rate 122 beats/min
Nutrition-Focused Physical Exam: Infant is in no acute distress, lying supine in an incubator. Continuous positive airway pressure (CPAP) in place (Figure 19.1). Moves extremities symmetrically. Palate intact, abdomen soft, not distended. Patent anus. Anterior fontanelles are open, soft, and flat. No dysmorphic features. Alert, active, normal tone for gestational age (GA). Pink skin, no rash, no petechiae noted.

Dietary Data:

Diet Prescription: NPO

Questions

1. What are Quinn's most significant nutrition risk factors?
2. What additional information would you like to obtain from Quinn's mom?
3. How would you assess Quinn's weight at birth? Is she ELBW, VLBW, or LBW?
4. How would you assess her growth? Is she SGA, AGA, or LGA?
5. Is her growth symmetrical or asymmetrical?
6. What prenatal factors could have contributed to Quinn's IUGR?

weights that chart between the 10th and 90th percentiles are **appropriate-for-gestational-age (AGA)**.[5–9] Neonates are symmetric SGA or LGA if their birth weight, length, and head circumference are all below the 10th percentile for age or above the 90th percentile, respectively.[10] If at least one of those measurements, but not all three, is below the 10th percentile or above the 90th percentile, the infants are considered to be asymmetric SGA or LGA, respectively.[10]

Infants that are born AGA or SGA may be at increased nutritional risk if they experienced **intrauterine growth restriction (IUGR)**. IUGR describes a fetus that had been tracking along a healthy growth curve throughout gestation and then starts to track at least one standard deviation below their curve because of problems in utero.[11,12] Because a drop in the standard deviation may still be well above the 10th percentile for age, not all neonates with IUGR are necessarily SGA. IUGR can occur because of problems relating to the biological mother, the fetus, or the placenta, all of which result in reduced tissue deposition due to a reduced nutritional supply from the utero-placental circulation.[11–13] Some maternal causes of IUGR include malnutrition or being underweight, hypertensive disorders, pre-gestational diabetes, hyperthyroidism, kidney disease, autoimmune disease, cardiac disease, cystic fibrosis, asthma, living at a high altitude or in nonindustrialized countries, low socioeconomic status, race, family history or previous pregnancy with IUGR, extremes of maternal age, short interval pregnancy, tobacco use, and substance use disorder.[13] Placental reasons include placental placement, placental abruption, decreased placental blood flow, or uneven perfusion.[11] Fetal causes include genetic diseases, infection, multiple gestation, and fetal malformations.[13]

Being part of a multiple gestation puts a neonate at increased nutritional risk because abnormal fetal growth is more common in these infants. It is also common for multiples to have a shorter gestational period than singletons, resulting in most multiples being preterm at birth.[14] Multiples are at increased risk of experiencing IUGR, and the rate and severity of growth restriction increases as the number of fetuses increases.[13] Because severe IUGR is so common in multiples, multiples are also at increased risk of being born SGA. Another common risk in multiples is **growth discordance**, which is a significant size or weight difference between the two fetuses of a twin pregnancy. Birth weight discordance in conjunction with IUGR is associated with increased rates of fetal demise and neonatal morbidity and mortality.[13] Mortality rates of the smaller twin or multiple increase with increasing discordance in the setting of SGA.[13] However, both the smaller and larger subsets of discordant multiples are at increased risk of morbidity and mortality. Nutritional issues arise because of uneven nutrient deposition, potentially leading to malnutrition, blood glucose instability, fluid and electrolyte shifts, and compromised gut perfusion. These issues can result in feeding issues and difficulty in providing adequate nutrition for the infants.

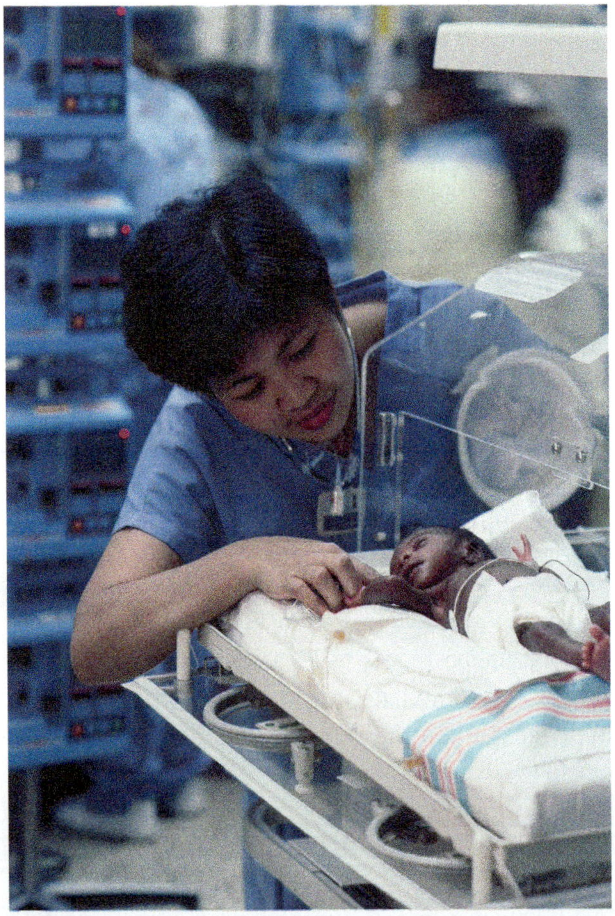

Premature Infant in the NICU

CORE CONCEPT 1

Infants that do not complete their full gestation are more susceptible to many physiological conditions that can impact their ability to feed, grow, and thrive, putting them at an increased nutritional risk.

PRACTICE POINT

The goal of nutrition management of premature infants is to achieve weight gain, growth, and development potential ex utero to match in utero growth potential.

Goals of Growth and Nutrition for Premature Infants

Fetal weight gain is the most rapid rate of growth that humans will experience in their lifetimes. If infants born prematurely do not achieve fetal rate of weight gain, they are at risk of growth failure.[15] Therefore, achieving rapid growth in the immediate postnatal period is essential. This is done through a mixture of parenteral nutrition (PN), human milk, and specific premature infant enteral nutrition (EN) formula products. Weight gain goals of premature infants have been established based on weight and gestational age at birth and change throughout the postnatal course until the infant reaches term PMA.[16,17] Ziegler et al. established goals of neonatal weight gain based on fetal weight gain standards.[17] These goals range from 14 to 21 grams per kilogram body weight per day (g/kg/day) and have an inverse relationship to the body weight of the infant.[17]

PRACTICE POINT

It is expected that the smallest neonates will gain the most weight per kilogram at the most rapid rate.

There are several options to assess neonatal anthropometrics at birth and also to track growth and weight gain throughout the neonatal course. Growth charts created by Lubchenco et al. and then by Babson and Benda became the standard for assessing fetal growth and weight gain at birth by establishing norms for fetal growth.[7,8,18] These charts have since been updated to include newer data and a larger sample size, especially for the purpose of tracking growth and weight gain over time ex utero.[5–9,18] The growth charts that have become the standard to track weight gain and catch-up growth from extreme prematurity (22 weeks GA) through term were published by Fenton in 2013 (**Figures 19.1** and **19.2**).[5,6]

PRACTICE POINT

The Fenton intrauterine growth charts have become the standard for tracking preterm neonatal growth throughout neonatal intensive care units and special care nurseries internationally.

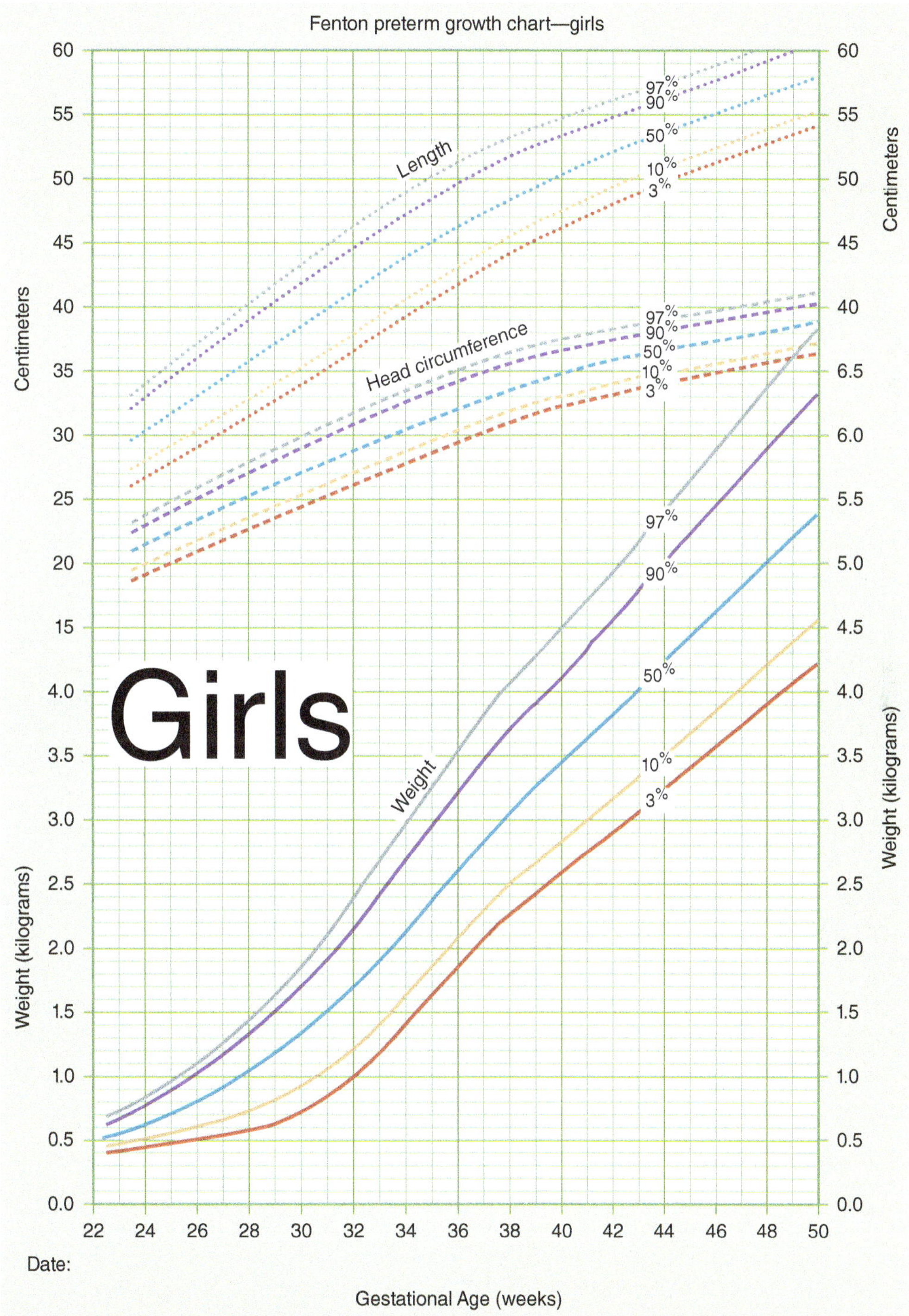

Figure 19.1 Fenton Preterm Growth Chart: Girls

Reproduced from Fenton TR, Kim JH. A systematic review and meta-analysis to revise the fenton growth chart for preterm infants. *BMC Pediatr*. 2013;13:59. doi:10.1186/1471-2431-13-59

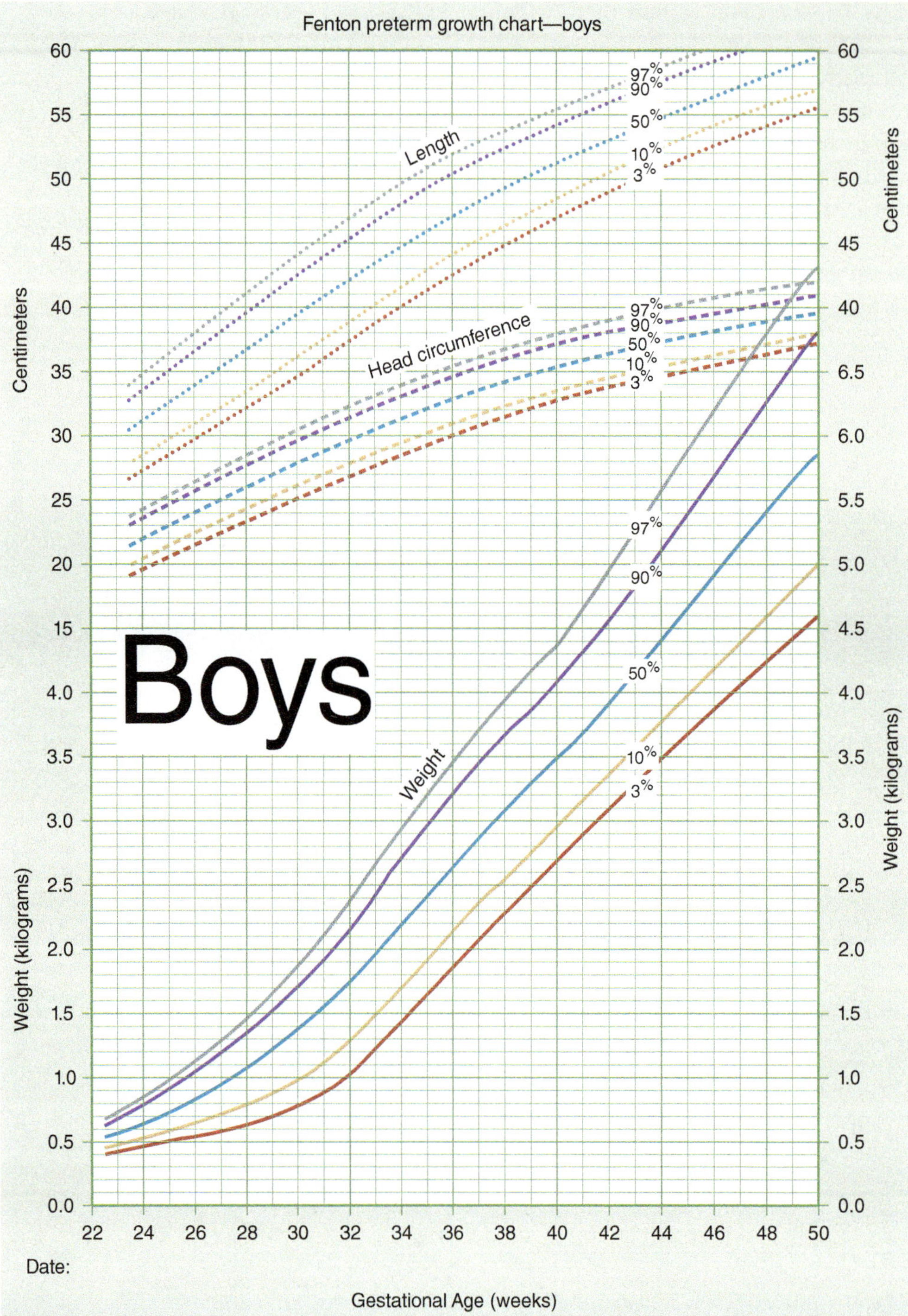

Figure 19.2 Fenton Preterm Growth Chart: Boys

Reproduced from Fenton TR, Kim JH. A systematic review and meta-analysis to revise the fenton growth chart for preterm infants. *BMC Pediatr*. 2013;13:59. doi:10.1186/1471-2431-13-59

Criteria for assessing malnutrition in the preterm and neonatal population were introduced in 2018 by Goldberg et al.[19] These criteria are intended for inpatient hospital use and in postdischarge settings for preterm infants prior to 37 weeks corrected age and for term infants up to 30 days old.[20] Nutrient intake is the preferred criterion for use within the first 2 weeks of life and can be used as a sole indicator.[19] The other criteria are recommended for use after the first 2 weeks of life.[19] Criteria that can be used with only one indicator after the first 2 weeks of life include weight gain velocity and decline in weight-for-age z-score.[19] Indicators that require at least two indicators to be used to identify malnutrition include linear growth velocity and decline in length-for-age z-score.[19] An additional indicator that requires two or more indicators is days to regain birth weight, and it is recommended for use in conjunction with nutrient intake.[19] Diagnosing malnutrition in the preterm and neonatal population allows those infants at the highest nutrition risk to be identified with the use of consistent criteria. It also establishes a mechanism to code for this higher level of care and increase reimbursement potential.[20] Of note, the recommended criteria are evidence informed and consensus driven by registered dietitians (RDs) with neonatal expertise, but the criteria have not been validated.[20]

Metabolism and Body Composition in Prematurity

Energy Requirements

It is estimated that preterm infants need about 105–130 kcal/kg/day when being enterally fed to maintain adequate growth and development, compared to 105–110 kcal/kg/day for their full-term counterparts. Basal metabolic rate accounts for the majority of calorie demand (40–45% of needs), followed by calories for growth (20% of needs).[21,22] Intermittent activity accounts for 10–15% of needs; metabolic stress of having to regulate and maintain normal body temperature, also known as "cold stress," and fecal losses account for 10% each of these needs; and the thermic effect of feeding makes up the final 5% of needs.[21] Placing preterm infants in an incubator will help minimize heat and evaporative water losses, thereby diminishing the energy cost of maintaining body core temperature (**Figure 19.3**). When the gastrointestinal (GI) tract is not being fed, there is no longer a calorie demand for fecal losses or the thermic effect of feeding, so the energy needs of neonates who are parenterally fed are generally lower than those being enterally fed.

CORE CONCEPT 2

Compared to term infants, premature infants have higher calorie needs.

PRACTICE POINT

Calorie needs for complete PN are about 15–20% less than those of enterally fed infants.

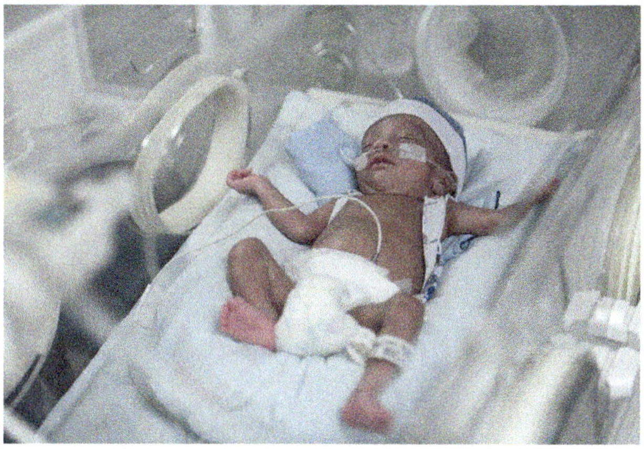

Figure 19.3 Preterm Infant in an Incubator

Protein Requirements

Because premature infants are born with virtually no or minimal energy stores, they are at high risk of becoming catabolic if not provided with an adequate provision of calories and protein soon after birth. If infants become catabolic, they will break down whatever limited amount of lean body mass they have to try to meet their energy and protein needs. The smaller and more immature an infant is, the greater the risk of accelerated protein losses.[16,23] Without adequate protein provision, preterm infants will lose an average of 0.6–1.2 grams protein/kg/day, which amounts to a loss of about 1.5% of total body protein loss per day.[16,23] Three days without adequate protein will result in a 10% loss of total body protein.[16,23] Ideally, premature infants should experience an accumulation of 2% total body protein per day.[16,23] Providing adequate protein to these infants is of extreme importance, but maintaining an optimal protein/energy ratio is also crucial for ensuring ideal protein accretion, with the highest ratio being required by the smallest preterm infants.[16]

Carbohydrate Requirements

The carbohydrate requirement for preterm infants is approximately 10–14 grams carbohydrate per kilogram per day (g/kg/day).[21] Glucose is the primary substrate used by the brain for energy and function. Carbohydrate is also a more effective energy substrate for preventing protein breakdown than fat. Late preterm infants have intestinal lactase activity; however, it is only about 30% as active as in term infants.[24] Despite this, lactose intolerance is rarely observed in premature infants. Lactose is the carbohydrate source in human milk and is typically well tolerated. This may be because premature infants are efficient at being able to hydrolyze carbohydrates in the small intestine.[24] Glucose polymers are well tolerated in preterm

CASE STUDY REVISITED

Quinn is now 24 hours old, DOL1. The neonatology team has asked you to provide recommendations for starting and advancing PN for Quinn. Her current labs are as follows:

Biochemical Data:

Sodium 143 (136–145 mEq/L)
Potassium 5.1 (3.5–5.0 mEq/L)
Chloride 113 (96–106 mEq/L)
Carbon dioxide 18 (22–31 mEq/L)
Blood urea nitrogen 25 (8–20 mg/dL)
Creatinine 0.55 (0.7–1.3 mg/dL)
Glucose 70 (70–139 mg/dL)

Clinical Data:

Urine Output: 4 mL/kg/hour

Questions

1. How would you assess Quinn's estimated energy needs?
2. Write two Problem/Etiology/Signs and Symptoms (PES) statements for Quinn.
3. Identify the nutrition interventions you would like to initiate for Quinn to address the problems identified in your PES statements.
4. What GIR would you provide and how much protein and fat (in g/kg/day) would you put in her initial PN?
5. At what rate would you advance each of these macronutrients?
6. What glucose, protein, and fat amounts (in g/kg/day) would you recommend for Quinn's final goal PN?
7. Considering Quinn's GA, labs, and urine output as a reflection of her postnatal diuresis, what are Quinn's fluid requirements?
8. How would you recommend her fluid intake from PN be advanced?
9. How would you assess her lab values?
10. Which electrolytes would you monitor closely?

CORE CONCEPT 3

Protein needs of premature infants are nearly 1.5–2 times higher than protein needs of term infants.

PRACTICE POINT

Premature infants will need approximately 3.5–4.5 grams protein/kg/day to achieve optimal growth rates ex utero, with an optimal protein/energy ratio of 2.7–4.1 grams protein per 100 kcals.

infants, likely because glucosidase enzymes for metabolizing glucose polymers are active in preterm infants.[21] For this reason, commercial preterm infant formulas provide about 50% of the carbohydrate as glucose polymers and about 50% as lactose.[25] The glucose polymers also contribute a lower osmotic load per unit weight than lactose, so this formulation can keep the osmolarity of the premature infant formula relatively low to improve GI tolerance.[21] Both the amount of carbohydrate and the balance of carbohydrate with the other macronutrients provided are important to a premature infant's metabolism. It is not uncommon for premature infants to have unstable blood glucose control because of their limited glycogen stores at birth. Providing them with an adequate amount of carbohydrate is essential to avoid hypoglycemia. It is equally important to avoid excessive carbohydrate. Feeding preterm infants an excessive amount of carbohydrate has been shown to lead to fat deposition in the liver, heart, and subcutaneous adipose tissue.[22] Overall, carbohydrate should be provided in adequate amounts along with adequate calories from fat and protein to help the infant with glucose control and stability.

CORE CONCEPT 4

Carbohydrate is a major energy source for infants, accounting for 30–40% of their daily calorie intake.

Fat Requirements

The daily fat requirement for preterm infants is approximately 5–7 g/kg.[21] Adequate fat provision is

Table 19.2 Macronutrient Requirements in Prematurity

Macronutrient	Premature Infant Requirements
Carbohydrate	10–14 g/kg/day
Protein	3.5–4.5 g/kg/day
Fat	5–7 g/kg/day

Data from Koletzko B, Poindexter B, Uauy R, eds. *Nutritional Care of Preterm Infants: Scientific Basis and Practical Guidelines*. Karger Medical and Scientific Publishers; 2014.

important for protein metabolism because optimal protein retention can be achieved when providing 30–40% of nonprotein calories as fat. Saturated fat, primarily triglycerides, is the major fat source of human milk. The saturated fat in human milk is easily digested, absorbed, and tolerated. This is due to the specific fatty acid chemical structure, compared to that of bovine milk, along with the lingual and gastric lipases in the GI tract of the preterm infant and bile salt–activated lipases within the breast milk.[21] These lipase activities compensate for the lack of pancreatic lipase and intraluminal bile salt concentration in preterm infants compared to their full-term counterparts. Because formula-fed infants do not benefit from the bile salt–activated lipases that are found in human milk, premature formulas contain 40–50% of their fat content as saturated fat and 40–50% as medium-chain triglyceride (MCT) oils.[14] MCT oil is readily absorbed from the GI tract because it is able to bypass the lymphatic system. Infants who receive feedings of preterm formula mixed with human milk have increased fat absorption compared to formula alone.[21] Human milk also contains small, yet well absorbed, amounts of the fatty acids docosahexaenoic acid (DHA) and arachidonic acid (ARA). Because these fatty acids are known to be beneficial for visual function and neurodevelopment, DHA and ARA are routinely added to premature infant formulas. **Table 19.2** summarizes macronutrient requirements for carbohydrate, protein, and fat in premature infants.

CORE CONCEPT 5

Fat is the primary energy source for preterm infants with 40–60% of their daily calories coming from fat.

Fluid Requirements

Fluid and electrolyte management is a critical part of the medical management of neonates, especially extremely premature infants. At the beginning of the third trimester (24 weeks gestation), the fetus is about 90% total body water (TBW).[15,22] Sixty-five percent of the TBW at this gestation is extracellular fluid (ECF) and 25% is intracellular fluid (ICF). As the fetus approaches term, TBW decreases to approximately 75%, with ECF accounting for 40% and ICF accounting for 35%.[15,22] In the days following delivery, the infant undergoes a contraction of ECF and expected physiological **postnatal diuresis**. This diuresis results in a loss of approximately 10–15% of birth weight gradually over the first 10–14 days of life for an extremely premature infant.[15] Expected losses are less and occur over a shorter length of time for neonates that are later in gestation and physiologically more mature. Comparatively, a term infant would be expected to experience a diuresis of 5–10% during the first week of life and regain birth weight by day of life (DOL) 7–10. The other major reasons for this difference are reduced insensible losses due to more mature skin and respiratory tract and reduced renal losses due to more mature kidneys of the term infant. These fluid losses should be accounted for when estimating fluid needs. Diuresis should not exceed 2–3% loss of birth weight per day, equating to a daily urine output of 1–3 mL/kg/hour, with a maximum of 5–7 mL/kg/hour. Fluid requirements may vary depending on physiological maturity, clinical conditions, and environmental factors. Generally, initial fluid requirements for neonates born at 24–25 weeks gestation will be approximately 100 mL/kg/day, 70–90 mL/kg/day for neonates born at 26–34 weeks gestation, and 60 mL/kg/day for infants born later than 34 weeks gestation.[26] Fluid needs may be higher for infants with abdominal wall defects or other GI losses, with high-output kidney failure, or receiving care under a radiant warmer or receiving phototherapy. Conversely, fluid needs may be lower for infants residing in a humidified incubator, infants with a **patent ductus arteriosus (PDA)**, which is a congenital heart defect causing abnormal blood flow between the arteries connecting to the heart, oliguric kidney failure, or brain injury. Indicators of overhydration may be excessive weight gain, edema, increased urine output, and normal or reduced urine output with hyponatremia. Indicators of dehydration may be excessive weight loss, decreased urine output with hypernatremia, hyperkalemia, azotemia, and metabolic acidosis. After the first few days of life, once diuresis rates and electrolyte losses begin to normalize, total fluid volumes may be advanced, typically by 10–20 mL/kg/day to a usual goal of 130–160 mL/kg/day based on weight, urine output, electrolytes, respiratory status, and cardiovascular status.[26] Infants with severe respiratory disease or a hemodynamically significant PDA may need their fluids restricted to 120–140 mL/kg/day.[26]

Electrolyte Requirements

During the diuresis period, electrolyte homeostasis should be maintained. This may be done with electrolyte supplementation in intravenous fluid, but, most commonly, electrolyte requirements are managed in PN solution for infants weighing less than 1500–1800 g. Maintaining electrolyte homeostasis may be challenging due to increased urinary losses of electrolytes via premature kidneys. In preterm kidneys, glomerular and tubular function is immature, resulting in a reduced glomerular filtration rate and a reduced capacity to resorb sodium, potassium, and bicarbonate. Immature kidneys also have decreased ability to concentrate and dilute urine, leading to serum sodium, potassium, and bicarbonate abnormalities, most readily found in ELBW infants. Thus, ELBW infants often receive PN solutions that minimize sodium and potassium and/or maximize acetate in the first few days of life during postnatal diuresis.

Sodium

In the first 24–72 hours of life, a premature neonate requires little to no exogenous sodium. Sodium restriction during this time period has been associated with reduced exacerbation of respiratory disease and reduced incidence of bronchopulmonary dysplasia (BPD), a form of chronic lung disease commonly found in premature infants caused by mechanical ventilation and long-term use of oxygen, later in life.[27] Also, hypernatremia may result from increased sodium intake. In some infants, sodium provision may be limited to less than 1 mEq/kg/day until postnatal diuresis is completed,[15] but some infants may require greater amounts of sodium during diuresis. After diuresis, sodium intake is typically advanced to 2–4 mEq/kg/day.[10,21] Some VLBW or ELBW infants may require more sodium, up to 10 mEq/kg/day, due to limited renal tubular sodium reabsorption resulting in increased losses through the kidney. To manage this, adjust fluid provision to maintain hydration and then adjust sodium intake by 1–2 mEq/kg/day as needed until serum sodium values are within normal limits.

Potassium

ELBW infants are at increased risk of developing nonoliguric hyperkalemia, usually within the first 72 hours of life, especially those who are born extremely premature, have blood group incompatibility with their biological mother, are catabolic, are bruised, have metabolic acidosis, or receive excessive potassium intake.[26] The incidence of this has decreased with earlier administration of amino acids in initial PN solutions and improved fluid management.[26] Potassium should not be provided until the infant is urinating regularly and serum potassium is normalized. Once this occurs, potassium can be introduced at 1 mEq/kg/day and advanced to 2–3 mEq/kg/day.[10,21] Further adjustments may be made as needed based upon changes in kidney function or serum levels, especially if diuretic therapy is being used.

Acid-Base Balance

Increased bicarbonate losses through immature kidneys of premature infants may result in shifts in acid–base balance, most commonly metabolic acidosis, in the first week or two of life. When this occurs, the infant will require alkalotic supplementation in the form of acetate.[26] Because acetate and chloride must be paired with cations in solution, intake of these anions should be restricted until the neonate is able to receive sodium and potassium as previously discussed.[26] Additional chloride supplementation may be required in neonates being treated with diuretic therapy, resulting in contraction alkalosis or an increase in blood pH due to fluid losses.

Calcium and Phosphorus

Approximately 80% of bone mineral stores are laid down during the last trimester of intrauterine development.[28] Calcium is readily transferred across the placenta during the third trimester of gestation, providing the fetus with optimal bone growth and calcium stores.[21] Infants born prior to completing their third trimester are born with a degree of hypocalcemia in direct correlation to how prematurely they are born. Low phosphate intake will cause the kidneys to retain phosphate, eliminating phosphate excretion in the urine and resulting in hypercalcemia and hypercalciuria.[14] Phosphate deficiency results in bone demineralization, further exacerbating osteopenia of prematurity.[14] Optimal provision of supplemental calcium and phosphorus is of extreme importance to optimize bone retention and growth.

A growing premature infant will require 3–4 mEq calcium/kg/day (60–90 mg/kg/day) and 1.3–2.25 mMol phosphorus/kg/day (40–70 mg/kg/day) via PN.[14] The ideal calcium-to-phosphorus (Ca:P) ratio to promote optimal mineral retention and bone growth is 1.3–1.7 mg elemental calcium to 1 mg phosphorus weight ratio (2.2–2.6 mEq Ca:1 mMol P).[26] VLBW infants on PN for longer than 2 weeks should receive increased monitoring for developing osteopenia. Increased losses of urinary calcium may result from certain medications, such as diuretics and steroids, especially with long-term use. This can lead to **nephrocalcinosis** (deposition of calcium in the kidney parenchyma) and an increased risk for metabolic bone disease. Infants who are SGA may have increased phosphorus requirements to prevent refeeding syndrome resulting from rapid growth and increases in lean tissue mass. Calcium and phosphorus provision may be limited in PN solutions due to limitations in solution stability and solubility. To optimize solubility, higher concentrations of amino acids and dextrose can be added, lipids should be given separately, and cysteine should be added to the PN solution. In addition, neonatal amino acid solutions are more acidic than standard solutions, which increase calcium and phosphorus solubility.

Relatively high amounts of calcium and phosphorus are also required for preterm neonates being enterally fed. Bovine or human milk–based multinutrient fortifiers that may be added to human milk are called **human milk fortifiers**. Human milk fortifiers are formulated for preterm infants and contain high amounts of calcium and phosphorus to meet the increased demand and support bone turnover and development. Commercial preterm infant formulas also contain more calcium and phosphorus than any other infant formulas to meet the needs of this population.

CORE CONCEPT 6

Neonates born prior to completing their third trimester are born relatively calcium deficient and are at higher risk of developing osteopenia.

Magnesium

The magnesium requirement for infants on PN is 0.2–0.5 mEq/kg/day.[14] Magnesium may be omitted from initial or transitional PN solution if the biological mother received significant amounts of magnesium sulfate prenatally to prevent premature labor or to treat preeclampsia. High amounts of circulating magnesium in a newborn may result in symptoms of increased tiredness or fatigue, sluggish GI motility, and constipation. Magnesium supplementation may be provided once the infant is passing stool normally. **Table 19.3** summarizes maintenance electrolyte requirements in premature infants.

Table 19.3 Maintenance Electrolyte Requirements in Prematurity

Electrolyte	Premature Infant Requirements
Sodium	2–4 mEq/kg/day
Potassium	2–3 mEq/kg/day
Calcium	3–4 mEq/kg/day (60–90 mg/kg/day)
Phosphorus	1.3–2.25 mMol/kg/day (40–70 mg/kg/day)
Magnesium	0.2–0.5 mEq/kg/day

Data from Corkins MR. *ASPEN Pediatric Nutrition Support Core Curriculum*. 3rd ed. Silver Spring, MD: American Society for Parenteral and Enteral Nutrition (ASPEN); 2025:692.

Nutrition Assessment

Nutrition assessment of preterm infants involves evaluation of anthropometrics, including weight, length, and head circumference plotted on appropriate growth charts. Regular measurements are important to track growth and assess the time to regain birth weight. Identify any conditions that may influence nutrition needs and the feeding plan, such as respiratory conditions requiring ventilatory or oxygen support. Evaluation of GI status is critical to determine appropriateness of and timing for enteral feed or parenteral nutrition. Fluid balance assessment is vital to evaluate postnatal diuresis as well as to ensure appropriate fluid administration. Biochemical assessment is needed to evaluate electrolyte balance, acid–base, and mineral status. Nutrition-focused physical examination is not typically included as a part of the nutrition assessment due to the fragility of the infant and need for a temperature-controlled environment.

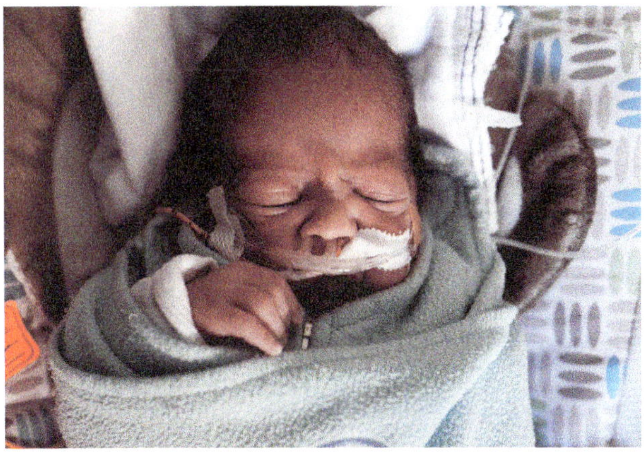

Premature Infant with a Feeding Tube and on Oxygen

Nutrition Intervention

Methods of Feeding

Parenteral Nutrition (PN)

Due to the extreme prematurity of the GI tract of VLBW neonates, meeting their high calorie demand enterally may be challenging, if not impossible, in the first days or weeks of life. The small stomach capacity, immaturity of the GI tract, and critical illness make advancing to full enteral feeds a slow and cautious process. PN has been a life-saving intervention not only for premature infants, but also for surgical infants who may have prolonged periods when they are unable to receive any nutrition via their GI tract. Providing PN is most critical for VLBW and ELBW infants. PN is used as a vehicle to maintain fluid requirements and deliver electrolytes the same way it would be done with intravenous fluids. Being able to meet the macronutrient and micronutrient needs of premature infants is what makes PN necessary for these patients to thrive.

CORE CONCEPT 7

Parenteral nutrition is a critical element of neonatal care in terms of the survival and development of premature infants.

Vascular Access

PN can be given whether a patient has central or peripheral access. Peripheral PN (PPN) is most useful in conjunction with EN to meet the nutrition needs of the patient. Because of the restrictions in osmolarity and dextrose concentration, PPN is not able to meet the nutrition needs of preterm infants alone. Current American Society of Parenteral and Enteral Nutrition (ASPEN) recommendations state that the maximum osmolality of a safe PPN is 900 mOsm/L and that dextrose concentration must not exceed 12.5%.[29] PPN is good for short-term use to supplement calorie and micronutrient needs but is not optimal for achieving nutrition needs for growth. PPN also carries the risks of intravenous infiltrates due to the hyperosmotic solution running through small vessels and the caustic nature of some of the PN additives, such as calcium. Running high volumes or high rates of fluid may also lessen the viability of a peripherally placed intravenous line.

Central PN (CPN) is the recommended delivery of PN in patients who will require PN for more than a few days. Larger vessels can tolerate a higher osmotic solution and higher dextrose concentrations. Complete nutrition and fluid needs can be met with CPN provided through centrally placed intravenous catheters. Central catheters will always carry the risk of sepsis; therefore, diligent line care is necessary to maintain safe access for long-term PN delivery.

Energy Requirements

Energy needs of parenterally fed preterm infants are 15–20% less than those of enterally fed infants because calorie expenditure of digestion and absorption loss does not occur when the nutritional provision bypasses the GI tract. Energy needs are based on body size, need for nutrient accretion, and losses to assure that postnatal growth will approximate the in utero growth of a normal healthy fetus of the same postconception age. ELBW infants have the lowest estimated resting energy expenditure (REE), while larger infants have a higher REE. Calorie requirement for ELBW on PN is estimated at approximately 90–95 kcal/kg/day.[16,17] VLBW infants are estimated to require 100–110 kcal/kg/day, while LBW infants require 110–115 kcal/kg/day while on PN.[16,17] It is generally accepted that estimated requirements for infants of these respective sizes are based on the above recommendations, regardless of whether the infant was born extremely premature or SGA. It is believed that infants born SGA did not acquire the necessary nutrient stores or develop to their full potential and, therefore, have catch-up growth needs. However, the necessity of catch-up growth for neonates, as well as the expectation that preterm infants will grow at the same velocity as their in utero counterparts, continues to be controversial.

Glucose

Glucose tolerance is limited in VLBW and smaller infants due to insufficient insulin production, relative insulin resistance, and the continued hepatic release of glucose from the starvation response triggered when placental transfer of nutrients is terminated. Glucose provision must be fairly low when initially administered and advanced slowly to prevent the reactive hyperglycemia caused by the physiological glucose intolerance. Hyperglycemic response will be lessened when dextrose is administered with amino acids, as amino acids stimulate insulin production and release. It is important to prevent hyperglycemia because glucose overload will impact the kidneys, causing osmotic diuresis potentially leading to dehydration. It is equally important to prevent hypoglycemia because glucose is the primary fuel to maintain brain function, growth, and development. Infants with IUGR are at increased risk of developing hyperglycemia due to delayed insulin production and response and increased risk of developing hypoglycemia due to increased metabolic demand of catch-up growth. In order to maintain blood glucose in a normal range, the glucose infusion rate must be closely monitored and controlled. **Glucose infusion rate (GIR)** is a function of the concentration of dextrose and the rate at which the dextrose is administered and is typically measured in milligrams of dextrose per kilogram per minute (mg/kg/min).

CORE CONCEPT 8

Carbohydrate, in the form of dextrose, providing 3.4 kcal/g, is the major energy source in parenteral nutrition.

PRACTICE POINT

Initial glucose infusion rate for premature infants must be between 4 and 6 mg/kg/min to maintain adequate glucose provision for the brain.

The demand for low GIR along with relatively high fluid requirements of ELBW infants may require the use of fluids with low dextrose concentration. The minimum dextrose concentration of fluids delivered should be 5% so that a hypotonic solution is not administered.

It is common practice in the neonate population to aim for a maximum GIR administration at 14–16 mg/kg/min. Excessive glucose intake may induce lipogenesis.[14,22] It may also negatively affect respiratory gas exchange by increasing carbon dioxide production, which the preterm infant has a harder time expelling, possibly exacerbating respiratory distress.[14,22]

PRACTICE POINT

Dextrose can be advanced, maintaining blood glucose levels above 50 mg/dL and below 120 mg/dL, by 1–2 mg/kg/min daily.

Amino Acids

While it has always been common to start premature neonates on dextrose-containing intravenous fluids soon after birth, the early administration of intravenous amino acids as a common practice is relatively recent.[22] Prior to this practice, amino acids were not given until several days after birth. It is now understood that protein provision promotes anabolism and weight gain. The type of amino acid solution used for infants contains high amounts of essential amino acids and emulates the serum amino acid profile of a breastfeeding infant.[26,30] Intravenous protein requirements are based on fetal requirements, amino acid delivery across the placenta throughout gestation, and the extrauterine environment after birth. In a fetal environment, 50% of amino acids passed across the placenta are utilized for energy, while the other half are used for protein synthesis.[22] Preterm infants have higher requirements than their fetal counterparts because of postnatal nitrogen excretion.

For preterm infants who were neither IUGR nor born SGA, 2.5 grams protein/kg daily, in conjunction with receiving 50 nonprotein kcal/kg/day, is the minimum dose needed to maintain positive nitrogen balance.[23] In order to achieve protein accretion and growth rates to match those of in utero growth rates, the premature infant needs 2.7–3.5 grams protein/kg/day and 70 nonprotein kcal/kg/day.[23] Early administration of amino acids can safely be initiated between 1.5 and 3 g/kg/day within the first few hours after birth to prevent catabolism and promote positive nitrogen balance. Most NICUs have a starter PN solution available that contains dextrose, amino acids, and sometimes calcium to initiate within hours of birth. Amino acids can be incrementally increased to 3.5–4 g/kg/day within the first few days of life.[31,32]

PRACTICE POINT

Providing up to 3.5–4 g/kg/day of amino acids is now common clinical practice and has been shown to be safe without clinically significant increases in azotemia, metabolic acidosis, or hyperaminoacidemia.

Monitoring for tolerance of amino acids is not typically necessary unless kidney dysfunction is present. Blood urea nitrogen (BUN) is not an effective monitoring tool of protein tolerance because amino acids are used for protein synthesis or oxidized for energy, which reflects metabolism. In the first few days to weeks of life, BUN is more reflective of hydration status rather than protein metabolism or tolerance. BUN levels as high as 40 mg/dL have been observed in neonates in the first week of life, whether or not they were receiving parenteral amino acids.

CORE CONCEPT 9

Provision of amino acids within the first hours of life prevents postnatal growth failure, reduces complications and morbidities, and promotes neurodevelopment even at low calorie intake.

Lipids

Long-chain fatty acids are necessary for newborn brain development. Essential fatty acid deficiency (EFAD) can develop in VLBW infants within the first week of life because of minimal fat tissue stores and high demand for rapid growth.[22] VLBW infants have minimal tissue stores of essential fatty acids, primarily linoleic acid; in utero, a fetus relies entirely on essential fatty acid transfer from the placenta.[15] Intravenous lipid emulsion (ILE), containing linoleic acid, can prevent essential fatty acid deficiency if provided at least at approximately 0.5 g/kg/day.[22,26] Lipids are also an important source of energy and are calorically dense. When given in greater volumes, lipids can balance the calorie breakdown of the macronutrient components of PN, lessening the demand to give excessive calories as carbohydrate.[15] This concentrated source of nonprotein calories promotes nitrogen retention.

Standard 20% lipid emulsions contain a lower phospholipid emulsifier to triglyceride ratio, which leads to more rapid lipid clearance than 10% lipid emulsions and therefore are preferable for use in the neonatal population.[15,26] Lipids can be safely initiated in the first 24–48 hours of life to aid in nitrogen balance and prevent EFAD. The initial dose recommendation is 0.5–1 g/kg/day.[22]

PRACTICE POINT

Provision of intravenous lipids is an essential component of neonatal PN.

PRACTICE POINT

Lipids should be advanced slowly each day, by 0.5–1 g/kg/day, and maximum dose should not exceed 3 g/kg/day to prevent ketosis.

For neonates, lipids should be administered over 20–24 hours for optimal clearance, although it is recommended that infusion of lipid emulsion alone hang for no more than 12 hours at a time.[26,33] Some institutions choose to change the lipid source and tubing every 12 hours in this population to accommodate a longer infusion time, while others opt to allow a 20- to 24-hour hang time in order to minimize additional manipulation of the lipid line to reduce potential contamination. Triglyceride levels should be monitored after advancing lipids to 2 and 3 g/kg/day to ensure normal serum levels. If serum triglyceride levels exceed 200 mg/dL, ILE should be reduced by 0.5–1 g/kg/day until serum triglyceride levels return to normal.[21]

Two formulations of 20% ILE are approved for routine use in neonates in the United States. One is exclusively soy oil based. The other is a blend of soy, fish, MCT, and olive oils. This fat blend has a more physiological mix of omega-3 and omega-6 fatty acids, balancing the proinflammatory and anti-inflammatory effects.[34,35] There is some concern regarding the high polyunsaturated fatty acid content of the ILE as linoleic acid (omega-6 fatty acids) from soybean oil ILE used in the United States. Linoleic acid can increase the production of inflammatory mediators, leading to the synthesis of prostaglandins, leukotrienes, and thromboxanes when converted to arachidonic acid.[15] These inflammatory agents have been identified in exacerbating pulmonary hypertension and increasing the risk of developing intestinal failure–associated liver disease (IFALD).[22] IFALD is clinically diagnosed by having a conjugated bilirubin level >2 mg/dL.[34] A third ILE has been developed from fish oil that contains the omega-3 fatty acids eicosapentaenoic acid and docosahexaenoic acid, which are anti-inflammatory.[36] This fat emulsion is currently used for patients who have a history of IFALD and is approved for use at 1 g/kg/day.

Plasma carnitine levels are low in premature infants and decrease further in the first 2 weeks of life if the infants are exclusively on PN. **Carnitine** is an amino acid derivative that aids in the oxidation of fatty acids. Studies have shown little, if any, clinical benefit to supplementing carnitine in PN as a means of improving fatty acid oxidation. However, it is commonly recommended to add carnitine to neonatal PN for patients who are exclusively receiving PN for longer than 2 weeks or if carnitine deficiency is determined.[15]

Electrolytes

Electrolytes are withheld or restricted in the first few days of life prior to the neonatal diuresis of initial fluid and to prevent exacerbation of pulmonary disease and later development of BPD. Once postnatal diuresis has occurred, sodium and potassium can be added to PN in limited amounts (1–2 mEq/kg/day) and advanced incrementally to meet physiologic needs. Neonatal needs during the first weeks of life will vary depending on kidney function, hydration status, and the use of systemic diuretics. While metabolic acidosis may be common during the first few weeks of life, requiring increased acetate provision in the PN, once the diuresis period is over, chloride can be added back into the PN to maintain optimal acid–base balance.

Minerals

Calcium and phosphorus supplementation are important parts of PN therapy. Premature neonates are at elevated risk of developing osteopenia of prematurity. Receiving PN with little or no calcium or phosphorus increases this risk further. Providing required amounts of calcium and phosphorus can be difficult due to solubility limitations and the high risk of precipitation. A severe fluid restriction will significantly decrease the ability to add appropriate amounts of calcium and phosphorus to the PN solution due to limitations related to solution concentration. Calcium and phosphorus will also need to be limited in PPN due to their high osmolalities and the risk of calcium causing intravenous infiltrates or extravasation. Neonatal amino acid solutions are more acidic compared to standard amino acid solutions. This increases the solubility of calcium and phosphorus, which may allow more to be added to the PN solution. The addition of cysteine hydrochloride and higher concentrations of amino acids and dextrose, and providing lipids as a separate infusion, helps to prevent the precipitation of calcium and phosphorus. Preterm infants, particularly LBW infants, receiving prolonged PN are likely to experience poor bone mineralization and should be monitored regularly. Serum calcium and phosphorus levels along with alkaline phosphatase, an enzyme that correlates with bone growth, should be checked every 1–2 weeks for patients requiring long-term PN. Although normal alkaline phosphatase levels are higher in preterm neonates (upwards of 500 IU/L) due to their rapid bone growth, levels above 800 IU/L require additional workup, including skeletal radiographs to look for bone demineralization and rickets.

Vitamins

All newborn infants are born with a relatively sterile GI tract. Without the colonization of appropriate bacteria, they are unable to synthesize their own vitamin K. Prenatal stores of vitamin K and initial dietary intakes are limited. Therefore, neonates are at increased risk of having hemorrhagic disease of the newborn from vitamin K deficiency. To prevent this, all neonates born in a U.S. hospital receive an intramuscular injection of vitamin K soon after birth.

Pediatric solutions of multivitamins are available and recommended for use in PN solution. Use of an adult multivitamin PN solution would put a neonate at increased risk of vitamin toxicities. All water- and fat-soluble vitamins are contained in the pediatric vitamin solution. Vitamins are photosensitive, putting them at risk of oxidation and degradation with light exposure on a PN bag. Protecting the PN bag and tubing with an opaque bag may aid in the preservation of these vitamins. In 2021, ASPEN recommended that all neonatal PN, ILE, and tubing be light protected, such as with an opaque bag or light protective or colored syringes or tubing.[37] There is also a relative risk of vitamins adhering to the plastic PN bag and tubing. Higher infusion rates and using the shortest IV tubing possible will help reduce this risk. Because VLBW infants have limited stores of vitamins, not receiving the full expected dose of vitamins due to these issues should be considered.

Vitamin A has been of particular interest for premature neonates in relation to the reduction of BPD. Premature neonates are born with low stores of vitamin A. Vitamin A has a role in tissue repair and cell differentiation and turnover. Supplemental vitamin A may be provided intravenously in addition to the multivitamin solution in the PN or by providing a high-dose intramuscular injection. While benefits have been shown in reducing the risk of BPD development with vitamin A supplementation in multiple studies,[38] individual neonatal intensive care units may choose to use or not use additional supplemental vitamin A depending on the BPD rates in their unit.

Trace Elements

Trace elements are required for all premature infants because adequate passage of trace elements across the placenta and storage do not occur without completion of gestation to term. Premature neonates also have increased demand due to rapid growth rates. These factors put them at increased risk of trace element deficiencies. Neonatal and pediatric multitrace solutions are available for addition to PN solution. Although due to supply chain shortages, trace elements may need to be added individually.

For infants with cholestatic jaundice, manganese can be reduced or removed in PN to prevent toxicity. However, zinc and selenium should always be provided. Inadequate selenium has been associated with increased risk of developing BPD and retinopathy of prematurity.[15] Zinc is required for energy metabolism,

CASE STUDY REVISITED

The neonatology team has stated that given the IUGR status of Quinn, they are feeling cautious about starting enteral feeds and are considering waiting until she is 3 days old before feeding her.

Questions

1. What recommendations would you provide to them about early enteral feeding?
2. When would you start MEN feeds for Quinn?

tissue accretion, and wound healing. VLBW infants have high requirements due to their rapid growth rates, so it is recommended that additional zinc sulfate be provided to PN solutions beyond what is provided in the multitrace solution.[15] This practice should also be considered for infants with increased losses from diarrhea, stomal losses, or severe skin disease.

While iron is not recommended for routine addition to PN, it may be added in limited amounts to PN solutions without lipids if a neonate is receiving the majority of their nutrition from PN for 2 months or longer. It may also be required if a neonate develops iron deficiency anemia while receiving PN. Recent red blood cell transfusions, which are also sources of iron, should be considered when evaluating the need for adding iron to a PN solution.

Enteral Nutrition

Enterally feeding infants, including preterm infants, is the preferred method of providing nutrition. Feeding the premature GI tract provides luminal nutrients to help the tissue mature, develop, and colonize appropriately. When the GI tract is not fed, it begins to atrophy, making it more susceptible to infections. One common, but serious, GI infection found primarily in the preterm population is **necrotizing enterocolitis (NEC)**, a condition characterized by inflammation and cell death within the intestinal wall. NEC is an acute ischemic condition that is a contributor to infant morbidity and mortality.[39] There are many risk factors associated with the development of NEC, including infants who have younger gestational age, are SGA, and/or VLBW. There are also maternal risk factors; Black parents are more likely than White parents to have premature infants who develop NEC.[40] Additionally, Black infants have a higher risk of death from NEC than White infants.[41] Breastfeeding and providing human milk has been consistently shown to be protective against NEC.[42] Infants fed formula demonstrated greater GI permeability than those provided human milk.[40] Human milk reduces but does not eliminate NEC risk in this population.[40]

Concern about GI immaturity may contribute to delays in enteral feeding. Early enteral feeding provides several benefits to the premature infant. For all ELBW infants and some VLBW infants, providing minimal enteral nutrition (MEN), or trophic feedings, will provide luminal nutrients and promote the secretion of gastric hormones and enzymes to prime the gut for larger volumes of enteral feeding. Stimulating the GI tract with MEN decreases PN-related problems, such as the development of PN-associated liver disease, and can help improve weight gain. MEN is defined as a subnutritional volume of enteral feeding, such as 10–20 mL/kg/day, provided for a predetermined length of time. Once the trophic feeding period is completed, advancing enteral feeds allows for achievement of full feeding volume and may facilitate weight gain. Many institutions have developed standardized methods of starting and advancing enteral feeds. Evidence has shown that developing and following a standardized feeding regimen can decrease the incidence of NEC in an institution.[43] Conditions that may delay the initiation and advancement of enteral feedings include hemodynamic instability, hypotension, indomethacin treatment, abnormal GI exam or GI dysfunction, severe metabolic acidosis, severe respiratory instability, hypoxia, or hypoxemia.[44]

PRACTICE POINT

Enteral nutrition should be started as soon after birth as possible, optimally in the first 24 hours of life.

Infants who lack the ability to suck, swallow, and breathe simultaneously need to be fed via a nasogastric or orogastric tube (**Figure 19.4**). Frequent intermittent or bolus feeding is the most physiological way to feed premature infants. This method allows for the natural rise and fall of gastric hormones and

CASE STUDY REVISITED

Quinn is now nearly 36 hours old. Her biological mother was sick from the preeclampsia after delivery. Despite her intentions of providing her milk to the baby, she has not been pumping as often as needed to establish an adequate supply. The medical team would like you to connect with the biological mother to establish a feeding plan with her so that feeds can be started for Quinn.

Questions

1. How would you educate Quinn's biological mother about nursing, expressing her milk, and the role of biological mother's milk and donor milk in feeding her preterm child?
2. What might you share with mom to encourage her to pump more regularly in order to be able to provide sufficient amounts of milk?

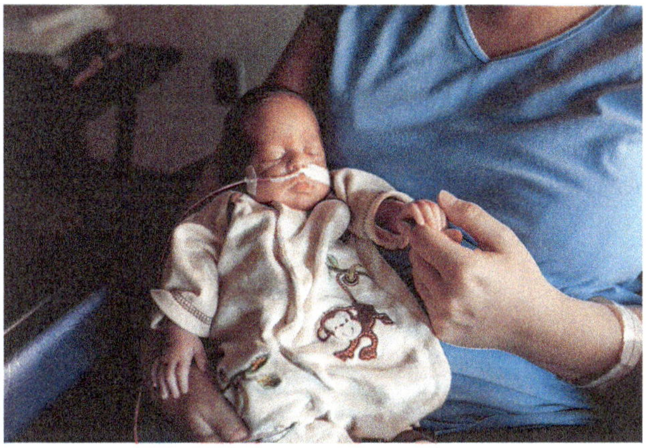

Figure 19.4 Preterm Infant with Nasogastric Tube

enzymes, aids in the development of hunger cues, and teaches the infants to wake at appropriate times to feed. Feeding small volumes more frequently (every 2 hours) has been shown to improve feeding tolerance compared to feeding larger volumes less frequently (every 4 hours). Feeding every 3 hours is common practice in this population. Bolus feeds delivered via gravity or via pump infusion decrease the nutrient loss observed with continuous feeding related to the adherence of fats, minerals, and vitamins by the extended dwell time of the milk or formula in the plastic tubing.[21] For this reason, bolus or intermittent feeding may promote better delivery of nutrients and may lead to improved weight gain for premature infants with intact, functional GI tracts compared to continuous feeding.[45] Once an infant reaches 32–34 weeks PMA, small oral feedings may be trialed. Transition to oral feeding should be initiated based on the infant's readiness cues, including waking or fussiness around the time of feeding, rooting, and putting hands near or around mouth.[46–48]

Continuous feedings may be advantageous for infants with severe lung disease, gastroesophageal reflux

PRACTICE POINT

Premature infants may lack the ability to feed orally on their own because of the inability to suck, swallow, and breathe simultaneously, which develops around 32–36 weeks gestational age.

(GER), malabsorption, hypoglycemia, poor motility, GI surgery, or severe or multiple episodes of feeding intolerance.[23,49,50] Continuous feeds may promote better absorption of nutrients and increased weight gain in infants with malabsorption as a result of short bowel syndrome or intestinal failure, or during recovery from NEC.[26,51] When feeding continuously, intragastric feeds are preferred to transpyloric or postpyloric feeding.[51] Transpyloric feeding has been associated with such complications as intestinal perforation and mortality. Transpyloric feedings should only be used as a last resort for infants who are at risk of aspiration, extremely severe GER, or severe respiratory compromise.[52]

Common issues that complicate enteral feeding are GER, emesis, and gastric residuals. All three occur commonly in premature infants and often lead to concerns of feeding intolerance. The premature GI tracts of preterm infants have an underdeveloped lower esophageal sphincter and gastroesophageal junction. Therefore, GER and mild emesis are common in premature infants and tend to resolve over time because these organ connections are not tight at birth and develop and tighten throughout infancy.[50] Most GER and emesis should not be concerning or indicate feeding intolerance.[52] GER becomes problematic when reflux is bilious or causes respiratory instability or aspiration. Emesis is concerning when the amount of emesis is 50% or more of the volume fed, if the amount of emesis is inhibiting weight gain, or if the emesis contains bile or blood.[15] Gastric residuals are

Clinical Controversy

Probiotics are live microorganisms that may be ingested to increase beneficial gut microflora and compete against pathogenic bacteria. The numerous types of strains and their benefits across population types continue to be researched.[1] Use of probiotics in preterm infants has been observed to reduce the risk of necrotizing enterocolitis (NEC), a condition in which damaged intestinal tissue causes bloating, diarrhea, inflammation, and infection. In this population, probiotics have been associated with decreased risk of NEC, reduced length of stay, improved short-term weight gain, and mortality, although more research is needed.[2,3] Recent safety concerns with respect to bacteremia have been raised by the Food and Drug Administration.[4] Since probiotics are live bacterial strains, they may enter the bloodstream, leading to sepsis and have been associated with the death of a preterm infant. The risk versus benefit of probiotic use in preterm infants is under debate with the European Society for Paediatric Gastroenterology, Hepatology and Nutrition calling for reconsideration of the warning.[5]

Questions

1. Outline the risks versus benefits of probiotic administration in preterm infants.
2. How might these risks be mitigated to reconsider introducing probiotics in this population?

References

1. He P, Yu L, Tian F, Chen W, Zhang H, Zhai Q. Effects of probiotics on preterm infant gut microbiota across populations: a systematic review and meta-analysis. *Adv Nutr*. 2024;15(6):100233. doi:10.1016/j.advnut.2024.100233
2. Batta VK, Rao SC, Patole SK. *Bifidobacterium infantis* as a probiotic in preterm infants: a systematic review and meta-analysis. *Pediatr Res*. 2023;94:1887-1905. doi:10.1038/s41390-023-02716-w
3. Panchal H, Athalye-Jape G, Rao S, et al. Growth and neurodevelopmental outcomes of probiotic-supplemented preterm infants: a systematic review and meta-analysis. *Eur J Clin Nutr*. 2023;77:855-871. doi:10.1038/s41430-023-01270-2
4. US Food and Drug Administration. FDA raises concerns about probiotic products sold for use in hospitalized preterm infants. News release. October 26, 2023. Accessed January 2, 2025. https://www.fda.gov/news-events/press-announcements/fda-raises-concerns-about-probiotic-products-sold-use-hospitalized-preterm-infants
5. van den Akker CHP, Embleton ND, Lapillonne A, et al. Reevaluating the FDA's warning against the use of probiotics in preterm neonates: a societal statement by ESPGHAN and EFCNI. *J Pediatr Gastroenterol Nutr*. 2024;78:1403-1408. doi:10.1002/jpn3.12204

also fairly common in infants and more common in preterm infants. Gastric residuals are more commonly observed in the setting of continuous feeds compared to bolus feedings, and do not likely indicate feeding intolerance if the abdominal exam is normal.

CORE CONCEPT 10

Feeding the gastrointestinal tract early has been shown to promote endocrine adaptation and to accelerate early motility patterns. Premature infants also have better tolerance of feeds, achieve full feeding volume sooner, and have a reduced risk of feeding aversion when fed early; all of which may lead to decreased length of hospital stay.

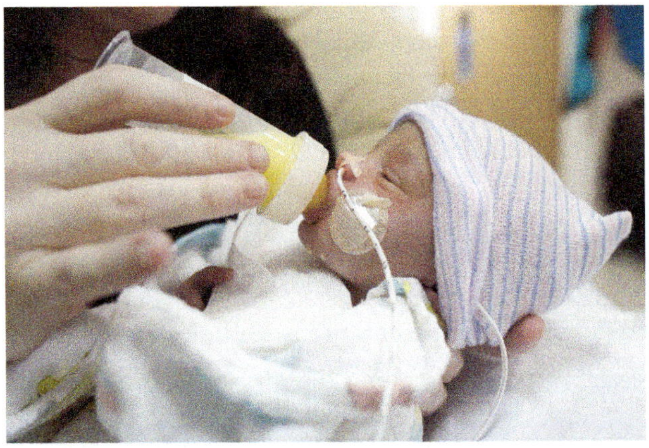

Figure 19.5 Preterm Infant with Nasogastric Feeding Tube in Place Being Bottle Fed with Human Milk

Feeding Selection

Breast Milk, Breastfeeding, and Donor Milk

For the premature infant, human milk is ideally used for enteral feeds. The options for human milk are biological mother's own milk or pasteurized donor human milk. Biological mother's own milk is the optimal choice compared to donor milk. Biological mothers can express their milk using a breast pump so that the milk can be fed to the premature infants in controlled volumes, at specific times, and via a feeding tube (Figure 19.5). During the first month of a premature infant's life, the composition of the biological mother's milk is slightly different than that of the milk of the biological mother of a term infant.[21] Preterm human milk contains higher amounts of protein and sodium compared to term human milk. After the first month of lactation, the milk produced by the biological mother of the preterm infant will transition to a composition more similar to term human milk.

There are several reasons why human milk is the preferred food for premature infants. Human milk contains many nonnutritive components that have been found to be protective or beneficial to the GI tract of premature infants. There are anti-infectious compounds, including lactoferrin, nucleotides, cytokines, and oligosaccharides, as well as immune cells such as neutrophils, macrophages, and T-lymphocytes.[22] Feeding the premature infant with human milk has been proven to decrease the incidence of NEC and sepsis, likely due to these components.[21] These immune-protective components have anti-inflammatory, antibacterial, antiviral, and prebiotic effects that help the GI tract develop a healthy microbiome.[22] Multiple types of growth factors and enzymes are found in human milk and likely contribute to the fact that preterm infants fed human milk tolerate their feeds better, are able to advance their feedings more rapidly, and achieve full enteral feeds earlier. This may lead to an earlier discharge from the hospital. Human milk also contains many different hormones that may contribute to better neurodevelopment. It has been suggested that these beneficial and protective effects of human milk are likely dose-dependent, with the most benefits observed in infants that receive exclusively human milk.[45,53–55]

PRACTICE POINT

The concentrations of macro- and micronutrients are lower in human milk when compared to infant formulas; however, the nutrients are more readily absorbed from human milk. This is especially true for zinc and iron, as well as fat due to the presence of lipases in breast milk.

PRACTICE POINT

Even with optimal absorption, the nutrient concentrations of human milk are insufficient to meet the high calorie demands and calcium and phosphorus needs of preterm infants to maintain rapid growth and bone mineralization rates.

Human milk fortifiers are often added to human milk to increase macro- and micronutrient concentrations. Human milk fortifiers are available in bovine milk–based versions and human milk–based versions. They all contain macro- and micronutrients, but in varying amounts. Bovine milk–based versions have particularly high amounts of calcium, phosphorus, and protein, which are hydrolyzed for improved tolerance, digestion, and absorption. These fortifiers can be added to human milk to increase the caloric density by 2 and 4 kcal/fl. oz. Human milk–based fortifiers are made by concentrating pasteurized human milk. Since pasteurization denatures or decreases the amounts of certain nutrients in the milk, infants receiving human milk feedings fortified with human milk–based fortifiers may require additional supplementation of sodium, chloride, protein, iron, or vitamins. Human milk–based fortifiers may be added to human milk to increase the caloric density by 2, 4, 6, 8, and 10 kcal/fl. oz. These fortifiers are not available for retail purchase. If growth is still inadequate after the addition of these fortifiers, modular products may be added such as liquid hydrolyzed protein, MCT oil, emulsified lipids, vegetable oils, or glucose polymers. A human milk-based cream product to add additional calories from fat is also available. It is important to try to use these modulars in appropriate ratios so the natural distribution of calories from carbohydrate, protein, and fat is not altered and the protein:energy ratio used to preserve optimal growth of lean body mass is maintained. Providing too much fat from an oil or cream-based modular may put the infant at risk of developing ketosis, providing too much carbohydrate from glucose polymers may promote lipogenesis, and providing too much protein fortifier may unnecessarily strain the premature kidneys. Infant formula powders or concentrates can also be used instead of modular products, although sterile liquids are preferred to nonsterile powders for premature infants.

Nursing and providing expressed human milk can be emotionally rewarding for the biological mothers of premature infants during a frightening and stressful time when the infants are in the hospital. Providing this type of nutrition promotes involvement in the infant's care and direct interaction with the infant at a time when the typical development of the biological mother–infant dyad is inhibited due to the complex care needs of the premature infant. Biological mothers who are interested in nursing are encouraged to do so as soon as possible for premature infants. After a biological mother expresses her milk (**Figure 19.6**), a premature infant may be put to the breast or chest for nonnutritive suckling, also referred to as "oral stimulation." This practice helps develop the oral skills of the infant, enhances biological mother's milk production, and encourages

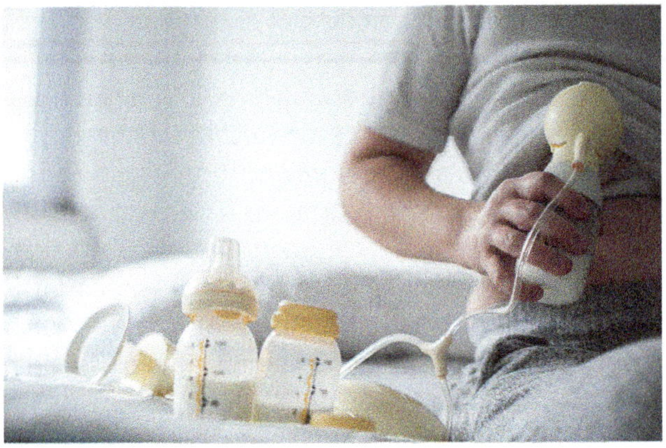

Figure 19.6 Biological Mothers of Babies in the NICU Are Encouraged to Breastfeed and Express Breast Milk.

biological mother–infant bonding. Pacifiers can also be used as oral stimulation. While controversial in term infants, a preterm infant sucking on a pacifier while receiving enteral feeds through an enteral feeding tube helps strengthen their suck strength, stimulate oral and gastric enzymes, and develop an association between suckling and being fed. Swabbing the inside of the preterm infant's mouth with milk or providing milk drops is another form of oral stimulation. This practice allows the infant to become familiarized with the taste and scent of human milk, also stimulates oral and gastric enzymes and secretions, and has the added benefit of helping reduce the risk of ventilator-associated pneumonia in infants who are intubated. Once the premature infant reaches 32–33 weeks PMA and is showing cues for oral feeding readiness, actual nursing prior to expressing milk may be started.[47,48] Because of the high metabolic demands of premature infants, supplemental high-calorie, fortified human milk or formula feeds are typically needed in conjunction with direct nursing.

There are some instances in which a biological mother may wish to provide human milk for her infant, but is unable. For these infants, especially the ones at highest risk of developing NEC, sepsis, or feeding intolerance, pasteurized donor human milk is available. Donor milk banks accept donations of human milk from bereaved biological mothers or biological mothers with a surplus milk supply. The donated milk is screened, pooled with the milk of several donors, and then pasteurized to eliminate bacteria and other infectious organisms. Milk banks are nonprofit entities and operate under the guidance and regulations of the Human Milk Banking Association of North America.[56] Donor milk is generally term milk from later in lactation; however, some milk banks collect and are able to supply preterm donor milk. Donor human milk is considered to be the second-best enteral choice for premature infants, following the biological mother's own milk. Evidence suggests that it may decrease the risk of developing NEC.[57] Growth and development rates of infants receiving donor milk tend to be slower. Donor milk typically has lower concentrations of protein, sodium, and chloride as a result of pasteurization, handling, and storage of donor breast milk.[58,59] The lower amounts of these nutrients may be why growth and development rates are lower in infants receiving donor milk.

Safe preparation, handling, and storage of human milk, both biological mother's own milk and donor milk, is critical. Milk preparation rooms, sometimes referred to as "Milk Labs," are dedicated areas within a hospital or NICU where human milk is stored and

⚠ Clinical Controversy

Some religious and cultural communities engage in the practice of milk sharing or wet nursing. Some parents also purchase expressed human milk via the internet. Informal milk sharing occurs when a lactating individual shares or sells their expressed milk directly with other parents who may be experiencing insufficient milk supply. Since it is shared directly from one family to another, this milk is typically not screened, tested, or pasteurized as it is when milk is donated to milk banks. For hospitalized infants, different hospitals choose to address this phenomenon in different ways.

Questions

1. What risks may informally shared human milk pose to a hospitalized infant? Are the risks different if the milk is shared from someone in the parents' community versus purchased on the internet?
2. What departments and professionals within the hospital may you engage to establish a policy on informal milk sharing?
3. If you suspect a family may be bringing in human milk that might not be their own, how would you approach the question with them in a culturally aware way?

Reference

1. Sriraman NK, Evans AE, Lawrence R, et al. Academy of Breastfeeding Medicine's 2017 position statement on informal breast milk sharing for the term healthy infant. *Breastfeed Med.* 2018;13(1):2–4.

prepared by specially trained milk preparation technicians. Milk preparation rooms can provide an aseptic area to ensure safe handling, avoid compromising the integrity of the milk, and reduce the likelihood of incorrect administration to the wrong patient. Centralized preparation of human milk can reduce the possibility of inaccurate measurements of additives and variable nutrient content that can contribute to feeding intolerance, delay advancement of enteral feeds, and possibly contribute to poor growth, and is considered best practice in milk handling.[60,61]

CORE CONCEPT 11

Human milk is the ideal choice for enterally feeding premature infants.

Preterm and Transitional Formulas

Because the nutritional needs and capabilities of the GI tract of premature infants are so different from that of term infants, commercial formula companies have developed infant formulas to meet the specific needs of this population. The protein formulation of these products is whey predominant, and the fat contained in the formula is 50% MCT oil for improved absorption and easier digestion.[62] The formulas are only available as ready-to-feed liquid and are made in concentrations of 20, 24, and 30 kcal/fl. oz.[62] These different calorie forms can be mixed with one another to create various calorie concentrations between 22 and 28 kcal/fl. oz. The 30 kcal/fl. oz concentrated preterm formula can also be used as a liquid fortifier for human milk. All preterm formulas are formulated to have a high concentration of vitamins and minerals, particularly vitamin A, vitamin D, calcium, and phosphorus to support eye health and bone mineralization. All premature infants born before 34 weeks gestation and born at a weight less than 1800 g who are not receiving breast milk or who need supplemental feeds with formula should receive preterm formula. These formulas are not available for retail purchase.

PRACTICE POINT

Preterm formulas contain higher amounts of protein, calcium, phosphorus, and vitamins to meet the high needs of preterm infants.

Specialty formulas have also been developed for infants who are born closer to term or for preterm infants once they reach at least 34 weeks PMA and weigh at least 2000 g. These transitional formulas come in a standard formulation of 22 kcal/fl. oz. They contain higher concentrations of nutrients than term infant formulas, but less than preterm formulas. This is specifically true for protein, calcium, phosphorus, and vitamins.[62] These formulas contain 25–30% MCT oil for improved digestion.[62] It is recommended that infants stay on this formula for the first 9–12 months of life or until the infant's weight-for-length is maintained above the 25th percentile. These formulas are available as powder or ready-to-feed. The powder form can be concentrated to make a formula of greater

Clinical Roundtable

Topic: New-to-Market Infant Formulas

Background: Infant formulas sold in the United States need to meet the Food and Drug Administration's (FDA) requirements for nutrient adequacy, packaging, and labeling. One of the major formula producers in the United States experienced a large-scale recall in 2022, resulting in a nationwide infant formula shortage. To respond to the shortage, European infant formulas derived from cow's milk or goat's milk, that met the FDA requirements, became available for purchase for the first time in the United States. These formulas are intended for use in healthy, term infants.

Roundtable Discussion

1. What nutrient(s) that are lacking in goat's milk would need to be supplemented in goat's milk-derived infant formula in order for the formula to meet the FDA requirements?
2. Aside from the nutrient content of the new formulas, what other labeling details should be reviewed to ensure safe preparation?
3. How would you help counsel parents who have questions about these new formulas? How would your counseling change if their infant was preterm?

References

1. DiMaggio DM, Du N, Scherer C, et al. Comparison of imported European and US infant formulas: labeling, nutrient, and safety concerns. *J Pediatr Gastroenterol Nutr*. 2019;69(4):480-486.
2. Dipasquale V, Serra G, Corsello G, Romano C. Standard and specialized infant formulas in Europe: making, marketing, and health outcomes. *Nutr Clin Pract*. 2020;35:273-281.

CASE STUDY REVISITED

Quinn is now 35 weeks PMA (about 1 month old). Her mom is noticing that her milk supply is starting to slow down. She would like to directly nurse Quinn as much as possible in order to stimulate her milk supply.

Questions

1. Is Quinn developmentally ready to start feeding by mouth?
2. If Quinn's biological mother's supply is still inadequate, what would you suggest as a backup option?
3. Quinn's biological mother is also asking when Quinn will be ready to come home. What goals will Quinn have to achieve to be discharged home from the hospital?

calorie density than 22 kcal/fl. oz if higher calories are needed to promote weight gain. The powder can also be added to the breast milk of late premature infants to increase the calorie density of the breast milk as the infant is getting ready to transition to home. Transitional formulas are available for retail purchase and, therefore, can be used outside of the hospital.

PRACTICE POINT

In order to be ready to go home, a premature infant must be able to take all of their feedings by mouth via a bottle, nursing, or a combination of both; be demonstrating adequate weight gain; wake for feedings every 2 and 4 hours; and maintain their body temperature without the use of an incubator.

Monitoring and Evaluation

Preparing for Discharge

It is common that premature infants will need increased calorie feedings upon discharge to continue to support their rapid growth rates and high metabolic demand. The method of how a premature infant feeds will impact discharge planning. In rare cases, an infant may be discharged with a feeding tube or may need to be woken up for feedings at least every 4 hours. It is important for all parents of premature infants to receive discharge teaching and education about the special needs and risks of bringing home a baby born prematurely.

The premature infant is still likely to be smaller than they would have been if born at term. These infants should be monitored closely once discharged. Many hospitals with NICUs also have a NICU graduates or follow-up outpatient clinic for continuity of care. These clinics target premature infants who are at highest risk for growth failure or developmental delay and follow up with them at least every 6 months for growth measurements, weight checks, and developmental testing. Home services are also available for high-risk infants that can provide physical and occupational therapy, speech therapy, and feeding therapy once per week or more. Premature infants are at risk of physical and cognitive developmental delays, and the risks are higher the more prematurely an infant is born. Intensive support, follow-up, and intervention may prevent or lessen delays in this population as they reach childhood and adulthood.

Chapter Summary

Nutritional management of the preterm population presents many challenges, including, but not limited to, increased nutrient needs and immature organ function. Appropriate utilization and timing of provisions of parenteral, enteral, and/or oral nutrition are necessary for successful growth. The achievement of extrauterine growth through specialized nutrition support is vital for the health and development of the premature neonate.

Key Terms

oligohydramnios, low birth weight (LBW), very low birth weight (VLBW), extremely low birth weight (ELBW), small-for-gestational-age (SGA), appropriate-for-gestational-age (AGA), large-for-gestational-age (LGA), intrauterine growth restriction (IUGR), growth discordance, postnatal diuresis, patent ductus arteriosus (PDA), nephrocalcinosis, human milk fortifiers, glucose infusion rate (GIR), carnitine, nectrotizing enterocolitis (NEC)

References

1. March of Dimes. 2023 Premature Birth Report Card. Accessed November 10, 2024. http://www.marchofdimes.org/report-card
2. The American College of Obstetricians and Gynecologists Committee on Obstetric Practice Society for Maternal-Fetal Medicine Committee Opinion No.579: Definition of term pregnancy. *Obstet Gynecol*. 2013;122(5):1139–1140.
3. American Academy of Pediatrics Committee on Fetus and Newborn: age terminology during the perinatal period. *Pediatrics*. 2004;114(5):1362–1364.
4. ACOG Committee on Obstetric Practice. *Guidelines for Perinatal Care*. AAP Books; 2012.
5. Fenton TR. A new growth chart for preterm babies: Babson and Benda's chart updated with recent data and a new format. *BMC Pediatr*. 2003;3(1):13.
6. Fenton TR, Kim JH. A systematic review and meta-analysis to revise the Fenton growth chart for preterm infants. *BMC Pediatr*. 2013;13:59.
7. Lubchenco LO, Hansman C, Boyd E. Intrauterine growth in length and head circumference as estimated from live births at gestational ages from 26 to 42 weeks. *Pediatrics*. 1966;37(3):403–408.
8. Lubchenco LO, Hansman C, Dressler M, Boyd E. Intrauterine growth as estimated from liveborn birth-weight data at 24 to 42 weeks of gestation. *Pediatrics*. 1963;32:793–800.
9. Olsen IE, Groveman SA, Lawson ML, Clark RH, Zemel BS. New intrauterine growth curves based on United States data. *Pediatrics*.2010;125(2):e214–e224.
10. Cloherty J, Stark A. Identifying the high-risk newborn and evaluating gestational age. *Manual of Neonatal Care*. Lippincott Williams Wilkins; 2010:41–58.
11. Cetin I, Alvino G. Intrauterine growth restriction: implications for placental metabolism and transport. *Placenta*. 2009;30:77–82.
12. Cetin I, Foidart J, Miozzo M, et al. Fetal growth restriction: a workshop report. *Placenta*. 2004;25(8):753–757.
13. Hendrix N, Berghella V. Non-placental causes of intrauterine growth restriction. *Semin Perinatol*. 2008;32(3):161–165.
14. Martin JA, Hamilton BE, Osterman MJ, Driscoll AK, Matthews TJ. Births: final data for 2015. *Natl Vital Stat Rep*. 2017;66(1):1–70.
15. Adamkin DH. *Nutritional Strategies for the Very Low Birthweight Infant*. Cambridge University Press; 2009.
16. Rigo J, Senterre J. Nutritional needs of premature infants: current issues. *J Pediatr*. 2006;149(5):S80–S88.
17. Ziegler EE. Nutrient requirements of premature infants. *Nestle Nutr Workshop Ser Pediatr Program*. 2007;59:161–172; discussion 172–176.
18. Babson SG, Benda GI. Growth graphs for the clinical assessment of infants of varying gestational age. *J Pediatr*. 1976;89(5):814–820.
19. Goldberg, DL, Becker, PJ, Brigham K, et al. Identifying malnutrition in preterm and neonatal populations: recommended Indicators. *J Acad Nutr Diet* 2018;118(9):1571–1582.
20. Goldberg DL, Becker PJ. Applying the recommended indicators for the diagnosis of preterm and neonatal malnutrition: answers to frequently asked questions. *Nutr Clin Pract*. 2022;37:50–58.
21. Kleinman RE, American Academy of Pediatrics. *Pediatric Nutrition Handbook*. 6th ed. Academy of Pediatrics; 2009: 1470.
22. Koletzko B, Poindexter B, Uauy R, eds. *Nutritional Care of Preterm Infants: Scientific Basis and Practical Guidelines*. Karger Medical and Scientific Publishers; 2014.
23. Ziegler EE. Protein requirements of very low birth weight infants. *J Pediatr Gastroenterol Nutr*. 2007;45 Suppl 3: S170–S174.
24. Tsang RC, Uauy R, Koletzko B, Zlotkin S. *Nutrition of the Preterm Infant: Scientific Basis and Practical Guidelines*. Digital Educational Publishing, Inc.; 2005.
25. Wirth Jr F, Numerof B, Pleban P, Neylan M. Effect of lactose on mineral absorption in preterm infants. *J Pediatr*. 1990;117(2):283–287.
26. Groh-Wargo S, Thompson M, Cox JH. *Pocket Guide to Neonatal Nutrition*. Academy of Nutrition and Dietetics; 2016.
27. Baumgart S, Costarino AT. Water and electrolyte metabolism of the micropremie. *Clin Perinatol*. 2000;27(1):131–146.
28. Nehra D, Carlson SJ, Fallon EM, et al. A.S.P.E.N. clinical guidelines: nutrition support of neonatal patients at risk for metabolic bone disease. *JPEN*. 2013;37(5):570–598.
29. Mirtallo J, Canada T, Johnson D, et al. Safe practices for enteral nutrition. *JPEN*. 2004;28:S39–70.
30. Helms RA, Christensen ML, Mauer EC, Storm MC. Comparison of a pediatric versus standard amino acid formulation in preterm neonates requiring parenteral nutrition. *J Pediatr*. 1987;110(3):466–470.
31. Robinson, DT, Calkins KL, Chen Y, et al. Guidelines for parenteral nutrition in preterm infants: The American Society for Parenteral and Enteral Nutrition. *JPEN*. 2023; 47:830–858.
32. Corkins MR. *ASPEN Pediatric Nutrition Support Core Curriculum*, 3rd ed. ASPEN; 2025:692.
33. Erratum for Guidelines for preventing catheter-related infections. *MMWR*. 2002;16:711.
34. Wales PW, Allen N, Worthington P, George D, Compher C. ASPEN clinical guidelines: support of pediatric patients with intestinal failure at risk of parenteral nutrition–associated liver disease. *JPEN*. 2014;38:538–557.
35. Tomsits E, Pataki M, Tolgyesi A, Fekete G, Rischak K, Szollar L. Safety and efficacy of a lipid emulsion containing a mixture of soybean oil, medium-chain triglycerides, olive oil, and fish oil: a randomised, double-blind clinical trial in premature infants requiring parenteral nutrition. *J Pediatr Gastroenterol Nutr*. 2010;51(4):514–521.
36. Gura KM, Duggan CP, Collier SB, et al. Reversal of parenteral nutrition-associated liver disease in two infants with short bowel syndrome using parenteral fish oil: implications for future management. *Pediatrics*. 2006;118(1):e197–201.
37. Robinson DT, Ayers P, Fleming B, et al. Recommendations for photoprotection of parenteral nutrition for premature infants: an ASPEN position paper. *Nutr Clin Pract*. 2021;36(5): 927–941. doi:10.1002/ncp.10747
38. Ding Y, Chen Z, Lu Y. Vitamin A supplementation prevents the bronchopulmonary dysplasia in premature infants: a systematic review and meta-analysis. *Medicine* (Baltimore). 2021;100(3):e23101. doi:10.1097/MD.0000000000023101
39. Wolf MF, Rose AT, Goel R, Canvasser J, Stoll BJ, Patel RM. Trends and racial and geographic differences in infant mortality in the United States due to necrotizing enterocolitis, 1999 to 2020. *JAMA Netw Open*. 2023;6(3):e231511. doi:10.1001/jamanetworkopen.2023.1511
40. Necrotizing Enterocolitis (NEC) in Preterm Infants Working Group of the National Advisory Council of Child Health

and Human Development (NACHHD) Report to Secretary, Department of Health and Human Services. September 16, 2024. Accessed December 18, 2024. https://www.nichd.nih.gov/sites/default/files/inline-files/2024.09.16_NEC_WG_report_FINAL.pdf

41. Seeman SM, Mehal JM, Haberling DL, Holman RC, Stoll BJ. Infant and maternal risk factors related to necrotising enterocolitis-associated infant death in the United States. *Acta Paediatr*. 2016;105(6):e240–e246. doi:10.1111/apa.13390
42. Lucas A, Cole TJ. Breast milk and neonatal necrotising enterocolitis. *Lancet*. 1990;336(8730):1519–1523. doi:10.1016/0140-6736(90)93304-8
43. Jasani B, Patole S. Standardized feeding regimen for reducing necrotizing enterocolitis in preterm infants: an updated systematic review. *J Perinatol*. 2017;37(7):827–833. doi:10.1038/jp.2017.37
44. Duggan C, Watkins JB, Walker WA. *Nutrition in Pediatrics: Basic Science, Clinical Applications*. Connecticut People's Medical Publishing House-USA; 2007.
45. Schanler RJ, Shulman RJ, Lau C, Smith EO, Heitkemper MM. Feeding strategies for premature infants: randomized trial of gastrointestinal priming and tube-feeding method. *Pediatrics*. 1999;103(2):434–439.
46. Kirk A, Alder S, King J. Cue-based oral feeding clinical pathway results in earlier attainment of full oral feeding in premature infants. *J Perinatol*. 2007;27(9):572–578.
47. Puckett B, Grover VK, Holt T, Sankaran K. Cue-based feeding for preterm infants: a prospective trial. *Am J Perinatol*. 2008;25(10):623–628.
48. McCain GC. An evidence-based guideline for introducing oral feeding to healthy preterm infants. *Neonatal Netw*. 2003;22(5):45–50.
49. Hwang ST, Shulman RJ. Update on management and treatment of short gut. *Clin Perinatol*. 2002;29(1):181–194.
50. Poets CF. Gastroesophageal reflux: a critical review of its role in preterm infants. *Pediatrics*. 2004;113(2):e128–e132.
51. Macdonald PD, Skeoch CH, Carse H, et al. Randomised trial of continuous nasogastric, bolus nasogastric, and transpyloric feeding in infants of birth weight under 1400 g. *Arch Dis Child*. 1992;67(4 Spec No):429–431.
52. Pereira GR. Nutritional care of the extremely premature infant. *Clin Perinatol*. 1995;22(1):61–75.
53. Meinzen-Derr J, Poindexter B, Wrage L, Morrow A, Stoll B, Donovan E. Role of human milk in extremely low birth weight infants' risk of necrotizing enterocolitis or death. *J Perinatol*. 2009;29(1):57–62.
54. Schanler R, Shulman R, Lau C. Feeding strategies for premature infants: beneficial outcomes of feeding fortified human milk versus preterm formula. *Pediatrics*. 1999;103:1150–1157.
55. Sisk P, Lovelady C, Dillard R, Gruber K, O'Shea T. Early human milk feeding is associated with a lower risk of necrotizing enterocolitis in very low birth weight infants. *J Perinatol*. 2007;27(7):428–433.
56. Human Milk Banking Association of North America. Accessed December 18, 2024. https://www.hmbana.org/find-a-milk-bank/overview.html
57. Parker MG, Stellwagen LM, Noble L, et al. Promoting human milk and breastfeeding for the very low birth weight infant. *Pediatrics*. 2021;148(5):e2021054272. doi:10.1542/peds.2021-054272
58. Ewaschuk J, Unger S, O'Connor D, et al. Effect of pasteurization on selected immune components of donated human breast milk. *J Perinatol*. 2011;31(9):593–598.
59. Moro GE, Arslanoglu S. Heat treatment of human milk. *J Pediatr Gastroenterol Nutr*. 2012;54(2):165–166.
60. Steele C, Collins E, eds. *Infant and Pediatric Feedings: Guidelines for Preparation of Human Milk and Formula in Health Care Facilities*. 3rd ed. Academy of Nutrition and Dietetics; 2019.
61. Rayyis SF, Ambalavanan N, Wright L, Carlo WA. Randomized trial of "slow" versus "fast" feed advancements on the incidence of necrotizing enterocolitis in very low birth weight infants. *J Pediatr*. 1999;134(3):293–297.
62. Klein CJ. Nutrient requirements for preterm infant formulas. *J Nutr*. 2002;132(6 Suppl 1):1395S–577S.

CHAPTER 20

Nutrition in Pediatrics

Jennifer Shiel
Kathy Prelack

CHAPTER OUTLINE

CORE CONCEPTS

1. Growth velocity and rates of gain in weight and length are well described, with the most rapid rates of gain during the first few months of life.
2. Body composition changes throughout childhood. Nutritional risk is greater in children 0–2 years of age due to a greater fat versus fat-free mass content and lower percentage of body protein.
3. Underweight is defined as low weight-for-age. Failure to gain weight may indicate acute or short-term deficits, history of insult, or long-term illness.
4. Stunting, or low height-for-age, may be indicative of long-term ongoing illness, genetic or endocrine abnormalities, or a history of insult.
5. Wasting refers to low weight-for-height or BMI-for-age and is an indication of recent and severe state of undernutrition. Wasting may be the result of disease and is responsive to nutrition intervention.
6. Growth charts are used to evaluate growth from birth to age 20 years. Serial measures of weight and height and their patterns can be used to determine nutritional status, as well as growth abnormalities and their potential etiology.
7. Energy and protein needs, per kilogram of body weight, are the highest at birth and plateau through early childhood, as a consequence of changes in growth.
8. Vitamins and minerals, especially calcium, iron, and vitamin D, provide essential nutrients for growth and development. Without adequate micronutrient status, children may have impaired growth.
9. At each stage, children should consume a well-balanced diet. Eating environment, parental modeling, and nutrition knowledge can all influence eating practices.
10. Growth faltering (or failure to thrive) must be addressed using an interprofessional approach, including feeding based on catch-up energy and nutrient requirements to prevent developmental delays and child mortality.
11. Nutrition support may be indicated in pediatric patients when oral feeding does not provide enough energy or nutrients. Timely initiation, particularly in children younger than 2 years of age, prevents rapid deterioration of nutritional status.

LEARNING OBJECTIVES

1. Compare and contrast body composition in different stages of growth and the implications for nutrition therapy.
2. Assess growth utilizing standardized growth charts, as appropriate for age.
3. Differentiate among patterns of growth abnormalities, including failure to gain weight, failure to grow, and stunting, and identify causal factors and etiology for each.
4. Assess malnutrition in children using anthropometric indices and standardized z-scores.
5. Relate introduction and progression of food with developmental cues in children.
6. Describe how pediatric macronutrient and micronutrient requirements change throughout childhood.
7. Identify common feeding problems among children and determine appropriate interventions.
8. Assess nutritional status using anthropometric, biochemical, clinical, dietary, and physical examination information.
9. Define growth faltering and its contributing factors.
10. Determine catch-up growth needs.
11. Develop an enteral nutrition care plan for the pediatric patient.
12. Describe parenteral nutrition needs of the pediatric patient.

Introduction

Childhood is a period of rapid growth and development. From birth to age 20 years, a child undergoes many physical, social, and developmental changes. Nutrition plays a vital role in this process. Assuring adequate nutritional status requires a multifaceted approach at each stage of development, with attention given to the role of increasing independence, peer influence, and environmental factors. When faced with disease and critical illness, children are vulnerable to altered growth and malnutrition. A comprehensive nutritional assessment and prompt initiation of nutrition intervention, including nutritional support, may be necessary to prevent complications such as dehydration and weight loss, as well as long-term consequences in growth.

As with adults, pediatric malnutrition is diagnosed using specific criteria. In children, growth velocity and z-scores for measures of weight, length, weight for length, or body mass index (BMI) are used to define malnutrition as well as growth as compared to reference standards.

This chapter will explore the foundations of pediatric nutrition. Child-specific nutrition assessment and normal nutrient requirements from birth to young adulthood will be discussed. The case study will prompt evaluation of growth trends and abnormalities, identification of common nutrition problems, and development of appropriate nutrition intervention strategies, including nutrition support therapy.

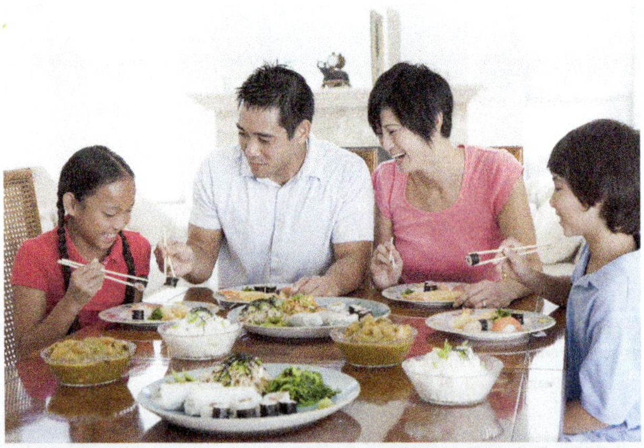

Growth and Development

Physical Growth and Its Characteristics

Growth is defined as an increase in physical size or mass of body tissues that occurs from infancy to adulthood. Growth is a defining process of childhood. It indicates more than just nutritional status because it can be a predictor of overall health and disease risk later in life. Growth is measured throughout childhood, beginning immediately after birth. Head circumference, recumbent length, and weight are key indices of growth among infants. As children grow older, the appropriate measures of growth become height and weight.

Children typically grow in **growth channels**, which are trajectories of growth. Although some deviations are expected, larger variations in growth can be a cause for concern. **Growth velocity** is the rate at which a child grows.[1] Growth velocity is greatest in the first year of life. The rate of growth then declines from age 1 to the onset of puberty. Once a child enters

CASE STUDY INTRODUCTION

Peter is a 4-month-old male infant referred to you by his pediatrician. Peter's family just moved to the area and are establishing care. During his initial routine visit, his parents express to the nurse practitioner their concern that he is not gaining enough weight. His mother reports that her first two children had hearty appetites and rapidly gained weight throughout the first few months of life. You are consulted to assess Peter's growth and meet with him and the family after the pediatrician examines Peter. As you screen for the medical record, you obtain the following information:

Anthropometric Data:

Age	Birth	3 months	4 months
Weight (kg)	3.3	5.2	5.4
Length (cm)	50	58	62

Biochemical Data:

None

Clinical Data:

Past Medical History: Peter was the product of a healthy, term pregnancy delivered via an uncomplicated vaginal delivery.

Social History: Parents married. Siblings: brother, 5 years of age, and a sister, 3 years of age. Mom is currently staying at home with children. Family has relocated to be closer to Dad's workplace.

Medications: He is not currently on any medications. He has had no previous ailments and is up to date with his vaccinations.

Vital Signs: Normal

Nutrition-Focused Physical Exam: Upon physical exam, you notice that Peter is difficult to arouse and appears thin. His lips are dry and slightly swollen. His eyes appear sunken and his abdomen is slightly distended.

Dietary Data:

Dietary History: For the past 4 months, Peter has been exclusively breastfed. His mother indicates that he normally feeds 8–10 times per day for approximately 45 minutes, sometimes up to an hour. She also reports that Peter tends to "spit up" after most feedings in significant amounts.

Questions

1. Identify Peter's anthropometric data at birth, 3 months, and 4 months on the correct growth chart. How might you classify Peter's pattern of growth?
2. What does your nutrition-focused physical exam reveal about Peter?
3. What are Peter's nutritional risk factors? Is Peter's feeding pattern adequate? What is concerning?
4. Write two Nutrition Diagnosis statements for Peter identifying the Problem/Etiology/Signs and Symptoms (PES) of Peter's active nutrition issues.
5. Identify the nutrition interventions you would like to initiate for Peter to address the problems identified in your PES statements.
6. What parameters will you monitor? What is Peter's expected daily weight gain?

puberty, they again experience greater rates of growth. Males and females grow at similar rates, with growth velocities diverging at the onset of puberty. This can be reflected in growth curves as children enter the adolescent years.

For pediatric patients, weight is assessed frequently. In newborns, weight is measured monthly during pediatrician visits. In newborns who are at nutritional risk, daily weight gain may be evaluated. Changes in length are not evident on a daily basis and are evaluated over a longer time span. The World Health Organization (WHO) provides statistical data by which growth can be assessed in children during early ages. **Table 20.1** shows the median weight gain during the first 60 days of life based on WHO data. Soon after birth, weight loss is expected; thereafter, the median daily weight increment ranges between 21–47 g/day in males and 14–39 g/day in females.

Table 20.1 Weight Velocity in the First 60 Days for Males and Females

	Boys			Girls		
Age (days)	Median (g/day)	25% (g/day)	5% (g/day)	Median (g/day)	25% (g/day)	5% (g/day)
0–7	21	5	−36	14	0	−29
7–14	36	19	−7	19	14	−7
14–28	47	38	25	39	32	21
28–42	40	32	21	35	27	18
42–60	34	28	18	39	22	15

Data from World Health Organization. *WHO Child Growth Standards*. November 2009. Data based on children with birthweight 2000–4000 g; values represent daily weight gain (g/day); median, 25th, and 5th percentiles.

Table 20.2 Weight and Length Velocity for Males and Females During the First Year in Life

Age (Months)	Weight Increment (g/day)	Range (g/day)	Length Increment (cm/3 months)	Range (cm/3 months)
Males				
0–3	36	23–50	11	9–14
3–6	19	10–30	6	4–9
6–9	11	4–21	4	3–6
9–12	9	1–18	4	2–6
Females				
0–3	31	19–46	11	8–13
3–6	18	10–28	6	4–8
6–9	11	4–20	4	3–6
9–12	8	1–17	4	2–6

Data from World Health Organization. *WHO Child Growth Standards*. November 2009. Values represent daily weight gain (g/day) with ranges based on ±2 standard deviations from the mean. Length is presented in 3-month increments (cm) with ranges based on ±2 standard deviations from the mean.

Thereafter weight and height decline as the child ages (**Table 20.2**). It is important to interpret growth according to the child's own trajectory and according to other factors such as ethnicity, parental size, and a child's natural growth disposition.[2]

CORE CONCEPT 1

Growth velocity and rates of gain in weight and length are well described, with the most rapid rates of gain during the first few months of life.

Body Composition During Growth

Body composition of children greatly differs from that of adults. In this respect, children are not just small adults. Generally, younger children have less lean body mass (LBM) as well as less fat mass but have far greater energy needs per kilogram of body weight than adults. In addition, in the early stages of life, LBM tends to be composed of less protein and more water. When injured or facing metabolic stress, this can put infants and young children at greater nutritional risk.

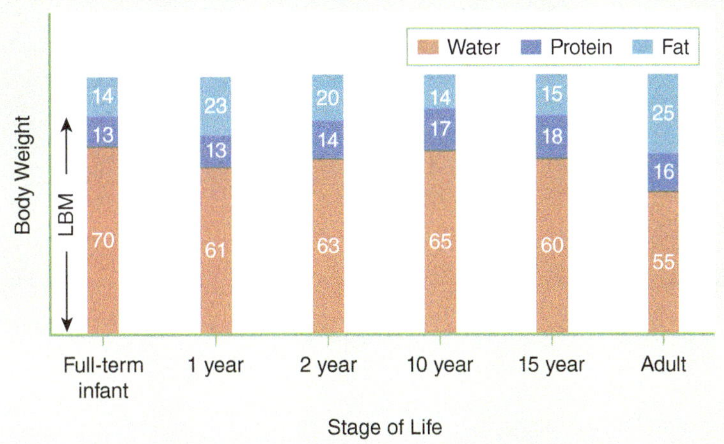

Figure 20.1 Changes in Body Composition During Growth

Body composition varies based on stage of development (**Figure 20.1**). At birth, the body composition of children is primarily composed of water (70%), with diminished lean body protein and fat masses. Preterm infants are at an even greater risk because they have marginal fat stores and LBM of poorer quality (meaning more water and less protein content). As they grow, infants gain proportionally more fat than LBM. Furthermore, the quality of their LBM with respect to protein content remains low, at approximately 13% throughout the first year of life.[3–5] Because infants preferentially rely on glucose versus fat as an energy source, they are at high risk for LBM depletion. In situations of stress that result in accelerated gluconeogenesis, LBM reserves are quickly exhausted. This can sometimes be masked by their abundant fat stores. Lastly, given their larger proportion of viscera and skin to overall body mass, infants are at greater risk for heat and evaporative water losses, making them prone to dehydration and electrolyte imbalance.[4]

CORE CONCEPT 2

Body composition changes throughout childhood. Nutritional risk is greater in children 0–2 years of age due to a greater fat versus fat-free mass content and lower percentage of body protein.

After 2 years of age, there is a gradual increase in the quantity and quality of LBM. Increases in both protein and bone mineral content take place. By age 10 years, a child's protein content is approximately 17% and bone mineral content is 4%. Combined with this is a diminished reliance on glucose as a primary energy source, making older children at lower risk for LBM depletion than infants.[4] Fat content as a proportion of body weight is less than that of infancy and young age. However, prolonged calorie deficits in prepubertal children are still harmful, because they result in an increased rate of fat mass depletion.

Between 6 and 8 years of age, there is a second rapid increase in body mass primarily in the form of adipose tissue. The timing of this **adiposity rebound** can be an indicator of adult body composition. Research has indicated that those who experience an early adiposity rebound are at a greater risk for adult obesity.[6] Adolescence is the next stage of development, which begins around age 10 years and continues until age 17–18 years in females and age 20 years in males. This is a time of increased growth velocity resulting in increases in body mass and height. Sexual dimorphism exists at this stage, where females gain more fat mass relative to lean tissue. Males demonstrate fat mass gain during pre-pubescence, followed by a rapid gain in LBM.[7,8] The fat-free mass plateaus around age 17 years for females and age 20 years for males. When faced with metabolic stress or illness, older adolescents are at a lower risk than younger children because they have greater energy reserves compared to their metabolic rate.[4]

Nutrition Screen

A nutrition screen helps to identify patients who may be at nutritional risk. It is the first step in identifying the presence of factors that can contribute to poor growth or intake as well as malnutrition. There are numerous nutrition screening tools (NSTs) that have been validated in the pediatric population (**Table 20.3**). Questions asked fall into the general categories of diminished intake or increased losses, impact of disease, clinical signs of muscle or fat wasting, and weight loss

Table 20.3 Nutrition Risk Screening Tools for Pediatric Patients

Screening Tool	Description	Intake and Losses	Clinical or Medical Diagnosis	Measures of Weight or Height
PNRS Pediatric Nutrition Risk Score	Developed for patients >1-month old at risk for malnutrition. Score of 0–5 with 4–5 high risk	X	Disease severity	Anthropometrics
PNST Pediatric Nutrition Screening Tool	Simplified screening tool with 4 basic yes/no questions. Two affirmative response indicates risk. Does not require measure of anthropometrics	X		
PMST Pediatric Malnutrition Screening Tool	For hospitalized children less than 2 up to 17 years; screens for both under- and overnutrition	X	Includes malnutrition points for BMI >85th and >98th percentile	Includes BMI
STAMP Screening Tool for the Assessment of Malnutrition	Validated in hospitalized children ages 0–16. Includes medical diagnosis, intake, and measured anthropometrics to determine malnutrition risk	X	Assesses nutritional implication of disease	Weight and height percentiles
STAMP(Mod) Screening Tool for the Assessment of Malnutrition in Pediatrics-Modified	STAMP(Mod) adapted for outpatient setting. Scoring generates lower points and risk. Also requires measured anthropometrics	X	Assesses nutritional implication of disease	Weight and height percentiles
STRONGkids Screening Tool for Risk on Nutritional Status and Growth	Allows for subjective assessment, includes questions on intake, losses, weight loss, or poor growth	X	Includes scoring for high-risk diseases	

Data from Academy of Nutrition and Dietetics. *Evidence Analysis Library. Nutrition Screening Pediatrics (NSP) Systematic Review (2017–2018).* Barriers to intake are assessed, including factors such as appetite, inability to eat, and pain. Losses most commonly refer to gastrointestinal losses due to vomiting and diarrhea..

or poor weight gain. Tools exist for both inpatient and outpatient settings as well as age and population types. For example, the Pediatric Nutrition Risk Score (PNRC) and Pediatric Nutrition Screening Tool (PNST) are designed to identify risk in hospitalized children greater than 1 year of age. Other screening tools for inpatients include the Screening Tool for Risk on Nutritional Status and Growth (STRONGkids), the Screening Tool for the Assessment of Malnutrition (STAMP), and the Pediatric Malnutrition Screening Tool (PMST). STAMP allows for reassessment and has also been modified to be used in an outpatient setting. STAMP and STRONGkids have shown to be the most reliable to date and are used in many different countries.[9,10]

Nutrition Assessment

Nutrition assessment is a process of evaluating several different components to determine nutritional risk and status, diagnose malnutrition if it exists, identify problems that need intervention, and establish a plan of care. Information is drawn from anthropometrics, biochemical data, medical history, nutrition-focused physical exam, diet history, and discussion with other healthcare team members. In children, obtaining laboratory values is less routine than in adults. Similarly, children typically have a brief medical history, if any. Therefore, anthropometrics, along with a detailed diet history and nutrition-focused physical exam, serve as the cornerstones of a nutrition assessment.

Anthropometric Measures

Anthropometrics are the measurement of physical characteristics of the human body. Anthropometric measurements include height, weight, head circumference, BMI, skin fold thickness, and arm circumference. These measures are used to evaluate the growth of a child and can also provide indicators of overall well-being and nutritional status. Accurate measurement of growth in children is critical for nutrition evaluations. Measures of weight and length or height should be taken at every hospital or physician office visit. Anthropometric data are most useful when **serial measures** are taken because they demonstrate patterns of growth and they allow for comparison to reference standards.[2] Patterns of growth can also help determine etiology and hence the appropriate intervention.

PRACTICE POINT

Measures of weight and length or height should be taken at every hospital admission.

Stature: Length or Height

In infants, recumbent length is used instead of height. Recumbent length is measured using a fixed headboard with a movable footboard. The child lies flat on the length board with their head positioned against the headboard and eyes looking straight up. Length is measured from the vortex to the soles of their feet. It is best to have two individuals taking this measurement because it can be difficult to have a child maintain a straight position while they are measured (**Figure 20.2**). Recumbent length is typically greater than height by about 0.5 cm. This is the most difficult measurement to accurately obtain in young children.

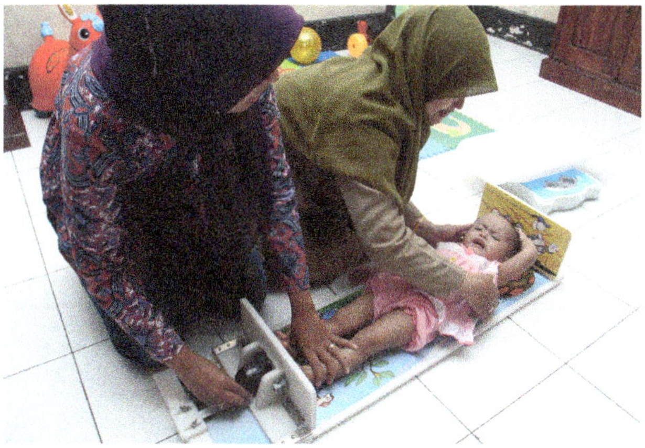

Figure 20.2 Two-Person Method of Measuring Length in an Infant Child

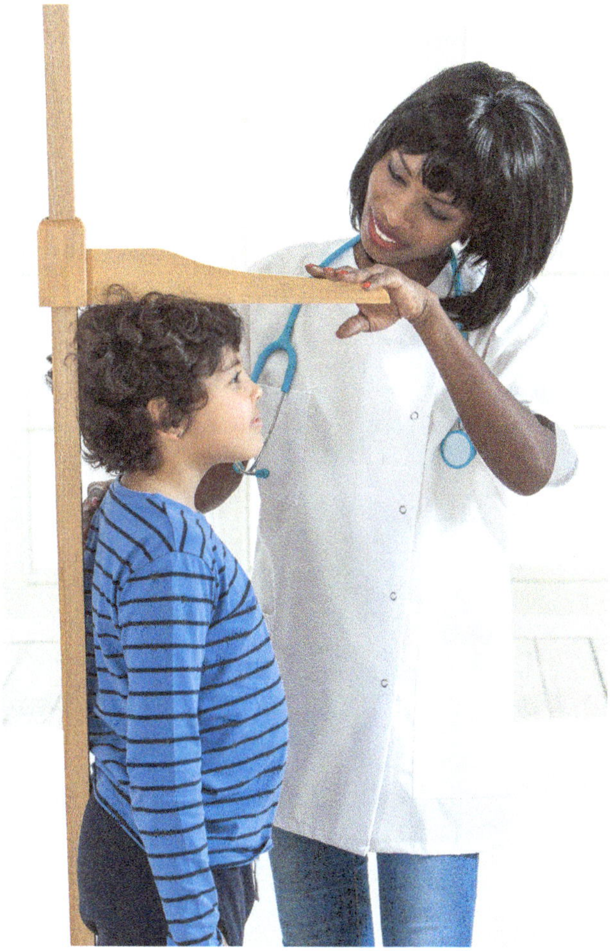

Figure 20.3 Measurement of Height in Older Child by Stadiometer

Once children are older and can stand up straight, their height is measured using a stadiometer, as displayed in **Figure 20.3**.

The height of a child when they are standing up can be referred to as their "stature." The child should stand in bare feet with their occipital part of the cranium, shoulder blades, and buttocks against the wall.

Another reference point of height is the **mid-parental height** of the child. This can provide an indication of how the child is expected to grow. It is important to note that if parents are unusually tall or short, the resulting mid-parental height can be a poor indicator of child stature. The target height, when estimated by mid-parental, is the parent's height ± 2 standard deviations, which is about 10 cm.[11]

For females

$$\text{Mid}-\text{parental Height} = \frac{(\text{Maternal Height (cm)} + \text{Paternal Height (cm)} - 13)}{2}$$

For males

$$\text{Mid}-\text{parental Height} = \frac{(\text{Maternal Height (cm)} + \text{Paternal Height (cm)} + 13)}{2}$$

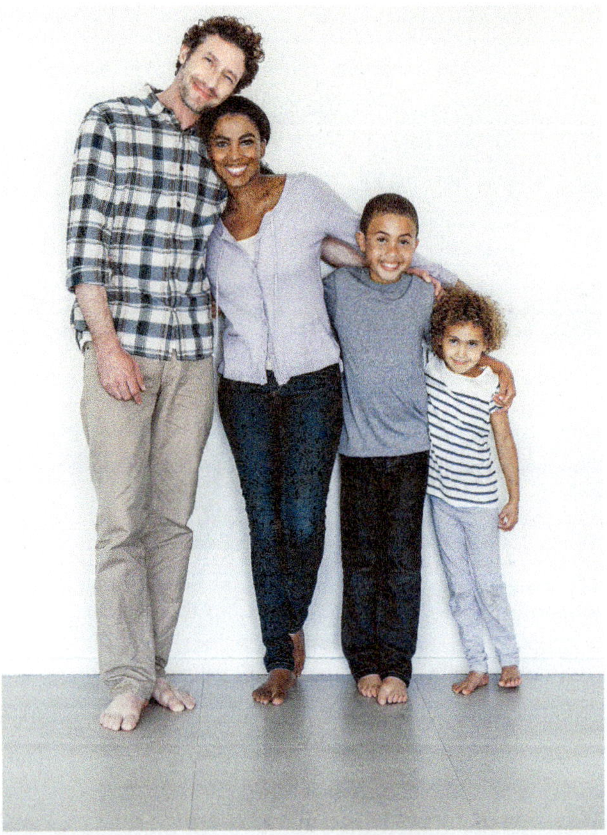

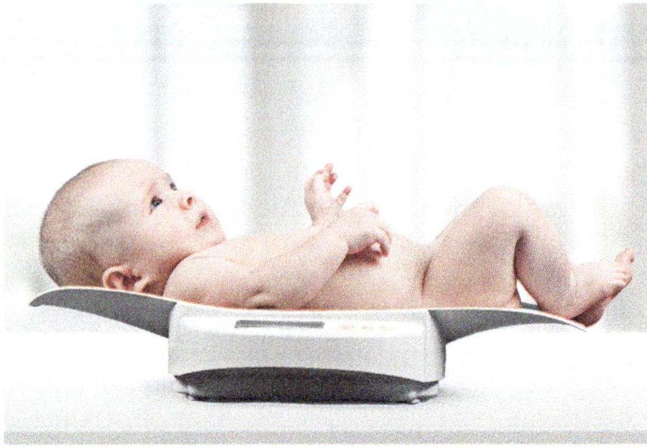

Figure 20.4 Measurement of Weight in Infant Child

Weight

Body weight is used as a basic indicator of nutritional status. It is most sensitive to changes in nutritional intake and health. Infants should be measured nude (**Figure 20.4**), while children can be weighed in light clothing. Although weight is a key component of assessment measures, it can be influenced by many factors. For example, weight is influenced by fluid status, fed or fasting state, scale accuracy, and interobserver error. It is best to control for some of these factors by taking serial measures using the same scale and the same trained observers.

Infants can also be measured using the tare method. Using this method, the parent first steps on the scale, which is then tared. Next, the parent holds the child and together they are weighed, and the weight recorded on the scale is that of the infant.

Head Circumference

Head circumference (HC) is taken by wrapping a tape measure around the most prominent area on the back of the head, immediately above the supraorbital ridge, to just above the patient's eyebrows. This will provide the greatest circumference (**Figure 20.5**). This measure is only performed up to 36 months of age. HC that is ± 2 standard deviations below the mean or below the 2nd percentile may indicate microcephaly. **Microcephaly** at birth can be due to a variety of genetic disorders. Normal HC at birth followed by a decline in HC is known as "acquired microcephaly," which can be the result of an infectious process such as meningitis and may indicate poor brain growth or development. **Macrocephaly** is when HC is more than ± 2 standard deviations larger than the mean.[12] HC is the least sensitive to undernutrition, and changes

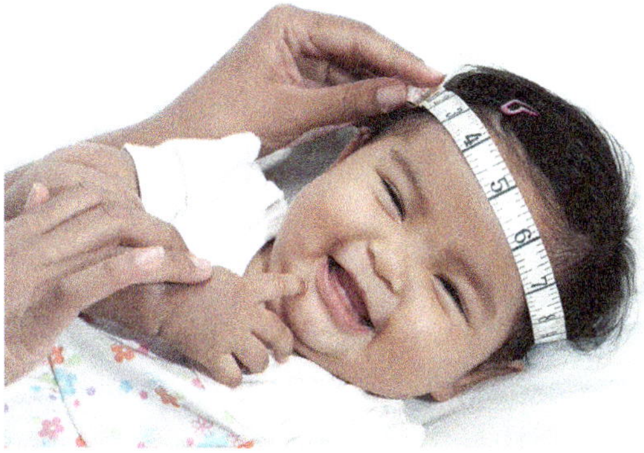

Figure 20.5 Measurement of Head Circumference in an Infant Child

in height and weight will occur before those in HC. Like height and weight, HC can be analyzed using a growth chart.

Body Mass Index

BMI is a key indicator used in nutrition assessment. It represents weight in kilograms divided by stature in meters squared. In essence, BMI is an index of weight relative to height. In younger children, weight-for-height is interpreted in a similar way and is used to define overweight and obesity in children younger than 2 years of age. BMI is calculated beginning at age 2 years (prior to age 2 years, weight-for-length is used) and is interpreted using BMI percentiles (BMI-for-age). BMI-for-age is useful in determining overweight and obesity, as well as wasting. Children with a BMI-for-age greater than the 95th percentile are considered obese. Those within the 85th–94th percentile are considered overweight.[13,14]

$$\text{BMI} = \frac{\text{Weight (kg)}}{\text{Stature (m)}^2}$$

Skinfold Thickness and Arm Circumference Measurements

Skinfold thickness (SFT) is used to estimate percent fat by measuring the skinfold at various parts of the body. Most commonly, SFT is measured using a skinfold caliper at the midpoint of the arm between the acromion and olecranon.[15] Measurements should be taken from the same arm each time, with the arm relaxed. A skinfold caliper is used to pull the layer of skin along with the subcutaneous fat tissue away from the muscle. Measurements are then recorded to 0.5 mm. Using predictive equations, the percentage of body fat can be determined. Caution should be used when predicting body fat mass from skinfold measurements in children. Use of the predictive equations should match the population being measured. In addition, these measurements should be taken carefully and repeated for accuracy. Effort should be made to ensure that the muscle layer is not included in the measurement. Lastly, the clinician should keep in mind changes in body composition that occur during growth, particularly fat distribution surrounding prepubertal and pubertal years.

Mid-upper arm circumference (MUAC) is another anthropometric measurement that can be used to determine nutritional status and identify malnutrition. Measures of MUAC represents a measure of muscle mass and can be compared to reference standard. Similar to SFT, the circumference is taken from the midpoint of the arm between the acromion and olecranon. Measures of MUAC and SFT combined can be used to determine another parameter: mid-upper arm muscle area (AMA). Reference comparative standards exist for all of these measures for children ages 1–20.[15,16]

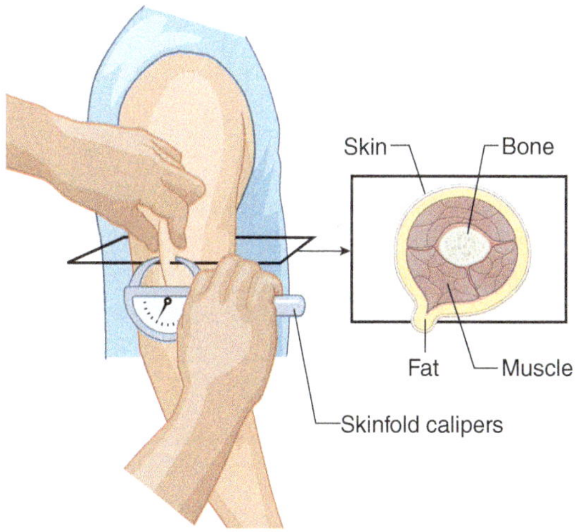

Skinfold Thickness

Evaluating Growth Using Standardized Growth Charts

Anthropometric measures are interpreted using **growth charts**. Use of growth charts dates back to the late 1800s.[1] Growth charts describe the normal or expected amount of growth based on well-child data. They depict the growth channels and velocity that correlate to patterns of growth in healthy children. There are two sets of charts: the WHO growth charts and the Centers for Disease Control and Prevention (CDC) growth charts.

WHO Growth Charts

In 1993, a review conducted by the WHO indicated that the existing growth curves developed based on National Center for Health Statistics (NCHS) and WHO data did not adequately describe early childhood growth. Soon after, the WHO Multicentre Growth Reference study, which included six different countries (Brazil, Ghana, India, Oman, Norway, and the United States), was initiated. The WHO charts begin at birth and describe growth of infants who were exclusively breastfed for the first 4–6 months (**Figure 20.6**). Infants in this sample then had complementary foods introduced at 6 months, in addition to human milk.[2]

The **WHO growth charts** are considered **growth standards**. They represent optimal growth or how typical children should grow when breastfed, which serves as the gold standard for feeding.[2] Compared to other growth data, the WHO data set is superior, compiled from more frequent serial measures from a significantly larger sample size, beginning at birth.[17] The WHO growth chart is the first to describe optimal growth for children.[2]

The WHO charts should be used from birth to age 2 years, according to the CDC and the American Academy of Pediatrics (AAP).[18] There are several parameters that can be evaluated on these charts, including weight-for-age, height-for-age, head-circumference-for-age, and weight-for-height, BMI, and growth velocity. Z-scores and percentiles exist for measures of tricep and subscapular skinfolds as well as arm circumference. Charts are sex-specific for males and females. Growth curves range from the 2nd to the 98th percentile.

CDC Growth Charts

The CDC charts were updated in May 2000 using NHANES II and NHANES III data.[19] The CDC charts also include data from Vital Statistics because the NHANES data do not include infants younger than 3 months. As a result, these charts fail to accurately capture the rapid weight gain that occurs during the first 6 months of life. In contrast to the WHO data, relatively few infants in this data set were exclusively breastfed for more than a few months. In addition, the data are more cross-sectional in design.[17]

The **CDC growth charts** are a **growth reference**. These charts describe growth in a specific time or place (**Figure 20.7**).[17] The CDC and AAP recommend that CDC charts are used to evaluate growth in children older than 2 years of age.[19] Like the WHO charts, they are sex-specific. There are several curves that can be used to evaluate a child's growth status, using percentiles or z-scores. These include weight-for-age, height-for-age, and BMI-for-age. BMI-for-age curves were developed when the CDC charts were updated in 2000. Due to the prevalence of obesity, in 2022, the CDC revised the BMI percentiles to further extend beyond the 97th percentile to include the 98th, 99th, 99.9th, and 99.99th percentiles.[20]

Application of z-Score Growth Charts to Evaluate Growth and Malnutrition

The WHO routinely applies **z-scores** to assess growth and nutritional status in children. A z-score can provide more specific information than the percentiles provided by growth charts for weight-for-age, height-for-age, BMI-for-age, and weight-for-height evaluations. The z-scores also enable a more precise assessment of change within an individual child's growth pattern or nutritional status. A z-score is a representation of the individual difference from the median.[21]

$$\text{z-score} = -\frac{\text{(Individual Anthropometric} \\ \text{Median Anthropometric)}}{\text{Standard Deviation}}$$

A z-score of 0 is considered normal, because it represents the median or the 50th percentile. The z-scores can range three standard deviations above or below the median. Positive z-scores indicate height, weight, or BMI that are above the median, whereas negative z-scores indicate height, weight, or BMI below the median.[21] It is recommended by the Academy of Nutrition and Dietetics (AND) and the American Society of Parenteral and Enteral Nutrition (ASPEN) that z-scores be used to classify children who are underweight, stunted, or wasted based on WHO standards (**Table 20.4**).[22] **Underweight** is defined as

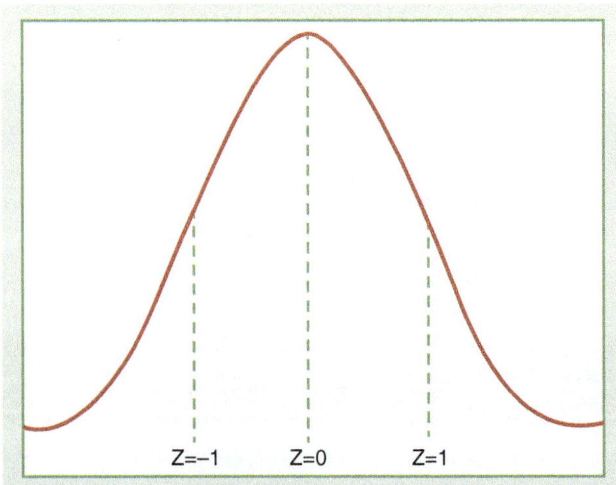

Z-Score

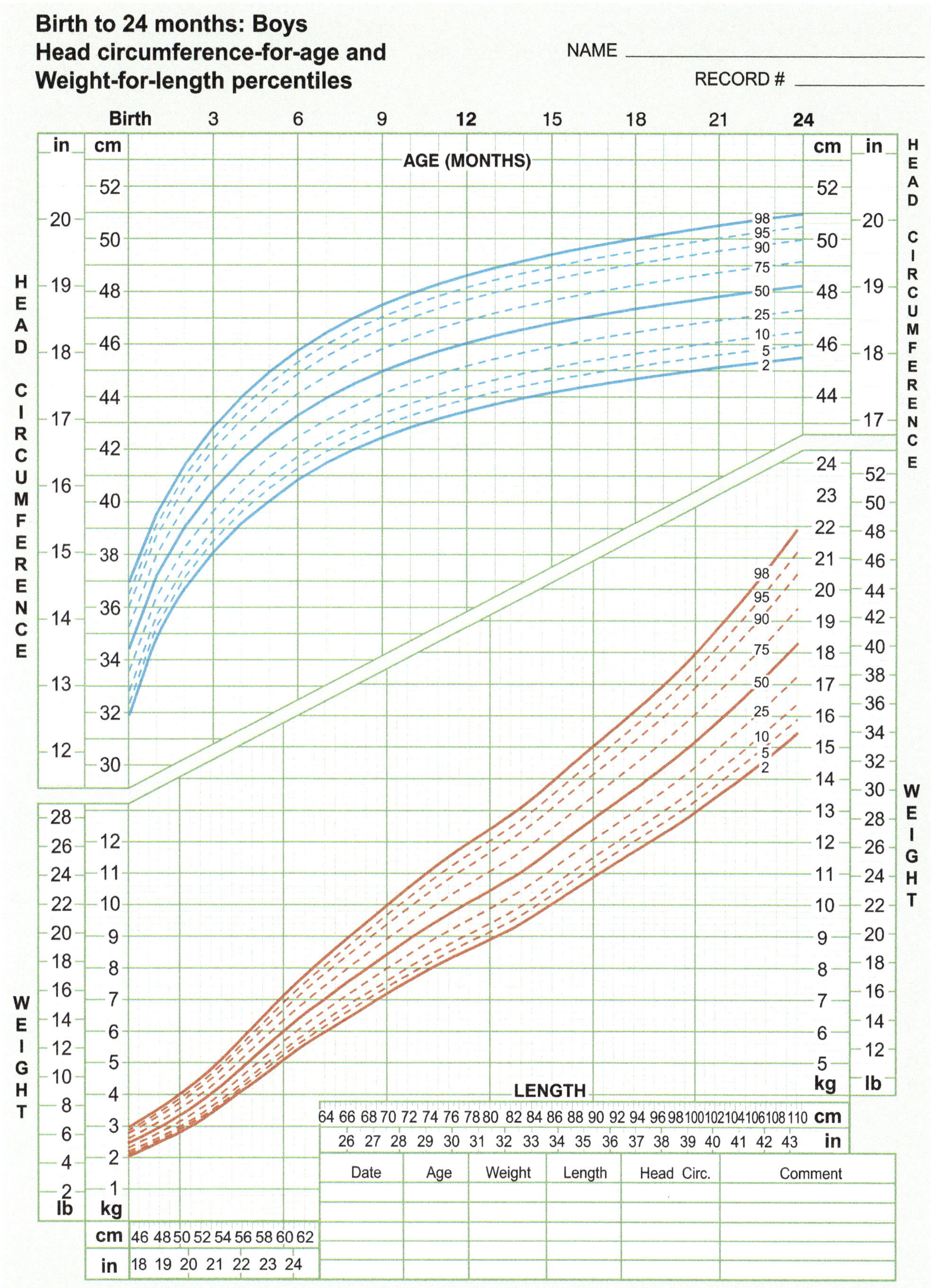

Figure 20.6 WHO Growth Charts for Weight for Age and Length for Age

Courtesy of the Centers for Disease Control and Prevention, November 1, 2009.

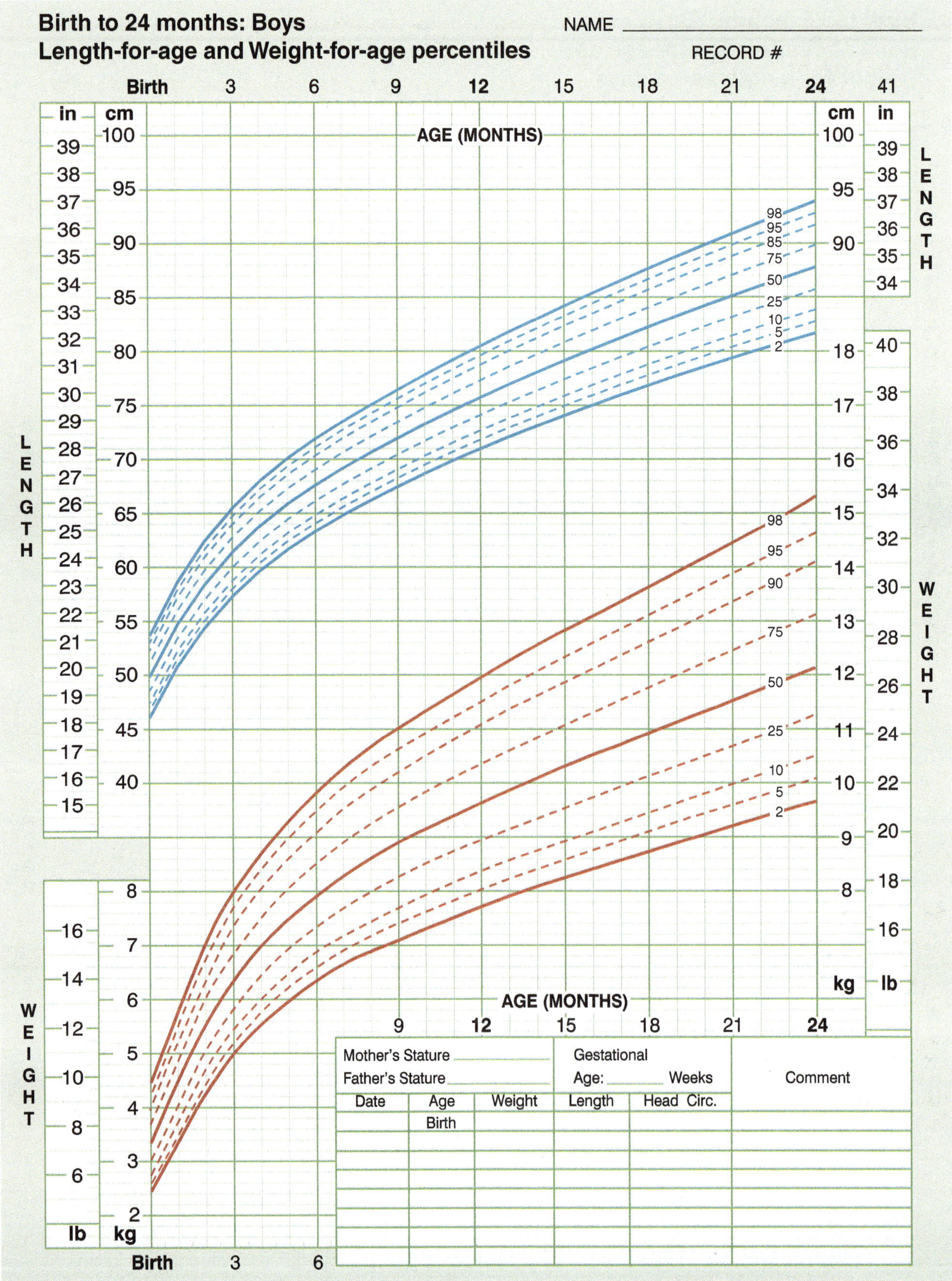

Figure 20.6 (continued)

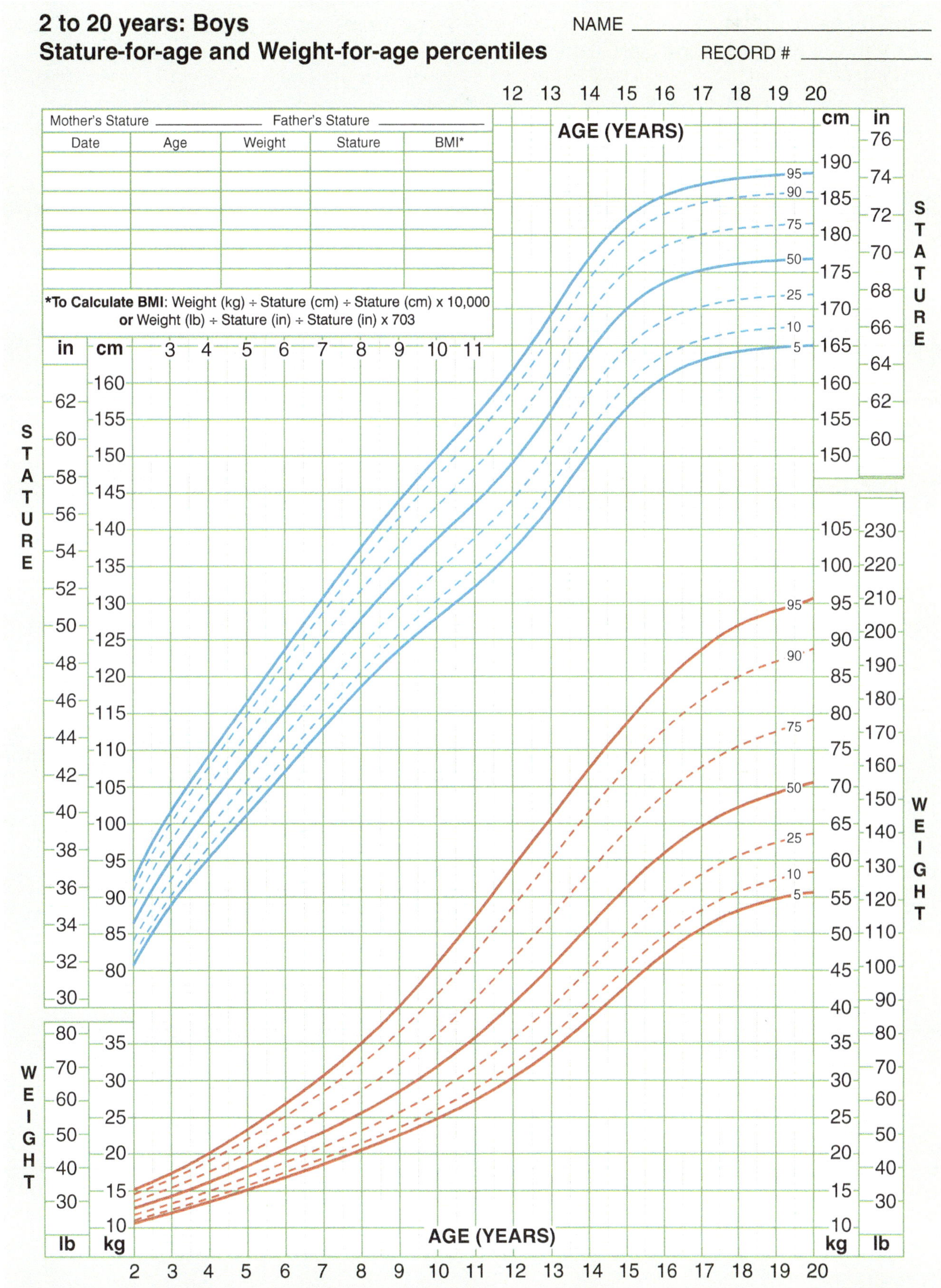

Figure 20.7 CDC Growth Charts for Weight for Age and Height for Age

Reproduced from Centers for Disease Control and Prevention. CDC growth charts: United States. Developed by the National Center for Health Statistics in collaboration with the National Center for Chronic Disease Prevention and Health Promotion; 2000. Accessed January 14, 2026. https://www.cdc.gov/growthcharts

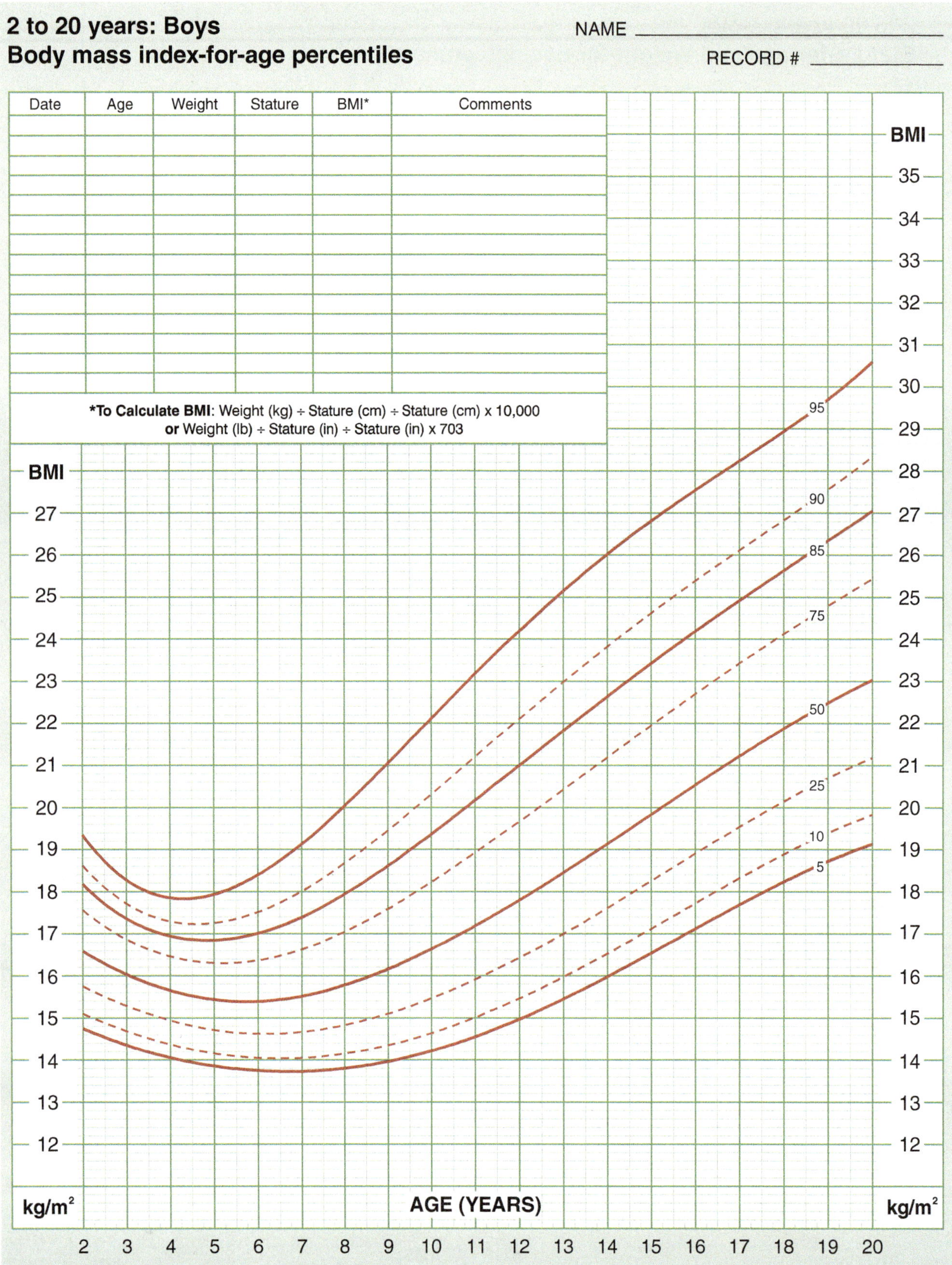

Figure 20.7 *(continued)*

Table 20.4 Interpretation of Z-Scores During Growth and Malnutrition

z-Score	Growth Indicators			
	Length/Height-for-Age	Weight-for-Age	Weight-for-Length/Height	BMI-for-Age
Above 3	Refer to note 1	Refer to note 2	Obese	Obese
Above 2			Overweight	Overweight
Above 1			Possible risk of overweight (refer to note 3)	Possible risk of overweight (refer to note 3)
0 (median)				
Below −1				
Below −2	Stunted (refer to note 4)	Underweight	Wasted	Wasted
Below −3	Severely stunted (refer to note 4)	Severely underweight (refer to note 5)	Severely wasted	Severely wasted

Notes:

1. A child in this range is very tall. Tallness is rarely a problem, unless it is so excessive that it may indicate an endocrine disorder such as a growth hormone–producing tumor. Refer a child in this range for assessment if you suspect an endocrine disorder (e.g., if parents of normal height have a child who is excessively tall for their age).
2. A child whose weight-for-age falls in this range may have a growth problem, but this is better assessed from weight-for-length/height or BMI-for-age.
3. A plotted point about 1 indicates possible risk. A trend toward the 2 z-score indicates definite risk.
4. It is possible for a stunted or severely stunted child to become overweight.
5. This is referred to as very low weight in IMCI training modules (*Integrated Management of Childhood Illness, In-Service Training*. WHO; 1997).

Reproduced from World Health Organization. *Training Course on Child Growth Assessment*. Geneva, Switzerland: World Health Organization; 2008.

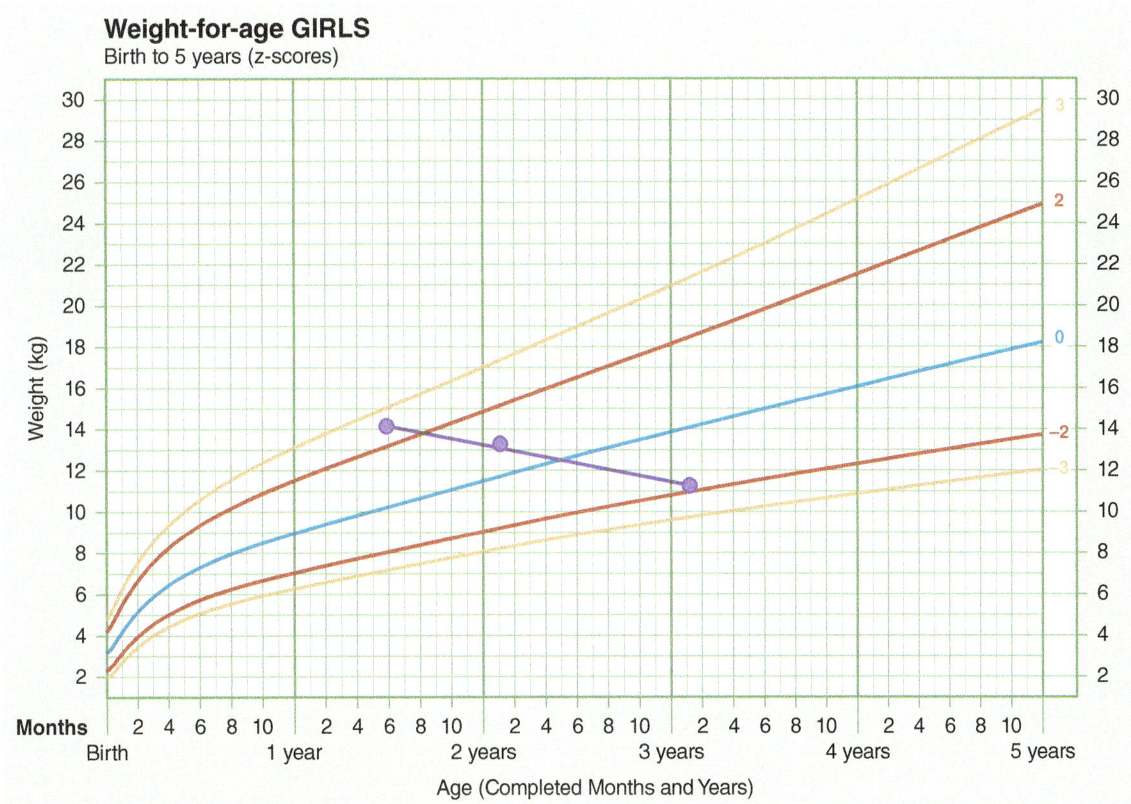

A

Figure 20.8 **A.** Using trends in z scores to evaluate growth. A-Z- scores show a downward trend in weight-for- age, crossing over 2 z score lines. **B.** A rapid transient decrease in weight-for -age representative of short term illness. Weight gain is restored eventually. **C.** This z score trend line demonstrate a decline in BMI-for-age over time. In cases of weight management, this may be a desirable outcome.

Reproduced from The WHO Child Growth Standards. Accessed at: http://www.who.int/childgrowth/standards/en/

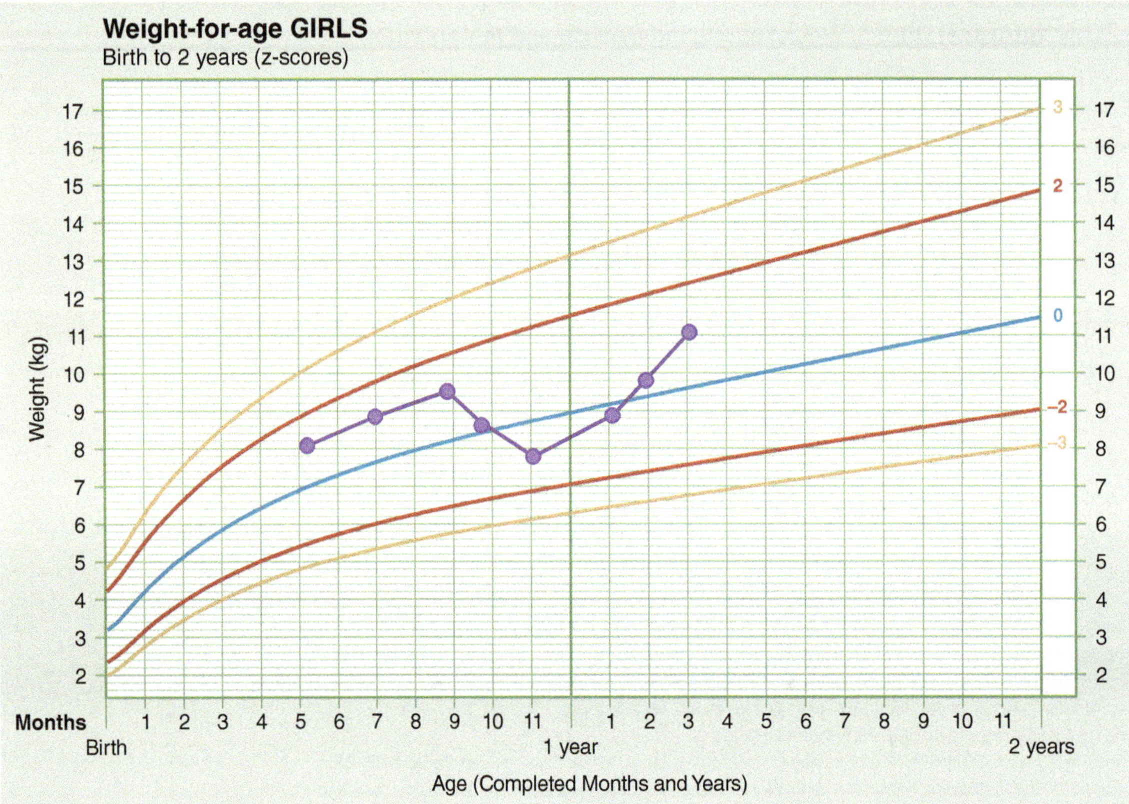

B

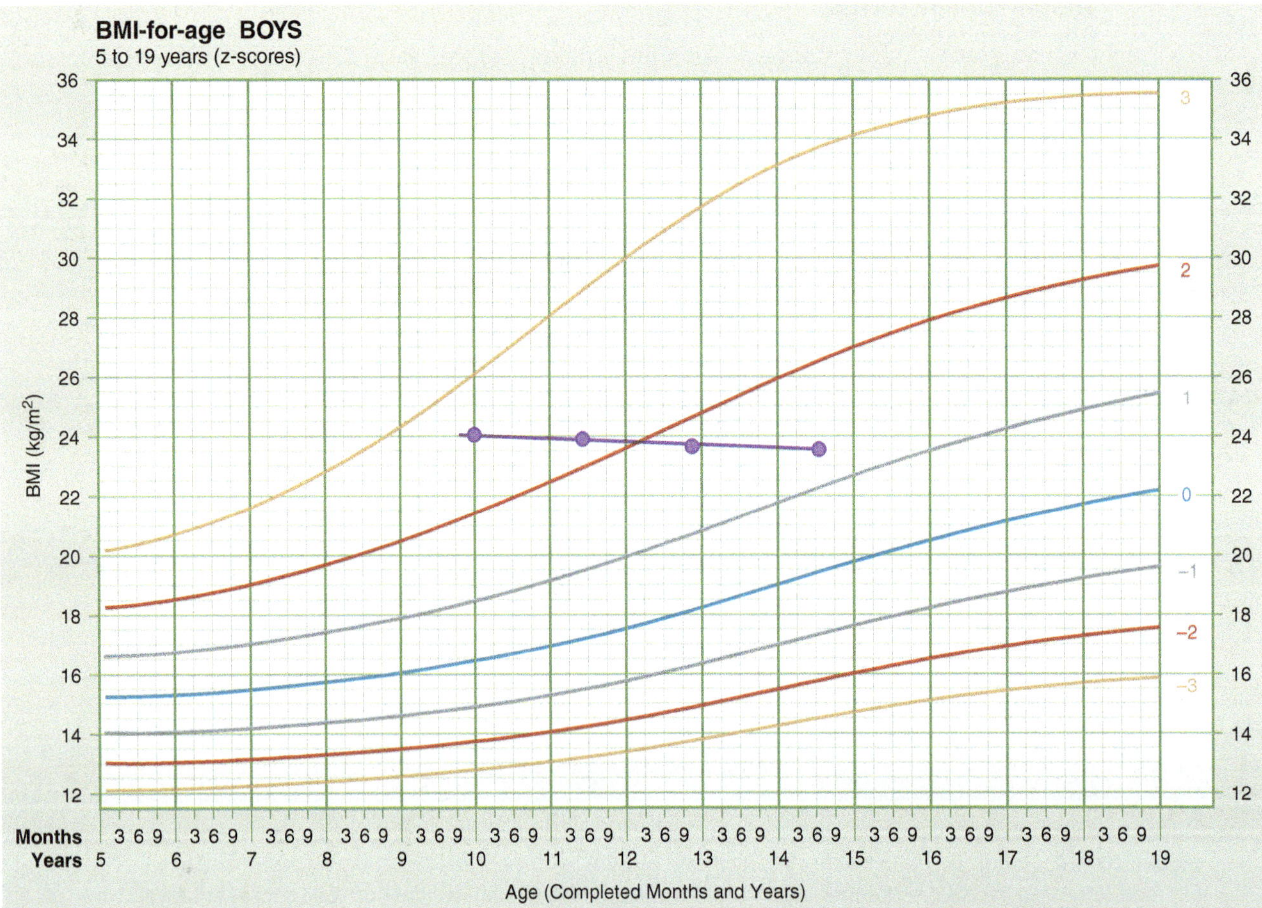

C

Figure 20.8 (continued)

a low weight-for-age, with a z-score less than −2, with severe underweight being defined as a z-score of less than −3. Stunting, defined as a low height-for-age, and wasting, defined as a low weight-for-height or low BMI-for-age, are similarly classified based on z-scores below the median. Z-scores can be calculated and are increasingly used to evaluate growth, often being included in the medical record.[13,22] Most healthy children will "track" along a certain z-score percentile. **Figure 20.8** shows how trends in z scores can be used to evaluate growth patterns. Patterns of concern include sharp increase or decline in trendline, crossing a z-score line, or a growth line that is flat (stagnation). Interpreting risk based on these trends requires consideration of many factors. For example, a rapid transient decrease in a trendline for weight may occur with short-term illness, whereas a gradual decline or a crossing of a z-score line can indicate chronic illness. On the other hand, children who are overweight may show a downward trendline in weight-for-height or BMI-for-age that is desirable.

Diet Interview and History

The goal of a diet history is to understand the overall pattern of eating and tolerance to food in a child. The focus of a diet interview and history will change based on the age and condition of the child. In newborns through infancy, emphasis is placed on frequency and duration of breast or formula feedings, tolerance to feedings, and introduction of complementary foods. Observing the infant feeding can provide useful information on adequacy of suck, positioning, tolerance to feeding, and comfort level of the caregiver (**Table 20.5**).

Diet interviews should screen for common nutritional problems during infancy such as diarrhea, constipation, gastroesophageal reflux (GERD), and colic (**Table 20.6**). Information on hydration and adequacy of intake can be assessed by determining frequency of wet diapers and stool patterns. Newborns can have up to 8–10 wet diapers or stools per day. Stool frequency varies and it is not unusual for babies to stool every 2–3 days, even up to a week in breastfed infants. Normal stools can be liquid or soft in earlier stages of life. Breastfed babies tend to have softer, more yellow stools than formula-fed infants. Constipation is a common problem and is useful to screen for during the interview. When identified, a proactive bowel regimen along with fiber and fluid intake can alleviate constipation. GERD occurs when food from the stomach refluxes into the esophagus. GERD often occurs when the lower esophageal sphincter is still immature. It usually resolves on its own and is rarely serious. However, anorexia, poor weight gain, and malnutrition can occur in some children, in which case medication is often then used. When GERD is refractory to medications and the baby is not growing, surgery may be indicated.

For children older than 6 months, a 24-hour diet recall or 3-day food record, similar to adults, can be taken. However, food type and quantity do not describe the full picture. There are many factors that influence the pediatric diet history, and these can change throughout childhood. As a child ages, information about introduction to foods, vitamin and mineral supplementation, and food intolerance or food allergies are important. At every age, it is necessary to understand the cultural and socioeconomic factors that influence a child's nutrition. The diet interview should address parental beliefs and knowledge, dietary customs, eating behaviors, and developmental cues to eating.

Table 20.5 Dietary Assessment of Breast feeding and Formula Intake in Infants

Feeding Method	Questions to Ask	General Guidelines
Breastfed	Frequency and duration Complementary feedings/foods Is the mother expressing her breast milk? Vitamin/mineral or other supplements?	On-demand feeding suggested Feed every 2–3 hours, or 8–12 feedings in 24 hours. *If feeds are shorter than 10 minutes* Possible insufficient breast milk *If feeds are longer than 50 minutes* Possible ineffective sucking, an anatomic cause, or low milk production
Formula fed	Formula intake and preparation Nipple used Complementary foods Vitamin/mineral supplementation	Approximately 2–3 oz (60–90 mL) per feeding for the first month (6–8 times per day) Individual variation; look for hunger and satiety cues Volume increases and frequency decreases

Data from CDC. Infant and Toddler Nutrition. https://www.cdc.gov/infant-toddler-nutrition/about/index.html

Table 20.6 Common Nutrition-Related Problems in Infants

Problem	Evaluation	Signs and Symptoms	Recommended Treatment
Stool patterns	Normal *Breastfed:* loose, soft to runny, seedy, yellow *Formula fed:* Thick, pasty consistency; green, tan, or yellow Stool frequency can vary from after each feed to 1 every 2 days	Diarrhea Difficult to define stool frequency can be high in first 1 month Decreases over 1 year Look for change in pattern to more frequent and watery Constipation Dry, hard, infrequent stools	Diarrhea Treat dehydration—normal diet if hydrated Fat restriction Lactose free Constipation Fluid Fiber
Colic	Babies usually cry if hungry or wet. Rule of Threes: Cries more than 3 h/d, 3 d/wk, for 3 weeks or more	Excessive crying or distress when otherwise healthy; predictable time of day or episodes; posture changes, such as clenched fists and abdominal tension	Short-lived, usually resolves over 3–6 months; parent may omit common allergens, hydrolyzed formula may help (avoid switching formula too much)
Gastroesophageal reflux (GERD)	Small amount of reflux several times per day is common in healthy babies	Symptoms include regurgitation, coughing, weight loss, anorexia, arching of the back when feeding	*Position changes:* Hold baby upright for 20–30 minutes after feeding; interrupt feeding to burp baby *Dietary changes:* Switch formula, thicken formula with rice cereal, use a different-sized nipple *Medications:* omeprazole or ranitidine

Data from *J. Pediatr. (Rio J.)* 92 (3 Suppl 1) • May–Jun 2016; https://doi.org/10.1016/j.jped.2016.02.008.

The diet interview in toddlers should recognize that most toddlers are able to eat on their own. Their eating practices are influenced by familial choices; therefore, asking about familial diet is useful.[23,24] Understanding a child's eating practices—how well they respond to newly introduced foods; their typical eating environment; and whether the child eats at the table with the family, in front of the television, or while playing—facilitates patient and parent education. A 3-day food record may be necessary because a child's eating habits vary from day to day. Information should be gathered about snack time, grazing between meals, and beverage consumption.

In children aged 3–10 years, diet interviews should focus on food eaten outside of the home, such as school lunch.[14] Nutrition knowledge, beliefs, and food intolerances or avoidances should be explored.[23,24] This concept extends to adolescence, where eating behavior is highly influenced by body image, peer pressure, home life, and eating environment.[25]

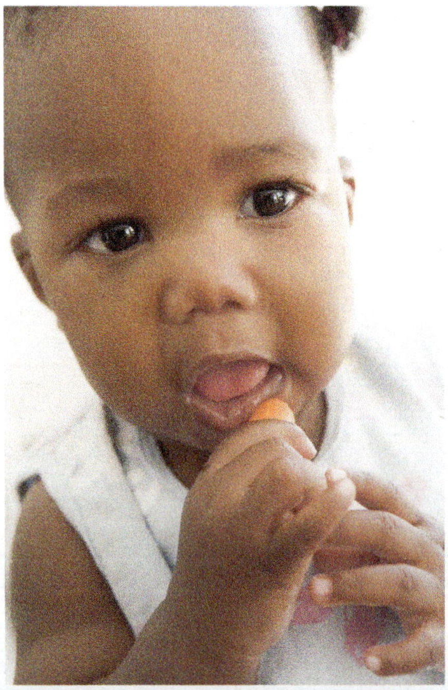

© Monkey Business Images/Shutterstock

Conferring with other clinicians can provide additional information on developmental milestones and social and environmental factors that arise in their individual assessments. An interprofessional approach to pediatric assessment lends itself to a better rounded, more comprehensive model of care and is considered best practice.

Nutrition-Focused Physical Exam

The physical exam is another vital piece of information for nutrition assessment. The physical exam should be completed in collaboration with the medical team. During the exam, the accuracy of anthropometric measures can be confirmed and signs of malnutrition can be detected.[10] The exam also provides the opportunity to developmentally assess the child. Development delays, such as an inability to hold the head up or hold utensils, may impact nutritional status and the child's ability to advance their diet. The nutrition-focused physical exam is critical in children because they are at the greatest risk for change in nutritional status and malnutrition.[10,26] Malnutrition can result in delays in growth and development if left undetected.

Physical examination of a pediatric patient uses similar techniques to those used in adults. Inspection is the visual examination of the patient, with particular emphasis on body color, symmetry, and shape. Palpation, or the touching and feeling of the patient, is another technique used to evaluate temperature, moisture, and tenderness. Percussion is a technique used on the abdomen to determine the presence of solids and air. The final technique used is auscultation, or listening to the sounds of the bowel using a stethoscope.

General Inspection

The first step of the exam is to inspect the patient. General inspection can confirm the patient's height and weight status, giving information beyond the actual anthropometric measure, particularly with respect to body composition and musculature. Overall appearance is important to assess, noting whether the child is restless, engaged, or lethargic. Look for signs of labored breathing or a fruity odor to the breath.

PRACTICE POINT

Assessing overall appearance provides useful information about the patient's overall health and disposition.

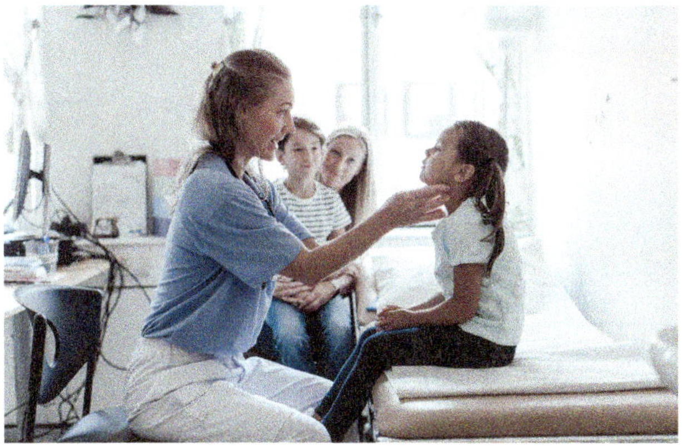

During this first step, it is important to monitor for signs of subcutaneous fat loss, muscle wasting, and edema.[10,26]

Head and Face

The next area to examine is the head and face. Inspect the head and face, assessing specifically for symmetry; temporal wasting, an indication of malnutrition; or puffiness of the eyes/eyelids, suggesting edema.[10,26] The patient's hair quality should be examined for fullness, texture, and symmetry. Hair quality may deteriorate with essential fatty acids, zinc, or biotin deficiency, as well as with insufficient protein or calorie intake. The examiner should also palpate the top of the head. Lack of closure in the anterior fontanelle by 18 months of age suggests that the infant may have a vitamin D deficiency.[26] A child's eyes should be inspected as part of the physical exam. Healthy eyes will appear shiny, bright, and clear with moist membranes. Abnormalities of the eyes can be related to vitamin A deficiency.

Oral Cavity

It is important to examine the oral cavity, which includes the lips, tongue, teeth, and gums, because many nutritional deficiencies can present in the mouth.[27] Many B vitamin deficiencies manifest in the oral cavity. Lips may appear dry and swollen.[27] A magenta coloration on the tongue may be an indication of folate, riboflavin, niacin, vitamin B_{12}, or iron deficiency.[26] Lesions discovered in the mouth should be noted because they may indicate iron or vitamin C deficiency. Vitamin C deficiency may also be indicated by bleeding gums. In addition to revealing micronutrient deficiencies, oral lesions may impair food intake. Children with stomatitis or soreness in the mouth may refuse to eat. Conditions such as GERD, bulimia, or celiac disease may result in the erosion of tooth enamel.[27]

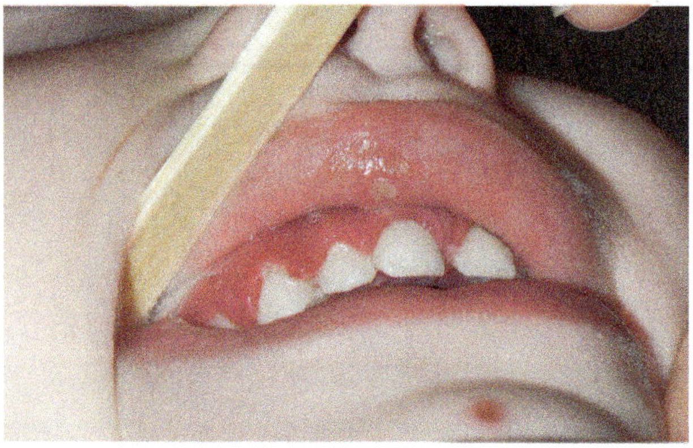

© Karen Grigoryan/Shutterstock

Skin and Nails

Skin integrity is clinically meaningful. Pallor, dry skin, or moist, clammy skin can be indicative of poor health or nutrition-related problems. Many micronutrient deficiencies first appear on the skin. The skin should be thoroughly examined for color, symmetry, marks or rashes, bruises, lacerations (cuts, scrapes, or tears), turgor, and flaking.[26] Skin abnormalities may be associated with iron, folate, vitamin B12, essential fatty acid, or zinc deficiency. Nails are easy to inspect and signal potential deficiencies of iron, protein, or vitamins A or C. Nails that are dull appearing, spoon shaped, or ridged, or that contain white spots, can be a sign of iron, protein, or other nutrient deficiencies.

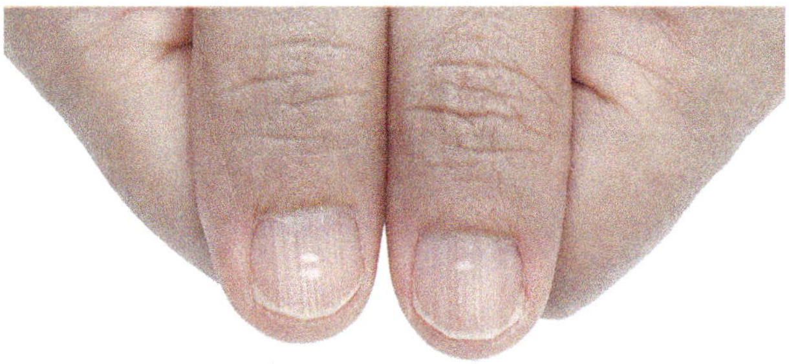

© Toa55/Shutterstock

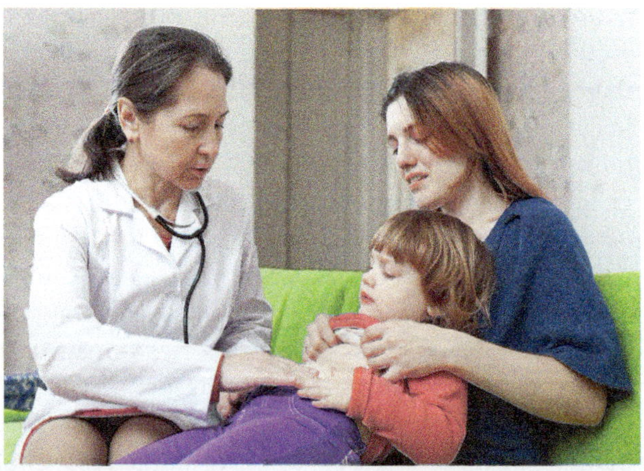

© Iakov Filimonov/Shutterstock

Abdominal Examination

The examination of the abdomen should begin with the practitioner standing over the child. The symmetries and delineation of the region should be examined. Next, observe the abdomen from the horizontal view in order to note the shape. A flat abdomen is considered to be normal and healthy. A scaphoid shape (sunken abdomen) indicates decreased subcutaneous fat stores, likely as a result of poor intake, whereas a protuberant abdomen is a sign of obesity.[26] Next, palpation of the area, feeling for texture, distention, and tenderness, is performed. The abdomen may feel firm or distended as a result of gas, fluid, or bowel obstruction.[26] Using the nondominant hand, gently tap over each quadrant of the abdomen and note the resulting sounds. A dull sound will result when the area above organs, fluid, or fecal matter is tapped. The last component of the nutrition-focused abdominal examination is auscultation of the bowel sounds. Using a stethoscope, gently press into the right lower quadrant of the abdomen. Bowel sounds can be defined in three categories: normal or high-pitched gurgling that occurs 5–35 times per minute, hypoactive or softer than normal, with decreased frequency, or hyperactive or loud rustling.[26] Bowel sound activity can help corroborate gastrointestinal symptoms related to motility, constipation, diarrhea, bacterial overgrowth, and reflux.[28]

Biochemical Data

Biochemical markers are highly disease dependent. As such, laboratory data can be quite useful for identifying nutritional deficiency, diet inadequacy, and disease. There are many different markers that can be analyzed to gain a better understanding of a patient's nutritional status. However, minimal lab work is done in pediatric patients unless history, signs, and symptoms indicate that it is necessary. For growing children, vitamin D, calcium, and iron are nutrients of concern; therefore, if their dietary intake suggests insufficient intake of these nutrients, it may be useful to check blood values. In children who are vegan, it is critical to ensure adequate vitamin B_{12} consumption through diet recall; here, additional lab work may be indicated. Research has indicated that children with obesity are at risk for certain nutrient deficiencies.[29] Similarly, concern over the long-term impact of obesity on health outcomes may prompt measurement of lipid profile and hemoglobin A1c (HbA1c) in this population. There is no benefit or harm to measuring a lipid profile in children.[30] The increase in type 2 diabetes mellitus (T2DM) among adolescents who are overweight or obese supports measuring HbA1c in this population. The risk of T2DM was found to be 9 times higher in children who were overweight with HbA1c of 5.9–6%, and up to 72-fold greater risk with HbA1c between 6.3% and 6.4% when compared to a baseline level below 5.5%.[31]

Electrolytes

Electrolytes such as sodium, potassium, chloride, glucose, calcium, magnesium, and phosphorus should be evaluated in children who are not eating or feeling well. Electrolytes can be an indication of hydration status, kidney function, and hemodynamics. For patients who are critically ill, analysis of electrolytes may indicate how well they are tolerating treatments and feeding.

Iron Status Indicators

Iron status should be checked in preschool- and school-aged children, as well as adolescents. Guidelines for screening iron can vary. The AAP recommends all babies to be screened for anemia at age 12 months. The CDC suggests babies at risk for anemia be screened at 9–12 months with a 6-month follow-up. Term infants who are fed non-iron-fortified formulas or who are still breastfeeding at 9 months or preterm infants not having received iron-fortified formula before the age of 3 months should be screened for anemia.[32] Hemoglobin, hematocrit, iron, total iron binding capacity, and mean corpuscular volume should be analyzed in the pediatric patient. Iron deficiency anemia and other types of anemia, such as macrocytic anemia, can be detected through these markers. **Table 20.7** lists the normal hemoglobin and hematocrit levels for children ages 2–18 years. Monitoring of iron status is especially important for children who follow vegetarian or vegan diets.[33]

Table 20.7 Normal Hemoglobin and Hematocrit Levels in Pediatric Patients, by Sex and Age Group

Hemoglobin and Hematocrit Levels by Age Group		
Age Range (Sex)	**Hemoglobin (g/dL)**	**Hematocrit (%)**
2–6 years (Both)	12.5	37
6–12 years (Both)	13.5	40
12–15 years (Female)	11.8	35.7
12–15 years (Male)	12.5	37.3
15–18 years (Female)	12	35.9
15–18 years (Male)	13.3	39.7

Modified from Academy of Nutrition and Dietetics. *Pediatric Nutrition Care Manual*. Accessed August 19, 2017. https://www.nutritioncaremanual.org/topic.cfm?ncm_category_id=12&lv1=144610&ncm_toc_id=144610&ncm_heading=&

Bone Health Markers

Vitamin D, calcium, and parathyroid hormone are three critical values to assess in pediatric patients. All three of these markers work together in bone mineralization. Sufficient amounts of vitamin D and calcium are necessary for growth. Currently there is no specific recommendation for testing vitamin D, calcium, and PTH in well children. Many older children do not consume the recommended amounts of calcium and vitamin D.[29,34] However, currently the AAP recommends monitoring only in children with low bone mass or history of fractures.[35]

PRACTICE POINT

There are no routine lab values monitored for pediatric patients, unless warranted by diet history or signs and symptoms.

Medical and Social History

Medical and social history help the healthcare team to better understand the patient. These data provide a more comprehensive picture of the patient.

Medical History

In the hospital setting, a patient's medical history will be a part of their medical record. This may include information about chronic illness, trauma, surgery, or infection. In addition, a child's birth history, any current illness or diagnosis, and medications will be listed. History of nausea, vomiting, and diarrhea; any problems with reflux; and stool patterns should be noted. It is important to review this information, because it can provide greater detail about the child's current state and guide further evaluation and discussion. In an outpatient setting, some of the medical history may be provided if the patient was referred by a physician. However, it may be necessary to consult the parent to get a complete history.

Social History

Social history is an essential component of a child's nutrition assessment. The social history will provide information about the child's family's education, values, and beliefs; family stressors; or other personal details. The Office of Disease Prevention and Health Promotion has defined social determinants of health (SDOH) in order to identify factors that may impact health outcomes. They include five domains: (1) economic stability,

CASE STUDY REVISITED

You next meet with Peter 5 months later at his 9-month visit. His anthropometric and diet history are as follows:

Anthropometric Data:

Age (months)	Birth	3	4	6	9
Weight (kg)	3	5.2	5.4	5.6	5.8
Length (cm)	50	58	62	63	64

Dietary Data:

Dietary History: Peter's mother has gone back to work and transitioned him to bottle feeds using a standard baby formula. He continues to spit up frequently and seems "colicky." On average, he feeds 5–6 times per day and drinks 4–6 oz per feed (although much is lost with spitting up). Peter continues to have difficulty finishing his bottles in under 30 minutes. At the end of the visit, his mother notes it has been difficult to keep up with the amount of formula he needs, and she has been worried they will run out.

Questions

1. How would you assess Peter's growth since you last saw him at 4 months? How would you describe his pattern of growth? What has changed?
2. What might you look for in a nutrition-focused physical exam?
3. What is your assessment of his dietary intake? Is it sufficient?
4. Assess Peter's PES statements from his initial visit. Identify if each statement remains an active issue or if the PES statement has been resolved. If the PES statement remains an active issue, has improvement in the issue been noted? If the issue has been resolved, write a new PES statement.
5. What might a dietary intervention be for Peter? What labs might you obtain? What referrals might you make?

(2) education access and stability, (3) healthcare access and stability, (4) social and community context, and (5) neighborhood and built environment (**Figure 20.9**).[36]

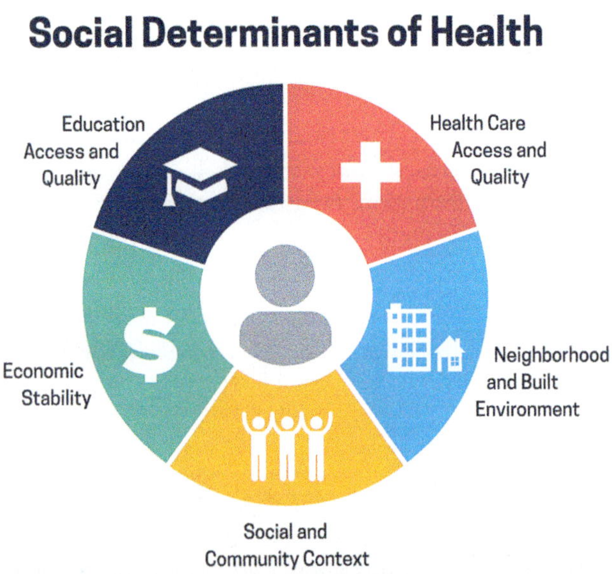

Figure 20.9 The Office of Disease Prevention and Health Promotion (OASH) Established the 5 Domains of Social Determinants of Health

Reproduced from *Healthy People 2030*, U.S. Department of Health and Human Services, Office of Disease Prevention and Health Promotion. Accessed January 5, 2025. https://health.gov/healthypeople/objectives-and-data/social-determinants-health.

In simple terms, where a child lives, goes to school, and plays, along with their home environment, can impact their health outcome. Assuring access to nutritious foods and opportunities for physical activity are two examples that relate to dietetics practice. Diet education on healthy food choices is not effective if access to grocery stores and nutritious foods is not available to the patient.

Assessing Patterns of Growth and Etiology

Plotting growth on percentile growth curves is the most common method of tracking growth in a hospital or clinical setting. Measures are more valuable when there are several data points to interpret. One data point is not as meaningful because it does not indicate a pattern of development. When analyzing growth data, it is important to consider the interval between measurements. Also, growth can occur in bursts and is not necessarily linear. If a value seems irregular, a repeat measurement should be requested. As discussed earlier, there are several different growth indices that can be interpreted by charting growth (**Table 20.8**).

Table 20.8 Diagnostic Interpretations of Growth Chart Analysis

	Growth Chart Interpretations		
Diagnosis	**Underweight (Low Weight-for-Height)**	**Stunted (Low Weight-for-Height)**	**Wasted (Low Weight-for-Height)**
Acute, short-term deficit	X		
Normal for ethnicity History of insult	X	X	
Long-term, ongoing illness	X	X	X
Genetic Endocrine		X	

Data from Training Course on Growth Assessment. WHO Child Growth Standards. https://iris.who.int/bitstream/handle/10665/43601/9789241595070_C_eng.pdf?sequence=3&isAllowed=y

Interpreting Changes in Weight-for-Age

Weight-for-age is a reflection of body mass for age. It represents how a child's weight compares to other children of the same age. Along with nutritional intake, weight-for-age is influenced by both ethnicity and genetics and is related to height and BMI. As previously stated, changes in weight are most sensitive to short-term alterations in nutritional status. Low weight-for-age or underweight may indicate acute or short-term deficits, history of insult, or long-term illness. For some ethnicities, low weight-for-age may be considered typical. Generally speaking, children who are low weight-for-age are defined as being underweight. However, an index of weight-for-age alone is difficult to interpret because it does not distinguish between overall size and weight status. A child who is small but of adequate proportional weight will have the same weight-for-age as a child who is tall, but extremely thin. Likewise, the duration and identification of any pattern of decline provides more meaningful information and insight on cause and treatment. Children who have a low weight-for-age, but track along that same percentile, are likely not to be at risk, as opposed to children who demonstrate a drop in their weight-for-age percentile channel. Minor changes in weight that are transient may represent a brief lapse in nutritional intake or overall health. Changes in weight-for-age are significant when they cross percentiles and continue over time. This is a cue to thoroughly assess diet history, because weight is strongly linked to caloric intake or an energy deficit due to increased energy expenditure or malabsorption. Monitoring changes in stature that accompany alterations provides valuable insight. A decline in weight-for-age without a drop in length or height can be defined as failure to gain weight (**Figure 20.10**). Weight-for-length in this instance will begin to fall. Failure to grow describes a drop in length or height without a drop in weight (**Figure 20.11**).[2,37]

CORE CONCEPT 3

Underweight is defined as low weight-for-age. Failure to gain weight may indicate acute or short-term deficits, history of insult, or long-term illness.

Interpreting Changes in Height-for-Age

Height-for-age represents a child's height compared to other children of the same age. Height is a less-sensitive indictor than weight in cases of inadequate intake. Thus, a drop in height-for-age is more indicative of long-term nutrition-related problems or chronic malnutrition.

Low height-for-age can also be a reflection of **stunting**. Stunting occurs when a child is below the 5th percentile in height-for-age or when they have a z-score less than 2 standard deviations below the median. Failure to reach linear growth suggests long-term insufficient nutrient intake or suboptimal health conditions, such as an infection or chronic disease. The cause of stunting is not always known and often prompts a medical workup. Certain disease states, environmental causes, repeated infections, or micronutrient deficiencies can all result in low height-for-age. Depending on the etiology of impaired linear growth, nutrition interventions may or may not be effective in reversing stunting.[2,37]

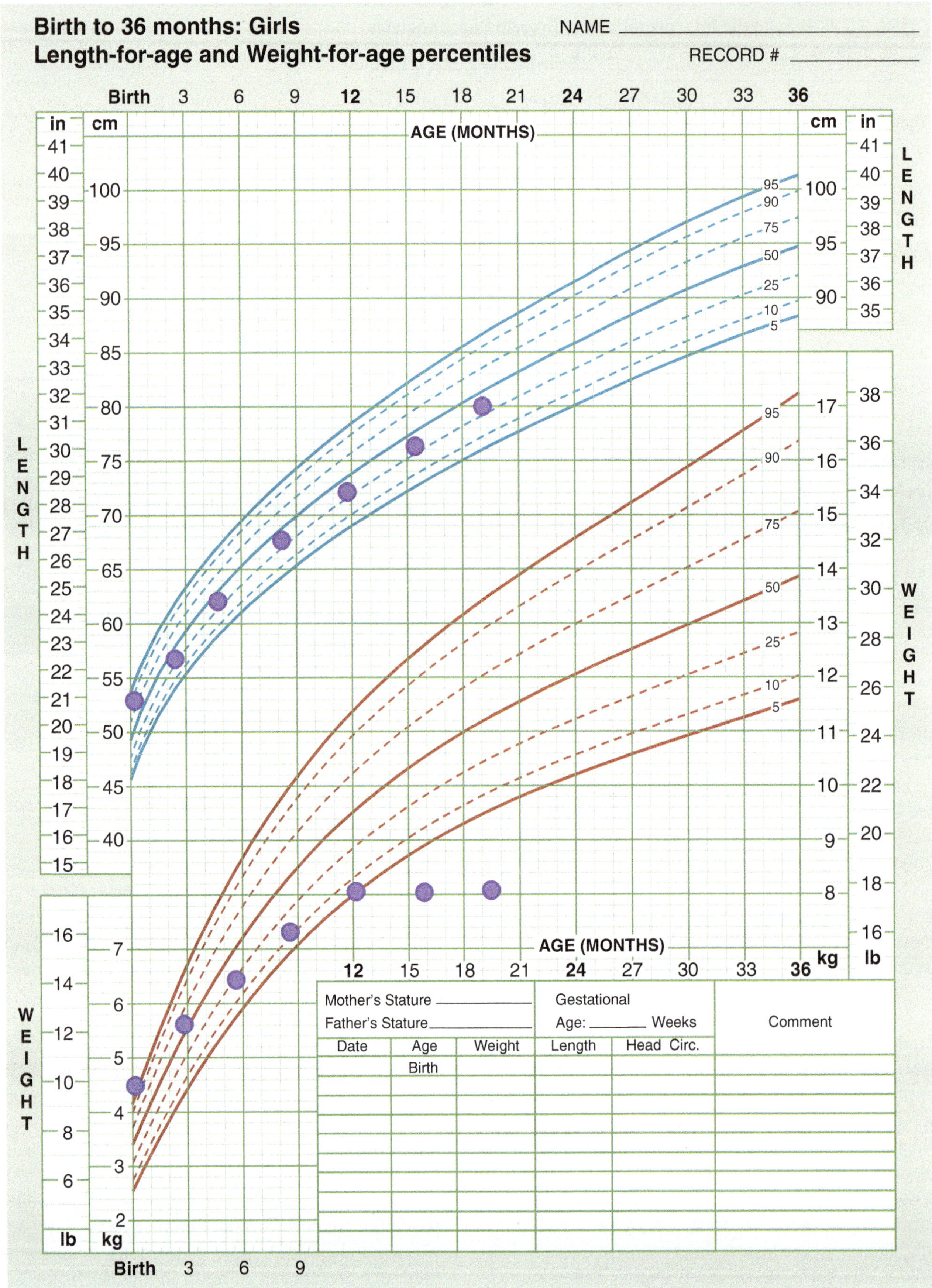

Figure 20.10 Failure to Gain Weight is Represented by a Decline in Weight but not Height or Length. Weight-for-Length will also Decline.

Reproduced from Centers for Disease Control and Prevention (CDC). Features of the CDC Growth Charts. (2015, April 30). Retrieved from https://www.cdc.gov/nccdphp/dnpao/growthcharts/training/overview/page3.html

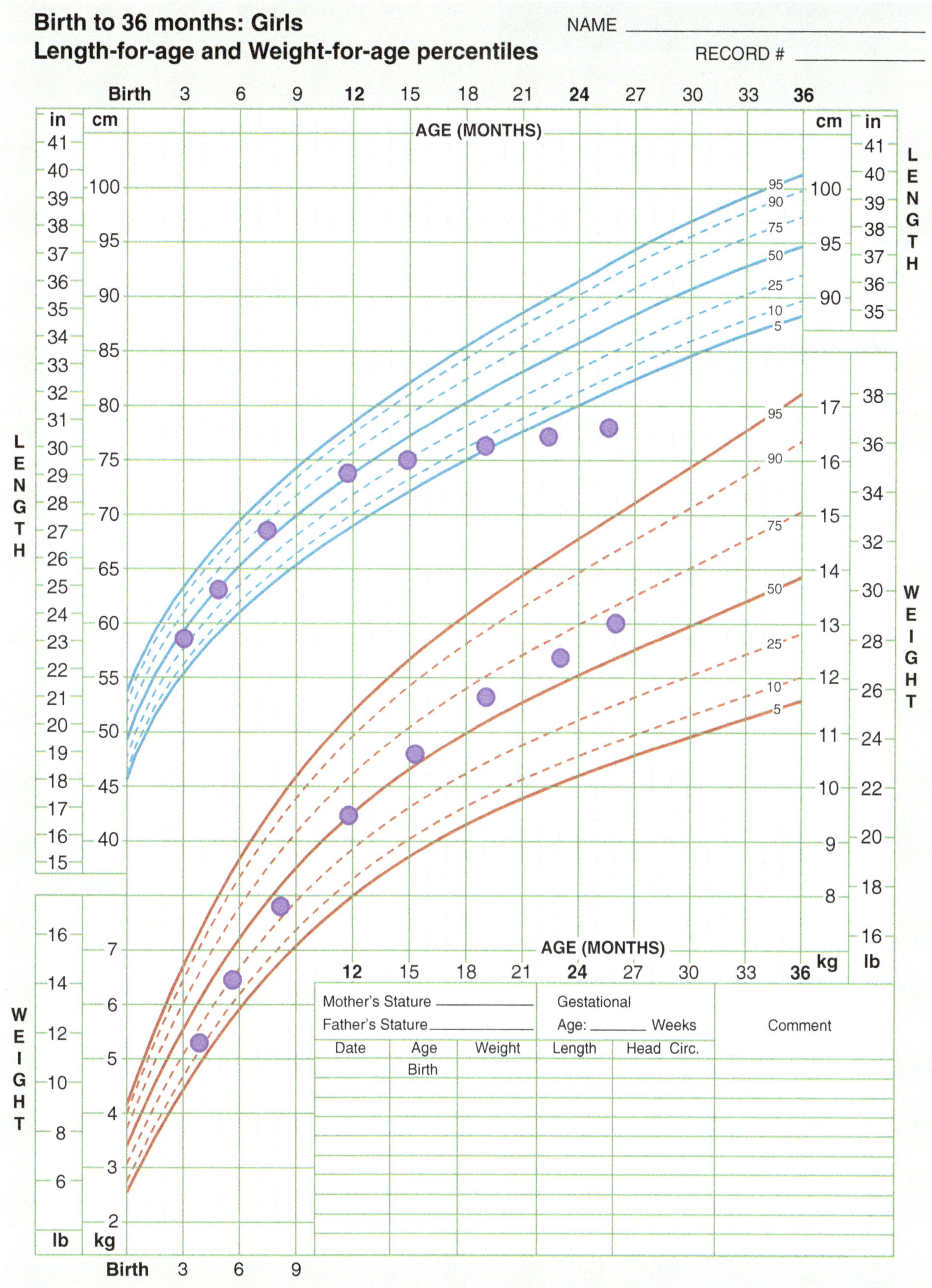

Figure 20.11 Failure to Grow Is Represented by a Decline in Stature Without a Decline in Weight. The Etiology May Relate to Non-nutritional Factors. In Patients Where Stunting Is Not Accompanied by a Decline in Weight-for-age, Overweight or Obesity Can Occur

Reproduced from Kuczmarski RJ, Ogden CL, Guo SS, et al. 2000 CDC growth charts for the United States: Methods and development. National Center for Health Statistics. *Vital Health Stat.* 11(246). 2002.

CORE CONCEPT 4

Stunting, or low height-for-age, may be indicative of long-term on-going illness, genetic or endocrine abnormalities, or a history of insult.

Interpreting Changes in Weight-for-Length or BMI-for-Age

Like height-for-age and weight-for-age, weight-for-length or BMI-for-age are analyzed based on percentiles in pediatric patients. BMI-for-age is similar to weight-for-height or length, the latter being the equivalent indicator in children younger than 2 years of age. BMI-for-age and weight-for-length, when plotted on the CDC growth charts, help identify children who are underweight, normal, overweight, or obese. Z-scores can also be used to classify BMI-for-age or weight-for-length. Children who have a z-score of one standard deviation above the median, which is equivalent to 25 kg/m^2 at 19 years of age, are considered overweight. Those with a z-score greater than two standard deviations are considered to be obese.[2] Pediatric obesity is often a predictor of adult obesity. BMI-for-age is one of the easiest methods to screen for overweight and obesity in children. High BMI-for-age may be an indicator of increased adiposity or overweight and obesity. BMI-for-age does not account for the differences between fat and fat-free masses. In some cases, high weight-for-height may not be an indication of obesity but a result of increased lean body mass. This may occur in child athletes.

Low BMI-for-age or **weight-for-height** (or length) is referred to as **wasting**, which is defined by

CASE STUDY REVISITED

At Peter's 1-year visit, it is determined that he has growth faltering. His information is below.

Anthropometric Data:

Age (months)	Birth	3	4	6	9	12
Weight (kg)	3	5.2	5.4	5.6	5.8	6.2
Length (cm)	50	58	62	63	64	65

Biochemical Data:

Iron 49 (50–160 mcg/dL)
Transferrin 395 (200–400 mg/dL)
Transferrin saturation 10.7% (20–50%)
Total iron binding capacity 455 (250–460 mcg/dL)

Clinical Data:

Past Medical History: Failure to gain weight, persistent GERD
Medications: Omeprazole
Vital Signs: Normal
Nutrition-Focused Physical Exam: Appears thin, slightly pale, lethargic

Dietary Data:

Diet Recall:
Breakfast: 4 oz low-fat milk, 1/4 pancake with syrup, 2 apple slices
Mid-Morning Snack: 10–15 Cheerios, 4 oz water
Lunch: 2 slices of turkey, 1 slice of cheese, juice box
Afternoon Snack: Refuses food, 4 oz chocolate milk (2%)
Dinner: Chicken or fish (1 oz), mashed potato or rice (2–3 tablespoons), corn or peas (1/3 cup)
Diet Prescription: Age appropriate

Questions

1. Assess Peter's current nutritional status. Using www.peditools.org, determine Peter's weight-for-age, length-for-age, and weight-for-length z-scores.
2. What are Peter's current nutritional problems?
3. Assess Peter's energy requirement for normal growth. Is Peter's dietary intake sufficient?
4. Determine Peter's needs for catch-up growth.
5. Provide recommendations to Peter's typical diet to help meet his needs for catch-up growth.

AND as a weight-for-height lower than 2 standard deviations below the median.[22] Wasting is not influenced by genetics or ethnicity. It is a strong predictor of mortality among children younger than 5 years of age. Low BMI-for-age or weight-for-height (or length) results from an acute short-term change in intake or the onset of disease. Those who present with wasting are likely to positively respond to nutritional intervention.

CORE CONCEPT 5

Wasting refers to low weight-for-height or BMI-for-age and is an indication of recent and severe state of undernutrition. Wasting may be the result of disease and is responsive to nutrition intervention.

CORE CONCEPT 6

Growth charts are used to evaluate growth from birth to age 20 years. Serial measures of weight and height and their patterns can be used to define wasting, stunting, and underweight status.

Table 20.9 Clinical Indicators of Pediatric Malnutrition When Only One Data Point Is Available

Mild Malnutrition	
■ Weight-for-length or BMI-for-age z-score ■ Mid-upper arm circumference	z-score of −1 to −1.9
Moderate Malnutrition	
■ Weight-for-length or BMI-for-age z-score ■ Mid-upper arm circumference	z-score of −2 to −2.9
Severe Malnutrition	
■ Weight-for-length or BMI-for-age z-score ■ Mid-upper arm circumference	z-score of −3 or lower

***Z*-scores** indicate how many standard deviations a measurement is from the mean. In other words, if comparing a malnourished child's weight-for-age to the CDC comparative data, a *z*-score will indicate how atypical this child's weight-for-age is compared to the average weight for children of their same age.

Use weight-for-length z-score for children <2 years of age.

Data from Becker PJ, Nieman Carney L, Corkins MR, et al. Consensus statement of the Academy of Nutrition and Dietetics/American Society for Parenteral and Enteral Nutrition: indicators recommended for the identification and documentation of pediatric malnutrition (undernutrition). *J Acad Nutr Diet*. 2014;114(12):1988–2000.

Pediatric Malnutrition

Pediatric malnutrition affects many children worldwide. ASPEN defines pediatric malnutrition as "an imbalance between nutrient requirement and intake resulting in cumulative deficits of energy, protein or micronutrients that may negatively affect growth, development, and other relevant outcomes."[22] In the United States, pediatric malnutrition is often secondary to disease, chronic illness, trauma, or surgery, and in children with special healthcare needs. Although hospitalized pediatric patients are at the greatest nutritional risk, children should be screened at their routine physical exams.[38,39] AND in conjunction with ASPEN have written a consensus statement on the indicators recommended for the identification and documentation of pediatric malnutrition. Indicators to be assessed when diagnosing pediatric malnutrition include food/nutrient intake, assessment of energy/protein needs, growth parameters, weight gain velocity, hand grip strength, and mid-upper arm circumference. Diagnosis of pediatric malnutrition can be made using either one or two indicators. **Table 20.9** shows the criteria used for diagnosis based upon one primary indicator, and **Table 20.10** shows the criteria used for diagnosis based upon two or more indicators. Note that a −3 z-score is indicative of severe pediatric malnutrition, regardless of which primary indicator is used. Prompt identification of pediatric malnutrition, and nutritional intervention, can help address nutritional concerns that could lead to worsening of illnesses or chronic conditions.[22] Addressing pediatric malnutrition may include use of high-calorie/protein foods, meal plans/schedules, oral nutrition supplements, supplemental nutrition support, or some combination of these interventions. Being mindful of refeeding syndrome is also important to note in this population, as the risks associated include significant electrolyte derangements, which can lead to severe consequences.

PRACTICE POINT

A −3 or lower z-score is indicative of severe malnutrition, regardless of which primary indicator is used.

Failure to Thrive or Growth Faltering

Failure to thrive (FTT) or **growth faltering (GF)** is defined as a slower rate of weight gain after the first 2 weeks of birth.[40,41] It is estimated that 5 out of

Table 20.10 Clinical Indicators of Pediatric Malnutrition When Two or More Data Points Are Available

Mild Malnutrition
1. Weight gain velocity (<2 years of age) less than 75% of normal expected weight gain
2. Weight loss (2–20 years of age) equal to 5% of usual body weight
3. Decline of 1 z-score for weight/length or BMI
4. Intake between 50% and 75% estimated energy/protein requirement
Moderate Malnutrition
Weight gain velocity (<2 years of age) less than 50% of normal expected weight gain
Weight loss (2–20 years) equal to 7.5% usual body weight
Decline of 2 z-score for weight/length or BMI
Intake between 25% and 75% of estimated energy/protein requirement
Severe Malnutrition
Weight gain velocity (<2 years of age) less than 25% of normal expected weight gain
Weight loss (2–20 years of age) equal to or greater than 10 % of usual body weight
Decline of 3 (or greater) z-score for weight/length or BMI
Intake between less than 25% estimated energy/protein requirement

***Z*-scores** indicate how many standard deviations a measurement is from the mean. In other words, if comparing a malnourished child's weight-for-age to the CDC comparative data, a *z*-score will indicate how atypical this child's weight-for-age is compared to the average weight for children of their same age.

Must choose two indicators from any one category of malnutrition. If indicators fall in two different categories of malnutrition, clinical judgment should be used.

Data from Becker PJ, Nieman Carney L, Corkins MR, et al. Consensus statement of the Academy of Nutrition and Dietetics/American Society for Parenteral and Enteral Nutrition: indicators recommended for the identifica-tion and documentation of pediatric malnutrition (undernutrition). *J Acad Nutr Diet*. 2014;114(12):1988–2000.

100 children experience FTT, which unfortunately can go undetected. FTT or GF increases the risk of infection, prolonged hospital stays, diminished skeletal muscle mass, and cognitive and behavioral difficulties.[42,43] GF is the preferred term over FTT since it represents a temporary variation from a child's expected growth pattern as opposed to "failure" to grow. GF can be described as a crossing of 2 percentile spaces in weight for age (WFA) when birth weight is between the 9th and 91st percentile WFA.[40] The WHO defines GF as a drop in WFA z-score of 1 or greater over a 1-month period.[41] Patients with GF may also meet the criteria for malnutrition if additional criteria are found. GF can be due to illness or non-illness-related etiologies. Illness-related etiologies generally point to disease or pathophysiology that results in inadequate intake, increased needs, or increased losses. Non-illness-related GF can include a complex interaction between environmental and socioeconomic factors such as food insecurity, alterations in feeding practices, and inadequate dietary intake. This is the most common cause of GF in low-income countries.[42,43]

Nutrition Interventions

Nutrient Requirements for Normal Growth

Nutritional needs are assessed in relation to growth and activity. Children have the highest energy and protein requirements per kilogram of body weight of any age group. Energy needs are significantly higher in this population due to the increased synthesis of new tissue, as well as storage of energy in the tissue. Micronutrient needs are also greatest to support growth and development.

Recommendations for a Healthy Eating Pattern

The US Department of Agriculture and US Department of Health and Human Services recently released the 2025 Dietary Guidelines for Americans (DGA) (**Table 20.11**). In their report, they recommend that children consume a diet that consists of quality protein, dairy, vegetables, fruits, healthy fats and whole grains. The guidelines

Table 20.11 **Comparison of Dietary Recommendations for Children According to 2020 and 2025 Dietary Guidelines for Americans (DGA)**

Food Category	2020 DGA	2025 DGA
Added Sugar Ages Under 2 years	Avoid added sugars	Avoid completely, no safe amount
Added Sugar Ages 2-10	Limit to < 10% of total calories	Avoid completely, no safe amount
Dairy Type	Fat-free, skim or 1% low fat	Whole and 2% milk
Protein Type	Choose lean protein	Choose high quality protein (meats, egg, fish) at every meal
Processed Foods	General advice to limit	Avoid all ultra-processed foods
Caffeine and energy drinks, sugary beverages	Limited guidance made for young children	Avoid completely for children up to age 10 years

Source: US Department of Health and Human Services, US Department of Agriculture. 2020-2025 Dietary Guidelines for Americans. 2020; U.S. Department of Agriculture and U.S. Department of Health and Human Services. *Dietary Guidelines for Americans*, 2025-2030. 10th Edition. January 2026. Available at Dietary Guidelines.gov.Academy of Pediatrics; 2025

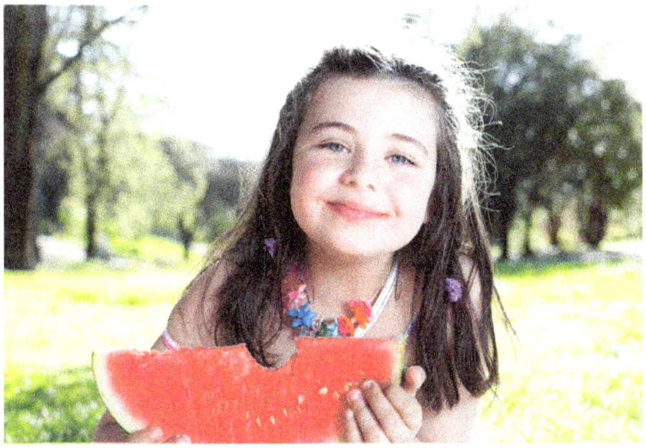

© JW LTD/DigitalVision/Getty Images

emphasize the importance of nutrient dense, minimally processed whole foods as part of a healthy meal pattern for children.[44] The 2025 DGA also provide stricter limits on added sugar, recommending zero tolerance for children less than 10 years of age. Along with the AAP, the 2025 DGA also recommend avoidance of caffeinated beverages and energy drinks suggesting water and unsweetened beverages instead.[44, 45]. It is the role of the dietitian to promote healthy eating in all settings.The AAP also suggests that fruit juice be limited to less than 4 ounces per day for children 1-3 years, 4-6 ounces for children ages 4-6 years and 8 ounces for children 7-18 years of age.[45]

Of note, the new guidelines represent a shift from previous editions with respect to dairy, encouraging full fat milk and yogurt after 2 years of age. The rationale for the new guideline states the importance of full fat dairy for meeting energy needs and to support brain development. While limiting saturated fat to 10% of total calories remains a goal, including a quality protein source such as meat, eggs and fish at each meal is also strongly emphasized. Limiting sodium intake while increasing intake of specific nutrients of concern such as iron, calcium and vitamin D is also advised. Children and adolescents are encouraged to participate in food shopping and meal preparation in order to develop healthy eating habits later in life.[44] Table 20.11 compares the current DGA with the 2020 DGA guidelines on several key aspects.[39] These patterns are intended for individuals of all ages to promote a healthy lifestyle and prevent chronic diseases such as obesity, T2DM, and cardiovascular disease.

Despite these recommendations, many children do not consume adequate amounts of fiber and key vitamins and minerals such as vitamin D, calcium, and potassium. In addition, children often have a positive energy balance; excessive intakes of fat, saturated fat, sugar, and sodium; and inadequate intakes of fruits, vegetables, whole grains, dairy, and seafood.[46]

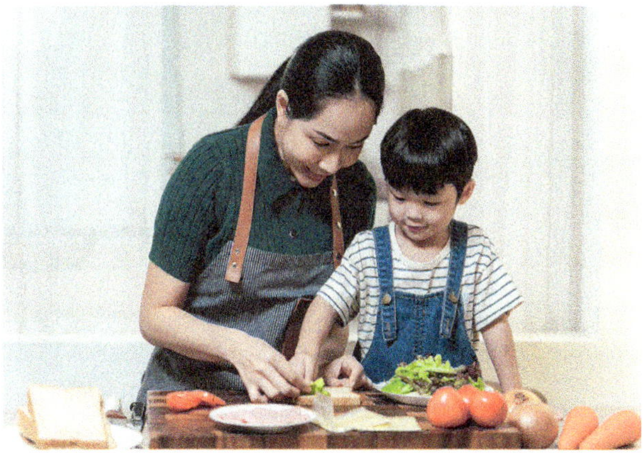

Reproduced from U.S. Department of Agriculture. ChooseMyPlate.gov.

Energy Requirements

Energy needs can be predicted for children using the Dietary Reference Intakes (DRIs), including the estimated energy requirements (EERs). EERs in the healthy child include the energy required for growth and tissue deposition, with the goal of adequate but not excessive intake. These requirements are based on studies of energy metabolism in the general population and incorporate additional needs for growth and physical activity (**Table 20.12**).[46] The DRIs are not appropriate for children with an altered clinical status such as acute or chronic diseases or critical illness. Instead, standardized equations must be used that account for relevant stress factors.

Protein

Protein is a critical nutrient for growth; in fact, 58% of dietary protein is used to support growth from 6 months to almost 13 years of age.[47] More protein per kilogram of body weight is therefore needed early on, compared to requirements in later stages of development. **Table 20.13** contains the recommended daily allowance (RDA) for protein, based on age range and sex.[42] Like energy requirements, males and females have identical requirements through middle childhood, which then differ at the time of adolescence. The differences in protein requirements occur as a result of the sex-specific changes in body composition. These standards account for tissue maintenance, tissue growth, variation in growth, and efficiency of utilization.[48] Additional protein may be needed in cases such as wound healing or for disease-specific concerns.

CORE CONCEPT 7

RDA protein intake goals account for tissue maintenance, tissue growth, variation in growth, and efficiency of utilization

Table 20.12 Summary Table of EER Equations by Age, Sex, Physical Activity, and Energy Cost of Growth in Children and Adolescents

Age	Male	Female
0–2.99 months	EER = −716.45 − (1.00 × age) + (17.82 × height) + (15.06 × weight) + 200	EER = −69.15 + (80.0 × age) + (2.65 × height) + (54.15 × weight) + 180
3–5.99 months	EER = −716.45 − (1.00 × age) + (17.82 × height) + (15.06 × weight) + 50	EER = −69.15 + (80.0 × age) + (2.65 × height) + (54.15 × weight) + 60
6 months to 2.99 years	EER = −716.45 − (1.00 × age) + (17.82 × height) + (15.06 × weight) + 20	EER = −69.15 + (80.0 × age) + (2.65 × height) + (54.15 × weight) + 20/15[a]
3–13.99 years	**Inactive EER** = −447.51 + (3.68 × age) + (13.01 × height) + (13.15 × weight) + 20/15/25[b] **Low active EER** = 19.12 + (3.68 × age) + (8.62 × height) + (20.28 × weight) + 20/15/25 **Active EER** = −388.19 + (3.68 × age) + (12.66 × height) + (20.46 × weight) + 20/15/25 **Very active EER** = −671.75 + (3.68 × age) + (15.38 × height) + (23.25 × weight) + 20/15/25	**Inactive EER** = 55.59 − (22.25 × age) + (8.43 × height) + (17.07 × weight) + 15/30[c] **Low active EER** = −297.54 − (22.25 × age) + (12.77 × height) + (14.73 × weight) + 15/30 **Active EER** = −189.55 − (22.25 × age) + (11.74 × height) + (18.34 × weight) + 15/30 **Very active EER** = −709.59 − (22.25 × age) + (18.22 × height) + (14.25 × weight) + 15/30
14–18.99 years	**Inactive EER** = −447.51 + (3.68 × age) + (13.01 × height) + (13.15 × weight) + 20 **Low active EER** = 19.12 + (3.68 × age) + (8.62 × height) + (20.28 × weight) + 20 **Active EER** = −388.19 + (3.68 × age) + (12.66 × height) + (20.46 × weight) + 20 **Very active EER** = −671.75 + (3.68 × age) + (15.38 × height) + (23.25 × weight) + 20	**Inactive EER** = 55.59 − (22.25 × age) + (8.43 × height) + (17.07 × weight) + 20 **Low active EER** = −297.54 − (22.25 × age) + (12.77 × height) + (14.73 × weight) + 20 **Active EER** = −189.55 − (22.25 × age) + (11.74 × height) + (18.34 × weight) + 20 **Very active EER** = −709.59 − (22.25 × age) + (18.22 × height) + (14.25 × weight) + 20

Notes: kcal/d = kilocalories per day; PAL = physical activity level; EER = estimated energy requirement. Age is in years, weight is in kilograms, and height is in centimeters.

[a] Energy cost of growth for girls: 6–11.99 months: 20 kcal/d; 12–35.99 months: 15 kcal/d.

[b] Energy cost of growth for boys: 3 y: 20 kcal/d; 4–8 y: 15 kcal/d; 9–13 y: 25 kcal/d.

[c] Energy cost of growth for girls: 3 y: 15 kcal/d; 4–8 y: 15 kcal/d; 9–13 y: 30 kcal/d.

Modified from the Institute of Medicine. 2005. *Dietary Reference Intakes for Energy, Carbohydrate, Fiber, Fat, Fatty Acids, Cholesterol, Protein, and Amino Acids*. Washington, DC: The National Academies Press. https://doi.org/10.17226/10490; National Academies of Sciences, Engineering, and Medicine. 2023. *Dietary Reference Intakes for Energy*. Washington, DC: The National Academies Press.

Table 20.13 RDA for Protein Based on Age Range and Sex

	RDA for Protein	
Age (Sex)	Grams of Protein/kg Body Weight	Grams of Protein/Day
0–6 months (Both)	1.52*	9.1*
7–12 months (Both)	1.2	11
1–3 years (Both)	1.05	13
4–8 years (Both)	0.95	19
9–13 years (Both)	0.95	34
14–18 years (Males)	0.85	52
14–18 years (Females)	0.85	46

*AI (adequate intake)

Data from Institute of Medicine. 2005. *Dietary Reference Intakes for Energy, Carbohydrate, Fiber, Fat, Fatty Acids, Cholesterol, Protein, and Amino Acids*. Washington, DC: The National Academies Press. https://doi.org/10.17226/10490

Micronutrients: Vitamins and Minerals

As children grow, they require vitamins and minerals for adequate development and cellular processes. A summary of the key nutrients required for children is provided in **Table 20.14**[9] and an overview of nutrients of concern and supplementation recommendations is provided in **Table 20.15**.[50] It should be noted that for children following a vegetarian or vegan diet, calcium, vitamin D, vitamin B_{12}, and iron are particular nutrients of concern because the major dietary sources of these nutrients are from animal products.

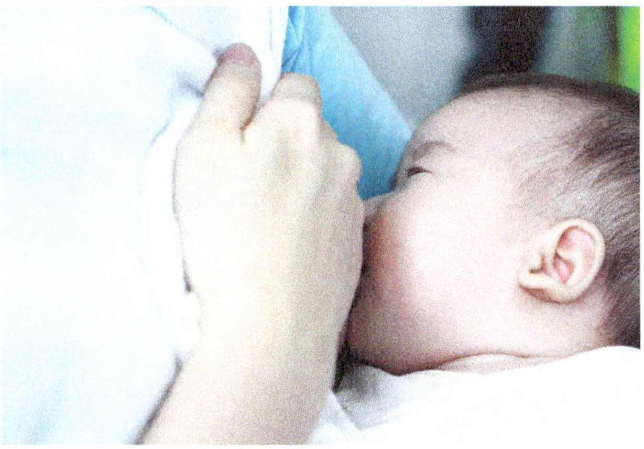

CORE CONCEPT 8

Vitamins and minerals, especially calcium, iron, and vitamin D, provide essential nutrients for growth and development. Without adequate micronutrient status, children may have impaired growth.

Full-term Infants

From birth through the first 4–6 months of life, infants are fed exclusively human milk and/or commercial baby formula. The AAP recommends that human milk be the sole source of infant nutrition from birth to approximately 6 months, because it provides specific energy and nutrients necessary for the developing infant.[51] It is recommended that breastfeeding be continued as long as mutually desired, for 2 years or beyond, along with the addition of complementary foods.

Human Milk. Human milk provides complete nutrition for the infant in their first months of life. Human milk is composed of fat, carbohydrate, and protein and contains approximately 20 kcal/oz. Fat makes up 40–55% of the total energy of milk. The majority of the fat is composed of triglycerides, of which approximately 17% are fatty acids.[51] Carbohydrates are in the human milk as lactose and oligosaccharides. Lactose is the primary carbohydrate in milk and fuels the high energy demands of the brain. Oligosaccharides also comprise a large portion of carbohydrates but are not able to be digested by the infant. Instead, they feed the gut microbiota, functioning as prebiotics.[52,53] Lastly, protein is present in three different classes: whey, casein, and mucins. Protein in the milk has an antimicrobial and immune-modulating effect, as well as a nutrient role. The concentration of these macronutrients changes throughout lactation to meet baby's changing needs.

Human milk is classified into three groups—**colostrum**, transitional milk, and mature milk—based on the changes in composition that occur throughout lactation. In the early stages, colostrum is produced, which has a very high concentration of whey protein. Colostrum is also highly bioactive, providing immunoglobulins to promote the development of the infant's immune system.[52] In addition, colostrum contains growth factors, which promote development in the newborn. From the 2nd to 7th month of lactation, the protein concentration decreases and ultimately levels off. In contrast, the fat concentration gradually increases. Carbohydrate content in breast milk is at its greatest concentration between 4 and 7 months. Mature human milk is approximately 55%

Table 20.14 Selected Vitamin and Mineral Recommended Daily Allowance, Birth to 18 Years

Age (Sex)	Select Recommended Daily Allowance											
	Vitamin A (ug/d)	Vitamin C (mg/d)	Vitamin D (ug/d)	Vitamin E (mg/d)	Vitamin K (ug/d)	Thiamin (mg/d)	Riboflavin (mg/d)	Niacin (mg/d)	Vitamin B_6 (mg/d)	Folate (ug/d)	Iron (mg/d)	Zinc (mg/d)
0–6 months (Both)	400	40	10	4*	2.0*	0.2	0.3	2	0.1*	65*	0.27*	2*
7–12 months (Both)	500	50	10	5*	2.5*	0.3	0.4	4	0.34*	80*	11	3
1–3 years (Both)	300	15	15	6	30*	0.5	0.5	6	0.5	150	7	3
4–8 years (Both)	400	25	15	7	55*	0.6	0.6	8	0.6	200	10	5
9–13 years (Female)	600	45	15	11	60*	0.9	0.9	12	1.0	300	8	8
9–13 years (Male)	600	45	15	11	60*	0.9	0.9	12	1.0	300	8	8
14–18 years (Female)	700	65	15	15	75*	1.0	1.0	14	1.2	400	15	9
14–18 years (Male)	900	75	15	15	75	1.2	1.3	16	1.3	400	11	11

Data from Office of Dietary Supplements, Dietary Supplement Fact Sheets for Health Professionals, 2021–2023.
*AI (adequate intake)

Table 20.15 Key Nutrients to Monitor According to Age Category

Age Range	Nutrients	Role	Recommendations for Potential Need for Supplementation
Full-term infants	Vitamin D Iron Fluoride	Bone development Brain development Red blood cell synthesis Strong tooth enamel	*Vitamin D:* within first few days after birth *Iron:* after 4–6 months for breastfeeding infant; for formula-fed infants, the AAP recommends use of an iron-fortified formula *Fluoride:* after 6 months
Preschool-aged children	Vitamin A Vitamin D/ Calcium Iron Zinc	Vision Immune function Skin Continued bone development Expansion of red blood cells Cognitive development Coenzyme in many metabolic activities Supports growth Immune function	If nutrient intake is low or varied, a vitamin supplement may be necessary Reduced iron intake with transition to cow's milk may indicate need for supplement Zinc may be needed if vegetarian; deficiency can result in increased infections
School-aged children	Vitamin D/ Calcium	Continued bone development	If nutrient intake is low or varied, a vitamin supplement may be necessary It is important to ensure that children in this age range consume a variety of calcium-rich foods
Adolescents	Vitamin A Vitamin D/ Calcium Folate Iron Magnesium	Sexual maturation (in addition to above) Continued bone accretion Coenzyme for DNA and RNA synthesis; transfers one-carbon units in many processes Supports academic performance Supports bone and muscle growth	If nutrient intake is low or varied, a vitamin supplement may be necessary Increased independence can result in unhealthy food choices Iron deficiency risk for girls during menarche Low magnesium intake commonly found in adolescents; risk of lower muscle mass

Data from What We Eat in America: NHANES Survey.

whey and 44% casein. The composition of milk is thought to be unique to each infant because it is associated with maternal characteristics such as age and diet, as well as the birth weight of the infant.[52]

In addition to its nutritional benefits, human milk contains many biologically active components that serve other roles. The immunoglobulins present in milk help to protect the newborn from illness while their immune system is still developing. Separately, human milk also functions to develop the infant's intestinal microbiota. Research indicates that breastfed infants have a more stable and less diverse microbiota with double the number of bacterial cells.[53]

PRACTICE POINT

Exclusive breastfeeding is recommended by the AAP for approximately 6 months after birth because it provides complete nutrition and changes in nutrient composition based on the infant's needs.

Infant Formula. Infant formulas are designed to provide infants with adequate nutrition throughout the first 6 months of life. They are formulated to mimic the effect that human milk has on the infant's growth and development, immunity, and microbiota.[49] There are many different formulas on the market, available as ready to use, liquid concentrate, and powder. They are composed of similar proteins and carbohydrates as human milk. Formulas are available in different varieties as well, including iron-fortified formulas, cow's milk–based formulas, and soy formulas, among others. Infant formulas typically provide 20 kcal/oz, when mixed at standard concentrations. Infant formulas can also be concentrated to provide 24 kcal, or higher, per ounce, for infants with suboptimal growth needing increased caloric intake. Refer to **Table 20.16**, which outlines the mixing instructions using a powdered infant formula, for achieving higher caloric density per ounce.

Table 20.16 Fortifying Formula to Higher Caloric Concentrations

Sample mixing instructions starting from standard 20 kcal/oz formula.
Using powdered formula

Step 1. Check the recipe chart for powdered formula below. Using a clear liquid measuring cup, measure the desired amount of water. Set the measuring cup on a flat surface, and check the level of the liquid at eye level.

Step 2. Add unpacked, level scoops of formula powder to the water. Use only the scoop provided in the formula can.

Step 3. Mix or shake well until all lumps are gone.

Calories per Ounce	Water	Powdered Formula	Final Volume
22	3.5 oz	2 scoops	4 oz
	7 oz	4 scoops	8 oz
	21 oz	12 scoops	24 oz
24	5 oz	3 scoops	5.5 oz
	8 oz	5 scoops	9 oz
	21 oz	13 scoops	24 oz
26	3 oz	2 scoops	3.5 oz
	9 oz	6 scoops	10.5 oz
	21 oz	14 scoops	24 oz
28	4 oz	3 scoops	4.5 oz
	200 mL	5 scoops	8 oz
	16 oz	12 scoops	18.5 oz

Data from Children's Minnesota. Patient & Family Education. Formula Adjustment (standard 20 kcal/oz formula). https://www.childrensmn.org/references/pfs/nutr/formula-adjustment-(standard-20-cal-oz).pdf

Cow's milk–based formulas provide 1.45–1.6 g/dL of protein, which is higher than the protein content in human milk. The protein sources in these formulas are casein and whey. Like human milk, lactose is the main source of carbohydrate.[54] Fat provides 40–50% of total calories. Vegetable oil, in a blend of palm, soy, coconut, safflower, and sunflower oils, is used as the fat source to provide essential fatty acids and improve digestibility.[55] Docosahexaenoic acid and arachidonic acid, as well as antioxidants, are often added to infant formulas. These are used to enhance the immune system and potentially aid in the development of the infant's vision and neurological development.[55]

Iron-fortified formulas contain 40–55% of total calories from carbohydrates, 5–6% of total calories from protein, and 50% of calories from fat. Iron-fortified formulas are indicated for preterm infants, as they help to replenish iron stores. The AAP recommends the use of iron-supplemented formulas in infants who are formula fed. The use of these formulas can have a positive effect on the long-term iron stores of the infant.[56] Despite this recommendation, some argue against iron fortification in formula because it far exceeds the concentration in human milk. Opponents of iron fortification suggest that the decreased iron concentration in human milk is an evolutionary adaptation.[57]

Infant formulas continue to evolve in other ways to better human breast milk. Additives such as prebiotics and probiotics are being used to enhance infant formulas with varying success as far as growth and clinical benefit.[58–61] Prebiotics can reduce respiratory infections in infants through the first 6 months of life.[60] However, formulas supplemented with prebiotics have not improved growth rates beyond that of non-prebiotic–fortified supplements.[61] While probiotics are proven to be safe, they do not offer any clinical advantage over non-probiotic formula in full-term infants. Probiotics may reduce necrotizing enterocolitis in preterm infants and are thought to also be beneficial for infants with GI distress, because they alter the gut microbiota.[58] Thus overall, despite their proposed benefits, research has not substantiated the clinical value in prebiotic and probiotic supplementation of infant formula.

PRACTICE POINT

Iron is a nutrient of concern in newborns, especially those receiving formula. An iron-fortified formula is recommended.

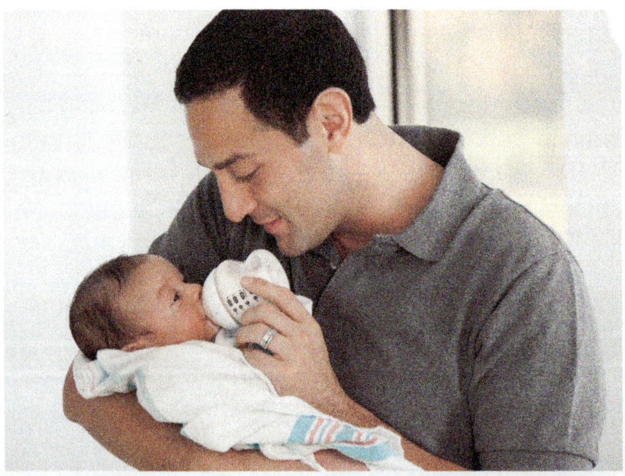

© Ariel Skelley/DigitalVision/Getty Images

Table 20.17 Introduction to Foods

Introduction to Foods			
Age Range	**Nutrition-Related Developmental Cues**	**Food Type Consumed**	**Feeding Behavior**
0–4 months	Sucking and tongue thrusting	Breast milk Infant formula	*Newborn:* feed every 1.5–2 hours *1–4 months:* feed every 2–3 hours
4–6 months	Mature sucking Munching pattern Steady head control Briefly sits independently	Continue to breastfeed or bottle-feed Baby cereal introduced Puree fruit/vegetables	Feed every 3–4 hours Messy spoon feeding, suckling motion on spoon
7–9 months	Normal gag reflex Sits alone for 3–5 minutes Holds bottle Steady head control (no bobbing)	Continue to breastfeed or bottle-feed Stage 1 baby food introduced Stage 2 introduced at 8 months Soft mashed table food at 9 months	Feed every 3.5–4 hours Hand-to-mouth play
10–12 months	Finger feeds Reaches for spoon Learning mature chewing; by 12 months, chewing skills advance	Continue to breast feed or bottle-feed Table foods Foods that dissolve introduced at 10 months Foods that are easily chewed introduced at 11 months	Feed every 4–6 hours Use food as toy, mouth play

Modified from *ASPEN Pediatric Nutrition Support Curriculum*. 2nd ed. 2015.

Introduction of Food and Developmental Cues

After 4–6 months of breastfeeding or formula feeding, it is necessary to begin to introduce the baby to solid foods. Breastfeeding and/or formula feeding alone is no longer sufficient to sustain the nutritional requirements of infants at this age. The AAP recommends introducing complementary foods at 6 months of age; however, the exact time when exclusive breastfeeding no longer provides adequate energy and nutrients is unknown.[62] Introducing new foods is guided by the development of the child. Grains and fruits are typically the first to be introduced because they are the least allergenic. **Table 20.17** summarizes the introduction of foods and corresponding developmental cues. Development is the key factor in determining readiness for solid foods; feeding a child solid foods before they are developmentally ready can delay additional feeding milestones. Of note, in recent years there has been increasing interest and attention to what is referred to as "baby-led weaning." This is a practice of offering infants the opportunity to self-feed family foods in their whole form.[63] Examples may include starting solid introduction with whole pieces of fruits such as strawberries or bananas, or choices such as pieces of toast or scrambled eggs. This differs from the more traditional approach of gradually increasing textures and only starting with smooth, pureed options. Potential benefits to the baby-led weaning feeding approach are increased variety and acceptance of foods, and motor skill development; however, care must be exercised to reduce choking risk. Further research is needed to assess risks and benefits.

As solid foods are introduced, it is necessary to postpone exposure to foods that may pose a risk to the infant. In the first year of life, both cow's milk and honey should be avoided. The AAP recommends that cow's milk be introduced only after 12 months.[64] Early introduction of cow's milk can diminish the iron status of the infant.[65] However, cow's milk products such as yogurt and cheese are encouraged. Avoidance of honey is important as consumption of honey in infants can result in botulism. Botulism results from ingestion of spores, which may be present in honey, that release a nerve-damaging toxin.[66] Foods that pose a choking hazard for infants, such as hot dogs, popcorn, grapes, nuts, and raisins, should also be avoided until the child has further developed their oral motor skills.

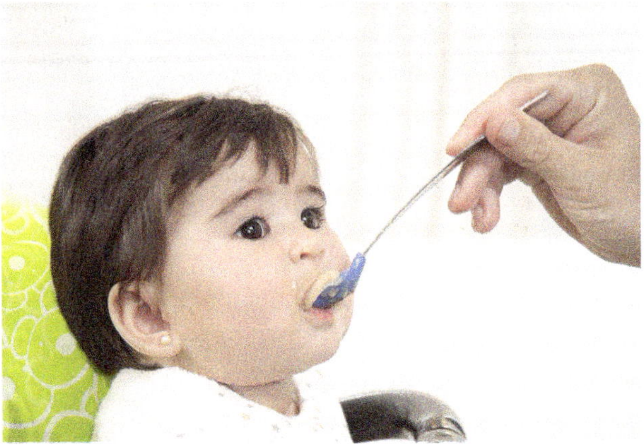

© Marcos Mesa Sam Wordley/Shutterstock

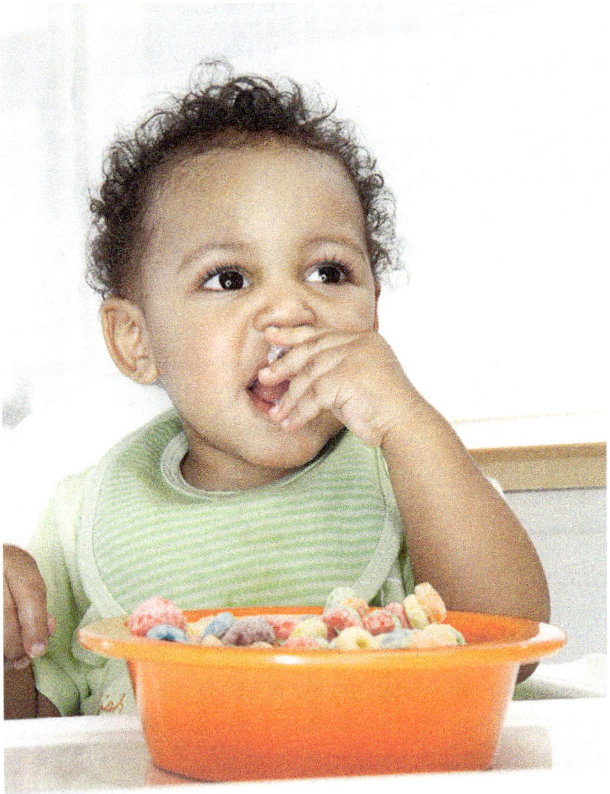

© James Woodson/Digital Vision/Thinkstock

Toddlers

Nutrition at this stage is important for the continuation of growth and development and maintenance of life long health. Toddlers are still continuing to develop oral motor skills. By 18 months of age, a toddler should be able to handle a cup, self-feed, and self-regulate. They begin to consume more textured foods but are cautious to accept new foods. It may take several attempts at introducing new foods before a toddler will try them. Parents should allow them to explore the look, smell, and taste of new foods to help gain acceptance.

Because toddlers have increased energy requirements but cannot eat large portions, they require smaller, more frequent meals. This can be in the form of three meals and two to three snacks or six smaller meals per day to meet their nutritional needs. It is important that children be allowed to learn to feed themselves and decide how much to eat in a comfortable yet structured atmosphere. However, like infants, toddlers are at risk for choking, because they are still developing their oral motor muscles. Most toddlers fail to eat the recommended amount of fruit and vegetables. Early introduction of fruits and vegetables is associated with greater consumption of fruits and vegetables later in life.[66–68]

PRACTICE POINT

Toddlers may need to be exposed to certain foods on numerous occasions to create familiarity before trialing it. Early introduction of healthy foods promotes life-long positive eating habits.

Preschool-Aged Children

Preschool-aged children, like toddlers, require multiple small meals each day to meet their energy requirements. It is recommended that they consume nutrient-dense foods and avoid consumption of excess sugar-sweetened beverages. To lower-fat foods, such as low-fat dairy products. At this age, children continue to learn how to self-regulate. Parents should practice division of responsibility as their child is able to feed themselves. Research has indicated that when

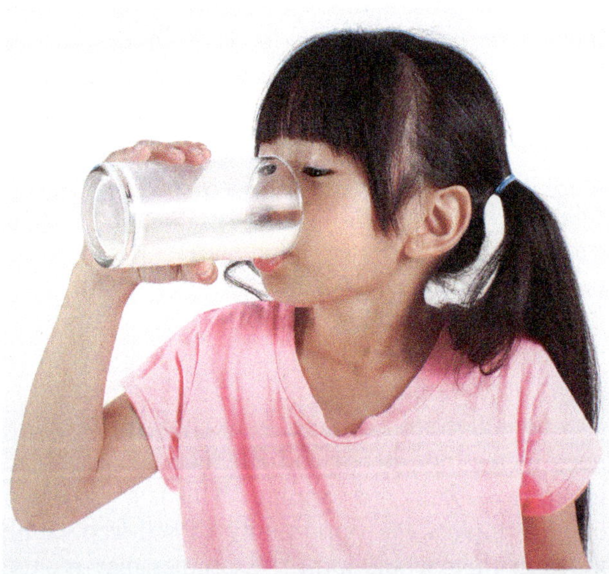

© paulaphoto/Shutterstock

children fill their own plates, they consume less food and begin to recognize their own satiety cues. Forceful or restrictive environments can have a negative impact on children. In these atmospheres, children are prone to overeating and later weight gain, because they are not able to exercise control. The intake of preschool-aged children is largely reflective of their parents' typical diets.

School-Aged Children

School-aged children begin to better understand and describe food. They are able to categorize food by their likes and dislikes, as well as if they are considered healthy. At the same time, school-aged children have the potential to consume more sugar-sweetened beverages and high-fat foods and less wholesome foods like fruits, vegetables, and whole grains. School-aged children who eat meals with their family are less likely to drink sugar-sweetened beverages.[69] Unlike toddlers and preschoolers, school-aged children consume a wider variety of foods. School-aged children also have lower energy needs, thus a balance between energy intake and activity becomes increasingly important. It is recommended by the AAP that school-aged children exercise for a minimum of 60 minutes/day. This should be a combination of aerobic exercise and muscle- and bone-strengthening activities.

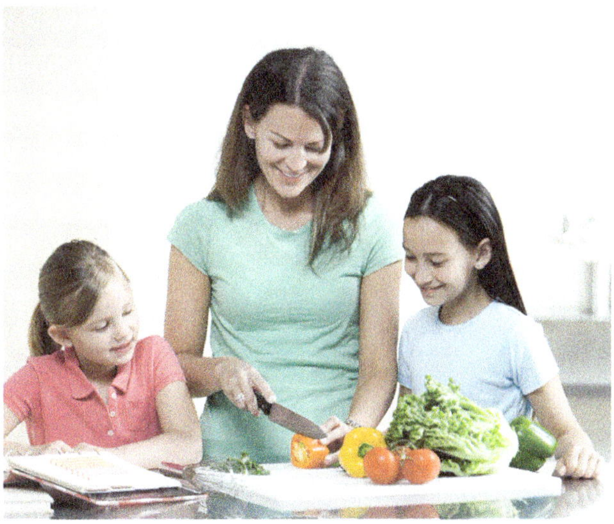

© Artemis Gordon/Shutterstock

There are many factors that influence a child's eating behavior, including their eating environment. As a dietitian, it is important to provide education about how the environment promotes the development of healthy eating practices. Children's early eating practices are highly affected by their parents. Family feeding practices can influence a child's perception of meal size and satiety.[68] As children grow and develop, their tastes develop as well. The eating environment is especially important as children try new foods. Enthusiastic modeling and repeated exposures can help a child to try new foods. A healthy home environment is most closely associated with healthy eating habits, such as increased fruit and vegetable consumption and decreased soda and snack food consumption.[66]

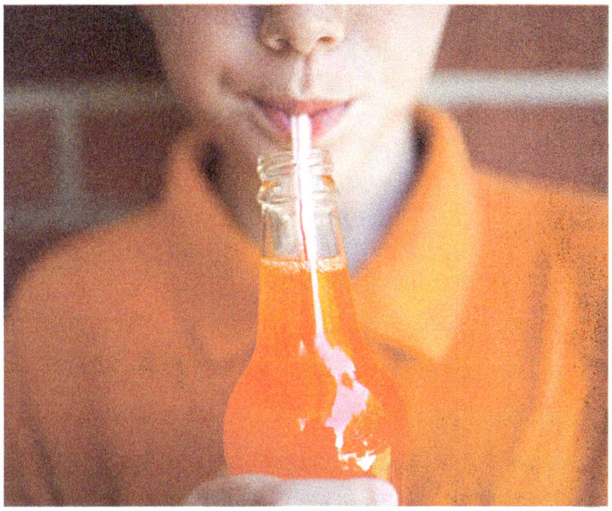

© Melissa Lomax Speelman/Moment/Getty Images

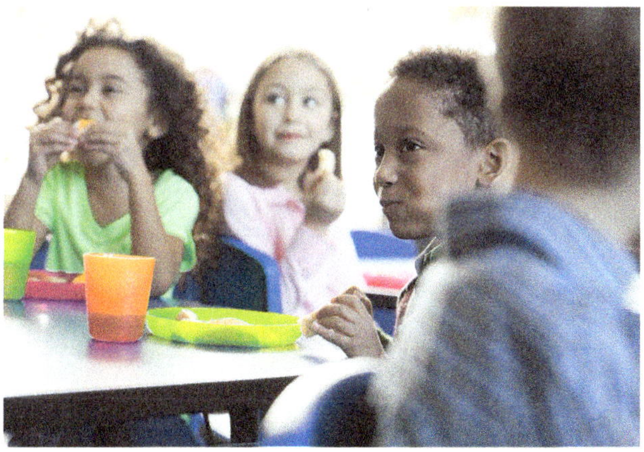

© Hero Images/Getty Images

Adolescents

Adolescents have increased energy and nutrient needs compared to preschool and school-aged children due to an increase in growth velocity. Older children's eating habits are largely influenced by their friends, often resulting in decreased consumption of nutrient-dense foods and increased intake of sugar-sweetened beverages and high-fat, nutrient-poor foods. Despite increased calorie intake, lack of certain nutrients such as calcium and iron is problematic for this age group. Adolescents are at increased risk for osteoporosis later in life due to suboptimal bone mineralization. Iron deficiency anemia, poor weight management, and chronic diseases such as T2DM and heart disease may also result from poor dietary habits. While older children should be encouraged to make their own healthy food choices, it is important to continue family meals. Assuring a good breakfast is associated with more healthful eating behaviors as well as better diet quality.[69–73]

As previously described, adolescents become increasingly aware of the changes in their bodies as they progress through the pubertal growth spurt. Thus, they are at increased risk for disordered eating patterns and poor weight management. Disordered adolescent eating patterns are also related to parenting styles.[74] Recognizing the signs and symptoms of an eating disorder may help to improve outcomes. Please refer to Chapter 23, *Nutrition in Eating Disorders*, for more information on identifying and working with individuals with eating disorders.

CORE CONCEPT 9

At each stage, children should consume a well-balanced diet. Eating environment, parental modeling, and nutrition knowledge can all influence eating practices.

PRACTICE POINT

Diet interview and education in pediatrics should include assessment of parenteral knowledge and attitudes as well as family meal patterns.

Nutrient Support During Illness or Chronic Disease

Management of Growth Faltering

The first step to managing GF is to identify the cause of the underlying problem and correct it. Because there are many causes and contributing factors to GF, this can involve several steps. With illness-related GF, nutrient prescriptions should be based on the macro- and micronutrient requirements associated with the specific disease state. For children with critical illness experiencing prolonged hospital stays, this involves use of a protein-enriched, calorically dense formula to support weight gain.[74] For children with medical conditions influencing their ability to suck or swallow, special bottles and nipples may be needed to facilitate intake. Evaluating feeding habits such as duration of feeds, latching, and milk supply can identify problem areas. It is important to look for signs of intolerance such as the baby arching, spitting up, coughing or gagging, or changes in stool pattern.[75] Maximizing nutrient quality of intake by fortifying human milk or including concentrated infant formulas is often required. In children no longer on formula, using high-calorie and high-protein foods and drinks is also effective. Homemade shakes can be made as desired using choices such as whole milk, ice cream, and added nut butters. If swallowing difficulties exist, modular thickening agents can be used to achieve the proper consistency. In addition, a high-calorie oral nutrition supplement can be helpful to maximize oral intake. In cases of severe undernutrition, supplemental nutrition support by feeding tube may be warranted. **Table 20.18** presents possible etiologies for GF and the appropriate intervention.

Children suffering from non-illness–related GF are likely to have a complexity of factors impacting growth. For infants, continuation of breastfeeding is highly recommended when possible; however, milk fortification may be needed to increase protein and calorie content. For formula-fed infants, concentrating formula can improve weight gain. It is important to educate parents on preparing formula properly, including a check back to assure they understand. Evaluation of the home environment with respect to food security, family stressors, structure of mealtimes, parental nutrition knowledge, and beliefs about eating should also be evaluated. Using an interprofessional team of specialists that includes medicine, nursing, speech, and/or occupational therapy, as well as a dietitian, is considered best practice.[72]

PRACTICE POINT

Human milk fortifiers and concentrated formula are often needed in patients with GF. Diet interviews should include how parents are preparing, mixing, and storing formula or human milk.

CORE CONCEPT 10

Growth faltering (or failure to thrive) can be the result of both illness and non-illness etiologies.

Catch-Up Growth. **Catch-up growth** describes increased growth velocity following recovery from an illness or a period of undernutrition.[73] Catch-up

Table 20.18 Factors Associated with Growth Failure

Illness Related	Inadequate Intake	Increased Energy Expenditure	Increased Losses or Altered Utilization
	Poor appetite due to disease/illness Eating disorder	Congenital heart or lung disease (includes cystic fibrosis, bronchopulmonary dysplasia)	Gastrointestinal disease (celiac, inflammatory bowel disease, cystic fibrosis)
	Impaired suck or swallow (cleft lip and palate)	Critical illness	Inborn errors in metabolism
	Dysphagia	Chronic infection	Food allergies
	Gastrointestinal symptoms (reflux, constipation)	Malignancy	Renal, endocrine disease
Non-Illness Related	**Socioeconomic**	**Parental Factors**	**Other Environmental**
	Low-income settings	Maternal depression/anxiety	Undiagnosed feeding problem
	Food insecurity	Parental knowledge, belief or attitudes	Neglect, deprivation
	Improper formula or food preparation	Family stressors	Food scarcity due to war, lack of water

Data from Smith AE, Shah M, Badireddy M. Failure to Thrive. [Updated 2023 Nov 12]. In: *StatPearls* [Internet]. Treasure Island (FL): StatPearls Publishing; 2025. Available from: https://www.ncbi.nlm.nih.gov/books/NBK459287/

growth is different from growth acceleration, which is spontaneous and occurs naturally at critical periods of development. While both result in an upward acceleration of percentile growth, catch-up growth only occurs after recovery from an illness or insult. Goals for energy and protein are generally estimated using the patient's ideal body weight. The median weight for age (or the 50th percentile) can be used. In patients with weight-for-age below the 3rd percentile, the 25th percentile weight for age or clinical judgment can be used. A high protein intake is critical for catch-up growth to occur.[73] Care should be taken when using modulars to supplement calories so as not to lower the protein-to-calorie ratio. **Table 20.19** presents calculation of energy and protein needs. The patient should remain on the fortified protein and energy diet until they reach their preinjury weight-for-age percentile.[42]

PRACTICE POINT

Ideal body weight (represented by median weight for age) should be used to determine energy and protein goals for catch-up growth.

Table 20.19 Calculating Catch-Up Growth Needs and Goal Volume of Formula Feed

Step 1: Calculate estimated energy requirement (EER) in 2-month-old female with growth faltering using ideal body weight (IBW).

Anthropometrics:

Weight: 4.0 kg 3rd % WFA; $z = -1.89$

Length: 56 cm 30th % LFA; $z = -0.52$

IBW (Median or 50th % WFA): 5.13

$$\begin{aligned} EER &= -69.15 + (80 \times age) + (2.65 \times height) + (54.15 \times weight) + 180 \\ &= -69.15 + (80 \times 0.167) + (2.65 \times 56) + (52.15 \times 5.13) + 180 \\ &= -69.15 + 13.36 + 148.4 + 267.5 + 180 \\ &= 540.11 \text{ or } 540 \text{ kcal/day} \end{aligned}$$

Step 2: Determine kcal/kg of actual weight.

EER = 540 kcal/day

Actual Weight: 4.0 kg

540/4.0 = 135 kcal/kg/day

Step 3: Determine formula volume to meet EER.

Using standard formula:

540/20 kcal/ oz = 27 oz/day

Data from Cooke R, Goulet O, Huysentruyt K, et al. Catch-up growth in infants and young children with faltering growth: expert opinion to guide general clinicians. *J Pediatr Gastroenterol Nutr*. 2023; 77(1):7–15. https://doi.org/10.1097/MPG.0000000000003784

Nutrition Support During Malnutrition or Illness. Children with chronic disease or illness are especially vulnerable to malnutrition. Because of their limited LBM stores, infants and younger children can become malnourished quickly. About 40–50% of hospitalized children are at risk for malnutrition.[76–78] Pediatric patients with critical illness are at the greatest risk due to impact of protein catabolism on LBM stores. Failure to provide optimal nutrition can impact clinical outcome. All children admitted into a pediatric intensive care unit (PICU) should have a proper nutritional screening and assessment.[78]

Nutrition support is a strategy used to minimize the risk of and treat malnutrition. Enteral nutrition (EN) and parenteral nutrition (PN) are the two forms of nutrition therapy that are used. The goal of nutrition therapy is to provide adequate nutrition to minimize LBM losses and minimize the long-term consequences of critical illness. Providing sufficient nutrients can improve the patient's immune response, prevent reduced gut function, and decrease the length of hospital stay.[78]

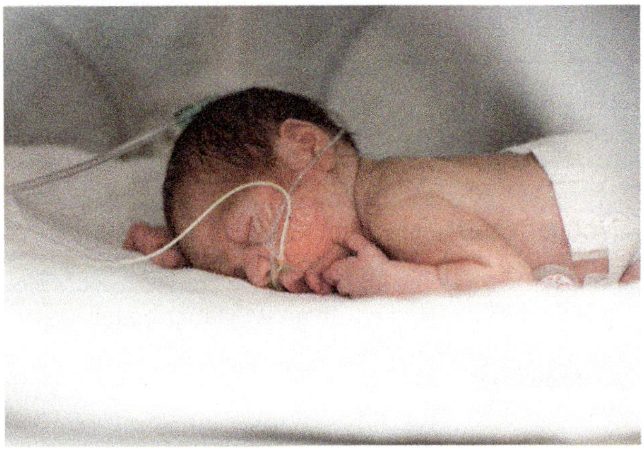

PRACTICE POINT

Enteral nutrition is the preferred mode of nutrition support in children.

Enteral and parenteral nutrition are both considered in the pediatric patient with critical illness. The enteral route is beneficial in maintaining mucosal immunity and is associated with improved mortality in children with critical illness.[78] However, PN should be used when EN is not tolerated, particularly in children at nutritional risk or if the gastrointestinal (GI) tract is dysfunctional. The current ASPEN guidelines on the provision of nutrition support state that while EN is the preferred modality, however delaying PN, as is common in adults, should not be broadly applied in the pediatric population. Timing and use of supplemental PN should be individually determined based on the status of the patient. Patients in the PICU who cannot receive EN during the first week of admission may receive supplemental PN. Patients with malnutrition or those at risk for rapid deterioration, such as in metabolic stress, should also receive PN if EN cannot be advanced beyond a low volume. **Table 20.20** presents the indications and contraindications for EN and PN in the pediatric patient.[65]

CORE CONCEPT 11

Nutrition support may be indicated in pediatric patients when oral feeding does not provide enough energy or nutrients. Timely initiation, particularly in children younger than 2 years of age, prevents rapid deterioration of nutritional status.

Enteral Nutrition

EN initiated within the first 24–48 hours following admission, and at rates up to two-thirds of goal, is associated with improved clinical outcomes in children.[78] In a critical care setting, there are many barriers to EN progression, such as use of vasoactive drugs, prolonged periods of holding feeds for procedures, and GI intolerance.[79–83] Use of stepwise algorithms to guide initiation and progression of EN is advised for safe and timely EN support (**Figure 20.12**).[78] Evaluation of nutritional risk based on malnutrition or the severity of disease and accompanying metabolic stress should be incorporated into this decision-making process. Given their decreased LBM, children 0–2 years of age should be presumed high risk.

PRACTICE POINT

Standard feeding algorithms should be used to guide nutrition support therapy, including parameters for bedside monitoring of feeding tolerance.

Enteral Access and Type of Delivery

EN support can be administered into the stomach (gastric) or into the small intestine (postpyloric). Gastric feeds are more physiologic and mimic normal nutrition, particularly when given as a bolus feed. Bolus feedings are generally preferred in ambulatory pediatric patients, as larger volumes of formula

Table 20.20 Indications and Contraindications for Enteral and Parenteral Nutrition

Enteral Versus Parental Nutrition		
	Indications	**Contraindications**
Enteral nutrition	**Inadequate oral intake** *Causes:* developmental, behavioral, or anatomical complications **Increased nutritional needs** *Causes:* chronic disease, malabsorption, metabolic disorders, inadequate intestinal function, increased energy expenditure, critical illness	**GI tract cannot be safely accessed** *Causes:* facial or esophageal injury **Gut is not functional** *Causes:* feedings cannot be advanced, excessive diarrhea, ileus, obstruction, fistulas **Hemodynamic instability** *Causes:* critical illness, as evidenced by vasopressor or extracorporeal membrane oxygenation utilization
Parenteral nutrition	GI tract is not functional or it cannot be accessed Nutrient needs exceed what can be provided by enteral nutrition and oral intake Premature infants: GI tract is not fully developed Certain disease states: congenital heart disease, congenital abnormalities, necrotizing enterocolitis, short bowel syndrome Critical illness Failure to thrive with diarrhea	Oral and enteral nutrition provides enough energy and nutrients Poor central line access Low nutritional risk

Modified from *ASPEN Pediatric Nutrition Support Core Curriculum*. 2nd ed. Corkins; 2015.

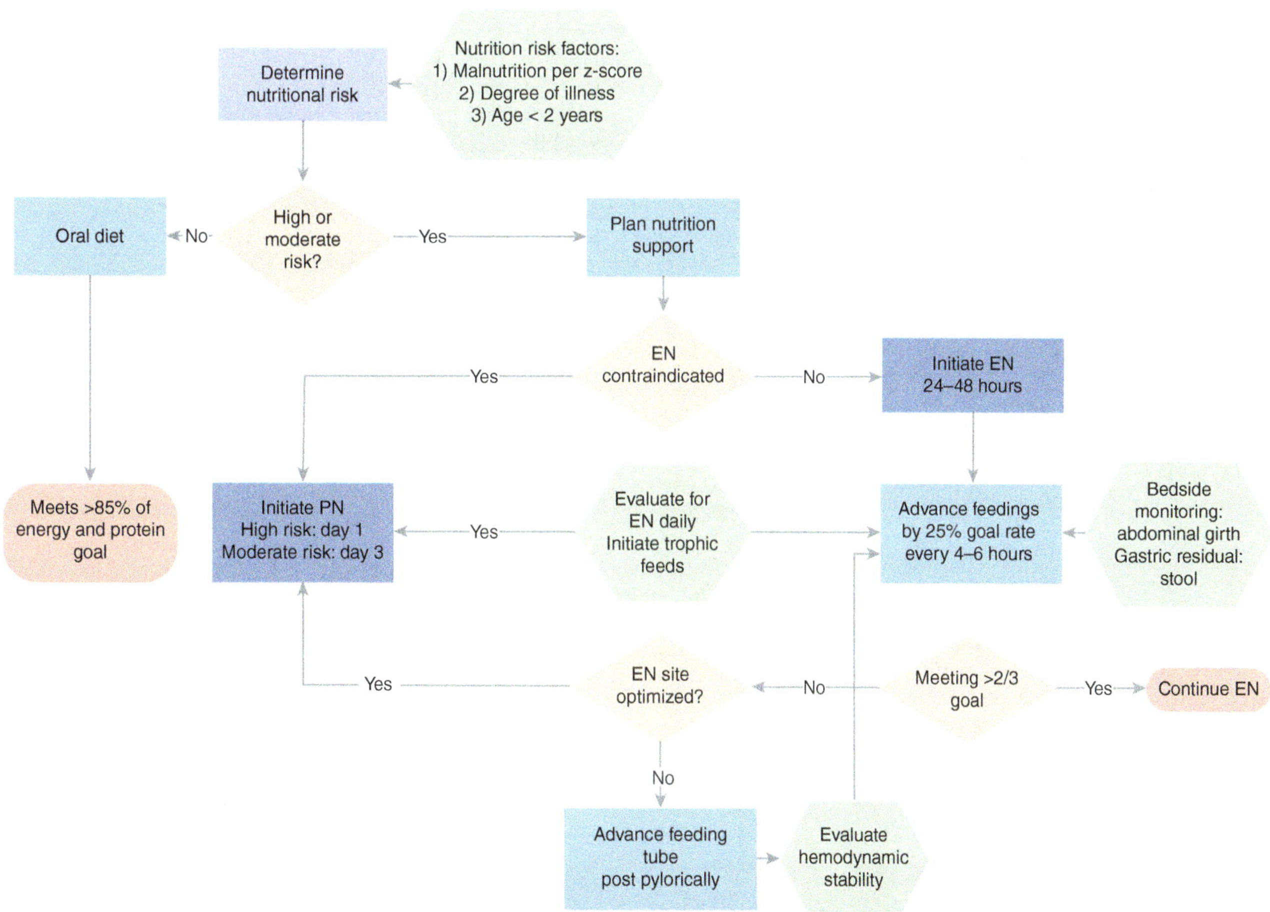

Figure 20.12 Example of an Algorithm for Nutrition Support Therapy in Children

can be administered at once without interruption to lifestyle.[80] Although less common in an acute setting, bolus feedings are well tolerated in hospitalized children.[81] More commonly, a continuous delivery of formula is provided for improved tolerance. In some patients, postpyloric feedings can overcome challenges with gastroparesis, reflux, or risk of aspiration.[82]

There are several different enteral access points. Feeding tubes such as nasogastric, nasojejunal, gastrostomy, percutaneous endoscopic gastrostomy (PEG), jejunostomy, and percutaneous endoscopic jejunostomy (PEJ) are all options for feeding the pediatric patient. Nasoenteric tubes can be used in the short term, for a maximum of 8 weeks, as they can cause nasal erosion and oral feeding aversion in children.[79]

Gastrostomy and PEG tubes are also commonly used in the pediatric patient when they require long-term EN or if they cannot have a nasoenteric feeding tube.[79] Gastrostomies are indicated when a patient will be fed through a tube for longer than 6–12 weeks. Gastrostomies feed directly into the stomach but differ in the techniques used to insert the tubes. PEG tubes are associated with greater complications in children, because there is potential to damage the bowel or create an obstruction; however, they are presumed safe in infants as small as 6 kg. Gastrostomy tubes are generally preferred by families because they maintain quality of life and are more aesthetically pleasing.[79] Jejunostomy and PEJ tubes are placed similarly to a gastrostomy tube. They can either be advanced or have the stoma created postpylorically. Because patients with jejunostomy tubes will be less tolerant to higher volumes or unable to receive bolus feedings, a schedule that works for the child and family will need to be established.

PRACTICE POINT

If enteral nutrition is expected to be used for longer than 6–12 weeks, a semi-permanent tube, such as a PEG, PEJ, gastrostomy, or jejunostomy, should be inserted instead of a nasoenteric tube.

Enteral Formulas

There are many factors, including growth and diet history, biochemical data, level of GI function, and current feeding regimen, that should be considered when choosing an enteral formula for a pediatric patient (**Table 20.21**). Age of the patient is also a consideration. For infants, concentrated infant formulas and

Table 20.21 Tube Feeding Formulas Used in Pediatric Patient

Formula Name	Pediasure*	Nutren Jr*	Kate Farms Peptide	Peptamen	Vivonex Pediatric	Promote*
Concentration (kcal/mL)	1.0	1.0	1.0	1.0	0.8	1.0
Protein g/1000 mL (% kcal)	30 (12)	30 (12)	36 (14)	40 (16)	24 (12)	62.5 (25)
Carbohydrate g/1000 mL (% kcal)	143 (54)	110 (40)	120 (47)	128 (51)	128 (63)	130 (32)
Fat g/1000 mL (% kcal)	38 (34)	50 (44)	44 (39)	33 (39.2)	23 (11)	26 (23)
Dietary fiber g/1000 mL	13	6	12	-	-	14
NCP:N ratio	183:1		149:1	133:1	185:1	75:1
Sodium/potassium mg/1000 mL	380/1310	460/1320	640/1520	560/1500	376/1092	1000/1980
Calcium/phosphorus mg/1000 mL	1055/84	1000/800	1120/880	800/700	856/720	1200/1200
Vitamin D (IU)	675	560	1200	528	576	400
Zinc (mg/L)/selenium (mcg/L)/copper (mg/L)	6.3/30/0.8	10.8/30/1	6/40/0.8	24/50/2	4.8/31/0.56	24/70/2
Description	Standard polymeric +/− fiber option	Standard polymeric +/− fiber option	Plant-based, hydrolyzed pea protein	Peptide-based, whey protein	Elemental, low fat, improved tolerance	Adult formula, high nitrogen

*Fiber content reported for fiber-containing version of formula

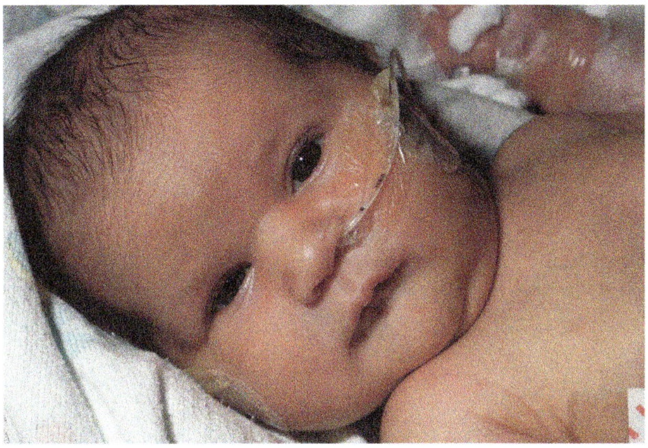

© Rick's Photography/Shutterstock

fortified breast milk are often necessary. Pediatric formulas are designed for patients aged 1–13 years. Adult formulations may be indicated for the adolescent population and are also well suited for younger patients with burns or trauma, as they are higher in protein and micronutrients that support wound healing.

The osmotic load of most adult formulas is likely acceptable for older children. In general, children require a lower renal solute load. Children younger than 4 years of age should receive formulas less than 400 mOsm/kg. Older children can tolerate slightly more concentrated formulas but should not exceed 600 mOsm/kg. Presence of abdominal distention, delayed gastric emptying, vomiting, and diarrhea may indicate that the osmotic load is too great for the patient.

PRACTICE POINT

Pediatric enteral formulas are appropriate to feed children during early childhood. After age 10 years, adult formulas should be considered because they can better meet the needs of the patient.

Types of Formulas. For infants younger than 1 year of age, infant formula can be provided through a feeding tube. It is common practice to concentrate infant formula from 24 to 30 cal/oz. This is done with alterations in mixing instructions of powdered infant formula. In addition, modular proteins, and/or fat, such as in the form of vegetable oil, can be added. Human milk can be given through a feeding tube as well. This is ideal, because it can promote continuation of breastfeeding once the child recovers. Human milk can also be fortified to meet the increased needs of a child during illness through the addition of fat sources, protein modular, infant formulas, or a combination of these.

After the age of one, standard polymeric formulas are available. There are three main classes of enteral formulas: polymeric, semi-elemental, and elemental. Pediatric formularies differ from adult ones, because there are not as many disease-specific formulas available for the pediatric population. In these situations, adult formulations may be necessary to provide a better nutrient composition or to promote recovery. Polymeric formulas can be used when the entire digestive tract is normally functioning. Polymeric formulas are characterized by the presence of intact protein. These formulas provide 30 kcal/oz, 12–15% of which are from protein, 44–53% from carbohydrate, and the remaining 35–45% from fat. Vitamins and minerals are also provided to reach 100% of the DRI when 1 L is provided. Polymeric formulas are available as standard, calorie dense, and fiber enriched. The variations in the formulations help individualize nutrition therapy based on patient needs and for different disease states. Fiber-enriched formulas typically contain 5–8 g/L of fiber. For example, a child who presents with diarrhea may benefit from the use of a polymeric fiber-enriched formula. Calorie-dense pediatric

Clinical Roundtable

Topic: Micronutrient Supplementation in Children Receiving Enteral Nutrition

Background: Children receiving nutritional support are often metabolically stressed, resulting in increased micronutrient losses and/or requirements. Despite a lack of evidence defining micronutrient needs in conditions of stress and illness, certain antioxidant nutrients such as selenium, vitamins C and E, and wound-healing trace elements zinc and copper can often be supplemented in high amounts. Some clinicians advocate that use of adult formulas, particularly in amounts needed to meet increased energy and protein requirements of children who are critically ill, will provide sufficient amounts of these micronutrients.

Roundtable Discussion

1. What are the risks associated with single-nutrient supplementation in high doses?
2. What are the advantages and disadvantages of using adult formulas to meet requirements in children younger than age 10 years?
3. Given the lack of evidence, how might you determine the best practice for meeting micronutrient requirements in children receiving nutrition support?

formulas are designed for children younger than age 10 years and are concentrated to 1.5 kcal/mL.

Semi-elemental formulas are specially designed to enhance nutrient absorption when the GI tract has been compromised. These formulas are indicated when children present with GI conditions due to malabsorption or maldigestion. Semi-elemental formulas contain proteins that have been broken down into peptides and amino acids. The macronutrient composition of these formulas is similar to that of the polymeric formulas. Calorically dense semi-elemental formulas can also be used when children do not tolerate large volumes of formula.

Elemental formulas are also indicated in several situations, such as a compromised GI tract, short bowel syndrome, malabsorption, and multiple protein allergies. These formulas contain only free amino acids. The macronutrient composition of elemental formulas varies greatly. Carbohydrates provide approximately 46–63% of total calories, fat contributes 25–45% of total calories, and protein adds the remaining 10–15% of calories. Elemental formulas are often provided in powdered form, which allows the osmotic load to be changed based on the energy concentration of the order. Elemental formulas typically have a greater osmolality than semi-elemental or polymeric options.

Monitoring of Enteral Tolerance

Patients receiving EN should be closely monitored. There are several complications that may result from enteral feeds; they can be related to tube function or GI intolerance. Signs of intolerance include presence of GI symptoms (abdominal distention, poor gastric emptying, constipation, diarrhea, nausea, vomiting), which may lead to an inability to receive sufficient volume to obtain necessary nutrients from EN.[82,83] Measurement of abdominal girth prior to starting enteral feedings and at every nursing shift is a useful way to anticipate the onset of tube feeding intolerance through monitoring of abdominal distention.

It is also important to evaluate all potential causes of intolerance to enteral feedings. Children may also have adverse reactions to some of the medications they are receiving. In addition, enteral supplementation of electrolytes such as sodium, potassium, or phosphorus via feeding tube can result in a high osmolality, contributing to signs of dumping syndrome. Patients on prolonged antibiotics may develop altered gut flora, resulting in diarrhea. It is useful to evaluate these contributing factors first before switching the formula.

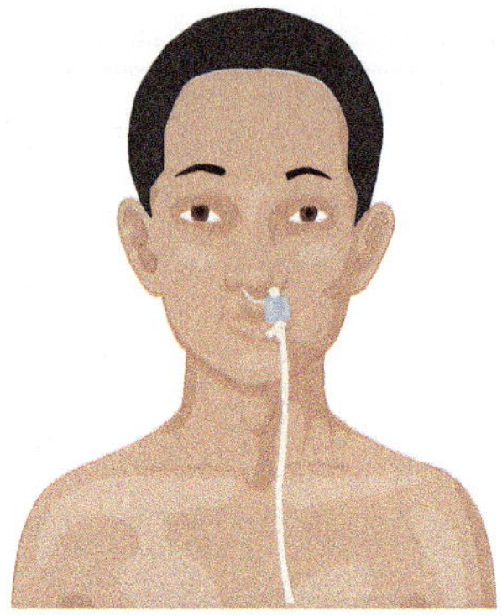

Figure 20.13 Nasal Bridle Used to Secure Nasoenteric Feeding Tube

Feeding tubes should be monitored for placement by marking the tube. Feeding tubes can migrate or be improperly placed, which can lead to aspiration and poor tolerance. The use of a nasal bridle to secure a nasoenteric feeding tube is often used in children to prevent migration and dislodgement (**Figure 20.13**). Feeding tubes may also become clogged and should be checked for signs of occlusion. Fine bore tubes that are placed nasoenterically are more comfortable for the patient but pose a greater risk for occlusion.

Patients who begin nutrition support after a period of decreased intake are at risk for refeeding syndrome. These patients are prone to hypophosphatemia, hypokalemia, hypomagnesemia, and thiamine deficiency. Physiologic alterations include tachycardia and fluid retention. Criteria exist for identifying pediatric patients at risk of refeeding syndrome, which essentially include indicators used to diagnose malnutrition such as weight loss, decreased weight/length or BMI/age z-scores, or physical signs of muscle wasting and fat loss. Inadequate intake for greater than 4 days and abnormally low serum levels of potassium, phosphorus, and magnesium (25–50% below normal values) are also considered when assessing refeeding risk.

Protocols for advancing diet in patients with refeeding risk should be followed. ASPEN recommendations for advancing feedings in pediatric patients with refeeding risk include starting at 40–50% of the energy goal. For patients receiving PN, initiating at a glucose infusion rate (GIR) between 4 and 5 mg of carbohydrate/kg/min and slowly advancing by 1–2 mg/kg/min is suggested. In older patients, it may be necessary to start at a lower GIR rate such as 3–4 mg/kg/min. Serum electrolytes should be measured prior to initiating feeds and then at least every 12 hours or more frequently depending on severity, repleting as necessary. A thiamine supplement of 1–2 mg/kg or 100–200 mg is recommended prior to starting feedings. This should continue for at least 5–7 days after starting feedings.[84]

Parenteral Nutrition

PN may be indicated in pediatric patients who are unable to feed orally and do not tolerate enteral feedings. There are a number of pediatric conditions where PN is indicated. The primary one is intestinal failure, with short bowel syndrome (SBS) being the most common cause.[85] Dysmotility disorders such as pseudo-intestinal obstruction, and congenital anomalies such as gastrochisis (when organs are born outside of abdominal wall), atresia, and malrotation are all conditions for which PN can be lifesaving. PN is also indicated in premature infants as their GI tract is underdeveloped. Children who are critically ill or those at nutritional risk may also require PN (**Table 20.22**). It is important to use clinical judgment with particular focus on preexisting nutritional status, malnutrition risk, and disease severity. Unlike adults, children (particularly younger children) have limited LBM stores and preferentially rely on glucose. In these cases, PN feedings should not be delayed if enteral intolerance occurs to avoid rapid erosion of LBM stores.[65,78.]

Parenteral Access

PN can be administered through a central or a peripheral line. A central venous catheter is placed with the catheter tip into the superior vena cava. Access through a main, central vein is often preferred as more concentrated solutions can be provided. Peripheral parenteral nutrition (PPN) is delivered via a smaller vein and is limited to 10–12% dextrose solutions. PPN cannot meet the nutritional needs of premature infants.

Timing and Dosing in Parenterally Fed Patients

PN dosing in terms of macro- and micronutrients is age and condition specific. In preterm infants with underdeveloped GI systems, PN is recommended soon after birth. In this population, the recommended minimum intake of protein is 3 g/kg with a maximum of 3.5 g/kg. Advancing intravenous lipid emulsion (ILE) to 3 g/kg/day is recommended to support growth.[86,87] Infants have a high capacity for glucose oxidation such that dextrose infusions providing up to 10–14 mg of carbohydrate (CHO)/kg/min are well tolerated. After 1 year of age, reliance on glucose declines such that dextrose infusion rates of 8–10 mg CHO/kg/m are recommended. After 10 years, glucose oxidation is similar to adults: 5–6 mg CHO/kg/min.[86] **Table 20.23** displays PN macronutrient dosing for preterm infants through adolescents.

Targets for Energy Provision

For pediatric patients who are critically ill, energy goals are set for maintenance, not growth. As such, pediatric patients can sometimes appear to have lower energy needs than when in health because they are not laying down new tissue or being physically active. During the acute phase of care, newborns requiring PN should receive at least 45–55 kcal/kg/day for homeostasis. From age 1 to 7 years, energy needs are slightly less at 40–45 kcal/kg. Ages 7–12 require 30–40 kcal/kg. For children ages 12–18 years, 20–30 kcal/kg is suggested. As patients become stable, or during the recovery phase, energy goals can be increased.[88]

Commonly, predictive equations are used to determine the energy requirements of children who are critically ill. However, as in adults, these equations do

Table 20.22 Pediatric Conditions Requiring Parenteral Nutrition

Intestinal Failure	Feeding Intolerance	Conditions with Risk of Mesenteric Ischemia
Short Bowel Syndrome (due to intestinal resection in gastrointestinal disease) Congenital GI Anomalies - Gastroschisis - Atresia Dysmotility Disorders - Pseudo-obstruction - Congenital enteropathy disease	Irretractable vomiting or diarrhea Radiation Enteritis Paralytic Ileus	Hemodynamic instability Extracorporeal membrane oxygenation (ECMO) Critical illness Necrotizing enterocolitis

Data from Mehta NM, Skillman HE, Irving SY, et al. Guidelines for the provision and assessment of nutrition support therapy in pediatric critically ill patient: Society of Critical Care Medicine and American Society for Parenteral and Enteral Nutrition. *J Parenter Enteral Nutr.* 2017;4(5):706–742.

Table 20.23 Parenteral Nutrition Macronutrient Dosing

	Preterm	Infants	Children age 1–10 years	Adolescence
Protein (g/kg)	3–3.5	2.5	1.5–2.5	0.8–2
Dextrose (mg/kg/min)	10–14	10–14	8–10	5–6
Fat (g/kg)	3 max 0.15 g/kg/h	3 max 0.15 g/kg/h	2–2.5	1–2

Data from *ASPEN Pediatric Nutrition Support Core Curriculum*. 2nd ed. Corkins. Silver Spring, MD;2015.

not accurately estimate energy needs, given that many disease states produce variable metabolic responses. This can be particularly concerning in parenterally fed patients, where overfeeding and underfeeding lead to serious respiratory and hepatic complications.[78] Thus, use of indirect calorimetry is considered to be the gold standard in determining the patient's energy expenditure.[78,88–91] Indirect calorimetry can estimate what substrates are being metabolized, as well as the resting energy expenditure of the individual.[89] ASPEN states that patients who do not meet their calorie goals, fail to wean off respiratory support, require increased respiratory support, need muscle relaxants for 7 days, are hypermetabolic, or have an expected length of stay longer than 4 weeks in the intensive care unit are candidates for indirect calorimetry. In this context, patient populations who would benefit from indirect calorimetry include those who are critically ill, ventilator-dependent, and/or burn-injured; patients who are underweight or overweight; patients with cancer; and those with neurological trauma.[78] If indirect calorimetry is not available, using the Schofield equation for REE with the appropriate factors for stress is recommended. Patients should receive two-thirds of their prescribed energy target by the end of 7 days.[78]

Carbohydrate. Glucose should be the primary carbohydrate source for patients receiving PN. It is a preferred fuel source for the brain, red and white blood cells, and wounded tissue. Provision of intravenous dextrose blunts gluconeogenesis, thereby minimizing erosion of lean body mass. As mentioned, children 0–2 years of age are highly reliant on glucose as their primary fuel source. Therefore, intravenous dextrose should comprise a majority of calories. Intakes of at least 50–60% of total energy requirement are suggested. Likewise, intake can be based on the GIR, which represents the amount of glucose that is oxidized. This varies according to age and weight of the child. The GIR is highest in young children, gradually declining to rates similar to adults by 2–5 years of age. The GIR must be about 2 mg/kg/min to prevent ketosis, but below 15 mg/kg/min to prevent hepatic steatosis and lipogenesis.[78,91]

Fat. ILEs offer the advantage of being energy dense and low in osmolality. Compared to dextrose as an energy source, they stimulate less carbon dioxide production. Lipid turnover and fatty acid oxidation are increased during critical illness in children, indicating that fat is a good source of energy in this setting. ILEs also provide essential fatty acids, linoleic, and linolenic fatty acids. As a general rule, these fatty acids should contribute to 5% of total energy intake in order to prevent fatty acid deficiency. In patients expected to be on long-term PN, 1 g/kg/day is sufficient for meeting essential fatty acid requirements without increasing risk for hepatic complications.[85] For pediatric patients receiving PN, fat in general accounts for approximately 30–40% of energy intake. Infants can receive as little as 25% of their total calories from fat, or 2–2.5 g/kg/day. Older children with decreased fat needs may receive a higher percentage, approximating 1–2 g/kg/day of fat.

Protein. Protein is provided as amino acids in PN solutions. In infants, pediatric-specific formulations contain amino acid compositions that simulate the amino acid composition of human milk and can stimulate growth in patients without critical illness. PN provision in neonates has added cysteine, which is conditionally essential in this population. A dose of 30 mg/day is recommended. Supplemental cysteine has been found to have no added benefit in older children.

Protein needs vary based on age as well as disease state. During critical illness, amino acids are redistributed from the skeletal muscle to the liver and other organs for wound healing, immunity, and overall recovery. Typically, during critical illness and the stress response, the rates of protein breakdown exceed synthesis, placing children at high risk for prolonged negative nitrogen balance and catabolism. When protein losses are profound and occur in critical organs such

Table 20.24 Electrolyte Requirements in Pediatric Patients

Electrolyte	Infants and Children	Adolescents >50 kg
Sodium	2–5 mEq/kg	1–2 mEq/kg
Potassium	2–4 mEq/kg	1–2 mEq/kg
Calcium	0.5–4 mEq/kg 500–600 mg/L	10–20 mEq/day 200–400 mg/L
Phosphorus	0.5–2 mmol/kg 400–450 mg/L	10–40 mmol/day 150–300 mg/L
Magnesium	0.3–0.5 mEq/kg 50–70 mg/L	10–30 mEq/day 20–40 mg/L

Data from *ASPEN Pediatric Nutrition Support Core Curriculum*. 2nd ed. Corkins. Silver Spring, MD;2015.

as the heart and lungs, clinical manifestations take place that can hinder breathing and weaning from the mechanical ventilator. The recommended minimum amount of protein in children with critical illness is 1.5 g/kg/day.[78] However, protein needs can be much higher, particularly in severe trauma or burn injury, rising to greater than 3–4 g/kg/day. Ultimately, protein targets should promote positive nitrogen balance. In neonates, 1.5–3 g/kg of protein is required. From ages 1–3 years, 2–3 g/kg of protein are necessary as a minimum, while older children require 1–2.5 g/kg of protein in PN solutions. Amino acid solutions should not exceed 4 g/kg to prevent azotemia.[78]

Fluid and Electrolytes. In PN solutions, fluid and electrolytes are provided based on the clinical condition of the patient. Often, requirements are determined based on the biochemical indices, hydration, and clinical condition. Electrolyte management is best managed in IV fluids outside of the PN solution to avoid wasting solution once abnormalities are corrected. **Table 20.24** summarizes the general electrolyte requirements in children.

Additives. There are many micronutrients and medications that can be administered through a PN solution. Vitamin and trace element solutions are added to formulas. In patients younger than 11 years, pediatric vitamin mixes are provided based on the weight of the child. Similar to typical pediatric patients, calcium and phosphorus are both nutrients of concern because they are required for bone mineralization; however, their amounts are limited due to risk of precipitation. Deficiencies in zinc, selenium, and copper are common in patients receiving PN. Adequate levels of these minerals are necessary for development, as well as wound healing and immunity. Carnitine, an amino acid derivative, is required for lipid oxidation in patients receiving PN for more than 4 weeks. It can also benefit patients who have high triglycerides. Carnitine should be provided at a rate of 2–5 mg/kg/day.

Administration of Parenteral Nutrition

PN can be administered continuously or cyclically. There are benefits and risks associated with both methods of administration. Continuous infusion of PN results in a continuous supply of glucose to the child, which causes constant release of insulin. It also allows for a lower osmotic load to be delivered to the patient. There are additional risks associated with continuous glucose infusion, however, such as the development of liver dysfunction, hepatomegaly, and parenteral nutrition–associated liver disease (PNALD).

Parenteral Nutrition-Associated Liver Disease

PNALD is a difficult condition that affects from 30% to 70% of infants on PN, which is far higher than its prevalence in adults.[92] PNALD presents most commonly as cholestasis in children. The prevalence of PN cholestasis is high among patients receiving PN for greater than one month.[93] In addition to PN duration, rates of cholestasis are increased in children following GI surgery, enteral nutrition starvation, or excessive carbohydrate intake.[94] Additional factors such as prematurity and low birth weight, short bowel syndrome, bacterial overgrowth, decreased enterohepatic circulation, and lack of certain amino acids may be to blame.[92] Intestinal failure–associated liver disease (IFALD) is the term used to define liver disease associated with intestinal failure and long-term reliance on PN.[85] Currently in the forefront of understanding the etiology and treatment of IFALD is the lipid source used in parenteral solutions. Traditional ILE is soybean oil (SO) based, which is high in omega-6 fatty acids and may be inflammatory. Use of fish oil (FO)-based ILE is proven to decrease the incidence of sepsis, cholestasis, and IFALD.[85,94–96] One mechanism appears to be a reduction in cytokines and inflammatory mediators, due to a higher omega-3 fatty acid content.[95] Reducing soybean ILE to a lower dose has also been proposed to avoid IFALD. However, low dosing of 1 g/kg/day may detrimentally impact neurodevelopment and growth.[96] At this time, there is no recommendation regarding the composition of ILE for preventing IFALD.[86]

PRACTICE POINT

Pediatric patients on PN support are at increased risk for PNALD. Monitoring of labs for cholestasis and liver function should occur regularly. Prolonged duration of PN and excessive carbohydrate intake should be avoided if possible.

Monitoring

Parenteral feeding needs to be closely monitored. In the pediatric patient with critical illness, overfeeding and underfeeding can both be problematic. Overfeeding is sometimes difficult to observe given the ease at which PN can be provided with few signs of intolerance that would otherwise be found with EN feedings. However, overfeeding of PN can negatively impact the liver, potentially resulting in hepatic steatosis. In addition, overfeeding results in increased carbon dioxide production, making it difficult to wean from the ventilator. Exacerbation of hyperglycemia, a common problem during metabolic stress, is another risk of overfeeding with PN. Underfeeding is equally problematic because patients present with a negative nitrogen balance, malnutrition, and impaired immunity. In addition, increased catabolism, accelerated loss of LBM, and respiratory muscle mass loss all result from underfeeding.[91,97,98] Clinicians wishing to avoid the negative consequences of overfeeding PN may be overly judicious in providing adequate

⚠ Clinical Controversy

IV Lipid Emulsions in Intestinal Failure-Associated Liver Disease

PN is required in children with intestinal failure (IF). IF can be caused by short bowel syndrome or a dysfunctional GI tract due to necrotizing enterocolitis and a number of congenital diseases of the GI l system. The incidence of IF in children is 3–5 per 100,000 cases. PN is necessary in supporting these children during bowel adaptation until enteral nutrition can be tolerated. Unfortunately, the process of bowel adaptation is lengthy and may take months to years to occur. During this time, IF-associated liver disease (IFALD) is a common complication. The primary consequence of IFALD is cholestasis, which in some patients leads to end-stage liver disease and the need for liver transplant. Research demonstrates that replacement of soybean oil (SO) with fish oil (FO) reduces the effects of IFALD. Several studies describe the potential benefits of FO ILE as decreased inflammation, improvement in the lipid panel, decreased bilirubin levels, and reversal of PNALD. Calkins et al.[1] reported that 75% of infants receiving FO versus 6% receiving SO have resolution of cholestasis. Researchers have looked at the efficacy of reducing the administration of SO ILE to less than 1 g/kg/day. Calkins et al.[2] demonstrated that giving low-dose SO at 1 g/kg/day versus conventional SO at 3 g/kg/day was also associated with decreased levels of conjugated bilirubin without impacting growth parameters. This raises the question of whether lower doses of SO ILE could be sufficient in treatment and prevention of ILALD. Given the cost and lack of FDA approval, this could be valuable therapeutic option for FO ILE.

The introduction of composite lipid emulsions that contain less soybean oil (30%) and inclusion of medium chain triglycerides (30%), olive oil (25%), and fish oil (15%) has brought yet another alternative for treating and preventing IFALD. Diamond et al.[3] demonstrated a reduction in IFALD in patients receiving composite lipid versus conventional SO ILE. This is contrary to the study by Ferguson et al.[4] where there was no difference in IFALD when comparing mixed oils that contain FO and SO. Controversy therefore remains as to whether the best treatment and prevention of IFALD lies in monotherapy with FO as the sole lipid source, reduction in SO lipid, or a combined approach where SO is reduced and FO is given.

Question

1. Evaluate the type and strength of the studies described above. What is your opinion on the ideal approach to treating and preventing IFALD in children with intestinal failure?

References

1. Calkins KL, Dunn JC, Shew SB, et al. Pediatric intestinal failure associated liver disease is reversed in 6 months with intravenous fish oil. *JPEN*. 2014;38(6):682–692.
2. Calkins KL, Havraneck T, Kelley-Quon LI, et al. Low-dose parenteral soybean oil for the prevention of parenteral associated liver disease in neonate with gastrointestinal disorders: a multicenter randomized controlled pilot study. *JPEN*. 2017;41(3):404–411.
3. Diamond IR, Grant RC, Pencharz PB, et al. Preventing the progression of intestinal failure-associated liver disease in infants using a composite lipid emulsion: a pilot randomized controlled trial of SMOFlipid. *JPEN*. 2017;41(5):866–877.
4. Ferguson CL, Perry C, Subramanian M, et al. Mixed oil-based lipid emulsions vs soybean oil-based lipid emulsions on incidence and severity of intestinal failure-associated liver disease in a neonatal intensive care unit. *JPEN J Parenter Enteral Nutr*. 2021;25:303-308.

Table 20.25 Biochemical Monitoring of Children Receiving PN

Biochemical Indices	Monitoring Schedule
Electrolytes Calcium (ionized), phosphorus, magnesium	Prior to PN; every 6 hours after the initiation of PN; then daily
Glucose	Prior to PN; every 6 hours after the initiation of PN; then daily *Requires more frequent monitoring with insulin therapy*
Liver function tests	Weekly
Triglycerides	Prior to initiating IVLE; then weekly
Urinary urea nitrogen	Weekly
Blood urea nitrogen, creatinine	Daily
Amylase, lipase	Weekly

Data from *ASPEN Pediatric Nutrition Support Core Curriculum*. 2nd ed. Corkins. Silver Spring, MD;2015.

calories. Likewise, given the risk of ILE as described above, lipids are sometimes omitted. Routine assessment of nutritional parameters such as weight, nitrogen balance, and healing is useful to ensure patients are being fed adequately.

Monitoring of electrolytes and other biochemical parameters is important in PN-fed children. **Table 20.25** presents a recommended schedule for patients receiving PN. Often, because these patients are critically ill, many of these parameters are monitored as part of acute care management. It is therefore important not to duplicate lab monitoring to avoid excess blood loss with multiple blood draws.

Immunonutrition Support in Children

Given the paucity of data and potential harm of immune-modulating nutrients as evidenced in adults, ASPEN currently does not recommend the use of immune-enhancing nutrients in children.[78] The most common nutrients studied, either alone or in combination, are glutamine, arginine, omega-3 fatty acids, and antioxidants such as selenium. An overview of the rationale for use and current findings is provided here.

Glutamine

Glutamine is involved in immune response, metabolic function, and tissue production; however, it is a conditionally essential amino acid during the inflammatory response. It is thought that glutamine may maintain GI function, decrease inflammatory markers, and improve outcomes when administered during critical illness.[99–102] In a meta-analysis, glutamine supplementation was not proven to have a benefit on pediatric patients with severe GI disease.[103] There is limited research to support the use of glutamine supplementation in nutritional support of the pediatric population at this time.

Arginine

Like glutamine, arginine plays a critical role in the body. Arginine is a precursor to growth hormone–promoting anabolism. It is also a precursor to nitric oxide, which in proper doses can be effective for bronchial dilation and respiratory mechanics.[104,105] Studies show that levels of arginine, glutamine, and citruline (an intermediary necessary for urea cycle function) are decreased in children with congenital heart disease following surgery.[106] In children with critical illness, decreased arginine and citrulline have also been reported, suggesting that arginine is a conditionally essential amino acid.[107] There is limited research to support the supplementation of arginine in children with critical illness. Because arginine has the potential to do harm in hemodynamically unstable patients, there may be negative consequences to supplementation, so it is not recommended for the critically ill pediatric population.[78]

Omega-3 Fatty Acids

Omega-3 fatty acids are hypothesized to have immune benefits for patients with critical illness. Apart from research described above in IFALD, the use of omega-3 fatty acids provided in combination with antioxidants and other immune-enhancing nutrients to children with respiratory failure, to date, does not show improved clinical outcome.[78]

Overall, the use of immunonutrition in pediatric nutrition support formulations is not consistently recommended. Research indicates that immune-enhanced formulas do not have an impact on key endpoints such as length of hospital stay or mortality. Further research needs to be done to better understand the impact of these factors on hard clinical outcomes.[78]

Chapter Summary

Childhood is a time of growth and development that requires adequate nutritional status. Nutrition assessment in the pediatric patient revolves around assessment of growth patterns and their etiology. Diet history and nutrition-focused physical exams are key components of nutritional assessment. Growth failure can be illness or non-illness related. Evaluating social factors, including parental education, nutrition beliefs, and socioeconomic status, can guide nutrition interventions. As children grow and develop, nutritional risk factors and concerns vary; however, a consistent focus on calcium, iron, and vitamin D is necessary.

As a result of the changes in body composition experienced during childhood, children are at the greatest risk for malnutrition. Nutrition support therapies such as enteral and parenteral nutrition can prevent and reverse signs of malnutrition in this population.

Key Terms

growth, growth channels, growth velocity, adiposity rebound, serial measures, anthropometrics, mid-parental height, head circumference, microcephaly, macrocephaly, growth charts, WHO growth charts, CDC growth charts, growth standards, growth reference, z-scores, underweight, weight-for-age, height-for-age, stunting, wasting, weight-for-height, colostrum, pediatric malnutrition, failure to thrive (FTT), growth faltering (GF), catch-up growth

References

1. Cole TJ. The development of growth references and growth charts. *Ann Hum Biol*. 2012;39(5):382–394.
2. de Onis M, Onyango A, Borghi E, Siyam A, Pinol A. *WHO Child Growth Standards: Growth Velocity Based on Weight, Length and Head Circumference: Methods and Development*. World Health Organization. Department of Nutrition for Health and Development; 2009.
3. Fomon SJ, Haschke F, Ziegler EE, Nelson SE. Body composition of reference children from birth to age 10 years. *Am J Clin Nutr*. 1982;35(suppl):1169–1175.
4. Forbes GE. Human body composition. *Growth, aging, nutrition, and activity*. 12th ed. Springer-Verlag; 2012.
5. Tori-Romos T, Paley C, Pi-Sunyer FX, Gallager D. Body composition during fetal development and infancy through the age of 5 years. *Nutrition*. 2015;69:1279–1289. doi:10.1038/ejcn.2015.117
6. Pomi AL, Pepe G, Aversa T, et al. Early adiposity rebound: predictors and outcomes. *Ital J Pediatr.* 2024; 50:98. doi:10.1186/s13052-024-01671-4
7. Abbassi V. Growth and normal puberty. *Pediatrics*.1998;102(2 Pt 3):507–511.
8. Weber DR, Leonard MB, Zemel BS. Body composition analysis in the pediatric population. *Pediatr Endocrinol Rev.* 2012;10(1):130–139.
9. Maciel JR, Nakano EY, Carvalho KM, Dutra ES. STRONGkids validation: tool accuracy. *J Pediatr.* 2020;96:371–378.
10. Teixeira AF, Viana KD. Nutritional screening in hospitalized pediatric patients: a systematic review. *J Pediatr*. 2016;92:343–352.
11. Wright CM, Cheetham TD. The strengths and limitations of parental heights as a predictor of attained height. *Arch Dis Child*. 1999;81(3):257–260.
12. Sniderman A. Abnormal head growth. *Pediatr Rev*. 2010;31(9):382:384.
13. Ogden CL, Flegal KM. Changes in terminology for childhood overweight and obesity. *Natl Health Stat Report*. 2010; 25:1–5.
14. Division of Nutrition, Physical Activity and Obesity, National Center for Chronic Disease Prevention and Health Promotion. Defining childhood obesity. Centers for Disease Control and Prevention. Updated September 10, 2024. Accessed January 7, 2025. https://www.cdc.gov/nccdphp/divisions-offices/about-the-division-of-nutrition-physical-activity-and-obesity.html
15. Addo OY, Himes JH. Reference curves for triceps and subscapular skinfold thicknesses in US children and adolescents. *Am J Clin Nutr.* 2010;91(3):635–642.
16. Addo OY, Himes JH, Zemel BS. Reference ranges for mid-upper arm circumference, upper arm muscle area, and upper arm fat area in US children and adolescents aged 1-20 y. *Am J Clin Nutr*. 2017;105(1):111–120. doi:10.3945/ajcn.116.142190
17. de Onis M, Garza C, Onyango AW, Borghi E. Comparison of the WHO child growth standards and the CDC 2000 growth charts. *J Nutr*. 2007;137(1):144–148.
18. Grummer-Strawn LM, Reinold C, Krebs NF, Centers for Disease Control and Prevention (CDC). Use of World Health Organization and CDC growth charts for children aged 0–59 months in the United States. *MMWR Rec Rep*. 2010;59(RR–9):1–15.
19. Ogden CL, Kuczmarski RJ, Flegal KM, et al. Centers for Disease Control and Prevention 2000 growth charts for the United States: improvements to the 1977 National Center for Health Statistics version. *Pediatrics*. 2002;109(1):45–60.
20. Centers for Disease Control. Growth Chart Training. Updated December 2022. Assessed December 1, 2025. https://www.cdc.gov/growth-chart-training/hcp/extended-growth-charts/index.html#:~:text=What%20changed,Optimize%20care%20for%20this%20group
21. Dibley MJ, Staehling N, Nieburg P, Trowbridge FL. Interpretation of Z-score anthropometric indicators derived from the international growth reference. *Am J Clin Nutr.* 1987;46(5):749–762.

22. Becker PJ, Nieman Carney L, Corkins MR, et al. Consensus statement of the Academy of Nutrition and Dietetics/American Society for Parenteral and Enteral Nutrition: indicators recommended for the identification and documentation of pediatric malnutrition (undernutrition). *J Acad Nutr Diet*. 2014;114(12):1988–2000.
23. Mahmood L, Flores-Barrantes P, Moreno LA, Manios Y, Gonzalez-Gil EM. The influence of parental dietary behaviors and practices on children's eating habits. *Nutrients*. 2021;13(4):1138. doi:10.3390/nu13041138
24. Scaglioni S, De Cosmi V, Ciappolino V, Parazzini F, Brambilla P, Agostoni C. Factors influencing children's eating behaviours. *Nutrients*. 2018;10(6):706. doi:10.3390/nu10060625
25. Loth KA, MacLehose RF, Fulkerson JA, Crow S, Neumark-Sztainer D. Are food restriction and pressure-to-eat parenting practices associated with adolescent disordered eating behaviors? *Int J Eat Disord*. 2014;47(3):310–314.
26. Green Corkins K. Nutrition-focused physical examination in pediatric patients. *Nutr Clin Pract*. 2015;30(2):203–209.
27. Radler DR, Lister T. Nutrient deficiencies associated with nutrition-focused physical findings of the oral cavity. *Nutr Clin Pract*. 2013;28(6):710–721.
28. Moshiree B, Drossman D, Shaukat A. AGA clinical practice update on evaluation and management of belching, abdominal bloating, and distention: expert review. *Gastroenterology*. 2023;165(3):791–800.
29. Calcaterra V, Verduci E, Milanta C, et al. Micronutrient deficiency in children and adolescents with obesity—a narrative review. *Children*. 2023; 10(4):695. doi:10.3390/children10040695
30. Guirguis-Blake JM, Evans CV, Coppola EL, Redmond N, Perdue LA. Screening for lipid disorders in children and adolescents: updated evidence report and systematic review for the US preventive services task force. *JAMA*. 2023;330(3):261–274. doi:10.1001/jama.2023.8867
31. Hoe FM, Darbinian JA, Greenspan LC, Lo JC. Hemoglobin A1c and type 2 diabetes incidence among adolescents with overweight and obesity. *JAMA Netw Open*. 2024;7(1):e2351322. doi:10.1001/jamanetworkopen.2023.51322
32. McDonagh M, Blazina I, Dana T, et al. Introduction. In: *Routine Iron Supplementation and Screening for Iron Deficiency Anemia in Children Ages 6 to 24 Months: A Systematic Review to Update the U.S. Preventive Services Task Force Recommendation*. Agency for Healthcare Research and Quality (US); 2015. https://www.ncbi.nlm.nih.gov/books/NBK285661
33. Gibson RS, Heath AL, Szymlek-Gay EA. Is iron and zinc nutrition a concern for vegetarian infants and young children in industrialized countries? *Am J Clin Nutr*. 2014;100 (Suppl 1):459S–468S.
34. Fiamenghi VI, de Mello ED. Vitamin D deficiency in children and adolescents with obesity: a meta-analysis. *J. Pediatr.* 2021;97 (3):273–279. doi:10.1016/j.jped.2020.08.006
35. Golden NH, Abrams SA, Committee on Nutrition. Optimizing bone health in children and adolescents. *Pediatrics*. 2014;134(4):e1229–1243. doi:10.1542/peds.2014-2173
36. Healthy People 2030, U.S. Department of Health and Human Services, Office of Disease Prevention and Health Promotion. Accessed January 5, 2025. https://health.gov/healthypeople/objectives-and-data/social-determinants-health
37. Nofal AA, Schwenk WF. Growth failure in children. A symptom or disease? *Nutr Clin Prac*. 2013;28(6):651–658.
38. Secker DJ, Jeejeebhoy KN. How to perform subjective global nutritional assessment in children. *J Acad Nutr Diet*. 2012;112(3):424–431.e6.
39. Holt KA. *Bright futures: nutrition*. 3rd ed. American Academy of Pediatrics; 2011:278.
40. National Guideline Alliance (UK). *Faltering Growth–Recognition and Management*. National Institute for Health and Care Excellence (NICE); 2017.
41. World Health Organization. *WHO Global Database on Child Growth and Malnutrition*. World Health Organization/Department of Nutrition for Health and Development; 2014:27.
42. Cooke R, Goulet O, Huysentruyt K, et al. Catch-up growth in infants and young children with faltering growth: expert opinion to guide general clinicians. *J Pediatr Gastroenterol Nutr*. 2023;77(1):7–15.
43. Atalay A, McCord M. Characteristics of failure to thrive in a referral population: implications for treatment. *Clin Pediatr*. 2012;51(3):219.
44. U.S. Department of Agriculture and U.S. Department of Health and Human Services. Dietary Guidelines for Americans, 2025-2030. 10th Edition. January 2026. Available at DietaryGuidelines.gov.Academy of Pediatrics; 2025
45. Kleinman RE, Greer FR, eds. Pediatric Nutrition. 9th ed. Itasca, IL: American Academy of Pediatrics.
46. National Academies of Sciences, Engineering, and Medicine. *Dietary Reference Intakes for Energy*. The National Academies Press; 2023. doi:10.17226/26818
47. Muth ND, Tanaka M. *The Clinician's Guide to Pediatric Nutrition*. 1st ed. American Academy of Pediatrics; 2023.
48. Institute of Medicine. *Dietary Reference Intakes for Energy, Carbohydrate, Fiber, Fat, Fatty Acids, Cholesterol, Protein, and Amino Acids*. The National Academies Press; 2005. doi:10.17226/10490
49. National Institutes of Health. Health Information. Office of Dietary Supplements. Dietary Supplement Fact Sheets. Vitamin and Mineral Fact sheets. Accessed January 13, 2025. https://ods.od.nih.gov/factsheets/list-all
50. What We Eat in America, NHANES 2013-2014, individuals 2 years and over (excluding breast-fed children), day 1. Accessed January 5, 2025. www.ars.usda.gov/nea/bhnrc/fsrg
51. Meek JY, Noble L. Section on breastfeeding. Policy statement: breastfeeding and the use of human milk. *Pediatrics*. 2022;150(1):e2022057988.
52. Andreas NJ, Kampmann B, Mehring Le-Doare K. Human breast milk: a review on its composition and bioactivity. *Early Hum Dev*. 2015;91(11):629–635.
53. Vandenplas Y, Zakharova I, Dmitrieva Y. Oligosaccharides in infant formula: more evidence to validate the role of prebiotics. *Br J Nutr*. 2015;113(9):1339–1344.
54. Lonnerdal B. Infant formula and infant nutrition: bioactive proteins of human milk and implications for composition of infant formulas. *Am J Clin Nutr*. 2014;99(3):712S–717S.
55. Joeckel RJ, Phillips SK. Overview of infant and pediatric formulas. *Nutr Clin Pract*. 2009;24(3):356–362.
56. Meek JY, Noble L. Section on breastfeeding; policy statement: breastfeeding and the use of human milk. *Pediatrics*. 2022;150(1):e2022057988. doi:10.1542/peds.2022-057988
57. Quinn EA. Too much of a good thing: evolutionary perspectives on infant formula fortification in the United States and its effects on infant health. *Am J Hum Biol*. 2014;26(1):10–17.
58. Mugambi MN, Musekiwa A, Lombard M, Young T, Blaauw R. Probiotics, prebiotics infant formula use in preterm or low birth weight infants: a systematic review. *Nutr J*. 2012;11:58.

59. Vandenplas Y, De Greef E, Veereman G. Prebiotics in infant formula. *Gut Microbes.* 2014;5(6):681–687.
60. Arslanoglu S, Moro GE, Boehm G. Early supplementation of prebiotic oligosaccharides protects formula-fed infants against infections during the first 6 months of life. *J Nutr.* 2007;137(11):2420–2424.
61. Ashley C, Johnston WH, Harris CL, Stolz SI, Wampler JL, Berseth CL. Growth and tolerance of infants fed formula supplemented with polydextrose (PDX) and/or galactooligosaccharides (GOS): double-blind, randomized, controlled trial. *Nutr J.* 2012;11:38.
62. Committee on Nutrition of the American Academy of Pediatrics. Complementary feeding. In: Kleinman RE, ed. *Pediatric Nutrition Handbook.* 6th ed. AAP; 2009:113.
63. Brown A, Jones SW, Rowan H. Baby-led weaning: the evidence to date. *Curr Nutr Rep.* 2017;6(2):148–156. doi:10.1007/s13668-017-0201-2
64. National Center for Chronic Disease Prevention and Health Promotion. Centers for Disease Control (CDC). Division of Nutrition, Physical Activity, and Obesity. Cow's Milk and Milk Alternatives. Last updated October 10, 2024. Assessed January 7, 2025. https://www.cdc.gov/infant-toddler-nutrition/foods-and-drinks/cows-milk-and-milk-alternatives.html
65. Corkins M, ed. *ASPEN Pediatric Nutrition Support Core Curriculum.* 2nd ed. ASPEN; 2015.
66. Cox N, Hinkle R. Infant botulism. *Am Fam Physician.* 2002;65(7):1388–1392.
67. Frankel LA, Hughes SO, O'Connor TM, Power TG, Fisher JO, Hazen NL. Parental influences on children's self-regulation of energy intake: insights from developmental literature on emotion regulation. *J Obes.* 2012;327259.
68. Fink SK, Racine EF, Mueffelmann RE, Dean MN, Herman-Smith R. Family meals and diet quality among children and adolescents in North Carolina. *J Nutr Educ Behav.* 2014;46(5):418–422.
69. Loth KA, MacLehose RF, Larson N, Berge JM, Neumark-Sztainer D. Food availability, modeling and restriction: how are these different aspects of the family eating environment related to adolescent dietary intake? *Appetite.* 2016;96:80–86.
70. Larson N, MacLehose R, Fulkerson JA, Berge JM, Story M, Neumark-Sztainer D. Eating breakfast and dinner together as a family: associations with sociodemographic characteristics and implications for diet quality and weight status. *J Acad Nutr Diet.* 2013;113(12):1601–1609.
71. Neumark-Sztainer D, Wall M, Fulkerson JA, Larson N. Changes in the frequency of family meals from 1999 to 2010 in the homes of adolescents: trends by sociodemographic characteristics. *J Adolesc Health.* 2013;52(2):201–206.
72. Woodruff SJ, Campbell K, Campbell T, Cole M. The associations of meals and snacks on family meals among a sample of grade 7 students from southwestern Ontario. *Appetite.* 2014;82:61–66.
73. Neumark-Sztainer D, Hannan PJ, Story M, Croll J, Perry C. Family meal patterns: associations with sociodemographic characteristics and improved dietary intake among adolescents. *J Am Diet Assoc.* 2003;103(3):317–322.
74. Eveleens RD, Dungen DK, Verbruggen SCAT, Hulst JM, Joosten KFM. Weight improvement with the use of protein and energy enriched nutritional formula in infants with a prolonged PICU stay. *J Hum Nutr Diet.* 2019;32:3–10. doi:10.1111/jhn.12603
75. Goodwin ET, Buel KL, Cantrell LD. Growth faltering and failure to thrive in children. *Am Fam Physician.* 2023;107(6):597–603 [Erratum in: *Am Fam Physician.* 2024;109(2):105–106].
76. Cole SZ, Lanham JS. Failure to thrive: an update. *Am Fam Physician.* 2011;83(7):829–834.
77. Prieto MB, Cid JL. Malnutrition in the critically ill child: the importance of enteral nutrition. *Int J Environ Res Public Health.* 2011;8(11):4353–4366.
78. Mehta NM, Skillman HE, Irving SY, et al. Guidelines for the provision and assessment of nutrition support therapy in pediatric critically ill patient: Society of Critical Care Medicine and American Society for Parenteral and Enteral Nutrition. *JPEN.* 2017;4(5):706–742.
79. Vermilyea S, Goh VL. Enteral feedings in children: sorting out tubes, buttons, and formulas. *Nutr Clin Pract.* 2016;31(1):59–67.
80. Brown AM, Fisher E, Forbes ML. Bolus vs continuous nasogastric feeds in mechanically ventilated pediatric patients: a pilot study. *JPEN.* 2019;43:750–758.
81. Martinez EE, Pereira LM, Gura K, et al. Gastric emptying in critically ill children. *JPEN.* 2017;41(7):1100–1109.
82. Blaser AR, Starkopf J, Kirsimagi U, Deane AM. Definition, prevalence, and outcome of feeding intolerance in intensive care: a systematic review and meta-analysis. *Acta Anaesthesiol Scand.* 2014;58(8):914–922.
83. Tume LN, Valla FV. A review of feeding intolerance in critically ill children. *Eur J Pediatr.* 2018;177(11):1675–1683. doi:10.1007/s00431-018-3229-4
84. da Silva JSV, Seres DS, Sabino K, et al. ASPEN consensus recommendations for refeeding syndrome. *Nutr Clin Pract.* 2020;35(2):178–195. doi:10.1002/ncp.10474 [Erratum in: *Nutr Clin Pract.* 2020;35(3):584–585. doi:10.1002/ncp.10491].
85. Duggan CP, Jasik T. Pediatric intestinal failure. *N Engl J Med.* 2017;377:666–675.
86. Robinson DT, Calkins KL, Chen Y, et al. Guidelines for parenteral nutrition in preterm infants: the American Society for Parenteral and Enteral Nutrition. *JPEN.* 2023;47:830–858. doi:10.1002/jpen.2550
87. Druyan ME, Compher C, Boullata JI, et al. Clinical guidelines for the use of parenteral and enteral nutrition in adult and pediatric patients. *JPEN.* 2012;36:77–80. doi:10.1177/0148607111420157
88. Joosten K, Embleton N, Yan W, et al. ESPGHAN/ESPEN/ESPR/CSPEN guidelines on pediatric parenteral nutrition: energy. *Clin Nutr.* 2018;37:2309–2314.
89. Dokken M, Rustoen T, Stubhaug A. Indirect calorimetry reveals that better monitoring of nutrition therapy in pediatric intensive care is needed. *JPEN.* 2015;39(3):344–352.
90. McClave SA, Lowen CC, Kleber MJ, McConnell JW, Jung LY, Goldsmith LJ. Clinical use of the respiratory quotient obtained from indirect calorimetry. *JPEN.* 2003;27(1):21–26.
91. Mehta NM, Bechard LJ, Leavitt K, Duggan C. Cumulative energy imbalance in the pediatric intensive care unit: role of targeted indirect calorimetry. *JPEN.* 2009;33(3):336–344.
92. Kumpf VJ. Parenteral nutrition-associated liver disease in adult and pediatric patients. *Nutr Clin Pract.* 2006;21(3):279–290.
93. Lauriti G, Zani A, Aufieri R, et al. Incidence, prevention, and treatment of parenteral nutrition-associated cholestasis and intestinal failure-associated liver disease in infants and children: a systematic review. *JPEN.* 2014;38(1):70–85.
94. Koseesirikul P, Chotinaruemol S, Ukarapol N. Incidence and risk factors of parenteral nutrition-associated liver disease in newborn infants. *Pediatr Int.* 2012;54(3):434–436.

95. Nandivada P, Fell GL, Gura KM, Puder M. Lipid emulsions in the treatment and prevention of parenteral nutrition-associated liver disease in infants and children. *Am J Clin Nutr*. 2016;103(2):629S–634S.

96. Calkins KL, DeBarber A, Steiner RD, et al. Intravenous fish oil and pediatric intestinal failure–associated liver disease: changes in plasma phytosterols, cytokines, and bile acids and erythrocyte fatty acids. *JPEN*. 2017. doi:10.1177/0148607117709196

97. Kyle UG, Arriaza A, Esposito M, Coss-Bu JA. Is indirect calorimetry a necessity or a luxury in the pediatric intensive care unit? *JPEN*. 2012;36(2):177–182.

98. Mehta NM, Bechard LJ, Dolan M, Ariagno K, Jiang H, Duggan C. Energy imbalance and the risk of overfeeding in critically ill children. *Pediatr Crit Care Med*. 2011;12(4):398–405.

99. Mok E, Hankard R. Glutamine supplementation in sick children: is it beneficial? *J Nutr Metab*. 2011:617597.

100. Zhou YP, Jiang ZM, Sun YH, Wang XR, Ma EL, Wilmore D. The effect of supplemental enteral glutamine on plasma levels, gut function, and outcome in severe burns: a randomized, double-blind, controlled clinical trial. *JPEN*. 2003;27(4):241–245.

101. Gholamalizadeh M, Tabrizi R, Rezaei S, et al. Effect of glutamine supplementation on inflammatory markers in critically ill patients supported with enteral or parenteral feeding. *JPEN*. 2022;46:61–68. doi:10.1002/jpen.2217

102. Jordan I, Balaguer M, Esteban ME, et al. Glutamine effects on heat shock protein 70 and interleukines 6 and 10: randomized trial of glutamine supplementation versus standard parenteral nutrition in critically ill children. *Clin Nutr*. 2016;35(1):34–40.

103. Brown JV, Moe-Byrne T, McGuire W. Glutamine supplementation for young infants with severe gastrointestinal disease. *Cochrane Database Syst Rev*. 2014;12:CD005947.

104. Argaman Z, Young VR, Noviski N, et al. Arginine and nitric oxide metabolism in critically ill septic pediatric patients. *Crit Care Med*. 2003;31(2):591–597.

105. Zhou M, Martindale RG. Arginine in the critical care setting. *J Nutr*. 2007;137(6 Suppl 2):1687S–1692S.

106. Navaei AH, Shekerdemian LS, Mohammad MA, et al. Derangement of arginine and related amino acids in children undergoing surgery for congenital heart disease with cardiopulmonary bypass. *Crit Care Explor*. 2020;2(7):e0150. doi:10.1097/CCE.0000000000000150

107. National Academies of Sciences, Engineering, and Medicine; Health and Medicine Division; Food and Nutrition Board. 4. Disease-Induced Deficiency and Conditionally Essential Nutrients in Disease. In: *Examining Special Nutritional Requirements in Disease States: Proceedings of a Workshop*. National Academies Press (US); 2018. https://www.ncbi.nlm.nih.gov/books/NBK525313

CHAPTER 21

Nutrition in Cystic Fibrosis

Laura Padula
Sara Hendrix

CHAPTER OUTLINE

CORE CONCEPTS

1. Cystic fibrosis is a disease in which nutrition is of utmost importance, and routine nutrition screening and assessments are essential in the care of every patient.
2. Energy needs are often high in a patient with cystic fibrosis due to an increased metabolic demand associated with breathing and malabsorption of fat due to exocrine pancreatic insufficiency.
3. Exocrine pancreatic insufficiency affects the majority of patients with cystic fibrosis. It results in malabsorption of fat without proper treatment with pancreatic enzyme replacement therapy. Patients who initially present with pancreatic insufficiency and are started on a cystic fibrosis transmembrane conductance regulator (CFTR) modulator at an early age should have routine assessment of pancreatic status via pancreatic elastase-1 (PE-1) testing to monitor for conversion to pancreatic sufficiency.
4. Treatment for exocrine pancreatic insufficiency is to provide pancreatic enzyme replacement therapy (PERT), taken by mouth with meals and snacks, to substitute for the enzymes the pancreas is not endogenously secreting. These enzymes contain lipase, protease, and amylase for the digestion of fat, protein, and carbohydrates.
5. Patients with cystic fibrosis and exocrine pancreatic insufficiency require supplementation of vitamins and minerals due to risk for malabsorption-related deficiencies. Serum fat-soluble vitamin levels should be assessed annually, because they are the primary nutrients at risk for deficiency.
6. Patients with cystic fibrosis have higher sodium needs than those of the general population due to increased sweat-related losses. Patients with cystic fibrosis are prescribed a high-salt diet to compensate for the additional losses.
7. If an adequate weight cannot be maintained with diet alone, oral supplements, and sometimes enteral nutrition support, are recommended to promote weight gain and optimize nutritional status.
8. Patients with cystic fibrosis are at increased risk for eating disorders, body image concerns, and with recent advances in treatment, for overweight, obesity, and weight stigma.

9. The introduction of cystic fibrosis transmembrane conductance regulator (CFTR) modulators has transformed nutrition care for people with cystic fibrosis, shifting focus toward individualized medical nutrition therapy that addresses evolving patient needs. Assessment of body composition and lipid profiles can be useful for providing individualized nutrition care.
10. Patients with cystic fibrosis are at risk for developing cystic fibrosis–related diabetes (CFRD), bone disease, and liver disease.

LEARNING OBJECTIVES

1. Identify the etiology of cystic fibrosis and the importance of good nutrition in maintaining lung health.
2. Explain the specific nutritional needs of a patient with cystic fibrosis.
3. Describe exocrine pancreatic insufficiency and its treatment in patients with cystic fibrosis.
4. Recognize specific vitamin and mineral deficiencies associated with cystic fibrosis.
5. Discuss the nutrition-related disease complications that may be associated with cystic fibrosis.

Introduction

This chapter will review cystic fibrosis and its associated nutritional complications. The importance of proper nutrition and strategies to improve the nutritional status of patients with cystic fibrosis will be discussed.

Cystic fibrosis (CF) is a life-threatening, autosomal recessive genetic disorder. It is the most common genetic disorder among White people and affects approximately 40,000 people in the United States.[1] CF is characterized by an abnormal **CF transmembrane conductance regulator (CFTR) protein** (Figure 21.1), which results in abnormal transport of sodium, chloride, and water throughout the cells of the body. This results in abnormally thick mucus that causes damage to the lungs, pancreas, and other organs. The mucus obstructs the airways, causing damage to the lungs, promoting bacterial infections that lead to progressive lung disease. The mucus also clogs the ducts of the pancreas, preventing digestive enzymes from being secreted into the small intestine and leading to exocrine pancreatic insufficiency (EPI) in about 85% of patients.[1] Treatment for those with CF aims to promote normal lung function, support normal growth throughout childhood and adolescence, and maintain optimal nutrition in adulthood. It is recommended that all patients with CF in the United States be treated under the care of a Cystic Fibrosis Foundation–accredited center. These centers include a multidisciplinary team, usually comprising a doctor, advanced practice provider, registered nurse, registered dietitian, social worker, physical therapist, respiratory therapist, pharmacist, and a variety of other subspecialists, to help care for the complex needs of a patient with CF.[2]

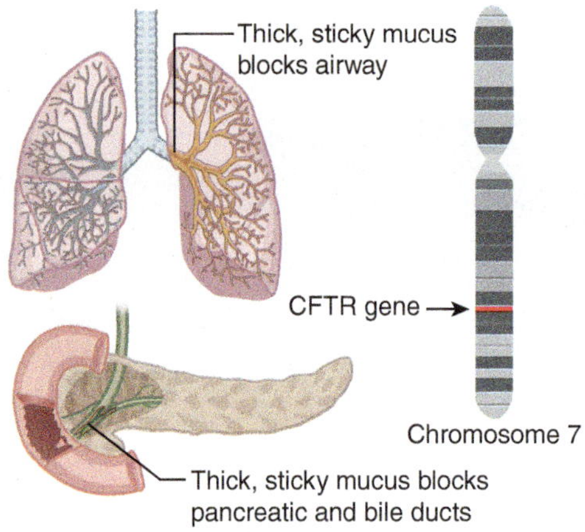

Figure 21.1 A Defect in the CFTR Gene Results in Thick Mucus Production in the Lungs and Pancreas

Diagnosis

Newborn screening for CF is now routinely performed in all 50 states. Prior to the development of newborn screening, patients were diagnosed with CF after showing signs and symptoms of disease, which may have included chronic cough, pneumonia, malnutrition, rectal prolapse, or steatorrhea. Presently, most patients in the United States initially present to a CF center because of an abnormal newborn screen. A **sweat test** is ordered to measure the amount of chloride in sweat. If elevated above 60 mmol/L, a diagnosis of cystic fibrosis can be made. If the sweat test is borderline and the newborn screen is positive, genetic testing may be used to determine whether the patient has any CFTR mutations that cause CF.[3]

Clinical Manifestations of Cystic Fibrosis

CF can present with various signs and symptoms and in varying degrees of severity. The disease-causing genetic mutations, if known, can often predict the pancreatic status of the individual. However, patients with the same two CF genotypes can present with different disease courses throughout the lifespan. The most common respiratory manifestations of the disease include chronic cough, chronic sinusitis, and repeated lung infections, along with **digital clubbing** (focal enlargement of the terminal ends of the fingers). Common gastrointestinal (GI) manifestations of the disease include malabsorption, steatorrhea, rectal prolapse, constipation, distal intestinal obstruction syndrome (DIOS), gastroesophageal reflux disease (GERD), and fat-soluble vitamin deficiencies. Some infants may present within 24 hours of birth with meconium ileus, an intestinal obstruction in the early newborn period that requires immediate medical and sometimes surgical intervention.

Cystic Fibrosis and the Lungs

The lungs can be visualized like an upside-down tree. The trunk represents the trachea, the main branches are the **bronchi**, **bronchioles** are the smaller branches, and finally the **alveoli** are the smallest twigs and branches (**Figure 21.2**). **Cilia** are hair-like structures within the lungs that normally remove bacteria.

Thick mucus in CF prevents the cilia from performing this function. Microorganisms become trapped in the mucus, leading to infection. An inflammatory immune response ensues, increasing white cell production. Tissue damage caused by infection and the immune response itself further contribute to thickened mucus. Inflammation, which constricts the passageways, makes it more difficult to clear mucus secretions. A cycle of inflammation, weakened immunity, and recurrent infections occurs (**Figure 21.3**).

The mainstay of medical management in CF includes a series of interventions aimed at airway clearance, fighting respiratory infections, and preserving lung function. **Bronchodilators** are oral and inhaled medications used to expand constricted passageways and improve breathing. **Mucolytics** help mobilize mucus and decrease sputum thickness. **Nebulizers**, which turn liquid medication into a mist, are commonly used (**Figure 21.4**). Airway clearance

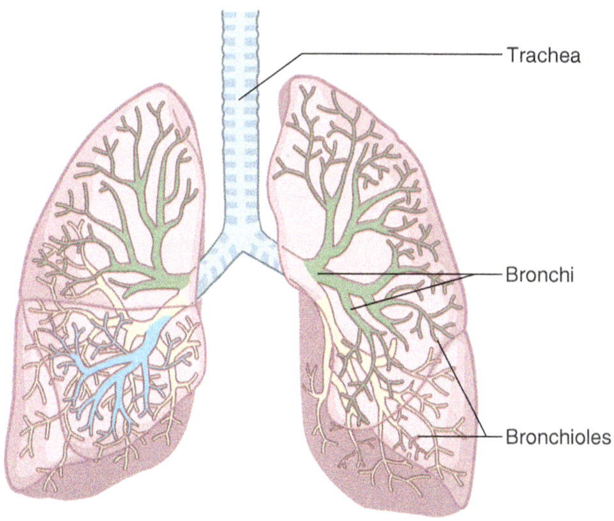

Figure 21.2 The Lungs

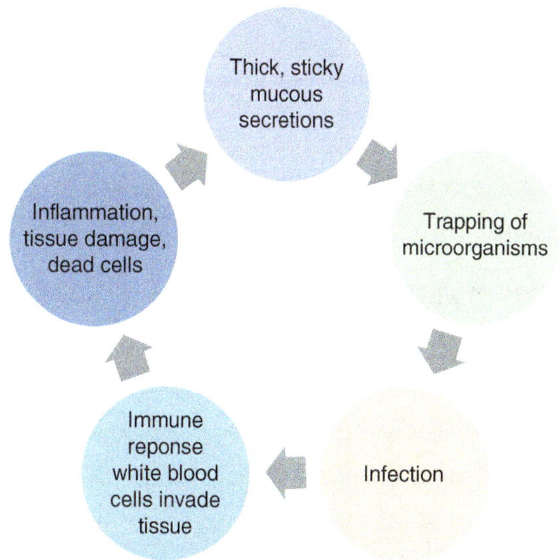

Figure 21.3 Cycle of Increased Mucus Production, Inflammation, and Recurrent Infections

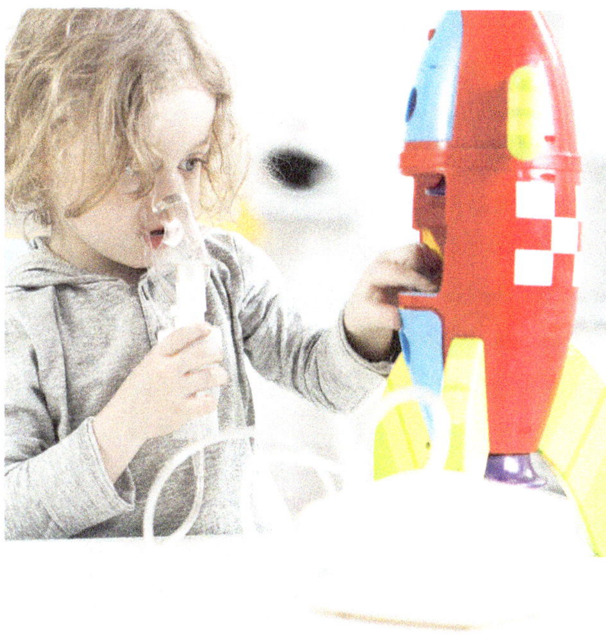

Figure 21.4 Use of a Nebulizer in a Child with CF

CASE STUDY INTRODUCTION

Lucy is a 4-month-old female with no significant medical history, seen by you for the first time for poor growth. Lucy was breastfed exclusively until 3 months of age and then maintained on a combination of breast milk and infant formula. Her parents report that Lucy is eager to feed and appears interested; however, she fails to gain weight. They are also concerned with her increasing stool pattern, which is foul smelling and appears to contain visible oil. Mom and Dad both work. Lucy has an older brother aged 3 years. They have support from extended family. Lucy's grandmother takes care of Lucy and is also present for the visit. Lucy's grandmother mentions that when she kisses Lucy, she has a salty taste to her skin.

Anthropometrics:

Length 59.5 cm
Weight 5.0 kg

Weight History

Age (months)	Weight (kg)	Length (cm)
Birth	3.4	52
1 month	4.0	55
2 months	4.8	57
3 months	5.0	58

Biochemical Data:

Sodium 123 (136–145 mEq/L)
Potassium 2.9 (3.5–5.0 mEq/L)
Chloride 73 (96–106 mEq/L)
Carbon dioxide 22 (22–31 mEq/L)
Pancreatic elastase-1: <15 mcg/g

Blood urea nitrogen 25 (8–20 mg/dL)
Creatinine 1.8 (0.7–1.3 mg/dL)
Glucose 78 (70–139 mg/dL)

Clinical Data:

Past Medical History: None
Medications: None
Vital Signs: Normal

Nutrition-Focused Physical Exams: Lucy is alert but appears distressed. When you observe her, she has a productive cough during the visit. She has a thin appearance.

Questions

1. What are Lucy's nutritional risk factors?
2. Describe the possible pathophysiologic etiology associated with Lucy's electrolyte abnormalities.
3. Describe Lucy's growth pattern.
4. Write two Nutrition Diagnosis statements for Lucy identifying the Problem/Etiology/Signs and Symptoms (PES) of Lucy's active nutrition issues.
5. Identify the nutrition interventions you would like to initiate for Lucy to address the problems identified in your PES statements.
6. What biochemical indices should be included in your monitoring and evaluation plan? Why?

techniques also include chest physical therapy; use of a **percussor** (a handheld device that helps mobilize bronchial secretions); use of therapeutic vests that provide high-frequency chest compression to remove mucus; and intrapulmonary percussive ventilation, a technique that uses compressed gas to deliver medications and loosen secretions. Anti-inflammatory medications are provided to decrease lung inflammation. Antibiotics given orally, inhaled, or intravenously are provided to treat infection. Most recently, CFTR modulators have become important medications in the treatment of CF. These medications are designed to correct the defective CFTR protein and are only effective in patients with specific genetic mutations that cause CF. There are four CFTR modulators currently available for patients with CF with more in the

Table 21.1 Categories of Medications Used to Treat Pulmonary Complications of CF

Treatment Category	Purpose	Administration	Examples of Common Medications
Bronchodilators	Open airway passages in the lungs by relaxing smooth muscle	Inhaler Oral Aerosol	Albuterol, theophylline, ipratropium
Mucolytics	Thin mucus, increase sputum secretion	Nebulizer	Dornase alfa, hypertonic saline
Anti-inflammatories	Decrease lung inflammation	Inhaler Oral Intravenous	Triamcinolone, flunisolide, prednisone, azithromycin
Antibiotics*	Treat bacterial infection	Oral Aerosol Intravenous	Ciprofloxacin, co-trimoxazole, inhaled tobramycin, IV tobramycin, IV cefepime
CFTR modulators	Target CFTR gene and restore function	Oral	Elexacaftor/tezacaftor/ivacaftor, tezacaftor/ivacaftor, lumacaftor/ivacaftor, and ivacaftor

*Antibiotics are prescribed according to infection type.
Data from Cystic Fibrosis Foundation. Medications. https://www.cff.org/Life-With-CF/Treatments-and-Therapies/Medications/.

development pipeline. These medications work directly on the defective CFTR gene to correct and/or potentiate the CFTR protein to improve its function. As a result, there is improved chloride flow across the cell surface, hydrating mucus throughout the body, which mitigates many of the symptoms of CF.[4] **Table 21.1** presents commonly used medications in CF.

Relationship Between Lung Function and Nutritional Status

CF is a disease in which nutrition is of utmost importance, and routine nutrition screening and assessments are essential in the care of every patient. Studies have been conducted to show a strong association between lung function and nutritional status, specifically body mass index (BMI).[5,6] According to data from the CF Foundation registry database, there is a direct correlation of **forced expiratory volume at 1 second (FEV_1)** and BMI.[1] In patients ages 6–20 years, the FEV_1 is optimized when the BMI-for-age reaches the 50th percentile (**Figure 21.5**). Similarly, the same trend is seen in adult patients, in which lung function is optimized at a BMI of 22 kg/m^2 for females and 23 kg/m^2 for males (**Figure 21.6**). As a result of these findings, the CF Foundation emphasizes the importance of optimizing nutritional status in the patient with CF to delay the progressive lung damage that results from the disease.

CORE CONCEPT 1

CF is a disease in which nutrition is of utmost importance, and routine nutrition screening and assessments are essential in the care of every patient.

CASE STUDY REVISITED

Following Lucy's diagnosis of CF, you are asked to provide energy and protein goals for Lucy.

Questions

1. What factors should be considered in determining energy and protein requirements?
2. What is your suggested intervention?
3. In addition, suggestions for micronutrient supplementation are requested. Provide your recommendations with appropriate rationale.
4. What nutritional indices will you monitor routinely?

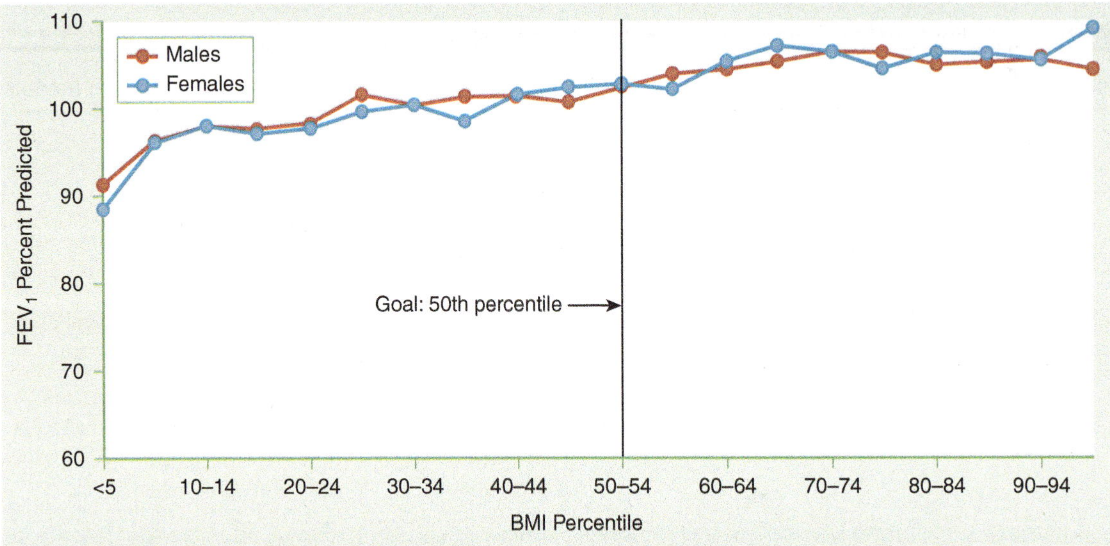

Figure 21.5 Positive Relationship Between FEV$_1$ Percentage Predicted and BMI/Age in Children

Reproduced from Cystic Fibrosis Foundation Patient Registry, 2023 *Annual Data Report, Bethesda,* Maryland ©2024 Cystic Fibrosis Foundation.

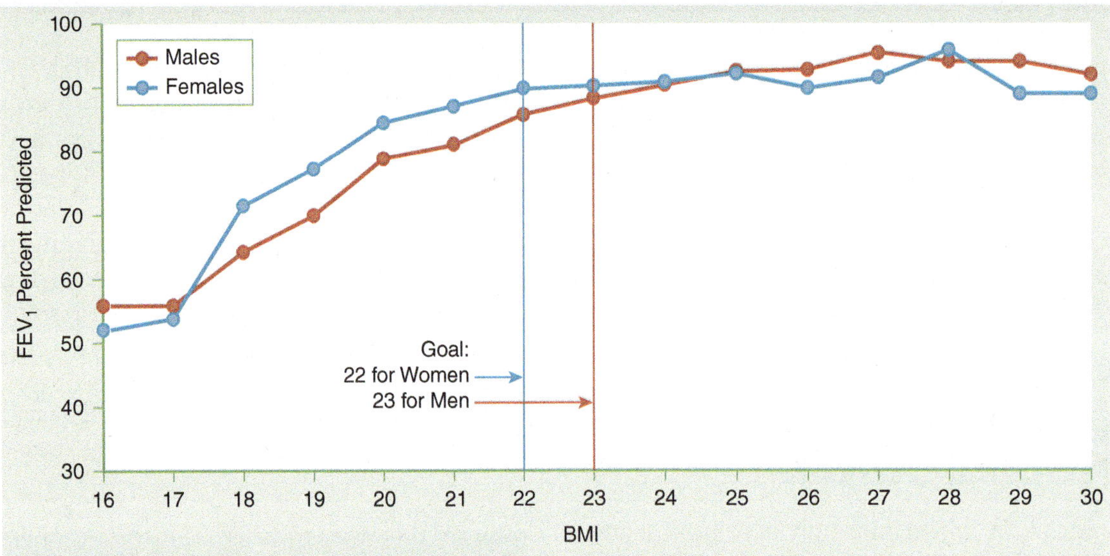

Figure 21.6 Positive Association Between FEV$_1$ Percentage Predicted and BMI in Adults

Reproduced from Cystic Fibrosis Foundation Patient Registry, 2023 *Annual Data Report, Bethesda,* Maryland ©2024 Cystic Fibrosis Foundation.

Nutrition Assessment

The relationship between nutritional status and the trajectory of CF cannot be overstated. Clinical manifestations of the disease impart significant risk factors to nutritional status and growth (**Table 21.2**). While the increased work of breathing and EPI are the most prominent determinants of nutritional status, inflammation associated with recurrent infections, other GI disturbances, altered appetite, and psychosocial factors can all influence nutritional adequacy. Conversely, malnutrition negatively impacts clinical outcomes in CF. As previously stated, a low BMI is associated with diminished lung function. Diminished fat-free mass impairs immune function, reduces exercise capacity, and lowers quality of life.[7] These factors make ongoing nutritional assessment and aggressive diet therapy a cornerstone of care for patients with CF.

Energy and Protein Needs

Children with CF are expected to gain weight and grow at the same rate as a child without CF. Additionally, adults with CF are expected to maintain a weight and BMI comparable to a healthy adult. As energy needs in many patients with CF are higher than

Table 21.2 Clinical Manifestations of CF and Their Impact on Nutritional Status

CF-Related Pathophysiology or Disturbance	Clinical Manifestation	Impact on Nutritional Status
Diminished pulmonary function	Increased work of breathing	Increased resting energy expenditure Weight loss
Recurrent respiratory infections	Pulmonary exacerbations and frequent hospitalizations	Systemic inflammation Interruption in normal nutritional intake
Gastrointestinal abnormalities	Exocrine pancreatic insufficiency	Steatorrhea and malabsorption Micronutrient deficiencies ▪ Essential fatty acids ▪ Fat-soluble vitamins Bone demineralization CF-related diabetes
	Gastrointestinal reflux, esophagitis, intestinal obstruction, nausea	Impaired nutrient intake
	Cholestatic liver disease	Altered nutrient metabolism
Psychosocial	Family stressors Depression Anxiety	Poor nutritional intake and compliance with therapy

Data from Patel D, Shan A, Mathews S, Sathe M. Understanding cystic fibrosis comorbidities and their impact on nutritional management. *Nutrients*. 2022 Feb 28;14(5):1028. doi: 10.3390/nu14051028. PMID: 35268004; PMCID: PMC8912424..

in those without CF, maintenance of good nutritional status often requires extra effort on the part of the patient and family. Energy expenditure is higher due to the higher metabolic demand required to breathe. Chronic pulmonary infections can cause an increased work of breathing and therefore an increased metabolic rate. Additionally, despite pancreatic enzyme replacement therapy aimed to treat EPI, there continue to be some losses of fat in the stool, contributing to a loss of calories. Although the mechanism is unknown, measured resting energy expenditure (REE) is increased with pancreatic insufficiency. Research indicates that children with CF and EPI have higher REEs than their pancreatic-sufficient counterparts. A negative linear relationship between pulmonary function, as measured by FEV_1, and REE exists with EPI.[8] Most patients with CF require 110–200% of the energy needs of a healthy individual of similar age, sex, and size.[6] Calorie needs are often estimated using REE multiplied by a factor to accommodate the physiologic impact of the disease and an activity factor. Equations for energy needs are not precise in CF given the variability in disease and symptom severity. Clinicians must evaluate the extent of diminished lung function, pancreatic insufficiency, physical activity, and current nutritional status when determining the proper factor to use. Energy needs and appropriateness of set targets are based on clinical outcomes of weight gain and growth.[9]

There are no specific recommendations for protein intake, and it is usually assumed that protein intake is adequate if energy needs are met. However, recognizing the importance of promoting anabolism and fat-free mass in patients with CF is advocated. Patients with low fat-free mass have reduced lung function, bone mineral loss, altered muscle function, and a high frequency of pulmonary exacerbations requiring hospitalization.[7]

CORE CONCEPT 2

Energy needs are often high in a patient with cystic fibrosis due to an increased metabolic demand associated with breathing and malabsorption of fat due to pancreatic insufficiency.

PRACTICE POINT

Patients with CF may have energy requirements equivalent to 110–200% of the energy needs of a healthy individual of similar age, sex, and size.

Clinical Controversy

Use of BMI-for-Age to Classify Nutritional Failure

The CF Foundation, based on a consensus report for children with CF, recommends that patients ages 2–20 years achieve a BMI-for-age at or above the 50th percentile. This classification, while useful for standardizing nutritional assessment and guidelines for initiation of nutrition-based interventions, has a number of shortcomings.

Konstan et al. showed that many children, despite BMI-for-age between the 25th and 50th percentiles, had weights and heights that were below the 10th percentile for age. The researchers emphasized that BMI-for-age fails to identify poor nutritional status in stunted children.

There are other patient subgroups that may not benefit from the standard BMI-for-age recommendation. Stephenson et al. showed that the benefit of increasing BMI on lung function was only clinically significant in underweight patients. The effect was much less in overweight patients. They concluded that the greatest benefit of improving BMI was in underweight, pancreatic-insufficient patients. The authors cautioned that given the risk of obesity, standard recommendations for increasing BMI, which do not make a distinction between under- and overweight patients, may have implications for overweight patients.

In a recent meta-analysis Nagy et al found that measures of fat free mass depletion may exist despite normal BMI in patients with CF. Furthermore, Fat free mass was more closely associated with lung function than BMI.

Questions

1. Using the reports referenced above, discuss the implications of relying on BMI-for-age alone to assess nutritional risk and dietary intervention for all patients with CF.

References

1. Konstan MW, Pasta DJ, Wagener JS, VanDevanter DR, Morgan WJ. BMI fails to identify nutritional risk in stunted children. *J Cystic Fibr*. 2017;(16):158–160.
2. Nagy R, Gede N, Ocskay K, et al. Association of Body Mass Index With Clinical Outcomes in Patients With Cystic Fibrosis: A Systematic Review and Meta-analysis. *JAMA Netw Open*. 2022;5(3):e220740. Published 2022 Mar 1. doi:10.1001/jamanetworkopen.2022.0740
3. Stephenson AL, Mannik LA, Walsh S, et al. Longitudinal trends in nutritional status and the relation between lung function and BMI in cystic fibrosis: a population-based cohort study, *AM J Clin Nutr*. 2013;97(4):872–877.

Anthropometrics

Weight and height should be measured, and BMI calculated at every visit. For children, all anthropometrics should be plotted on the growth chart appropriate for age and sex. The CF Foundation, based on consensus reports, recommends that all children ages 2–20 years achieve a BMI-for-age at or above the 50th percentile. For children and infants younger than 2 years of age, attaining a weight-for-length percentile at or above the 50th percentile for age is recommended. For adults with CF, a BMI of 22 kg/m^2 is recommended for females and a BMI of 23 kg/m^2 for males. It is also important to ensure children with CF are growing within their genetic height potential because chronic malnutrition can result in stunting.[6]

Biochemical Assessment

As part of the nutrition assessment, routine labs should be monitored annually per the recommendations of the CF Foundation.[9] At approximately 2 months after starting vitamin supplementation and annually thereafter, serum vitamin A (retinol), vitamin E (alpha-tocopherol), and 25-hydroxy vitamin D levels should be measured to assess vitamin status.[10] Protein Induced by Vitamin K Absence or Antagonist-II (**PIVKA-II**) is the laboratory test of choice to assess vitamin K status. If this test is unavailable, prothrombin time can be used in the setting of a patient without liver dysfunction. Elevated prothrombin time can indicate vitamin K deficiency, although it is not as sensitive a marker as PIVKA-II.[11] Hemoglobin and hematocrit should be measured yearly to evaluate iron status. Liver function tests are monitored to follow for any signs of CF-related liver disease. All patients with CF, starting at the 10 years of age, should complete a 2-hour oral glucose tolerance test to screen for the development of CF-related diabetes.[12] In special circumstances, other laboratory tests may be completed. Additionally, for patients with concerns for poor bone health, a dual-energy x-ray absorptiometry

PRACTICE POINT

At approximately 2 months after starting vitamin supplementation and annually thereafter, serum vitamin A (retinol), vitamin E (alpha-tocopherol), 25-hydroxy vitamin D, and vitamin K via either PIVKA-II or prothrombin time should be measured to assess vitamin status.

(DXA) scan can be completed starting at 8 years of age to monitor bone status and should be completed no later than 18 years of age for patients with CF with no risk factors for bone disease.[13,14]

Diet Assessment

Every patient with CF should be evaluated by a registered dietitian (RD) at least once per year. In patients who are struggling to maintain a healthy nutrition status, more frequent nutrition assessment should be completed. It is important to evaluate fluid, calorie, sodium, and calcium intake to ensure the diet is meeting the needs of the patient. A 24-hour diet recall or a 3-day food record can be used to better evaluate the patient's usual dietary intake. The nutrition assessment should also include any oral supplements, tube feeds, and vitamin supplements that the patient may be taking to augment their dietary consumption. Laboratory values should be reviewed and adjustments to the vitamin regimen should be made based on results. Stool pattern should also be evaluated to assess for any signs or symptoms of malabsorption. The RD should also note any medications that the patient may be taking that may have drug–nutrient interactions.

Food insecurity can pose a significant barrier to adequate nutritional intake, particularly for those with lower incomes or without paid employment. According to a 2019 study, approximately 33% of people with CF in the United States are food insecure: three times the national average. The financial strain of CF-related medical costs exacerbates difficulties in maintaining a nutritious diet, and food insecurity can severely impact health outcomes. Given the increased need for optimal nutrition in CF, regular screening for food security and access to community resources like SNAP benefits and food banks are crucial components of CF care.[15]

PRACTICE POINT

Patients with CF should be evaluated by an RD at least once per year. In patients who are struggling to maintain healthy nutrition status, more frequent nutrition assessment should be completed.

Exocrine Pancreatic Insufficiency

Approximately 85% of all patients with CF have exocrine pancreatic insufficiency (EPI), a loss of the exocrine function of the pancreas.[1] EPI results in the pancreas's inability to secrete lipase, protease, and amylase, the digestive enzymes needed to break down and utilize the nutrients from food. Untreated EPI results in malabsorption of macronutrients and can contribute to poor nutritional status and fat-soluble vitamin deficiencies. Some patients may present initially with normal function of the pancreas (pancreatic sufficiency) and may convert to **pancreatic insufficiency** over time. Pancreatic status can often be determined by reviewing the mutations causing CF because many mutations are associated with pancreatic disease. All patients presenting with CF should have a stool test to measure pancreatic elastase-1 (PE-1). PE-1, a digestive enzyme secreted exclusively by the pancreas, is a fecal marker used to assess exocrine pancreatic function. If the result is <200 mcg/g stool, **pancreatic enzyme replacement therapy (PERT)** should be initiated.[9] Additionally, the CF Foundation recommends initiating PERT before the results of a stool test in a patient with two known CFTR mutations that are known to cause EPI, or in a patient presenting with signs and symptoms of malabsorption upon diagnosis.[9] Although EPI was once thought to be irreversible in CF, evidence indicates that CFTR modulator therapy has the potential to improve pancreatic function. Some patients may achieve pancreatic sufficiency with PE-1 levels increasing above 200 mcg/g while on modulator therapy, particularly in those who started modulators at an early age. These findings support routine PE-1 testing in children receiving CFTR modulators.[16]

CORE CONCEPT 3

Exocrine pancreatic insufficiency affects the majority of patients with cystic fibrosis. It results in malabsorption of fat without proper treatment with pancreatic enzyme replacement therapy. Patients who initially present with pancreatic insufficiency and are started on a cystic fibrosis transmembrane conductance regulator (CFTR) modulator at an early age should have routine assessment of pancreatic status via pancreatic elastase-1 (PE-1) testing to monitor for conversion to pancreatic sufficiency.

Most pancreatic enzymes currently on the market are in capsule form and contain small microspheres or microtablets that are each enterically coated to protect them from the acidic environment of the stomach. The enteric coating is designed to dissolve in the alkaline pH of the duodenum, where digestion and absorption of nutrients occur. Historically, acid blockers in the form of H_2 antagonists or proton pump inhibitors (PPIs) have been prescribed to

CASE STUDY REVISITED

Lucy is now 3 years old. She is not eligible for any of the CFTR modulators. Her weight is 12 kg and her height is 91 cm. Her steatorrhea has improved with PERT; however, she remains substantially underweight. Her mother gives her enzymes immediately following all meals and snacks. Her enzyme dose has not been adjusted recently, and she is currently receiving 500 units lipase/kg/meal.

Questions

1. Assess Lucy's growth.
2. Describe the adequacy of Lucy's enzyme dose.
3. How might Lucy's nutritional status and symptoms be improved?
4. If you give Lucy four capsules of an enzyme that contains 6000 units lipase each, what is her enzyme dose per kg per meal?
5. Assess Lucy's previous PES statements. Identify if each statement remains an active issue or if the PES statement has been resolved. If the PES statement remains an active issue, has improvement in the issue been noted? If the issue has been resolved, write a new PES statement.

assist in decreasing the acidity of the duodenum to possibly aid in enzyme efficacy.[17] This practice is still utilized in practice; however, there is limited evidence in clinical trials to demonstrate that the reduction of gastric acidity by acid blockers effectively improves fat absorption in patients with CF.[18] All brands and dosages of pancreatic enzymes, generically known as "pancrealipase," on the market today are approved by the U.S. Food and Drug Administration (FDA), and no generic forms should be used.[19] Additionally, there is one non-enteric-coated product in tablet form normally prescribed for patients with chronic pancreatitis that is sometimes used off-label in patients with CF who are receiving enteral feeds.[19]

CORE CONCEPT 4

Treatment for exocrine pancreatic insufficiency is to provide pancreatic enzyme replacement therapy, taken by mouth with meals and snacks, to substitute for the enzymes the pancreas is not endogenously secreting. These enzymes contain lipase, protease, and amylase for the digestion of fat, protein, and carbohydrates.

Recommendations for weight-based dosing of PERT are available from the CF Foundation; however, dosages must be individualized to the patient. It is important to closely monitor the dose of pancreatic enzymes because extremely high lipase doses have been associated with fibrosing colonopathy or bowel wall thickening. For infants, the recommended starting dose is 2000–5000 units lipase per 120-mL feeding.[9] In patients who are diagnosed after infancy, enzymes can be dosed based upon weight, with a starting dose of 1000 units lipase/kg/meal for patients younger than 4 years of age and 500 units lipase/kg/meal for those older than 4 years.[20] Enzyme doses for snacks are generally half of the usual meal dose. Enzyme doses can be adjusted upward based on clinical assessment of stools, weight gain, and growth. The maximum recommended dose is 2500 units lipase/kg/meal, with a maximum daily dose of 10,000 units lipase/kg/day.[20] If signs of malabsorption are still present after the maximum enzyme dose has been reached, the method of administration, adherence to the enzyme regimen, timing of enzymes with meals, and the method of enzyme storage should be assessed.

Example PERT calculation:

Patient weight = 8 kg

Meal dose: 3 capsules of pancrealipase 5000

3 caps × 5000 units lipase = 15,000 units lipase/meal

15,000 units/8 kg = 1875 units lipase/kg/day

PRACTICE POINT

For infants, the recommended starting dose is 2000–5000 units lipase per 120-mL feeding. In patients who are diagnosed outside of the period of infancy, enzymes can be dosed based upon weight, with a starting dose of 1000 units lipase/kg/meal for patients younger than 4 years of age and 500 units lipase/kg/meal for those older than age 4 years.

Clinical Roundtable

Topic: Recovery of Pancreatic Function on CFTR Modulators

Background: The majority of patients with CF have EPI and require PERT to treat their underlying malabsorption of fat. PERT is typically started shortly after birth and continued for life if the PE-1 test is low (<200 mcg/g). The addition of CFTR modulators as a treatment option for some patients with CF has changed the thought that EPI is a lifelong condition and has made recovery of exocrine pancreatic function a possibility.

The first studies to document this recovery of pancreatic function were the trials of the first CFTR modulator, ivacaftor, in children <5 years. The KIWI (2–5 years) and the ARRIVAL (12–4 months) trials both showed statistically significant improvements in PE-1 values of 99.8 and 164.7 mcg/g, respectively, after treatment with ivacaftor for 24 weeks. The PROMISE study observed children on elexacaftor/tezacaftor/ivacaftor aged 12 years and older with different results. This study did not show a significant change in the PE-1 values and conversion to pancreatic sufficiency, demonstrating that it is likely that early initiation of CFTR modulators prior to age 12 years makes recovery of pancreatic function more likely than initiation after the age of 12.

The interval of time on CFTR modulators needed before patients with CF to convert to being pancreatic sufficient can vary and is not firmly known; however, the majority of the data in the literature demonstrates improvement within 6 months of therapy. While there is no agreed upon method of rechecking PE-1, it has been suggested to test the stool at 6–12 months post-initiation of any CFTR modulator using >200 mcg/g as a cutoff for pancreatic sufficiency. A PE-1 should also be checked anytime a patient with CF on a CFTR modulator develops pancreatitis, demonstrates excessive weight gain, or is routinely missing PERT without symptoms of malabsorption. Until further research is completed, discontinuation of PERT should be individualized for each patient. Consider reducing the enzyme dose by 50% if pancreatic sufficiency is confirmed. If no malabsorption symptoms are noted on 50% dosing for 1–2 weeks, consider discontinuing PERT while monitoring for any recurrence of malabsorption symptoms.

Roundtable Discussion

1. What factors would you consider before reducing the enzyme dose?
2. What symptoms would you monitor after reduction or discontinuation of PERT?

References

1. Davies JC, Cunningham S, Harris WT, et al. Safety, pharmacokinetics, and pharmacodynamics of ivacaftor in patients aged 2–5 years with cystic fibrosis and a CFTR gating mutation (KIWI): an open-label, single-arm study. *Lancet Respir Med*. 2016;4(2):107-115.
2. Rosenfeld M, Wainwright CE, Higgins M, et al. Ivacaftor treatment of cystic fibrosis in children aged 12 to <24 months and with a CFTR gating mutation (ARRIVAL): a phase 3 single-arm study. *Lancet Respir Med*. 2018;6(7):545-553.
3. Schwarzenberg SJ, Vu PT, Skalland M, et al. Elexacaftor/tezacaftor/ivacaftor and gastrointestinal outcomes in cystic fibrosis: report of promise-GI. *J Cyst Fibros*. 2023;22(2):282-289.
4. Stephenson KG, Lingle AJ, Baumberger KA, Dellon EP, Esther CR Jr, Meier EM, Oermann CM, Shenoy VK, Smith NR, Wimmer NS, Duehlmeyer SR, Kam CW, McKinzie CJ, Poisson MO, Elson EC. Changes in fecal elastase-1 following initiation of CFTR modulator therapy in pediatric patients with cystic fibrosis. *J Cyst Fibros*. 2023 Nov;22(6):996-1001.

Pancreatic enzymes should be taken immediately prior to any meal containing fat or protein so that the enzymes reach the duodenum before any food. For infants and small children unable to swallow pills, the capsules should be opened and the beads mixed with a small amount of acidic, pureed food, such as applesauce, and given via spoon. As soon as the patient is able, the capsules can be swallowed whole.

PRACTICE POINT

Pancreatic enzymes should be taken immediately before any meal containing fat or protein so that the enzymes reach the duodenum before any food.

When patients are receiving enteral feeds, they require enzymes for proper absorption. RELiZORB® is an FDA-cleared cartridge containing lipase that connects to a patient's feeding tube, and as formula passes through, fats are hydrolyzed into absorbable fatty acids and monoglycerides (**Figure 21.7**).[21] Studies show improvement in GI symptoms, growth, and fatty acid absorption in patients with CF and pancreatic insufficiency with RELiZORB use.[22] RELiZORB is designed for use with both enteral feeding pumps and syringe bolus feeds. Although PERT was formulated for oral intake, in cases where patients are unable to access RELiZORB, oral PERT may need to be utilized in conjunction with enteral feeds. The most common method to provide oral enzymes for these feeds is to

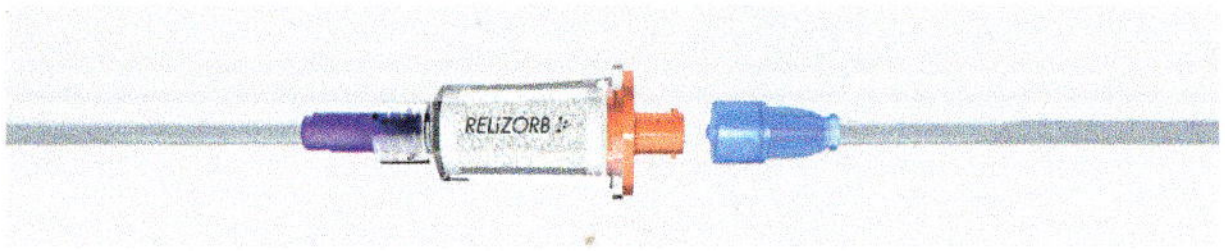

Figure 21.7 RELiZORB Digestive Enzyme Cartridge

administer enzymes by mouth before and after overnight feeds, or prior to a bolus feed. However, in some instances, patients with CF are physically unable to take their enzymes by mouth. Examples include intubation during critical illness or oral aversion. Many CF centers have developed methods by which to give enzymes through a tube if RELiZORB is unavailable or not appropriate for use. The most common method is to use a non-enteric-coated enzyme called Viokace®. To use this method, Viokace tablets are crushed into a fine powder and the powder is added directly to the enteral formula.[19] This method allows the macronutrients in the enteral formula to be predigested prior to administration of the enteral feed. Other methods have also been described. One is to dissolve the enteric-coated enzyme beads into a bicarbonate solution and add the enzyme/bicarbonate solution to the enteral formula or bolus directly prior to formula administration.[23] Another described method is to mix the enteric-coated enzyme beads into nectar-thick fruit juice and administer into a 10 French or larger feeding tube prior to administering formula.[24] Enteric-coated beads should not be administered directly via feeding tube due to the risk of clogging the tube. When using any of the above methods, enzyme dosing should be calculated by the grams of fat that the formula contains. Dosing ranges from 500 to 4000 units lipase/g fat, with usual dosing of approximately 2000 units lipase/g fat.[20]

The stool pattern of the patient should be assessed at every visit to determine adequacy of the enzyme dose. Signs and symptoms of malabsorption may include increased frequency of stools, bulky stools, foul-smelling stools, stool that floats in the toilet, presence of oil in diaper or toilet, increased gassiness, or frequent rectal prolapse.

CASE STUDY REVISITED

Lucy is now 9 years old. She is doing well with minimal steatorrhea. Her BMI-for-age is still below recommended CF standards. The medical team advises that if she cannot improve her weight gain from the oral route, then a feeding tube would be recommended.

Anthropometric Data:

Height: 129 cm
Weight: 25 kg

Clinical Data:

Meds: albuterol, dornase alfa, budesonide/formoterol, CF-specific multivitamin chewable tablet, pancrealipase

Dietary Data:

Dietary Recall:
Breakfast (7:30 am): Orange juice, Shredded wheat (1 cup) with 6 oz skim milk, 1 slice toast with jelly
Lunch (11:30 am): Apple juice, garden salad with hard-boiled egg, and tuna with low-fat dressing or a turkey sandwich with mustard
Dinner (5 pm): Spaghetti with marinara sauce
Dessert (5:30 pm): Frozen yogurt

Questions

1. How might Lucy improve the caloric density of her diet?
2. What macronutrient would you emphasize? Why?
3. Are there any other medications you could consider adding to help increase Lucy's caloric intake?
4. Assess Lucy's previous PES statements. Identify if each statement remains an active issue or if the PES statement has been resolved. If the PES statement remains an active issue, has improvement in the issue been noted? If the issue has been resolved, write a new PES statement.

Nutrition Intervention

Macronutrients

In general, patients with CF require a high-calorie diet for proper weight gain and growth. Historically, it was recommended to restrict fat in the diet to avoid the symptoms of fat malabsorption. Now, with adequate PERT, the diet of patients should be individualized for the patient and fat can be added to the diet without restriction.[25,26]

PRACTICE POINT

When given adequate PERT, fat restriction is not indicated; diet and macronutrient distribution should be individualized for each patient.

Infants

As a result of newborn screening, infants are commonly diagnosed with CF in the first few weeks to months of life. Human milk is recommended as the infant's primary source of nutrition due to its widely recognized benefits. If human milk is not available, standard infant formula should be used.[10] Hydrolyzed protein formulas have not shown a benefit over standard formulas when proper pancreatic enzyme replacement is used.[27] Introduction of solid foods should be initiated per standard recommendations by the American Academy of Pediatrics. Some infants may require fortified human milk or calorie-dense infant formulas due to the high metabolic demands of CF. Once solids are introduced to the infant's diet, purees and table foods can be made more energy-dense with the addition of fats. These adjustments in diet should be done only in infants who are demonstrating poor weight gain and growth.[10]

Micronutrients

Patients with CF and EPI require supplementation of vitamins and minerals due to the risk of deficiencies because of malabsorption. Fat-soluble vitamin (vitamins A, E, D, and K) deficiencies are often present at diagnosis and are normally corrected once PERT and vitamin supplements are initiated.[28] There are many vitamin supplements available today that are specifically designed for patients with CF. These supplements contain higher amounts of fat-soluble vitamins in addition to water-soluble vitamins and zinc. Infants are started on these vitamins upon diagnosis of CF and EPI.[9] Dosages of CF-specific vitamins are adjusted based on results of serum vitamin levels drawn annually as part of routine CF care. Some patients require single-nutrient supplementation of vitamins A, E, D, or K if deficiency of a particular vitamin persists despite supplementation with a CF-specific multivitamin. The CF Foundation has published consensus guidelines specifically on the treatment of vitamin D deficiency. In summary, the CF Foundation recommends all patients maintain a 25-OH vitamin D level greater than 30 ng/mL and that all low levels be treated with vitamin D3 (cholecalciferol).[29] These guidelines should be referred to when treating a patient with a low vitamin D level because they differ based on the patient's age and vitamin D level. All patients should be counseled that their vitamins should be taken with a fat-containing food or beverage in conjunction with PERT to ensure adequate absorption.

CORE CONCEPT 5

Patients with cystic fibrosis and exocrine pancreatic insufficiency require supplementation of vitamins and minerals due to risk for malabsorption-related deficiencies. Serum fat-soluble vitamin levels should be assessed annually, because they are the primary nutrients at risk for deficiency.

In addition to fat-soluble vitamins, some mineral deficiencies may be present in CF. Zinc losses occur in the stool prior to initiation of enzyme therapy or in patients whose enzyme regimen is not optimized.[30] Zinc deficiency is difficult to diagnose because serum zinc is not a good predictor of zinc stores in the body. In patients in whom a zinc deficiency is suspected, 1 mg elemental zinc/kg weight can be prescribed for 6 months in addition to a regular CF-specific multivitamin.[31]

Dietary intake of calcium should be assessed regularly due to the higher risk for bone disease in CF. With the risk for vitamin D deficiency apparent, calcium intake must be adequate in the diet.[32] If dietary intake of calcium is poor, calcium supplements should be recommended.

Sodium Chloride

Patients with CF have higher sodium needs than those of the general population. This is due to increased sodium losses in their sweat.[33] Liberal salt intake is recommended in CF. For infants, the CF Foundation guidelines recommend 1/8 teaspoon of salt (12.5 mEq sodium) daily upon diagnosis and through 6 months of age.[10] The salt should be added in small, frequent amounts throughout the day in bottles or in the applesauce used to administer enzymes. At 6 months, 1/4 teaspoon salt (25 mEq sodium) should be given daily not to exceed 4 mEq/kg/day.[10] After the child is eating a variety of table foods, salt should be added liberally to foods. Special attention is needed when the patient is participating in strenuous activity, where sweating may increase sodium losses.

CORE CONCEPT 6

Patients with cystic fibrosis have higher sodium needs than those of the general population due to increased sweat-related losses. Patients with CF are prescribed a high-salt diet to compensate for the additional losses.

PRACTICE POINT

Cystic Fibrosis Foundation guidelines recommend 1/8 teaspoon of salt daily upon diagnosis and through 6 months of age. The salt should be added in small, frequent amounts throughout the day in bottles or in the applesauce used to administer enzymes. At 6 months, 1/4 teaspoon salt should be given daily.

Nutrition Support

Adequate nutrition status and BMI are essential to maintaining normal lung function in CF. If an adequate weight cannot be maintained with a high-calorie diet alone, high-calorie oral supplements are often prescribed. Patients and families may choose to make their own high-calorie shakes due to the high cost of commercial supplements or due to taste preference.

Oral supplements may not be sufficient in promoting weight gain and normal growth, and in those cases enteral feeds may be recommended.[6] Enteral feeds are typically given at a continuous rate overnight during sleep. The patient eats and drinks normally throughout the day and receives additional calories overnight. Most patients choose to have a gastrostomy tube inserted; however, nasogastric feeds can be used if the feeds are thought to be only needed on a short-term basis. Both intact protein and semi-elemental formulas can be used, but both formulas require RELiZORB or PERT for proper absorption.[34] Postpyloric feeds are rarely needed, although they may be beneficial in patients with severe reflux or those who are intubated and ventilated. Parenteral nutrition is not routinely used in CF but may be required in circumstances where the GI tract cannot be used or when enteral feeds are not tolerated.

Prior to prescribing enteral feeds, a trial of appetite stimulants may be indicated. If oral supplements are not sufficient or are not tolerated by the patient and inadequate calories are suspected, appetite stimulants may stimulate hunger enough to promote adequate weight gain.[35] Other causes of poor weight gain, such as malabsorption or increased energy expenditure due to respiratory illness, should be ruled out before appetite stimulants are prescribed. Cyproheptadine hydrochloride is a common appetite stimulant used in CF.[36] It is an antihistamine with a secondary effect of

CASE STUDY REVISITED

Lucy is now 18 years of age. She is admitted to evaluate new-onset CF-related diabetes. She also experienced a wrist fracture last summer while playing softball. Her clinical information is as follows:

Anthropometrics:

Height: 162 cm
Weight: 56 kg

Biochemical Data:

Electrolytes normal
2-hour glucose on glucose tolerance test 204 (<200 mg/dL)
HbA1c 8.9 (4.3–5.6%)
Vitamin D 14 (20–100 ng/mL)

Questions

1. What is Lucy's BMI-for-age, and how would you describe her nutritional status at this point?
2. How do you interpret Lucy's biochemical data at this visit? How might this relate to her CF?
3. Write a new PES statement for Lucy related to her recent complication.

appetite stimulation. It is often used due to its low side effect profile, but it may initially cause fatigue in some patients. Megestrol acetate is successful in promoting weight gain; however, it must be used with caution due to its risk of causing adrenal suppression and diabetes.[37,38] Dronabinol (Marinol™) has also been described as helpful in patients with severe lung disease, as the medication can improve appetite and nausea.[39]

CORE CONCEPT 7

If an adequate BMI cannot be maintained with diet alone, oral supplements, and sometimes enteral nutrition support, are recommended to promote weight gain and optimize nutritional status.

Nutrition Monitoring

Monitoring of patients with CF should be done routinely in a multidisciplinary manner. During infancy, routine visits (monthly or more frequently) are needed to assess growth and dietary intake. Screening for malnutrition is essential with adjustments in diet intervention as needed. Understanding pulmonary function and incidence of respiratory infections is needed to assess their impact on energy expenditure and weight status. Evaluation of PERT efficacy should be done during nutrition assessment via diet history, signs of malabsorption, and growth, with adjustment in enzyme dosing as indicated. Due to the risk of fat malabsorption, measures of vitamin D and other fat-soluble vitamins should be done routinely. Assessment of sodium and calcium intake should be completed routinely to assure adequate intake given increased sodium losses through sweat and increased risk of bone disease. Specific monitoring of nutrition-related conditions and complications of CF should also be done (provided below).

Body Image, Disordered Eating, and Weight Stigma

Individuals with CF are at heightened risk for eating disorders and body image issues, which can negatively impact their weight gain, lung function, and overall mortality. The unique challenges of CF, including EPI, high energy demands, an intense focus on BMI, lack of control in a chronic disease, and the potential for medication manipulation, contribute to these disorders.[40] Moreover, as CF treatment has advanced in recent years, issues of overweight and obesity have surfaced, often accompanied by stigma and its associated negative psychological impacts, such as increased stress, depression, and decreased motivation to adopt healthier behaviors.[41] Clinicians should be equipped to identify potential eating disorders and body image issues and take a sensitive and empathetic approach when discussing overweight and obesity. Implementation of improved screening and monitoring practices, and involving multidisciplinary support from RDs, mental health professionals, and social workers, is essential to provide comprehensive care and enhance patient outcomes.[42]

CORE CONCEPT 8

Patients with cystic fibrosis are at increased risk for eating disorders, body image concerns, and with recent advances in treatment, for overweight, obesity, and weight stigma.

Individualized Nutrition in the Era of Modulators

The introduction of CFTR **modulators** in recent years has transformed nutrition care for people with CF, offering improved symptom management, longer lifespans, and a reduced risk of undernutrition. With these advancements, nutrition strategies are shifting from reliance on high-energy, nutrient-poor diets toward individualized medical nutrition therapy (MNT). RDs should continue regular nutrition screenings, adapting MNT based on factors such as disease severity, body composition, laboratory values, and physical activity. A healthy, balanced diet emphasizing nutrient-dense foods such as fruits, vegetables, whole grains, seafood, eggs, beans and peas, nuts and seeds, dairy products, and meats and poultry should be encouraged, with oral or enteral supplements introduced when needed to support growth and to maintain a healthy weight.[25]

During routine assessment of bone mineral density using DXA, body composition may also be assessed if software allows. If DXA is not feasible or indicated, assessment of body composition using skinfold measures or bioelectrical impedance analysis (BIA) may be used with caution over time, considering that prediction equations using these methods may over- or underestimate fat and fat-free mass in patients with CF. Nutrition status can be further assessed using mid-upper arm circumference and/or nutrition-focused physical examination.[25]

Cardiovascular health should also be monitored, with fasting lipid profiles recommended at least once between ages 10 and 20 years, and every 4–6 years thereafter. In all cases, MNT should be adapted as patient needs evolve, ensuring that optimal nutrition supports long-term health outcomes.[25]

CORE CONCEPT 9

The introduction of CFTR modulators has transformed nutrition care for people with CF, shifting focus toward individualized medical nutrition therapy that addresses evolving patient needs. Assessment of body composition and lipid profiles can be useful for providing individualized care.

Nutrition-Related Complications of Cystic Fibrosis

Gastrointestinal Complications

Gastroesophageal reflux is common in patients with CF, and it must be treated effectively to prevent additional damage to the lungs.[43,44] Untreated reflux can result in inadequate oral intake and poor weight gain and can also exacerbate lung disease.[45] Constipation is also a common complication of CF. This is a result of poor CFTR function in the GI tract, causing the stool to become dehydrated and difficult to pass.[46] Untreated constipation can result in distal intestinal obstruction syndrome (DIOS) that may require surgical intervention if left untreated.[47] It is important to prevent constipation in CF with adequate hydration and salt intake. Often, stool softeners such as polyethylene glycol are used as a maintenance medication to prevent constipation.[47]

Patients with CF who remain pancreatic sufficient are at risk for developing pancreatitis. These patients may go on to become pancreatic insufficient and should be closely monitored with an annual pancreatic elastase. Patients with CF are also at risk of developing CF-related liver disease. This may progress to end-stage liver disease, in which a liver transplant may be indicated. Liver function tests and other imaging studies are recommended on a yearly or every other year schedule to monitor the liver for damage related to progression of disease.[48]

CF-Related Diabetes

Patients with CF are at risk for developing **CF-related diabetes (CFRD)**. CFRD has similarities to both type 1 and type 2 diabetes.[12] The major problem is a shortage of insulin, but insulin resistance can also play a role in hyperglycemia.[12] The risk of developing CFRD increases with age.[49–51] Hyperglycemia can also occur without a diagnosis of CFRD during times of illness or when patients are receiving corticosteroid therapy. CFRD is usually diagnosed by a 2-hour oral glucose tolerance test completed annually starting at age 10 years.[12] A 2-hour value >200 mg/dL is diagnostic for CFRD. Other diagnostic criteria include a fasting glucose ≥126 mg/dL, a HbA1c ≥6.5%, or a random glucose ≥200 mg/dL. HbA1c should not be used exclusively as a screening tool for CFRD due to increased red blood cell turnover in patients with CF.[12]

Treatment for CFRD is usually insulin, and oral hypoglycemic medications are typically not used. Insulin regimens should be individualized for every patient by an endocrinologist who is familiar with CFRD. A high-calorie diet should continue to be recommended if indicated, and carbohydrates should not be restricted.[12] Proper treatment with insulin and normal blood sugar control is vital to maintaining adequate nutrition status.

CF-Related Bone Disease

Patients with CF are at a greater risk of developing bone disease.[52] Mainly, malabsorption of fat results in fat-soluble vitamin deficiencies, specifically vitamin D. Additionally, chronic malnutrition and frequent use of corticosteroids may contribute to poor bone health. By the age of 18 years, all patients with CF should have a DXA scan according to recommendations of the CF Foundation. Based on the results, patients should have a repeat scan every 1–5 years. It is recommended that children with CF who have strong risk factors for bone disease should receive a DXA scan prior to 18 years of age.[53–55] For abnormal DXA scans, it is important that calcium, vitamin D, and vitamin K are optimized in the diet and/or supplements are used.

CORE CONCEPT 10

Patients with cystic fibrosis are at risk for developing CF-related diabetes (CFRD), bone disease, and liver disease.

PRACTICE POINT

All patients with CF should have a dual-energy x-ray absorptiometry (DXA) scan by age 18 years. Children at high risk may need to receive one prior to 18 years of age.

Summary

Cystic fibrosis is a genetic disease associated with the abnormal transport of sodium, chloride, and water at the cellular level, resulting in abnormally thick mucus leading to organ damage. Nutritional management of CF involves promoting normal growth during childhood and adolescence and maintaining optimal nutrition in adulthood. Malabsorption due to EPI occurs in most individuals with CF. Treatment of EPI involves the use of PERT to provide exogenous lipase, protease, and amylase to assist in macronutrient digestion. Due to the prevalence of malabsorption, individuals with CF should be monitored for fat-soluble vitamin deficiencies and receive supplementation as appropriate. If an adequate BMI cannot be achieved or maintained, oral supplements or enteral nutrition support may be indicated. Management of CF-related comorbidities such as gastroesophageal reflux, constipation, liver disease, CF-related diabetes, and CF-related bone disease is important to maintain optimal health and nutritional status. The introduction of CFTR modulators to the care of patients with CF has improved symptom management, lifespan, and nutrition status for many people with CF. Individualized nutrition care is essential to addressing evolving patient needs.

Key Terms

Cystic fibrosis, CF transmembrane conductance regulator (CFTR) protein, pancreatic insufficiency, sweat test, digital clubbing, bronchi, bronchioles, alveoli, cilia, bronchodilators, mucolytics, nebulizers, percussor, forced expiratory volume at 1 second (FEV_1), PIVKA-II, pancreatic enzyme replacement therapy (PERT), CF-related diabetes (CFRD), modulators

References

1. Cystic Fibrosis Foundation. *Cystic fibrosis foundation patient registry*. [2023 Annual Data Report to the Center Directors]. 2024.
2. Brown RF, Close CT, Mailes MG, et al. Cystic Fibrosis Foundation position paper: redefining the cystic fibrosis care team. *J Cyst Fibros*. 2024;23(6):1045–1054.
3. Farrell PM, White TB, Ren CL, et al. Diagnosis of cystic fibrosis: consensus guidelines from the Cystic Fibrosis Foundation. *J Pediatr*. 2017;181S:S4–S15.
4. Landess L, Prieur MG, Brown AR, Dellon EP. Exploring perceptions of and decision-making about CFTR modulators. *Pediatr Pulmonol*. 2024;59(6):1614–1621.
5. Yen EH, Quinton H, Borowitz D. Better nutritional status in early childhood is associated with improved clinical outcomes and survival in patients with cystic fibrosis. *J Pediatr*. 2013;162(3):530–535.e1.
6. Stallings VA, Stark LJ, Robinson KA, Feranchak AP, Quinton H. Evidence-based practice recommendations for nutrition-related management of children and adults with cystic fibrosis and pancreatic insufficiency: results of a systematic review. *J Am Diet Assoc*. 2008;108(5):832–839.
7. Engelen MP, Com G, Deutz NE. Protein is an important but undervalued macronutrient in the nutritional care of patients with cystic fibrosis. *Curr Opin Nutr Metab Care*. 2014;17(6):515–520.
8. Moudiau T, Galli-Tsinopoulou, Vamvakoudis E, Nousia-Arvanitakis S. Resting energy expenditure in cystic fibrosis as an indicator of disease severity. *J Cystic Fibr*. 2007;6:131–136.
9. Borowitz D, Baker RD, Stalling VD. Consensus report on nutrition for pediatric patients with cystic fibrosis. *J Pediatr Gastroenterol Nutr*. 2002;35(3):246–259.
10. Borowitz D, Robinson KA, Rosenfeld M, et al. Cystic Fibrosis Foundation evidence-based guidelines for management of infants with cystic fibrosis. *J Pediatr*. 2009;155(6):S73–S93.
11. Sankararaman S, Hendrix SJ, Schindler T. Update on the management of vitamins and minerals in cystic fibrosis. *Nutr Clin Pract*. 2022;37(5):1074–1087.
12. Moran A, Brunzell C, Cohen RC, et al. Clinical care guidelines for cystic fibrosis-related diabetes: a position statement of the American Diabetes Association and a clinical practice guideline of the Cystic Fibrosis Foundation, endorsed by the Pediatric Endocrine Society. *Diabetes Care*. 2010;33(12):2697–2708.
13. Aris RM, Merkel PA, Bachrach LK, et al. Guide to bone health and disease in cystic fibrosis. *J Clin Endocrinol Metab*. 2005;90(3):1888–1896.
14. Putman MS, Anabtawi A, Le T, Tangpricha V, Sermet-Gaudelus I. Cystic fibrosis bone disease treatment: current knowledge and future directions. *J Cyst Fibros*. 2019;18 Suppl 2:S56–S65.
15. Seyoum S, Regenstein M, Nolan L. Risk indicators of food insecurity in the CF population. *Health Policy and Management Issue Briefs*. 2021;59. https://hsrc.himmelfarb.gwu.edu/sphhs_policy_briefs/59
16. Stephenson KG, Lingle AJ, Baumberger KA, et al. Changes in fecal elastase-1 following initiation of CFTR modulator therapy in pediatric patients with cystic fibrosis. *J Cyst Fibros*. 2023;22(6):996–1001.
17. Liu C, Bach TR, Farrell PM, et al. Impact of acid blocker therapy on growth, gut microbiome, and lung disease in young children with cystic fibrosis. *J Pediatr Gastroenterol Nutr*. 2024;79(6):1124–1133. doi:10.1002/jpn3.12389
18. Ng SM, Jones AP. Drug therapies for reducing gastric acidity in people with cystic fibrosis. *Cochrane Database Syst Rev*. 2003;(2):CD003424.
19. Berry AJ. Pancreatic enzyme replacement therapy during pancreatic insufficiency. *Nutr Clin Pract*. 2014;29(3):312–321.

20. Borowitz DS, Grand RJ, Durie PR. Use of pancreatic enzyme supplements for patients with cystic fibrosis in the context of fibrosing colonopathy. *J Pediatr*. 1995;127(5):681–684.
21. Alcresta Therapeutics. RELiZORB (immobilized lipase). Accessed September 15, 2024. https://www.relizorb.com/
22. Stevens J, Wyatt C, Brown P, Patel D, Grujic D, Freedman SD. Absorption and Safety with Sustained Use of RELiZORB Evaluation (ASSURE) study in patients with cystic fibrosis receiving enteral feeding. *J Pediatr Gastroenterol Nutr*. 2018;67(4):527–532.
23. Nicolo M, Stratton KW, Rooney W, Boullata J. Pancreatic enzyme replacement therapy for enterally fed patients with cystic fibrosis. *Nutr Clin Pract*. 2013;28(4):485–489.
24. Ferrie S, Graham C, Hoyle M. Pancreatic enzyme supplementation for patients receiving enteral feeds. *Nutr Clin Pract*. 2011;26(3):349–351.
25. McDonald CM, Alvarez JA, Bailey J, et al. Academy of Nutrition and Dietetics: 2020 Cystic Fibrosis Evidence Analysis Center Evidence-Based Nutrition Practice Guideline. *J Acad Nutr Diet*. 2021;121(8):1591–1636.
26. McDonald CM, Bowser EK, Farnham K, Alvarez, JA, Padula L, Rozga M. Dietary macronutrient distribution and nutrition outcomes in persons with cystic fibrosis: an evidence analysis center systematic review. *J Acad Nutr Diet*. 2021;121(8):1574–1590.
27. Ellis L, Kalnins D, Corey M, Brennan J, Pencharz P, Durie P. Do infants with cystic fibrosis need a protein hydrolysate formula? A prospective, randomized, comparative study. *J Pediatr*. 1998;132(2):270–276.
28. Feranchak AP, Sontag MK, Wagener JS, Hammond KB, Accurso FJ, Sokol RJ. Prospective, long-term study of fat-soluble vitamin status in children with cystic fibrosis identified by newborn screen. *J Pediatr*. 1999;135(5):601–610.
29. Tangpricha V, Kelly A, Stephenson A, et al. An update on the screening, diagnosis, management, and treatment of vitamin D deficiency in individuals with cystic fibrosis: evidence-based recommendations from the Cystic Fibrosis Foundation. *J Clin Endocrinol Metab*. 2012;97(4):1082–1093.
30. Easley D, Krebs N, Jefferson M, et al. Effect of pancreatic enzymes on zinc absorption in cystic fibrosis. *J Pediatr Gastroenterol Nutr*. 1998;26(2):136–139.
31. Krebs NF. Update on zinc deficiency and excess in clinical pediatric practice. *Ann Nutr Metab*. 2013;62(suppl 1):19–29.
32. Ross AC, Manson JE, Abrams SA, et al. The 2011 report on dietary reference intakes for calcium and vitamin D from the Institute of Medicine: what clinicians need to know. *J Clin Endocrinol Metab*. 2011;96(1):53–58.
33. Arvanitakis S, Lobeck C. Metabolic alkalosis and salt depletion in cystic fibrosis. *J Pediatr*. 1973;82(3):535–536.
34. Durie P, Newth C, Forstner G, Gall D. Malabsorption of medium-chain triglycerides in infants with cystic fibrosis: Correction with pancreatic enzyme supplements. *J Pediatr*. 1980;96(5):862–864.
35. Nasr SZ, Drury D. Appetite stimulants use in cystic fibrosis. *Pediatr Pulmonol*. 2008;43(3):209–219.
36. Homnick DN, Homnick BD, Reeves AJ, Marks JH, Pimentel RS, Bonnema SK. Cyproheptadine is an effective appetite stimulant in cystic fibrosis. *Pediatr Pulmonol*. 2004;38(2):129–134.
37. Eubanks V, Koppersmith N, Wooldridge N, et al. Effects of megestrol acetate on weight gain, body composition, and pulmonary function in patients with cystic fibrosis. *J Pediatr*. 2002;140(4):439–444.
38. Marchand V, Baker SS, Stark TJ, Baker RD. Randomized, double-blind, placebo-controlled pilot trial of megestrol acetate in malnourished children with cystic fibrosis. *J Pediatr Gastroenterol Nutr*. 2000;31(3):264–269.
39. Anstead M, Kuhn R, Martyn D, Craigmyle L, Kanga J. Dronabinol, an effective and safe appetite stimulant in cystic fibrosis. *Pediatr Pulmonol*. 2003;36:323.
40. Darukhanavala A, Merjaneh L, Mason K, Le T. Eating disorders and body image in cystic fibrosis. *J Clin Transl Endocrinol*. 2021;26:100280.
41. Bailey J, Krick S, Fontaine KR. The changing landscape of nutrition in cystic fibrosis: the emergence of overweight and obesity. *Nutrients*. 2022;14(6):1216.
42. Leonard A, Bailey J, Bruce A, et al. Nutritional considerations for a new era: A CF foundation position paper. *J Cyst Fibros*. 2023;22(5):788–795.
43. Mousa HM, Woodley FW. Gastroesophageal reflux in cystic fibrosis: current understandings of mechanisms and management. *Curr Gastroenterol Rep*. 2012;14(3):226–235.
44. Bongiovanni A, Manti S, Parisi GF, et al. Focus on gastroesophageal reflux disease in patients with cystic fibrosis. *World J Gastroenterol*. 2020;26(41):6322–6334.
45. Cucchiara S, Santamaria F, Andreotti MR, et al. Mechanisms of gastro-oesophageal reflux in cystic fibrosis. *Arch Dis Child*. 1991;66(5):617–622.
46. van der Doef, Hubert PJ, Kokke FT, van der Ent, Cornelis K, Houwen RH. Intestinal obstruction syndromes in cystic fibrosis: meconium ileus, distal intestinal obstruction syndrome, and constipation. *Curr Gastroenterol Rep*. 2011;13(3):265–270.
47. Colombo C, Ellemunter H, Houwen R, Munck A, Taylor C, Wilschanski M. Guidelines for the diagnosis and management of distal intestinal obstruction syndrome in cystic fibrosis patients. *J Cystic Fibrosis*. 2011;10(Suppl 2):S24–S28.
48. Sellers ZM, Assis DN, Paranjape SM, et al. Cystic fibrosis screening, evaluation, and management of hepatobiliary disease consensus recommendations. *Hepatology*. 2024; 79(5):1220–1238.
49. Moran A, Dunitz J, Nathan B, Saeed A, Holme B, Thomas W. Cystic fibrosis-related diabetes: current trends in prevalence, incidence, and mortality. *Diabetes Care*. 2009; 32(9):1626–1631.
50. Solomon MP, Wilson DC, Corey M, et al. Glucose intolerance in children with cystic fibrosis. *J Pediatr*. 2003;142(2):128–132.
51. Lanng S, Hansen A, Thorsteinsson B, Nerup J, Koch C. Glucose tolerance in patients with cystic fibrosis: five year prospective study. *BMJ*. 1995;311(7006):655–659.
52. Anabtawi A, Le T, Putman M, Tangpricha V, Bianchi ML. Cystic fibrosis bone disease: pathophysiology, assessment and prognostic implications. *J Cyst Fibros*. 2019;18 (Suppl 2):S48–S55.
53. Putman MS, Anabtawi A, Le T, Tangpricha V, Sermet-Gaudelus I. Cystic fibrosis bone disease treatment: Current knowledge and future directions. *J Cyst Fibros*. 2019;18 (Suppl 2):S56–S65.
54. Aris RM, Merkel PA, Bachrach LK, et al. Guide to bone health and disease in cystic fibrosis. *J Clin Endocrinol Metab*. 2005;90(3):1888–1896.
55. Marquette M, Haworth CS. Bone health and disease in cystic fibrosis. *Paediatr Respir Rev*. 2016;20 Suppl:2–5.

CHAPTER 22

Nutritional Management of Pediatric Obesity

Yujia (Sandra) Zhang

CHAPTER OUTLINE

CORE CONCEPTS

1. The medical and psychosocial comorbidities associated with pediatric obesity present unique challenges to the healthcare provider in the prevention, diagnosis, and treatment of this disease.
2. Pediatric obesity is associated with many of the risk factors for cardiovascular disease, including hypertension, dyslipidemia, and poor glycemic control that could eventually lead to diabetes.
3. Children who are overweight or obese are at an increased risk for multiple risk factors associated with cardiac dysfunction, increasing the likelihood of cardiovascular disease progression with age.
4. Type 2 diabetes in children and adolescents is associated with early onset of micro- and macrovascular complications and increased risk of mortality with aging, making prevention of this disease extremely important.
5. Children and adolescents with obesity who seek medical treatment for obesity have demonstrated elevated rates of depressive disorder, anxiety disorder, social anxiety, loneliness, and preference for isolative activities.
6. The etiology of pediatric obesity is multifactorial; individual factors, social factors, and environmental factors all play a role in a child's health status.

7. For successful weight loss, it is recommended to introduce children to healthy eating and behavioral patterns instead of placing them on calorie-restricted diets, which may set them up for failure and future weight gain.
8. Behavioral change in children can be achieved by employing motivational interviewing during counseling, providing positive reinforcement from the child's support system, and identifying cues that lead to unhealthy behaviors.
9. Several weight loss pharmacotherapy options are available for pediatric patients 12 years and older to consider while implementing lifestyle changes. There are side effects associated with different medications.
10. Two metabolic and bariatric procedures are recommended for weight loss in adolescents: the Roux-en-Y gastric bypass and the sleeve gastrectomy.
11. Although federal agencies implement nutrition programs at school to provide low-cost or free and healthy meals to most school-aged children, children may not consume proper nutrition at school due to various reasons.

LEARNING OBJECTIVES

1. Define pediatric obesity and list the available indicators used by health practitioners to assess obesity, along with the advantages and disadvantages of each.
2. Explain the pathophysiology of pediatric obesity and related medical comorbidities.
3. Recognize the potential psychological effects that obesity and weight gain can have on children.
4. Describe the etiology of pediatric obesity and the interplay of multifactorial aspects, particularly with the growing field of nutrigenomics.
5. Explore the different models of nutritional care and intervention used for pediatric obesity.
6. Identify the different techniques used for behavioral intervention with children with obesity and the correlation between BMI and the development of mental health conditions.
7. Discuss the significance of pediatric obesity prevention and the most recent Centers for Disease Control and Prevention (CDC) guidelines.
8. Specify the different types of weight loss medications and surgical procedures that are safe and available for children.
9. Identify the current guidelines and challenges in the school environment for tackling pediatric obesity.

Introduction

Pediatric obesity is a significant health problem in the United States and a major focus of many public health efforts. The medical and psychosocial comorbidities associated with pediatric obesity present unique challenges to the healthcare provider in the prevention, diagnosis, and treatment of this disease. The etiology of pediatric obesity varies among individuals; however, numerous genetic and environmental factors have been identified as key risk factors for this disease. Medical nutrition therapy is indicated in the prevention, treatment, and management of pediatric obesity.

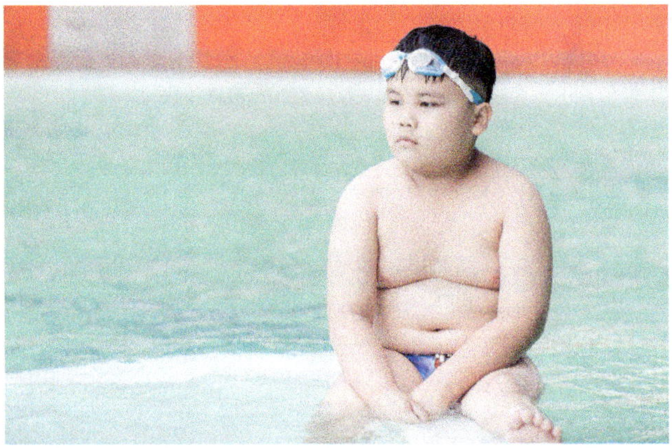

©kwanchai.c/Shutterstock

CORE CONCEPT 1

The medical and psychosocial comorbidities associated with pediatric obesity present unique challenges to the healthcare provider in the prevention, diagnosis, and treatment of this disease.

Prevalence

Pediatric obesity is one of the most common chronic diseases in children and adolescents. From 2021 to 2023, the prevalence of obesity among U.S. children and adolescents was 21.1%, and the prevalence of severe obesity was 7.0%.[1] **Figure 22.1** displays the prevalence of obesity in children and adolescents from

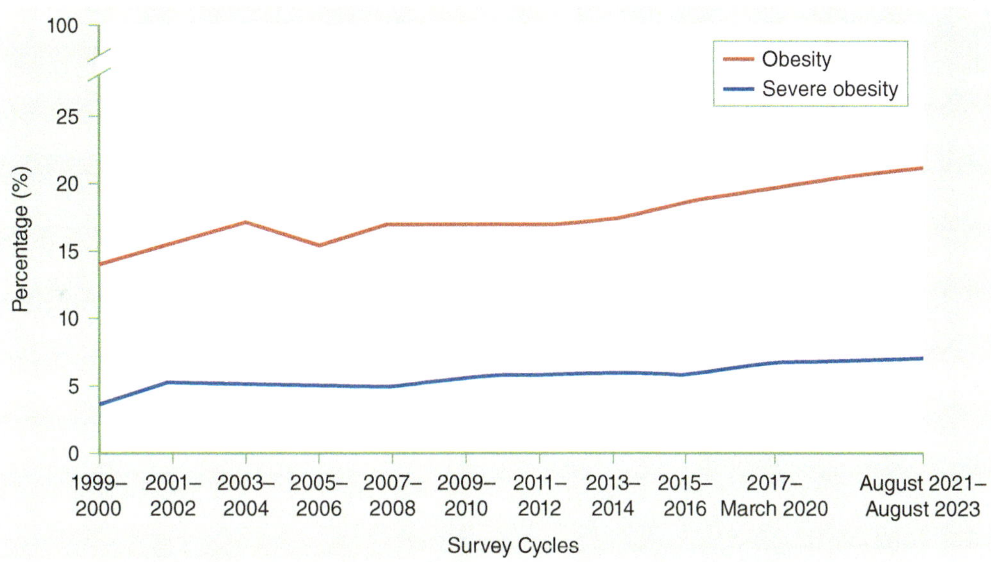

Figure 22.1 Prevalence of Obesity and Severe Obesity Among Persons Aged 2–19 Years—United States, 1999–2000 Through 2021–2023

Reproduced from CDC/NCHS. QuickStats: Prevalence of Obesity and Severe Obesity Among Persons Aged 2–19 Years – United States, 1999–2000 Through 2021–2023. *MMWR Morb Mortal Wkly Rep* 2024;73:936. DOI: http://dx.doi.org/10.15585/mmwr.mm7341a

CASE STUDY INTRODUCTION

Nora is a 14-year-old female referred for medical nutrition therapy by her primary care provider (PCP). Nora has gained over 9 kg this past year. Her PCP is concerned that with continuous weight gain and high low-density lipoprotein (LDL) cholesterol and triglyceride levels, Nora will develop type 2 diabetes and cardiovascular disease. Nora arrived at her initial appointment with her mother, who has class 3 obesity. At the initial meeting, Nora explains that her favorite foods include fast-food options and processed desserts such as cream-filled cake snacks and cinnamon buns. Nora does little physical activity during the week and reports that she does not find any enjoyment from exercise.

Anthropometric Data:

Height: 165 cm
Weight: 85 kg
BMI: 31 kg/m^2
Waist Circumference: 101.6 cm

Biochemical Data:

Total Cholesterol 275 mg/dL (Desirable: <200 mg/dL)
LDL-Cholesterol 145 mg/dL (Desirable: <100 mg/dL)
HDL-Cholesterol 22 mg/dL (Desirable: ≥40 mg/dL)
Triglycerides 220 mg/dL (Desirable: <150 mg/dL)
HbA1c 6.0% (4.3–5.6%)
Fasting blood sugar 115 mg/dL (70–99 mg/dL)

Clinical Data:

Past Medical History: asthma, prehypertension, prediabetes
Medications: corticosteroids (asthma), sertraline (anxiety disorder)
Vital Signs: Blood pressure 140/90 mm Hg, Temperature 97.5°F, Heart rate 80 beats/min
Nutrition-Focused Physical Exam: Appears well nourished. Adiposity consistent with android body type. Oral exam, hair, and nails appear normal. Skin is warm and intact. No evidence of acanthosis nigricans. Abdominal exam unremarkable. No evidence of lower or upper extremity edema.

Dietary Data:

24-Hour Diet Recall:

Breakfast (7 am): 2 bowls of chocolate sweetened cereal, whole milk, 1 cup of orange juice, 1 toaster pastry

Snack (10 am): 1 bag of trail mix, 8 to 10 mini cookies, 8 oz of chocolate milk

Lunch (12:30 pm): 1 hamburger with bun with ketchup and mayonnaise, French fries, steamed peas and carrots, 1 oz bag of potato chips, 1 medium soda (Nora receives school lunch)

Snack (4 pm): 2 chocolate chip waffles (no syrup), 1 mini bag of cheese crackers

Dinner (7 pm): 2 bowls of boxed macaroni and cheese, 1 roll, steamed green beans, 1 can regular soda, 1 brownie for dessert

Pre-bedtime snack (9 pm): 1 bowl of vanilla ice cream with whipped cream and 1 Tbsp chocolate chips

Questions

1. Plot Nora's data on the Centers for Disease Control and Prevention (CDC) growth chart for girls. In what percentile is her weight-for-age? Height-for-age? BMI-for-age?
2. Does this information classify Nora as underweight, normal weight, overweight, or obese?
3. What risk factors does Nora have for diabetes and cardiovascular disease (CVD)?
4. Access Nora's diet recall. Write two Problem/Etiology/Signs and Symptoms (PES) statements for Nora identifying Nora's active nutrition issues.
5. Identify the nutrition and lifestyle interventions you would like to initiate for Nora to address the problems identified in your PES statements.
6. What indices are included in your monitoring and evaluation plan? Why?

1999/2000–2021/2023. The U.S. Preventive Services Task Force recommends that clinicians screen for obesity in children 6 years or older with intensive behavioral interventions to promote weight regulation, when indicated.[2]

Defining Pediatric Obesity

A unique challenge presented in the pediatric population when considering obesity is how to identify and define it. The screening of obesity for children in the United States is typically made using the 2000 Centers for Disease Control and Prevention (CDC) body mass index (BMI) sex- and age-specific charts. (Refer to Chapter 20, *Nutrition in Pediatrics*, for more information on pediatric nutrition.) These BMI charts illustrate the distribution of BMI in U.S. children aged 2 to 20 years using percentile curves, allowing healthcare providers to track an individual's height and weight over time.[3] Providers can calculate growth velocity and interview families on events and external factors that may have impacted the patient's growth at specific times.

When BMI is calculated, it is plotted on one of the sex-specific CDC BMI-for-age growth charts. Age- and sex-specific percentiles are used in children and adolescents because body fat percentage changes with age and differs between sexes. Weight classifications are as follows: 5th to 85th percentile is considered normal weight, 85th to 95th percentile is considered overweight, and greater than 95th percentile is considered obese.[4] Pediatric obesity is further divided into three classes, with 100–120% of the 95th percentile defined as class 1 obesity, 120–140% of the 95th percentile as class 2 obesity, and more than 140% of the 95th percentile as class 3 obesity.[5] Class 2 and class 3 pediatric obesity is also called "severe pediatric obesity."[5] Children's height and weight should be measured at least annually to assess any upward or downward trends in growth. The CDC has developed the Extended BMI-for-age Growth Charts for providers to monitor high BMI values.[6] When Extended BMI-for-age Growth Charts are not available, z-scores are useful in assessing the patient's growth trend as they are the deviation of the value for an individual from the mean value of the reference population divided by the standard deviation for the reference population.[7]

While BMI-for-age is a useful tool to screen for and diagnose overweight and obesity, it is not the best indicator of total excess body adiposity.[8] BMI-for-age also cannot accurately assess adiposity in different racial and ethnic groups. For children and adolescents with high fat-free mass, BMI-for-age may incorrectly classify them as overweight or obese.

Waist circumference (WC), skinfold thickness, hip circumference, waist/hip ratio, and waist/height ratio are alternative measurements used to assess body fat.[9] Measurements of skinfold thickness have proven to be more accurate predictors of adiposity in children than BMI. However, measuring height and weight in children is a much simpler process than measuring skinfold thickness, which often can be inaccurate due to human error. Thus, BMI continues to be the preferred measurement when identifying children with overweight or obesity.

Measuring WC is an inexpensive method that has been highly effective in measuring body fat and predicting the development of obesity-related chronic disease in adults. WC measurements are used less often in the pediatric population, although it is an important assessment method that may predict future adverse health complications. Emerging evidence suggests that central obesity is increasing at an even faster rate than BMI.[10] An upward trend in WC is seen even when BMI is stabilized, which is alarming as substantial evidence suggests that measurements of central adiposity may be a better predictor of adverse health outcomes than overall adiposity. The CDC provides guidelines for clinicians to use when measuring WC (refer to **Table 22.1**).

To implement appropriate interventions, it is necessary to assess and classify the weight status of an individual. Establishing a consistent and effective way to do this in the pediatric population is highly important. Currently, use of BMI age- and sex-specific growth charts is the method most often used in the United States. Measurement of WC should be considered due to its effectiveness in predicting the likelihood of health complications in the future. Pediatric obesity is associated with many of the risk factors for cardiovascular disease (CVD), including hypertension, dyslipidemia, and poor glycemic control that could eventually lead to type 2 **diabetes** mellitus (T2DM). As the rates of pediatric obesity continue to be high, so too are the medical comorbidities that accompany this disease.[11]

CORE CONCEPT 2

Pediatric obesity is associated with many of the risk factors for cardiovascular disease, including hypertension, dyslipidemia, and poor glycemic control that could eventually lead to type 2 diabetes.

PRACTICE POINT

Use BMI as the general screening tool when identifying pediatric obesity. Further measurements that may be beneficial to include in the assessment are measuring waist circumference, skinfold thickness, hip circumference, waist/height ratio, and waist/hip ratio.

Table 22.1 CDC Waist Circumference Measurements for Assessing Childhood Obesity

Male				
	Percentile Centimeters			
Age	**5th**	**85th**	**90th**	**95th**
12	58.6	87.6	89.9	98.6
13	62.0	93.9	100.7	na
14	64.3	95.8	102.0	111.4
15	64.3	94.4	103.4	114.9
16	68.8	101.7	104.7	117.1
17	69.5	95.8	105.8	120.9
18	69.5	101.2	105.5	119.0
19	69.9	102.2	na	na
Female				
	Percentile Centimeters			
Age	**5th**	**85th**	**90th**	**95th**
12	59.2	92.0	98.7	108.0
13	61.9	87.9	97.6	100.1
14	66.0	93.9	97.2	101.3
15	67.1	98.5	104.4	108.4
16	65.7	101.8	108.8	na
17	67.5	101.3	102.2	114.5
18	67.0	97.6	112.2	na
19	67.4	101	117.2	123.2

Data from National Health and Nutrition Examination Survey, United States, 2011–2014. https://www.cdc.gov/nchs/data/series/sr_03/sr03_039.pdf

Pediatric Obesity Comorbidities

Given the current prevalence of pediatric obesity, there is concern that children with overweight and obesity will become adults at high risk for CVD. It has been predicted that the number of additional cardiovascular events related to obesity in adolescence will be more than 100,000 by 2035. As unsettling as these predictions are, perhaps most unsettling are the reports of cardiovascular abnormalities in children with obesity, suggesting cardiovascular dysfunction may not only be a concern in the future for these children, but a concern to be dealt with at present.[11]

Left Ventricular Hypertrophy, Hypertension, and Epicardial Fat

Obesity is associated with increased metabolic demand due to greater adipose tissue and lean mass, increased blood volume, and increased preload to the heart. **Left ventricular hypertrophy (LVH)** is a disease in which the muscle of the left ventricle becomes thickened and enlarged (**Figure 22.2**). LVH is caused by the increase in workload that the heart experiences as a response to hypertension. It has been well documented as a risk factor for the development of CVD morbidity and mortality in adults, and it has been shown that, on average, children and adolescents with obesity have greater left ventricular mass than their counterparts of the same sex and age without obesity. This increase in LVH is of particular concern for children and adolescents with hypertension, because this combination of CVD risk factors has demonstrated an increased risk of cardiovascular events.[11,12]

The clustering of risk factors that have been identified in pediatric metabolic syndrome may also be

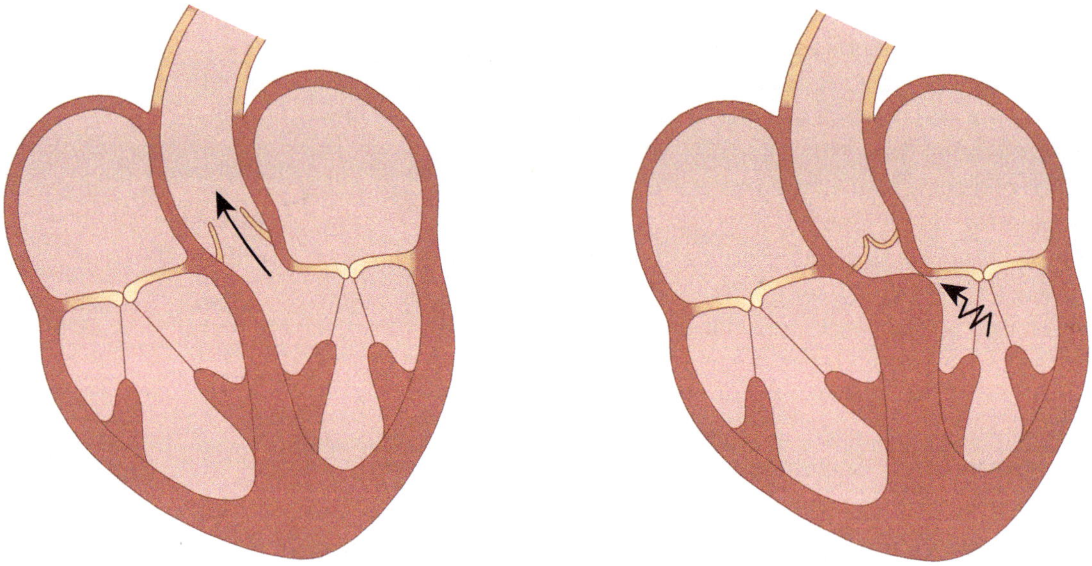

Figure 22.2 Left Ventricular Hypertrophy. Hypertrophy of the Left Ventricle Leads to Obstructed Blood Flow

CASE STUDY REVISITED

Nora reports feeling "exhausted" no matter what time she falls asleep. Nora's mother says she snores loudly, and the doctor notices Nora is having increased work of breathing sitting in the PCP's office.

Biochemical Data:

Triglycerides 220 (Desirable: <150 mg/dL)
Total Cholesterol 275 (Desirable: <200 mg/dL)
LDL-Cholesterol 145 (Desirable: <100 mg/dL)
HDL-Cholesterol 22 (Desirable: ≥40 mg/dL)

Clinical Data:

Vital Signs: Blood pressure 140/90 mm Hg

Questions

1. What comorbidities are associated with obesity that Nora might be experiencing?
2. Based on Nora's biochemical and clinical data, for which conditions is she at risk?

significant for the acceleration of atherosclerosis in adolescents. Observations from autopsy studies by the Bogalusa Heart Study,[13] a long-term epidemiologic study of cardiovascular risk factors from birth through age 38 years, have demonstrated a strong relationship between coronary atherosclerosis and cardiovascular risk factors in young people. Elevated BMI was reported to have been significantly related to the extent of atherosclerotic lesions in adolescents, along with other identified risk factors including increased systolic blood pressure, high serum low-density lipoprotein (LDL) cholesterol, increased serum triglyceride concentration, and smoking. Although the development of atherosclerosis is not often documented as clinically significant before adulthood is reached, the development of fatty streaks and thickening of the arterial media begin in the obese pediatric population.[14]

In addition to the clustering of risk factors for CVD mentioned above, children with obesity have been observed to have greater epicardial fat deposition as compared to their peers with a BMI within the normal range. **Epicardial fat** is a fat deposit that surrounds the heart and is enclosed by the visceral pericardium. Epicardial fat has multiple important functions, such as acting as an endocrine and paracrine gland and providing an energy reservoir for cardiomyocytes. Although epicardial fat is necessary for numerous metabolic and bodily functions, increased epicardial fat deposition has been associated with insulin resistance, coronary artery disease, carotid intima-media thickness, and arterial stiffness.[15]

Children who are overweight or obese are at an increased risk for multiple risk factors associated with cardiac dysfunction, increasing the likelihood of CVD progression with age. Establishing standardized values to evaluate measures of cardiovascular risk in the pediatric population will be an important consideration because this population would benefit from early intervention to slow or stop the progression of CVD into adulthood.

CORE CONCEPT 3

Children who are overweight and obese are at an increased risk for multiple risk factors associated with cardiac dysfunction, increasing the likelihood of cardiovascular disease progression with age.

Metabolic Syndrome

Metabolic syndrome in adults is identified when an individual has three or more of the following metabolic risk factors: increased WC, high systolic or diastolic blood pressure, elevated fasting glucose and triglyceride levels, and low high-density lipoprotein (HDL) cholesterol (**Figure 22.3**). Threshold values determining high and low risk levels for these components were established in the National Cholesterol Education Program's Adult Treatment Panel III guidelines. Meeting the criteria for metabolic syndrome indicates increased risk for CVD, T2DM, liver steatosis, gallstones, asthma, and sleep disturbances.[16]

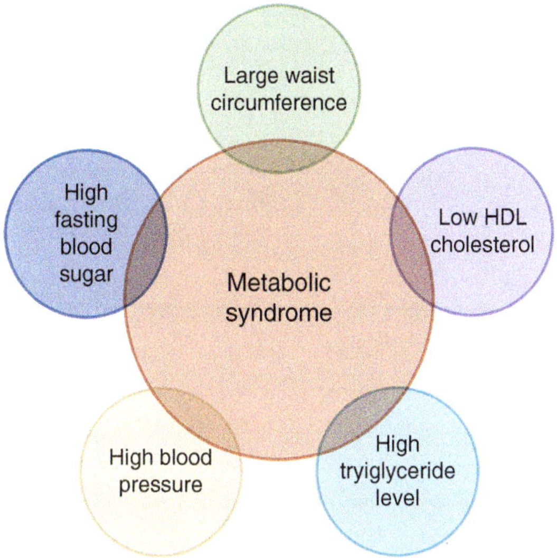

Figure 22.3 Factors Contributing to Metabolic Syndrome

In the past decade, there has been a greater focus on defining metabolic syndrome as it relates to the pediatric population. Pediatric metabolic syndrome has been defined in over 27 different pediatric studies, and over 40 varying definitions have been established.[17] There is currently no clear definition of metabolic syndrome in the pediatric population, but a similar clustering of risk factors has been shown in children as compared to adults. Additionally, studies of populations have found the prevalence of metabolic syndrome in children and adolescents with obesity may be as high as 30%, and note increases in BMI to correlate with increased risk for metabolic syndrome in children.[11] Studies have also shown that measuring WC is a better predictor than BMI when identifying the presence of metabolic syndrome and cardiovascular disease in children.[18] A large WC is reflective of the total body fatness and the excess visceral abdominal fat, which increases the risks of developing CVD and T2DM.[19]

Insulin Resistance and Type 2 Diabetes

Insulin resistance occurs when peripheral tissues are insensitive to insulin action, resulting in increased insulin production by the pancreatic beta cells. When the beta cells are no longer able to compensate for the lack of insulin sensitivity in the tissues, high levels of glucose remain in the blood and hyperglycemia results. This increased demand on the pancreatic beta cells to hypersecrete insulin influences the progressive beta cell failure that is characteristic of T2DM.[20]

T2DM was rarely diagnosed in children before the 1990s, which is why it was often referred to as "adult-onset" diabetes, whereas type 1 diabetes (T1DM) was referred to as "juvenile-onset" diabetes.[20] "Adult-onset" is no longer an accurate depiction of T2DM, because it now accounts for 45% of new-onset diabetes in adolescents, with the highest rates observed among underrepresented population aged 15 to 19 years.[21]

Inflammation in the setting of obesity has been associated with insulin resistance. Increased **intramyocellular lipid deposition** has been linked to decreased uptake of glucose; adolescents with impaired glucose tolerance (IGT) often present with increased intramyocellular lipid content and increased visceral fat deposition. Impaired glucose tolerance may then lead to prediabetes and eventually T2DM in adolescence, making early intervention essential in this population.[21]

Prediabetes in adults is characterized by impaired glucose tolerance and/or impaired fasting glucose. Increased prevalence of prediabetes among adolescents and children characterized by IGT has been documented.[19] IGT has been reported in children and adolescents with obesity, indicating prevalence of prediabetes in this population.[18]

If insulin resistance and IGT are detected early, it is possible to stop the progression of and even reverse T2DM. Screening is not universally performed, however, and there are relatively few reports on the epidemiology and history of complications in adolescents with T2DM. As the rates of obesity and T2DM in this population increase, screening may become an important tool to prevent progression of this disease.[20] The gold standard method to measure insulin resistance in this population is a hyperinsulinemic-euglycemic clamp, which requires an overnight fast followed by constant infusion of insulin and glucose with periodic sampling of insulin and glucose concentrations. Use of this test is rare because it is not well suited for the outpatient setting.

T2DM in children and adolescents is associated with early onset of micro- and macrovascular complications and increased risk of mortality with aging, making prevention of this disease extremely important.[22] Prevention should be directed toward preventing or delaying the onset of T2DM and targeting glucose control. This can be achieved through lifestyle and dietary changes. Weight management programs incorporating nutrition, exercise, and behavior modification have been found to improve insulin resistance.[20]

When behavior change is difficult to achieve, adolescents with T2DM may require pharmacologic therapy early on. Metformin with insulin is the first choice in combination therapy; metformin is approved by the U.S. Food and Drug Administration (FDA) to treat T2DM in children 10 years or older. It decreases hepatic glucose production while improving insulin resistance. Combination treatments of metformin, insulin therapy, and lifestyle intervention have proven to be most effective in the treatment of T2DM in the pediatric population.[20]

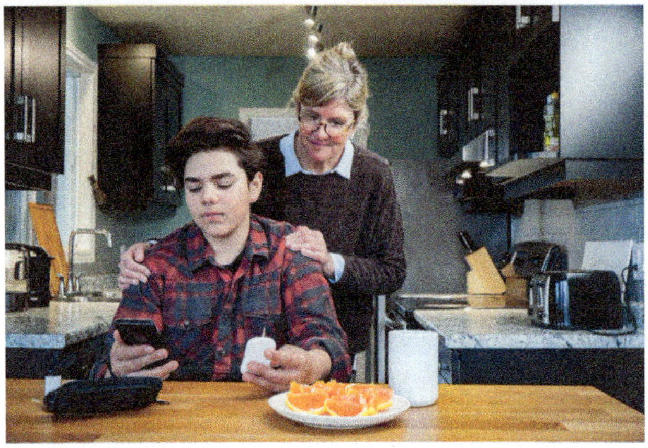

CORE CONCEPT 4

Type 2 diabetes in children and adolescents is associated with early onset of micro- and macrovascular complications and increased risk of mortality with aging, making prevention of this disease extremely important.

PRACTICE POINT

Type 2 diabetes prevention for children should be directed toward preventing or delaying the onset of diabetes and targeting glucose control. This can be achieved through dietary changes and weight management programs that incorporate nutrition, exercise, and behavioral modifications.

Asthma

As the rate of pediatric obesity has risen over the years, so too have the rates of asthma, making overweight/obesity and asthma two of the most significant health problems worldwide. Asthma affects about 9.1% of children in the United States. Prevalence has been attributed to air pollution, tobacco smoke, and dietary or lifestyle choices, and now a link between obesity and asthma is being suggested.[23]

Excess body fat affects the free movement of air and compresses the lungs. In addition, lack of deep breathing resulting from restricted lung movements and obesity can cause reduction of bronchial smooth muscle expansion and consequential airway narrowing. It has been hypothesized that obesity can cause asthma because these are both inflammatory diseases; adipose tissue produces proinflammatory cytokines that could possibly lead to airway inflammation, although this relationship has yet to be confirmed.[24] What is known, however, is that obesity can lead to increased asthma symptoms. The literature also suggests that children and adolescents who are overweight or obese may experience a unique type of asthma that is resistant to steroid treatments, requires higher medication use, and results in more hospitalizations as compared to the asthma in children within the healthy BMI range.[23] Weight loss has demonstrated improvement in pulmonary function, and research suggests possible benefits of an anti-inflammatory diet connected to relief of asthma symptoms.[24,25]

Sleep Apnea

Sleep apnea has been documented in 4% of children who are obese and 17% of children who are overweight.[26] As defined by the American Thoracic Society, **obstructive sleep apnea** is "a disorder of breathing during sleep characterized by prolonged partial upper airway obstruction and/or intermittent complete obstruction that disrupts normal ventilation during sleep and normal sleep patterns."[27] Evidence supports adult obesity as a risk factor for sleep apnea; a link between pediatric obesity and sleep apnea has also been established. Fatty infiltration of upper airway structures, subcutaneous fat deposits in the anterior neck region promoting pharyngeal collapse, and increased respiratory load secondary to increased adipose tissue in the abdominal wall and cavity may result in decreased lung volumes and increased work of breathing during sleep.[28] Obstructive sleep apnea is associated with cardiovascular complications and can lead to systemic hypertension, increased ventricular mass, and diastolic dysfunction, further adding to the health complications already associated with pediatric obesity. A common treatment of sleep apnea is continuous positive airway pressure (CPAP), which helps keep the airway open during sleep (**Figure 22.4**).

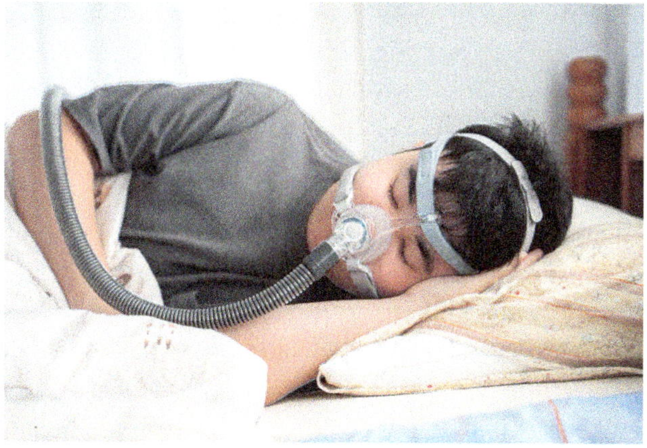

Figure 22.4 Continuous Positive Airway Pressure (CPAP) Is a Machine That Is Often Used to Treat Sleep Apnea

Improvement in obstructive sleep apnea has been demonstrated with weight loss, making lifestyle intervention an important part of prevention and treatment of this disorder. Weight loss may be particularly challenging for this population because increased daytime sleepiness and changes in appetite and eating patterns are often a result of obstructive sleep apnea and can promote weight gain and severity of obesity.[11]

Other Comorbidities: Orthopedic, Dental, and Steatotic Liver Disease

The medical comorbidities associated with pediatric obesity are vast. In addition to those mentioned, children and adolescents with obesity are at risk for orthopedic problems because of excess weight and stress on the musculoskeletal system, dental caries, and **metabolic dysfunction–associated steatotic liver disease (MASLD)**.[20,29]

MASLD, formerly known as "nonalcoholic fatty liver disease (NAFLD)," is one of the most common causes of chronic liver diseases in children and adolescents in the United States.[30,31] MASLD is a condition where macrovesicular fat accumulates in hepatocytes, resulting in the enlargement of the liver. Along with liver fat accumulation, MASLD causes the liver cells to become damaged and inflamed.[32] The development of MASLD in children can lead to cirrhosis, a disease that can eventually lead to liver failure. MASLD is caused by an array of conditions, such as metabolic syndrome, obesity, high levels of total cholesterol and LDL cholesterol, and insulin resistance.[23] MASLD is more prevalent in boys than girls due to the absence of estrogen, which has been found to reduce lipid peroxidation in lipoproteins.[32] Specific ethnicities, ages, and genetic factors can also have an impact on the development of MASLD in children. The only treatment recommended for children with MASLD is a healthy lifestyle and weight loss, as weight loss can reduce fibrosis and fat deposition in the liver. There are currently no recommended medications for treating pediatric MASLD alone without lifestyle changes, and thus improving diet and increasing exercise levels is the main treatment for this condition. Medications that are approved for weight loss in pediatric patients may lead to an improvement in MASLD as the patient loses weight, but currently there is no established relationship between weight loss medications and MASLD outcomes.

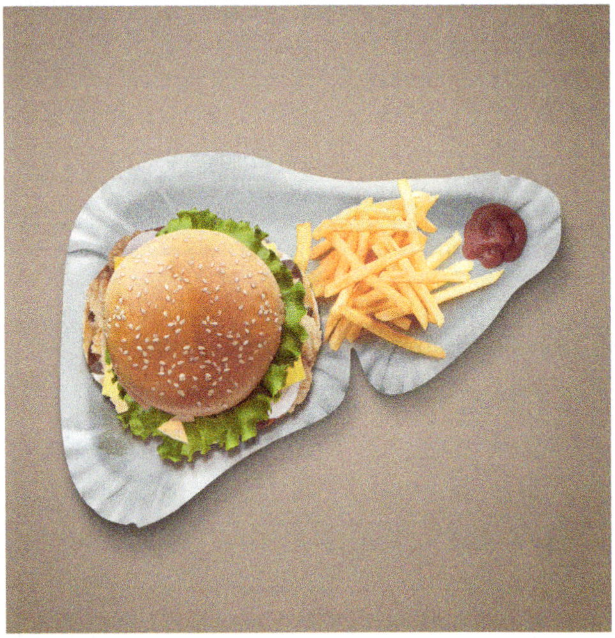

© PW creative design/Shutterstock

Psychological Effects of Pediatric Obesity

Along with the medical comorbidities that accompany pediatric obesity, there are also many psychological comorbidities to consider. Children who are overweight or obese often face stigma and prejudice from their peers that can lead to serious psychological damage.[33]

Depressive Disorder, Weight Stigma, and Eating Disorders

Children and adolescents with obesity who seek medical treatment for obesity have demonstrated elevated rates of depressive disorder. Rates of children who meet depressive disorder criteria in those seeking obesity treatments through bariatric surgery have been reported as high as 45%.[34] These rates greatly exceed that of the general pediatric population. According to the 2015 Scientific Statement from the American Heart Association, longitudinal studies have shown that pediatric obesity increased the risk for major depressive disorder and vice versa.[35]

Psychological complications may result from teasing and weight stigma. Children who are overweight or obese often face negative stereotypes from their peers, educators, and parents.[36] Weight stigma has been associated with adverse effects on self-esteem and body image. In addition, weight stigma may contribute to weight gain because it can lead to a decreased desire to participate in physical activity, lower academic achievement, and perpetuation of adverse eating habits such as skipping meals and binge eating.[34] Healthcare professionals should use weight-neutral terms such as "fast weight gain" or "healthy weight" rather than "obese" or "ideal body weight" when addressing weight history with pediatric patients.

Eating disorders such as binge eating disorders or restrictive eating disorders are prevalent in the pediatric population with obesity. More than one-quarter of pediatric patients who are overweight or obese are estimated to experience binge and loss of control eating.[37] Adolescent girls with obesity are especially vulnerable to binge eating episodes because this population is more likely to experience weight stigma and have overconcern about weight and body shape.[38] Without appropriate medical and nutritional guidance and support, pediatric patients who attempt to lose weight are at risk for developing a disordered eating pattern or disordered beliefs around food that can increase risks of developing eating disorders later in adulthood. It is also important to note that pediatric patients with obesity along with a disordered eating pattern can develop malnutrition and nutritional deficiencies.

Peer Relationships

Bullying by peers of youth who are overweight or obese has been associated with self-reported depressive disorders, anxiety disorders, social anxiety disorders, loneliness, and preference for isolative

CASE STUDY REVISITED

Through communicating with Nora and her mother, you notice a strained relationship between the two. Nora seems depressed and has mentioned a couple of times the bullying she experiences in school. She wants to start losing weight, and she wants to do it fast!

Questions

1. What are the risks associated with attempting to lose weight quickly without clinical guidance, especially in adolescent girls?
2. How would you approach behavioral interventions with Nora to help her achieve her goal? Outline the components of the lifestyle education that should be provided to Nora.

activities.[18] Peer relationships during adolescence have proven to be essential; healthy social and cognitive development depends on interactions with peers. Literature has shown that adolescents with obesity may have poor social functioning and have a more difficult time making friends with peers.[39]

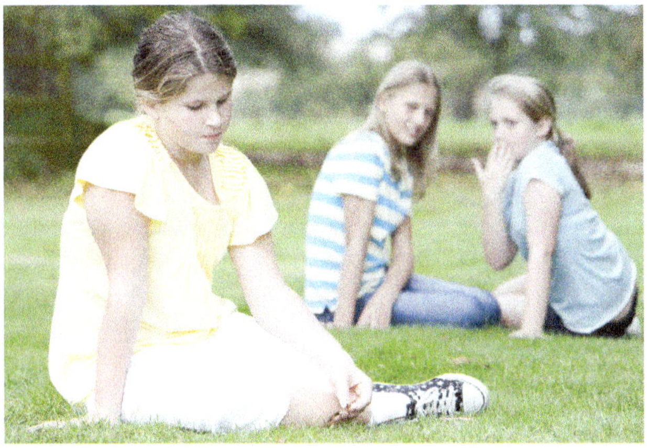

Family Relationships

Parents are important role models for children, and their participation in pediatric obesity intervention and prevention is essential for success. A support system provided by parents and siblings is key as a child adopts a healthier lifestyle. It can be difficult for parents to realize that if their child is overweight or obese, there is an increased risk of comorbidities. Often, parents of children who are overweight or obese may deny that their child's weight is a problem; it is the role of the health professional to help the parents understand the connection between the child's dietary pattern and risks of metabolic diseases.

Cognitive Impairment

Early onset of obesity is associated with cognitive impairments. Children with early-onset severe obesity displayed lower levels of cognitive functioning than their siblings without obesity. Research suggests that obesity and/or a high-fat diet lead to local inflammation within the hypothalamus that alters synaptic plasticity, contributes to neurodegeneration, and even initiates brain atrophy.[39] Youth with obesity have also been found to have significantly more negative behaviors and poor adaptive functioning.[11] Interventions to treat obesity and central inflammation have proven effective in improving some aspects of cognitive function.[36]

CORE CONCEPT 5

Children and adolescents with obesity who seek medical treatment for obesity have demonstrated elevated rates of depressive disorders, anxiety disorders, social anxiety disorders, loneliness, and preference for isolative activities.

PRACTICE POINT

To gain a better understanding of the psychological factors impacting the patient, it is recommended to assess how the peer and parental relationships present in the patient's life affect the patient's dietary pattern.

Health-Related Quality of Life

The Pediatric Quality of Life Inventory is a tool designed to measure health-related quality of life for children and adolescents; using this tool to assess measures of fatigue in pediatric patients revealed that those with obesity experience fatigue comparable with pediatric patients receiving cancer treatments.[40] Patients who are overweight or obese often experience difficulty with completing daily tasks or engaging in physical activity. When impairment of everyday functioning occurs, the child's quality of life may suffer greatly; the likelihood of quality of life impairment in individuals with obesity was found to be 5.5 times greater than that of a child who is at a healthy weight.[34] When tasks of daily living become difficult for the child, it is often at that time that parents and adolescents seek weight management therapy.[34]

Factors Associated with Pediatric Obesity

The etiology of pediatric obesity is multifactorial; genetic factors, behavioral factors, social factors, and environmental factors all play a role in a child's health status. Understanding the main reasons that a child is overweight or obese is extremely important for planning effective treatment and management.

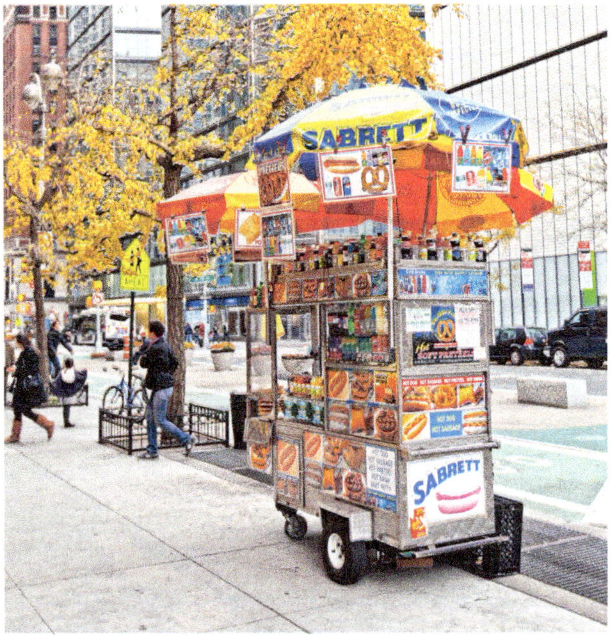

© Stuart Monk/Shutterstock

Low Socioeconomic Status

There is an association between low family income and a higher percentage of youth who are overweight or obese. Children living in communities with lower mean annual income are more likely to have decreased physical activity, increased time engaging with television, and a steady consumption of school lunches that are frequently energy dense.[41] Low-income communities often have lower access to supermarkets with fresh and affordable produce and lower access to recreational parks and youth exercise programs. Low-income communities also have significantly more fast-food chain restaurants, street food vendors, and convenience stores than higher-income neighborhoods,[41] leading to greater consumption of lower cost, higher-calorie foods.[42]

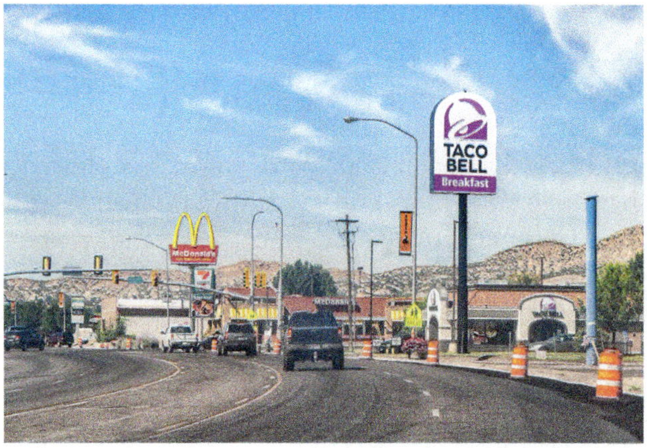

© krblokhin/iStock Editorial/Getty Images Plus/Getty Images

According to the Healthy People 2030 Initiative, the definition of **food insecurity** is "household-level economic and social condition of limited or uncertain access to adequate food."[40] Living with food insecurity can cause stress in children and adolescents to engage in healthy lifestyle behaviors and impact the parental ability to provide proper nutrition. The COVID-19 pandemic exacerbated food insecurity in many countries as financial constraints worsened. In 2020, 10.5% of U.S. households struggled with food insecurity.[43] Obesity is one of the many negative outcomes of food insecurity in children. Federal nutrition programs such as the Supplemental Nutrition Assistance Program (SNAP) have been shown to be not effective in supporting healthy living patterns in low-income populations.[44] Parents using SNAP benefits may purchase the most financially efficient products to provide food to children. Children on SNAP are less likely to eat three meals a day, as skipping meals is a hallmark of food insecurity. When families cycle between food insecurity and relative stability, they may binge when food is abundant.[45] Accessibility of food impacts food consumption behavior in children and adolescents and may lead to a disordered eating pattern that can contribute to weight gain. There have been many initiatives implemented to address the concern of diet quality among participants receiving nutrition assistance, such as providing incentives for healthy foods (Health Bucks NYC) and limiting allowance to purchase sugar-sweetened beverages with SNAP benefits. However, food insecurity continues to be a significant barrier for treating pediatric obesity. Providers caring for patients with pediatric obesity should screen, assess for, and consider food insecurity among patients when recommending lifestyle changes to families.

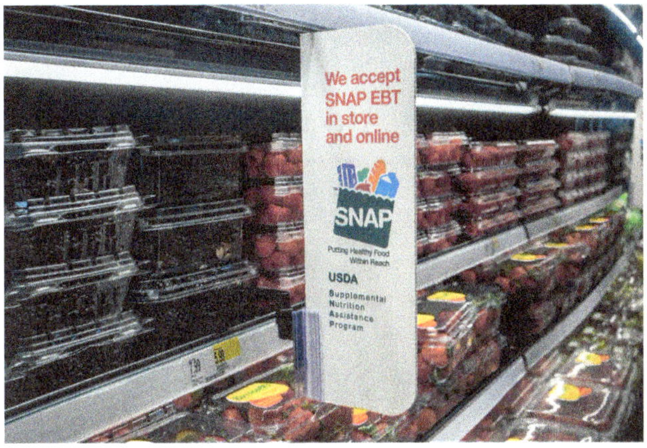
We accept
SNAP EBT
in store
and online
SNAP
USDA
Supplemental
Nutrition
Assistance
Program

© rblfmr/Shutterstock

Family Patterns

The family environment is an important factor in a child's development and lifestyle habits. Children often mirror their parents' lifestyle choices, and they are affected by exposure to certain foods, portion sizes provided, and family routines. Children who grow up in sedentary households are less likely to engage in physical activity. Part of the caregiver's role is to provide young children with nutrient-dense foods and encourage physical activity. As children grow, develop, and mature, they will be able to make their own decisions regarding diet and exercise habits, although they are still likely to mirror their parents' actions. Thus, it is the responsibility of the parents to act as role models.[20]

Parenting style can influence a child's eating patterns.[20] Authoritative feeding style, which is characterized by parental sensitivity and high expectations for child self-control, has shown to be effective in promoting healthy eating behaviors and increased consumption of fruits and vegetables.[46] Evidence indicates that encouragement to try fruits and vegetables is effective, whereas pressure to do so is often ineffective. In similar fashion, restriction of some unhealthy food items to promote a healthy food environment is often beneficial, while extreme restriction has proven to facilitate unhealthy eating behaviors and disordered relationships with food.[46]

Genetic Factors and Nutrigenomics

Genetic factors can play a strong role in the development of pediatric obesity. Parental obesity has a large impact on the trajectory of a child's BMI and future health status. When both parents are overweight, their children have an 80% chance of becoming obese, whereas obesity prevalence reduces by 14% when both parents have a BMI in the normal range.[47]

The interaction between genes and the environment is a rapidly progressing field of research. It is estimated that genetic factors account for greater than 40% of population variation in BMI.[48] With the discovery of leptin, a hormone that decreases appetite derived from the adipose tissue, the identification of the proposed number of obesity-susceptible genes is growing. Mutations in the genes that code for leptin and leptin receptors have been linked to human obesity.[49] In children, increased sleep duration resulted in lower fasting leptin levels, decreased appetite, and decreased weight. Conversely, ghrelin levels were not affected.[50] Both leptin and ghrelin, the hunger hormone, are hereditary and also increase the probability of pediatric obesity.[51] The regulation of leptin and ghrelin is outlined in **Figure 22.5**.

Nutrigenomics, the study of how genes and nutrients interact, is another factor that can contribute to pediatric obesity. Numerous studies have demonstrated that consumption of specific macronutrients and micronutrients control gene expression in various ways. The research of nutrigenomics focuses on the association between single-nucleotide polymorphisms (SNPs), a specific genetic code that varies among people, and how they are altered by the consumption of specific nutrients.[52] These SNPs act as biological markers in research to help determine which genes are associated with specific diseases. For example, studies have shown that certain SNPs (rs9939609) in the FTO (fat mass and obesity-related) gene region are associated with T2DM and increased BMI.[53] This correlation is observed in children from the age of 7 and in adults up to the age of 74. Furthermore, the association between these SNPs and T2DM is mediated through BMI. Children who inherit the FTO gene with the SNPs are more likely to struggle with obesity and T2DM.

CORE CONCEPT 6

The etiology of pediatric obesity is multifactorial; individual factors, social factors, and environmental factors all play a role in a child's growth.

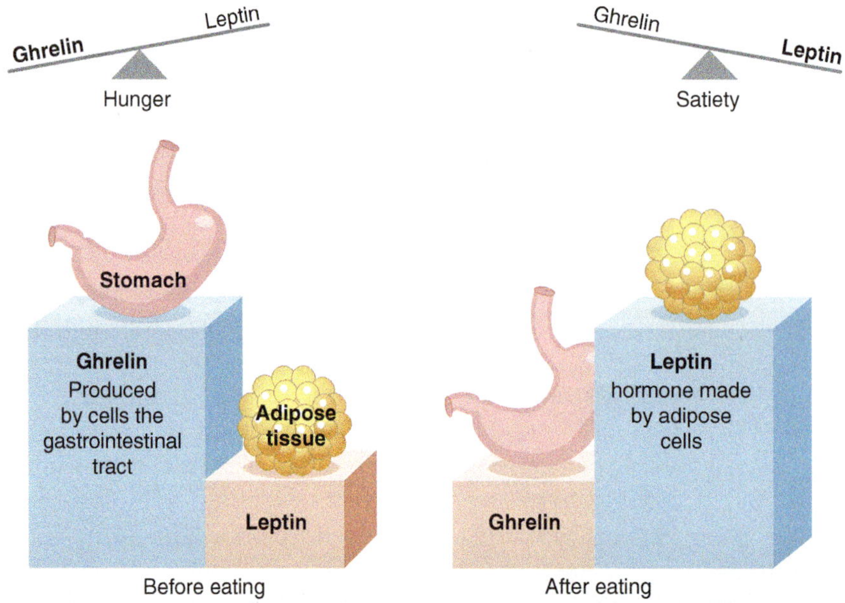

Figure 22.5 Hormone Regulators of Appetite. Before eating, ghrelin is produced to stimulate hunger. The increase in ghrelin increases appetite and food intake. After eating, leptin levels are increased to promote satiety.

PRACTICE POINT

When children are frustrated with the hardships that come with losing weight, it is important to teach them about the genetic and social factors that can contribute to weight gain. This conversation can help pediatric patients recognize the areas where they have the ability to improve their health (i.e., physical activity, dietary changes) as opposed to certain genetic and social factors that are beyond their control.

Nutrition Assessment in Pediatric Obesity

The American Medical Association Expert Committee has established guidelines for assessing pediatric obesity. At every primary care visit, the pediatric patient's height and weight should be measured, and their BMI should be plotted on the CDC BMI sex- and age-specific charts (**Figure 22.6**). The child's medical risk (i.e., child history and exam, parental obesity, and family history), behavior risk (i.e., sedentary time, dietary habits, and physical activity), and attitudes (i.e., family and patient motivation) should be assessed. For those children with a BMI in the 85th to 94th percentiles, classified as overweight, laboratory values should be assessed as needed. For the patient charting greater than or equal to the 95th percentile, classified as obese, laboratory values should be collected and assessed.[54] Refer to Figure 22.6 for the Extended BMI-for-age percentile growth charts for girls and boys 2–20 years of age.

PRACTICE POINT

For children with a BMI classified as overweight or obese, collect and monitor laboratory values to assess early signs of hypertension, diabetes, cardiovascular disease, and liver disease.

Nutrition Intervention

Primary and Secondary Prevention: Approaches to Weight Loss

As seen in adult populations, primary strategies for weight maintenance or weight loss for children focus on energy balance; energy intake should be equal to energy expended. In their position paper on interventions for prevention and treatment of pediatric obesity, the Academy for Nutrition and Dietetics identified key areas for primary prevention, which include integrating education with supportive environment change in school and childcare settings, including physical activity and caregiver engagement.[55] As for secondary prevention, for children who are overweight and obese, a staged approach based on BMI percentiles is recommended.

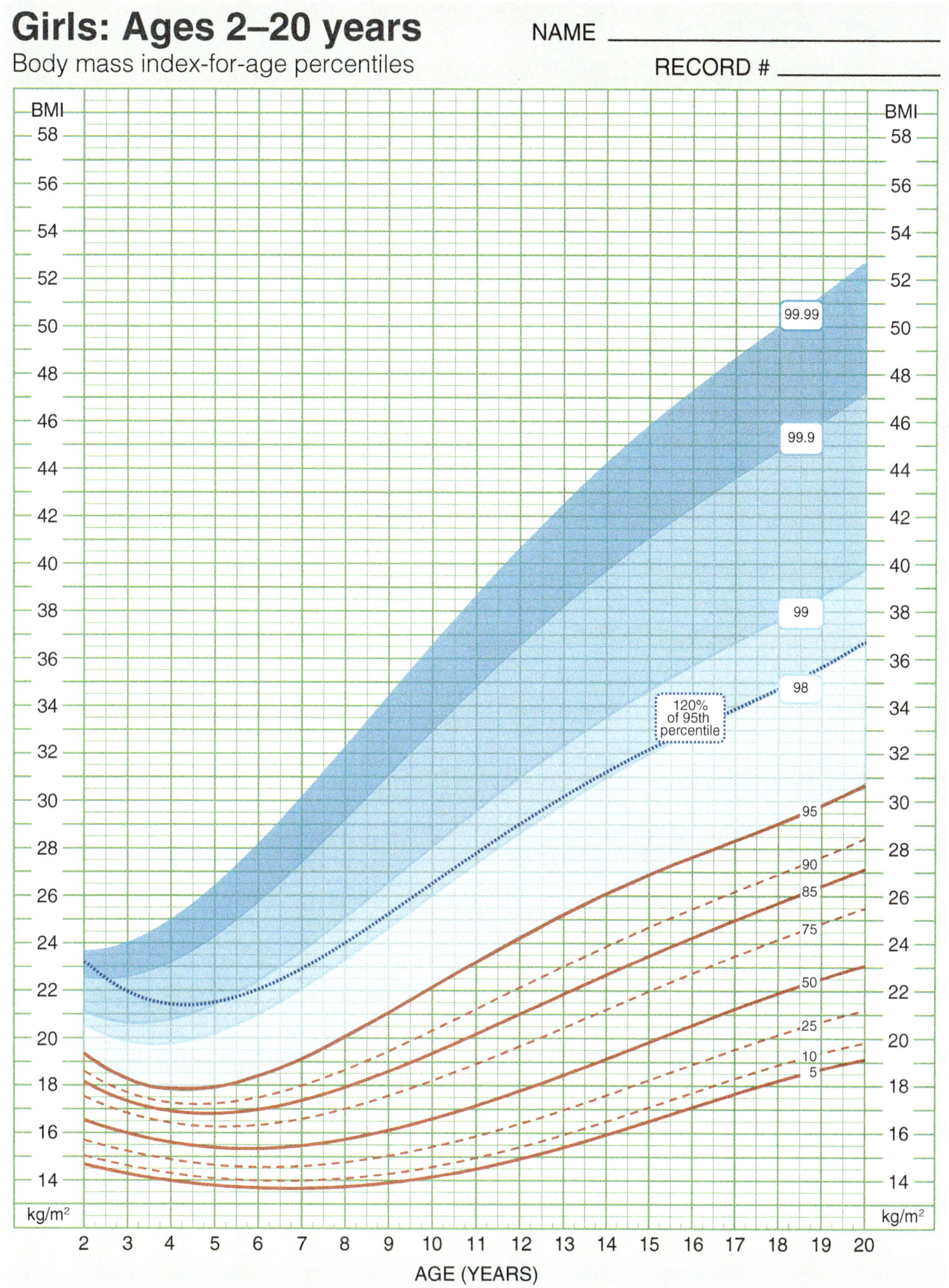

A

Figure 22.6 Body Mass Index-for-Age Percentiles: (**A**) Girls and (**B**) Boys Ages 2 to 20 Years[5]

A: Reproduced from National Center for Health Statistics in Collaboration with National Center for Chronic Disease and Health Promotion, 2000. www.cdc.gov/growthCharts. https://www.cdc.gov/growthcharts/data/extended-bmi/BMI-Age-percentiles-BOYS.pdf

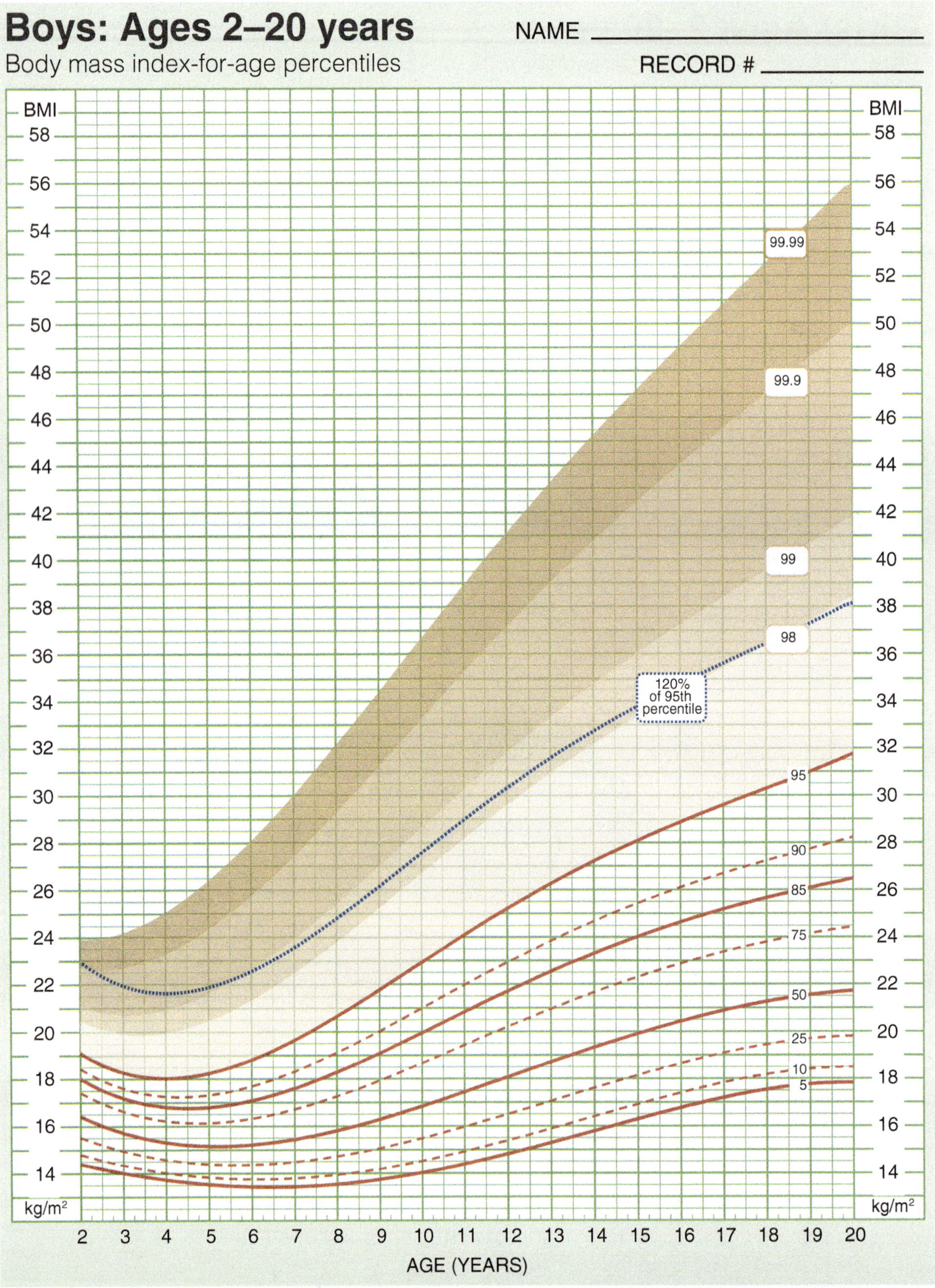

B

Figure 22.6 *(continued)*

B: Reproduced from National Center for Health Statistics in Collaboration with National Center for Chronic Disease and Health Promotion, 2000. www.cdc.gov/growthCharts.https://www.cdc.gov/growthcharts/data/extended-bmi/BMI-Age-percentiles-GIRLS.pdf

Table 22.2 Institute of Medicine Daily Energy Recommendations (in Calories)

Gender	Age (Years)	Sedentary	Moderately Active	Active
Male	2–3	1000–1200	1000–1400	1000–1400
Male	4–8	1200–1400	1400–1600	1600–2000
Male	9–13	1600–2000	1800–2200	2000–2600
Male	14–18	2000–2400	2400–2800	2800–3200
Female	2–3	1000	1000–1200	1000–1400
Female	4–8	1200–1400	1400–1600	1400–1800
Female	9–13	1400–1600	1600–2000	1800–2200
Female	14–18	1800	2000	2400

Data from Institute of Medicine. 2005. *Dietary Reference Intakes for Energy, Carbohydrate, Fiber, Fat, Fatty Acids, Cholesterol, Protein, and Amino Acids*. Washington, DC: The National Academies Press. https://doi.org/10.17226/10490. https://nap.nationalacademies.org/read/10490/chapter/7#176

Each stage increases in intensity based on obesity risk. Stages 1 to 3 focus primarily on behavioral changes, while Stage 4 is a tertiary-based intervention that can include a combination of dietary, behavioral, pharmacological, and surgical interventions.[55]

For children considered overweight or obese, intervention goals can include slowing the rate of weight gain, stopping weight gain, or losing weight. For safe and sustainable weight loss, it is recommended to introduce children to healthy eating and behavioral patterns instead of placing them on a calorie-restricted diet, which may set them up for failure and future weight gain.[56] While restrictive dieting is not recommended for children, success in weight loss has been seen in children who were introduced to the concepts of calories and portion control. The Institute of Medicine (IOM) provides calorie guidelines for children and parents that are based on age, sex, and the child's level of physical activity (**Table 22.2**).[57] Other governmental organizations also offer various suggestions and tools regarding weight loss and living a healthy lifestyle for children.

Children and adolescents experience periods of rapid growth, and as height continues to increase, interventions related to portion control and healthy eating should result in a decrease in BMI. For many children who are overweight, it is recommended that the child maintain their weight and allow for growth in height to normalize their BMI. Children experience an adiposity rebound period, which is an increase in BMI at approximately 5–7 years of age after an initial decrease in BMI after age 1 year. An earlier adiposity rebound often predicts persistence and adulthood obesity. Similarly, the pre- and early pubertal periods of adolescence cause dramatic changes in body composition and metabolism. It is during these periods that weight surveillance and intervention may be most beneficial.[54]

CORE CONCEPT 7

For safe and sustainable weight loss, it is recommended to introduce children to healthy eating and behavioral patterns instead of placing them on a calorie-restricted diet, which may set them up for failure and future weight gain.

PRACTICE POINT

The NIH daily caloric recommendations chart is a great reference for registered dietitians (RDs) to use when estimating the calories that a child should consume to achieve weight loss. While strict calorie diets have been found to be unsuccessful for children, the daily caloric recommendations can be a guide for parents when deciding which foods to offer their children for meals.

Behavioral Intervention

Components of a successful weight management program for children and adolescents will focus on healthy eating habits, incorporation of physical activity, and minimization of sedentary behavior. Goal setting, self-monitoring, group-based interventions involving the family, and stimulus control have all proven to be successful behavioral interventions for this population.[20]

When providing an intervention, it is important to remember the population you are trying to reach and the reasons they may find it difficult to follow through with healthy lifestyle changes. Pediatric patients may not realize the significance of the health complications they may face in the future when making changes that will be difficult and uncomfortable for them in the present. Cardiovascular risks are invisible to youth and their parents; symptoms are often not felt and thus even the presentation of elevated laboratory values may not be effective.

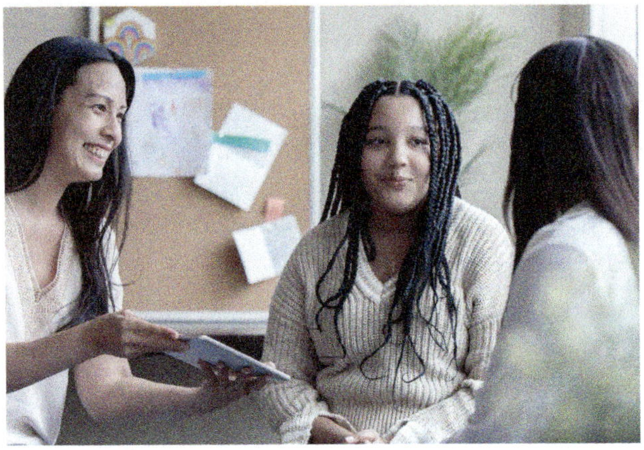

Dietary Intervention

The dietary approach to pediatric obesity that is recommended by most healthcare providers is a moderate energy restriction. The goal is to encourage a healthy relationship with food; over-restriction may lead to sneaking behaviors and subsequent weight gain. The goals of intervention should focus on developing nutritionally balanced and portion-controlled eating that is age appropriate. To assess the best dietary approaches for weight management in children, the Academy of Nutrition and Dietetics systematically reviewed the efficacy of the Stop Light Diet for Children, the Low Carbohydrate diet, and the Reduced Glycemic Load diet. The impact on outcome was inconsistent, leading the Academy of Nutrition and Dietetics Expert Committee to conclude that a variety of dietary approaches may be useful. Of note, studies indicate that emphasis on increasing intake of healthy foods is more effective in reducing weight and preventing rebound as is reducing intake of high-energy foods. This finding correlates with less parental restriction on eating behaviors and less focus on a child's weight.[55]

Examples of dietary intervention extracted from the Position of the Academy of Nutrition and Dietetics include:[55]

- Macronutrient-balanced, portion controlled, with an emphasis on promoting intake of high-fiber foods, such as fruits, nonstarchy vegetables, and whole-grain products to help manage hunger
- Reduced glycemic load
- Calorie-defined plan
- Unbalanced macronutrient (e.g., high protein, low carbohydrate, or low-fat)
- Mediterranean diet (ages 12 and older)
- DASH b—Child 1 version
- Meal replacement
- Mindful eating (self-regulation of stomach hunger/satisfaction/fullness; identifying nonstomach hunger triggers for eating [e.g., emotional eating]; slowing down the rate of eating and savoring what is eaten)
- Healthy Nutrition Guidelines targeting specific changes in eating habits (e.g., reducing intake of sugary drinks; establishing a regular meal and snack pattern; eating age-appropriate portions of protein sources and starchy foods; selecting healthier snacks; eating more fruit and nonstarchy vegetables; selecting healthier options when eating out, etc.)
- Parenting/caregiver support with eating that is developmentally appropriate (e.g., providing structure around eating, division of responsibility, etc.)

PRACTICE POINT

Several dietary approaches may be effective in promoting a healthy weight in children. A focus on eating healthy food, as opposed to energy restriction, may be more effective and sustainable.

Physical Activity

Sedentary behaviors, such as engaging with TV, playing video games, or using the computer, should be limited. These sedentary activities may take the place of physical activity in a child's routine and, most importantly, can lead to excess caloric intake. Media plays a big role in the pediatric obesity epidemic, as children are bombarded with ads promoting high-energy, high-sugar foods that can act as triggers to consume these food items. The American Academy of Pediatrics recommends limiting screen time and taking special care to eat meals away from the TV, to limit distractions.[58] A common recommendation is to limit screen time to a maximum of 2 hours daily.[59,60]

Increasing physical activity level is an important part of a weight management program **(Box 22.1)**. Studies have shown that structured or programmed aerobic exercises are less effective than increasing the activity of everyday living. Walking to school, taking the stairs, and helping with chores are examples of daily living tasks that increase physical activity.[61] Recent guidelines for physical activity recommend at least 60 minutes of activity on most days of the week.[62] Children should be encouraged to make small changes that incorporate more activity throughout the day. **Table 22.3** provides examples of aerobic, muscle-strengthening, and bone-strengthening activities for children. Healthcare professionals can also provide community resources to support the child's interest in certain sports or exercises. Physical activity has been shown to improve lipid and glucose metabolic profiles, insulin resistance, and respiratory function, and reduce adiposity.[63]

Table 22.3 Aerobic, Muscle and Bone Strengthening Exercises in Children

Exercise	Examples
Moderate-to-Vigorous Aerobic 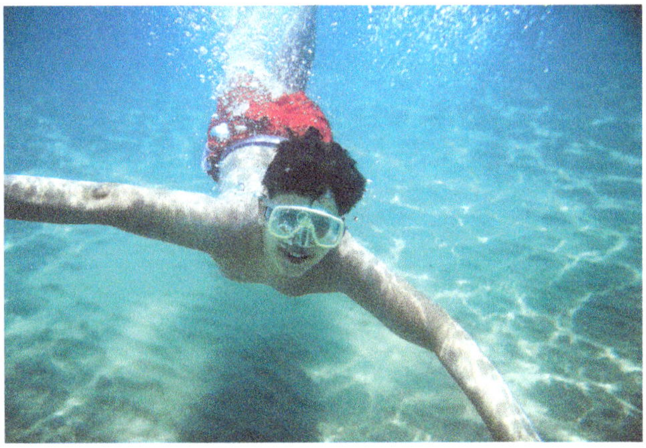 © Constantinis/E+/Getty Images	Moderate intensity: brisk walking, biking, hiking, swimming, catching and throwing, house and yard work Vigorous intensity: running, jumping rope, martial arts, team sports, vigorous dancing
Muscle-Strengthening Activities 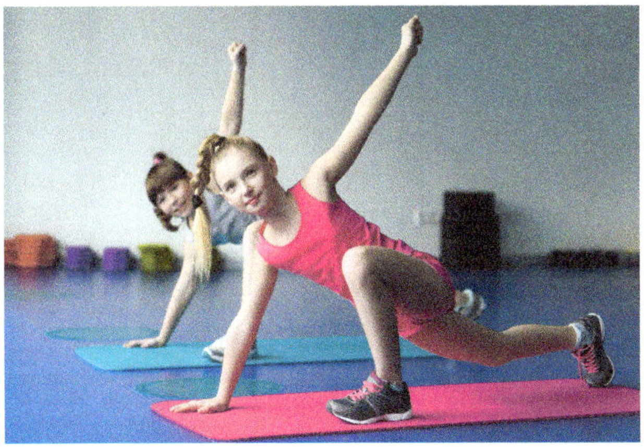 © Dreams Come True/Shutterstock	Yoga, resistance exercises using body weight or resistance bands, rope climbing, games such as tug of war

(continues)

Table 22.3 Aerobic, Muscle and Bone Strengthening Exercises in Children (continued)

Exercise	Examples
Bone-Strengthening Activities 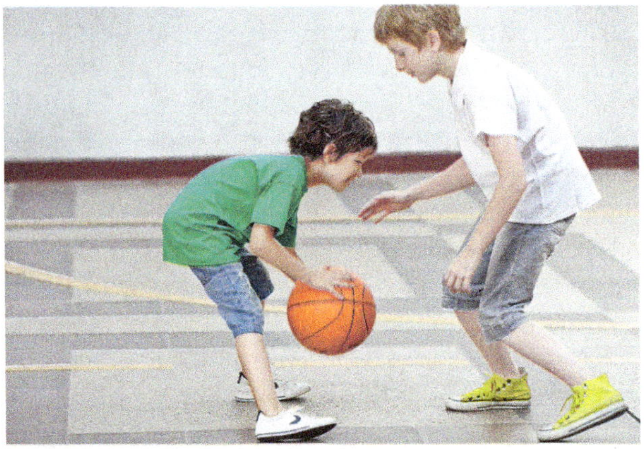 © Robert Kneschke/Shutterstock	Jumping, hopping, skipping, and running Sports such as basketball, tennis, and volleyball

Data from CDC Youth Physical Activity Guidelines, 2024. Retrieved from: https://www.cdc.gov/physical-activity-basics/adding-children-adolescents/what-counts.html

Intervention Approaches

Group Based

Family-based behavioral intervention that focuses on dietary and physical activity changes has been shown to be effective for long-term weight management. Parental influence on children and adolescents as role models is often overlooked, but these relationships are extremely important for weight management.[19]

Intensive Health Behavior and Lifestyle Treatment (IHBLT)

Intensive Health Behavior and Lifestyle Treatment (IHBLT) is an evidence-based framework of implementing a multidisciplinary approach to treat pediatric obesity in the primary care setting.[8] Its successful implementation requires involvement of professionals from different lifestyle-related fields, engagement and participation of families, and sufficient frequency and intensity of visits beyond the routine primary care visits. According to the American Academy of Pediatrics, the most effective IHBLT program delivers 26 or more hours of face-to-face, family-based counseling on nutrition and physical activity over at least a 3- to 12-month period. IHBLT can be implemented in primary care settings, obesity specialty clinics, and community entities.[8]

Motivational Interviewing

Motivational interviewing is a counseling style that is patient centered and can elicit behavior change by having the patient identify a behavior change they would like to make and come up with their own solutions on how to enact.[8,20] Motivational interviewing can be successful in the older pediatric population because it allows the patient to be in charge of their own behavior changes. There are four stages of motivational interviewing (refer to **Table 22.4**).

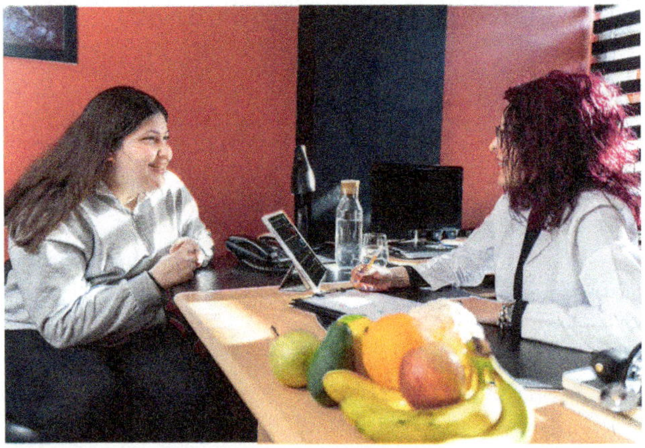

© Phynart Studio/E+/Getty Images

Positive Reinforcement

Positive reinforcement, such as praise and acknowledgment, has been demonstrated to be effective in promoting behavior changes. Rewards unrelated to food and rewards that encourage extra physical activity, such as a trip to the park or a new piece of sports equipment, can be effectively used.[20]

Stimulus Control

The focus of this behavioral intervention is to minimize the cues for undesirable behavior and promote the cues for desirable behavior. This approach

Box 22.1 CDC Youth Physical Activity Guidelines

Children and adolescents should have 60 minutes (1 hour) or more of physical activity daily.

- Aerobic: Most of the 60 or more minutes a day should be either moderate- or vigorous-intensity aerobic physical activity and should include vigorous-intensity physical activity at least 3 days a week.
- Muscle-strengthening: As part of their 60 or more minutes of daily physical activity, children and adolescents should include muscle-strengthening physical activity on at least 3 days of the week.
- Bone-strengthening: As part of their 60 or more minutes of daily physical activity, children and adolescents should include bone-strengthening physical activity on at least 3 days of the week.

Reproduced from CDC. 2018 Physical Activity Guidelines for Americans. Retrieved from: https://health.gov/our-work/nutrition-physical-activity/physical-activity-guidelines/current-guidelines

Table 22.4 Key Concepts of Motivational Interviewing

Express empathy: It is important for the healthcare provider to show the patient and family understanding about their situation; this helps them to feel comfortable and be more willing to be attentive to suggestions made by the healthcare provider.
Develop discrepancy: Being attentive for inconsistencies between future goals and current behavior can help the patient make connections as to how their current behavior is hindering their future progress toward achieving their goal.
Roll with resistance: Using different ways to confront resistance from the patient about making a behavior change that do not include arguing with the patient. These approaches might include shifting focus away from the area of contention, establishing patient control over choices, or restating the patient's concern from a new perspective.
Support self-efficacy: Building the patient's confidence in their ability to make the behavior change.

Data from Miller WR, Moyers TB. Motivational interviewing and the clinical science of Carl Rogers. *J Consult Clini Psychol*. 2017; 85(8): 757–766.

Clinical Roundtable

Topic: The Influence of Media Use in Pediatric Obesity

Background: The ease of accessing various forms of media is one of the main factors that promotes sedentary behaviors and the development of pediatric obesity. Children are spending more hours sitting in front of electronic devices than engaging in physical activity. Not only does media consumption foster sedentary behaviors, but it also encourages unhealthy eating patterns through constant food commercials for fast-food restaurants and undesirable processed foods. The World Health Organization has established guidelines to protect children from the harmful impact of food marketing.[1] The guideline calls for mandatory policies to restrict marketing of foods high in saturated fat, trans fat, added sugars, and/or salt. Such policies should protect children of all ages. Although there has been systematic success in reducing food marketing exposure on television to younger children,[2] regulating food marketing on social media platforms such as YouTube, TikTok, and Instagram remains a challenge.[3]

Roundtable Discussion

Consider the use of media when developing nutrition interventions for children with obesity.

1. Identify examples of ways to incorporate electronic devices and social media with beneficial nutrition interventions for children?
2. What are some challenges that can come with this development?

References

1. Data from World Health Organization. Policies to protect children from the harmful impact of food marketing: WHO guideline. Geneva: World Health Organization; 2023.
2. Powell LM, Leider J, Schermbeck RM, Vandenbroeck A, Harris JL. Trends in children's exposure to food and beverage advertising on television. *JAMA Netw Open*. 2024;7(8):e2429671. doi:10.1001/jamanetworkopen.2024.29671
3. Coates AE, Hardman CA, Halford JCG, Christiansen P, Boyland EJ. Food and beverage cues featured in YouTube videos of social media influencers popular with children: An exploratory study. *Front Psychol*. 2019;10:2142. doi:10.3389/fpsyg.2019.02142

CASE STUDY REVISITED

Nora returns in 2 years for a check-up. Her BMI is now 35 kg/m^2, and she is charting at the 99th percentile for her sex and age. Nora is now 17 years old and has been seeing an RD for the past year, but she has not been able to lose more than 9 kg before quickly putting it back on. Her lab values have not improved. Nora is inquiring about the possibility of pharmacotherapy.

Questions

1. Assess Nora's PES statements from her initial visit. Identify if each statement remains an active issue or if the PES statement has been resolved. If the PES statement remains an active issue, has improvement in the issue been noted? If the issue has been resolved, write a new PES statement.
2. Identify the nutrition interventions you would like to initiate for Nora to address the problems identified in your PES statements.
3. Is Nora a candidate for weight loss medications? If so, which weight loss medications would be appropriate for Nora?
4. What indices are included in your monitoring and evaluation plan? Why? How would you approach the follow-up nutrition visits with Nora if she initiates pharmacotherapy?

recommends the removal of certain foods from the home so that the temptation to eat unhealthy foods is no longer present. Similarly, having healthy foods readily available and in clear view can trigger healthful eating.[20]

Goal Setting

Patients who set clear and achievable goals have been proven to have more success following through with a behavior change than those who did not set goals or who set goals that were too broad. Small, specific goals encourage slow and steady changes that are likely to be more sustainable as well as increase self-efficacy in the child. An example of a small, specific goal would be recommending the child to "walk the dog for 30 minutes, 5 times per week," as opposed to the broader goal of "get more exercise."[20]

CORE CONCEPT 8

Behavioral change in children can be achieved by employing motivational interviewing during counseling, providing positive reinforcement from the child's support system, and identifying cues that lead to unhealthy behaviors.

Pharmacotherapy

For pediatric patients 12 years and older with severe obesity, pharmacotherapy may be recommended to aid in weight loss if behavioral changes alone are not effective.[8] A multidisciplinary approach is necessary to ensure safe and effective usage of medications and lifestyle changes in adjunct to the medications. However, pharmacotherapy options are limited to pediatric patients by costs and availability. Information on long-term use of weight loss medications for adolescents is also lacking. Families that are considering initiating pharmacotherapy for weight loss should consider long-term management and potential reliance on medications to maintain a healthy weight in younger patients.

GLP-1 Receptor Agonists

Semaglutide is a GLP-1 (glucagon-like peptide-1) agonist that mimics the actions of GLP-1 naturally produced in the small intestine. It increases insulin secretion, decreases glucagon secretion, slows gastric emptying, and impacts the regulation of appetite and satiety in the brain. Semaglutide helps manage T2DM and reduce food intake, leading to weight loss. This medication is approved by the FDA for adjunct therapy with a reduced-calorie diet and increased physical activity in pediatric patients over 12 years of age with a BMI in the 95th percentile or higher for age and sex.[64] This medication is administered weekly through subcutaneous injection (**Figure 22.7**). Adverse reactions in pediatric patients include nausea, vomiting, diarrhea, abdominal pain, constipation, dyspepsia, hypoglycemia, headache, acute pancreatitis, and acute kidney injury.[65]

Liraglutide is also a GLP-1 agonist that mimics the actions of GLP-1. It is approved by the FDA for

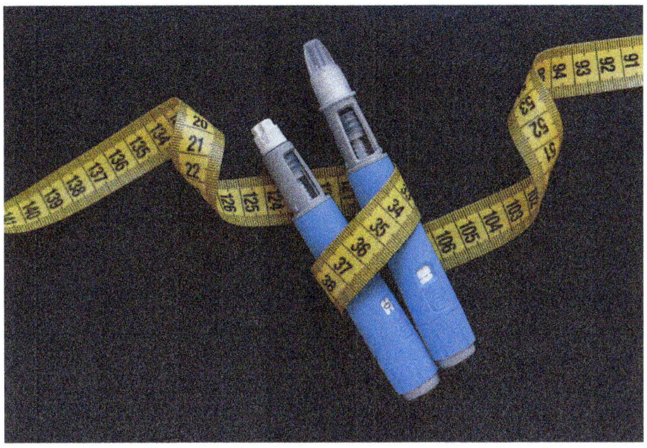

Figure 22.7 Pharmacotherapy May Be Offered in Certain Situations to Aid in Weight Loss if Lifestyle Modifications Have Been Unsuccessful

weight loss in pediatric patients over 12 years of age and older with obesity. It is also used for treatment of T2DM when administered at a lower dose. Liraglutide is less efficacious for weight loss and may cause more gastrointestinal side effects than semaglutide.[64,66] It also requires daily subcutaneous injections, leading to a more challenging treatment course and lower compliance among pediatric patients.

Phentermine-Topiramate

This combination of phentermine and topiramate is approved for adjunct treatment of obesity in patients 12 years and older.[67] Phentermine is a norepinephrine reuptake inhibitor and amphetamine agonist that reduces appetite and may increase energy expenditure by stimulating the hypothalamus to release norepinephrine. Topiramate is primarily used for epilepsy and migraine treatment, but it also has effects on appetite suppression and satiety enhancement. This combination treatment may cause adverse effects that are sympathomimetic and neuropsychiatric. It is usually not the first-line treatment for obesity in adult and pediatric patients.

Other Medications

Setmelanotide, phentermine, metformin, and orlistat are other less common medications used in treatment of pediatric obesity.[8] Setmelanotide is approved for children 6 years and older who have been genetically tested for leptin and leptin receptor deficiency that contributed to obesity. Phentermine alone is approved for children 16 years and older and for short-term use only. Metformin can be used in children 10 years and older who have developed T2DM. Orlistat, which causes fat malabsorption, can be used in children 12 years and older.

CORE CONCEPT 9

Several weight loss pharmacotherapy options are available for pediatric patients 12 years and older to consider while implementing lifestyle changes. There are side effects associated with different medications.

Surgical Intervention

For pediatric patients with severe obesity, behavioral interventions alone are sometimes not effective. If a pharmacological approach is also not effective or contraindicated, surgical interventions may be considered. The long-term effectiveness and degree of risk that weight loss surgery has on children remains controversial.

Indications for Surgical Intervention

Guidelines for surgical intervention in the pediatric population vary in medical literature. The American Academy of Pediatric 2023 Clinical Practice Guideline for Pediatric Obesity outlined that the severe form of pediatric obesity is eligible for consideration for metabolic and bariatric surgery.[8] Criteria for evaluation for pediatric metabolic and bariatric surgery include class 2 obesity (BMI $\geq$35 kg/m^2 or 120% of the 95th percentile for age and sex, whichever is lower) with a comorbidity or class 3 obesity (BMI $\geq$40 kg/m^2 or 140% of the 95th percentile for age and sex, whichever is lower) without a comorbidity requirement.[8] Weight loss surgery is safe and effective for eligible pediatric patients in bariatric settings that are experienced with pediatric populations. Patients must demonstrate that they understand the significant lifestyle changes they will have to make regarding diet and physical activity postoperatively. Often, an interprofessional team approach is used to guide these patients through a multistep process and evaluate their readiness for this life-changing operation.

PRACTICE POINT

Prior to the weight loss procedure, it is important for the patient to understand the health risks and benefits of the surgery. The parents and interprofessional team determine whether the patient is mature enough and with a sufficient support system to have surgical procedure.

Weight Loss Procedures

Weight loss surgical approaches are similar in pediatric and adult populations. Laparoscopic Roux-en-Y gastric bypass and vertical sleeve gastrectomy are both performed in pediatric patients.[8] Longitudinal studies have demonstrated that adolescents who have undergone **Roux-en-Y gastric bypass** or **sleeve gastrectomy** have demonstrated sustainable weight loss, maintained resolution of comorbidities, and unaltered growth.[68,69] Laparoscopic adjustable gastric band procedures have declined in use in both adult and pediatric patients because of its suboptimal long-term effects and higher complication rates. Refer to Chapter 7, *Weight and Health*, for details of the metabolic and bariatric surgical procedures.

CORE CONCEPT 10

Two metabolic and bariatric procedures are recommended for weight loss in adolescents: the Roux-en-Y gastric bypass and the sleeve gastrectomy.

PRACTICE POINT

The following criteria indicate when weight loss surgery is appropriate and recommended for pediatric patients: patient age is 12–18 years and BMI is >35 kg/m^2, or 120% of the 95th percentile for age and sex with serious comorbidities or BMI is >40 kg/m^2, or 140% of the 95th percentile for age and sex.

Nutritional Considerations

Postoperative nutritional management is similar in pediatric and adult patients. Lifelong daily supplementation is needed after metabolic and bariatric surgery due to dietary vitamin and mineral intake restriction and possible malabsorption. Patients will also need to consume high-protein and small-volume foods as well as adequate hydration around meals. Refer to Chapter 7, *Weight and Health*, for details of postoperative management.

Due to the reduction of the gastric reservoir size, **dumping syndrome** is a common condition that often develops after bariatric surgery. Dumping syndrome is a condition where large particles of food rapidly travel from the stomach to the small intestine, making it difficult for the small intestine to digest and absorb nutrients. The dietary measures recommended for patients with dumping syndrome include delaying the intake of any liquids until 30 minutes after the meal, consuming six small meals per day, and eliminating rapidly absorbed carbohydrates from the diet. Refer to Chapter 10, *Nutritional Management of Gastrointestinal Maldigestion*, for details related to dumping syndrome.

Follow-up with an RD is important to help the patient make positive dietary changes and improve or maintain nutritional status following surgery. RDs can work with the pediatric patient to understand the micronutrient deficiencies they are at risk for, as well as help develop a plan for dietary intervention. Patients may experience symptoms such as nausea,

Clinical Controversy

Is Bariatric Surgery Safe and Effective for Children?
As pediatric obesity rates continue to rise nationwide, there is a growing need to determine the appropriate forms of intervention available for chronic diseases associated with obesity. Metabolic and bariatric surgery is a controversial solution that has been found to help with weight loss and decrease long-term risks associated with severe obesity. While some studies have proven the effectiveness of metabolic and bariatric surgery for children, others have stated that these procedures can leave children with long-term medical and psychological complications and thus bariatric surgery is not recommended.[1] Dr. Joan C. Han, the director of Pediatric Obesity Program at the National Institutes of Health, discusses in her article that the risks of metabolic and bariatric surgery for children and long-term efficacy is an area where more research needs to be developed and thus should be only recommended to children with extreme caution.[2]

A prospective study completed in Australia compared the weight loss that adolescents experienced after a lifestyle intervention program (reduced energy intake, behavioral intervention, and increased physical activity) with metabolic and bariatric surgery.[3] Fifty participants aged 14–18 years, with a BMI ≥35 kg/m^2 and existing medical complications of hypertension, asthma, or metabolic syndrome, were randomized to participate in either the gastric banding program or the lifestyle program. The participants in the gastric banding program underwent adjustable lap band gastric surgery and were given detailed dietary recommendations by dietitians and advised to be physically active for 30 minutes each day after recovery. The participants in the lifestyle program were given individualized diet plans (800–2000 kcal/day), recommended physical activity schedules, and behavioral modifications. While successful weight loss was found in both groups, 84% of the participants in the gastric banding group lost more than 50% of their excess weight versus 12% of participants in the lifestyle program. In addition, participants in the gastric banding program had higher scores in the quality-of-life assessment and also saw their metabolic syndrome and insulin resistance completely resolved.

The Medical University of Vienna conducted a follow-up study regarding the lives of 10 adolescents who participated in an original study on obesity in adolescents and metabolic and bariatric surgery.[4] The 10 participants in this study were ages 14–20 years, had a BMI of ≥49 kg/m^2, and were unsuccessful in previous forms of weight loss interventions. Although weight loss was found 24 months after the procedure, 6 out of the 10 patients regained the weight 3 years later. Participants also felt exhausted and weak and experienced abdominal pain 44 months post procedure. In addition, 40% of the participants experienced rheumatic pain, and 60% reported daily drowsiness, palpitations, and chest pain. Participants turned to food when coping with emotional stress, experienced a negative body image, and received high scores on the depressive disorder screening tools.

Questions

1. Describe the conflicting issues related to the use of metabolic and bariatric surgery in the pediatric population with obesity.
2. What are the strengths and weaknesses of both studies?
3. What recommendation might you make for initiation of a metabolic and bariatric surgery program at your institution?

References

1. Inge TH, Zeller MH, Lawson, ML, Daniels SR. A critical appraisal of evidence supporting a bariatric surgical approach to weight management for adolescents. *J Pediatr.* 2005,147(1):10–19.
2. Han JC, Lawlor DA, Kimm SYS. Pediatric Obesity—2010: Progress and Challenges. *Lancet*. 2010;375(9727):1737–1748. doi:10.1016/S0140- 6736(10)60171-7
3. O'Brien PE, Sawyer SM, Laurie C, et al. Laparoscopic adjustable gastric banding in severely obese adolescents. A randomized trial. *JAMA*. 2010;303(6):519–526. doi:10.1001/jama.2010.81
4. Dietrich S, Widhalm K, Prager G, Silberhummer G, Orth D. Bariatric surgery in morbidly obese adolescents: a 4 years follow-up of ten patients. *Aktuelle Ernährungsmedizin*. 2008;33(03). doi:10.1055/s-2008-1079394

vomiting, or diarrhea. The RD can help address these symptoms by providing targeted medical nutrition therapy.

Postoperative Care

Postoperatively, patients should follow an interprofessional program that encourages follow-up with different members of the medical team.[70] The team should include a pediatrician, psychologist, RD, bariatric surgeon, and program coordinator. A strong postoperative program that offers ample support for these patients is important for long-term success and maintenance of weight loss.[63]

Healthy Eating at School

School meals play an essential role in the nutrition status and health of school aged children. According to the CDC, schools should educate families about school meals, encourage students to start their day with the school breakfast, allow students to have adequate time for meals, promote healthy eating habits throughout the day, and incorporate nutrition education in curriculums.[71] Among these areas of nutrition intervention at school, what food items are provided or accessible at school has the greatest influence on students' dietary choices. Although policies and standards are in place to regulate what nutritious foods should be offered at school meals, research has shown that the most popular food items among students include sandwiches and pizzas.[72] Because students have full autonomy during school meals to decide what items they will consume, nutrition education and motivational counseling may be effective to facilitate building balanced meals in this population. On the other hand, students may skip meals for a variety of reasons including inadequate seated time and lack of interest in the foods provided. Skipping meals is a behavior that contributes to a worsened nutritional profile and prevalence of obesity among children as it leads to increased appetite and promotes overconsumption later in the day.[73] For families experiencing food insecurity, skipping free meals at school further hinders the child's access to nutritious foods. Motivational counseling and troubleshooting types of intervention can help pediatric patients find solutions in navigating external factors that influence their meal patterns at and after school. RDs can help families with building a pantry with healthy snacks or shopping on a budget. The USDA Nutritional Standards for School Meals 2024 are as follows:[74]

- Offer fat-free or low-fat milk, flavored and unflavored
- If meals meet weekly calorie limits, schools can offer menu items high in added sugar
- Sodium amount allowed per meal is limited according to age group
- At least 80% of the weekly grains offered must be whole grain-rich (at least 50% whole grains)

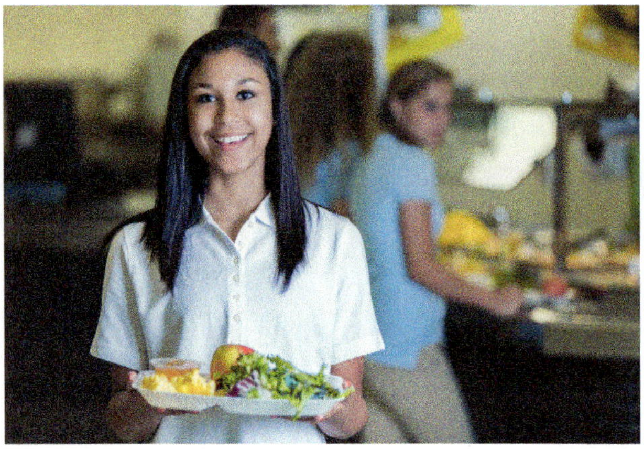

CORE CONCEPT 11

Although federal agencies implement nutrition programs at school to provide low-cost or free and healthy meals to school-aged children, children may not consume proper nutrition at school due to various reasons.

Monitoring and Evaluation

Monitoring pediatric obesity includes periodic measurement of height and weight, diet records, eating and physical activity behaviors and attitudes, and laboratory data or vital signs, as indicated if comorbidities exist. Following growth trends is also critical to ensure any weight loss is not interfering with growth. For older adolescents, monitoring of health habits will need to consider changes in school and occupation, participation in sports, and other influencers of food intake such as social factors, including access to care, peer influence, and food choices away from home. Primary care providers should routinely monitor psychosocial status of patients 12 years and older.[8] As the patient approaches 21 years of age, transition of care to adult primary care should also be initiated. Frequency of follow-up should be determined based upon individual circumstances, such as severity of comorbidities or intensity of and response to treatments.

Chapter Summary

Rates of pediatric obesity are following a concerning upward trend, and as rates of obesity in children and adolescents increase, so do the related comorbidities. Children are now facing serious health complications, such as T2DM, metabolic syndrome, hypertension, obstructive sleep apnea, and cardiac dysfunction that had previously only been seen in adulthood.

A standardized method to assess and evaluate these children and adolescents who are overweight or obese should be established. Currently, BMI and age- and sex-specific growth charts are the most common ways to assess for overweight and obesity. Individuals considered overweight or obese should be evaluated for comorbidities, and interventions should be implemented as early as possible so that the patient does not carry adverse health complications into adulthood. Behavioral interventions can be used to address dietary and physical activity lifestyle changes. In some individuals, behavioral changes may not be effective, and pharmacological and/or surgical intervention can then be considered.

Pediatric obesity is associated with medical and psychological comorbidities that can affect almost all

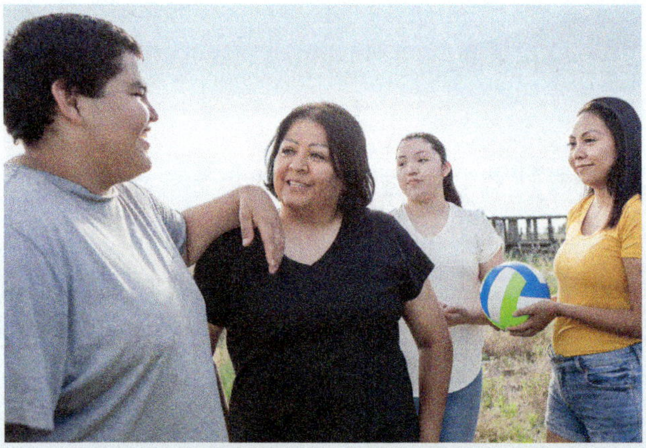

aspects of a child's life. Health professionals should attempt to identify trends of overweight and obesity early to implement an intervention plan as soon as possible since early intervention is associated with reduced health complications and progression of obesity into adulthood.

Key Terms

pediatric obesity, left ventricular hypertrophy (LVH), epicardial fat, metabolic syndrome, insulin resistance, intramyocellular lipid deposition, obstructive sleep apnea, metabolic dysfunction-associated steatotic liver disease (MASLD), food insecurity, nutrigenomics, semaglutide, liraglutide, Roux-en-Y gastric bypass surgery, sleeve gastrectomy, dumping syndrome, school meals

Acknowledgments

The author acknowledges Adi Goldberg and Ashley Abbott for contributions to the previous version of this chapter.

References

1. National Center for Health Statistics, National Health and Nutrition Examination Survey, 1999–2000 through August 2021–August 2023. Updated October 17, 2024. Accessed December 3, 2024. https://www.cdc.gov/nchs/nhanes/index.htm
2. US Preventative Service Task Force, Grossman DC, Bibbins-Domingo K, et al. Screening for obesity in children and adolescents: US Preventive Services Task Force Recommendation Statement. *JAMA*. 2017;317(23):2417–2426. doi:10.1001/jama.2017.6803
3. Centers for Disease Control and Prevention. Growth charts. September 2, 2024. Accessed November 16, 2024. https://www.cdc.gov/growthcharts/index.htm
4. Division of Nutrition, Physical Activity and Obesity, National Center for Chronic Disease Prevention and Health Promotion. Defining childhood obesity. CDC. 2015. Updated August 20, 2024. Accessed November 16, 2024. https://www.cdc.gov/nccdphp/dnpao/data-trends-maps/help/npao_dtm/definitions.html#OWS1
5. Kelly AS, Barlow SE, Rao G, et al. Severe obesity in children and adolescents: identification, associated health risks, and treatment approaches: a scientific statement from the American Heart Association. *Circulation*. 2013;128:1689–1712. doi:10.1161/CIR.0b013e3182a5cfb3
6. Centers for Disease Control and Prevention, National Center for Health Statistics. Last updated October 19, 2023. Accessed November 16, 2024. https://www.cdc.gov/growthcharts/Extended-BMI-Charts.html
7. Centers for Disease Control and Prevention, National Center for Health Statistics. Last updated October 19, 2023. Accessed November 16, 2024. https://www.cdc.gov/growthcharts/information-for-healthcare-professionals.htm
8. Hampl SE, Hassink SG, Skinner AC, et al. Clinical practice guideline for the evaluation and treatment of children and adolescents with obesity. *Pediatrics*. 2024;153(1):e2023064612.
9. Freedman DS, Wang J, Ogden CL, et al. The prediction of body fatness by BMI and skinfold thicknesses among children and adolescents. *Ann Hum Biol*. 2007;34(2):183–194. doi:10.1080/03014460601116860
10. Griffiths C, Gately P, Marchant PR, Cooke CB. A five year longitudinal study investigating the prevalence of childhood obesity: comparison of BMI and waist circumference. *Public Health*. 2013;127(12):1090–1096.
11. Daniels SR. Complications of obesity in children and adolescents. *Int J Obesity*. 2009;33:S60. doi:10.1038/ijo.2009.20
12. Berenson GS, Srinivasan SR, Bao W, Newman WP, Tracy RE, Wattigney WA. Association between multiple cardiovascular risk factors and atherosclerosis in children and young adults. *N Engl J Med*. 1998;338(23):1650–1656. doi:10.1056 NEJM199806043382302
13. Wattigney WA, Webber LS, Srinivasan SR, Berenson GS. The emergence of clinically abnormal levels of cardiovascular disease risk factor variables among young adults: the Bogalusa Heart Study. *Prev Med*. 1995;24(6):617–626. doi:10.1006/pmed.1995.1097
14. DeBoer MD. Obesity, systemic inflammation, and increased risk for cardiovascular disease and diabetes among adolescents: a need for screening tools to target interventions. *Nutrition*. 2013;29(2):379–386.
15. Salazar J, Luzardo E, Mejías JC, et al. Epicardial fat: physiological, pathological, and therapeutic implications. *Cardiol Res Prac*. 2016;2016;1291537. doi:10.1155/2016/1291537
16. Grundy SM, Brewer HB, Cleeman JI, Smith SC, Lenfant C, for the Conference Participants. Definition of metabolic syndrome: report of the National Heart, Lung, and Blood Institute/American Heart Association conference on scientific issues related to definition. *Circulation*. 2004;109(3):433–438. doi:10.1161/01.CIR.0000111245.75752.C6
17. Schubert CM, Sun SS, Burns TL, Morrison JA, Huang TT. Predictive ability of childhood metabolic components for adult metabolic syndrome and type 2 diabetes. *J Pediatr*. 2009;155(3):S6.e1–S6.e7.
18. Sarría A, Moreno LA, Garcí-LIop LA, Fleta J, Morellón MP, Bueno M. Body mass index, triceps skinfold and waist circumference in screening for adiposity in male children and adolescents. *Acta Paediatrica*. 2007. http://onlinelibrary.wiley.com/doi/10.1111/j.1651-2227.2001.tb00437.x/full
19. Després J-P. Cardiovascular disease under the influence of excess visceral fat. *Crit Pathways Cardiol*. 2007; 6(2):51–59. doi:10.1097/hpc.0b013e318057d4c9
20. Kim G, Caprio S. Diabetes and insulin resistance in pediatric obesity. *Pediatr Clin North Am*. 2011;58(6):1355–1361.
21. D'adamo E, Caprio S. Type 2 diabetes in youth: epidemiology and pathophysiology. *Diabetes Care*. 2011;34:S161. doi:10.2337/dc11-s212

22. Craig ME, Huang C. Type-2 diabetes in childhood: incidence and prognosis. *Pediatr Child Health.* 2009;19(7):321–326. doi:10.1016/j.paed.2009.03.011
23. Pulgarón ER. Childhood obesity: a review of increased risk for physical and psychological comorbidities. *Clin Ther.* 2013;35(1):A18–A32. doi:10.1016/j.clinthera.2012.12.014
24. Rance K, O'Laughlen M. Obesity and asthma: a dangerous link in children: an integrative review of the literature. *J Nurse Pract.* 2011;7(4):287–292. doi:10.1016/j.nurpra.2010.06.011
25. Papoutsakis C, Priftis KN, Drakouli M, et al. Childhood overweight/obesity and asthma: is there a link? A systematic review of recent epidemiologic evidence. *J Am Nutr Diet.* 2013;113(1):77–105. doi:10.1016/j.jand.2012.08.025
26. Verhulst SL, Schrauwen N, Haentjens D, et al. Sleep-disordered breathing in overweight and obese children and adolescents: prevalence, characteristics and the role of fat distribution. *Arch Dis Child.* 2007;92:205–208.
27. Lumeng J, Chervin R. Epidemiology of pediatric obstructive sleep apnea. *Proc Am Thorac Soc.* 2008;5:242. doi:10.1513/pats.200708-135MG
28. Tauman R, Gozal D. Obesity and obstructive sleep apnea in children. *Paediatr Respir Rev.* 2006;7(4):247–259. doi:10.1016/j.prrv.2006.08.003
29. Cummings DE, Shannon MH. Roles for ghrelin in the regulation of appetite and body weight. *Arch Surg.* 2003;138(4):389–396. doi:10.1001/archsurg.138.4.389
30. Shneider BL, González-Peralta R, Roberts EA. Controversies in the management of pediatric liver disease: hepatitis B, C and NAFLD: summary of a single topic conference. *Hepatology.* 2006;44(5):1344–1354. doi:10.1002/hep.21373
31. Rinella ME, Lazarus JV, Ratziu V, et al. A multisociety Delphi consensus statement on new fatty liver disease nomenclature. *Hepatology.* 2023;78(6):1966–1986. doi:10.1097/HEP.0000000000000520
32. Spengler EK, Loomba R. Recommendations for diagnosis, referral for liver biopsy, and treatment of NAFLD and NASH. *Mayo Clinic Proc.* 2015;90(9):1233–1246. doi:10.1016/j.mayocp.2015.06.013
33. Dockray S, Susman EJ, Dorn LD. Depression, cortisol reactivity, and obesity in childhood and adolescence. *J Adolesc Health.* 2009;45(4):344–350. doi:10.1016/j.jadohealth.2009.06.014
34. Dreyer ML, Egan AM. Psychosocial functioning and its impact on implementing behavioral interventions for childhood obesity. *Prog Pediatr Cardiol.* 2008;25(2):159–166. doi:10.1016/j.ppedcard.2008.05.007
35. Goldstein BI, Carnethon MR, Matthews KA, et al. Major depressive disorder and bipolar disorder predispose youth to accelerated atherosclerosis and early cardiovascular disease: a scientific statement from the American Heart Association. *Circulation.* 2015;132(10):965–986. doi:10.1161/CIR.0000000000000229
36. Vander Wal JS, Mitchell ER. Psychological complications of pediatric obesity. *Pediatr Clin North Am.* 2011;58(6):1393–1401.
37. He J, Cai Z, Fan X. Prevalence of binge and loss of control eating among children and adolescents with overweight and obesity: an exploratory meta-analysis. *Int J Eat Disord.* 2017;50(2):91–103. doi:10.1002/eat.22661
38. Sonneville KR, Grilo CM, Richmond TK, et al. Prospective association between overvaluation of weight and binge eating among overweight adolescent girls. *J Adolesc Health.* 2015;56(1):25–29. doi:10.1016/j.jadohealth.2014.08.017
39. Miller AA, Spencer SJ. Obesity and neuroinflammation: a pathway to cognitive impairment. *Brain Behav Immun.* 2014;42:10–21. doi:10.1016/j.bbi.2014.04.001
40. U.S. Department of Agriculture, Economic Research Service. (n.d.). Definitions of food security. Retrieved March 10, 2022, from https://www.ers.usda.gov/topics/food-nutrition-assistance/food-security-in-the-u-s/definitions-of-food-security/This link is external to odphp.health.gov
41. Hilmers A, Hilmers DC, Dave J. Neighborhood disparities in access to healthy goods and their effects on environmental justice. *Am J Public Health.* 2012;102(9):1644–1654. doi:10.2105/AJPH.2012.300865
42. Eagle TF, Sheetz A, Gurm R, et al. Understanding childhood obesity in America: linkages between household income, community resources, and children's behaviors. *Am Heart J.* 2012;163(5):836–843. doi:10.1016/j.ahj.2012.02.025
43. Office of Disease Prevention and Health Promotion. Food insecurity. Health.gov. Published October 2022. Accessed September 13, 2024. https://health.gov/healthypeople/priority-areas/social-determinants-health/literature-summaries/food-insecurity
44. Andreyeva T, Tripp AS, Schwartz MB. Dietary quality of Americans by supplemental nutrition assistance program participation status: a systematic review. *Am J Prev Med.* 2015;49(4):594–604. doi:10.1016/j.amepre.2015.04.035
45. Tester JM, Rosas LG, Leung CW. Food insecurity and pediatric obesity: a double whammy in the era of COVID-19. *Curr Obes Rep.* 2020;9(4):442–450. doi:10.1007/s13679-020-00413-x
46. Blissett J. Relationships between parenting style, feeding style and feeding practices and fruit and vegetable consumption in early childhood. *Appetite.* 2011;57(3):826–831.
47. Lifshitz F. Obesity in children. *J Clin Res Pediatr Endocrinol.* 2008;1(2):53–60. doi:10.4008/jcrpe.v1i2
48. Hjelmborg JVB, Fagnani C, Silventoinen K, et al. Genetic influences on growth traits of BMI: a longitudinal study of adult twins. *Obesity.* 2008;16(4):847–852.
49. Cheung WW, Peizhong M. Recent advances in obesity: genetics and beyond. *ISRN Endocrinol.* 2012;2012:536905. doi:10.5402/2012/536905
50. Hart CN, Carskadon MA, Considine RV, et al. Changes in children's sleep duration on food intake, weight, and leptin. *Pediatrics.* 2013;6(2):1–10.
51. Aznar LM, Pigeot I, Ahrens W. *Epidemiology of obesity in children and adolescents: prevalence and etiology.* Springer; 2011.
52. Mead MN. Nutrigenomics: the genome–food interface. *Environ Health Perspect.* 2007;115(12):A582–A589.
53. Frayling TM, Timpson NJ, Weedon MN, et al. A common variant in the FTO gene is associated with body mass index and predisposes to childhood and adult obesity. *Science.* 2007;316(5826):889–894.
54. Barlow SE, for the Expert Committee. Expert committee recommendations regarding the prevention, assessment, and treatment of child and adolescent overweight and obesity: summary report. *Pediatrics.* 2007;120(suppl 4):S164–S192.
55. Hoelscher DM, Kirk S, Ritchie L, Cunningham-Sabo L, for the Academy Positions Committee. Position of the Academy of Nutrition and Dietetics: interventions for the prevention and treatment of pediatric overweight and obesity. *J Acad Nutr Diet.* 2013;113:1375–1394.
56. Tanofsky-Kraff M, Faden D, Yanovski SZ, Wilfley DE, Yanovski JA. The perceived onset of dieting and loss of control eating behaviors in overweight children. *Int J Eating Disord.* 2005;38(2):112–122. doi:10.1002/eat.20158

57. Institute of Medicine. *Dietary Reference Intakes for Energy, Carbohydrate, Fiber, Fat, Fatty Acids, Cholesterol, Protein, and Amino Acids.* The National Academies Press; 2005. doi .org/10.17226/10490
58. American Academy of Pediatrics. *Policies on Children and Media Beyond Screen Time: A Parent's Guide to Media Use.* Updated February 23, 2021. Accessed December 3, 2023. https://www.aap.org/en/patient-care/media-and-children /policies-on-children-and-media
59. Poorolajal J, Sahraei F, Mohamdadi Y, Doosti-Irani A, Moradi L. Behavioral factors influencing childhood obesity: a systematic review and meta-analysis. *Obes Res Clin Pract.* 2020;14(2):109–118. doi:10.1016/j.orcp.2020.03.002
60. Council on Communications and Media. Media use in school-aged children and adolescents. *Pediatrics.* 2016; 138(5):e20162592. doi:10.1542/peds.2016-2592
61. Centers for Disease Control and Prevention. Aerobic, Muscle- and Bone-Strengthening: What Counts? Accessed November 16, 2024. https://www.cdc.gov/physicalactivity/basics/children /what_counts.htm.
62. Centers for Disease Control and Prevention. *Physical Activity Guidelines for Americans.* 2nd ed. Accessed December 3, 2024. https://odphp.health.gov/sites/default/files/2019-09 /Physical_Activity_Guidelines_2nd_edition.pdf
63. Lenders CM, Gorman K, Lim-Miller A, Puklin S, Pratt J. Practical approaches to the treatment of severe pediatric obesity. *Pediatr Clin North Am.* 2011;58(6):1425–1438. doi:10.1016/j .pcl.2011.09.013
64. In brief: Semaglutide (Wegovy) for weight loss in children. *Med Lett Drugs Ther.* 2023;65(1670):31–32. doi:10.58347 /tml.2023.1670d
65. U.S. Food and Drug Administration. Wegovy. FDA Label. Published August 24, 2022. Accessed September 13, 2024. https://www.accessdata.fda.gov/drugsatfda_docs/label/2022 /215256s005lbl.pdf
66. Kelly AS, Auerbach P, Barrientos-Perez M, et al. A randomized, controlled trial of liraglutide for adolescents with obesity. *N Engl J Med.* 2020;382(22):2117–2128. doi:10.1056 /NEJMoa1916038
67. Dhillon S. Phentermine/topiramate: pediatric first approval. *Paediatr Drugs.* 2022;24(6):715–720. doi:10.1007 /s40272-022-00532-z
68. Alqahtani AR, Elahmedi M, Abdurabu HY, Alqahtani S. Ten-year outcomes of children and adolescents who underwent sleeve gastrectomy: weight loss, comorbidity resolution, adverse events, and growth velocity. *J Am Coll Surg.* 2021;233(6):657–664. doi:10.1016/j.jamcollsurg.2021 .08.678
69. Wu Z, Gao Z, Qiao Y, et al. Long-term results of bariatric surgery in adolescents with at least 5 years of follow-up: a systematic review and meta-analysis. *Obes Surg.* 2023;33(6):1730–1745. doi:10.1007 /s11695-023-06593-4
70. Brei MN, Mudd S. Current guidelines for weight loss surgery in adolescents: a review of the literature. *J Pediatr Health Care.* 2014;28(4):288–294. 10.1016/j.pedhc.2013.04.005
71. Centers for Disease Control and Prevention. Eating healthier. Published September 30, 2020. Accessed September 13, 2024. https://www.cdc.gov/healthyschools/features/eating _healthier.htm
72. Ensaff H, Russell J, Barker ME. Meeting school food standards - students' food choice and free school meals. *Public Health Nutr.* 2013;16(12):2162–2168. doi:10.1017 /S1368980012005575
73. Ricotti R, Caputo M, Monzani A, et al. Breakfast skipping, weight, cardiometabolic risk, and nutrition quality in children and adolescents: a systematic review of randomized controlled and intervention longitudinal trials. *Nutrients.* 2021;13(10):3331. doi:10.3390/nu13103331
74. Food and Nutrition Service. School nutrition standards updates. USDA. Published June 15, 2021. Accessed September 13, 2024. https://www.fns.usda.gov/cn/school -nutrition-standards-updates.

CHAPTER 23

Nutrition in Eating Disorders

Natalie F. Pirolli

CHAPTER OUTLINE

CORE CONCEPTS

1. The etiologies of eating disorders generally comprise a complex interaction of genetic, biological, behavioral, psychological, and social factors, requiring that diagnosis and treatment incorporate an interprofessional team of psychiatric, medical, and nutrition professionals.
2. Eating disorders are spectral disorders because they exist on a continuum of severity and often become more severe the longer they are present.
3. Research has shown that when cessation of disturbed eating behaviors and physical restoration occur early in the treatment process, better responses to psychotherapy and improved overall prognosis result.
4. In the eating disorder community, laboratory values within normal limits do not reflect nutrition stability; conservation mechanisms, like the body's adaptive ability to maintain visceral protein metabolism in chronic starvation mode, can initially hide nutrient deficiencies.
5. Individuals with eating disorders can present with fluid and electrolyte abnormalities secondary to purging methods, fluid restriction or overload, metabolic changes, or a combination of these.
6. Medical nutrition therapy guidelines for eating disorders are largely based on clinical experience.
7. Changes in resting energy expenditure must be considered during the refeeding process because the reintroduction of food causes a dramatic increase in diet-induced thermogenesis, or the thermic effect of food.
8. Indirect calorimetry is the best method to determine whether a patient with an eating disorder is hypometabolic or hypermetabolic.

9. Refeeding syndrome is a serious and potentially fatal condition that can result from the metabolic and electrolyte shifts that occur following the reintroduction and/or increase of nutrition after a period of decreased or absent caloric intake. This reintroduction of nutrition may be in the form of oral diet, enteral nutrition, parenteral nutrition, or intravenous dextrose.

LEARNING OBJECTIVES

1. Describe the interprofessional approach needed to diagnose and treat individuals with eating disorders and the role of the registered dietitian (RD) in detection and treatment.
2. Specify the signs and clinical complications of anorexia nervosa and bulimia nervosa and their subtypes.
3. Define binge eating disorder and explain its treatment.
4. Recognize the signs and three major complications of the female athlete triad.
5. Define refeeding syndrome, specify those at risk, and state the serum shifts that are characteristic of the syndrome.
6. Identify the treatment goals for each eating disorder.
7. Describe obstacles that clinicians may encounter in treating patients with eating disorders.

Introduction

An **eating disorder (ED)** is a psychiatric illness characterized by chronic disturbances of eating habits and weight control behaviors that debilitate both physical health and psychological functioning. EDs are clinically diagnosed mental health disorders classified by the criteria of the *Diagnostic and Statistical Manual of Mental Disorders* (DSM). The manual's fifth edition, the DSM-5 categorizes eight EDs, including three of the most widely known, anorexia nervosa (AN), bulimia nervosa (BN), and binge eating disorder (BED), along with pica, rumination disorder, avoidant/restrictive food intake disorder (ARFID), and two additional categories of EDs, "other specified feeding or eating disorder" (OSFED) and "unspecified feeding or eating disorder."[1]

EDs affect individuals of all genders, races, ethnicities, sexual orientations, and body shapes and sizes. Given the secretive nature of the disorder and barriers to receiving treatment, prevalence estimates of EDs are difficult to accurately calculate and may reflect only a small portion of those affected. In 2020, a comprehensive report from the Academy of Eating Disorders, the Strategic Initiative for the Prevention of Eating Disorders (STRIPED), and Deloitte Access Economics estimated overall lifetime prevalence of EDs as 8.6% among females and 4.07% among males in the United States.[2] It also estimated that 28.8 million Americans will experience an ED at some point in their lives, and 1.9 million of the future ED cases will occur in children and adolescents under 20 years of age.[2] Rates of EDs are steadily increasing, as a 3.5% increase was seen between 2000 and 2006, and a 7.8% increase was seen between 2013 and 2018.[3] Social media use is identified as a plausible risk factor to ED development and has been linked to body dissatisfaction and poor mental health related to the comparison to "thin/fit" body ideals.[4]

EDs have the second highest mortality rate of any psychiatric illness, with opioid addiction being the first. EDs represent a large public health issue due to their life-threatening nature and potentially long-lasting implications on health. The etiologies of EDs are multifactorial, comprising a complex interaction of genetic, biological, behavioral, psychological, and social factors. Thus, diagnosis and treatment must incorporate an interprofessional team of psychiatric, medical, and nutrition professionals. Due to the complex nature of EDs, it is imperative for team members to work together and coordinate care plans to provide consistent and efficacious care during treatment.

CORE CONCEPT 1

The etiologies of eating disorders generally comprise a complex interaction of genetic, biological, behavioral, psychological, and social factors, requiring that diagnosis and treatment incorporate an interprofessional team of psychiatric, medical, and nutrition professionals.

Background and Etiology

Anorexia Nervosa

Anorexia nervosa (AN) is characterized by an intense fear of weight gain that leads to over-restriction of dietary intake, significantly low body weight, and a distorted self-perception of body weight or shape. The lifetime prevalence of AN in the United States ranges from 0.9% to 1.42% among females and 0.12% to 0.53% among males.[1,2,5] Higher incidences of AN are commonly seen in post-industrialized, high-income countries such as the United States, New Zealand, Australia, Japan, and many European countries, and appear to be increasing in Asia and the Middle East.[1] Onset typically begins in adolescence or young adulthood, with a documented increase among 15- to 19-year-olds worldwide since the 1930s.[6] However, recently, the incidence of AN is increasing in individuals under age 15, and onset has been documented over age 40 as well. Of those affected, only 33.8% are receiving treatment.[5]

AN develops as one of two subtypes: the restrictive type or the binge–purge type. Individuals with the restrictive type achieve a low body weight through extreme dietary restraint. Excessive exercise is often characteristic of this subtype. Exercise is considered excessive when it occurs at inappropriate times or settings, continues despite injury, or when it significantly interferes with important activities and/or daily life. Individuals with the binge–purge type have recurrent episodes of binge eating followed by compensatory behaviors that may include self-induced vomiting; misuse of laxatives, enemas, or diuretics; or a combination of these. Both subtypes share an intense fear of gaining weight and a distorted perception of body shape (**Figure 23.1**). Crossover between the two subtypes is common, as patients may start with the restrictive type and adopt binge–purge behaviors over time.[6,7]

Patients with AN are often described as having a weight deficit or being of "significantly low body weight." The DSM-5 defines significantly low as a weight that is less than minimally "normal" for adults or less than minimally expected for children and adolescents. The World Health Organization classifies

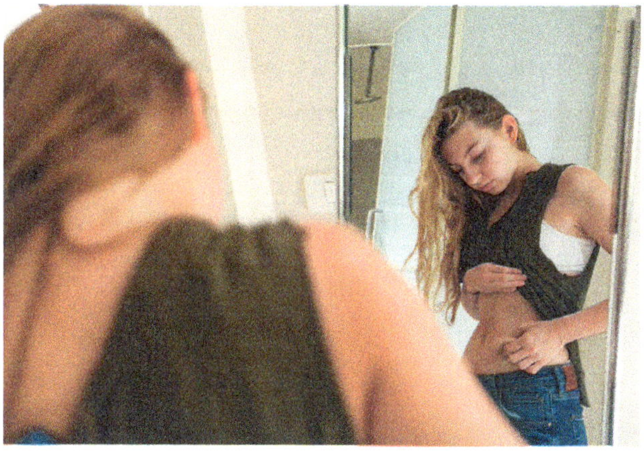

Figure 23.1 Individuals with Eating Disorders Often Have a Distorted Self-Perception of Body Weight or Shape

CASE STUDY INTRODUCTION

Emma is a 22-year-old female with anorexia nervosa. Her disordered eating habits started at age 20, during her second year of college. Her senior year of college brought on more stress as she finished difficult classes, searched for jobs, and ended a relationship with her long-term partner. For the last few months, Emma reported eating fewer than 600 calories per day and performing cardiovascular exercise for 1 to 2 hours daily. She states that she has not menstruated for the past 6 months. Emma presents to the emergency department for suspected dehydration after fainting in class.

Anthropometric Data:

Height: 167.7 cm
Weight: 45 kg
BMI: 16 kg/m^2

Weight history
56.8 kg 2 years ago
50 kg 6 months ago
Lowest adult weight: current weight of 45 kg

Biochemical Data:

Sodium 148 (136–145 mEq/L)
Potassium 3.4 (3.5–5.0 mEq/L)
Chloride 94 (96–106 mEq/L)
Carbon dioxide 32 (22–31 mEq/L)
Blood urea nitrogen 33 (8–20 mg/dL)
Creatinine 0.8 (0.7–1.3 mg/dL)

Phosphorus 3.4 (2.5–4.5 mg/dL)
Magnesium 1.9 (1.5–2.7 mg/dL)
Glucose 70 (70–139 mg/dL)
Total cholesterol 202 mg/dL (Desirable<200 mg/dL)
Albumin 3.5 (3.5–5.5 g/dL)
Vitamin B12 150 (200–950 pg/mL)

Clinical Data:

Past Medical History: Anorexia nervosa

Medications: None

Vital Signs: Blood pressure 93/55 mm Hg (sitting), 70/50 mm Hg (standing); Temperature 96.7°F; Heart rate 50 beats/min

Nutrition-Focused Physical Exam: Skin appears pale and dry. Lips appear dry with cracked, reddened corners of the mouth. Clavicular muscle wasting, thin extremities, and mild bruising on lower extremities noted. Hands and feet are cold to touch. Hair appears thin, dry, with noted thinning on scalp. Nails are thin and brittle. Mild abdominal distention noted.

Dietary Data:

Dietary History: Follows a vegetarian, low-fat diet. Limits dairy intake, although eats yogurt. Drinks water and black coffee daily.

Questions

1. How would you identify Emma's nutritional status?
2. What are your nutrition priorities for Emma during her inpatient hospitalization?
3. Write two Problem/Etiology/Signs and Symptoms (PES) statements for Emma.
4. Identify the nutrition interventions you would like to initiate for Emma to address the problems identified in your PES statements.
5. What indices are included in your monitoring and evaluation plan? Why?

adult thinness as mild, moderate, severe, and extreme as body mass index (BMI) values greater than or equal to 17, between 16 and 16.99, between 15 and 15.99, and less than 15, respectively.[1] Per the DSM-5-TR (text-revised version), individuals with a BMI of 19 or greater would not meet the criteria for "significantly low body weight" and instead should be diagnosed with OSFED.[1] It is important to note that an individual's weight history, body frame, and experienced physiological disturbances should be considered and may better indicate a weight deficit than a BMI value. Failure to maintain one's growth trajectory may indicate significantly low body weight for children and adolescents, even for those above the 5th percentile for BMI-for-age, which the Centers for Disease Control and Prevention (CDC) suggests as underweight.

Many risk factors are thought to play a role in the development of AN. Drug or alcohol misuse and psychiatric disorders such as anxiety disorders, panic disorder, and obsessive-compulsive disorder are some of the psychosocial factors associated with AN.[1] Influential social factors include cultural settings where thinness is valued, and criticism of one's weight or shape, especially from peers, parents, coaches, or significant others.[8] Professions that encourage a lean physique, such as modeling or elite athleticism, can also be instrumental in the development of an ED. Personality traits such as rigid and inflexible thinking, lack of spontaneity, perfectionism, low self-esteem, and need for control are characteristic of AN as well. Unintentional weight loss, for example, from illness, or adoption of new dietary or physical activity habits (e.g., becoming vegan/vegetarian, participating in organized sports), can also trigger ED behaviors.

The genetic component of the disorder is unclear; however, it has been shown that the likelihood of developing an ED is significantly increased in first-degree biological relatives of individuals with EDs. There is also a higher concordance rate of AN in monozygotic twins versus dizygotic twins. Alterations in brain serotonin levels, neuropeptide systems, and brain neurocircuitry are also thought to be components of ED etiology.[6,7]

Bulimia Nervosa

Bulimia nervosa (BN) is an ED characterized by recurrent episodes of binge eating followed by one or more compensatory behaviors to avoid weight gain. A binge is defined as the consumption of an unusually large amount of food within a discrete period of time, generally within 2 hours.[1] Feelings of loss of control over binging and purging behaviors and an intense sense of body dissatisfaction are central to diagnosis.[9] Patients generally maintain a body weight at or above minimally normal, as defined by BMI value,

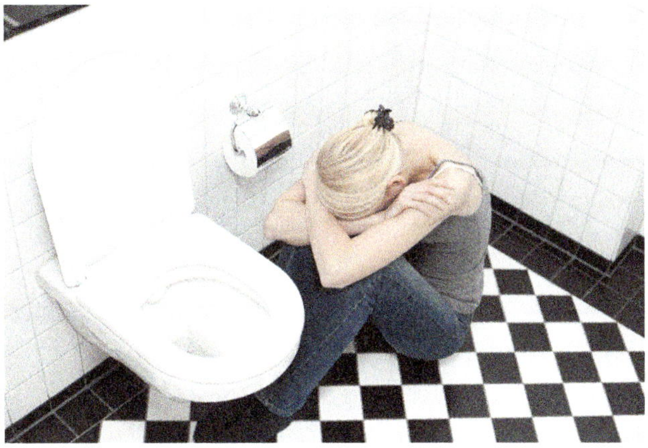

Figure 23.2 Individuals with Bulimia Nervosa Use Compensatory Behaviors, such as Self-Induced Vomiting, Misuse of Laxatives/Diuretics, Fasting, and/or Excessive Exercise

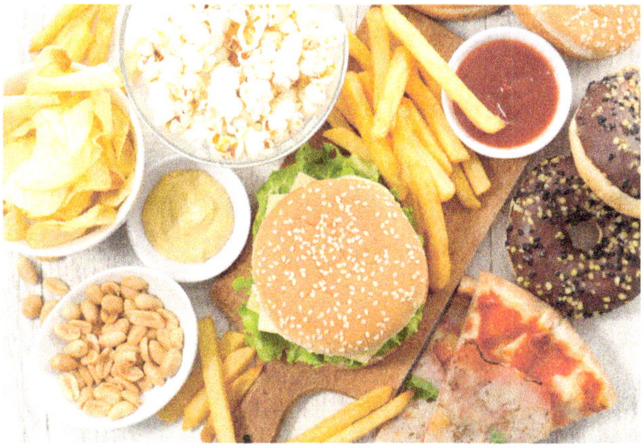

Figure 23.3 Foods That Are Consumed During a Binge Typically Include Energy-Dense Snacks and Desserts That Individuals Would Normally Avoid

differentiating this disorder from the binge–purge type of AN. The lifetime prevalence ranges from 0.46 to 1.5% among females and 0.05% to 0.24% among males in the United States, and only 43.2% of those affected are receiving treatment.[1,2,5,10] Like AN, the highest occurrences are in post-industrialized, high-income countries.[1]

The compensatory behaviors employed in BN are used to categorize individuals into one of two subtypes: purging type and non-purging type. Purging behaviors include self-induced vomiting (**Figure 23.2**) and laxative, enema, and/or diuretic misuse. Non-purging behaviors include excessive exercise and fasting. Individuals with type 1 diabetes mellitus (T1DM) and BN may reduce or omit insulin doses as a compensatory behavior in an attempt to decrease the uptake and utilization of carbohydrates consumed during a binge, a disordered behavior pattern coined "diabulimia."[1,8] Binging is central to the diagnosis of BN. Episodes of binge eating usually take place in secrecy and are accompanied by feelings of guilt and shame. Foods that are consumed during a binge vary on an individual basis, but typically include energy-dense snacks and desserts that the individual would normally avoid (**Figure 23.3**). Certain "triggers" may stimulate binge eating episodes, such as interpersonal stressors, dietary restraint, boredom, and negative feelings related to body shape, weight, and food.[11]

Like AN, there are many potential contributing factors to the development and course of BN. Psychosocial factors such as feelings of low self-esteem and anxiety; parental obesity and substance misuse; and childhood experiences such as sexual or physical assault, early pubertal maturation, and obesity are associated with BN. Individuals with BN tend to have a strong desire to lose weight and may have attempted to diet many times in the past. They may also experience adverse emotional states like anxiety, frustration, and labile mood, and may have psychiatric issues such as depression, personality disorders, and social anxiety disorders.[1]

PRACTICE POINT

Patients with BN generally maintain a body weight at or above minimally normal, which differentiates this disorder from the binge–purge type of anorexia nervosa.

Binge Eating Disorder

Binge eating disorder (BED) is characterized by recurrent binge eating episodes that are not followed by compensatory purging or non-purging behaviors. The lifetime prevalence of BED ranges from 1.25% to 3.5% among females and 0.42% to 2% among males in the United States.[1,5] BED is similarly prevalent among different racial and ethnic groups. Children and adolescents are less likely than adults to meet the criteria for the disorder; however, they may still experience some of the symptoms such as loss of control overeating.[12] Individuals with BED are generally overweight or obese and may be seeking weight loss treatment, particularly those interested in bariatric surgery.[7]

Binge eating episodes must be accompanied by a sense of lack of control, cause marked distress, and occur at least once a week for 3 months to be classified as BED.[1] Binges are typically characterized by rapid eating and eating when not physically hungry, eating alone due to embarrassment for the amount of food consumed, and are followed by feelings of guilt, disgust, and shame. Comparable to BN, individuals with BED tend to feel powerless over their eating behaviors and unhappy with their weight or body shape. BED may arise from multiple biological, psychological, social, and cultural factors. BED seems to occur in families, and has a heritability estimate of 41–57%.[6] Other risk factors for BED include substance misuse, childhood obesity, family weight concerns and eating issues, and physical or sexual assault. Food insecurity is associated with 1.67 higher odds of BED or subclinical BED and 1.31 higher odds of binge eating symptoms in early adolescence.[13] Adolescents who have experienced racial or ethnic discrimination are three times more likely to have BED than those who have not experienced racial or ethnic discrimination.[14]

PRACTICE POINT

Individuals with BED are generally overweight or obese and may be seeking weight loss treatment, particularly those interested in bariatric surgery

Other Specified Feeding or Eating Disorder

The DSM-5 defines OSFED as "presentations of characteristics of feeding and eating disorders that cause clinically significant distress or impairment in social, occupational, or other areas of functioning," but do not meet the full criteria for any other disorder in the feeding and ED diagnostic class.[1] Lifetime prevalence of individuals with OSFED has been found to be higher than that of AN, BN, and BED, with overall lifetime prevalence estimated at 3.82% among females and 1.61% among males in the United States.[2]

Night eating syndrome (NES) falls under this category of EDs and is a disordered eating pattern characterized by morning anorexia, evening hyperphagia, and insomnia.[15] NES is comparable to BED in that both disorders are characterized by episodes of hyperphagia or binging and occur in individuals with body shape, weight, and eating concerns. NES is also associated with psychiatric issues such as anxiety and depression.[15] Individuals with NES differ in that they experience nocturnal anxiety, which is not symptomatic of BED. Crossover between the two disorders often occurs and approximately 9% of individuals with BED have NES as well.[16]

Other disorders classified as OSFED include individuals that meet criteria for BED or BN except for the frequency or duration of binging and purging behaviors. Atypical AN is also classified as OSFED and occurs when individuals meet the criteria for AN, but are of normal or above normal weight, per BMI value, despite significant weight loss. Purging disorder is another example where individuals engage in purging behaviors to influence weight or shape, but do not engage in binge eating behaviors.[1]

Unspecified Feeding or Eating Disorder

The diagnosis of unspecified feeding or eating disorder is used when a clinician chooses not to specify the reasons an individual does not meet the full criteria for a specific ED. This could be used in situations when the clinician lacks sufficient information to make a more specific diagnosis. For instance, if the patient is in an emergency room setting, or unwilling to provide information, the clinician may be unable to formulate an accurate diagnosis.[1]

Avoidant/Restrictive Food Intake Disorder

Avoidant/restrictive food intake disorder (ARFID) is defined by the DSM-5 as a persistent disturbance in eating resulting in failure to meet appropriate nutritional and/or energy needs, leading to significant clinical consequences, such as one of more of the following: weight loss (or inadequate weight gain or growth in children and adolescents), significant nutrient deficiencies, dependence on enteral feedings or oral supplements, and/or impaired psychosocial functioning (such as an inability to eat with others).[1] The primary symptoms of ARFID include lack of interest in food or eating, food avoidance due to sensory characteristics of food, and fear of potential aversive consequences associated with food intake (e.g., choking or vomiting). Patients are typically diagnosed with ARFID in childhood or adolescence; however, it can also affect adults, with either adult onset or persistence through childhood.[17] Prevalence information on ARFID is limited. Unlike other categories of eating disorders, occurrence appears to be equally common in females and males (**Figure 23.4**). However, it is greater in males when ARFID is comorbid with autism spectrum disorder. ARFID differs from AN in that the preoccupation with body weight and shape is not the driving force of restrictive behaviors.[1]

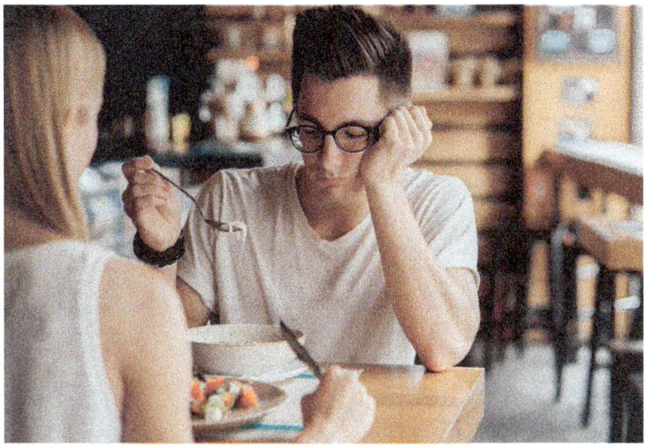

Figure 23.4 Both Females and Males Struggle with Eating Disorders

Orthorexia and Disordered Eating

EDs differ from disordered eating in that eating disorders are clinically diagnosed mental health disorders that significantly impact one's quality of life. Disordered eating may include similar behaviors to EDs like restrictive or compulsive eating, food or weight preoccupation, rigid food and exercise rules, and compensatory behaviors, but differ in frequency and severity. Although not clinically recognized as an ED, disordered eating behaviors should not be dismissed by healthcare professionals as they can still adversely affect one's physical and mental health and quickly evolve into a clinical eating disorder.

Orthorexia is a form of disordered eating that describes a pathological preoccupation with healthy eating. It may begin as an attempt at healthy eating and turn into an obsession with food-related topics, the quality of food in the diet, and rigid beliefs about food. Disordered behaviors may include compulsive checking of food ingredient lists, avoidance of several foods or food groups, consumption of only foods deemed "healthy" or "clean," and distress when accepted foods are unavailable or "unhealthy" foods are consumed. While these characteristics are similar to those of EDs, individuals with orthorexia differ in that their behaviors are not driven by the fear of weight gain, and/or preoccupation with weight loss. This pathological fixation on health-conscious eating behaviors is not recognized in the DSM-5 as a clinical diagnosis.[18]

Prognosis

EDs are associated with significant medical complications, physical and psychological morbidities, relapse, and mortality. They are considered spectral disorders because they exist on a continuum of severity and often become more severe the longer they are present. Even with psychiatric treatment and nutritional rehabilitation, relapses are common in EDs. Approximately one-third of individuals with EDs will experience relapse, with rates ranging from 40% to 50% in AN, and 30% in BN and BED.[19]

CORE CONCEPT 2

Eating disorders are spectral disorders because they exist on a continuum of severity and often become more severe the longer they are present.

Anorexia Nervosa

The course and outcome of AN are extremely variable. The average age of onset is 19 years and is generally associated with a stressful life event, such as leaving home for college.[1] Many individuals adopt a new eating behavior, such as vegetarianism, prior to developing the disorder.[20] Such changed behaviors may serve as a red flag for clinicians to intervene.[10] During the course of the disorder, crossover between the AN subtypes often occurs. For instance, individuals with the restricting type may begin to engage in binge eating and purging behaviors. Crossover between subtypes post-ED treatment is even more likely to occur.[21]

PRACTICE POINT

Many individuals develop a new eating behavior, such as vegetarianism, prior to developing anorexia nervosa.

Clinical Complications

Many physiological changes can occur during the course of AN. These may include development of brittle hair and nails; **lanugo** or soft, downy hair growth on the face and body; ketotic breath caused by ketosis; cyanosis of the extremities; hypercarotenemia, or the presence of orange pigment in the skin typically related to overconsumption of carotenoid-containing foods (**Figure 23.5**); and hypothermia, and/or cold intolerance. Protein-energy malnutrition often results from inadequate intake, causing a loss of adipose tissue and somatic protein stores. Resultant cachectic and prepubescent-appearing bodies are distinct features of AN.[9] Serious cardiac complications such as bradycardia, arrhythmias, and orthostatic or postural hypotension, which is a drop in blood pressure that

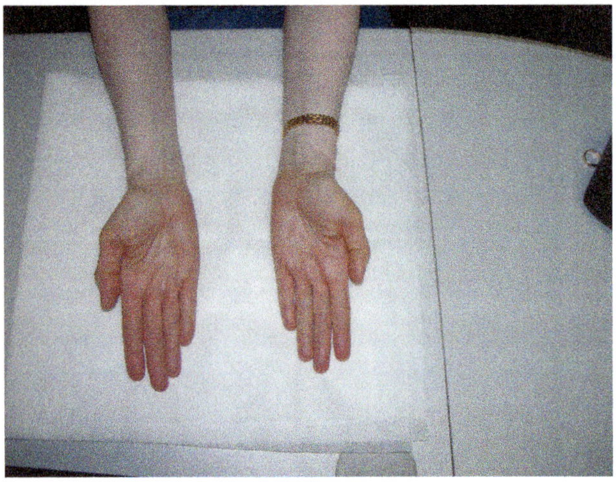

Figure 23.5 Individuals Who Consume a Diet Excessively High in Carotenoid-Containing Foods May Develop Orange Pigment in the Skin

Reproduced with permission from *Atlas Dermatológico*. Accessed January 14, 2026. http://www.atlasdermatologico.com.br/disease.jsf?diseaseId=69

occurs upon standing from a sitting or lying down position, are often found in AN, but are largely reversible with restoration and correction of dietary deficiencies.[11] Gastrointestinal (GI) issues that can result include delayed gastric emptying, severe constipation, and decreased small bowel motility. Peripheral edema can also occur from cessation of diuretics that may have been used in the binge–purge type.[20]

A decrease in resting energy expenditure (REE) will occur secondary to weight loss, decreased lean body mass, energy restriction, and decreased leptin levels. As patients refeed and restore weight, REE increases and often results in hypermetabolism.[22] Physical activity can account for up to 50% of total energy expenditure in patients with AN due to decreased REE.[23]

Postmenarcheal women with AN may develop **amenorrhea**, which is the absence of three consecutive menstrual cycles. Prepubescent males and females can experience sexual maturation arrest, in which males may develop a testosterone deficiency, and females may experience primary amenorrhea or delayed menarche, which is not achieving first menses by age 15 years. Low leptin levels are a key feature of AN and reflect a low body fat mass, as adipocytes secrete this hormone in proportion with the body's adipose stores. Leptin helps regulate the oscillating levels of luteinizing hormone and estradiol, thus low levels of estradiol are characteristic to AN as well.[7] Other hormonal alterations, like a decrease in the thyroid hormone triiodinethyroxine (T3), known as T3 syndrome, can occur and may alter metabolic functioning.

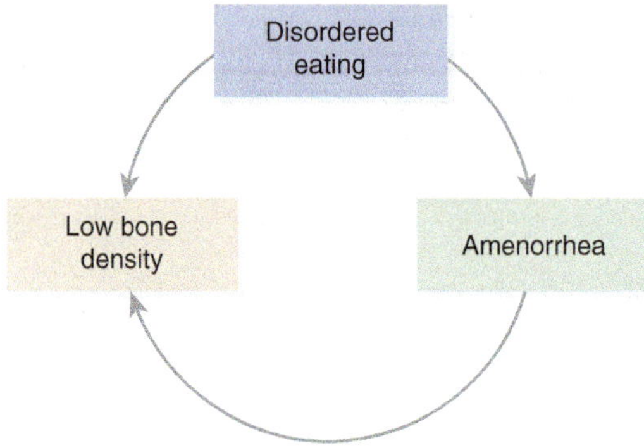

Figure 23.6 The Female Athlete Triad

Bone mineral density significantly decreases early in the course of illness and may not be fully reversed by recovery. In a state of starvation, bone metabolism will favor resorption, which impedes bone formation.[24] In an 8-year follow-up of patients with AN, it was found that low body weight was associated with low bone mineral density in the spine, and 2 or more years of amenorrhea was associated with reduced bone mineral density in the hip and spine.[25] Bone mineral loss and hormonal alterations are two key features of a syndrome known as **female athlete triad**, which consists of disordered eating habits, osteoporosis, and menstrual disorders (**Figure 23.6**). These females typically utilize at least one unhealthy weight control method and exhibit characteristics of perfectionism, competitiveness, and high self-motivation. Female athletes may have classifiable eating disorders, but not all meet the criteria for AN. The term "anorexia athletica," is often used to distinguish the disrupted eating behaviors associated with training and sports performance from pathological AN.[26]

The three areas of this triad are interrelated through physiological and psychological mechanisms. Psychological pressures for elite performance are often perceived as requiring low body mass, which may lead to high-volume training and low energy intake. Chronic low energy intake can temporarily pause the menstrual cycle to conserve energy; low body weight, excessive exercise, and stress can halt the cycle as well. Resultant amenorrhea causes a decrease in the production of estrogen, a major hormone required for maintaining bone mineral density. Hypoestrogenic states are associated with low bone mineral density and high osteoporosis risk.[26]

AN is associated with cerebral changes, such as significant loss of gray and white matter, cerebral atrophy, and enlarged ventricles. The severity of cerebral changes is related to the amount of weight loss.[8] Psychosocial symptoms of AN may include social withdrawal, irritability, insomnia, and depressed

CASE STUDY REVISITED

Emma is admitted to the hospital, and the medical team immediately provides intravenous fluids of D5W at 125 mL/hour to treat her dehydration. She starts on a regular diet and is provided oral nutrition supplements at mealtimes.

Questions

1. What physiological complications of AN does Emma exhibit?
2. How would you interpret Emma's labs?
3. How might you expect her labs to change after she receives intravenous fluids?
4. Is her REE expected to be high or low at this time, and why?
5. How would you expect her REE to change during the weight restoration process?

mood. Substance misuse, suicidal ideation, self-hatred, and self-harm behaviors may also occur. Patients may also be perfectionistic and extremely focused on work or schoolwork. Cognitive symptoms may include dichotomous thinking, difficulty in thinking clearly or concentrating and making decisions, and distorted body image where patients often experience themselves as being in much larger bodies than they are in reality. Patients also may exhibit obsessive-compulsive features, both related and unrelated to food. Preoccupation with food and weight-related thoughts might manifest as a desire to cook for others, collect recipes, or hoard food. The Minnesota Starvation Experiment, a well-known study conducted by Ancel Keys during World War II, suggested a link between these obsessive and compulsive behaviors and undernutrition.[27,28] Refer to the Clinical Roundtable for more information about the Minnesota Starvation Experiment.

Relapses and Mortality

Disordered cognition about food and eating behaviors can be difficult to overcome, making relapses in AN common. Predictors of AN relapse include age, psychosocial functioning, preoccupation with and misperception of body weight or shape, and individual psychotherapy.[21] Sometimes, relapse may involve a brief return of ED behaviors that self-resolve; other times, relapse may be more severe, requiring the patient to seek medical treatment again. Hospital readmissions for AN have been significantly associated with three major factors: prior admission to the hospital, length of initial hospital stay, and rapid regain of weight.[29]

The crude mortality rate for AN is approximately 5% per decade.[1,21] Mortality rate and suicide risk are higher for individuals with AN compared to other EDs.[30] Mortality risk is higher in individuals with poor psychosocial functioning, low body weight, substance misuse, and a longer duration of illness.[31]

Bulimia Nervosa

The average age of onset for BN is 20 years and is typically initiated during or after an attempt at dieting for weight loss or multiple stressful events.[1,5] Disordered eating patterns associated with BN generally occur for several years and exhibit either a chronic or intermittent course. Crossover from BN to AN occurs in 10% to 15% of cases and usually results in the return of BN behaviors. Other individuals may continue to binge eat, but no longer engage in compensatory behaviors at a certain point.[1]

Clinical Complications

Individuals with BN are usually of normal weight, as defined by BMI classification, and often keep their ED behaviors secretive, making clinical detection difficult. When vomiting is the compensatory mechanism utilized, certain signs and symptoms can help identify the disorder, such as eroded dental enamel, increased incidence of dental caries, gingivitis, enlarged parotid glands, and **Russell's sign** (the scarring by teeth of the lower dorsum of the hand from repeated use to stimulate the gag reflex). Chronic vomiting can result in dehydration, alkalosis, and hypokalemia, and can manifest as a sore throat, esophagitis, subconjunctival hemorrhage, and mild hematemesis. More serious complications include **Mallory-Weiss tears**, or tears in the mucosa at the stomach–esophagus junction; esophageal rupture; and acute gastric dilation. Laxative misuse may result in dehydration, elevated serum aldosterone and vasopressin levels, rectal bleeding, abdominal cramps, and intestinal atony. Individuals that misuse laxatives may experience rectal prolapse or become dependent on laxatives to stimulate bowel movements.[7,9]

Compensatory behaviors put individuals with BN at increased risk for serious electrolyte abnormalities. Hypokalemia, one of the most common abnormalities observed with self-induced vomiting, can lead to atrial and ventricular arrhythmias. It has been found that generally 40% of individuals who purge twice or more daily are hypokalemic.[11] Individuals who utilize ipecac syrup, an emetic agent typically used to induce vomiting after ingestion of poison, as a compensatory behavior are at risk for cardiomyopathy due to emetine, a cardiac toxin found in ipecac. Death from ventricular arrhythmias or congestive heart failure can occur when excessive amounts are consumed.[11] **Figure 23.7** outlines the clinical complications observed in both AN and BN.

The effect of compensatory behaviors on REE is not entirely clear. Some studies have shown that purging decreases metabolic rate, while other studies have shown that its effects are insignificant.[32,33] Dietary restriction, found in both AN and BN, is thought to decrease REE by putting the body into semi-starvation mode, while binge eating behaviors may partially compensate this reduction.[34] Psychosocial characteristics include drug or alcohol misuse, social irregularities such as alternation between withdrawal and erratic need for social contact, low self-esteem, self-disgust, and depression. Inability to identify and/or express feelings, obsessive or perfectionistic qualities, and self-harm behaviors are also common.[8]

Relapse and Mortality

Patients who experience full remission for 1 year after treatment have better long-term outcomes than those that relapse within the first year. Some predictors of relapse have been identified as level of psychosocial functioning; anxiety about weight or body shape; lower scoring on the Global Assessment Functioning Scale, a numeric scale used by mental health clinicians to subjectively rate an individual's social, occupational, and psychological functioning; and higher mania scoring on the Psychiatric Status Rating Scale, a rating scale used by mental health clinicians to evaluate degree of mental illness.[21] Like AN, suicide risk is also elevated for individuals with BN. The crude mortality rate is 2% per decade, and individuals with BN are considered to have a significantly elevated risk for mortality.[1]

Binge Eating Disorder

Little is known about the development and course of BED, as it has more recently begun to gain empirical attention. The average age of onset is 25 years, with onset typically occurring in adolescence or young adulthood, although onset later in adulthood has been documented as well.[1,5] Unlike BN, attempts at dieting often follow the development of the disorder rather than preceding it. BED is a relatively persistent disorder, and its course is generally comparable to BN in terms of severity and duration.[1]

Clinical Complications

BED is associated with increased risk for weight gain and development of obesity. Obesity and obesity in BED are two distinct conditions in that most individuals with obesity do not engage in binge eating behaviors and on average consume fewer calories than individuals with obesity and BED.[1] This puts individuals with BED at a significantly higher risk for

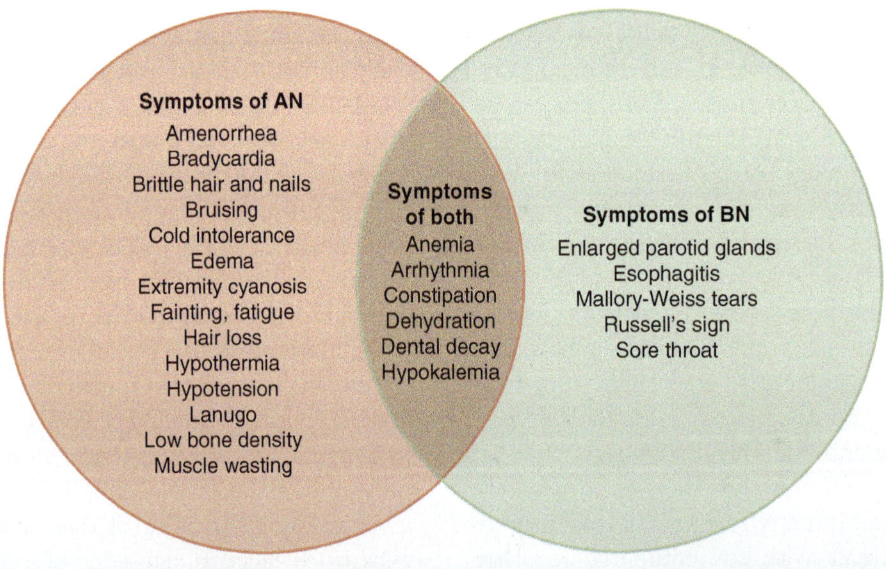

Figure 23.7 Comparison of Clinical Complications of AN and BN

Clinical Roundtable

Topic: The Minnesota Starvation Experiment

Background: During World War II, Ancel Keys and his colleagues conducted a prospective, randomized controlled trial to gain insight in to the physical and psychological effects of semi-starvation and the obstacles involved in refeeding in order to better understand how to refeed civilians who had been starved during the war. The findings of this landmark study demonstrated how starvation and nutrition dramatically impact the mind as well as the body. The study has been helpful in understanding the implications of food deprivation on both physiological and cognitive functioning in individuals with AN and BN.

At a Minnesota lab in 1944, 36 male volunteers, many of whom were conscientious objectors who wanted to contribute to the war effort, were observed at baseline for 3 months, during a semi-starvation phase for 6 months, and in a nutrition rehabilitation phase for 3 months. The research protocol was designed to have volunteers lose 25% of their normal body weight by following a hypocaloric meal plan. Additionally, participants expended energy walking 22 miles/week and tending to various duties like housekeeping, laboratory work, and participating in university classes and activities. Measurements of physical strength, body weight, and endurance were taken in addition to clinical monitoring that included laboratory measures and electrocardiograms.

Some of the side effects reported during the semi-starvation state were physical symptoms such as decreased stamina and libido, intolerance to cold temperatures, hair loss, and dizziness. Participants also reported experiencing fatigue, apathy, introversion, irritability, and decreased ability to concentrate. Some participants began reading and collecting cookbooks; hoarding or hiding food instead of eating it; and savoring food by eating slowly, taking small bites, or adding water to meals to increase volume. Some participants would "cheat" from their diet; for instance, on a trip into town, one participant demonstrated binge-like behaviors where he consumed milkshakes and ice cream sundaes in excess instead of following the hypocaloric meal plan. Excessive gum chewing and caffeine intake also emerged for some during this malnourished stage, with reports of up to 40 packs of gum per day and 15 cups of coffee per day between meals. Participants also experienced distorted body image, not seeing themselves as excessively thin despite appearing cachectic.

In the 3-month rehabilitation phase, calorie increases were distributed among four subgroups: initially an additional 400, 800, 1200, and 1600 kcal/day each. It was found that vitamin and protein supplements were ineffective for weight gain at this stage and only abundant calories aided restoration. Keys found a positive effect when 800 kcal/day were added to each group and concluded that around a total of 4000 kcal/day for some months was necessary for rehabilitation.

Almost 60 years after the experiment, 18 of the participants were interviewed about their experience in the Minnesota study. They all felt it took longer than 3 months of rehabilitation to feel back to normal, and that there were some lingering aftereffects of the study. They all spoke passionately about what made them volunteer for the study and that even after going through the grueling experience, they would make the sacrifice again.

Roundtable Discussion

The Minnesota Experiment participants and Keys may not have known the insight this experiment would provide in the treatment and understanding of EDs.

1. How might the physical side effects experienced by the participants be similar to symptoms observed in AN?
2. One of the surprising findings of the study was the psychological impact of the hypocaloric diet. How do the psychological side effects described by the Minnesota Experiment correlate with EDs in general and AN in particular?
3. Describe how Keys's findings of the refeeding process help us to understand hypermetabolism in the refeeding process and caloric requirements necessary to restore weight.

References

1. Franko DL, Keshaviah A, Eddy KT, et al. A longitudinal investigation of mortality in anorexia nervosa and bulimia nervosa. *Am J Psychiatry*. 2013;170(8):917–925.
2. Kalm FL, Semba RD. They starved so that others be better fed: remembering Ancel Keys and the Minnesota Experiment. *J Nutrition*. 2005;135(6):1347–1352.

developing type 2 diabetes mellitus and cardiovascular diseases such as coronary artery disease, hypertension, and hyperlipidemia.[12] Other comorbidities such as gastroesophageal reflux disease (GERD), obstructive sleep apnea, and hypothyroidism may be common.[35] Compared to obese, BMI-matched controls, individuals with BED experience greater functional impairment, lower quality of life, and increased health-care utilization. They also experience a higher lifetime prevalence of substance misuse problems and psychological comorbidities like major depressive disorder, personality disorders, substance use disorder, anxiety disorder, and disruptive behavior disorder such as attention-deficit/hyperactivity disorder.[1,35] Psychosocial symptoms of BED are similar to BN and may also include negative affect regulation, alterations in reward processing, and inhibitory control issues.[35]

Relapse and Mortality

Those who seek treatment for BED tend to be older than those seeking treatment for other EDs. Many times, weight that was lost during treatment is regained within the first year. Like AN and BN, BED increases the risk for medical morbidities and mortality. Remission rates are higher for BED than for AN or BN and crossover from BED to other EDs is uncommon.[1]

The Interdisciplinary Team

The complex nature of EDs calls for a collaborative approach to treatment by an interdisciplinary team (IDT). The IDT traditionally consists of a medical provider (e.g., primary care physician, internist, nurse practitioner, physician assistant), psychiatrist or psychiatric nurse practitioner, mental health counselor (e.g., psychotherapist, licensed social worker), and nutrition counselor. Members of the team may vary based on the patient's needs; for example, there may not be a psychiatrist if treatment does not include prescribed medication.

Medical providers are required for the treatment and management of medical complications related to eating disorders. This includes medical monitoring, such as obtaining and evaluating vital signs, throughout the course of treatment. As a patient becomes more physically stable, medical monitoring will become less frequent, and the focus of the medical provider may shift to more preventative primary care.[8] Psychiatrists or psychiatric nurse practitioners may diagnose mental health disorders and provide medication to help treat them. Mental health counselors address mental, behavioral, and emotional disorders. They provide support and psychoeducation for patients with EDs and potentially for a patient's family or support system. Their role becomes more involved as a patient becomes better nourished, making counseling sessions more accessible and efficacious. For example, patients may become better equipped to learn and utilize coping skills in a nourished versus malnourished state. Nutrition counselors, or RDs, provide nutrition assessments, interventions, and continued monitoring and evaluation directed toward treatment goals (e.g., correcting nutrient deficiencies, weight restoration, weight maintenance, ceasing of binge eating behaviors, etc.). This includes, but is not limited to, meal planning, normalizing eating behaviors, expanding food choices, providing nutrition education, and counseling to help decrease ED thoughts related to food, eating, body image, and weight.

It is imperative that the IDT work collaboratively, aligning in their treatment goals and philosophy, and communicating regularly throughout the course of treatment. The medical provider and RD may collaborate on weight-related goals while the psychiatrist, mental health counselor, and medical provider collaborate on medications. The RD and mental health counselor may collaborate on approaches to body image issues and food fears. Both the RD and mental health counselor may collaborate with patients' families on meal planning and family issues, respectively. Different team members may come together to address various aspects of treatment while collectively working toward the same treatment goals.

Regular communication and collaboration amongst the entire IDT can help to prevent *splitting*, a term used to describe patients' attempts at creating discord across the treatment team. This might include communicating with one provider that they dislike another provider on the team or being dishonest about a team member's recommendations during treatment. For instance, a patient may share with their RD that their medical provider will clear them for exercise as long as the RD is also in agreement. They may do this in an attempt to receive clearance on exercise from the RD, meanwhile they have not in fact received it from their medical provider. In this situation, the RD should contact the medical provider directly to confirm before providing clearance.

RDs are often the first point of contact for patients seeking help for an ED, or often the first to recognize ED behaviors in an individual who sought counseling for an unrelated reason. It is important for RDs to convey that an IDT approach is the standard of care for ED treatment.[7] Patients with undiagnosed EDs may be unaware of their need for more support. RDs may approach the topic of assembling an IDT by reflecting statements made by the patient; for example, how a mental health provider may provide support for their identified anxiety with eating.[8] For pediatric patients, RDs may inform their parents of ED concerns and receive consent for assembling an IDT.

RDs may obtain consent to speak with a patient's current mental health counselor or medical provider, such as the patient's primary care physician, to share their concerns and begin to collaborate care. Medical and mental health providers without training or experience working with ED populations may not feel qualified to collaborate on the treatment of a patient's ED, and the RD may need to assist with finding new providers for the patient to ensure adequate care. Resources such as the National Alliance for Eating Disorders and the National Association of Anorexia Nervosa and Associated Disorders (ANAD) provide a directory of treatment centers and ED providers across the United States. It is ideal for the IDT to be experienced in ED treatment, and also to be kind, empathetic, and firm in their approach, taking EDs seriously and understanding the dynamics of working with this patient population.

Individuals with EDs may respond differently to the recommendation of establishing an IDT. Some may welcome it and provide consent for the RD to assist. Others may deny the severity of their ED warranting the need for additional support. RDs may require that a patient with an ED have an IDT in order to continue nutrition counseling. Additionally, RDs in the outpatient setting may need to deny care if a patient presents with symptoms requiring a higher level of care. It is also important to note that while the typical patient with an ED and nutrition counselor relationship can be challenging at times, sometimes patient–counselor relationships may just not be a good fit. If an RD feels that a patient may be better served working with a different nutrition counselor, whether it be due to expertise or approach, they should honor that and make a referral.[8]

Psychological Treatment

EDs are complex psychiatric illnesses that require ongoing psychological treatment. Nutrition education and physical restoration alone do not constitute recovery; cognitive and emotional restoration must be achieved in treatment as well. Research has shown that when cessation of disturbed eating behaviors and physical restoration occur early in the treatment process, better responses to psychotherapy and improved overall prognosis result.[7] Family-based treatment, **cognitive behavioral therapy (CBT)**, interpersonal psychotherapy, and **dialectical behavioral therapy (DBT)** are forms of psychotherapeutic treatment that have been shown to be effective in the treatment of EDs.

CORE CONCEPT 3

Research has shown that when cessation of disturbed eating behaviors and physical restoration occur early in the treatment process, better responses to psychotherapy and improved overall prognosis result.

The **Maudsley approach** or Maudsley method, also known as "family-based treatment," has been shown to be an effective treatment for adolescents with AN and BN.[36,37] This approach empowers parents to take on the responsibility of weight restoring their child, transform their relationship to involve issues other than food, and help their child resume normal adolescent behavior without having an ED.[38] Involving family members in treatment may also provide a more reliable recollection of a patient's history of weight loss, dietary intake prior to ED onset, and other features of the illness, as patients with EDs generally deny or lack insight to their disorder.[1]

The Maudsley approach consists of three phases: weight restoration, returning control over eating to the adolescent, and establishing a healthy adolescent identity.[39,40] The first phase focuses on empowering parents to disrupt the ED and support their adolescent by taking charge of their eating; parents are responsible for providing meals and snacks that ensure nutritional needs are met to aid weight restoration and cease binge and purge behaviors. Parents may follow a meal plan created by their adolescent's RD at this stage.[8] This stage also helps parents to see their adolescent's ED behaviors as separate from their adolescent. The second phase of treatment focuses on restoration of physical health and the transition of control overeating back to the adolescent. The third phase occurs when a healthy, stable weight is achieved, binge and purge behaviors have ceased, and focuses on the ways the family can help to address the effects of the ED on adolescent developmental processes, family dynamics, and individuation.[8,39,40] It is important for the IDT to determine if their patient and patient's family would be appropriate for family-based therapy, as this approach may not be suitable for all patients and families.

CBT is regarded as the first-line treatment for BN.[30] CBT is a highly structured therapy that identifies and replaces maladaptive behaviors and cognitive processes with more suitable ones (e.g., discrimination between physical symptoms, such as bloating, with resumption of food intake and body weight changes).[7] Interpersonal psychotherapy has also been shown to be efficacious in BN treatment. This form of therapy may reduce the risk of a setback by helping patients recognize and cope with psychosocial stressors that contribute to their disordered eating. Both CBT and interpersonal therapy have been effective in decreasing binge eating habits for individuals with BED.[21,41] A combination of CBT and behavioral treatments (e.g., weight management programs or counseling) has shown positive results in BED treatment as well.[41]

DBT is designed to help individuals change unhelpful patterns of behavior by identifying triggers and applying new coping skills. When used in ED treatment, it involves teaching new coping skills, replacing ED behaviors with more constructive ones, and enhancing self-respect. This method holds potential for decreasing episodes of binge eating, which may be influenced by emotional dysregulation and used as a maladaptive coping skill.[7]

Pharmacotherapy

Pharmacotherapy for treatment of EDs is an area of ongoing research. Recent trials have shown that olanzapine, an atypical neuroleptic agent, improved both weight and dysfunctional thinking in patients with AN.[42,43] Medications such as **selective serotonin reuptake inhibitors (SSRIs)** may also be prescribed to patients with AN to alleviate mood symptoms or reduce anxiety; however, they have demonstrated low efficacy in treatment of AN. It is important to note that SSRIs may not be effective in the severely malnourished.[42] Fluoxetine, a type of SSRI, is currently the only U.S. Food and Drug Administration (FDA) approved drug to treat BN.[7] Tricyclic antidepressants and SSRIs have been found to alleviate some symptoms of BN and BED.[41,44] Lisdexamfetamine, a stimulant, is FDA approved for the treatment of BED.[35] Certain antiepileptic medications have been efficacious in suppression of binge eating episodes and reduction of body weight as well.[44] It is important to note that medication is typically used as adjuvant therapy to nutrition and mental health counseling and physiological monitoring and interventions; it should not be considered a standalone treatment.

Nutrition Assessment

The nutrition assessment will depend on the stage of illness and treatment setting, but will generally include measuring anthropometrics, evaluating dietary and fluid intake, assessing eating behaviors and attitudes, interpreting biochemical data, and applying a nutrition diagnosis to create a treatment plan for nutritional rehabilitation.

Anthropometric Assessment

Anthropometric assessment in the ED population includes measurement of body weight, height, and fat percentage. Height should be assessed to confirm accuracy of reported value and account for any losses that could result from osteoporosis. Regular height measures should be obtained for pediatric and adolescent patients every 3–6 months. For patients with AN, a daily preprandial weight should be taken gowned, post-void, and first thing in the morning for patients in an inpatient setting. Outpatients who are weight restoring should also be weighed post-void and gowned, if possible. Street clothes may be worn for weight measurement in the outpatient setting, removing shoes, pocket items, and outer layers or jackets. Street clothes typically account for 2–4 pounds (0.9–1.8 kg).[8] It is important to be cautious that patients may attempt to produce false weights by withholding bowel movements, waiting to void, drinking excessive fluids, or hiding weighted objects on themselves.

Taking a blind weight is a common practice in ED treatment and may be taken by having the patient step backwards onto the scale facing away from the reading, or on a scale where the reading is not visible to the patient. This weight check method may be preferred by patients and beneficial early on in treatment as it can help to reduce weight-related anxiety, potentially increasing the patient's ability to engage in treatment and aiding the weight restoration process. Blind weights are thought to also promote tolerance of weight uncertainty and help patients to become less focused on the scale. As treatment progresses, viewed weights may be better tolerated. Practitioners can routinely conduct viewed weights or discuss weight trends to help desensitize patients to knowing their weight.[45] Patient preference and treatment program protocols regarding blind or viewed weights may vary per patient and facility. Estimation of body fat percentage may be required for malnourished clients in an inpatient setting and can be obtained from skinfold measurements taken from the tricep, bicep, subscapular, and suprailiac regions.[9]

PRACTICE POINT

Patients with eating disorders may try to produce false weights by withholding bowel movements, waiting to void, drinking excessive fluids, or hiding weighted objects on themselves.

Dietary Assessment

In obtaining diet history, the RD should assess the patient's overall energy intake, macronutrient distribution, and fluid consumption.[7] Patients with AN tend to overestimate their caloric intake and fail to recognize that their eating habits are extremely restrictive. The distributions of macronutrients consumed are affected as a result. Aversion of high-fat foods and adoption of a vegetarian diet are common; reasons for following a vegetarian diet should be evaluated by the RD to determine if they are being used as a guise to limit intake.[9]

Micronutrient intake generally parallels macronutrient intake: fat-restricted diets may result in deficiencies of fat-soluble vitamins and essential fatty acids (EFA). Avoidance of fats puts individuals at greater risk for EFA deficiencies. Vegetarian diets are commonly low in protein, vitamin B12, iron, and zinc, while vegan diets may additionally be low in calcium, iodine, and vitamin D. B vitamin deficiencies, particularly riboflavin, vitamin B6, thiamine, folic acid, and vitamin B12, are commonly reported in EDs, especially in lower weight patients with AN. Both insufficient intake of meat and carbohydrates and alcohol use disorder can cause or intensify these deficiencies.[46] A deficiency in vitamin B6 can exacerbate EDs due to its effects on serotonin and appetite.

Fluid intake should also be assessed to identify whether the patient is restricting intake to avoid feeling full or drinking excessively to ward off hunger. Water loading, or excessive water intake, may be utilized as a weight manipulation method prior to weigh-ins to produce a falsely elevated weight. A urine-specific gravity level below 1.010 may indicate water loading.[7]

A 24-hour dietary recall may not provide an accurate diet representation for individuals with BN and BED, since chaotic eating patterns ranging from restrictive, to adequate, to binge eating are common in this population. Assessing intake over a week and averaging the total caloric intake over 7 days would provide a more accurate depiction of diet. Despite reports of feeling "empty" after compensatory behaviors used in BN, such as self-induced vomiting and laxative misuse, the majority of calories consumed prior are retained, making these behaviors ineffective for weight loss. Evidence has shown that up to 1200 calories are retained after a binge, whether that binge was 1500 or 3500 calories.[47] Laxative misuse also has minimal effects on the removal of calories as it has been shown to reduce calorie absorption by only up to 12%.[48]

RDs can begin to assess the patient's eating habits, behaviors, and attitudes while obtaining the diet history. Eating habits include the pattern of intake

⚠ Clinical Controversy

Vegetarianism and Eating Disorders

While many individuals adopt a vegetarian lifestyle due to environmental awareness, health concerns, and/or animal rights, some may use the diet as a tactic for weight loss or masking of an ED. Given the stigma of eating disorders, one may report adopting a vegetarian diet for animal rights as this would appear as a more socially acceptable reason to avoid or restrict foods than for weight control motives. Bardone-Cone et al. found that women with EDs are four times more likely to be vegetarian than women without EDs. It also found that more than 52% of women with a history of EDs had been vegetarians at one point in their lives, of which 42% were motivated by weight-related reasons and 68% perceived their vegetarianism to be related to their ED. In a systematic review by Sergentanis et al., a correlation between vegetarianism and the presence of EDs, particularly AN was found. This correlation was marked for adolescents, where an interconnection was reported between vegetarianism and ED behaviors for weight control. Common nutrient deficiencies associated with vegetarianism can impact appetite and mood, for example, B vitamins, vitamin D, omega-3 fatty acids, and zinc, potentially contributing to the onset or exacerbation of EDs. Timko et al. sought to identify whether various types of vegetarian diets (vegan, vegetarian, and semi-vegetarian) were related to the development of an ED. This study found that semi-vegetarians, but not full vegetarians or vegans, were most likely to engage in disordered eating behaviors and that vegans and vegetarians appeared to have the healthiest attitudes toward food.

Questions

1. Given the contradictory findings, how might clinicians interpret vegetarianism and eating pathology?
2. Should individuals at high risk of eating disorders be discouraged from following a vegetarian diet?
3. How might the adoption of various forms of vegetarianism guide a clinician in assessing dietary intent?
4. How would you determine whether it is appropriate to allow ED clients to continue their vegetarian lifestyle?

References

1. Bardone-Cone AM, Fitzsimmons-Craft EE, Harney MB, et al. The inter-relationships between vegetarianism and eating disorders among females. *J Acad Nutr Diet*. 2012;112(8):1247–1252.
2. Timko Ca, Hormes JM, Chubski J. Will the real vegetarian please stand up? An investigation of dietary restraint and eating disorder symptoms in vegetarians versus non-vegetarians. *Appetite*. 2012;58(3):982–990.
3. Sergentanis TN, Chelmi M-E, Liampas A, et al. Vegetarian diets and eating disorders in adolescents and young adults: a systematic review. *Children*. 2021;8(1):12.

(i.e., number of meals per day, time and duration of meals, eating environment, etc.), avoidance of specific food groups, amount of variation in the diet, and fluid intake. A common intake pattern among EDs is to be restrictive in the morning, saving the majority of caloric intake for later in the day. Patients with EDs may also have an eating cut-off time where they are fearful to take in calories past a certain hour. Duration of meals varies among EDs, in that patients with BN and BED tend to eat quickly, demonstrating their difficulty with satiety cues, while those with AN may eat slowly to avoid eating too much. The amount of variation in the diet is typically low in EDs, and patients tend to consume the same foods in the same-sized portions every day.[7,9] It is common for accepted or "safe" foods and portion sizes to continually decrease over time.

PRACTICE POINT

Dietary variety is typically low in patients with eating disorders, and the same foods in the same-sized portions tend to be consumed every day.

Many ritualistic, atypical behaviors are exhibited in EDs. Ritualistic behaviors include cutting food into small pieces, eating food in a certain order, not allowing different food items to touch, and moving food around the plate to avoid consumption. Patients may also use atypical seasonings like lemon juice and spices to avoid salt and may use excessive amounts of artificial sweeteners knowing they do not have caloric value. Unusual combinations of food and unusual use of utensils or fingers to eat are also characteristic in EDs.[7]

Attitudes about food include dichotomous thinking about foods that trigger binges as well as distorted ideas about portion sizes. Patients with EDs tend to view certain foods as being "good" or "bad," or foods that feel safe versus unsafe to eat. Foods that are higher in fat, sugar, or starch are often regarded as "bad," while fruits, vegetables, and lean proteins are regarded as "good." Patients with AN tend to avoid "bad" foods similarly to how individuals with BN and BED may try to avoid foods that trigger binge eating episodes. For some, over-restriction of "bad" foods can lead to intense cravings for them, causing them to trigger episodes of binging when encountered. Portion sizes of foods also tend to be inaccurately estimated in patients with EDs. Individuals with BN, for example, have been shown to overestimate the portion size of foods by more than 125% to 700%.[49]

Biochemical Assessment

It is generally accepted in the ED treatment community that laboratory values within normal limits do not reflect nutrition stability. The etiology behind this phenomenon relates to the metabolic changes that occur during starvation. During periods of low energy intake, there is a greater reliance on fatty acids and ketones as a source of energy to decrease use of protein for gluconeogenesis to spare lean body mass. If dietary protein is also lacking, amino acid recycling is increased, with reprioritization toward visceral protein synthesis. This conservation mechanism, which supports the body's adaptive ability to maintain visceral protein metabolism in chronic starvation mode, can initially hide nutrient deficiencies.[50] In addition, dehydration may mask serum albumin levels, making them appear normal. It may not be until the refeeding process begins, when metabolic activity improves and tissue repair and cell turnover start utilizing already low nutrient stores, that true deficiencies will be revealed.[46]

CORE CONCEPT 4

In the eating disorder community, laboratory values within normal limits do not reflect nutrition stability; conservation mechanisms, like the body's adaptive ability to maintain visceral protein metabolism in chronic starvation mode, can initially hide nutrient deficiencies.

Despite generally low-fat intake, abnormal lipid values are a common feature of EDs. Malnutrition may affect the functionality of the liver, resulting in high serum cholesterol levels. A low intake of EFAs may also be related to elevated cholesterol levels. Elevated liver function tests AST and ALT can be found due to liver dysfunction.[8] Postprandial hypoglycemia is another clinical feature of AN due to depleted hepatic glycogen reserves. Without these reserves, the liver is unable to normalize blood glucose levels following the elevated release of insulin that occurs in response to increased food intake.[20] Blood glucose levels may be decreased from poor nutrition intake or elevated in patients with diabetes from insulin omission. Low thyroid-stimulating hormone and low T3 levels may also result as an adaptation to fasting, starvation, and protein-energy malnutrition.

Low zinc and vitamin B12 levels are common in EDs and can result from insufficient energy intake, avoidance of red meat, or adoption of a vegetarian diet.[7] Zinc deficiency may also exacerbate EDs due

CASE STUDY REVISITED

On hospital day (HD) 2, you meet with Emma to complete a nutrition assessment. You start by getting additional information about her diet prior to admission.

Dietary Data:

Usual diet recall for 2 months prior to admission:
Breakfast (7 am): 24 oz black coffee with artificial sweetener
Lunch (12 pm): 1 apple, 1 veggie burger (no roll), 12 baby carrots, 12 oz water
Snack (3 pm): 6 oz fat-free plain Greek yogurt, 8oz black coffee with artificial sweetener
Dinner (6 pm): Salad with 2 cups romaine lettuce, 1 cup baby spinach, 1 tomato, 1 green pepper, ¼ chopped onion, ½ cup black beans, 3 Tbsp balsamic vinegar, 12 oz water
Snack (8 pm): 1 cup popcorn, 12 oz water

In collecting Emma's diet history, she reveals that she became vegetarian as an attempt to lose weight 2 years ago. She privately discloses that she has engaged in purging behaviors (self-induced vomiting) on days when she felt she "overate." Emma shares that since admission, she has mainly been drinking oral nutrition supplements because she has not yet been able to choose her meals from a hospital menu. She has been avoiding the food on her trays because they have been mainly "fear foods" such as pasta, white bread, butter, peanut butter, and dairy. She shares that she prefers to eat low-calorie, high-volume foods, such as raw vegetables, and asks if she can remain on a vegetarian diet in the hospital. Emma's mother enters the room at the end of your meeting and requests that her daughter start an iron supplement given her meat avoidance for the past 2 years.

Questions

1. How would you address Emma's vegetarianism and her mother's request?
2. How could incorporating more animal proteins potentially help with food volume? Would you encourage Emma to do this?
3. Considering her diet history and the nutrition-focused physical exam findings during her admission assessment, in addition to iron, what other micronutrients may Emma be lacking?
4. Given the information Emma provided about fear of food and difficulty eating, how might you help her increase her food intake?

PRACTICE POINT

Abnormal lipid levels are a common feature in EDs. Patients with AN who are malnourished can present with elevated cholesterol levels secondary to impaired liver functioning.

to its effects on the sense of taste and symptoms of depression.[46] Low vitamin D levels are often reported for patients with EDs related to decreased dairy intake and are also linked to mental health symptoms like anxiety and depression. Inadequate calcium intake is also common; however, it is unlikely to be reflected in serum calcium levels. A food frequency questionnaire or dietary recall would more accurately reveal low calcium intake. Iron deficiency anemia is common in women of childbearing age, with or without EDs. Patients who follow vegetarian or vegan diets are also at increased risk for deficiency, as well as patients with excessive exercise due to red blood cell hemolysis.[46]

Fluid and electrolyte abnormalities secondary to purging methods, fluid restriction or overload, metabolic changes, or a combination are normally present in EDs. Elevated blood levels of sodium, potassium, blood urea nitrogen, and creatinine may reflect dehydration, while overhydration or water loading may be reflected by low sodium and low chloride levels. GI losses from purging most commonly appear as hypokalemia but may also be revealed by decreased chloride and elevated bicarbonate and amylase levels. Laxative misuse may be reflected by elevated bicarbonate and decreased chloride levels as well.[7,46] Low levels of magnesium may result from laxative misuse and poor nutrition.

CORE CONCEPT 5

Individuals with eating disorders can present with fluid and electrolyte abnormalities secondary to purging methods, fluid restriction or overload, metabolic changes, or a combination of these.

Nutrition Intervention

Medical Nutrition Therapy

There is no professional consensus on restoring health and weight in AN, stopping binge–purge behaviors in BN, or modifying the disturbed thoughts and attitudes about food and body weight central to all EDs. Medical nutrition therapy guidelines for EDs are largely based on clinical experience. RDs provide medical nutrition therapy for the normalization of nutritional status and play an essential role in the treatment team.[5] Communication among the IDT members is imperative to ensure coordination of care, consistency of and adherence to treatment plans, and avoidance of drug–nutrient interactions. RDs may also act as a resource of nutrition education for other healthcare professionals and family members of patients.

CORE CONCEPT 6

Medical nutrition therapy guidelines for eating disorders are largely based on clinical experience.

Treatment for EDs may begin at one of five levels of care: inpatient hospitalization, residential treatment centers, partial hospitalization/full-day treatment, intensive outpatient, and outpatient.[49] The level of care required may depend on several factors, including severity of malnutrition and ED behaviors, degree of medical and psychiatric instability, weight percentage of ideal body weight (IBW), amount of structure and support needed for restoring weight and ceasing binge/binge–purge behaviors, geographic availability, and accessibility to treatment (i.e., health insurance coverage, affordability of care). Patients with EDs may require treatment at multiple levels of care. Whether a patient begins at an outpatient level of care and eventually requires inpatient stabilization, or gradually moves from higher to lower levels of care, it is common for patients with EDs to require more than one level of care throughout their course of treatment. It is also important to note that treatment may not be linear—it can fluctuate up and down in the level of care and amount of support needed as the severity of a patient's ED can vary over time.

Goals and Guidelines

Anorexia Nervosa

Nutrition rehabilitation goals for AN are to restore body weight and normalize eating patterns. Weight restoration is essential for recovery and will generally require supervision in a residential ED treatment program or specialized hospital unit for those who are severely malnourished. Treatment plans generally include a targeted weight gain of 2–3 lbs. (0.9–1.4 kg) per week in an inpatient setting, and 0.5–1 lb. (0.2–0.5 kg) per week in an outpatient setting.[51] It is important to note common weight fluctuations in AN. Body water loss can occur simultaneously with the depletion of glycogen stores and loss of lean tissue, while edema can occur secondary to constipation, malnutrition, and refeeding. Even in the most cautious approaches to refeeding, fluid retention will occur at first.[20] Sustained weight gain greater than 3 lbs. (1.4 kg) per week may indicate binge eating behavior, edema, bowel impaction, or weight manipulation.[8]

Goal weights, which may also be referred to as IBWs or **biologically appropriate weights (BAWs)**, may be established as a range instead of a specific number of pounds or kilograms and should be determined on an individual level. BAW refers to a person's genetically determined natural weight, or a weight at which a person is healthy, and can maintain with normal eating and exercise behaviors. Ranges should be individualized based on age, height, pubertal stage, premorbid weight and weight trends, and previous growth trajectories. Return of menses provides an objective measure of health in postmenarcheal females; however, BAWs for females are typically higher than the minimum weight required for menses.[8,42]

Growth charts containing multiple points of reference provide crucial information for expected growth trajectories and can be used to set a BAW (i.e., a more accurate, individualized IBW) for patients up to 20 years old. For example, setting IBW at the population average BMI-for-age (50th percentile) would not be a realistic expectation for an adolescent who previously trended between the 10th to 25th percentile, or the 75th to 90th percentile, BMI-for-age prior to ED onset. Research has shown that when IBW was set using a patient's growth charts to estimate BMI-for-age versus the standard 50th percentile BMI-for-age, it more closely estimated the weight at which menses returned in adolescents.[52] Growth charts also paint a picture of weight history prior to ED onset. Input from the treatment team and parents is crucial in setting weight goals for children and adolescents, because an IBW set too low may perpetuate EDs. For children, energy needs and weight goals must be readjusted every 3–6 months to account for growth.[7,42]

Adult goal weight ranges are more of a state of health that the treatment team can assess based on endocrine status, laboratory values, cognitive improvements, and overall nutrition status.[7] Some indicators that an individual has reached their BAW include absence of ED behaviors, adequate responses to hunger and fullness cues, absence or significant reduction in the intensity and frequency of ED thoughts, consistent and stable weight, normalized testosterone levels or regular menses, and absence of cold hands and feet.[8] There is limited research on setting a goal weight for adult patients. IBW calculations can vary in their estimated weights up to 15 lbs. (6.8 kg) for females and 25 lbs. (11.4 kg) for males depending on the formula used and may not estimate a BAW for an individual. For example, the Hamwi method would estimate an IBW of 125 lbs. (57 kg) for a 65-inch-tall female patient; however, her weight history may reflect that she was healthy and consistently stable around 140 lbs. (64 kg) prior to ED onset. Her weight history indicates that around 140 lbs. (64 kg) would be her BAW, and to use the IBW of 125 lbs. (57 kg) may perpetuate ED behaviors. Best practices include obtaining a detailed weight history to determine where a patient's weight and medical status was previously stable when nourished and healthy prior to use of ED behaviors. Nutrition counselors can create a weight timeline from gathering information such as the highest and lowest recent body weights, weight at menses, and weights associated with times of stress, illness, good health, and stability. Additionally, knowledge about a patient's family's weights and body shapes is helpful to consider.[8]

PRACTICE POINT

Goal weights, which may also be referred to as ideal body weights (IBWs) or biologically appropriate weights (BAWs), may be established as a range instead of a specific number of pounds or kilograms and should be determined on an individual level. Ranges should be individualized based on age, height, pubertal stage, premorbid weight, and previous growth trajectories.

Changes in REE must be considered during the refeeding process. The reintroduction of food causes a dramatic increase in diet-induced thermogenesis (DIT), or the thermic effect of food. In healthy individuals, DIT can account for 14–16% of REE and up to 30% of energy expenditure in patients with AN during the refeeding process.[53] As the body shifts from a starvation state to fed state, it shifts from energy conservation to increased energy utilization as it rebuilds tissues and muscles and carries out its various biochemical processes. Thus, during refeeding, REE begins to increase, and patients can become hypermetabolic, causing them to lose weight easily and require increasing amounts of energy to gain weight. REE eventually normalizes as food intake becomes adequate and weight and lean body mass are restored, although individuals may remain hypermetabolic for 3–6 months after weight restoration.[7,53] Additionally, energy intake may convert to heat before it can be used to build tissue, which can manifest as night sweats. These effects are obstacles to weight gain, and ongoing adjustments in caloric intake should be made to account for them. Cessation of physical activity will likely be necessary in the initial phases of treatment to promote weight gain, maintain or improve cardiac health, or normalize laboratory values. If a patient is medically stable, gentle movement such as stretching, yoga, tai chi, and short walks may be appropriate and provide some relief from GI discomfort.

CORE CONCEPT 7

Changes in resting energy expenditure must be considered during the refeeding process because the reintroduction of food causes a dramatic increase in diet-induced thermogenesis, or the thermic effect of food.

Prescribed daily caloric intakes should be individualized and involve vigilant clinical and laboratory monitoring to promote weight gain and prevent refeeding syndrome. Indirect calorimetry is the best method to determine whether the patient is hypometabolic or hypermetabolic; however, this is not always available for use. REE equations such as the Mifflin–St Jeor and Dietary Reference Intake for age may overestimate calorie needs in the initial stages of restoration and underestimate needs in the later stages of restoration, because increasingly more energy is needed to maintain the same rate of weight gain.[54] For instance, compared to individuals without EDs, patients with AN require higher caloric intake to maintain and restore weight. In order to maintain weight, 25–30 kcal/kg body weight/day, on average, is required for healthy individuals, while individuals with AN, over time, may require between 60 and 100 kcal/kg body weight/day to restore weight.[53,55] There is no general consensus on how to best estimate energy needs in patients with AN as clinical literature suggests there are significant variations among individuals, genders, and ED subtypes. For example, patients with AN typically require higher calorie meal plans to restore weight than patients with the AN binge–purge subtype.[8] The American Psychiatric Association recommends an initial caloric prescription of 1000–1600 kcal/day or 30–40 kcal/kg body weight per day.[51] A more individualized approach is to add 200–300 calories to a patient's current estimated caloric intake as a starting point.[8,51] For example, if a patient's estimated intake is 900 kcal/day, their recommended initial intake or meal plan would be prescribed at 1100–1200 kcal/day. To continue to aid weight restoration, an increase of 200–300 calories is prescribed when weight plateaus, and an increase of 500 calories is prescribed when weight decreases.[8] For example, if a patient's weight did not increase following a 1200 kcal/day meal plan, it would be increased to 1400–1500 kcal/day or increased to 1700 kcal/day if weight had been lost. Meal plans often require regular caloric increases to adjust to increasing REE and promote continued weight restoration. Males and females generally peak at 4000 and 3500 kcal/day, respectively, with meal plans ranging from 1850–4500 kcal/day.[8,20,51]

It is important to observe and address eating behaviors during times of high energy intake to confirm that patients are not discarding or hiding food or engaging in compensatory behaviors like vomiting or being secretly active. Behaviors such as excessive standing, pacing, and fidgeting to exert energy or weight manipulation tactics may increase as patients are required to consume higher calorie meal plans.

CORE CONCEPT 8

Indirect calorimetry is the best method to determine whether a patient with an eating disorder is hypometabolic or hypermetabolic.

The amount of empirical data regarding optimal food choices to support weight gain is limited. Increased dietary variety has been associated with better weight restoration and increases the probability of meeting macro- and micronutrient needs.[7,53] Currently, there are no specific recommendations for macronutrient distribution for patients with EDs. RDs can promote nutritional adequacy by creating meal plans that incorporate an appropriate balance of macronutrients.

Fat intake is crucial during refeeding to replenish depleted lipids and correct lipid alterations. Lipids play a key role in neuronal wiring between brain regions. EFAs are present in high concentrations in the brain and appear to play a role in memory, brain performance, and mental well-being. Deficiency of omega-3 fatty acids has been linked to psychiatric disorders like depression and psychological traits such as hostility.[1,56] Due to their high fat content, fatty fish and oils, such as canola and flaxseed, which are rich sources of omega-3 fatty acids, are likely to be avoided by patients with AN.

Vegetarian and vegan diets may need to be discouraged during the initial phases of refeeding to promote adequate EFA intake and high biological value (HBV) sources of protein.[7] Adequate protein intake from a mix of HBV sources and vegetable sources can increase the rate at which nutrient status is restored.[53] It may be helpful to initially incorporate "safer" HBV sources like fish or chicken when reintroducing animal proteins, because individuals with AN may be uncomfortable consuming red meat. Patients may find HBV sources more appealing because they can reduce meal volume, as it typically takes a larger volume of a vegetable protein to provide the same amount of protein provided from an animal source. For example, it would require about two cups of beans to provide the same amount of protein in about three ounces of chicken (about 25 g). As meal plans increase to match rising energy needs, lower volume food options are ideal to reduce GI discomfort. Intake of HBV sources of protein, such as red meat, will also increase zinc intake. Zinc needs are higher in children and adolescents for proper growth, making this a particular micronutrient of concern in young adults who are vegetarians.

Promoting adequate fluid intake is also important to correct electrolyte imbalances and further assist any problems with constipation. Fiber intake may promote early satiety and increase GI discomfort.[11] High-fiber foods should be introduced slowly with appropriate water intake to prevent GI discomfort. Use of non-stimulant laxatives, such as polyethylene glycol, may be a more appropriate treatment for constipation in this population. Supplementation with a 100% Recommended Daily Allowance multivitamin—with the exception of iron, as iron can exacerbate constipation as well—is recommended for patients with AN in the initial weight restoration phase.[7]

Oral feeding is the first choice of treatment because it provides a safer, less invasive, and more therapeutic form of refeeding. Use of high-energy oral nutrition supplements may be prescribed in combination to an oral diet to aid weight restoration and can help to reduce the total volume of food needed to meet higher calorie needs. Refractory cases may require enteral nutrition support during treatment. Multiple failed attempts at oral feeding, life-threatening weight loss

CASE STUDY REVISITED

It is HD 7 and Emma has been tolerating the volume of meals since agreeing to reintroduce chicken and fish. She has been following her meal plan consistently for 1 week and her weight has increased. She shares that she is feeling bloated and "puffy" and has not had a bowel movement in 4 days.

Anthropometric Data:

Weight: 46.4 kg increased from admission weight of 45 kg   BMI: 16.5 kg/m^2

Questions

1. Could other factors in addition to true restoration be contributing to this weight increase?
2. Is this an appropriate rate of weight restoration in the inpatient setting?
3. If not, what adjustments would you make to her meal plan?
4. How can Emma's constipation be addressed?

of more than 40% below IBW, and a worsening or severe psychological or physical state are indicators for nutritional support. Enteral nutrition (EN) supplying 1–1.5 kcal/mL of polymeric formula via nasogastric tube is typically the first choice for nutrition support in such situations.[20] Nocturnal EN may be beneficial in assisting weight gain in patients who have plateaued or continued to restore at a slow rate. Parenteral nutrition (PN) is prescribed for severe and refractory cases only. PN increases risk for catheter-related infections and could result in an air embolism if an agitated patient refusing nutrition support attempted removal of the intravenous line. Medical teams must use utmost discretion around PN use in patients with AN.[20]

Refeeding syndrome (RS) is a serious and potentially fatal condition that can result from the metabolic and electrolyte shifts that occur following the reintroduction and/or increase of nutrition after a period of decreased or absent caloric intake. This reintroduction of nutrition may be in the form of oral diet, EN, PN, or intravenous dextrose.[57] As the body transitions from starvation to refeeding, it transitions from a catabolic to anabolic state. This metabolic shift causes increased cellular uptake and utilization of glucose, thiamine, and electrolytes potassium, phosphorus, and magnesium, resulting in low serum concentrations.[58,59] Electrolyte depletion is further compounded by extracellular losses when purging methods such as vomiting, laxative misuse, and excessive exercise leading to excessive perspiration take place.

These serum shifts, particularly hypophosphatemia, are hallmarks of RS. Left untreated, this electrolyte imbalance can progress into acute fluid overload due to sodium and water retention, respiratory compromise due to hypophosphatemia, cardiac involvement due to hypokalemia and hypomagnesemia, and/or neurologic complications due to thiamine deficiency.[60] Refer to Chapter 2, *Biochemical Assessment*, for more information on RS.

Due to the complex nature of RS and limited high-quality scientific data on the condition, it has previously lacked a universally accepted definition and prevention and treatment guidelines. The American Society for Parenteral and Enteral Nutrition's (ASPEN) 2020 consensus report provides guidance for recognizing RS risk as well as avoiding and treating RS in both adult and pediatric patient populations.[57] For the purposes of this text, the adult risk factors, diagnostic criteria, and avoidance and treatment recommendations will be reviewed.

ASPEN has outlined criteria for adult patients' risk factors, which are categorized as a moderate or significant risk for RS:

Moderate Risk (two criteria needed):

- BMI 16–18.5 kg/m^2
- Weight loss of 5% in 1 month
- None or negligible oral intake for 5–6 days, or <75% of estimated energy requirement for >7 days during an acute illness or injury, or <75% of estimated energy requirement for >1 month
- Abnormal serum concentrations of potassium, phosphorus, or magnesium: either minimally low levels or normal current levels and recent low levels that necessitated minimal or single-dose supplementation
- Evidence of moderate subcutaneous fat loss
- Evidence of mild or moderate muscle mass loss
- Moderate comorbidities*

Significant Risk (one criterion needed):

- BMI <16 kg/m^2
- Weight loss of 7.5% in 3 months or >10% in 6 months
- None or negligible oral intake for >7 days, or <50% of estimated energy requirement for >5 days during an acute illness or injury, or <50% of estimated energy requirement for >1 month
- Abnormal serum concentrations of potassium, phosphorus or magnesium: Either moderately/significantly low levels or minimally low or normal levels and recent low levels that necessitated significant or multiple-dose supplementation
- Evidence of severe subcutaneous fat loss
- Evidence of severe muscle mass loss
- Severe comorbidities*

*ASPEN has identified several comorbidities/diseases and clinical conditions associated with increased risk of RS, such as cancer, chronic alcohol and drug use, eating disorders (e.g., anorexia nervosa), food insecurity and homelessness, post-bariatric surgery, and prolonged fasting, among others. It is important to note that RS can occur in patients with elevated BMI levels, as individuals of all weights and body shapes can experience malnutrition.[57]

ASPEN has outlined diagnostic criteria for RS as follows:

- A decrease in any 1, 2, or 3 of serum phosphorus, potassium, and/or magnesium levels:
  - by 10–20% (Mild RS)
  - by 20–30% (Moderate RS)
  - or by >30% and/or organ dysfunction resulting from these deficiencies and/or due to thiamine deficiency (Severe RS)
- And occurring within 5 days of reinitiating or substantially increasing energy provision

CORE CONCEPT 9

Refeeding syndrome is a serious and potentially fatal condition that can result from the metabolic and electrolyte shifts that occur following the reintroduction and/or increase of nutrition after a period of decreased or absent caloric intake. This reintroduction of nutrition may be in the form of oral diet, enteral nutrition, parenteral nutrition, or intravenous dextrose.

Recommendations to avoid RS and to treat or avoid worsening of RS are often the same and focus on electrolyte and thiamine repletion, and conservative caloric administration with gradual advancement.

The ASPEN consensus recommendations for the avoidance and treatment of RS in adults include:

- Close monitoring of potassium, phosphorus, and magnesium both before initiating nutrition and regularly after initiation, such as every 12 hours in high-risk patients, and repleting when needed.
- Thiamine supplementation of 100 mg prior to initiation of feeding or IV dextrose.
- Conservative calorie initiation such as 10–20 kcal/kg for the first 24 hours, advancing by 33% of total caloric goal every 24–48 hours.
- Holding calorie initiation until electrolyte levels have normalized from supplementation in those severely at risk for RS.

The focus of treatment for RS should be correcting electrolyte abnormalities and may additionally include a reduction of calories or slowing of the advancement of calories. A patient's tolerance and physiological response to refeeding, such as serum electrolyte levels and cardiac output, should be monitored closely. Overall, an individualized approach to refeeding patients is recommended, as patients may present and respond to nutrition reintroduction differently. Of note, ASPEN recommends less conservative caloric recommendations for refeeding pediatric patients with AN, as nutrient deprivation may have a more profound effect than it does on adults due to the metabolic demands of growth and development.[57]

PRACTICE POINT

Recommendations to avoid causing RS and to treat or avoid worsening of RS are often the same and focus on electrolyte and thiamine repletion, and conservative caloric administration with gradual advancement.

Bulimia Nervosa

Goals for nutrition rehabilitation in BN typically include weight maintenance or restoration, cessation of binge–purge cycle, restoration of normal eating behavior, correction of nutrient deficiencies, balance of electrolyte levels, and recognition of hunger and satiety cues. Although weight loss may be the intention of the patient's purging behaviors and may be an appropriate long-term goal for some individuals above their BAW, it should not be the initial goal of intervention and should not be explored until after treatment. RDs can provide adequate calorie prescriptions, information related to correcting electrolyte abnormalities and nutrient deficiencies, and nutrition education while assisting in the establishment of a normal eating pattern. Additional guidelines for medical nutrition therapy include meal planning to provide adequate macro- and micronutrient intake and establishing a meal pattern to promote dietary structure.[10]

Like AN, changes in REE must be considered when calculating calorie prescriptions in BN. Generally, patients with BN will require lower calorie intake to restore or maintain weight than patients with AN.[8,53] Clinical signs of hypometabolism, such as cold intolerance or low T3 levels, are also useful assessments of metabolic efficiency. Body weight should be monitored and caloric adjustments made accordingly to support weight maintenance or restoration goals. Weight fluctuations due to purging are common because weight loss may initially result from dehydration, followed by weight gain from rebound fluid retention. Individuals who abruptly stop purging may experience significant fluid retention or rebound edema for several weeks, resulting in short-term weight gain typically between 2 and 6 lbs. (0.9 and 2.7 kg).[8,51] Patients who have a significantly low weight and are purging multiple times per day tend to experience more severe rebound fluid retention, which may reach up to 10 lbs. (4.5 kg). Edema, fluid retention, and swollen salivary glands that can result from purging behaviors may be mistaken as true weight gain. It is important to educate patients on this side effect to potentially prevent an increase in compensatory behaviors triggered by this presumed weight gain.

Patients may be resistant to meal plans, or structured food plans, at first. Typically, fasting for the first half of the day to avoid contributing to caloric intake consumed during binges later, or as a means of restriction following a binge the previous day, is common. Restricting intake below energy needs can trigger binge eating episodes, as dietary restraint is identified as the most direct cause of binging.[8] A structured meal plan that avoids long periods of fasting by providing three meals and snacks daily along with a balanced intake of macronutrients can decrease cravings and promote satiety and nutritional adequacy. This approach helps reduce the likelihood of binging by providing multiple eating opportunities so that adequate nourishment may be achieved. The consistency of eating regularly throughout the day prevents long periods of fasting, which can also trigger binges. This also promotes regular digestion, return of hunger and fullness cues, and matches the liver's capacity to maintain blood glucose levels with glycogen.[8] Satiety and satisfaction can be achieved through a balance of macronutrients at meals and snacks. Incorporation of adequate protein is helpful as it has been shown to be the most satiating macronutrient.[8] Menu planning and self-monitoring have been shown to be effective in decreasing binge–purge behaviors. Additionally, meal and snack consistency and cessation of binge–purge behaviors together can help to strengthen hunger and satiety cues in these patients.[7]

During treatment for BN, patients will require a great deal of encouragement to follow a structured dietary plan and cease purging and non-purging compensatory behaviors. Patients who exercise excessively begin to decrease the frequency and/or duration of physical activity, and an increase in restrictive eating habits can result as a means of making up for the decrease in calories burned. Patients should be reminded that restrictive eating increases the likelihood of binge eating, a behavior that was unhelpful for weight loss in the past and can perpetuate the binge–restrict cycle.[7] Patience and support are crucial for facilitating positive changes in patients with BN.

Binge Eating Disorder

The goals of BED treatment include interrupting binge eating behaviors, improving body image and nutrition status, increasing physical activity, and promoting self-acceptance. A combination of dietary counseling and psychotherapy is generally used to treat BED and can lead to the most desirable outcomes.[61] An RD's role includes helping identify patients with the disorder, evaluating their nutrition requirements, and educating them on normal eating habits to prevent future binges. Similar recommendations for structured, balanced meal planning to reduce binge eating episodes that are helpful in BN are effective in BED treatment as well. Also, like BN, weight loss may be an appropriate long-term goal, but the initial emphasis of treatment should be on reduction of binge eating episodes. Creating a calorie deficit for weight loss would be counterproductive in reducing triggers to binge eating. Self-monitoring of eating behaviors can help to provide insight into binge triggers. RDs may encourage patients to record food intake in a journal or smartphone app that can later be reviewed in counseling sessions. Some patients may find food logging unhelpful or contributory to ED behaviors. RDs should assess whether self-monitoring is appropriate on an individual basis.

CASE STUDY REVISITED

It is now HD 12. The nutrition therapy goals for Emma are to correct nutrient deficiencies and work toward a weight restoration goal of being within 10% of her ideal body weight.

Current Anthropometric Data:

Weight: 47.2 kg increased from 46.4 kg on HD 7 BMI: 16.8 kg/m^2

Biochemical Data:

	Normal Range	HD 1	HD 3	HD 5	HD 7	HD 9	HD 11
Sodium	136–145 mEq/L	148	132	138	142	141	141
Potassium	3.5–5 mEq/L	3.4	3.1	3.6	3.6	3.7	3.8
Chloride	96–106 mEq/L	94	95	100	100	99	99
CO_2	22–31 mEq/L	33	32	29	28	29	28
BUN	8–20 mg/dL	33	13	15	17	16	17
Phosphorus	2.5–4.5 mg/dL	3.4	2.1	2.9	3.3	3.2	3.4
Magnesium	1.5–2.7 mg/dL	1.9	1.2	1.5	1.6	1.7	1.7
Albumin	3.5–5.5 g/dL	3.5	—	—	—	—	2.9

Questions

1. Did Emma meet the risk factors for refeeding syndrome according to ASPEN guidelines? Why or why not?
2. How might you explain Emma's biochemical data trends? What other factors might have played a role in her labs increasing or decreasing?
3. On HD 12, approximately how many calories might Emma be consuming in her meal plan?
4. What would Emma's next steps in treatment consist of after the inpatient level of care?
5. What questions can you ask Emma to assess her attitude and approach to food and eating as she progresses through the weight restoration process?

Nutrition Counseling

Not all individuals with EDs will be ready to change or willing to participate in treatment because they may not be ready to let go of their ED or want recovery. For example, individuals with AN may interpret their disorder as an identity that is more meaningful to them than the disorder's detrimental health effects, potentially including death.[62] Providing nutrition recommendations and counseling for this patient population can be quite difficult. RDs should always provide support and positive reinforcement when counseling patients with EDs (**Figure 23.8**). Training in motivational interviewing can be beneficial for the treatment process as this client-centered counseling method can help clinicians determine individuals' motivation or readiness for making health behavior changes. It also allows for a collaborative approach to treatment, which enhances individuals' intrinsic motivation to change.[7]

Weight restoration and fluctuations during treatment can be extremely difficult, both physiologically and psychologically. Symptoms of delayed gastric emptying, constipation, fluid retention, and edema are uncomfortable and can impair the ability to meet nutritional needs, especially in patients with AN who may be consuming large amounts of food to restore weight. For some patients, weight may initially be restored in the abdominal region.[62] While the weight will redistribute over time, the abdominal region tends to be a particularly sensitive area or focus of negative body image for patients with AN, making this change

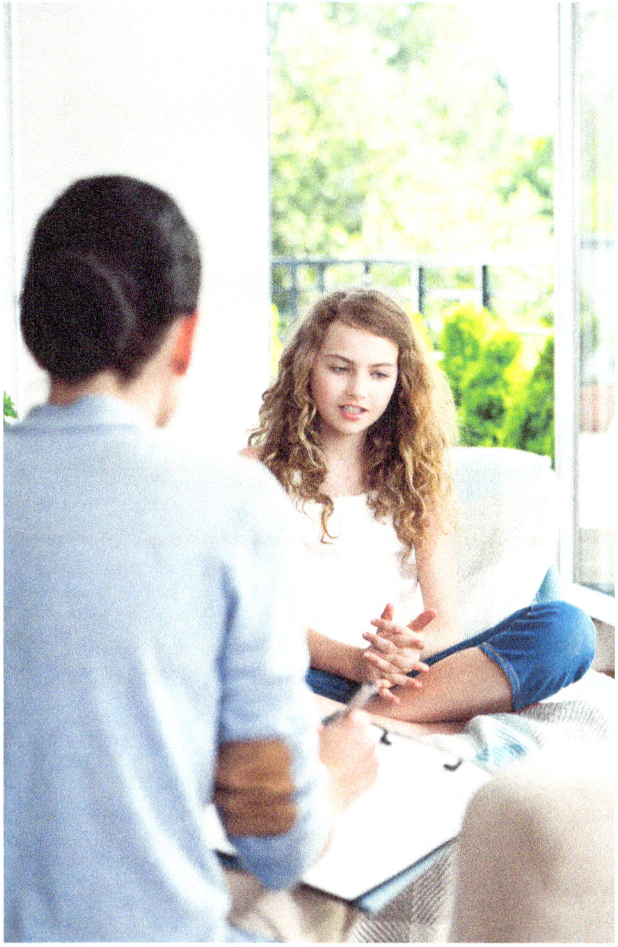

Figure 23.8 Providing Support and Positive Reinforcement When Counseling Patients with EDs Is Critical

incredibly difficult. As they notice changes in their body weight or shape, they may experience increased symptoms of anxiety, depression, irritability, and, for some, thoughts of suicide. With sustained weight gain and maintenance, these mood symptoms improve.[51] In AN, weight restoration is associated with improved cognitive and physical symptoms and is essential for psychotherapy. It is important to be thoughtful of these changes during the refeeding process and offer education and support around them during nutrition counseling.

RDs and other members of the treatment team should be aware of the various pro-anorexia ("pro-ana") and pro-bulimia ("pro-mia") websites that glorify EDs. These sites view EDs in a positive light, as something that takes great strength, determination, and self-control. Thinness is depicted as an ideology, with pictures of extremely thin models and encouraging messages to continue working toward this valued goal. They also provide tips for achieving this goal such as extremely low-calorie diet plans, ways to ward off hunger without eating, and secretive purging methods. It is important for RDs to understand the content of these sites because they can provide insight in to strategies used by their patients to continue ED habits during treatment.[7] Social media influencers that seemingly promote health and fitness may also be promoting disordered eating behaviors. RDs can play a key role in helping clients identify social media accounts that are unhelpful for their body image and self-esteem, and challenge or fact-check the nutrition advice these non-experts are sharing.

Other topics for nutrition counseling may include exposures to fear foods, expanding food variety, identifying binge triggers and tactics to prevent binge eating episodes, improving body image and self-acceptance, incorporating healthy exercise or joyful movement, and exploring mindful and/or intuitive eating. It is important for RDs to assess a patient's readiness and stage of recovery to determine whether a specific education topic or area of counseling is appropriate.

Nutrition education is an essential part of treatment and is most helpful after malnutrition is corrected when the ability to process new information is no longer impaired. Some patients with EDs may already spend significant amounts of time learning about nutrition-related topics, but their ED or lack of sound resources may cause them to misinterpret the information. Topics to consider during treatment include guidelines for balanced eating; the impact of malnutrition on growth, development, behavior, fertility, and mood; set-point theory; hunger and satiety cues; the effects of restrictive diets on metabolism; the ineffectiveness of compensatory behaviors and their physiological effects; and exercise and energy balance. An RD may need to consult with the IDT before providing certain education topics. Topics like sports nutrition and healthy eating while dining out may not be appropriate until the patient is in remission.[7,9]

PRACTICE POINT

Nutrition education is an essential part of treatment and is most helpful after malnutrition is corrected, when the ability to process new information is no longer impaired.

Monitoring and Evaluation

Monitoring methods for ED treatment include measurements of height and weight, resting and postprandial energy expenditure, diet records, eating behaviors and attitudes, and laboratory data, if indicated. Daily weights should be taken for patients in the hospital, and weekly weights should be taken for those receiving outpatient treatment. A baseline height should be obtained in adults and measured every 3–6 months in children and adolescents. Anthropometric skinfold tests should be monitored as medically indicated for both inpatients and outpatients. Food records for outpatients with AN, BN, or BED should include fluid intake, physical activity, and eating behaviors. Individuals with BN and BED should also include feelings experienced while eating, types of foods consumed during binges, and for those with BN, the time and method of compensatory behaviors.[7]

Screening tools may be helpful for identifying patients with suspected EDs. The SCOFF (Sick, Control, One stone [equal to 14 lbs. or 6.4 kg], Fat, Fear) questionnaire is a validated, simple screening tool that can be used in adjunct with physical examination and laboratory studies.[11] The Eating Disorder Examination Questionnaire (EDE-Q) is widely used to assess the change in ED symptoms over the course of treatment, and has been found to be reliable in assessing ED attitudes.[63] RDs working with candidates for bariatric surgery should be mindful that individuals with BED often seek weight loss surgery. Screening for this major contraindication of surgery and educating individuals with BED on the role it plays in nutrition and lifestyle, both pre- and post-surgery, can be used to address this disordered eating behavior.[7]

Early detection and prevention of EDs are the best treatment practices and can be achieved through patient monitoring. Being cautious of red flags (e.g., an individual recently adopting a restrictive or vegetarian diet or a patient with T1DM skipping insulin doses with the intention of weight control) during counseling sessions can help the RD to address disordered eating habits before they develop into a serious ED.

The main focus of nutrition counseling sessions with all individuals should support health-centered behaviors rather than weight-centered behaviors, also known as a "Health at Every Size® approach," to decrease the risk of ED development.[64] Incorporating the concepts of intuitive eating, a non-diet approach that honors both physical and mental well-being, challenges society's thin ideal, exposes the adverse effects of restrictive dieting, and encourages individuals to make peace with food and honor their bodies through eating and exercising in healthy ways they enjoy, is also helpful.[65] Intuitive eating aligns with a Health at Every Size® approach in that both help reduce weight stigma and the risk of EDs. RDs can help to prevent EDs and disordered eating while encouraging health and well-being utilizing these two approaches in their practice.

PRACTICE POINT

Early detection of eating disorders is one of the best treatment practices and can be achieved through patient monitoring. Be cautious of red flags in counseling sessions such as recent adoption of a vegetarian diet or a patient with T1DM skipping insulin doses with the intention of weight control.

Additional Information and Resources

Certified Eating Disorder Specialist

Dietitians working with the ED population may apply for certification to become a Certified Eating Disorder Specialist (CEDS). Certification is regulated by the International Association of Eating Disorder Professionals (IAEDP). The certification process includes a minimum of 2500 hours of eating disorder-specific practice, 24 hours of consultation provided by an IAEDP-approved consultant (CEDS-C), completion of course work provided by IAEDP, and passing of the CEDS exam among other requirements. Certification must be upheld through renewal every 2 years and completion of continuing education hours. Fees are typically associated with supervision, exam preparation and registration, and certification renewal.

Certification is not required for RDs to work with ED populations. Some dietitians feel that the credential is beneficial for marketing and establishing a private practice with an ED niche and may distinguish them from other local RDs. RDs with or without the CEDS certification can benefit from networking with other ED treatment providers and general medical and mental health providers sharing their expertise with this patient population and availability for referrals.

Additional Information

Additional resources for nutrition counseling:

Nutrition Counseling in the Treatment of Eating Disorders by Marcia Herrin and Maria Larkin

Nourish: How to Heal Your Relationship with Food, Body, Self by Heidi Schauster

Intuitive Eating by Evelyn Tribole and Elyse Resch

Body Respect by Linda Bacon and Lucy Aphramor

Health at Every Size by Linda Bacon

Association for Size Diversity and Health: asdah.org

Organizations for ED information, treatment and provider directories, and resources for patients, caregivers, and providers:

National Eating Disorder Association (NEDA): neda.org

National Association of Anorexia Nervosa and Associated Disorders (ANAD): anad.org

National Alliance for Eating Disorders: allianceforeatingdisorders.com

For CEDS Certification:

International Association of Eating Disorder Professionals (IAEDP): iaedpfoundation.com

Chapter Summary

EDs are multifactorial conditions associated with significant physical and psychological morbidities that require management through an interprofessional approach. Disordered thoughts and behaviors related to food and eating can be extremely difficult to overcome and relapse is common. Medical nutrition therapy is essential for nutritional rehabilitation. The refeeding process can lead to significant physiological changes, and a gradual reintroduction of the provision of energy can reduce the risk of refeeding syndrome as well as corresponding fluid and electrolyte abnormalities. Treatment of EDs may include various types of inpatient and/or outpatient care. The restoration of body weight and the normalization of eating patterns are essential for successful outcomes and prognosis.

Key Terms

eating disorder (ED), anorexia nervosa (AN), amenorrhea, bulimia nervosa (BN), binge eating disorder (BED), night eating syndrome (NES), avoidant/restrictive food intake disorder (ARFID), orthorexia, lanugo, female athlete triad, Russell's sign, Mallory–Weiss tears, Maudsley approach, cognitive behavioral therapy (CBT), dialectical behavioral therapy (DBT), selective serotonin reuptake inhibitors (SSRIs), refeeding syndrome (RS), biologically appropriate weights (BAWs)

References

1. American Psychiatric Association. *Diagnostic and statistical manual of mental disorders, Text Revision: DSM-5-TR*. 5th ed. American Psychiatric Association; 2022.
2. Academy of Eating Disorders, STRIPED, Deloitte Access Economics. *Social and Economic Cost of Eating Disorders in the United States of America: A Report for the Strategic Training Initiative for the Prevention of Eating Disorders and the Academy for Eating Disorders*. June 2020.
3. Galmiche M, Déchelotte P, Lambert G, Tavolacci MP. Prevalence of eating disorders over the 2000–2018 period: a systematic literature review. *Am J Clin Nutr*. 2019;109(5):1402–1413. doi:10.1093/ajcn/nqy342
4. Dane A, Bhatia K. The social media diet: a scoping review to investigate the association between social media, body image and eating disorders amongst young people. *PLOS Glob Public Health*. 2023;3(3). doi:10.1371/journal.pgph.0001091
5. Hudson J, Hiripi E, Pope H, Kessler R. The prevalence and correlates of eating disorders in the National Comorbidity Survey Replication. *Biol Psychiatry*. 2007;61:348.
6. Keski-Rahkonen A, Hoek HW, Susser ES, et al. Epidemiology and course of anorexia nervosa in the community. *Am J Psychiatry*.2007;164(8):1259–1265.
7. Ozier AD, Henry BW. Position of the American Dietetic Association: nutrition interventions in the treatment of eating disorders. *J Am Diet Assoc*. 2011;111(8):1236–1241.
8. Herrin M, Larkin M. *Nutrition Counseling in the Treatment of Eating Disorders*. Brunner-Routledge, 2013.
9. Luder E, Schebendach J. Nutrition management of eating disorders. *Top Clin Nutr*. 1993;8(3):48–63.
10. Swanson SA, Crow SJ, Le Grange D, Swendsen J, Merikangas KR. Prevalence and correlates of eating disorders in adolescents: results from the National Comorbidity Survey Replication Adolescent Supplement. *Arch Gen Psychiatry*. 2011;68(7): 714–723. doi:10.1001/archgenpsychiatry.2011.22
11. Trent SA, Moreira ME, Colwell CB, Mehler PS. ED management of patients with eating disorders. *Am J Emerg Med*. 2013;31(5):859–865.
12. Iacovino JM, Gredysa DM, Altman M, Wilfley DE. Psychological treatments for binge eating disorder. *Curr Psychiatry Rep*. 2012;14(4):432–446. doi:10.1007/s11920-012-0277-8
13. Simone M, Telke S, Anderson LM, Eisenberg M, Neumark-Sztainer D. Ethnic/racial and gender differences in disordered eating behavior prevalence trajectories among women and men from adolescence into adulthood. *SSM*. 2022;294:114720. doi:10.1016/j.socscimed.2022.114720

14. Raney JH, Al-Shoaibi AA, Shao IY, et al. Racial discrimination is associated with binge-eating disorder in early adolescents: a cross-sectional analysis. *J Eat Disord*. 2023;11(1):139. doi:10.1186/s40337-023-00866-0
15. Fischer S, Meyer AH, Hermann E, Tuch A, Munsch S. Night eating syndrome in young adults: delineation from other eating disorders and clinical significance. *Psychiatry Res*. 2012;200(2-3):494–501.
16. Berner LA, Allison KC. Behavioral management of night eating disorders. *Psychol Res Behav Manag*. 2013;6:1–8.
17. Białek-Dratwa A, Szymańska D, Grajek M, Krupa-Kotara K, Szczepańska E, Kowalski O. ARFID—Strategies for dietary management in children. *Nutrients*. 2022;14(9):1739. doi:10.3390/nu14091739
18. Gramaglia C, Brytek-Matera A, Rogoza R, et al. Orthorexia and anorexia nervosa: two distinct phenomena? A cross-cultural comparison of orthorexic behaviours in clinical and non-clinical samples. *BMC Psychiatry*. 2017;17:75. doi:10.1186/s12888-017-1241-2
19. Sala M, Keshishian A, Song S, et al. Predictors of relapse in eating disorders: a meta-analysis. *J Psychiatric Res*. 2023;158:281–299. doi:10.1016/j.jpsychires.2023.01.002
20. Mehler P, Winkelman A, Andersen D, Gaudiani J. Nutritional rehabilitation: practical guidelines for refeeding the anorectic patient. *J Nutr Metab*. 2010;2010. doi:10.1155/2010/625782
21. Keel PK, Dorer DJ, Franko DL, Jackson SC, Herzog DB. Postremission predictors of relapse in women with eating disorders. *Am J Psychiatry*. 2005;162(12):2263–2268.
22. Forman-Hoffman VL, Ruffin T, Schultz SK. Basal metabolic rate in anorexia nervosa patients: using appropriate predictive equations during the refeeding process. *Ann Clin Psychiatry*. 2006;18(2):123–127.
23. Melchior J. From malnutrition to refeeding during anorexia nervosa. *Curr Opin Clin Nutr Metab Care*. 1998;1(6):481–485.
24. Swenne I, Stridsberg M. Bone metabolism markers in adolescent girls with eating disorders and weight loss: effects of growth, weight trend, developmental and menstrual status. *Arch Osteoporos*. 2012;7(1-2):125–133. doi:10.1007/s11657-012-0090-3
25. Halvorsen I, Platou D, Hoiseth A. Bone mass eight years after treatment for adolescent-onset anorexia nervosa. *Eur Eat Disorders Rev*. 2012;20(5):386–392. doi:10.1002/erv.2179
26. Birch K. Female athlete triad. *BMJ*. 2005;330(7485):244-246.
27. Kalm LM, Semba RD. They starved so that others be better fed: remembering Ancel Keys and the Minnesota Experiment. *J Nutr*. 2005;135(6):1347–1352.
28. Tucker T. *The Great Starvation Experiment: Ancel Keys and the Men Who Starved for Science*. University of Minnesota Press; 2007.
29. Willer MG, Thuras P, Crow SJ. Implications of the changing use of hospitalization to treat anorexia nervosa. *Am J Psychiatry*. 2005;162(12):2374–2376.
30. Touyz S, Le Grange D, Lacey H, et al. Treatment for severe and enduring anorexia nervosa: a review. *Aust N Z J Psychiatry*. 2012;46(12):1136–1144. doi:10.1017/S0033291713000949
31. Franko DL, Keshaviah A, Eddy KT, et al. A longitudinal investigation of mortality in anorexia nervosa and bulimia nervosa. *Am J Psychiatry*. 2013;170(8):917–925.
32. Kotler LA, Devlin MJ, Matthews DE, et al. Total energy expenditure as measured by doubly-labeled water in outpatients with bulimia nervosa. *Int J Eat Disord*. 2001;29(4):470–476. doi:10.1002/eat.1044
33. Obarzanek E, Lesem MD, Goldstein DS, et al. Reduced resting metabolic rate in patients with bulimia nervosa. *Arch Gen Psychiatry*. 1991;48(5)456–462.
34. Castellini G, Castellani W, Lelli L, et al. Association between resting energy expenditure, psychopathology and HPA-axis in eating disorders. *World J Clin Cases*. 2014;2(7):257–264. doi:10.12998/wjcc.v2.i7.257
35. Mars JA, Iqbal A, Rehman A. Binge eating disorder. *StatPearls*. StatPearls Publishing; 2024. https://www.ncbi.nlm.nih.gov/books/NBK551700/
36. Le Grange D, Lock J, Agras WS, Bryson SW, Jo B. Randomized clinical trial of family-based treatment and cognitive-behavioral therapy for adolescent bulimia nervosa. *JAACAP*. 2015;54(11):886–894.e2. doi:10.1016/j.jaac.2015.08.008
37. Hay P. A systematic review of evidence for psychological treatments in eating disorders: 2005–2012. *Int J Eat Disord*. 2013;46(5):462–469. doi:10.1002/eat.22103
38. Attia E, Walsh BT. Anorexia nervosa. *Am J Psychiatry*. 2007;164(12):1805–1810.
39. Lock J, Le Grange D, Agras WS, Dare C. *Treatment Manual for Anorexia Nervosa: A Family-Based Approach*. Guilford Press; 2001.
40. Le Grange D, Lock J. *Treating Adolescent Bulimia: A Family-Based Approach*. Guilford Press; 2007.
41. Monteleone AM, Pellegrino F, Croatto G, et al. Treatment of eating disorders: a systematic meta-review of meta-analyses and network meta-analyses. *Neurosci Biobehav Rev*. 2022;142(142):104857. doi:10.1016/j.neubiorev.2022.104857
42. Rosen DS and the Committee on Adolescence. Clinical report identification and management of eating disorders in children and adolescents. *Pediatrics*. 2010;126(6):1240–1253. doi:10.1542/peds.2010-2821
43. Han R, Bian Q, Chen H. Effectiveness of olanzapine in the treatment of anorexia nervosa: a systematic review and meta-analysis. *Brain Behav*. 2022;12(2). doi:10.1002/brb3.2498
44. Mitchell JE, Roerig J, Steffen K. Biological therapies for eating disorders. *Int J Eat Disord*. 2013;46(5):470–477. doi:10.1002/eat.22104
45. Froreich FV, Ratcliffe SE, Vartanian LR. Blind versus open weighing from an eating disorder patient perspective. *J Eat Disord*. 2020;8(39). doi:10.1186/s40337-020-00316-1
46. Setnick J. Micronutrient deficiencies and supplementation in anorexia and bulimia nervosa: a review of literature. *Nutr Clin Pract*. 2010;25(2):137–142. doi:10.1177/0884533610361478
47. Kaye WH, Weltzin TE, Hsu LK, et al. Amount of calories retained after binge eating and vomiting. *Am J Psychiatry*. 1993;150(6):969–971. doi:10.1176/ajp.150.6.969
48. Bo-Linn GW, Santa Ana CA, Morawski SG, et al. Purging and calorie absorption in bulimic patients and normal women. *Ann Intern Med*. 1983;99(1):14–17.
49. Stang JS, Story M, Zollman M. Food risk ratings and food portion size estimations among women with bulimia nervosa. *Top Clin Nutr*. 1997;12(4):50–57.
50. Jensen GL, Bistrian B, Roubenoff R, Heimburger DC. Malnutrition syndromes: a conundrum vs continuum. *JPEN*. 2009;33(6):710–716.
51. Yager, J, Devlin, M, Halmi, K, et al. Practice guideline for the treatment of patients with eating disorders, third edition. *Am J Psychiatry*. 2006;163:1–128.
52. Harrison ME, Obeid N, Fu MCY. Growth curves in short supply: a descriptive study of the availability and utility of growth curve data in adolescents with eating disorders. *BMC Family Practice*. 2013;14:134.
53. Marzola E, Nasser JA, Hashim SA. Nutritional rehabilitation in anorexia nervosa: review of the literature and implications for treatment. *BMC Psychiatry*. 2013;13:290.

54. Scalfi L, Marra M, DeFilippo E, et al. The prediction of basal metabolic rate in female patients with anorexia nervosa. *Int J Obes.* 2001;25:359–364. doi:10.1038/sj.ijo.0801547
55. Width M, Reinhard T. *The Essential Pocket Guide for Clinical Nutrition.* Jones & Bartlett Learning; 2020.
56. Iribarren C, Markovitz JH, Jacobs Jr DR, et al. Dietary intake of n-3, n-6 fatty acids and fish: relationship with hostility in young adults—the CARDIA study. Eur J Clin Nutr. 2004;58(1):24–31.
57. da Silva JSV, Seres DS, Sabino K, et al. ASPEN Consensus Recommendations for Refeeding Syndrome. *Nutr Clin Pract.* 2020;35(2):178–195. doi:10.1002/ncp.10474
58. National Institute for Health and Clinical Excellence. *Nutrition Support in Adults.* National Collaborating Center for Acute Care. London, The Royal Surgeons of England; 2006.
59. Rio A, Whelan K, Goff L, et al. Occurrence of refeeding syndrome in adults started on artificial nutrition support: prospective cohort study. *BMJ Open.* 2013;3. doi:10.1136/bmjopen-2012-002173
60. Solomon SM, Kirby DF. The refeeding syndrome: a review. *JPEN.* 1990;14:90–97.
61. Wonderlich SA, de Zwaan M, Mitchell JE, Peterson C, Crow S. Psychological and dietary treatments of binge eating disorder: conceptual implications. *Int J Eat Disord.* 2003;34. doi:10.1002/eat.10206
62. Cockfield A, Philpot U. Symposium 8: Feeding size 0: the challenges of anorexia nervosa managing anorexia from a dietitian's perspective. *Proc Nutr Soc.* 2009;68:281–288. doi:10.1017/S0029665109001281
63. Rose JS, Vaewsorn A, Rosselli-Navarra F, et al. Test-retest reliability of the eating disorder examination-questionnaire (EDE-Q) in a college sample. *J Eat Disord.* 2013;1:42.
64. Bacon L. *Health at Every Size: The Surprising Truth about Your Weight.* Benbella Books; 2010.
65. Tribole E, Resch E. *Intuitive Eating: A Revolutionary Program That Works.* St Martins Essentials; 2020.

CHAPTER 24

Nutrition in Developmental Disabilities

Jennifer Shiel
Kathy Prelack

CHAPTER OUTLINE

CORE CONCEPTS

1. Developmental disabilities are lifelong conditions that can present along a wide spectrum within the same condition.
2. Developmental disabilities are associated with a variety of medical and nutritional complications, of which the potential for obesity is present for all and can further complicate care.
3. Prader Willi syndrome is a genetic condition that occurs due to a chromosomal microdeletion.
4. The hallmark characteristic of Prader Willi syndrome is hyperphagia, which persists despite many attempts at intervention.
5. Weight management is one of the biggest challenges in caring for a patient with Prader Willi syndrome.
6. Spina bifida is a neural tube defect that can be prevented, in part, through folate supplementation.
7. Myelomeningocele is the most common form of spina bifida and is characterized by incomplete fusion of the spine, often resulting in swallowing, gastrointestinal, and bladder dysfunction.
8. Patients with cerebral palsy are classified based upon type of movement and limbs affected, with the main distinctions being between spastic and athetoid (also known as dyskinetic).
9. Muscle tone and ambulatory status can vary within patients with cerebral palsy and can greatly impact energy assessment.
10. Down syndrome is a developmental disability that can occur as a result of chromosomal alterations.
11. Patients with Down syndrome have a higher prevalence of celiac disease compared to their peers without Down syndrome.
12. Autism spectrum disorder is a group of disorders that impact behavior, communication, and development.
13. Food selectivity can be one of the biggest challenges in caring for a patient with autism spectrum disorder.

LEARNING OBJECTIVES

1. Discuss the similarities and differences among each of the presented developmental disabilities.
2. Describe potential nutritional issues secondary to a patient's developmental disability.
3. Identify how nutrition assessment differs in a patient with each of these developmental disabilities.
4. Assess and develop nutrition care plans unique to each disability.
5. Formulate education plans and strategies for dietary management in each of the developmental disabilities.

Introduction

A **developmental disability** is a condition that becomes evident at birth or early childhood and has varying impacts on the individual throughout the life cycle. The prevalence of any developmental disability in children ages 3–17 years in the United States during 2015–2018 was 17.8%, with children living in rural areas being more likely to be diagnosed compared to those living in urban areas (19.8% vs. 17.4%).[1] The developmental disabilities covered in this chapter are common and have the most frequent secondary medical and nutritional issues within the category of developmental disabilities. While each condition faces its own unique challenges, the common nutritional themes of developmental disabilities are feeding difficulties, weight challenges, and the need for consistent long-term follow-up throughout the life cycle. These include Prader Willi syndrome, spina bifida, cerebral palsy, Down syndrome, and autism spectrum disorder.

CORE CONCEPT 1

Developmental disabilities are lifelong conditions that can present along a wide spectrum within the same condition.

Prader Willi syndrome is a genetic condition whose main symptom is hyperphagia leading to obesity, which necessitates the need for nutritional counseling and interventions.[2] Spina bifida is a neural tube defect that occurs as a result of the failure of spinal closure in the first month of fetal life, and can result in a variety of specific defects, each with unique medical and nutritional challenges.[3] Cerebral palsy is a neurological disorder that affects muscle tone, movement, and coordination; it presents on a wide spectrum from mild to severe.[4] Down syndrome and autism spectrum disorder each present with distinctive nutritional needs, the management of which can be complicated by cognitive and behavioral challenges.

The tools of nutrition assessment are important to revisit, because they play a large part in the care of this patient population. In cases of patients with developmental disabilities, it is important to look for and assess potential medical and nutritional complications unique to each condition, and to continue to reassess over time for changes. Practitioners should note the variations within each condition and assess each patient as an individual, while screening for risk factors. It may also be necessary to additionally interview parents or caretakers to ensure accuracy when collecting patient information.

Common topics to assess and discuss in this population include any recent weight changes or history of unplanned weight loss/gain, previous or current feeding and swallowing issues, any supplemental enteral needs past or present, and any previous work with a feeding team. In addition, gastrointestinal (GI) management is a topic that may need further questioning to adequately assess potential issues. Another important point to consider is whether the client has previously worked with a registered dietitian (RD), to assess what their learning needs are and what they may have been taught by another provider.

An important comorbidity that can impact patients with any type of developmental disability is obesity. The prevalence of obesity in adults with disabilities by most recent estimates is approximately 40%.[5] This is largely due to physical limitations and immobility, dietary habits, medications, and lack of resources. Children with developmental disabilities have much higher rates of obesity than children without disabilities, with adolescents being 1.8 times more at risk than typically developing adolescents.[6,7] Health risks associated with obesity such as heart disease and diabetes are the same in patients with developmental disease, suggesting that these conditions will worsen with any excess weight challenges.[7]

CORE CONCEPT 2

Developmental disabilities are associated with a variety of medical and nutritional complications, of which the potential for obesity is present for all and can further complicate care.

In general, it is important to ask the standard nutrition and nutrition-related questions when assessing a patient with a developmental disability. Client history is an essential part of a full nutrition assessment and can encompass a variety of topics. Client history can set the framework for determining previous and current nutrition issues, as well as methods that have led to success in the past. Obtain information about birth and early history, including any feeding challenges, growth issues, and any growth faltering or malnutrition history, as well as trends along growth charts, such as changes in percentiles. Additionally, learning about any previous feeding practices, any previous

CASE STUDY INTRODUCTION

Mario is an 8-year-old male referred for outpatient nutrition counseling by his pediatrician after a diagnosis of Prader Willi syndrome. Mario was referred due to a recent dramatic increase in weight over the past 3 months, now above the 99th percentile on the CDC growth charts. His parents report that Mario is constantly asking for food and snacking throughout the day, and he has started sneaking food into his room at night.

Anthropometric Data:

Visit	Weight (kg)	Weight/Age Percentile (%)	Height (cm)	Height/Age Percentile (%)	Body Mass Index (BMI) (kg/m²)	BMI/Age Percentile (%)
3 months ago	30	76	120	4	20.8	96
Today	40	97	120	3	27.8	99

Biochemical Data:

HbA1c 6.5 (4.3–5.8%)

Clinical Data:

Past Medical History: None
Medications: recombinant growth hormone (rGH)
Vital Signs: Blood pressure 130/68 mm Hg
Nutrition-Focused Physical Exam: Patient appears obese consistent with android body type. Hair and nails appear normal. Skin is pale, warm, and intact. Exam is limited due to patient's irritability.

Dietary Data:

24-Hour Diet Recall:
Breakfast: Bacon, eggs, pancakes, orange juice
Snack: Granola bar, milk, fruit
Lunch: Sandwich (turkey/cheese), chips, pickles, crackers, cookie, milk
Snack: Cheese, crackers, juice
Dinner: Macaroni and cheese, peas, bread and butter, chicken, milk, water
Snack: Ice cream, candy

Questions

1. What are Mario's nutritional risk factors?
2. Write two Nutrition Diagnosis statements for Mario identifying the Problem/Etiology/Signs and Symptoms (PES) for Mario's active nutrition issues.
3. Identify the nutrition interventions you would like to initiate for Mario to address the problems identified in your PES statement.
4. What are Mario's calorie goals?
5. What nutrition education might you provide for Mario and his family?

work with an RD, food allergies, medications, and dietary supplements taken are all points to highlight in a patient interview. It may also be important to have input from parents/guardians in addition to the patient report to ensure accuracy. Having background knowledge about the common issues seen in each condition will help to determine which questions may need further exploration and probing.

Prader Willi Syndrome

Prader Willi syndrome (PWS) is a genetic condition first described in 1956 by Prader, Labhart, and Willi. PWS was determined in 1981 to be a condition that occurs as a result of genomic imprinting, which means that the gene expression is altered based on which parent passed on the gene.[8] The majority of PWS patients, roughly 70%, have PWS due to the deletion on the 15q11-q13 area in chromosome 15 from the paternal region.[9] PWS is a prime example of genomic imprinting, because were this deletion to occur on the maternal side, it would result in Angelman Syndrome and not PWS.[9] Most of the remaining cases of PWS are found to be caused by maternal uniparental disomy, which is when two copies of the maternal side are included.[9] Rarely (fewer than 5% of cases) is the cause due to other imprinting center defects such as a deletion or epimutations.[10]

CORE CONCEPT 3

Prader Willi syndrome is a genetic condition that occurs due to a chromosomal microdeletion.

PWS occurs in 1 in 10,000 to 30,000 live births,[11] although the prevalence is thought to be underestimated due to potential late diagnosis. A clinical indicator that would lead to testing for PWS in an infant is central hypotonia (**Figure 24.1**). A typical presentation of a baby with PWS and central hypotonia will include lethargy, poor sucking ability, weak cry, and decreased movement, with the potential to develop growth failure as a result of these symptoms.[10–12] Other facial characteristics include almond-shaped eyes, thin upper lip, and hypopigmentation of hair and skin compared to other family members.[10] Healthcare workers diagnose PWS by assessing for the presence of major and minor clinical criteria. In children younger than 3 years of age, they must have at least one minor criterion, and at least four major criteria for a PWS diagnosis. For children over 3 years of age, they must have at least three minor criteria and at least five major criteria for a diagnosis.[12] Please refer to **Table 24.1** for relevant criteria. If PWS is suspected, genetic testing will be completed to determine the cause of the deletion and confirm the diagnosis. This involves methylation analysis, which, if positive, will prompt FISH (fluorescence in situ hybridization) testing.[10]

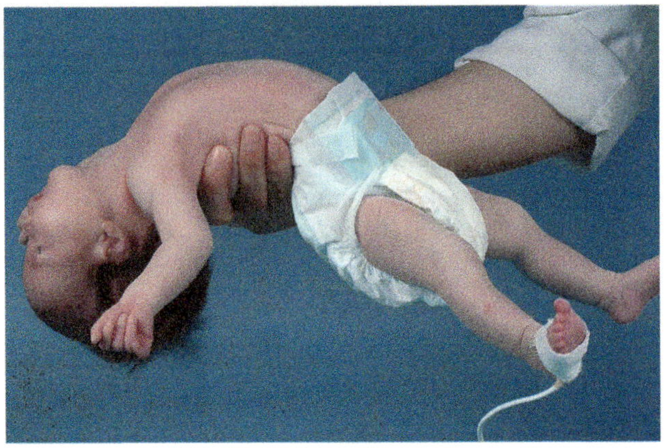

Figure 24.1 Infant Born with Prader Willi Syndrome and Hypotonia

Reproduced from Munné-Miralvés, C., Brunet-Llobet, L., Cahuana-Cárdenas, A. et al. Oral disorders in children with Prader-Willi syndrome: a case control study. *Orphanet J Rare Dis 15*, 43 (2020). https://doi.org/10.1186/s13023-020-1326-8. https://ojrd.biomedcentral.com/articles/10.1186/s13023-020-1326-8/figures/1. Open Access copyright information https://creativecommons.org/licenses/by/4.0/

Table 24.1 Clinical Criteria for Prader Willi Syndrome (PWS) Diagnosis

Major Clinical Criteria of PWS	Minor Clinical Criteria of PWS
▪ Developmental delays—mild-to-moderate intellectual disability ▪ Feeding difficulties/growth failure ▪ Difficulty sucking (in first few months) ▪ Extremely weak muscles in body torso ▪ Beginning of rapid weight gain between ages 1 and 6 resulting in severe obesity ▪ Excessive, uncontrollable overeating ▪ Facial features: narrow forehead, downturned mouth ▪ Reduced development of genital organs	▪ Decreased movement and fatigue in infancy ▪ Sleep disruption/daytime sleepiness ▪ Short stature ▪ Small feet, small and narrow hands ▪ Nearsightedness ▪ Thick saliva ▪ Behavioral problems (temper tantrums) ▪ Poor pronunciation ▪ Picking of skin ▪ Light color of hair, skin, eyes

Data from US Department of Health and Human Services, National Institutes of Health, Eunice Kennedy Shriver National Institute of Child Health and Human Development. Prader-Willi Syndrome (PWS). NIH Fact Sheet. Updated December 29, 2021. Accessed January 17, 2025. https://www.nichd.nih.gov/health/topics/factsheets/prader-willi

PRACTICE POINT

Presenting symptoms of PWS in infancy can include lethargy, decreased movement, weak suckling ability, and faint cry.

Generalized hypothalamic insufficiency occurs in all patients with PWS; hence growth hormone (GH) insufficiency is considered to be universally present. As patients grow, they are often characterized by short stature, small hands and feet, low IQ, and behavioral challenges.[10–12]

Common nutrition issues that can present include growth failure until about age 2 years, followed by increasing weight gain related to hyperphagia, often leading to eventual overweight and obese status if left uncontrolled. **Hyperphagia** (insatiable hunger) is a hallmark symptom of PWS, also thought to occur because of a hypothalamic abnormality.[8,10–13] PWS is the most common syndromic cause of life-threatening obesity. The same comorbidities associated with obesity, such as diabetes mellitus and cardiovascular disease, can also be observed over time with increasing weight gain in PWS.[13] **Figure 24.2** indicates an adult male with PSW.

Additionally, these patients can present with GI issues, typically constipation, which may be due to a combination of dietary choices, inactivity, or medications, and will require consistent management. Typical medical nutrition therapy strategies should be used, with education on the importance of a high fiber and fluid diet, as well as encouraging increased activity. This may be difficult for patients to follow, so the use of medications (stimulants, laxatives) may be needed.[14] Patients with PWS may also experience issues with osteopenia and osteoporosis.[10] While there are a multitude of nutritional and medical issues that require attention, a large part of this condition is behavioral and psychological, stemming from the hyperphagia and cognitive impairment. Common behavioral issues that arise are obsessive-compulsive disorder, food-seeking behavior, temper tantrums, and skin picking. Persistent hyperphagia can lead patients with PWS to go through extreme lengths to obtain food, and they may seek out and eat nonfood items such as garbage or pet food.[8]

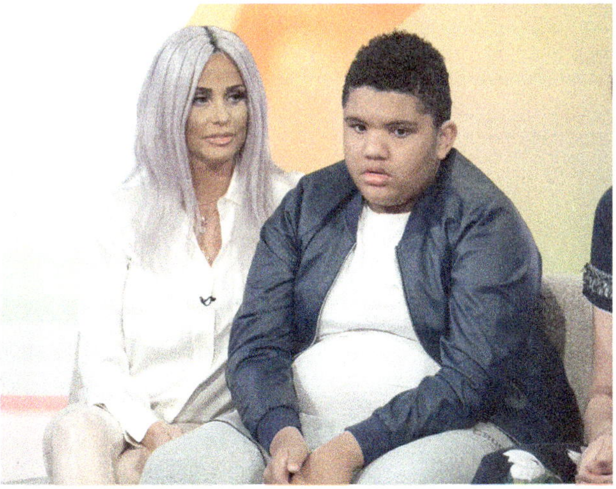

Figure 24.2 Harvey Price, son of famous model and media personality, Katie Price, and focus of a documentary series on PWS

CORE CONCEPT 4

The hallmark characteristic of Prader Willi syndrome is hyperphagia, which persists despite many attempts at intervention.

Nutrition Assessment: Anthropometrics

As previously mentioned, patients with PWS typically have initial feeding problems that can impact growth and, if not addressed, can suffer from growth failure, which is then followed by eventual obesity. All of this makes the collection and monitoring of anthropometric data essential to adequately monitor the patient. For patients with PWS, short stature is commonly noticed, which is important to keep in mind when taking anthropometrics and assessing growth charts.[11] Analysis of growth patterns reveals that the 50th percentile of height for children with PWS generally falls below the 5th percentile for typically growing children by ages 12–14 years.[9]

When assessing the growth of children with PWS, it is recommended to use the typical World Health Organization (WHO)/Centers for Disease Control and Prevention (CDC) growth charts, but to also keep in mind the growth expectations for potential use of recombinant growth hormone therapy (rGH) and how this may affect a patient's growth trajectory.[15] There are no standardized growth charts available. Further research is needed in this area, and for now, it is recommended to use the traditional growth charts, with the PWS-specific ones potentially as a supplement.[15]

Biochemical and Clinical

Proper diagnosis of PWS will require genetic testing for confirmation and to determine the cause of microdeletion. During the first year, measures of plasma insulin-like growth factor, thyroxine, and thyrotropin levels should be obtained in addition to a complete blood count and basic metabolic panel, including calcium. Radiography of the left hand and wrist to determine bone age should also be performed.[10] As patients age, should there be suspicion of osteopenia or osteoporosis, patients may receive a bone mineral density scan as well as measurements of vitamin D to determine the course of action.[9] Furthermore, as they start to transition to adulthood, obtaining HbA1c and a lipid panel to screen for comorbidities such as diabetes and hyperlipidemia is recommended.[10]

Diet History

Obtaining feeding history is essential throughout the stages of growth and development in patients with PWS. During infancy, mode of feeding including breastfeeding versus bottle feeding, preparation and use of formula, and frequency and volume of intake should be carefully assessed. These along with identifying GI intolerance and abnormal stool patterns allow for the proper intervention early on. Acquisition of feeding skills should be evaluated throughout the child's development. This often requires a multidisciplinary approach that includes speech, occupational, and physical therapy.[15] Screening for a weak suck in infancy, acceptance of textures and temperature as the diet transitions, as well as the ability to self-feed is important. As children get older, evaluating dietary intake using diet recall, food frequency questionnaires, and food diaries can be used to determine energy balance, potential for nutrient deficiencies, and food-seeking behaviors.[10,13–15]

Assessment of Energy Needs

Energy needs of patients with PWS will change with age. As an infant, patients should be prescribed standard age-appropriate recommendations unless there is a diagnosis of growth failure, in which case the infant will need to be placed on a higher-calorie formula or fortified breast milk to promote weight gain. As patients age, there are specific guidelines on energy-needs assessment for the PWS population. For weight maintenance, it is recommended to prescribe 10–11 calories/cm of height. For a patient who needs weight reduction, 8–9 calories/cm are recommended.[13,15] Both recommendations are listed in **Table 24.2**. These recommendations are lower than the standards used for the average population to account for hyperphagia, shorter stature, and obesity found in these patients. It is also important to note that because recommendations are for fewer calories than average patients, vitamin and mineral intake should be monitored to ensure patients are still achieving adequate amounts despite overall recommended lower energy intakes.[15]

Nutrition Intervention

Medical nutrition therapy for age-appropriate weight maintenance and weight loss should be used to help to curb weight gain that can often occur due to the hyperphagia experienced by these patients. A well-balanced healthy, low-calorie diet full of fruits, vegetables, lean proteins, and whole grains should be encouraged. Lower calorie options for foods and drinks should be explored in combination with adequate fiber and protein for promotion of satiety.[15]

Table 24.2 Prader Willi Syndrome Calorie Goals

Weight maintenance	10–11 calories/cm height
Weight reduction	8–9 calories/cm height

Data from Academy of Nutrition and Dietetics. *Pediatric Nutrition Care Manual*: Developmental Disabilities. Prader-Willi Syndrome. Accessed January 17, 2025. https://www.nutritioncaremanual.org/topic.cfm?ncm_category_id=13&lv1=144620&lv2=144745&ncm_toc_id=144745&ncm_heading=Nutrition%20Care%20home%20page

CASE STUDY REVISITED

Mario returns to the clinic 1 month after his initial visit, and he continues to gain weight. His parents report that Mario continues to frequently request food throughout the day, and he has escalated his habit of sneaking and hiding food.

Questions

1. Assess the status of your nutrition diagnosis/PES statement(s) for Mario (e.g., resolution of PES, any new or continued problems?)
2. What strategies and/or nutrition education would you use to help Mario and his family based upon your current PES statement?
3. What other practitioners would you want to get involved, and why?

Consuming smaller, more frequent meals can be a helpful strategy in dealing with hyperphagia and repetitive requests for food. Physical activity should be encouraged as tolerated to help combat weight gain. A plan for monitoring weight trends should be instituted to determine when food changes and activity are no longer enough to prevent excessive weight gain.

Due to the growth issues identified in PWS, the general consensus is that rGH is an appropriate part of the treatment plan for PWS when combined with other therapies such as dietary and lifestyle changes.[16,17] Studies have shown significant benefit from using rGH, including increased rate of linear growth, adolescent growth spurt, and improvement in body composition with decreased fat mass and increases in lean body mass.[11,13,16,17] Patients have also shown improvements in motor development and cognitive function.[8,13,16] rGH therapy can normalize growth and improve body composition; however, it does not help control hyperphagia.[11,14] Possible side effects include sleep apnea, joint pain, and peripheral edema, but the reported rate of these side effects is low.[16,17]

PRACTICE POINT

Recombinant growth hormone therapy can be used in the PWS population as part of a treatment plan.

Given that obesity is the leading cause of morbidity and mortality in PWS, bariatric surgery has become a treatment option in patients who fit specific criteria based on body mass index (BMI) and comorbidities.[13,18] A recent meta-analysis looking at outcomes in patients with PWS who underwent bariatric surgery demonstrated a significant reduction in BMI that was sustained for up to 7 years depending on the type of surgery.[18] However, the quality and paucity of research is limiting.[13,18] More studies are needed as well as development of data registries to better understand the long-term effects of bariatric surgery in this population.[13] Consideration should be given to the social, ethical, and psychological aspects of performing this surgery on patients with intellectual disabilities, and ensuring that they have adequate support.[13,18]

Another clinical topic of interest is the potential use of weight-loss medications in the PWS population. Various medications have been trialed in order to enhance weight loss and energy expenditure, but have been shown to be unsuccessful in short-term trials.[13,16,17] Antiepileptics, specifically topiramate, have been used in attempts to affect food-seeking behavior, but clinical trials are lacking, and there is a potential for many adverse side effects.[13] Additionally, anorexigenic agents have shown no benefit in treating hyperphagia, but research is limited.[2] Insufficient study data and lack of efficacy found in prior research necessitate the need for further research to evaluate pharmacotherapy's role in the treatment plans for patients with PWS. A list of possible medications to be used in treatment of PWS is listed in **Table 24.3**.

Table 24.3 Pharmacologic Approaches in Prader Willi Syndrome

Medication	Proposed Use	Implications/Evidence for Use
Recombinant Growth Hormone	Improve body composition	▪ Consensus agreement on use as early as the first year of life. ▪ Does not abate hyperphagia
Antiepileptics (topiramate)	Alter food-seeking behavior	▪ Numerous potential negative side effects such as confusion, dizziness, fatigue ▪ Potential role in behavior control of hyperphagia but no impact on weight loss
Anorexigens (phentermine)	Appetite control	▪ No benefit found to appetite control or weight status for PWS patients
Somatostatin	Suppress ghrelin Reduce hyperphagia	▪ No benefit found to appetite or weight status for PWS patients
Lipase Inhibitors (orlistat)	Inhibit pancreatic lipase (prevent some fat absorption)	▪ Known gastrointestinal side effects ▪ Evidence of some weight loss

Data from Casamitjana L, Blanco-Hinojo L, Giménez-Palop O, et al. One year of recombinant human growth hormone treatment in adults with Prader–Willi syndrome improves body composition, motor skills, and brain functional activity in the cerebellum. *J Clin Med.* 2022;11(7):1831.; Deal CL, Tony M, Höybye C, Allen DB, Tauber M, Christiansen JS; 2011 Growth Hormone in Prader-Willi Syndrome Clinical Care Guidelines Workshop Participants. Growth Hormone Research Society workshop summary: Consensus guidelines for recombinant human growth hormone therapy in Prader-Willi syndrome. *J Clin Endocrinol Metab.* 2013;98(6):E1072–E1087. doi:10.1210/jc.2012-3888

Clinical Controversy

Use of bariatric surgery procedures to manage obesity in the PWS population continues to be a topic for debate. Some small studies have shown that it is effective for weight loss. However, questions about safety remain. The risk of complications associated with the surgery, such as GI perforation, nutritional anemia, osteopenia, and even death, as well as limited weight reduction, are all reasons to avoid surgery and instead focus on treatment with exercise, diet, and behavior modification. Although more research is needed, some patients with PWS have had successful surgeries.

Questions

1. Discuss the use of bariatric surgery in the Prader Willi population.
2. What are the pros and cons to its use?
3. What is your opinion on use of bariatric surgery in this population?

References

1. Soomro FH, Razzaq A, Siddiq G. Effects of restrictive bariatric surgery on congenital Prader-Willi Syndrome: a case report. *Cureus*. 2022;14(8):e27955. doi:10.7759/cureus.27955
2. Liu SY, Wong SK, Lam CC, Ng EK. Bariatric surgery for Prader-Willi syndrome was ineffective in producing sustainable weight loss: long term results for up to 10 years. *Pediatr Obes*. 2020;15(1):e12575. doi:10.1111/ijpo.12575

CORE CONCEPT 5

Weight management is one of the biggest challenges in caring for a patient with Prader Willi syndrome.

PRACTICE POINT

Many patients will resort to eating nonfood items because of their hyperphagia, which necessitates the need for interventions from a multidisciplinary team to help manage behaviors.

Long-Term Monitoring and Evaluation

There is no cure for PWS, so patients within this population will require lifelong education and support to manage associated problems. Patients in this population often continually struggle with feeding difficulties and weight challenges. It is often difficult for patients to maintain weight or prevent weight gain due to hyperphagia. Practitioners will need to follow weight trends over time to assess adequacy of nutritional management and make any needed changes. Monitoring the lipid panel, HbA1C, and vitamin D should also be done routinely. Behavioral management is another large piece of a patient with PWS and their long-term management that will require consistent work, reassessment, and follow-up. Managing a patient's hyperphagia and weight will likely be the biggest challenges for the medical team in the long-term care of a patient with PWS.[13,15]

Spina Bifida

Both genetic and environmental factors play a role in spina bifida (SB), a primarily neurological condition that can often result in orthopedic complications.[19,20] By most recent statistics, SB occurs in 1 out of every 2,875 births in the United States each year.[21] The prevalence of SB has been declining in North America due to improved prenatal diagnosis and the dietary fortification of many foods with folate. In 1998, the Food and Drug Administration (FDA) began requiring manufacturers to fortify grain products with folic acid to help increase intake.[19] This was done because of the association between low folate intake and increased risk of children being born with neural tube defects, although the exact mechanism for this is still unknown.[19]

CORE CONCEPT 6

Spina bifida is a neural tube defect that can be prevented, in part, through folate supplementation.

There are four classifications of SB: myelomeningocele (the most common form, at 80-90% of all births), meningocele, closed neural tube defects, and occulta.[20,21] The differences among these are based on the impact to the spine and are listed in **Table 24.4**. **Myelomeningocele** is the most common form of SB and is an incompletely fused spine from which there is a protrusion of the spinal cord, including nerves. Meningocele also results in an incomplete fusion but does not include any

Table 24.4 Classification of Spina Bifida

Myelomeningocele	■ Most common ■ Most severe ■ Spinal cord and nerves extend through part of the spine ■ Possible nerve damage, hydrocephalus, and other disabilities
Meningocele	■ Exposed meninges and spinal fluid ■ Fewer disabilities/overall lower severity due to lack of nerve exposure
Occulta	■ Least severe form ■ Malformation of one or more vertebrae ■ Typically minimal to no symptoms
Closed neural tube defects	■ Malformations of bone, fat, or meninges ■ Wide range of symptoms and severity ■ Example: Lipomeningocele (fatty tissue deposit)

Data from Centers for Disease Control and Prevention. Spina Bifida: About Spina Bifida. Updated January 2, 2025. Accessed January 18, 2025. https://www.cdc.gov/spina-bifida/about/index.html

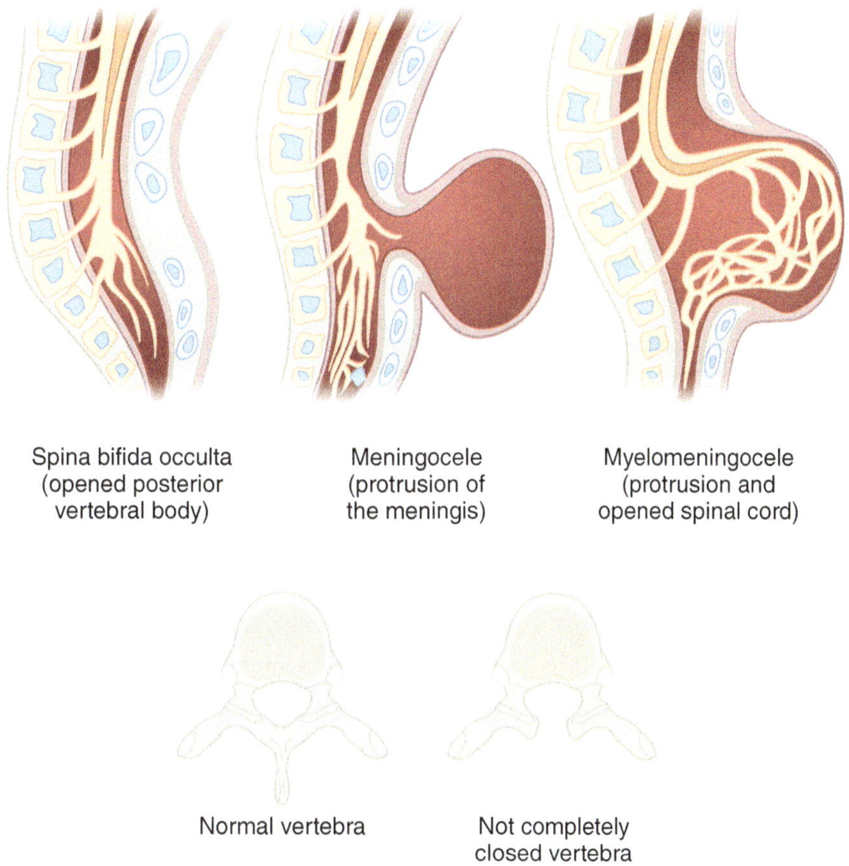

Figure 24.3 Comparison of Occulta, Meningocele, and Myelomeningocele

nerves—only spinal fluid—which makes this a less-severe form of SB.[21] Closed neural tube defects are a result of bone, meninges, or fat malformations.[21] **Figure 24.3** indicates a comparison of the three classifications. An example of a closed defect is **lipomeningocele**, which is the deposition of fatty tissue tumors. Lastly, occulta, which tends to be an asymptomatic form of SB, is often not detected until a patient presents with specific back or urologic problems.[20]

CASE STUDY INTRODUCTION

Olivia is a 6-year-old female with spina bifida who comes to the outpatient nutrition clinic after a referral from her pediatrician. Olivia is wheelchair-user and her parents are interested in a nutrition appointment because Olivia's pediatrician noted she is now overweight and has decreased interest in activities, which has decreased her mobility.

Anthropometric Data:

N/A

Biochemical Data:

None

Clinical Data:

Past Medical History: Spina bifida, constipation
Vital Signs: Normal
Medications: Colace, multivitamin (gummy), senna

Dietary Data:

24-Hour Diet Recall:
Breakfast: 1 bowl of cereal, whole milk (6 oz)
Snack: 6 peanut butter crackers
Lunch: Tuna sandwich, 1 small bag of chips, whole milk (6 oz)
Snack: 2 oatmeal cookies, whole milk (4 oz)
Dinner: 1 bowl of pasta with 2 meatballs, water
Snack: 1 cup ice cream

Questions

1. What are Olivia's nutritional risk factors?
2. Write two Nutrition Diagnosis statements for Olivia identifying the Problem/Etiology/Signs and Symptoms (PES) of Olivia's active nutrition issues.
3. Identify the nutrition interventions you would like to initiate for Olivia to address the problems identified in your PES statements.
4. How would you obtain anthropometrics for Olivia? Describe the pros and cons of various alternative methods.
5. How would you educate her parents about energy balance and adjustments in Olivia's diet?

Medical and Surgical Management

Chiari II malformation, also known as "Arnold–Chiari malformation" (**Figure 24.4**), is more often noticed in patients with myelomeningocele-type SB than in other types of SB.[22–25] This malformation is an extension of the cerebellar and brain stem tissue into the foramen magnum with the cerebellar vermis (connecting the two halves of the cerebellum) appearing as incomplete or damaged.[25] These malformations result in a change in pressure to the brain stem, potentially leading to blockages of cerebrospinal fluid and altering functions controlled by these areas, such as swallowing. Potential causes for this malformation can include genetic mutations, structural defects, or vitamin/mineral deficiencies (e.g., folic acid).[25] Patients can be asymptomatic or can appear with a variety of symptoms such as neck pain, balance issues, poor feeding, headaches, and drooling. Roughly 5% of patients with myelomeningocele have a severe malformation and initially present with symptoms such as apnea, growth failure, and **cyanosis** (bluish coloring of the skin).

The necessity of surgical intervention is dependent upon the type of SB, with early surgery needed only for patients with open defects. The typical clinical path has been for surgery to be performed in the first few days of life to close the defect, and to then provide lifelong care for associated disabilities. Recent advances in in utero surgery at 19–25 weeks gestation may reduce

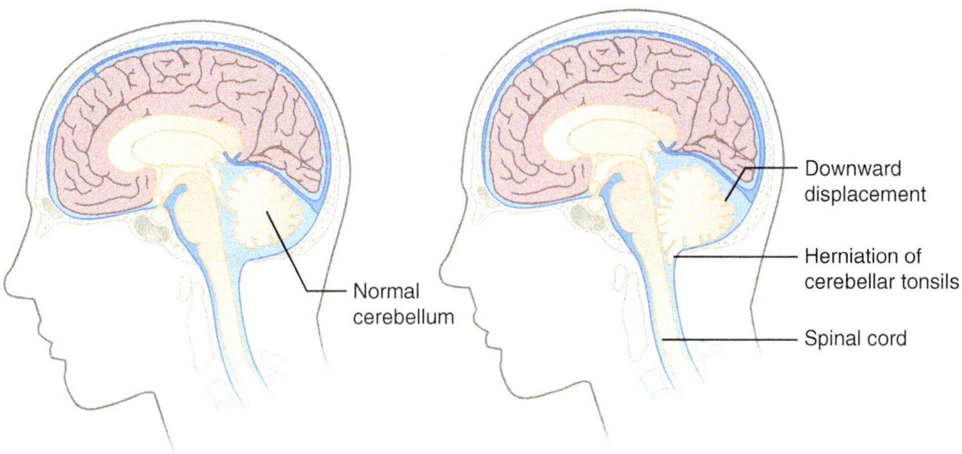

Figure 24.4 Arnold–Chiari Malformation

the occurrence of Chiari malformation and need for **ventriculoperitoneal (VP) shunting**. In addition, improved overall neuromotor function has been found with such procedures. In utero surgery for SB repair by hysterotomy is not without potential risks including membrane rupture and preterm delivery. More recently, fetoscopic open SB repair approaches have been shown to have equally beneficial outcomes while reducing maternal and fetal/neonatal risks.[23]

Some patients may need surgical management of potential complications such as hydrocephalus. Signs of this can be observed in the neonatal period, including enlarged head circumference and bulging anterior fontanel.[24] Hydrocephalus can be managed through VP shunting, which drains excess cerebrospinal fluid into a peritoneal space to alleviate pressure and prevent progression of hydrocephalus.[24]

In addition to the typical surgical interventions used in patients with SB, there is also the potential for many other associated conditions, each with their own unique challenges that need to be managed. Approximately 15–20% of patients with SB will experience seizures, occurring more often in patients with shunts.[24] Management for this will likely require antiepileptic medication. Rates of scoliosis are approximately 15–20% in patients with SB, which often need surgical correction.[24] Patients with SB may face challenges with other orthopedic issues such as club foot, which occurs in approximately 50% of patients.[24] Club foot management requires physical and occupational therapy, potential casting, releases, and/or splinting, with the possibility of further surgical management around age 1–2 years. An infant with club foot is presented in **Figure 24.5**.

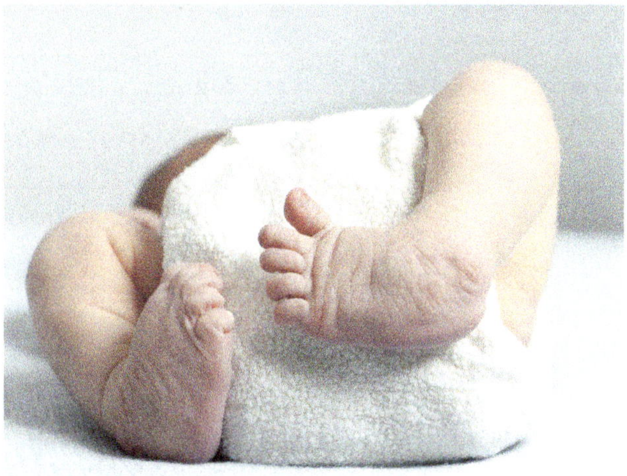

Figure 24.5 Infant with Club Foot

CORE CONCEPT 7

Myelomeningocele is the most common form of spina bifida and is characterized by incomplete fusion of the spine, often resulting in swallowing, gastrointestinal, and bladder dysfunction.

Nutrition Assessment: Anthropometrics

Anthropometrics can be difficult to obtain due to potential physical limitations of patients, in which case a variety of alternative methods may have to be used. For weight measurements, the first option is to use the standard digital or balance beam scale. However, if patients are unable to stand on the scale,

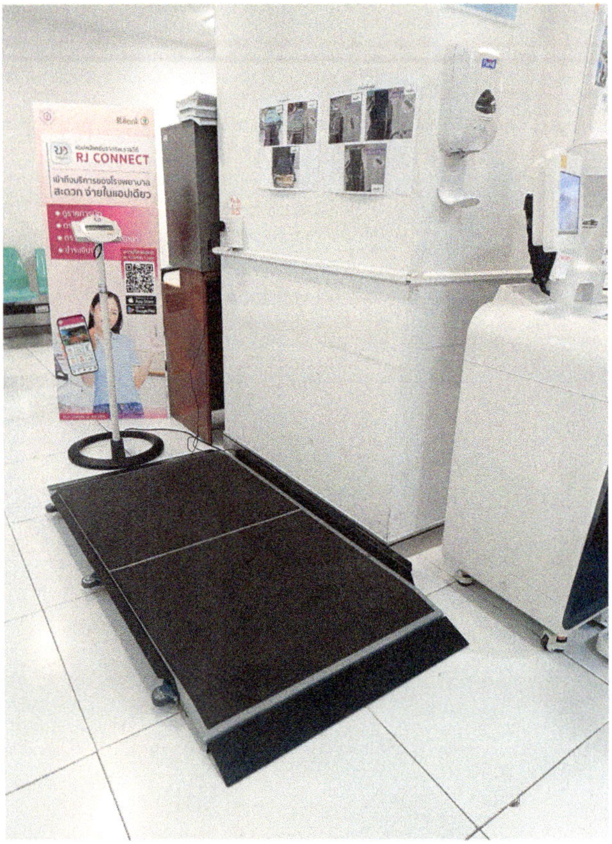

Figure 24.6 A Platform Scale is Used for Measuring Weight in Patients Who Require Use of a Wheelchair

there are a few alternatives. Patients who are small enough can be held by their parent on the scale, with parent's weight then subtracted. Additionally, a pan/bucket scale, bed scale, or platform scale in which a wheelchair can be placed are all viable options.[26] A platform scale for use in patients who require a wheelchair is displayed in **Figure 24.6**. It is also important to note the mode of weight measurement on the growth chart for consistency. For children who are unable to stand to obtain a traditional height measurement, alternatives include use of a length board, sitting height measurement, and arm span measurements.[26] Selecting a mode of height measurement should be done based upon specific needs of the child as well as the competency of the clinician in obtaining height through alternative methods. As with weight, it is important to note the method used to obtain height to maintain consistent and accurate measurements. Additionally, attention to presence of braces or assistive devices the patient may be wearing and how this might impact anthropometric measures is necessary. Standard CDC growth charts should be used to plot and track anthropometrics, as there are no available standardized growth charts for this population.

PRACTICE POINT

Accurate and consistent measurement of weight is important, preferably taken using the same measurement techniques over time. Large aberrations in weight should be verified by rechecking.

Biochemical and Clinical

The most commonly encountered nutrition-related issues with patients who have SB include GI problems such as constipation and incontinence, and under- or overweight status. Swallowing difficulties can also occur as a result of Chiari II malformation, which is present in 80–90% of patients with myelomeningocele SB.[20] Specific biochemical measurements obtained and medical procedures performed will depend on the patient, their age, any secondary conditions or issues, and their unique needs.

Two conditions that tend to be common and challenging for this population are neurogenic bladder and bowel. **Neurogenic bladder**, often present in the myelomeningocele form of SB, occurs when patients are unable to perceive bladder fullness and lack coordination between contraction and relaxation.[24] **Neurogenic bowel** is found in most patients with SB and results in decreased GI motility leading to constipation. The decreased motility, in turn, necessitates the need for the establishment of a bowel regimen. Methods for management can include stimulation, suppositories, enemas, and/or work with an RD for medical nutrition therapy for constipation, highlighting the importance of adequate fiber and fluids.[27] Given the inherent nature of constipation in patients with SB, nutrition interventions alone are unlikely to be sufficient to manage these problems.

PRACTICE POINT

Chiari II malformation can be found in patients with myelomeningocele form of SB, with the potential for severe symptoms such as apnea, cyanosis, and failure to thrive.

Diet History

Patients with SB, as with other developmental disabilities, have the potential to experience feeding difficulties. As mentioned, specific to SB are feeding problems due to a Chiari II malformation, which can cause swallowing problems.[24] Patients who present with frequent respiratory problems or history of pneumonia should have their swallowing ability assessed. Diet interview should assess for frequency of coughing, particularly when ingesting fluids.[22] Since children with swallowing difficulty may avoid drinking liquids, it is important to ask about food refusal and overall fluid intake. Other factors to assess include mouth movement and head positioning. These challenges may lead to regression of feeding skills and alterations in food choice. Diet history can be used to identify inadequate intake of fiber, iron, and protein.[22]

Assessment of Energy Needs

Patients with SB may have significantly lower energy needs than children without SB due to diminished lean body mass.[28] Additionally, any motor paralysis can lead to decreased caloric expenditure and presents the potential for obesity.[24] Obesity can be prevalent in this population, not due to the SB diagnosis itself, but as a result of comorbidities.[28–31] For these reasons, alternative methods to estimate the energy needs of patients with SB are available and based on height. Recommendations are for 9–11 kcal/cm for weight maintenance, or 7 kcal/cm for weight loss.[30] These recommendations, listed in **Table 24.5**, are lower than what a child of the same age without SB would receive using the traditional energy needs assessment.

PRACTICE POINT

Patients with spina bifida have lower energy needs than peers their age.

Nutrition Intervention

In infancy, supporting adequate growth, which may be interrupted due to difficulty feeding and surgical interventions, should be the primary focus of nutrition care. Patients who present with swallowing difficulties may require thickened liquids and texture modifications (refer to Chapter 18, *Nutrition in Neurology*, for guidelines on managing dysphagia). As the child ages, overweight and obesity may result due to typical factors related to diet and exercise. The diagnosis of SB presents unique challenges on top of the usual patient experience when it comes to energy balance. These patients may be less active than reference populations; inactivity increases risk of obesity, which, in turn, may negatively impact whatever mobility the patient has and serve as a risk factor for other comorbidities.[24] RDs will need to employ typical practices of medical nutrition therapy with changes made to counseling style or goal setting to fit individual patients as needed and to accommodate any challenges as a result of SB. Working with not only the patient but the caregiver/family for support with goals for weight management or weight loss should improve results over time. Additionally, a multidisciplinary team is helpful for managing care of the patient as a whole, including input from RDs, physical and occupational therapists, surgeons, and general practitioners. Constipation management is one of the main interventions needed in this population.[29] Poor adherence to fluid modifications can challenge goals for increased fluid intake that is needed to help treat constipation. Specific recommendations for constipation management are listed in **Table 24.6**.

Table 24.5 Energy Needs of Patients with Spina Bifida

Low energy needs	7–9 kcal/cm
Moderate energy needs	9–11 kcal/cm
High energy needs	12–15 kcal/cm

Data from Bunting K, Mills J, Philips S, Ramsey E, et al. Alternative methods to determine energy needs, energy requirements in children with developmental disabilities. In: *Pediatric Nutrition Reference guide*. 9th ed. Houston, TX: Texas Children's Hospital; 2010:21–22.

Long-Term Monitoring and Evaluation

Long-term monitoring includes evaluation of growth, feeding and swallowing issues, need for a consistent GI management program, and potential for overweight and obesity management. Additionally, dealing with any secondary health issues that come with normal aging, while taking into account the SB diagnosis and its unique challenges, is important.

Cerebral Palsy

Cerebral palsy (CP) is one of the most common disabilities, affecting approximately 3 live births out of every 1000 in the United States.[32] CP is largely a disorder of movement and posturing due to nonprogressive brain injury or abnormalities during birth.[33] Potential causes of CP include prematurity, brain malformations, in utero stroke, hypoxic ischemic encephalopathy, meningitis, anoxic insult, and accidental head trauma.[34]

The different CP classifications listed in **Table 24.7** are made based on the type of movement and limbs affected. **Spastic** CP is the most common form

Table 24.6 Recommendations for Constipation

Infancy

- Fiber may be introduced at 6 months of age in children developmentally ready for solids
- Limit infant cereal to once per day
- Use homemade baby food from lightly cooked or steamed fruits and vegetables
- Consider prune or pear juice for their laxative effect

Toddlers and young children

- Increase fruit consumption as primary approach
- Encourage 6–8 servings of fruits and vegetables per day
- Nuts and seeds can be introduced in ages 3 and older

For ages 4 years and older

- 0.5 g/kg fiber daily is recommended
- Increase fiber intake by eating more fruits, vegetables, and whole grains
- Consider the use of psyllium and methylcellulose

All Ages

- Increase fluid intake in addition to fiber, to avoid worsening constipation.
- Encourage water or other low or zero calorie beverages.

Data from Academy of Nutrition and Dietetics. *Pediatric Nutrition Care Manual:* Gastrointestinal Disease. Constipation. Nutrition Intervention. Accessed January 20, 2025. https://www.nutritioncaremanual.org/topic.cfm?ncm_category_id=13&lv1=144625&lv2=144769&lv3=270739&ncm_toc_id=270739&ncm_heading=Nutrition%20Care%20home%20page

Table 24.7 Cerebral Palsy Classifications

Type	Description
Spastic	■ General: Increased muscle tone ■ Most common type ~80% of people with cerebral palsy
Spastic diplegia/ diparesis	■ Muscle stiffness primarily in legs rather than arms ■ Tight hip and leg muscles causes legs to turn inward and cross at knees (scissoring)
Spastic hemiplegia	■ Unilateral upper and lower extremity involvement ■ Usually arm and leg of same side affected
Spastic quadriplegia	■ Involvement of all four extremities, trunk, and face ■ Involves intellectual disabilities, seizures ■ Problems with vision, speech, and hearing
Athetoid/Dyskinetic	■ Dystonia—slow rotational movement of torso, arms, and legs ■ Corea—sudden involuntary movements, especially in fingers and toes ■ Face and tongue may be involved resulting in difficulty sucking, swallowing, and talking
Ataxic	■ Difficulty with balance and coordination
Mixed	■ More than 1 type of cerebral palsy ■ Most common is spastic-dyskinetic

Data from My Child at Cerebral Palsy.Org. Prevalence of Cerebral Palsy. Accessed January 20, 2025. https://www.cerebralpalsy.org/about-cerebral-palsy/prevalence-and-incidence; Centers for Disease Control and Prevention. Cerebral Palsy: About Cerebral Palsy. Accessed January 20, 2025. https://www.cdc.gov/cerebral-palsy/about/index.html

representing approximately 80% of patients with CP. Patients with spastic CP have increased muscle tone that can present as hemiplegia (unilateral involvement), diplegia (disproportionate lower extremity movement), and quadriplegia (whole body involvement).[32] Athetoid or dyskinetic CP is a lack of ability to control movement, which can present in a variety of ways, such as dystonia (low postural tone) or ataxia (unbalanced walking), and chorea (sudden, involuntary movements). Mixed CP is a combination of characteristics of more than one type of CP, spastic-dyskinetic being the most common in this category.[34]

CORE CONCEPT 8

Patients with cerebral palsy are classified based upon type of movement and limbs affected, with the main distinctions being between spastic and athetoid (also known as dyskinetic).

Management of spasticity is important for overall quality of life for the patient, and there are various methods, including medications.[35–38] One class of medications used is benzodiazepines, which serve as anti-spasticity medications to reduce spasms by affecting gamma-aminobutyric acid (GABA) receptors. Note that potential side effects include increased secretions and/or salivation, as well as constipation

CASE STUDY INTRODUCTION

Ali, a 4-year-old female with cerebral palsy, is new to the nutrition clinic and is admitted for your evaluation. Her parents report she has been losing weight, and her status overall has been declining. They also report they were previously told that their daughter would likely need enteral nutrition support through tube feeding.

Anthropometric Data:

Weight: 12 kg, <3 percentile weight/age (CDC growth chart)
Height: 95 cm, 10 percentile height/age (CDC growth chart)
Weight/height: <3% (CDC growth chart)
BMI: 13.6 kg/m^2, <3 percentile BMI/age (CDC growth chart)

Biochemical Data:

Hemoglobin 8 (12.0–15.5 g/dL)

Clinical Data:

Past Medical History: Cerebral palsy, non-spastic
Nutrition-Focused physical exam: Appears pale and thin. Skin noted to be dry with poor skin turgor. No wounds noted. Oral exam notable for a dry tongue and mucosa. Hypotonic muscle tone observed.

Dietary Data:

24-Hour Diet Recall:
Breakfast: 2 oz whole milk (to thickened consistency), 1 silver dollar pancake, 3 tbsp vanilla yogurt
Lunch: ½ grilled cheese sandwich, apple juice (to thickened consistency)
Dinner: 1 small bowl of pasta with tomato sauce, 1 turkey meatball, 3 oz whole milk (to thickened consistency)
Snack: Chocolate pudding
Diet Prescription: IDSSI Level 3 thick liquids and Level 6 Soft bite sized food, high calorie/protein diet

Questions

1. What are Ali's nutritional risk factors?
2. Write two Nutrition Diagnosis statements for Ali, identifying the Problem/Etiology/Signs and Symptoms (PES) of Ali's active nutrition issues.
3. Identify the nutrition interventions you would like to initiate for Ali to address the problems identified in your PES statements.
4. What criteria are used in the decision about the necessity of a gastric feeding tube?
5. What would you recommend to her family and Ali about the plan moving forward?

and urinary retention.[35] Baclofen, which also acts by affecting GABA receptors, can be used as an oral medication or by insertion of a pump to deliver this medication.[35] Baclofen has been used to act as a muscle relaxant to help with spasticity and reduce muscle tone, which supports its use in this population. The potential benefits of choosing provision through a pump mechanism rather than orally are potential improved salivation, communication, and speech in addition to the improvements in spasticity. Another medication that can be used to combat spasticity in patients with CP is botulinum toxin, which has been used in this population since 1988. Studies show this medication can help improve comfort and ease of care of the patient who has spastic CP while also increasing fine motor function and improving upper limb spasticity.[35]

Neurological impairment is a major component of CP that can manifest as seizure disorders, deficits in learning and cognition, vision and hearing impairment, respiratory problems, GI disturbances, and orthopedic issues.[38] Seizures are present in up to 30% of patients; typical treatment will include use of anti-epileptics.[4] GI problems, specifically with poor gastric motility, often present as a result of the nature of CP and its effect on muscles, leading to issues with reflux and

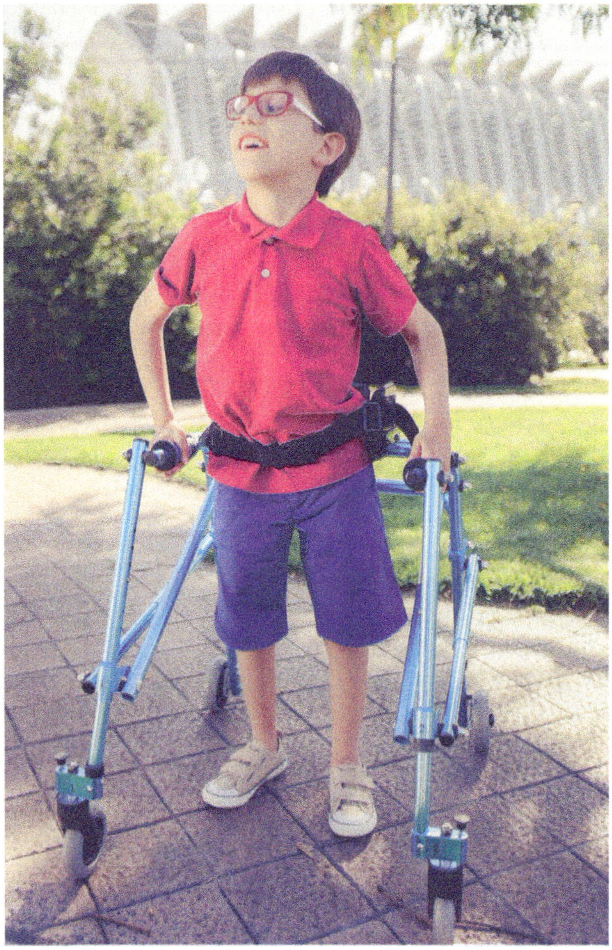

Figure 24.7 Walking Frame for Assistance with Movement

constipation.[4,39] Lastly, patients with severe CP have mobility issues, many of them needing to use special equipment to walk; some may have limited or no walking ability, requiring lifelong care.[33] A walking frame for assistance with movement is present in **Figure 24.7**.

PRACTICE POINT

Medications can be helpful in the management of spasticity, and the ones most often used for this population at this time include baclofen, botulinum toxin, or benzodiazepines.

Nutrition Assessment: Anthropometrics

Patients with CP often have issues with poor growth and are at risk for malnutrition, which can negatively affect overall health and well-being. Collection and monitoring of anthropometrics is essential in providing care for these patients. Unfortunately, measurement of weight and height is difficult, and established criteria for diagnosing malnutrition in the general pediatric population may not apply to patients with CP.[39]

Currently, it is recommended that CDC sex-specific growth charts should be used in assessing growth of children with CP. Of note, there are multiple specialized growth charts available that are categorized depending upon type of CP, with various distinctions that can be used to assess growth. However, these growth charts are more for a descriptive purpose and should be used with caution.[39,40] Patients will likely need alternative methods to measure weight and height based on the extent of the disability. Alternative methods can include a bed scale, weight with a parent and subtracting parent weight, platform scale, chair scale (if patient can sit alone), or another adaptive device for assistance.[40] An accurate height/length can also be difficult to obtain due to potential contractures and/or inability to stand. In these cases, alternatives include crown to rump length, sitting height, arm span, and tibia length or knee height.[40] It is also important to note the type of alternative measuring method used and to continue using the same method, which will provide further accuracy in assessing growth and show more meaningful trends in growth charts. In addition to using the same method to measure weight and height, braces or assistive devices the patient may wear should be kept in mind. Use of triceps skinfold thickness can be useful for assessing fat stores in patients with CP, as BMI/age will most likely not be a useful measure due to alterations in growth with CP. Proper tools for assessing nutritional status in this population are sorely needed.[39]

PRACTICE POINT

Alternative methods for obtaining anthropometrics are necessary for accurate assessment of a patient with CP, and noting which method was used is important for follow-up measurements and long-term monitoring.

Biochemical and Clinical

The collection of biochemical and clinical data will depend on the patient, their age, and any secondary conditions or issues, with particular focus on medication management. An important consideration in using anti-epileptics in children is that use of these drugs can negatively impact bone mineral density, making children more susceptible to fractures.[35-38] Patients taking anti-epileptic medications are also at risk for decreased levels of folic acid and other essential B vitamins.[37] Lastly, use of anti-spasticity medications, which can cause constipation, should be identified.[35,36]

Diet History

There are a variety of potential feeding difficulties that could arise in a patient with CP. Most commonly, patients may present with oromotor problems, which can lead to risk of aspiration, prolonged feeding times, and if left untreated, malnutrition. Increased risk of dysphagia in this population has the potential to present with silent aspiration, which is why proper assessment of feeding safety is important.[4,39,40] Obtaining a comprehensive diet history that includes assessment of food refusal, small volume feeding, coughing, and vomiting can help identify such problems. A diet interview should also include an assessment of GI problems such as stool patterns and reflux, which are common in this population.

Assessment of Energy Needs

There are several equations available to estimate the energy needs of a patient with CP, each with a different point of focus. One energy estimation equation by Holland recommends basing energy needs for children on height, with different ranges based on low-to-high energy needs.[29] Similarly, another equation uses height plus the presence or absence of motor dysfunction to determine a similar range of calorie needs. Krick recommended a different approach, estimating energy needs in children by taking into account multiple factors such as muscle tone, activity, and growth.[41] The starting equation used for an estimate with this method is as follows:

$$\text{Resting energy expenditure} \times \text{muscle tone} \times \text{activity} + \text{growth factors} = \text{kcal/day}$$

Note that although this equation is broader in scope than some others, it runs the risk of inaccuracies due to potential errors in estimating each factor. Clinical judgment should be used in deciding which equation to use, and any adjustments needed based upon each individual patient and their unique needs. **Tables 24.8** and **24.9** provide further considerations of muscle tone and ambulatory status when estimating energy needs in this population.

CORE CONCEPT 9

Muscle tone and ambulatory status can vary within patients with cerebral palsy and can greatly impact energy assessment.

Table 24.8 Energy Needs Adjustment by Muscle Tone and Ambulatory Status

Low muscle tone	Subtract 10%
Normal muscle tone	No adjustment
High muscle tone	Add 10%
Bedridden	Add 15%
Wheelchair- user	Add 20%
Ambulatory	Add 30%
Growth	Add 5 kcal/kg for expected/desired growth or catchup growth

Data from Krick J, Miller P. Nutritional implications in children with cerebral palsy. *Nutrition Focus*. 2003;18(3).

Table 24.9 Energy Needs in Cerebral Palsy

Low energy needs	7–9 kcal/cm
Moderate energy needs	9–11 kcal/cm
High energy needs	12–15 kcal/cm

Data from Holland M, Murray M. Diet and nutrition. In: Lucas BL, Feucht SA, Grieger LE, eds. *Children with Special Health Care Needs: Nutrition Care Handbook*. Pediatric Nutrition Practice Group and Dietetics in Developmental and Psychiatric Disorders, American Dietetic Association; 2004.

PRACTICE POINT

An interprofessional team approach, consisting of an RD, speech-language pathologist, occupational therapist, physician, and other healthcare professionals, is necessary to fully treat a patient and their unique feeding problems.

Nutrition Intervention

Medical nutrition therapy is individualized based on the patient's type of CP and its manifestations. The most common nutrition interventions are centered around addressing feeding and swallowing difficulties, GI problems, and underweight status.[39,42,43] Patients will need to work with appropriate resources, which may include speech–language pathologists and occupational therapists, to assess swallowing function and to ensure feeding is safer and easier. Many patients will require food texture modification, which may include thickened liquids.[43] Tools such as adaptive feeding devices can be instituted to improve feeding

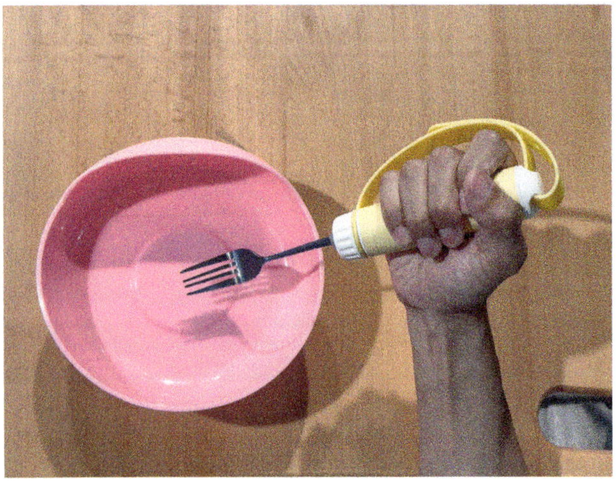

Figure 24.8 Adaptive Feeding Devices Help Meet the Individual Needs of the Patient

ability. This can include the use of specialized utensils, cups, and bowls; handcuffs for holding special tools; and seating devices. Adaptive feeding devices are patient-specific and tailored to their individual needs and abilities.[42] **Figure 24.8** provides an example of an adaptive feeding utensil.

Diet education plays a central role in managing dysphagia, GI problems such as reflux and constipation, as well as for maintaining appropriate weight. In children who are underweight, use of energy-dense foods and addition of calories and protein through added fats and powdered skim milk or protein powders can be helpful. Use of oral nutritional supplements can also be used.[42] If patients continue to struggle with meeting their nutritional needs orally, or if it is deemed unsafe to do so, consideration of nutrition support is appropriate. Gastric tube placement for feeding support is appropriate for severe cases in which patients are unable to safely feed (determined by failed speech/swallow evaluation), prolonged feeding times, and/or inadequate intake to maintain nutritional status.[44] Evidence exists that patients can gain weight after feeding-tube placement, but there are no clear data on improvements in overall growth.[44]

For patients working on overweight status, use of behavior modification techniques, portion control, and general healthy eating tips should be considered. For patients on both sides of the spectrum, nutritional education and goal setting, as well as monitoring of weight trends to assess progress, will be vital. Studies have shown that overweight status is increasing in ambulatory patients, while non-ambulatory and more severe patients are on the lower side of the weight spectrum.[45] Recent studies have shown that patients with less severe CP have fewer feeding issues, are more mobile, and are at risk for overweight just like peers within the same age group.[46] Recommendations for nutritional management of these patients will include individualized nutritional care plans to meet unique needs.

Finally, clinicians should ensure patients are achieving adequate intake from dietary or supplemental sources. Micronutrient supplementation of calcium, vitamin D, folate, and other B vitamins based on medications used may be needed to prevent deficiencies associated with medication therapy.[35-37]

Long-Term Monitoring and Evaluation

CP is a lifelong condition, and there is no cure, so patients within this population will require continued education and support to manage this condition as well as associated problems. Practitioners will need to follow weight trends over time to assess the adequacy of nutritional management and make any needed changes. Patients with more severe forms of CP will require long-term follow-up for nutritional support management as well as management of bowel regimens. Long-term work with other practitioners, especially physical and occupational therapy, will be important to best meet the goal of function and mobility.

Clinical Roundtable

Topic: Calculating Growth and Energy Needs for Patients with Cerebral Palsy

Background: Use of traditional formulas for estimating energy requirements in pediatric patients is imprecise in patients with cerebral palsy (CP). Differences in body composition, mainly decreased muscle mass, and activity render these formulas inaccurate. Multiple equations have been developed for the calculation of growth and energy requirements in patients with CP. However, patients will differ, particularly based on muscle spasticity and ambulatory status.

Roundtable Discussion

1. Based on the different classifications of CP (Table 24.7), how would you adjust your energy needs using the Krick model (Table 24.8)?
2. How would you determine whether you are using the proper calculation?

CASE STUDY REVISITED

Ali returns 2 months later with further weight loss. The decision is made to start supplemental tube feeding.

Anthropometric Data:

Weight: 11.5 kg, <3 percentile weight/age (CDC growth chart)
Height: 95 cm, 5 percentile height/age (CDC growth chart)
BMI: 12.7 kg/m^2 <3 percentile BMI/age (CDC growth chart)

Questions

1. Write an updated Nutrition Diagnosis/PES statement for Ali
2. Identify the nutrition intervention you would like to initiate for Ali to address the problem identified in your PES statement.
3. What would you recommend as a nutrition regimen?
4. What goals for oral intake would you recommend for the patient?
5. What parameters might you monitor?

Down Syndrome

Down syndrome (DS), also known as "trisomy 21," is a developmental disability with approximately 5700 infants born with this condition in the United States each year, making it the most common chromosomal condition diagnosed.[47] There are three types of DS that can occur: trisomy 21, translocation DS, and mosaic. The majority of DS cases (95%) present as trisomy 21, in which there is an extra copy of chromosome 21, making for a total of three rather than the typical two chromosomes. Translocation DS represents 3% of cases and occurs as a result of the translocation of extra chromosome 21 material onto another chromosome, rather than remaining independent as observed in classic trisomy 21. Lastly, mosaic makes up approximately 2% of cases and occurs when there is a mixture of typically formed pairs of chromosome 21 as well as trios.[47]

Although there are variations, patients with DS typically present with a certain grouping of physical characteristics. These can include almond-shaped eyes, short neck, flattened face, small hands and feet, short stature, and small ears (**Figure 24.9**).[47-49] Children with DS have developmental challenges such as being slower to learn to speak than their peers. Associated health problems for people with DS can include congenital heart disease (40–50%), hearing and vision problems (60–75%), obstructive sleep apnea (50–75%), celiac disease (5%), ASD (1%), and Hirschsprung disease (<1%).[48]

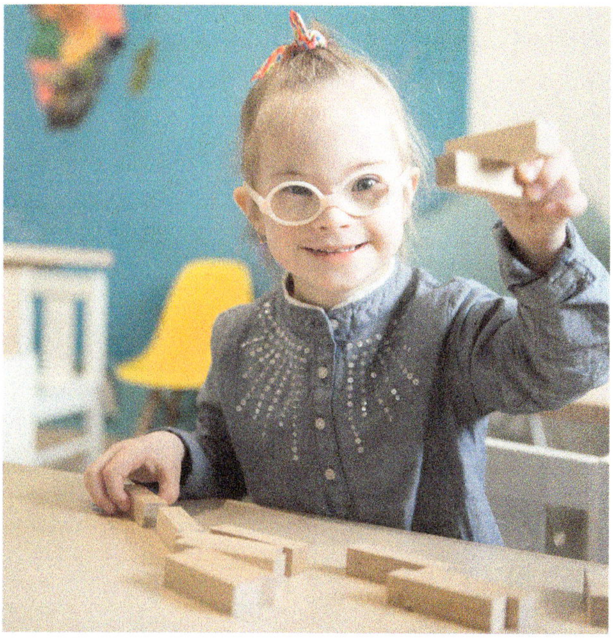

Figure 24.9 Child with Down Syndrome

Risk of DS increases as the mother's age during pregnancy increases, with higher prevalence found in mothers older than age 35 years.[47] Diagnosis of DS can be completed either during pregnancy or after birth. During pregnancy, the first step is to conduct standard screening tests, which can include an ultrasound and blood work, to be used for an initial assessment for DS. If there are findings consistent with DS, the next step would be to perform a diagnostic test, which

CASE STUDY INTRODUCTION

Teddy is a 5-year-old male with Down syndrome who has been referred by his pediatrician to visit an RD due to a recent diagnosis of celiac disease. Teddy presents as slightly underweight, and his parents report issues with finding foods he will like that are gluten free.

Anthropometric Data:

Weight: 15 kg, 5% weight/age (CDC growth chart)
Height: 109 cm, 50% height/age (CDC growth chart)
Weight/height: <3% (CDC growth chart)
BMI: 12.6 kg/m^2, <3% BMI/age (CDC growth chart)

Biochemical Data:

tTG-IgA result positive for celiac disease

Clinical Data:

Medications: Miralax PRN, multivitamin
Nutrition-Focused Physical Exam: Thin appearing, but otherwise normal for age; healthy-looking hair and skin. Abdominal exam notable for mild distention. No edema noted.

Dietary Data:

Dietary History: Previously eating a regular diet for age, but with reported GI symptoms when eating various carbohydrates (pasta, bread).

Questions

1. What nutritional risk factors does Teddy have?
2. How would you assess Teddy's energy needs?
3. Write two Nutrition Diagnosis statements for Teddy identifying the problem/etiology/signs and symptoms (PES) for Teddy's active nutrition issues.
4. What type of education is necessary for this family?
5. How would you adapt education based upon his diagnosis of Down syndrome?

could include amniocentesis, percutaneous umbilical cord testing, or chorionic villus sampling,[47] which all look for changes in chromosomes consistent with DS. Diagnosis after birth can be made through physical examination in combination with blood testing for alterations in chromosomal patterns.[47]

CORE CONCEPT 10

Down syndrome is a disability that can occur as a result of chromosomal alterations.

Nutrition Assessment: Anthropometrics

In general, people with DS tend to be of shorter stature and grow slower than their peers.[49] DS growth charts were created in 1988 after a study done by Cronk et al. showed that these differences in growth were true to this population, with growth rates in infancy almost 20% lower for children with DS.[50] A later study compiled a data set of over 600 children with DS to try and create a disease-specific growth chart. In this study, children were found to have better initial weight gain from birth to age 3 years and increases in height for both males and females.[51] However, with medical advances and increased life expectancy, these charts are not widely used, and current recommendations are instead to monitor growth via standard CDC and WHO growth charts based on sex.[49]

PRACTICE POINT

Down syndrome–specific growth charts are available, but current recommendations are to use CDC/WHO growth charts to monitor growth.

Biochemical and Clinical

Specific biochemical measurements obtained will depend on the patient, their age, any secondary conditions or issues, and their unique needs. One of the biggest concerns is that 50% of infants with DS are born with a congenital heart defect. The most commonly occurring cardiac defects are atrioventricular septal defects and ventricular septal defects.[52] The standard of care is to perform an echocardiogram on all infants with DS to assess for heart defects, even if this was done during pregnancy. Another medical complication that is associated with DS is Hirschsprung disease. While only affecting about 1% of patients with DS, the impact of this condition can be significant.[52] **Hirschsprung disease** is a blockage of the large intestine that is a result of missing nerves in the GI tract that function to move material through. This is treated through surgical repair, but studies have found that many patients with DS will still suffer from residual GI problems even after repair.[53] This can include incontinence, soiling, constipation, and even enterocolitis, all of which have the potential for long-term management needs.[53]

Obesity can become a problem for people with DS, because they have reduced resting metabolic rates compared to their peers, likely due to reduced fat-free mass and/or cellular metabolism abnormality.[54] The combination of lower metabolic rates and slower growth rates can contribute to development of obesity. Studies have shown that people with DS are more likely to be overweight or obese and additionally have a higher prevalence of secondary health problems compared to peers at a lower weight.[55] Close monitoring of growth charts and trends is important in combination with a healthy diet, regular physical activity, and limiting sedentary activities to help prevent obesity.[52]

An increased prevalence of celiac disease has been identified in patients with DS compared to the general population. Some studies estimate that roughly 6% of people with DS will develop celiac disease, often with delayed diagnosis.[56] Current recommendations from the American Academy of Pediatrics suggest a discussion of celiac disease and its symptoms and presentation at child's well visits to assess the potential for celiac disease.[48] If patients are exhibiting known signs of celiac such as abdominal pain/bloating, constipation, diarrhea, or growth changes, then testing should be done to confirm a diagnosis. There is currently no consensus on whether or not testing should be done in patients with DS who are non-symptomatic, even with the increased prevalence.[48] A positive diagnosis of celiac disease will mean following a gluten-free diet (avoidance of wheat, barley, and rye) in order to help alleviate and manage symptoms.

CORE CONCEPT 11

Patients with Down syndrome have a higher prevalence of celiac disease compared to their peers without Down syndrome.

Assessment of Needs

As previously mentioned, patients with DS have lower resting energy expenditure and growth rates relative to their peers. As a result, energy estimates and caloric needs for DS can be lower than average. Patients can have increased energy needs, especially in infancy, as a result of cardiac issues, poor growth, or decreased feeding abilities.[57] Estimates for energy needs can be made using equations specifically for this population; for children with DS, aged 5–11 years, starting estimates are 16.1 kcal/cm (males) and 14.3 kcal/cm (females).[57] More research is needed to help determine guidelines for this patient population, especially for other age groups.

CASE STUDY REVISITED

Teddy has overall been following the dietary instructions provided at the last appointment on gluten-free eating quite well. His family reports improved symptoms and intake. Anthropometrics today show a 1 kg weight gain, placing him at roughly the 10th percentile for weight.

Questions

1. Assess the status of your nutrition diagnosis/PES statement(s) for Teddy (e.g., resolution of PES, any new or continued problems).
2. What would be your educational focus for this appointment?
3. What goals would you set, keeping in mind the potential for growth slowing and future obesity in this population?

PRACTICE POINT

Calorie estimates based on height can be used to estimate energy needs of some patients with Down syndrome.

Nutrition Intervention

Nutritional interventions are centered around healthy eating and energy balance. Nutrition care should incorporate family members. Focus on offering a variety of foods and maintaining consistency at mealtimes is recommended. Managing the eating environment to decrease distraction, offer structure, and maintain communication during mealtimes can be beneficial. Foods that are lower in energy but high in nutrient quality should be encouraged. Modification of portion sizes and increased level of physical activity can help maintain energy balance for the DS population.[57]

For those patients who are diagnosed with celiac disease, diet education and assistance with developing strategies for a gluten-free diet are needed. The current market has numerous gluten-free options that can help ease the transition, which, combined with nutrition education and a focus on fruits, vegetables, and lean proteins, should lead to improvements in symptoms.

Long-Term Monitoring/Evaluation

Long-term monitoring for the DS population will include the potential cardiac issues in the future, even without issues in childhood; obesity; potential for celiac disease; vision/hearing problems; and the typical problems or comorbidities that can occur with aging such as diabetes, hypertension, or dyslipidemia. Also important to note is that advances in medicine have greatly impacted the life expectancy for patients with DS. Life expectancy has increased dramatically from 25 years of age in 1983 to 60 years of age in 2015.[58]

Autism Spectrum Disorders

Autism spectrum disorder (ASD) is a group of disorders that impact behavior, communication, and development. ASD prevalence has been increasing over the past 15 years and affects 1 in 36 children in the United States, occurring roughly four times more often in boys.[59] The current DSM, 5th edition, has standardized criteria from which a diagnosis of ASD can be made.[60] For a diagnosis to be made, a child must have persistent deficits in each of the three areas of social interaction and communication, and additionally have at least two of the four types of repetitive, restricted behaviors (refer to **Table 24.10** for diagnosis criteria).[60] ASD manifestations are largely heterogeneous, ranging from individuals with limited intellectual ability and communication skills to highly intelligent with above average language ability but poor social communication.[61] Typical features of ASD include inflexibility with behavior or other restrictive/repetitive behaviors, difficulty coping with change, and impairments with communication and social interactions. ASD is thought to have multiple etiologies that include both genetic and environmental factors. Treatment includes behavioral/education interventions and sometimes medications to manage corresponding diagnoses such as depression, anxiety,

Table 24.10 Diagnostic Criteria for Autism Spectrum Disorder

Persistent deficits in social communication and social interaction across multiple contexts (Must have all 3 for diagnosis)	Restricted, repetitive patterns of activities, interests, or behaviors (Must have at least 2 for diagnosis)
1. Deficits in social emotional reciprocity, such as abnormal social approach, reduced sharing of emotions, interests, or affect, failure of normal back-and-forth conversation 2. Deficits in developing, understanding, and maintaining relationships 3. Deficits in nonverbal communicative behaviors for social interaction (e.g., body language deficits or abnormalities in eye contact, lack of facial expressions)	A. Inflexible adherence to routines, difficulty with changes, insistence on sameness (e.g., eating the same foods every day) B. Repetitive motor movements, use of objects or speech (example: lining up toys, or flipping objects) C. Hypo- or hyperreactivity to sensory input or in aspects of the environment (e.g., fixation on lights/movements, excessive smelling) D. Fixated interests with abnormal intensity or focus

Data from Centers for Disease Control and Prevention. Autism Spectrum Disorder: Clinical Testing and Diagnosis for Autism Spectrum Disorder. Accessed January 20, 2025. https://www.cdc.gov/autism/hcp/diagnosis/index.html

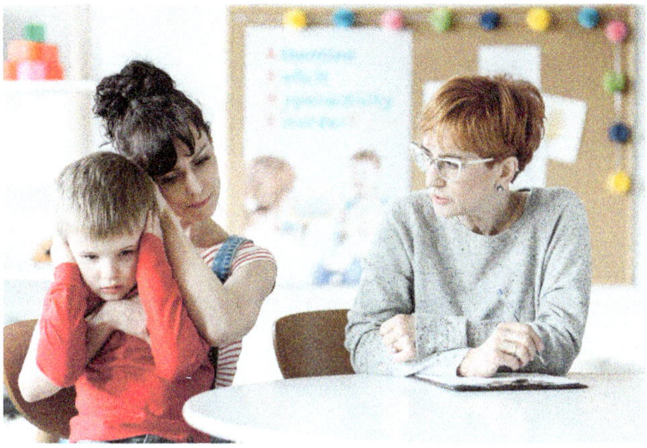

Figure 24.10 Child with Autism

or obsessive-compulsive disorder, but there are no specific medications to treat or manage ASD itself.[61] **Figure 24.10** presents a child with ASD.

CORE CONCEPT 12

Autism spectrum disorder (ASD) is a group of disorders that impact behavior, communication, and development.

Health problems commonly found in this population include GI issues, psychiatric disorders, and sleep difficulties. GI issues can include chronic diarrhea, constipation, esophageal reflux, bloating, and abdominal pain with potential contributing risk factors including diet, geography, medical conditions, medications, BMI, and genetics. Children with ASD are five times more likely to develop feeding problems such as poor intake, food selectivity, and food refusals.[62,63] Psychiatric disorders, in particular anxiety, are common in this population, impacting upwards of 70% of patients with an ASD diagnosis. Challenges with anxiety have also been showing to have an impact on GI issues such as constipation. Sleep difficulties can be common in patients with ASD, such as reduced sleep duration, and may also be associated with existing psychiatric disorders.[62]

Nutrition Assessment: Anthropometrics

There are no specialized growth charts for monitoring the growth of children with ASD, as this does not typically impact normal growth. Monitoring of growth in this population will include using standard CDC growth charts on a routine basis and use of BMI/age to assess weight status and trends.[64] Identified issues of under- or overweight status can be treated with the appropriate medical nutrition therapy. Of note, research has shown that there is a high prevalence of obesity in children with ASD, particularly in older children with ASD. The reason for increased likelihood of overweight and obesity in this population is likely multifactorial and due to potential issues with food selectivity/preferences, limited physical activity, and possible use of medications with side effects of weight gain.[65]

Biochemical and Clinical

Currently there is a lack of knowledge about the biological basis of ASD. Pharmacological interventions are limited. Risperidone and aripiprazole, which have dopaminergic and serotonergic antagonistic effects, are approved by the FDA for use in patients with ASD exhibiting irritability and aggressive behaviors. While they may be effective, these medications can lead to hyperglycemia, dyslipidemia, and weight gain.[61]

Diet History

Evaluating food intake is a key element in the nutritional assessment of patients with ASD. Diet history should include a combination of diet recall, food frequencies, and assessment of food-related behaviors.[66,67] Diet interview should help identify specific food aversions, hypersensitivities to texture, smell, and/or taste, and sensory issues.[68–70] Avoidant/restrictive food intake disorder (ARFID) is common in patients with neurodevelopment disorders, including those with ASD. Poor tolerance to sensory-related aspects of certain foods, fear of adverse consequences of food, and limited interest in foods (defining features of ARFID) also occur in ASD.[71] Selectivity with foods can lead to potential alterations in both macronutrient and micronutrient intake. Micronutrient deficiencies, including calcium, vitamin D, zinc, iron, folate, and vitamin B12, are dictated by which foods are included on a routine basis and which are avoided.[63,68] Patients with ASD have a tendency for food preferences that are high in refined carbohydrates, while dietary intakes of fiber and protein are lacking.[63,67,68] Increased intake of sweets can also lead to dental caries.[63] Identifying adherence to specific diets or foods avoided can help guide clinical decision-making.

A diet history should also screen for GI problems such as gastroesophageal reflux, constipation, and diarrhea. In children who cannot communicate well, these challenges can translate into irritability and aggressive behaviors.[63] Mealtime is also a social activity, which can be difficult for individuals with ASD. Gaining a better understanding of mealtime dynamics is important to help develop strategies for improvement.

CASE STUDY INTRODUCTION

Nick is a 4-year-old male, diagnosed with autism spectrum disorder 1 year prior, who has been referred to the RD from his pediatrician due to "picky eating" and selectivity with food choices. Nick is reported to have been growing appropriately despite challenges with his intake.

Anthropometric Data:

Weight: 16 kg, 45% weight/age (CDC growth chart)
Height: 100 cm, 30% height/age (CDC growth chart)
Weight/height: 59% (CDC growth chart)
BMI: 16 kg/m^2, 62% BMI/age (CDC growth chart)

Biochemical Data:

Labs within normal limits, including vitamin D level of 35 ng/mL (20–100 ng/mL)

Clinical Data:

Medications: Gummy multivitamin daily
Nutrition-Focused Physical Exam: Well appearing. Oral exam, hair, and nails appear normal. Skin is warm and intact. Abdominal exam unremarkable.

Dietary Data:

24-Hour Diet Recall:
Breakfast: Chocolate milk (8 oz), 2 medium pancakes with syrup, 1 vanilla yogurt
Lunch: Chocolate milk (8 oz), turkey sandwich (turkey, cheese, mayo), small bag potato chips
Snack: 4 vanilla wafer cookies, vanilla yogurt
Dinner: Chocolate milk (8 oz), 1 large bowl macaroni and cheese, 2 breadsticks

Questions

1. What are Nick's nutritional risk factors?
2. How would you assess Nick's energy needs?
3. Write two Nutrition Diagnosis statements for Nick identifying the Problem/Etiology/Signs and Symptoms of Nick's active nutrition issues.
4. Identify the nutrition interventions you would like to initiate for Nick to address the problems identified in your PES statements.
5. What indices should be included in your monitoring plans (e.g., anthropometrics, relevant labs)?

CORE CONCEPT 13

Food selectivity can be one of the biggest challenges in caring for a patient with autism spectrum disorder.

Assessment of Energy and Nutrient Needs

Estimation of energy and protein needs should be calculated by using standard energy estimation equations that are age appropriate. No condition-specific caloric estimates are established for this population. Goals should be based on weight status or other medical issues that impact energy needs. It is important to also consider the potential impact of selectivity or specificity in food changes and how this might translate into over- or undernutrition in regard to certain macro- and micronutrients.

PRACTICE POINT

There are currently no ASD-specific energy equations or growth charts.

Nutrition Intervention

Because there is no definitive form of treatment for ASD, parents will often seek complementary alternative medicine options such as following restrictive diets, taking nutritional supplements, or using alternative treatments such as yoga or chiropractors.[61] Use of restrictive diets to try and improve behavioral symptoms includes gluten/casein-free, ketogenic, food additive avoidance, and other **elimination diets**.[72]

Gluten-free or casein-free diets (GFCF) are often used in this population with the thought that eliminating these proteins from the diet will improve ASD symptoms. Research is mixed as to whether a GFCF diet can improve behavioral and ASD-related outcomes. Most studies are limited by small sample sizes, insufficient wash-out periods, and lack of long-term follow-up. Among the studies finding positive outcomes, the improvements were minor.[63,70,72,73] Nutrition education is necessary for patients who will be following these diets to ensure good nutritional status when eliminating foods with these nutrients. Patients eliminating these foods can risk calcium, vitamin D, and vitamin B deficiencies.[67]

The ketogenic diet (KD) is most recognized for its use in patients with epilepsy, but interest has grown in the use of this diet for patients with ASD, specifically for those with ASD who experience seizures. The KD involves high fat consumption (ranging from 60% to 89% of caloric needs), moderate protein, and low carbohydrate, so that the body will burn fat for fuel. Release of ketone bodies can cross the blood–brain barrier, having a neuroprotective effect.[74] Animal models have shown that the KD can inhibit inflammatory cytokines and levels of oxidative species.[74,75] In human studies, the KD was shown to improve communication and reduce the prevalence of attention-deficit/hyperactivity disorder, compulsive behavior, and abnormal sleep patterns.[63,67,70]

The link between behavioral issues in ASD and the gut microbiota is another area of research. This link is explained by the gut–brain axis, where the role of microbiota becomes significant. In this model, the production of short-chain fatty acid metabolites, typically known to be beneficial for gut health, also has neuromodulating effects, which may affect behavior in patients with ASD.[69] Studies are limited, but promising, with preliminary evidence showing that prebiotics, probiotics, and synbiotics can improve GI symptoms, decrease inflammation, and reduce the severity of ASD behavioral symptoms in children and young adults.[76,77] The Candida diet is based on the principle that *Candida* spp. has negative effects on immune function, brain, and behavior in children with ASD. In fact, numerous studies have shown an overgrowth of *Candida* spp. in stool of children with ASD. Probiotics such as *Saccharomyces boulardii* and *Lactobacillus* spp. may induce changes in the intestinal microflora leading to a decrease in *Candida* spp.[63]

Several other diets have been proposed for ASD. Most of these are focused on the elimination of foods.[78] The Feingold diet, named after Dr. Benjamin Feingold, is based on the theory that low-molecular-weight dyes added to foods result in behavioral problems in children. The aim of the diet is to eliminate food additives, artificial coloring and sweeteners, aspartame, and food preservatives, with the idea that these food additives have the potential to contribute to hyperactivity, GI problems, and behavior changes. Foods containing phenols and salicylates, such as tomatoes, peppers, peanuts, almonds, peaches, honey, and milk, among others, are also eliminated.[79] The Special Carbohydrate Diet (SCD) is a diet once proposed for celiac disease to decrease GI symptoms. In this diet, carbohydrates can be labeled as "legal" or "illegal" based on their content. Illegal or prohibited carbohydrates include all cereals (including maize, wheat, wheat germ, oats, barley, and rice), sugar, beans, potatoes, and all processed foods. The foods are thought to contribute to increased intestinal yeast and bacteria, and subsequently undesired GI symptoms. Similarly, the Low Sugar Diet (LSD) is believed to reduce the possible negative effect of sugar within the intestine, which is thought to contribute to an increase in harmful bacteria. The LSD may also improve balance of blood glucose levels. The LSD may decrease hyperactivity, irritability, and anxiety, while improving attention and cognition. It is important to highlight that these diets do not prevent, treat, or cure ASD, but may improve ASD-related symptoms in some children. Note that any recommendation to provide a restricted diet should be considered in light of a patient's baseline diet. If a patient already consumes a limited diet (due to picky eating, sensory issues, celiac disease, etc.), further restriction may risk development of a compromised nutritional status. **Table 24.11** presents some of the common diets used in patients with ASD.[63]

Long-Term Monitoring and Evaluation

Long-term monitoring will include evaluation of growth, food acceptance, potential need for a GI management program, and the potential for overweight and obesity. Additionally, dealing with any secondary health issues that come with normal aging while considering an ASD diagnosis and its unique challenges will be important.

PRACTICE POINT

There is currently insufficient scientific evidence to support the use of restrictive or elimination diets for patients with ASD.

CASE STUDY REVISITED

Nick and his family have returned for a follow-up appointment. His diet recall remains mostly the same, and his parents report that Nick is still resistant to trying any fruits and vegetables. They also report that he has recently been experiencing worsening issues with constipation.

Questions

1. Write an updated PES statement for Nick.
2. Identify the nutrition intervention you would like to initiate for Nick to address the problem identified in your PES statement.
3. What other healthcare providers might you consult?

Table 24.11 Therapeutic Diets Prescribed for Autism Spectrum Disorder

Diet	Diet Description	Possible Symptom Improvement
Gluten-Free and/or Casein-Free Diet	▪ Exclusion of gluten or gluten content of <20 mg/kg ▪ Exclusion of casein- dairy and other foods containing dairy or lactose products	▪ Cognition ▪ Language/communication ▪ Diarrhea ▪ Social interaction/understanding ▪ Sensory sensitivity ▪ Desire for sameness
Ketogenic Diet	▪ High fat—up to 90% of energy needs, low carbohydrate, moderate or high protein	▪ Attention and cognition ▪ Anxiety ▪ Language/communication ▪ Social interaction and understanding Constipation ▪ Seizures ▪ Lethargy ▪ Depression
Feingold Diet	▪ Elimination of food additives and preservatives; foods containing phenols and salicylates	▪ Hyperactivity ▪ Irritability ▪ Aggression ▪ Sensory sensitivity ▪ Falling sleep and staying asleep
Special Carbohydrate Diet	▪ Gluten free ▪ Excludes milk and milk products, sugars, beans, potatoes, processed foods, fructooligosaccharides	▪ Hyperactivity ▪ Aggression ▪ Irritability
Low-Sugar Diet	▪ Low in added sugars ▪ Limits sugary drinks and processed foods including sweets and pastries	▪ Hyperactivity ▪ Aggression ▪ Irritability ▪ Attention ▪ Cognition

Data from Matthews JS, Adams JB. Ratings of the effectiveness of 13 therapeutic diets for autism spectrum disorder: Results of a national survey. *J Pers Med.* 2023;13(10):1448. doi:10.3390/jpm13101448

Chapter Summary

Developmental disabilities are a group of conditions that are both diverse in nature but share similarities in secondary complications and necessary management. Each patient should be treated as a unique individual, using an interprofessional approach to help with management of care across the life span. As there is the potential for a variety of secondary complications with each developmental disability, it is important to know the hallmarks of each condition and work with a team approach to ensure all aspects of care are addressed.

Key Terms

developmental disability, hyperphagia, myelomeningocele, lipomeningocele, ventriculoperitoneal (VP) shunting, neurogenic bladder, neurogenic bowel, Chiari II malformation, spastic, cyanosis, Hirschsprung disease, autism spectrum disorder (ASD), elimination diets

References

1. Zablotsky B, Black LI. Prevalence of children aged 3-17 years with developmental disabilities, by urbanicity: United States, 2015-2018. *Natl Health Stat Report*. 2020;(139):1–7.
2. Goldstone A, Holland A, Hauffa B, Hokken-Koelega A, Tauber M. Recommendations for the diagnosis and management of Prader-Willi syndrome. *J Clin Endrocinol Metabol*. 2008;93(11):4183–4197.
3. National Institute of Neurological Disorders and Stroke. Spina bifida. Reviewed January 8, 2025. Accessed January 20, 2025. https://www.ninds.nih.gov/health-information/disorders/spina-bifida
4. Dodge NN. Cerebral palsy: Medical aspects. *Pediatr Clin North Am*. 2008;55(5):1189–1207.
5. Townsend MJ, Claridy MD, Bajaj SS, Tu L, Stanford FC. Obesity and eligibility for obesity treatments among adults with disabilities in the U.S. *Am J Prev Med*. 2022 Oct;63(4):513–520. doi:10.1016/j.amepre.2022.04.003
6. Bandini L, Danielson M, Esposito LE, et al. Obesity in children with developmental and/or physical disabilities. *Disability Health Jl*. 2015;8(3):309–316.
7. Maiano C, Hue O, Morin AJ, Moullec G. Prevalence of overweight and obesity among children and adolescents with intellectual disabilities: a systematic review and meta-analysis. *Obes Rev*. 2016;17(7):599–611.
8. Schwartz L, Caixàs A, Dimitropoulos A, et al. Behavioral features in Prader-Willi syndrome (PWS): consensus paper from the International PWS Clinical Trial Consortium. *J Neurodevelopment Disord*. 2021;13:1–3.
9. Butler MG. Prader-Willi syndrome: Obesity due to genomic imprinting. *Curr Genomics*. 2011;12(3):204–215.
10. McCandless SE. Committee on Genetics. Clinical report-health supervision for children with Prader-Willi syndrome. *Pediatrics*. 2011;127(1):195–204.
11. Bohonowych J, Miller J, McCandless SE, Strong TV. The global Prader-Willi syndrome registry: development, launch, and early demographics. *Genes (Basel)*. 2019;10(9):713. doi:10.3390/genes10090713
12. US Department of Health and Human Services. National Institutes of Health. Eunice Kennedy Shriver National Institute of Child Health and Human Development. Prader-Willi Syndrome (PWS). NIH Fact Sheet. Accessed January 17, 2025. https://www.nichd.nih.gov/health/topics/factsheets/prader-willi. Updated 12/29/21
13. Barrea L, Vetrani C, Fintini D, et al. Prader-Willi syndrome in adults: an update on nutritional treatment and pharmacological approach. *Curr Obes Rep*. 2022;11(4):263–276. doi:10.1007/s13679-022-00478-w
14. Kuhlmann L, Joensson IM, Froekjaer JB, Krogh K, Farholt S. A descriptive study of colorectal function in adults with Prader-Willi Syndrome: high prevalence of constipation. *BMC Gastroenterol*. 2014;14:63. doi:10.1186/1471-230X-14-63
15. Academy of Nutrition and Dietetics. Developmental disabilities. Prader Willi syndrome. In: *Pediatric Nutrition Care Manual*. Accessed January 17, 2025. https://www.nutritioncaremanual.org/topic.cfm?ncm_category_id=13&lv1=144620&lv2=144745&ncm_toc_id=144745&ncm_heading=Nutrition%20Care%20home%20page
16. Casamitjana L, Blanco-Hinojo L, Giménez-Palop O, et al. One year of recombinant human growth hormone treatment in adults with Prader–Willi syndrome improves body composition, motor skills, and brain functional activity in the cerebellum. *J Clin Med*. 2022;11(7):1831. doi:10.3390/jcm11071831
17. Deal CL, Tony M, Höybye C, Allen DB, Tauber M, Christiansen JS, 2011 Growth Hormone in Prader-Willi Syndrome Clinical Care Guidelines Workshop Participants. Growth hormone research society workshop summary: consensus guidelines for recombinant human growth hormone therapy in Prader-Willi syndrome. *J Clin Endocrinol Metab*. 2013;98(6):E1072–E1087. doi:10.1210/jc.2012-3888
18. Wolfe G, Salehi V, Browne A, et al. Metabolic and bariatric surgery for obesity in Prader Willi syndrome: systematic review and meta-analysis. *Surg Obes Related Dis*. 2023;19(8):907–915.
19. US Preventive Services Task Force. Folic acid supplementation for the prevention of neural tube defects: US Preventive Services Task Force recommendation statement. *JAMA*. 2017;317(2):183–189. doi:10.1001/jama.2016.19438
20. Fletcher JM, Brei TJ. Introduction: Spina bifida—A multidisciplinary perspective. *Dev Disabil Res Rev*. 2010;16(1):1–5.
21. CDC. Spina Bifida. About Spina Bifida. Updated January 2, 2025. Accessed January 18, 2025. https://www.cdc.gov/spina-bifida/about/index.html
22. Cortes MS, Chmait RH, Lapa DA, et al. Experience of 300 cases of prenatal fetoscopic open spina bifida repair: report of the International Fetoscopic Neural Tube Defect Repair Consortium. *Am J Obstetr Gynecol*. 2021;225(6):678-e1.
23. National Institute of Neurological Disorders and Stroke. Chiari Malformations. Last Reviewed July 19, 2024.

Accessed January 18, 2025. https://www.ninds.nih.gov/health-information/disorders/chiari-malformations
24. Tubbs RS, Oakes WJ. Treatment and management of the Chiari II malformation: an evidence-based review of the literature. *Child's Nervous System*. 2004;20(6):375–381.
25. Akbari SHA, Limbrick DD Jr, Kim DH, et al. Surgical management of symptomatic Chiari II malformation in infants and children. *Child's Nervous System*. 2013;29(7):1143–1154.
26. Academy of Nutrition and Dietetics. Spina bifida: anthropometrics. In: *Pediatric Nutrition Care Manual*. Accessed January 18, 2025. https://www.nutritioncaremanual.org/topic.cfm?ncm_category_id=13&lv1=144620&lv2=144744&lv3=269958&ncm_toc_id=269958&ncm_heading=Nutrition%20Care%20home%20page
27. Academy of Nutrition and Dietetics. Gastrointestinal disease. Constipation. Nutrition intervention. In: *Pediatric Nutrition Care Manual*. Accessed January 20, 2025. https://www.nutritioncaremanual.org/topic.cfm?ncm_category_id=13&lv1=144625&lv2=144769&lv3=270739&ncm_toc_id=270739&ncm_heading=Nutrition%20Care%20home%20page
28. Liusuwan RA, Widman LM, Abresch RT, Styne DM, McDonald CM. Body composition and resting energy expenditure in patients aged 11 to 21 years with spinal cord dysfunction compared to controls: comparisons and relationships among the groups. *J Spinal Cord Med*. 2007;30(suppl 1):S105–111.
29. Holland M, Murray M. Diet and nutrition. In: Lucas BL, Feucht SA, Grieger LE, eds. *Children with Special Health Care Needs: Nutrition Care Handbook*. Pediatric Nutrition Practice Group and Dietetics in Developmental and Psychiatric Disorders. American Dietetic Association; 2004.
30. Bunting K, Mills J, Philips S, Ramsey E, et al. Alternative methods to determine energy needs, energy requirements in children with developmental disabilities. In: *Pediatric Nutrition Reference Guide*. 9th ed. Texas Children's Hospital; 2010:21–22.
31. Reinehr T, Dobe M, Winkel K, Schaefer A, Hoffmann D. Obesity in disabled children and adolescents: an overlooked group of patients. *Dtsch Arztebl Int*. 2010;107(15):268–275.
32. My Child at Cerebral Palsy.Org. Prevalence of Cerebral Palsy. Accessed January 19, 2025. https://www.cerebralpalsy.org/about-cerebral-palsy/prevalence-and-incidence
33. Sørensen SJ, Brekke G, Kok K, et al. Nutritional screening of children and adolescents with cerebral palsy: a scoping review. *Dev Med Child Neurol*. 2021;63:1374–1381. doi:10.1111/dmcn.14981
34. Centers for Disease Control and Prevention. Cerebral Palsy. About Cerebral Palsy. Updated May 2024. Accessed January 19 2025. https://www.cdc.gov/cerebral-palsy/about/index.html
35. Verrotti A, Greco R, Spalice A, Chiarelli F, Iannetti P. Pharmacotherapy of spasticity in children with cerebral palsy. *Pediatr Neurol*. 2006;34(1):1–6.
36. Sheth RD, Binkley N, Hermann BP. Progressive bone deficit in epilepsy. *Neurology*. 2008;70(3):170–176.
37. Sener U, Zorlu Y, Karaguzel O, Ozdamar O, Coker I, Topbas M. Effects of common anti-epileptic drug monotherapy on serum levels of homocysteine, vitamin B12, folic acid and vitamin B6. *Seizure*. 2006;15(2):79–85.
38. Finbråten A, Syversen U, Skranes J, Andersen G, Stevenson R, Vik T. Bone mineral density and vitamin D status in ambulatory and non-ambulatory children with cerebral palsy. *Osteoporosis Int*. 2014:1–10.
39. Oftedal S, McCormack S, Stevenson R, Benfer K, Boyd RN, Bell K. The evolution of nutrition management in children with severe neurological impairment with a focus on cerebral palsy. *J Hum Nutr Diet*. 2025;38:e13277. doi:10.1111/jhn.13277
40. Academy of Nutrition and Dietetics. Cerebral palsy: anthropometrics. In: *Pediatric Nutrition Care Manual*. Accessed January 18, 2025. https://www.nutritioncaremanual.org/topic.cfm?ncm_category_id=13&lv1=144620&lv2=144742&lv3=269925&ncm_toc_id=269925&ncm_heading=Nutrition%20Care%20home%20page
41. Krick J. A proposed formula for calculating energy needs of children with cerebral palsy. *Dev Med Child Neurol*. 1992;34:481–487.
42. Academy of Nutrition and Dietetics. Cerebral palsy: Nutrition intervention. *Pediatric Nutrition Care Manual*. Accessed January 18, 2025. https://www.nutritioncaremanual.org/topic.cfm?ncm_category_id=13&lv1=144620&lv2=144742&lv3=269927&ncm_toc_id=269927&ncm_heading=Nutrition%20Care%20home%20page
43. Kamal S, Kamaralzaman S, Sharma S, et al. A review of food texture modification among individuals with cerebral palsy: the challenges among cerebral palsy families. *Nutrients*. 2022;14(24):5241. doi:10.3390/nu14245241
44. Rogers B. Feeding method and health outcomes of children with cerebral palsy. *J Pediatr*. 2004;145(2):S28–S32.
45. Hurvitz EA, Green LB, Hornyak JE, Khurana SR, Koch LG. Body mass index measures in children with cerebral palsy related to gross motor function classification: a clinic-based study. *Am J Phys Med Rehabil*. 2008;87(5):395–403.
46. Rogozinski BM, Davids JR, Davis RB, et al. Prevalence of obesity in ambulatory children with cerebral palsy. *J Bone Joint Surg*. 2007;89(11):2421–2426.
47. Centers for Disease Control and Prevention. Birth Defects: Down Syndrome. Reviewed May 16, 2024. Accessed August 5, 2024. https://www.cdc.gov/birth-defects/about/down-syndrome.html
48. Bull MJ, Committee on Genetics. Health supervision for children with Down syndrome. *Pediatrics*. 2011;128(2):393–406.
49. Academy of Nutrition and Dietetics. Down syndrome: anthropometrics. In: *Pediatric Nutrition Care Manual*. Accessed December 3, 2017. https://www.nutritioncaremanual.org/topic.cfm?ncm_category_id=13&lv1=144620&lv2=144743&lv3=269940&ncm_toc_id=269940&ncm_heading=Nutrition%20Care%20home%20page
50. Cronk C, Crocker AC, Pueschel SM, et al. Growth charts for children with Down syndrome: 1 month to 18 years of age. *Pediatrics*. 1988;81(1):102–110.
51. Zemel BS, Pipan M, Stallings VA, et al. Growth charts for children with Down syndrome in the United States. *Pediatrics*. 2015;136(5):e1204–1211.
52. Bull MJ, Trotter T, Santoro SL, et al. Health supervision for children and adolescents with Down syndrome. *Pediatrics*. 2022;149(5).
53. Friedmacher F, Puri P. Classification and diagnostic criteria of variants of Hirschsprung's disease. *Pediatr Surg Int*. 2013;29(9):855–872.
54. Murray J, Ryan-Krause P. Obesity in children with Down syndrome: background and recommendations for management. *Pediatr Nurs*. 2010;36(6):314.
55. Rimmer JH, Yamaki K, Davis BM, Wang E, Vogel LC. Obesity and overweight prevalence among adolescents with disabilities. *Prev Chronic Dis*. 2011;8(2):A41.

56. Du Y, Shan LF, Cao ZZ, Feng JC, Cheng Y. Prevalence of celiac disease in patients with Down syndrome: a meta-analysis. *Oncotarget*. 2017;9(4):5387–5396.
57. Academy of Nutrition and Dietetics. Down syndrome: nutrition therapy efficacy. In: *Pediatric Nutrition Care Manual*. Accessed January 19, 2025. https://www.nutritioncaremanual.org/topic.cfm?ncm_category_id=13&lv1=144620&lv2=144743&ncm_toc_id=144743&ncm_heading=Nutrition%20Care%20home%20page
58. National Down Syndrome Society. Down Syndrome Facts. Accessed December 3, 2017. http://www.ndss.org/Down-Syndrome/Down-Syndrome-Facts
59. Centers for Disease Control and Prevention. Autism Spectrum Disorder (ASD): Data and Statistics. Reviewed May 16, 2024. Accessed August 5, 2024. https://www.cdc.gov/autism/data-research/index.html
60. Centers for Disease Control and Prevention website. Autism Spectrum Disorder: Clinical Testing and Diagnosis for Autism Spectrum Disorder. Reviewed May 16, 2024. Accessed August 5, 2024. https://www.cdc.gov/autism/hcp/diagnosis/index.html.
61. Hirota T, King BH. Autism spectrum disorder: a review. *JAMA*. 2023;329(2):157–168. doi:10.1001/jama.2022.23661
62. Madra M, Ringel R, Margolis KG. Gastrointestinal issues and autism spectrum disorder. *Child Adolesc Psychiatr Clin N Am*. 2020;29(3):501–513. doi:10.1016/j.chc.2020.02.005
63. Önal S, Sachadyn-Król M, Kostecka M. A review of the nutritional approach and the role of dietary components in children with autism spectrum disorders in light of the latest scientific research. *Nutrients*. 2023;15(23):4852. doi:10.3390/nu15234852
64. Academy of Nutrition and Dietetics. Autism spectrum disorders (2024): anthropometrics. In: *Pediatric Nutrition Care Manual*. Accessed January 25, 2025. https://www.nutritioncaremanual.org/topic.cfm?ncm_category_id=13&lv1=144620&lv2=275629&lv3=275632&ncm_toc_id=275634&ncm_heading=Nutrition%20Care%20home%20page
65. Sammels O, Karjalainen L, Dahlgren J, Wentz E. Autism spectrum disorder and obesity in children: a systematic review and meta-analysis. *Obes Facts*. 2022;15(3):305–320. doi:10.1159/000523943
66. Academy of Nutrition and Dietetics. Autism spectrum disorders: feeding skills. In: *Pediatric Nutrition Care Manual*. Accessed August 23, 2024. https://www.nutritioncaremanual.org/topic.cfm?ncm_category_id=13&lv1=144620&lv2=145108&lv3=269988&ncm_toc_id=269988&ncm_heading=Nutrition%20Care%20home%20page
67. Molina-López J, Leiva-García B, Planells E, Planells P. Food selectivity, nutritional inadequacies, and mealtime behavioral problems in children with autism spectrum disorder compared to neurotypical children. *Int J Eat Disord*. 2021;54(12):2155–2166. doi:10.1002/eat.23631
68. Narzisi A, Masi G, Grossi E. Nutrition and autism spectrum disorder: between false myths and real research-based opportunities. *Nutrients*. 2021;13(6):2068. doi:10.3390/nu13062068
69. Rodop BB, Başkaya E, Altuntaş I, Erbaş O. Nutrition effect on autism spectrum disorders. *J Experiment Basic Med Sci*. 2021;2(1):7–17.
70. van der Wurff I, Oenema A, de Ruijter D, et al. A scoping literature review of the relation between nutrition and ASD symptoms in children. *Nutrients*. 2022;14(7):1389. doi:10.3390/nu14071389
71. Farag F, Sims A, Strudwick K, et al. Avoidant/restrictive food intake disorder and autism spectrum disorder: clinical implications for assessment and management. *Dev Med Child Neurol*. 2022;64(2):176–182. doi:10.1111/dmcn.14977
72. Yu Y, Huang J, Chen X, et al. Efficacy and safety of diet therapies in children with autism spectrum disorder: a systematic literature review and meta-analysis. *Front Neurol*. 2022;13:844117. doi:10.3389/fneur.2022.844117
73. González-Domenech PJ, Diaz-Atienza F, Gutiérrez-Rojas L, Fernández-Soto ML, González-Domenech CM. A narrative review about autism spectrum disorders and exclusion of gluten and casein from the diet. *Nutrients*. 2022;14(9):1797. doi:10.3390/nu14091797
74. Li Q, Liang J, Fu N, Han Y, Qin J. A ketogenic diet and the treatment of autism spectrum disorder. *Front. Pediatr.* 2021;9:650624. doi:10.3389/fped.2021.650624
75. Olivito I, Avolio E, Minervini D, et al. Ketogenic diet ameliorates autism spectrum disorders-like behaviors via reduced inflammatory factors and microbiota remodeling in BTBR T+ Itpr3tf/J mice. *Experiment Neurol*. 2023;366:114432.
76. Mitchell LK, Davies PS. Pre-and probiotics in the management of children with autism and gut issues: a review of the current evidence. *European J Clin Nutr*. 2022;76(7):913–921.
77. Soleimanpour S, Abavisani M, Khoshrou A, Sahebkar A. Probiotics for autism spectrum disorder: an updated systematic review and meta-analysis of effects on symptoms. *J Psychiatr Res*. 2024;179:92–104.
78. Matthews JS, Adams JB. Ratings of the effectiveness of 13 therapeutic diets for autism spectrum disorder: results of a national survey. *J Personal Med*. 2023;13(10):1448. doi:10.3390/jpm13101448
79. Smith M. Historical and social science perspectives on food allergy. *Clin Experiment Allergy*. 2023;53(9):902–910.

Glossary

24-hour dietary recall A retrospective tool that requires the client to recite all food intake within the previous 24 hours

A

Abscess Occurs when an area of tissue becomes infected, characterized by swollen tissue and accumulation of pus

Absorption The movement of digested food particles from the external environment and into the cells of the gastrointestinal tract, to be utilized by the body

Acetoacetic acid Ketone produced from the metabolism of fat

Acetone Ketone produced from the metabolism of fat

Acidemia Blood pH lower than 7.35

Acidosis The process that raises the hydrogen ion concentration

Activities of daily living (ADLs) Routine activities of daily life that are performed independently, including feeding, moving, toileting, and bathing

Activity energy expenditure (AEE) The energy expenditure associated with physical activity

Actual body weight (ABW) The unadjusted sum of all body compartments without distinction between fat and fat-free mass

Acute decompensated heart failure (ADHF) A rapid onset of heart failure symptoms that requires immediate treatment

Acute hepatitis Liver inflammation lasting up to 6 months

Acute kidney injury (AKI) A rapid decline in kidney function

Acute liver failure Massive hepatic necrosis with the onset of hepatic encephalopathy and coagulopathy within 6 months of known liver disease

Acute pancreatitis (AP) Short-term inflammation of the pancreas, most often the result of a biliary tract obstruction or chronic alcoholism

Acute respiratory distress syndrome (ARDS) A type of hypoxemic respiratory failure characterized by acute development of bilateral lung infiltrates that are visible on chest x-ray, an arterial oxygen tension to fraction of inspired oxygen ratio (PaO_2/FiO_2) less than 300 mm Hg, and a systemic inflammatory response

Acute wounds Injuries that heal through a normal sequence of events, usually between 5 and 10 days, or at least within 30 days

Acute-phase proteins Also known as acute-phase reactants; plasma proteins whose synthesis and circulating concentrations are regulated in inflammation, infection, and trauma

Acute-phase reactants Inflammation markers that change significantly (increase or decrease) during infection, trauma, inflammation, or surgery

Adaptation Changes in small intestinal structure and function to adapt to disease or damage

Adaptive hyperfiltration In cases of reduced nephrons, the remaining functional nephrons take on more pressure from the systemic circulation

Adipokines Cell-signaling proteins released by adipose tissue

Adipose Fat tissue

Adiposity rebound Increases in fat mass that occur during adolescence

Adjusted body weight Algorithm-derived weight used to determine energy expenditure in patients with extremes of body weight

Adjusted edema-free body weight (aBWef) A calculation of body weight in patients undergoing dialysis with edema who are either obese or underweight

Adverse reactions to food (ARF) Any abnormal physiological responses that occur following the ingestion of food

Aerophagia Excessive swallowing of air

Air embolism Embolism caused by the introduction of air into a vessel

Air displacement plethysmography (ADP) Body composition measure in which the volume of displaced air is measured to determine body volume

Alcohol-related hepatitis (AH) Steatohepatitis in alcohol-related liver disease

Alcohol-related liver disease (ALD) Liver disease caused by excessive consumption of alcohol

Alkalemia Blood pH higher than 7.45

Alkalosis The process that lowers the hydrogen ion concentration

Allergic rhinitis Nasal inflammation, sneezing, congestion, runny nose, and/or itchy eyes due to an allergic reaction; also known as "hay fever"

Allogeneic HSCT Stem cell transplant using donor cells

Alpha-gal syndrome (AGS) An immune response to galactose-alpha-1,3-galactose (alpha-gal), a carbohydrate found in the glycolipids and glycoproteins of mammals but absent in poultry, humans, and higher primates

Alternative medicine Medical products and practices used instead of standard medicine treatment (e.g., herbs and botanicals)

Alveoli Tiny sacs within the lungs that allow oxygen and carbon dioxide to exchange between the respiratory space and the bloodstream

Amenorrhea The bsence of three consecutive menstrual cycles

Amniotic fluid A complex fluid that cushions the fetus, provides immunological protection, and supports growth and development

Amniotic sac A double-membraned covering that encloses the fetus and amniotic fluid

Amyloid-β peptides Key components of amyloid plaques found in the brains of people with Alzheimer's disease

Amylorrhea Starch excretion in the feces

Anastomosis The site at which resected sections of intestine are reattached to each other

Anemia A reduction in erythrocytes per unit of blood volume or a decrease in hemoglobin of blood to below the level of physiologic needs

Anemia of chronic disease (ACD) Anemia caused by chronic inflammatory or infectious disorders

Angina pectoris Stable chest pain

Angioedema Swelling of the eyelids, face, or lips

Angiogenesis The formation of new blood vessels

Angiogram A radiographic procedure used to visualize blood flow and detect blocked, narrowed, or damaged vessels, often using contrast dye

Ankyloglossia The result of a short, tight, lingual frenulum causing difficulty in speech articulation due to limitation in tongue movement, also called "tongue-tie"

Anorexia Partial or complete loss of interest in food

Anorexia nervosa (AN) An eating disorder characterized by an intense fear of weight gain that leads to overrestriction of dietary intake, significantly low body weight, and a distorted self-perception of body weight or shape

Anorexigenic Appetite suppressing

Anthropometrics The measurement of physical characteristics of the human body

Anthropometry The assessment of measures and proportions of the human body

Anticariogenic foods Prevents plaque from recognizing cariogenic foods

Antidiuretic hormone (ADH) The hormone that controls the amount of urine formed

Anuria The absence of urine formation

Apolipoprotein B100 A dominant cholesterol that causes atherosclerosis

Apolipoproteins Protein molecules that are a component of the outer layer of lipoproteins

Appliance The plastic pouch that connects to a colostomy to collect stool

Appropriate-for-gestational-age (AGA) Infants born with weights that chart between the 10th and 90th percentiles for their gestational age

Arginine A conditionally essential amino acid required for cell growth, protein synthesis, and collagen deposition

Arterial blood gases (ABGs) Blood gas values used to assess the lungs' ability to oxygenate blood

Ascites Fluid in the abdomen

Asepsis The absence of bacteria, viruses, or other microorganisms

Aspiration The movement of liquid into the patient's lungs

Aspiration pneumonia Lung infection due to inhaling food or fluid

Asthma A chronic disease where the bronchial tubes of the lungs become inflamed and tighten

Asymmetric macrosomia Fetal overgrowth, may be associated with maternal diabetes

Atherosclerosis The hardening and narrowing of arteries due to plaque build-up

Atherosclerotic cardiovascular disease Coronary heart disease or coronary artery disease, cerebrovascular disease, and peripheral artery disease depending on the location of the plaque

Atopic dermatitis An inflammatory skin condition causing itching and redness

Atrophic gastritis Chronic inflammation of the stomach mucosa that is characterized by a partial loss of parietal cell mass

Auscultation The assessment of sounds that reflect movement of fluid or air through organs and viscera using a stethoscope

Autism spectrum disorder (ASD) A group of disorders that impact behavior, communication, and development

Autologous HSCT Stem cell transplant from the patient's own bone marrow, peripheral blood, or umbilical cord

Avoidant/restrictive food intake disorder (ARFID) A persistent disturbance in eating that leads to significant clinical consequences, such as weight loss, inadequate growth, significant nutrient deficiencies, and/or impaired psychosocial functioning such as an inability to eat with others

Azotemia Nitrogenous waste accumulation in the blood

Azotorrhea Excess nitrogen in the urine or feces

B

Baker's asthma A form of IgE-mediated wheat allergy associated with repeated exposure to inhaling wheat flour

Basal metabolic rate (BMR) Energy expenditure associated with maintaining the metabolic activities of the body's cells and tissues

Basic metabolic panel (BMP) Blood test that measures glucose, sodium, potassium, carbon dioxide, chloride, blood urea nitrogen, and creatinine

β-hydroxy-β-methylbutyrate (HMB) A metabolite of leucine that may prevent or delay muscle breakdown, increase cell proliferation and protein synthesis, and improve nitrogen balance

β-hydroxybutyric acid Ketone produced from the metabolism of fat

Binge eating disorder (BED) An eating disorder characterized by recurrent binge eating episodes that are not followed by compensatory purging or nonpurging behaviors

Bioelectrical impedance analysis (BIA) A test of the resistance of a high-frequency, low-amplitude electrical current passed through the body; used to make a distinction between fat-free mass and total body water

Biologically appropriate weight (BAW) Identification of an individualized healthy weight range for an individual, rather than adhering to predetermined ideals

Biotherapy A cancer therapy that stimulates or suppresses the body's immune system to kill cancer cells; also known as biological therapy

Blood-brain barrier (BBB) A semi-permeable membrane that separates the blood from the brain tissue

Body cell mass (BCM) All metabolically active tissue

Body mass index (BMI) An anthropometric comparison of body weight to body height independent of frame size; calculated as weight in kilograms divided by the square of height in meters

Bolus A ball of food or single dose of liquid or medication

Bolus feeding A specific volume of feeding is delivered for a specific time interval for a short period of time

Bowman's capsule A capsule-shaped structure in the kidney nephron that encloses the glomerulus

Braden Scale for Predicting Pressure Sore Risk A multifactorial scale for predicting the risk of ulcer development; includes sensory perception, moisture, activity, mobility, friction and shear, and nutrition

Brain death Irreversible cessation of all brain activity

Branched chain amino acids (BCAA) Amino acids, including leucine, isoleucine, and valine, that account for 40% of the essential amino acids and are primarily catabolized by skeletal muscle

Bronchi Large air passages that lead from the trachea to the lungs

Bronchioles Small branches in which the bronchus divides

Bronchodilators Oral and inhaled medications used to open up constricted passageways and improve breathing

Brush border Microvilli covered surface of epithelial cells found in certain locations such as the gastrointestinal tract

Bulbar neurons Motor neurons responsible for speech and swallow

Bulimia nervosa (BN) An eating disorder characterized by recurrent episodes of binge eating followed by one or more compensatory behaviors to avoid weight gain

C

Cachexia General wasting and malnutrition usually associated with chronic disease

Calf circumference (CC) Measurement of the girth of the calf taken at the widest part of the calf, which can provide information about muscle mass

Cancer cachexia A multifactorial syndrome characterized by an ongoing loss of skeletal muscle mass in people with cancer that cannot be fully reversed by conventional nutritional support

Carcinoma Type of solid malignancy that originates in the skin or tissues that line or cover internal organs

Cardiac cachexia An uncontrollable loss of weight in heart failure patients

Cardiac catheterization A procedure where a catheter is inserted into a large blood vessel leading to the heart to measure heart function

Cardiac output A measure of blood pumped per minute that is calculated by multiplying the stroke volume by the heart rate

Cardiac rehabilitation Physician-supervised multimodal behavioral and medical rehabilitative program that aims to improve cardiovascular health as a secondary prevention method for those with established or at risk for cardiovascular disease

Cardiogenic shock A severe, life-threatening condition of systemic hypoperfusion

Cardiopulmonary bypass A technique that temporarily takes the place of the function of the heart and lungs

Cardiovascular disease (CVD) Disease affecting the heart and blood vessels

Cariogenic foods Caries promoting

Cariogenicity The caries-promoting properties of a diet or food

Cariostatic foods Not contributing to decay

Carnitine An amino acid derivative that aids in the oxidation of fatty acids

Catabolic stress response Significant alterations in physiology, immune function, and metabolism in response to injury, propagated by inflammatory mediators

Catabolism Breakdown of body tissues for energy in response to lack of other energy sources

Catch-up growth Nutritional requirements necessary to achieve ideal body weight

Catecholamines Neurotransmitters that mediate the aberrations found in cell function and physiology; include epinephrine and norepinephrine

Catheter embolism Embolism caused by a fragment of a broken or damaged catheter

Catheter occlusion The inability to infuse, flush, and/or aspirate on the venous access device

Catheter-related bloodstream infection (CRBSI) Systemic infection that enters the body via the catheter or insertion site; see *central line–associated bloodstream infection (CLABSI)*

Catheter-related complications (CRCs) Mechanical (infectious or noninfectious) or metabolic complications of catheter use

Catheter-related venous thrombosis (CRVT) The creation of a thrombus as platelets and fibrin coagulate in a vessel damaged by catheter insertion

CDC growth charts Growth charts utilizing data on the growth rates of infants from the United States, starting at age 3 months

Celiac disease (CD) An autoimmune disorder characterized by inflammatory injury to the intestinal mucosa following gluten ingestion

Central line–associated bloodstream infection (CLABSI) Systemic infection that enters the body via the catheter or insertion site; see *catheter-related bloodstream infection (CRBSI)*

Central nervous system (CNS) The part of the nervous system that includes the brain and spinal cord

Central PN (CPN) Parenteral nutrition delivered via access to a central vessel; namely, the superior or inferior vena cava or right atrium

Central venous catheter (CVC) A sterile flexible tube inserted into a large vein in the chest, neck, or groin for delivery of parenteral nutrition or intravenous fluids

CF transmembrane conductance regulator (CFTR) protein A protein that functions as a channel across the membrane of cells producing mucus, sweat, saliva, tears, and digestive enzymes

CF-related diabetes (CFRD) A type of diabetes found in persons with cystic fibrosis; while it shares similarities with both type 1 and type 2 diabetes, it is its own separate type

Chemotherapy The use of antineoplastic drugs, used as a single agent or in combination with other agents, that disrupt the reproductive cycle of cancer cells

Chiari II malformation An extension of the cerebellar and brain stem tissue into the foramen magnum, with the cerebellar vermis (which connects the two halves of the cerebellum) appearing as incomplete or damaged

Child-Pugh score A scoring system used to classify the severity of liver disease and prognosis of individuals with cirrhosis. The categories include class A, B, or C, with class C being the most severe

Cholelithiasis Gallstones

Cholestasis Reduced bile flow

Cholestatic liver disease Liver disease caused by inhibition of bile flow

Choline A nutrient that is important for neurodevelopment, lipid metabolism, and brain development

Chronic hepatitis Liver inflammation lasting greater than 6 months

Chronic kidney disease (CKD) A decline in kidney function over time

Chronic obstructive pulmonary disease (COPD) A progressive, systemic disease marked by airflow obstruction; generally encompasses chronic bronchitis, emphysema, and small airways disease

Chronic pancreatitis (CP) Long-term, progressive inflammation of the pancreas, leading to loss of exocrine and endocrine function

Chronic wounds Injuries that persist longer than 6 weeks or frequently reoccur and are typically associated with underlying conditions that lead to tissue breakdown, inadequate tissue perfusion, and chronic inflammation

Chylomicrons Spherical vesicles that are part of the class of lipoproteins consisting of a triglyceride core surrounded by apoproteins and cholesterol

Chyme Partially digested food that passes from the stomach to the small intestine

Cilia Hair-like structures within the lungs that normally remove bacteria

Cirrhosis The final stage of liver fibrosis, in which fibrotic tissues form nodules that permanently alter the structure of the liver

Closed tube feeding system A ready-to-use container or bag of formula is connected to the patient's feeding access

Coagulopathy Any condition in which the blood's ability to clot is compromised

Cognitive behavioral therapy (CBT) A highly structured therapy that identifies and replaces maladaptive behaviors and cognitive processes with more suitable ones

Collagen The most abundant protein in the human body; the primary component of the extracellular matrix

Colostomy Removal of the rectum and connecting a portion of the colon as the stoma

Colostrum The first breast milk produced

Complementary medicine Medical products and practices that are not part of standard medical care but are used along with standard medicine (e.g., acupuncture)

Complete blood count Blood test that provides a count of the cells in the blood and a description of red blood cells

Comprehensive metabolic panel (CMP) Blood test that measures all the elements in a basic metabolic panel, plus albumin, total protein, alkaline phosphatase, alanine transaminase, aspartate transaminase, and bilirubin

Computed tomography (CT) An imaging modality that utilizes x-ray technology to provide quantitative data on muscle composition and distribution

Continuous ambulatory peritoneal dialysis (CAPD) A form of peritoneal dialysis that requires three to five exchanges daily

Continuous cycling peritoneal dialysis (CCPD) A form of peritoneal dialysis that uses a machine to carry out the exchanges overnight while the patient sleeps

Continuous feeding A slow drip of feedings into the stomach or small intestine on an hourly basis

Continuous infusion Infusion performed for over 24 hours

Continuous renal replacement therapy (CRRT) A type of dialysis utilizing hemofiltration, hemodialysis, or both

Correction factor Sensitivity factor; defines the number of points one unit of insulin will lower the blood glucose

Coronary artery bypass graft (CABG) Surgical procedure in which arterial stenosis is bypassed with the placement of an artificial or saphenous vein graft

Coronary artery disease (CAD) Atherosclerosis affecting the arteries that supply blood to the heart

Counterregulatory hormones Hormones that oppose the effects of insulin such as glucagon, cortisol, epinephrine, and norepinephrine

Cow's milk allergy (CMA) One of the most common IgE-mediated food allergies observed in early childhood

Cow's milk protein allergy An immune-mediated allergic reaction to protein (casein/whey) in milk

Creatinine height index (CHI) Measurement of creatinine excretion as a percentage

Crohn's disease A form of inflammatory bowel disease characterized by transmural inflammation that can affect any organ of the gastrointestinal tract from mouth to anus

Cross-contamination The passage of pathogens indirectly from one source to another due to the improper use of sterilization procedures, unclean instruments, or recycling of products

Cyanosis Bluish coloring of the skin from a lack of oxygen

Cyclical infusion Infusion performed for 10–12 hours per day

Cytokines Cell-signaling molecules that aid in cell-to-cell communication in immune responses and stimulate the movement of cells toward sites of inflammation, infection, and trauma

Cystic fibrosis A life-threatening, autosomal recessive genetic disorder characterized by abnormal transport of sodium, chloride, and water throughout the cells of the body resulting in abnormally thick mucus that causes damage to the lungs, pancreas, and other organs

D

De Ritis ratio The serum AST to ALT ratio

Debridement The removal of dead or damaged tissue

Decompensated cirrhosis See *end-stage liver disease (ESLD)*

Defined diets Dietary regimens based on an underlying theory or ideology of how food interacts with the body

Delayed lactogenesis II Milk production does not begin within 72 hours postpartum

Dementia A neurodegenerative condition that includes loss of memory, language, problem-solving, and/or other thinking abilities that are severe enough to impact activities of daily living

Demineralization The chemical process by which minerals are removed from the teeth

Dental caries Cavities

Dentin The bony tissue forming the bulk of a tooth beneath the enamel

Desensitization A temporary elevation in the threshold of allergen required to provoke an allergic reaction, contingent upon continuous allergen exposure

Developmental disability A condition that becomes evident at birth or early childhood and has varying impacts on the individual throughout the life cycle

Diabetes distress The intense stress related to the experience of living with diabetes

Diabetic ketoacidosis A condition where excessive ketone bodies cause the blood pH to drop to dangerous levels; can quickly lead to death

Dialectical behavioral therapy (DBT) Therapy that is designed to help individuals change unhelpful patterns of behavior by identifying triggers and applying new coping skills

Diastole Stage of the heartbeat where ventricles are relaxed and blood flows from the atria to refill the ventricles

Diastolic blood pressure The force that pushes against the blood vessels when the heart is at rest

Differential count A complete blood count for white blood cells

Digestion The mechanical or enzymatic breakdown of food into its constituents

Digital clubbing Focal enlargement of the terminal ends of the fingers

Direct calorimetry Direct measurement of heat produced or lost

Disaccharide Sugar made up of two monosaccharides

Diverticulosis The accumulation of pouches in the colon

Donation after cardiac death (DCD) Donation of organs after a patient is deceased by means of cardiac death

Doubly labeled water (DLW) A form of indirect calorimetry based on the assumption of an exponential disappearance of hydrogen and oxygen isotopes from the body

Dry weight An estimated weight in patients with fluid overload (from edema, overhydration, ascites, etc.); determined by subtracting the estimated fluid weight from the actual body weight

Dual energy x-ray absorptiometry (DXA) A scan used to differentiate bone, lean mass, and bone-free tissues; often used for measuring bone density

Dumping syndrome A range of symptoms that occur when stomach contents are released too quickly and in too large of a volume into the small intestine

Duodenum The proximal portion of the small intestine

Dysbiosis Disruption and imbalance in the gut microbiome where beneficial bacteria are reduced and harmful bacteria are increased

Dysgeusia Altered taste perception

Dyslipidemia Alterations in the normal transport of lipids and lipoproteins

Dysphagia Difficulty swallowing

Dyspnea Difficulty breathing

E

Early childhood caries (ECC) The presence of at least one decayed tooth, a missing tooth, or a tooth surface that has been filled in any primary tooth in a child 6 years or younger

Early enteral nutrition (EEN) The initiation of enteral nutrition within 48 hours of illness or traumatic event

Eating disorder (ED) A psychiatric illness characterized by chronic disturbances of eating habits and weight control behaviors that debilitate both physical health and psychological functioning

Eclampsia Severest form of pregnancy-induced hypertension, characterized by convulsions, seizure, proteinuria, and edema

Edentulism Tooth loss

Ejection fraction (EF) The amount of blood being pumped out of the ventricle each time it contracts

Electrocardiogram Diagnostic tool used to measure the heart's electrical activity by placing electrodes on the body surface

Electrolytes Substances that dissolve into ions in solution

Elemental formula A nutritional formula that provides nutrients in predigested forms that are thought to be absorbed within the first few feet of the small intestine

Elimination diet Systematically removing elements of a diet to determine what foods are contributing to symptoms, with the end goal of eliminating offending foods and reintroducing "safe" foods

Embolism A blood clot that breaks free and travels to another area of the body

Enamel The hard, mineralized surface of teeth

Enamel hypoplasia An enamel deficiency that increases tooth vulnerability to damage

End-stage liver disease (ESLD) A condition in which the body is unable to make up for the functional deterioration of the liver, resulting in life-threatening complications

End-stage kidney disease (ESKD)/End-stage renal disease (ESRD) The most advanced form of chronic kidney disease; also known as Stage 5 kidney or renal disease

Endotoxin Lipopolysaccharide; a toxin produced by Gram-negative bacteria

Engorgement Distention of a body part with fluid or other material

Enteral nutrition (EN) The delivery of nutrients into the gastrointestinal tract either by mouth or through a feeding tube

Enterocytes Intestinal absorptive cells

Epicardial fat A fat deposit that surrounds the heart and is enclosed by the viscera pericardium

Erythematous rashes Skin rash caused by inflammation

Erythrocyte A red blood cell

Erythematous rash Red, inflamed skin condition

Erythropoietin (EPO) The hormone that promotes red blood cell production in bone marrow upon detection of low oxygen levels

Eosinophilic esophagitis (EoE) An allergic immune-mediated disease characterized by an increased presence of eosinophils in the esophageal lining, causing inflammation, dysfunction, and damage

Eosinophilic gastrointestinal disorders (EGIDs) An inflammatory condition characterized by an increased presence of eosinophils in the GI tract

Estimated glomerular filtration rate (eGFR) An estimate of the amount of plasma filtered through the glomeruli within a given period, calculated through the use of various formulas

Euglycemia Normal blood sugar levels in the blood

Exit site The point where the catheter exits the body

Extravasation Leakage of fluids from an intravenous line into the surrounding tissue

Extremely low birth weight (ELBW) Infants born weighing less than 1000 grams

F

Failure to thrive (FTT) See growth faltering

Familial hypercholesterolemia (FH) A genetic disorder caused by defective LDL-C receptors that leads to LDL-C levels greater than the 95th percentile for age and gender

Fat-free mass (FFM) The body compartment that includes muscles, bones, organs, ligaments, tendons, and water

Feeding cues A baby's ability to signal hunger and fullness through signs such as crying, or sucking fingers or fists

Female athlete triad A syndrome comprising disordered eating habits, osteoporosis, and menstrual disorders, often observed in female athletes who utilize at least one unhealthy weight-control method

Fetal alcohol syndrome A range of conditions, including irreversible brain damage and growth problems, caused by excessive alcohol consumption during pregnancy

Fetal macrosomia A newborn that is significantly larger than normal

Fetus Unborn baby

Fiberoptic endoscopic evaluation of swallow (FEES) A diagnostic procedure in which a thin tube with a camera is used to visualize the throat during a swallow to assess safety

Fibrosis A buildup of connective tissue or scar tissue

Fibrostenosis Narrowing of the bowels

Fistula An abnormal tunnel-like connection between the hollow space of an organ and the body

Fluorapatite A crystalline structure that is a naturally occurring form of calcium, phosphorus, and fluoride; it is more resistant than hydroxyapatite

Fluoride A natural element that is important to the integrity of bone and teeth

Fluoroscopic tube placement Using x-ray imaging as a guide when placing the feeding tube into the gastrointestinal tract

Fluorosis Defective tooth mineralization resulting from excessive fluoride ingestion during pre-eruptive tooth mineralization

Foam cells Cells that are laden with fat and macrophages, often the hallmarks of atherosclerotic lesion formation

Food allergy An adverse immunological response to a food protein, which can be immunoglobulin E (IgE) mediated, non-IgE-mediated, or a mix of IgE/non-IgE-mediated mechanisms

Food frequency questionnaire (FFQ) A retrospective tool that requires the client to complete a survey about food intake over a specific period of time in an attempt to depict "usual" intake

Food insecurity Uncertainty about one's food supply, along with insufficient food intake with or without physical hunger

Food intolerance A food reaction that predominantly affects the digestive system, is dose-dependent, and typically has a delayed onset

Food protein-induced allergic proctocolitis (FPIAP) A non-IgE-mediated food allergy in infants, usually identified within the first 6 months, presenting as rectal bleeding, and triggered by ingested protein by the infant for formula-fed infant or by the breastfeeding mother for breastfed infants

Food protein-induced enterocolitis syndrome (FPIES) A non-IgE-mediated adverse reaction to food that typically manifests within the first year of life, usually following the introduction of the first foreign food protein in an infant's diet

Food records diary A method of acquiring data on nutritional intake; requires the client to record food intake for a specific time period

Forced expiratory volume at 1 second (FEV_1) The amount of air a person can exhale during forced breathing

Foremilk The first milk released during a feeding

Frailty A geriatric syndrome characterized by age-related declines in multiple organ systems due to the cumulative effects of disease, inactivity, stress, poor nutritional intake, altered physiology, and impaired homeostatic reserve

Fulminant liver failure Liver failure that occurs within 8 weeks of the onset of known liver disease

Functional assay Laboratory test that measures the specific biochemical or physiological functioning of a nutrient, rather than just the quantity of the nutrient

G

Galactagogues Substances believed to enhance milk production in lactating women

Galactosemia A rare genetically inherited metabolic disorder associated with the inability to metabolize the sugar galactose properly

Gastrectomy Surgical removal of part or all of the stomach

Gastric residual The volume of liquid that remains in the stomach during enteral feeding

Gastric stasis Delayed gastric emptying as a result of the elimination of vagus innervation

Gastroesophageal reflux disease (GERD) A digestive disorder in which the lower esophageal sphincter is relaxed or weakened and remains open, allowing reflux of gastric acid into the esophagus

Gastroparesis Delayed gastric emptying in the absence of a mechanical gastric outlet obstruction

Geriatric nutrition Medical nutrition therapy for older adults

Gestation The time between conception and birth

Gestational diabetes mellitus (GDM) Increased glucose intolerance that is first discovered during the second or third trimester

Gestational hypertension Systolic blood pressure equal to or greater than 140 mm Hg or a diastolic blood pressure equal to or greater than 90 mm Hg that occurs without proteinuria after 20 weeks' gestation

Gestational weight gain The amount of weight gained during pregnancy, which can impact both fetal and maternal health

Ghrelin Appetite-inducing gastrointestinal hormone that increases gastrointestinal motility and decreases insulin secretion

Gingiva Gums

Glasgow Coma Scale (GCS) A scoring system that rates traumatic brain injury based on eye opening, verbal response, degree of confusion and orientation, and motor response to command or painful stimulus

Glomerular filtration rate (GFR) The amount of plasma filtered through the glomeruli within a given period

Glomerulus A mass of capillaries that are specifically responsible for producing the ultrafiltrate

Gluconeogenesis Synthesis of glucose from noncarbohydrate sources, usually amino acids

Glucose infusion rate (GIR) A function of the concentration of dextrose and the rate at which the dextrose is administered

Glutamate A neurotransmitter and a nonessential amino acid

Glutamine The most abundant amino acid in the plasma; necessary for protein synthesis, lymphocyte proliferation, and wound healing

Glycemic index (GI) The quantity and rate at which different carbohydrate foods influence blood glucose response

Glycemic load (GL) The digestibility rate of foods balanced against the amount of carbohydrate they contain

Glycogenolysis Breakdown of glycogen stores for glucose

Graft Any tissue or organ used for implantation or transplantation

Graft thrombosis Obstruction of blood flow to a graft

Graft versus host disease (GVHD) An immune response designed to eliminate the foreign tissue in the recipient of an allogeneic HSCT, wherein the donor's cells recognize the host's cells are foreign

Granulomas A collection of monocytes and/or macrophages and other inflammatory cells with or without giant cells

Gravida The number of times a female has been pregnant

Growth An increase in physical size or mass of body tissues that occurs from infancy to adulthood

Growth channels Describes growth on or between growth percentiles

Growth charts Data that describe the normal or expected amount of growth based on well-child data

Growth discordance A significant size or weight difference between the two fetuses of a twin pregnancy

Growth faltering (GF) Also known as failure to thrive; a slower rate of weight gain after the first 2 weeks of birth

Growth reference Charts that describe growth in a specific time or place

Growth standards Charts that demonstrate optimal growth or how normal children should grow when breastfed

Growth velocity The rate at which a child grows

Gut-brain axis The intricate relationship between the gastrointestinal tract and the brain

Gut-liver axis The intricate relationship between the gastrointestinal tract and the liver

Gut-lung axis The intricate relationship between the gastrointestinal tract and the lung that involves a bidirectional exchange of microbiota and their metabolites

H

Half arm span (HAS) The length between the middle of the sternal notch and tip of the middle finger; measured with the patient's arm horizontal and in line with the shoulders; also known as arm length

Handgrip dynamometer A tool used to test handgrip strength

Handgrip strength (HCS) An assessment of muscle strength used to estimate nutritional status

Hang time The amount of time an enteral formula can safely be at room temperature

Head circumference (HC) A measure of head size, taken around the most prominent area on the back of the head, immediately above the supraorbital ridge, to just above the patient's eyebrows

Heart failure (HF) The final stage of cardiovascular disease

Height Also known as stature; how tall a person is

Height-for-age The plotting of a child's height according to the distribution of height for children of the same age and gender on a growth chart

Helicobacter pylori A bacterial infection that colonizes the stomach by moving through the mucosal lining, attaching to gastric epithelial cells, and sending out cytotoxins to allow for generation of more bacteria

HELLP syndrome A variant of severe preeclampsia characterized by hemolysis, elevated liver enzymes, and low platelet count

Hematemesis The vomiting of blood

Hematologic malignancy Cancer that originates in the blood-forming tissue, such as bone marrow (leukemias) or in the cells of the immune system (lymphomas and myelomas), and can be classified as acute or chronic

Hematopoietic stem cell transplant (HSCT) The infusion of stem cells to treat patients whose bone marrow or immune system is defective or damaged, such as in hematological cancers

Hemochromatosis An autosomal recessive disease characterized by accumulation of iron in the liver, pancreas, heart, adrenals, testes, pituitary, and kidneys

Hemoconcentration Increased red blood cell concentrations and low plasma levels

Hemodialysis (HD) Medical treatment in which blood is removed from the body and processed through a machine containing a dialysis membrane, which acts as an artificial kidney

Hemodilution Decreased red blood cell concentrations and high plasma levels

Hemodynamic instability Inadequate organ and tissue perfusion throughout the body; characterized by hypotension

Hemolysis Breakdown of red blood cells

Hemorrhagic stroke A stroke caused by bleeding within the brain due to a ruptured blood vessel, leading to pressure and damage to brain tissues

Hepatic encephalopathy (HE) A neuropsychiatric disorder characterized by personality changes, altered levels of consciousness, and cognitive impairment

Hepatic function panel Biochemical measures used to assess liver function; typically includes alanine aminotransferase, albumin, alkaline phosphatase, aspartate aminotransferase, direct bilirubin, total bilirubin, and total serum protein

Hepatic steatosis The accumulation of fat in the liver

Hepatocellular liver disease Liver disease caused by liver cell injury

Hepatorenal syndrome (HRS) Progressive kidney failure among people with liver disease

Hindmilk The last milk released during a feeding

Hirschsprung disease A blockage of the large intestine that is a result of missing nerves in the bowel that function to move material through

Home parenteral nutrition (HPN) Parenteral nutrition provided in the home, as opposed to a hospital or other healthcare institution

Human milk fortifier A nutritional supplement formulated for preterm infants which is added to human milk to increase macro- and micronutrient concentrations

Hydrogen breath test (HBT) A noninvasive diagnostic tool for lactose intolerance that measures hydrogen levels in a breath sample after consuming a lactose-containing solution; operates on the principle that undigested lactose fermented by intestinal bacteria produces gas, including hydrogen

Hydroxyapatite A crystalline structure that is a naturally occurring form of calcium and phosphorus

Hypercalcemia High calcium levels in the blood

Hypercapnia Increased carbon dioxide in the blood

Hyperchloremia High chlorine levels in the blood

Hyperemesis gravidarum (HG) Persistent nausea and vomiting resulting in dehydration, muscle wasting, electrolyte imbalances, ketonuria, nutritional deficiencies, and weight loss of greater than 5% of pre-pregnancy weight

Hyperglycemia High blood sugar levels

Hyperkalemia High potassium levels in the blood

Hypermagnesemia High magnesium levels in the blood

Hypermetabolic Referring to the physiologic state of increased rate of metabolic activity characterized by an abnormal increase in the body's basal metabolic rate

Hypernatremia High sodium levels in the blood

Hyperphagia Insatiable hunger

Hyperphosphatemia High phosphate levels in the blood

Hypertension (HTN) Chronic high blood pressure

Hypertriglyceridemia Elevated fasting serum triglyceride levels

Hypertonic Having a greater osmolarity than another solution

Hypervolemia Volume overload

Hypocalcemia Low calcium levels in the blood

Hypochloremia Low chlorine levels in the blood

Hypoglycemia Low blood sugar levels

Hypokalemia Low potassium levels in the blood

Hypomagnesemia Low magnesium levels in the blood

Hyponatremia Low sodium levels in the blood

Hypophosphatemia Low phosphate levels in the blood

Hypotonic Having a lower osmolarity than another solution

Hypovolemia Volume depletion

Hypoxemia Low blood oxygen

I

Ideal body weight (IBW) An adjusted weight-for-height, based on the weights associated with the lowest mortality for a given height

Ileal brake The delay of gastric emptying and slowing of transit time in the proximal portions of the small intestine, allowing extended contact time between nutrients and the mucosa

Ileocecal (IC) valve The valve that separates the ileum of the small intestine from the cecum of the large intestine

Ileostomy Removal of the colon and the rectum and connecting the distal end of the ileum as the stoma

Ileum The distal portion of the small intestine

Immunonutrition The effect of nutrients, including macronutrients, vitamins, minerals, and trace elements, on inflammation, the formation of antibodies, and the resistance to disease

Immunosenescence The gradual deterioration of the immune system that occurs with aging

Immunosuppression Suppression of the immune response by drugs or radiation

Indirect calorimetry Measure of respiratory gas exchange

Inflammation The body's initial response to injury; characterized by redness, warmth, swelling, pain, and loss of function; the first phase of wound healing

Inflammatory bowel disease (IBD) A group of chronic, relapsing-remitting immune disorders that originate in the gastrointestinal tract

Insensible water loss The loss of water through the skin and respiration

Inspection The visual observation of color, shape, texture, and size

Instrumental activities of daily living (IADLs) Activities that are not required for daily functioning, but are necessary for independent living, such as shopping, food preparation, managing finances, and using the telephone

Insulin resistance The inability of cells to uptake insulin for use in glucose metabolism

Insulin-to-carbohydrate ratio (ICR) The amount of carbohydrate processed by one unit of insulin

Integrative medicine A total approach to medicine that combines standard medicine with complementary and alternative practices

Intermittent feeding Feeding is delivered over a 20- to 60-minute interval, four to six times per day

International Dysphagia Diet Standardization Initiative (IDDSI) Internationally standardized terms and definitions to characterize thickened liquids and texture-modified foods

Intestinal failure The inability to maintain nutritional autonomy

Intestinal failure-associated liver disease (IFALD) Previously referred to as parenteral nutrition– associated liver disease (PNALD), hepatobiliary disorder associated with long-term parenteral nutrition therapy

Intestinal leakage The release of digestive contents into the peritoneum via a hole in the stomach, gallbladder, or small or large intestines

Intestinal permeability (IP) Also known as leaky gut; increased intestinal permeability

Intra-aortic balloon pump (IIABP) A surgical procedure that provides short-term mechanical support to increase cardiac output via a balloon placed in the aorta via the femoral artery

Intradialytic parenteral nutrition (IDPN) Parenteral nutrition provided via hemodialysis tubing during each hemodialysis treatment

Intramyocellular lipid deposition A condition where macrovesicular fat accumulates in hepatocytes, resulting in the enlargement of the liver

Intrauterine growth restriction (IUGR) The condition in which the fetus is unable to grow and develop normally, putting it at high risk of serious consequences after birth

Intravenous lipid emulsion (ILE) Intravenous fat administration to provide calories and essential fat

Intrinsic AKI Acute kidney injury caused by diseases within the renal parenchyma

Intrinsic factor A glycoprotein produced by the parietal cells of the stomach essential for B_{12} absorption

Involution The final state of mammary gland development, in which the mammary glands return to their pre-pregnancy state

Iron deficiency anemia Anemia caused by a lack of iron in the blood

Irritable bowel syndrome (IBS) A functional gastrointestinal disorder characterized by recurrent abdominal pain and altered bowel habits

Ischemic cardiomyopathy A type of heart failure in which the left ventricle is enlarged because of decreased blood supply to the heart muscle

Ischemic heart disease See *coronary artery disease*

Ischemic stroke A stroke characterized by a blockage of blood flow to the brain either by a clot or plaque in the arteries

Isolate Intact, natural form of protein

Isotonic Having the same osmolarity as another solution

Isotope dilution technique A classic method of measuring total body water using isotopes of oxygen or water (as deuterium or tritium), which are exchanged in the body similarly to water

J

Jejunostomy Connecting the distal jejunum as the stoma

Jejunum The middle portion of the small intestine

K

Kayser-Fleischer ring A brownish or gray-green ring at the rim of the cornea

Ketogenic diet (KD) A high-fat, low-carbohydrate, low-protein diet which, due to its macronutrient distribution, induces a metabolic state that mimics starvation

Ketone production The production of ketones that typically occurs when carbohydrate intake is low

Kidney Disease Improving Global Outcomes (KDIGO) A group of nephrology experts that provides a source of consolidated, evidence-based clinical practice guidelines to be used in all aspects of kidney disease

Kidney Disease Outcome Quality Initiative (KDOQI) A program by the National Kidney Foundation that develops and publishes evidence-based clinical practice guidelines for the diagnosis and treatment of all stages of kidney disease

Knee height A measurement taken from the sole of the foot to the anterior surface of the thigh while the lower limb is flexed; used to estimate standing height in nonambulatory patients

Kupffer cells Macrophages dedicated to the liver

Kussmaul's respirations Abnormally deep breathing associated with metabolic acidosis

Kwashiorkor Malnutrition, with or without caloric depletion, that results in depletion of visceral protein

L

Lactation Secretion of milk from the breasts

Lactogenesis I The process of converting inert breast cells to milk-producing cells

Lanugo Soft, downy hair growth on the face and body

Laparoscopic adjustable gastric band (LAGB) A metabolic and bariatric procedure that physically restricts the stomach by use of an inflatable band that, when filled with saline, squeezes and decreases the size of the stomach

Laparoscopy Using small ports placed on the abdominal wall so that the peritoneal cavity can be accessed

Large-for-gestational-age (LGA) Infants with birth weights that chart above the 90th percentile for their gestational age

Leaky gut Also known as intestinal permeability; increased intestinal permeability

Lean body mass (LBM) The portion of the body that includes body cell mass as well as extracellular mass, which includes bone and extracellular fluid

Left ventricular assist device (LVAD) A surgically implanted mechanical pump that supports heart function by pumping blood from the left ventricle to the aorta to circulate oxygen-rich blood throughout the body

Left ventricular hypertrophy (LVH) A disease in which the muscle of the left ventricle becomes thickened and enlarged

Leptin A hormone produced by white adipose tissue that inhibits appetite

Let down The release of breast milk

Lewy bodies Unusual clumps of proteins called alpha-synuclein that develop inside the neuron

Lipid panel Biochemical measures used to screen for dyslipidemia; typically includes total cholesterol, low-density lipoprotein (LDL)-cholesterol, high-density lipoprotein (HDL)-cholesterol, and triglycerides

Lipomeningocele A type of closed neural tube defect characterized by deposition of fatty tissue tumors

Lipoprotein(a) Lipoprotein having similar size and structure as LDL cholesterol that is atherogenic and prothrombotic

Lipoproteins Molecules responsible for the transport and delivery of fatty acids

Liraglutide A glucagon-like peptide-1 (GLP-1) agonist that mimics the actions of GLP-1 by increasing insulin secretion, decreasing glucagon secretion, slowing gastric emptying, and affecting the regulation of appetite and satiety in the brain. It is FDA approved for weight loss in pediatric patients over 12 years of age with obesity

Long-chain triglycerides A chain of fatty acids 14 carbons or more

Low birth weight (LBW) Infants born weighing less than 2500 grams

Low FODMAP diet A diet low in short-chain carbohydrates (fermentable oligo-, di-, and monosaccharides and polyols)

M

Macrocephaly A condition where a baby's head circumference is significantly larger than expected for their age and sex

Macrocytic anemia Large cell anemia; defined as a mean corpuscular volume of greater than 100 fL

Magnetic resonance imaging (MRI) An imaging modality utilizing what is referred to as a "free-ionizing radiation technique"

Malabsorption The result of defective mucosal uptake or transport of inadequately digested nutrients

Malassimilation The combination of maldigestion and malabsorption

Maldigestion Failure of the enzymatic processes of digestion

Mallory-Weiss tears Tears in the mucosa at the stomach–esophagus junction

Malnutrition A subacute or chronic state of nutrition, in which a combination of varying degrees of overnutrition or undernutrition and inflammatory activity has led to a change in body composition and diminished function

Malnutrition Screening Tool (MST) A nutrition screen tool that was created based on the need for a framework that used routinely available data, was noninvasive and convenient for nondietetics staff, and could be employed across a heterogeneous adult population

Malnutrition Universal Screening Tool (MUST) A nutrition screen tool that utilizes a simple five-step process to arrive at an overall score for risk of malnutrition—either low, medium, or high risk

Marasmus Malnutrition associated with severe caloric depletion, in which the body conserves visceral protein levels

Masticatory function The process of chewing

Mastitis Inflammation of breast tissue

Mature milk The final stage of breast milk produced, starting from 2 to 4 weeks postpartum until the end of breastfeeding

Maudsley approach A family-based treatment for eating disorders in adolescents, based on empowering parents to take on the responsibility of restoring weight to their child

Mean arterial pressure (MAP) The average pressure that pushes blood through the arteries during a cardiac cycle

Medium-chain triglyceride (MCT) A chain of fatty acids 6-12 carbons long

Melena Dark tarry stools associated with upper gastrointestinal bleeding

Metabolic acidosis A disorder characterized by a low pH, a low HCO_3^- concentration, and a compensatory hyperventilation that contributes to a decreased $PaCO_2$

Metabolic alkalosis A disorder characterized by a high pH, a high bicarbonate concentration, and compensatory hypoventilation that contributes to an increased $PaCO_2$

Metabolic and bariatric surgery Weight loss surgery

Metabolic dysfunction-associated steatohepatitis (MASH) The progression of metabolic dysfunction–associated steatotic liver disease into steatohepatitis

Metabolic dysfunction-associated steatotic liver disease (MASLD) Hepatic steatosis related to metabolic syndrome without significant alcohol consumption

Metabolic syndrome A syndrome in which an individual has three or more of the following metabolic risk factors: large waist circumference, high systolic or diastolic blood pressure, high fasting glucose and triglyceride levels, and low high-density lipoprotein cholesterol

Metallothionein A protein that binds to copper absorbed into the enterocyte, preventing its absorption

Micelles A combination of digested lipids, phospholipids, and bile acids formed during normal fat absorption

Microcephaly A condition where a baby's head circumference is significantly smaller than expected for their age and sex

Microcytic anemia Small cell anemia; defined as a mean corpuscular volume of less than 80 fL

Mid-arm muscle circumference (MAMC) A surrogate measure of lean body mass; cannot be measured directly, but can be estimated using mid-upper arm circumference and triceps skinfold data

Mid-parental height A child's projected adult height based on the height of their parents

Mid-upper arm circumference (MUAC) A measure of total arm circumference that provides a measure of both muscle and fat area

Migrating motor complex (MMC) The source of peristaltic motion in the small intestine

Mini Nutritional Assessment Screening tool used to assess nutritional status in the geriatric population

Microalbuminuria Low albumin output; greater than 30 mg but less than 300 mg daily of albumin in the urine

Micronutrients Essential nutrients, typically vitamins and minerals, needed in small amounts in the body

Model for End-Stage Liver Disease (MELD) A scoring system used to classify the severity of liver disease and prognosis of individuals with cirrhosis. The score ranges from 1 to >40, with higher scores predicting a higher 90-day mortality

Modulators Medications used in the treatment of cystic fibrosis that work directly on the defective CFTR gene to correct and/or potentiate the CFTR protein to improve its function

Monosaccharide Simple sugar

Mucolytics Medications that help mobilize mucus and decrease sputum thickness

Myelin A combination of proteins and fatty acids that cover and protect the nerve fibers

Myelomeningocele The most common form of spina bifida, in which there is an incompletely fused spine, from which there is a protrusion of the spinal cord, including nerves

Myocardial infarction (MI) A blockage in one or more of the arteries that supply blood to the heart; also known as a heart attack

Myocardium Middle layer of the heart

Myocytes Heart cells

N

Nasoduodenal tube A tube that is placed from the nose, through the stomach, to the duodenum of the small intestine

Nasoenteric See *nasogastric*

Nasogastric Going through the nose to the stomach

Nasogastric tube A tube that is entered through the nose or mouth and is placed directly to the stomach

Nasojejunal Going through the nose to the jejunum

Nasojejunal tube A tube that is placed from the nose and advanced to the jejunum of the small intestine

Nausea and vomiting of pregnancy (NVP) Nausea and vomiting that is common and typical during the early stages of pregnancy

Nebulizers Medical equipment that utilizes pressurized oxygen to turn liquid medication into a mist for inhalation

Necrotizing enterocolitis (NEC) An acute ischemic condition characterized by inflammation and cell death within the intestinal wall that is associated with significant morbidity and mortality in the neonatal population

Negative acute-phase protein Proteins that decrease during inflammation, such as serum albumin, prealbumin, retinal binding protein, and transferrin

Nephrocalcinosis Deposition of calcium in the kidney parenchyma

Nephrons The functional units of the kidney

Nephropathy Damage to the kidneys due to diabetes

Nephrotic syndrome A loss of protein through the glomerular membrane

Net secretory response The excretion of more water and sodium than can be ingested

Neural tube A hollow tube that houses the brain, spinal cord, and other neural tissue and eventually differentiates into the respective organs of the central nervous system

Neural tube defect A condition in which the neural tube closes prior to full development, resulting in birth defects

Neurodegenerative disease An incurable progressive condition involving the loss of neurons in the brain or peripheral nervous system. Examples include Alzheimer's disease, Parkinson's disease, and amyotrophic lateral sclerosis (ALS)

Neurogenic bladder Patients are unable to perceive bladder fullness and lack coordination between contraction and relaxation

Neurogenic bowel Decreased bowel motility leading to constipation

Neuroinflammation Inflammatory response in the brain or spinal cord

Neuron A nerve cell and the basic unit of the nervous system

Neuropathy Damage to the nerves

Neurotraumatic injury An injury involving the brain, spine, or nerves, commonly resulting from accidents, falls, or sports. Examples include traumatic brain injury and spinal cord injury

Neutropenia An abnormally low level of neutrophils in the blood

New-onset diabetes after transplant (NODAT) The development of diabetes in a patient who was not diabetic prior to organ transplantation surgery

Night eating syndrome (NES) A disordered eating pattern characterized by morning anorexia and evening hyperphagia and insomnia

Nissen Fundoplication A procedure where the top portion of the stomach is wrapped around the lower esophagus to improve the integrity of the lower esophageal sphincter and reduce reflux

Nitrogen balance Where nitrogen intake (oral, enteral, or parenteral) is equal to nitrogen excretion (urinary, fecal, or wound drainage)

Nitrogenous waste The end products of protein metabolism (urea, creatinine, and ammonia)

Non-celiac gluten sensitivity (NCGS) Clinical condition characterized by both GI and extraintestinal symptoms that manifests after the ingestion of gluten-containing foods in individuals without celiac disease–related antibodies or elevated specific IgE levels

Non-celiac gluten sensitivity (NCGS) Gastrointestinal symptoms without inflammation of the gut after consumption of gluten

Normalized protein nitrogen appearance (nPNA) PNA normalized to a function of body weight

Normocytic anemia Normal cell anemia; defined as a mean corpuscular volume between 80 and 99 fL

NPO Nil per os; nothing by mouth

Nutrigenomics The study of how genes and nutrients interact

Nutrition Care Process and Model (NCPM) A systematic framework to recognize, diagnose, and intervene upon nutrition-related problems for which a nutrition intervention is the primary treatment

Nutrition Care Process Terminology (NCPT) Standardized terminology used as part of the Nutrition Care Process and Model

Nutrition impact symptoms Nutrition-related side effects of disease

Nutrition-focused physical exam (NFPE) A system-based examination of each region of the body that aids in the evaluation of nutrition status by identifying markers of malnutrition and/or nutrient deficiencies

Nutrition Screening The process of identifying patients, clients, or groups who may have a nutrition diagnosis and benefit from nutrition assessment intervention by a registered dietitian (RD)

O

Obesity A medical condition in which an individual has excess body fat for a given height

Obesity paradox The protective effect of elevated body mass index in patients with heart failure

Obstructive sleep apnea A breathing disorder that occurs during sleep, characterized by airway obstruction that disrupts normal ventilation during sleep and normal sleep patterns

Odynophagia Pain with swallowing

Oligohydramnios Insufficient amniotic fluid

Oligosaccharides Carbohydrates made up of monosaccharides (more than two)

Oliguria Low urine volume

Open tube feeding system Formula from a can or package is poured into a separate container that is then attached to the patient's feeding access point

Open tube placement Placement of a gastrostomy tube in which a small incision is made on the abdomen so that the gastrostomy tube can enter

Oral allergy syndrome (OAS) A hypersensitivity reaction to certain plant-based foods, typically manifesting as itching, tingling, or swelling in the oropharyngeal region

Oral food challenge (OFC) A diagnostic test to determine the presence of a food allergy through the gradual introduction of the suspected food under strict medical supervision to monitor for adverse reactions

Oral immunotherapy (OIT) A medical treatment for IgE-mediated food allergies that involves administering progressively larger doses of an allergenic food

Oral propulsive phase The phase of swallowing in which the tongue facilitates the movement of the bolus (or liquid) through the oral cavity into the oropharynx

Oral rehydration solutions (ORS) Dilute glucose–water mixtures containing electrolytes

Order-writing privileges Clinical privileges that allow healthcare professionals to act within their scope of practice to order treatments without a physician co-signature

Orexigenic Appetite inducing

Oroenteric Leading from the mouth to the stomach

Oropharyngeal dysphagia (OD) The difficulty in forming or moving an alimentary bolus safely from the oral cavity to the esophagus

Orthorexia An excessive preoccupation with healthy eating

Orthotopic Something that occurs in the normal or usual place in the body

Osmolality A measure of osmotic pressure that represents the number of osmotically active particles per kilogram of solvent

Osmolarity A measure of the number of dissolved particles per liter of solution; reported as mOsm/L

Osmotic demyelination syndrome (ODS) A neurological condition in which the myelin sheath in the brainstem is destroyed, often triggered by the rapid correction of hyponatremia

Osmotic pressure The pressure needed to maintain equilibrium with no net movement of solvent

Osteodystrophy Abnormal development of bone

Osteoporosis A bone disease characterized by low bone mass and bone density

Ostomy The surgical procedure to create a stoma

Oxalate nephrolithiasis Kidney stones

P

Palpation The use of touch to assess texture, size, temperature, tenderness, and mobility

Pancreatic enzyme preparations (PEP) A mixture of the digestive enzymes amylase, lipase, and protease

Pancreatic enzyme replacement therapy (PERT) Giving of exogenous pancreatic enzymes as treatment for pancreatic exocrine insufficiency

Pancreatic exocrine insufficiency (PEI) A reduction in pancreatic enzyme activity below the threshold necessary for normal digestion

Pancreatic insufficiency The inability for digestive enzymes to be secreted into the small intestine from the pancreas

Pancreatitis Inflammation of the pancreas

Paracentesis Aspiration of fluid from peritoneal cavity

Parenteral nutrition (PN) A type of nutrition support that relies on the intravenous administration of nutrients to patients who are unable or unwilling to take adequate nutrition orally or enterally

Parenteral nutrition-associated liver disease Also known as intestinal failure–associated liver disease (IFALD); a hepatobiliary disorder associated with long-term parenteral nutrition therapy

Parietal cells Located in the gastric glands within the fundus that secrete hydrochloric acid and intrinsic factor

parity The number of times a female has given birth

Parvalbumin Protein found across various fish species, known for its stability even when heated or cooked

Patent ductus arteriosus (PDA) A congenital heart defect where the ductus arteriosus, a temporary fetal blood connecting the aorta and pulmonary artery, fails to close after birth, leading to abnormal blood flow between the arteries

Pediatric malnutrition Nutritional deficits that may negatively affect growth, development, and other relevant outcomes

Pediatric obesity A condition where a child is significantly overweight for their age and height

Percent ideal body weight (%IBW) The actual body weight divided by the ideal body weight, multiplied by 100; used to compare current and ideal body weights

Percent usual body weight (%UBW) The actual body weight divided by the usual body weight, multiplied by 100; the percentage of the current body weight as related to the normal weight

Percent weight change (%weight change) The amount of weight change divided by the usual body weight, multiplied by 100; the percentage change in body weight between two points in time

Percussion The tapping of fingers against body surfaces for sounds that reflect solids, fluids, or gas

Percussor A handheld device that helps mobilize bronchial secretions

Percutaneous Through the skin

Percutaneous coronary intervention (PCI)/Percutaneous transluminal coronary angioplasty (PTCA) A surgical procedure to correct arterial stenosis by inserting and expanding a balloon-tipped catheter at the site of the narrowing and placing a stent to hold the artery open

Percutaneous endoscopic gastrostomy (PEG) tube A tube that is placed into the stomach via needle puncture into the skin guided by endoscopy

Percutaneous endoscopic jejunostomy (PEJ) A tube that is placed into the jejunum via needle puncture into the skin guided by endoscopy

Periodontal disease Gum disease

Peripheral artery disease (PAD) Atherosclerotic narrowing of the arteries that deliver blood to the legs, arms, stomach, or kidneys

Peripheral PN (PPN) Parenteral nutrition delivered via access to a peripheral vessel, such as the vessels of the forearm

Peripherally inserted central catheter (PICC) Access where the catheter is inserted into the subclavian, jugular, femoral, cephalic, or basilic veins, and threaded through the vasculature until the tip reaches the vena cava or right atrium

Peristalsis Contraction of smooth and striated muscles within the gastrointestinal system to allow for the passage of food particles

Pernicious anemia Anemia associated with B_{12} deficiency

Peritoneal dialysis (PD) A form of dialysis that uses the peritoneum as a natural semipermeable membrane

Pharyngeal phase The phase of swallowing during which the bolus moves through the oropharynx into the esophagus

Phenylketonuria The condition in which an individual is unable to metabolize the amino acid phenylalanine that is found in human milk

Phlebitis Inflammation of the vein

Phlegmon A spreading diffuse inflammatory process associated with the formation of pus

Phosphate binders Medications used to reduce the small intestinal absorption of phosphorus from foods

physiochemical incompatibility Physical or chemical instabilities (such as precipitation) often considered in terms of medications and intravenous infusions

physiologic anemia of pregnancy Anemia in pregnant women caused by the greater increase in plasma compared to red blood cells (hemodilution)

Pica A condition marked by the consumption of nonfood items

PIVKA-II The laboratory test of choice to assess vitamin K status

Placenta A blood-rich structure that develops in the uterus and is responsible for transferring nutrients and gasses from the mother to the fetus via the umbilical vein

Placental insufficiency The state in which oxygen, glucose, and amino acid transport through the umbilical vein is hindered

Plaque Colonized bacteria on tooth surfaces

Pneumothorax Air accumulation in the pleural space

Polycystic kidney disease (PKD) An inherited disorder causing cysts on the kidneys

Polydipsia Thirst

Polyols Sugar alcohols

Polyphagia Hunger

Polyuria Frequent urination

Porcine-derived pancreatic enzymes Exogenous enzymes taken to treat pancreatic insufficiency

Portal hypertension Pressure greater than 10 mm Hg in the portal vein

Portosystemic shunting The redirection of blood to veins in the esophagus, stomach, and rectum, which have lower venous pressure

Positive acute-phase protein Proteins that increase during inflammation, such as C-reactive protein, ferritin, and cerulosplasmin

Postnatal diuresis Body's natural elimination of excess fluid through urine, which occurs after birth

Postpartum pulmonary embolism (PE) A blood clot that blocks the pulmonary artery, preventing blood flow to the lung during the postpartum period

Postprandial hyperemic response Increased blood flow to the gastrointestinal tract after enteral feeding

Postrenal AKI Kidney injury caused by urinary tract obstruction

Prebiotics Energy sources for the beneficial bacteria in the colon

Preconception health The physical and nutritional health of both men and women in relation to reproduction

Prediabetes Blood glucose levels that are elevated above what is normal, but not elevated enough to be classified as diabetes

Preeclampsia High blood pressure in pregnancy

Pregnancy Complex stage of life during which a mother serves as the sole source of nourishment to support fetal growth and development

Prerenal AKI Acute kidney injury caused by inadequate renal perfusion

Pressure injury A localized injury of the skin and/or underlying tissue as a result of pressure, or pressure in combination with friction

Primary (essential) HTN High blood pressure that is not the result of another disease

Primary hypertension Also known as essential hypertension; high blood pressure that is not the result of another disease

Probiotics Live microorganisms sold as dietary supplements or as components of foods that are intended to have health benefits through interaction with the body's normal flora

Prokinetics Medications that promote motility by increasing small intestine contractions

Prolamin A major storage protein in some grains; avoidance of the prolamins of wheat, barley, and rye is recommended in celiac disease

Proliferation An increase in the number of cells; the second phase of wound healing

Protein-energy malnutrition Malnutrition resulting from an energy deficit concurrent with protein deficit or condition of increased protein need

Pruritus Persistently itchy skin

Pseudohyponatremia A false biochemical finding where serum sodium appears low despite a normal serum sodium concentration; can occur due to hyperlipidemia or hyperproteinemia

pseudopolyps Inflammatory polyps

Purkinje fibers Tissues throughout the right and left ventricles that carry the heart's electrical impulse

Pyloroplasty A surgical procedure to enlarge the pyloric sphincter

R

Radiation therapy The use of high-energy radiation from x-rays, gamma rays, or other sources used to kill cancer cells and shrink tumors

Refeeding syndrome The effects of depletion, repletion, and compartmental shifts in electrolytes, fluids, and other substrates in response to excessive nutritional resuscitation; a serious and potentially fatal condition that can occur in severely malnourished patients

Rejection An immune reaction against grafted tissue that results in failure of the graft to survive

Remineralization The body's natural repair process for non-cavitated carious lesions; the rebuilding of enamel on teeth

Remodeling The final phase of wound healing, in which new epithelium and final scar tissue are formed

Renal function panel Biochemical measures used to assess kidney function; typically includes albumin, BUN, BUN:creatinine ratio, calcium, carbon dioxide, chloride, creatinine, glucose, phosphorus, potassium, and sodium

Renal replacement therapy (RRT) A treatment that replaces the normal blood-filtering function of the kidneys used to remove waste and fluid while kidney function is impaired

Respiratory acidosis A disorder characterized by low pH, high $PaCO_2$, and a variable increase in plasma HCO_3^- concentration

Respiratory alkalosis A disorder characterized by a high pH, low $PaCO_2$, and a variable decrease in plasma HCO_3^- concentration

Respiratory quotient (RQ) A measure of VCO2/VO2 that is useful for the interpretation of both composition and adequacy of feeds

Resting energy expenditure (REE) Energy derived from oxygen uptake when the body is awake, rested, at least 4-6 hours after eating or after engaging in physical activity

Retinopathy Damage to the eyes

Rhinorrhea Nasal congestion, including complete blockage of the nares

Root caries Decay on the root surface of the tooth

Roux-en-Y gastric bypass surgery (RYGB) A metabolic and bariatric surgical procedure that results in a small gastric pouch that severely restricts intake and bypasses the distal stomach, duodenum, and part of the jejunum, resulting in malabsorption

Russell's sign Tooth-induced scarring on the lower dorsum of the hand used to stimulate the gag reflex

S

Salvage absorption The normal flora will ferment any unabsorbed carbohydrates that enter the colon to short-chain fatty acids, which are subsequently absorbed and utilized

Sarcoma Type of solid malignancy that originates in the bone, cartilage, fat, muscle, blood vessels, or connective or supportive tissue

Sarcopenia The loss of lean body mass

Sarcopenic obesity The coexistence of age-related loss of skeletal mass and strength and excess body fat

School meals Meals provided to students at school typically during the school day

Secondary brain insult Brain damage from a traumatic brain injury that follows the initial brain injury

Secondary hyperparathyroidism Excessive secretion of parathyroid hormone in response to hypocalcemia

Selective serotonin reuptake inhibitor (SSRI) Antidepressant medications prescribed to alleviate mood symptoms and reduce anxiety disorder

Selective vagotomy Surgery to eliminate innervation from the vagus nerve to the parietal cells of the proximal stomach to decrease secretion of gastric acid and reduce cellular response to gastrin

Self-reported height (SRH) Height information provided by the patient

Semaglutide A glucagon-like peptide-1 (GLP-1) agonist that mimics the actions of GLP-1 by increasing insulin secretion, decreasing glucagon secretion, slowing gastric emptying, and affecting the regulation of appetite and satiety in the brain. It is used to treat type 2 diabetes and obesity

Sensitization The development of sensitivity to food allergens that can occur through various routes, including the gastrointestinal (GI) tract, compromised skin barriers, or through airway mucosa

Sepsis A condition in which the body's normal inflammatory response to infection is amplified

Serial measures Repeated measurements taken over time

Serum-specific IgE testing Quantitative assessment of food-specific IgE antibodies; measures the amount of IgE antibodies specific to particular foods in the blood

Shock liver Acute liver failure as the result of ischemic hepatocellular injury

Short-chain fatty acids Products of soluble fiber fermentation in the colon that promote water and electrolyte absorption

Short bowel syndrome (SBS) Any malabsorption related to decreased absorptive surface area and/or loss of functional capacity in the small intestine

Short Nutritional Assessment Questionnaire (SNAQ) A nutrition screening tool intended for use during admission to an acute care facility

Sinus tracts A narrow elongated channel in the body that allows the escape of fluid

Skin prick test (SPT) A rapid, safe, and sensitive diagnostic tool for identifying IgE-mediated food allergies

Skinfold anthropometry Skinfold thickness; measure of one or more anatomical sites using a skinfold caliper device to estimate body fat stores

Skinfold thickness (SFT) Measurement of subcutaneous fat in different segments of the body using skinfold calipers

Sleeve gastrectomy (SG) A metabolic and bariatric surgical procedure in which portions of the stomach are removed

Small intestinal bacterial overgrowth (SIBO) Where a disproportionate number of bacteria invade the small intestine, competing with the body for ingested nutrients and possibly impairing the individual's nutritional status

Small-for-gestational-age (SGA) Infants born with weights that chart less than the 10th percentile for their gestational age

Somatic protein Protein within skeletal muscle that makes up most of the total body protein pool

Somatization Complaint of recurrent medical symptoms of unknown cause

Spastic Increased muscle tone

Spirometry A pulmonary function test that measures how well lungs work by quantifying the amount of air inhaled and exhaled

Spontaneous bacterial peritonitis (SBP) Infection of the ascitic fluid without an apparent source

Stadiometer A piece of equipment designed to measure height constructed of a ruler and a sliding horizontal headpiece adjusted to rest on the top of the head

Standard body weight (SBW) The patient's actual body weight expressed as a percentage of a defined normal body weight for Americans of a similar frame size, gender, height, and age

Starvation Severe deficiency of caloric intake

Static assay Laboratory test used to measure the actual level of a nutrient in a specimen

Steatohepatitis Necroinflammation of the liver

Steatorrhea Greasy, foul-smelling diarrhea

Steatosis Accumulation of fat in the liver

Stellate cells Hepatic cells that are responsible for collagen formation and hold 90% of the body's vitamin A stores

Stoma An artificial opening in the skin

Stress A metabolic response characterized by increased energy expenditure, increased glucose production where glucose is used as a primary fuel source, fatty acid oxidization and recycling to triglycerides, amino acid release, and lean body mass erosion

Stroke A medical condition in which the blood supply to the brain is interrupted or reduced

Stroke volume The amount of blood pumped per heartbeat

Stunting Low height-for-age

Subjective Global Assessment (SGA) A clinical evaluation of a patient's nutritional status, including the patient's weight history, dietary intake, gastrointestinal symptoms, and functional capacity, as well as a physical exam of subcutaneous fat, muscle wasting, edema, and ascites

Sustained unresponsiveness (SU) A longer-lasting state of tolerance that persists even after oral immunotherapy maintenance treatment is discontinued

Sweat test A test to measure the amount of chloride in sweat; at levels about 60 mmol/L, it is diagnostic for cystic fibrosis

Systemic immune response Physiologic changes characterized by hypermetabolic macrophage activation and the subsequent release of proinflammatory mediators due to infection, trauma, inflammation, or surgery

Systemic inflammatory response syndrome (SIRS) An inflammatory response that occurs throughout the body in response to infection, inflammation, trauma, and burns

Systole The stage of the heartbeat that involves the active pumping of blood out of the heart by the ventricles

Systolic blood pressure The force caused when the heart is actively pumping blood

T

Tau proteins Reinforcing compounds that bind to microtubules, a class of structural proteins, that ultimately act to maintain the structural integrity of cells

Texture-modified diets (TMDs) Food and liquid that have altered consistency to reduce the risk of choking in individuals with dysphagia

Thermic effect of food (TEF) The production of heat associated with the digestion and metabolism of food; also known as diet-induced thermogenesis

Third spacing The accumulation of fluid in the interstices (edema) or in the potential fluid spaces (effusion) between body cavities

Thromboembolism The blockage of an artery by a thrombus that has detached and traveled to a point elsewhere in the circulatory system

Thrombophlebitis An inflammatory process that causes blood to clot and block one or more veins

Thrombosis A blood clot that interferes with normal blood flow

Thrombotic occlusion Blockage of a blood vessel by a thrombus

Total arm span (TAS) The length between the middle of the sternal notch and the tip of either middle finger, doubled; measured with the patient's arm horizontal and in line with the shoulders

Total energy expenditure (TEE) A 24-hour energy expenditure that includes the sum of basal metabolic rate, diet-induced thermogenesis, and activity

Total nutrient admixture (TNA) A preparation method that allows for extended hang time of parenteral nutrition

Total parenteral nutrition The provision of all nutrients intravenously

Total peripheral resistance Resistance of blood flow in systemic circulation

Total (truncal) vagotomy A surgical procedure wherein parietal cell innervation is severed and the portion of the vagus nerve that controls gastric emptying is eliminated

Toxic megacolon Colonic diameter >6 cm or cecal diameter >9 cm in the presence of systemic toxicity

Trace elements Minerals present in minute amounts that perform a variety of structural, regulatory, and catalytic roles in the body

Transitional milk The second stage of breast milk produced, usually within the 2 weeks between colostrum and mature milk

Transjugular intrahepatic portosystemic shunt (TIPS) A procedure used to reduce portal hypertension and its complications including variceal bleeding

Triceps skinfold (TSF) Skinfold anthropometry measured at the triceps

Tubules The part of the nephron that reabsorbs ultrafiltrate

Tumor necrosis factor-alpha (TNF-α) A proinflammatory cytokine produced by the liver

U

Ulcerative colitis (UC) A form of inflammatory bowel disease characterized by inflammation that is limited to the mucosal layer of the colon

Ultrafiltrate The substance remaining after the kidneys have filtered the waste from the blood

Ultrasound (US) A noninvasive imaging technique that can estimate adipose tissue and muscle thickness

Umbilical cord A membranous sheath through which nutrients and oxygenated blood are delivered to the fetus and waste and deoxygenated blood are removed

Underfill hypothesis A theory explaining the pathogenesis of ascites related to liver disease, in which peripheral arteriolar vasodilation and splanchnic vasodilation result in fluid accumulation in the peritoneal cavity

Underweight A state of having weight that is less than the median for children of similar age or height

Urea kinetic modeling (UKM) A method to evaluate the effectiveness of hemodialysis using Kt/V, where K stands for dialyzer clearance in mL/min, t stands for the amount of time spent on treatment, and v stands for the patient's total body water volume

Urea reduction ratio (URR) The reduction in the amount of urea as a result of treatments such as dialysis

Ureters The organs of the genitourinary system that carry urine to the bladder so that it can then be released from the body

Urticaria Itchy, raised red or skin-colored welts; also known as hives

Usual body weight (UBW) A patient's normal weight range; usually self-reported

V

Vagus nerve The longest cranial nerve passing through the neck and thorax to the abdomen

Varices Extremely dilated submucosal veins

Vascular access device (VAD) A catheter inserted into a blood vessel for the delivery of intravenous solutions, including parenteral nutrition

Vasopressor Medication that constricts blood vessels, thereby increasing blood pressure

Venipuncture The point where the catheter enters the vasculature

Venous blood gases (VBGs) Blood gas values used to assess tissue oxygenation

Ventriculoperitoneal (VP) shunting The draining of excess cerebrospinal fluid into a peritoneal space to alleviate pressure and prevent progression of hydrocephalus

Very low birth weight (VLBW) Infants born weighing less than 1500 grams

Videofluorographic swallowing study (VFSS) Also known as a modified barium swallow; radiographic visualization of the swallowing process

Viral hepatitis A systemic infection that damages the liver

Visceral hypersensitivity Describes the experience of pain within the inner organs often associated with irritable bowel syndrome

Visceral protein An assessment that directly measures protein stores by assessing the proteins made by the viscera, namely, organs (primarily the liver)

Vulnerable plaque A thin-cap fibroatheroma that is at risk for rupture

W

Waist circumference An indicator of fat mass around the waist, used to assess health risk

Waist-hip ratio (WHR) The waist circumference value divided by the hip circumference value

Wasting Low BMI or weight-for-height (or length)

Weight-for-age The plotting of a child's weight according to the distribution of weights for children of similar age and gender on a growth chart

Weight-for-height The plotting of a child's weight relative to their height on a growth chart

Wet voice A voice that sounds gurgly or wet, which may be a sign of aspiration

Wheat-dependent exercise-induced anaphylaxis (WDEIA) A rare condition typically triggered by the consumption of wheat accompanied by exercise; also known as omega-5-gliadin allergy

WHO growth charts Growth charts utilizing data on the growth rates of infants from six countries who were exclusively breastfed for the first 4–6 months of life

Wilson's disease An autosomal recessive disorder characterized by excessive deposition of copper in the liver and brain

Wound Damage to the structure and function of tissue

X

Xanthomas Yellow patches on the skin caused by deposits of excess lipids

Xerostomia Reduced or absent saliva flow

Z

Z-scores Representations of individual differences from the median

Index

A

B

C

D

E

F

G

H

I

J

K

L

M

P

Q

R

T

U

V